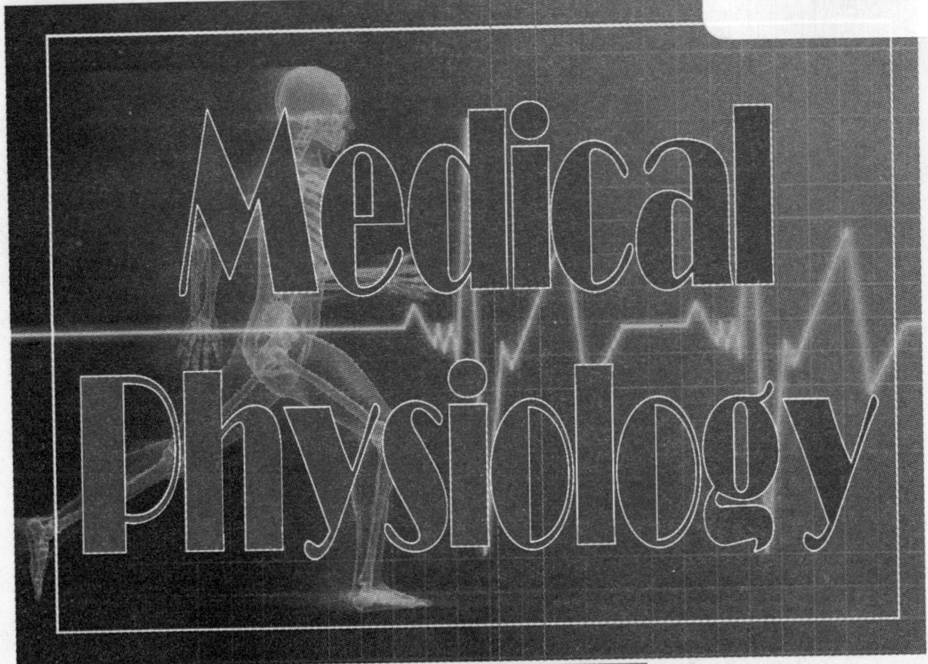

THIRD EDITION

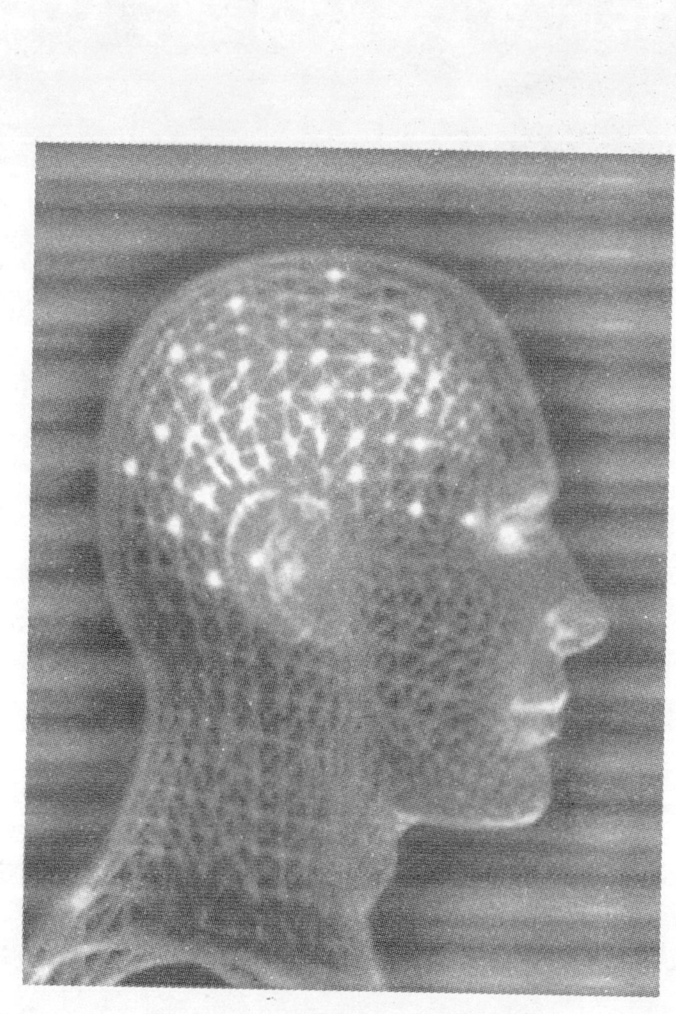

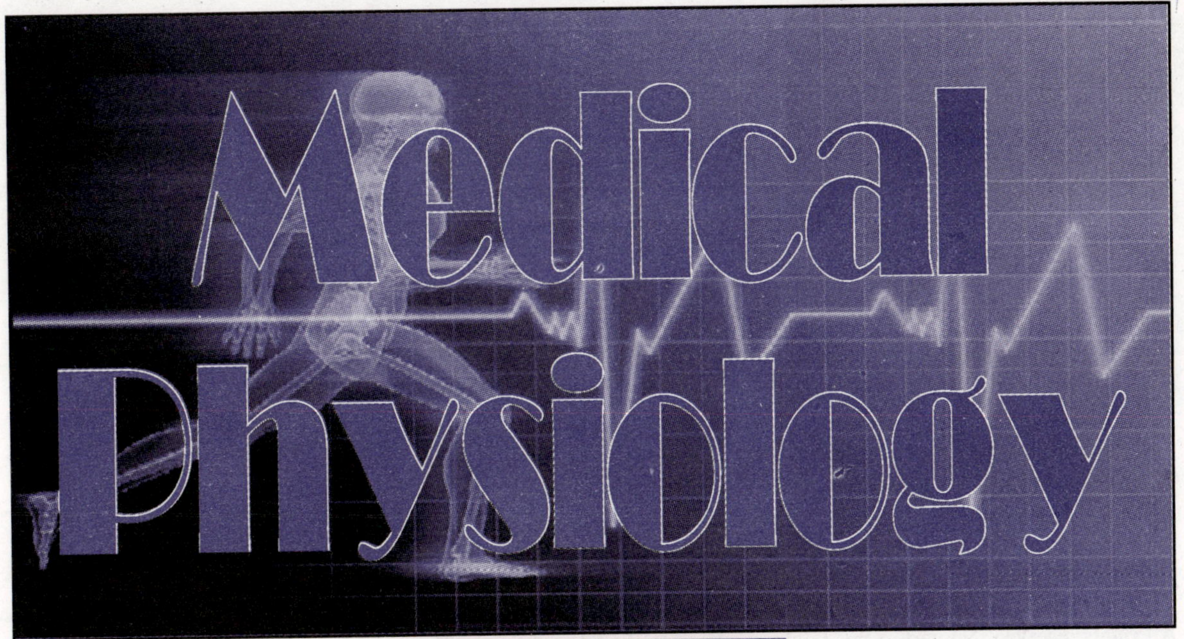

Medical Physiology

THIRD EDITION

R.K. Marya

Professor and Head of Unit of Physiology
Faculty of Medicine
AIMST University
Bedong, Kedah Darul Aman
Malaysia

Former

Professor and Head, Department of Physiology
Pt. B.D. Sharma Postgraduate Institute of Medical Sciences, Rohtak, Haryana

Professor, Department of Physiology, Faculty of Medicine
Al-Arab Medical University, Benghazi (Libya)

Professor and Head, Department of Physiology
S.S.R. Medical College, Belle Rive (Mauritius)

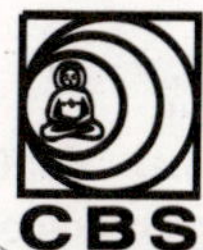

CBS Publishers & Distributors Pvt Ltd

New Delhi • Bangalore • Pune • Cochin • Chennai

ISBN : 978-81-239-1847-1

First Edition : 1997
Second Edition : 2003
Third Edition : 2010
Reprint : 2012

Published by Satish Kumar Jain and produced by V.K. Jain for
CBS Publishers & Distributors Pvt. Ltd.,
CBS Plaza, 4819/XI Prahlad Street, 24 Ansari Road, Daryaganj,
New Delhi - 110002, India. • Website: www.cbspd.com
e-mail: delhi@cbspd.com, cbspubs@airtelmail.in
Ph.: 23289259, 23266861, 23266867 • Fax: 011-23243014

Branches:

- ***Bengaluru:*** Seema House, 2975, 17th Cross, K.R. Road, Bansankari 2nd Stage, Bengaluru - 560070 Ph.: +91-80-26771678/79 • E-mail: cbsbng@gmail.com, bangalore@cbspd.com
- ***Pune:*** Bhuruk Prestige, Sr. No. 52/12/2+1+3/2, Narhe, Haveli (Near Katraj-Dehu Road By-pass), Pune - 411051 Ph.: +91-20-64704058/59, 32342277 • E-mail: pune@cbspd.com
- ***Kochi:*** 36/14, Kalluvilakam, Lissie Hospital Road, Kochi - 682018, Kerala • Ph.: +91-484-4059061-65 Fax: +91-484-4059065 • E-mail: cochin@cbspd.com
- ***Chennai:*** 20, West Park Road, Shenoy Nagar, Chennai - 600030 Ph.: +91-44-26260666, 26208620 E-mail: chennai@cbspd.com

Printed at :
Dynamic Print Grafix, Delhi

to

my wife,

Veena

who gave me

encouragement and inspiration

to write this book

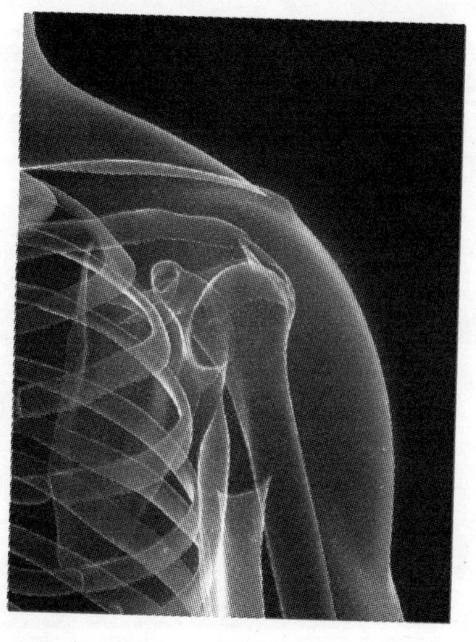

Preface to the Third Edition

In this edition, almost the entire book has been rewritten to bring it up-to-date. Moreover, in line with the latest recommendations of the Medical Council of India, this edition of the book has been given still greater clinical orientation. These changes have made it the most appropriate physiology textbook for the medical students. Greater stress is given to physiological concepts applicable to clinical studies rather than enumerating useless information with no clinical significance. In this way, the book remains short, but provides sound basis for understanding the situations the would-be doctor shall face as a clinician. Some of the important changes made in the third edition of *Medical Physiology* are given below.

In Section II (Blood), topics of erythropoiesis, red cell metabolism, polycythemia, jaundice, leucopoiesis, autoimmune disorders, plasma proteins, haemostasis, fibrinolytic system, interleukins, von Willebrand disease have been updated.

In Sections III and IV (Heart and Circulation), the topics of functional anatomy of the heart, nodal tissue, electrophysiology of myocardium, cardiac catheterization, heart sounds and murmurs, arterial pulse, cardiac output regulation, cardiac arrhythmias, arterial blood pressure, venous return, regulation of regional blood flow, coronary artery disease and pulmonary circulation have been rewritten.

In Section V (Respiration), topics of neural and chemical control of respiration, carbon monoxide poisoning, cyanosis, dyspnoea, Cheyne-Stokes breathing, high altitude pulmonary oedema, oxygen toxicity, emphysema, mechanical ventilators have been rewritten.

In Section VI (Nerve and Muscle), topics of neuronal transport system, nerve impulse conduction, neuroglial cells, neurotrophins, peripheral nerve injuries, muscle proteins, disuse atrophy, myasthenia gravis, and denervation hypersensitivity have been rewritten.

In Section VII (Central Nervous System), topics of inhibitory neurons, sensory receptors, neuropathic pain, central analgesia system, role of sensory information in motor activity, clinical aspects of reflexes, vestibule-ocular reflex, cerebellum, cerebral plasticity, extrapyramidal tracts, spinal cord lesions, thalamic syndrome, sleep, synaptic plasticity, regulation of food intake, pheromones, hypothermia, autonomic failure, blood–brain barrier have been rewritten.

In Section IX (Gastrointestinal tract), regulation of gastric secretion, pathophysiology of peptic ulcer and achalasia have been revised. Pathophysiology of a common disorder, gastro-oesophageal reflux disease, has been added.

In Section X (Nutrition), in view of their clinical importance, iron metabolism and obesity have been discussed in greater detail. Other important topics rewritten include glomerular filtration rate and pathophysiology of micturition (Section XIV) and theories of ageing (Section XVI). The index has also been revised.

In this edition, a large number of illustrations have been replaced and many are new. Twenty coloured figures, of which 15 are new, shall give greater depth to the understanding of many topics. All these changes have increased the bulk of the book by approximately 85 pages, but the book retains its hallmark—brevity and simplicity of presentation.

I would like to thank CBS Publishers and Distributors Pvt Ltd, New Delhi, for their ever-available cooperation. I would like to acknowledge the special contribution of Mr. Y.N. Arjuna, Senior Director—Publishing, for the beautiful layout of the book.

R.K. Marya
AIMST University, Malaysia
email: rkumarmarya@yahoo.com

Preface to the First Edition

In the recent years, medical textbooks have become highly voluminous and formidable. With limited time at their disposal, medical students find these books extremely tedious. This textbook of Medical Physiology has been written keeping in mind this problem of the students. Each topic has been presented in such a lucid manner that the students can easily understand the fundamentals of physiology. Consequently, the learning of the subject is expected to become a pleasurable pursuit rather than a boring and dreadful task.

This book is primarily meant for undergraduate MBBS and BDS students. The material given in the book shall provide a comprehensive base for the study of para-clinical and clinical subjects. In additions, the book has been written keeping in mind the requirements of students appearing in competitive postgraduate entrance tests.

At the end of each chapter pathophysiology of some of the related clinical disorders has been briefly discussed. Principles of important laboratory tests for the assessment of the deranged function of the organs have also been provided. The discussion helps to underline the fact that knowledge of physiology would be essential for the diagnosis and treatment of a disease on scientific basis. In addition, it provides greater insight into the basic concepts of physiology.

Children and aged individuals constitute over 50% of the population in most of the countries. Yet, all the textbooks of physiology are concerned with the physiology of adults only. A fairly detailed discussion of the physiological aspects of these two age-groups constitutes an important feature of this book.

I gratefully acknowledge the cooperation extended by all the colleagues in the Department of Physiology, Pt. B.D. Sharma Postgraduate Institute of Medical Sciences, Rohtak, particularly by Professor (Mrs.) K.K. Mahajan and Associate Professors, Dr. V. Raghunandanan, Dr. (Mrs.) Sushma Sood and Dr. (Mrs.) Indu Khurana. I am specially thankful to Dr. Sharmila Chhabra, a postgraduate student, for going through the whole text and providing useful suggestions from the angle of a student preparing for postgraduate entrance examinations.

I would like to thank many others who have helped in the publication of this book. Credit for the figures in the text goes to Miss Monica and Dr. Sandeep Maken. Dr. D.S. Mishra, Professor of Radiology, has been kind enough to provide the X-ray pictures. I owe special thanks to Mr. Dharmvir for giving valuable technical advice regarding the publication. I would also like to thank the publishers, CBS Publishers & Distributors Pvt Ltd, New Delhi, for their cooperation and keen interest in the publication of this book.

Some imperfections are likely to be noticed by the readers. Suggestions for the improvement of the book from the teachers and the students are most welcome.

R.K. Marya

Contents

Section III: The Heart

6 The Physiology of Cardiac Muscle

7 The Heart as a Pump

8 Electrocardiography

Section IV: The Circulation

9 Basic Principles of Pressure, Flow and Resistance

10 Pressure and Flow in Different Segments of Circulatory System

11 Regulation of Systemic Arterial Blood Pressure

12 Regulation of Blood Flow in the Tissues

13 Regional Circulations

14 Cardiovascular Homeostasis in Health and Disease

Section V: Respiration

15 Pulmonary Ventilation

16 Pulmonary Diffusion

17 Transport of Gases

18 Regulation of Respiration

19 Respiratory Adjustments in Health and Disease

Section VI: Nerve and Muscle

20 The Nerve

21 The Muscle Physiology

Section VII: Central Nervous System

22 Synaptic Transmission

23 Somesthetic Sensory System

24 Somatic Motor Activity: Regulation of Posture

25 The Cerebellum and the Basal Ganglia

26 The Motor Cortex

27 The Thalamus, Reticular Activating System, EEG and Sleep

28 Higher Functions of the Cerebral Cortex

29 The Limbic System and the Hypothalamus

30 The Cerebrospinal Fluid

31 The Autonomic Nervous System

Section VIII: The Special Senses

32 Vision

33 Hearing

34

Section IX: The Gastrointestinal Tract

35 Functional Organization of GI Tract

36 The Mouth and Oesophagus

37 The Stomach

38 The Pancreas, Liver and Gallbladder

39 The Intestines

40 Digestion and Absorption

Section X: Metabolism and Nutrition

41 Carbohydrate Metabolism

42 Lipid Metabolism

43 Protein Metabolism

44 Nutrition

Section XI: Endocrines

45 Mode of Action of Hormones

46 The Pituitary Gland

47 The Thyroid Gland

48 The Adrenal Gland

49 The Endocrine Pancreas

50 Hormonal Control of Calcium Metabolism

51 Endocrine Function of the Heart, Kidneys and Pineal Gland

Section XII: Reproduction

52 The Male Reproductive System

53 The Female Reproductive System

54 Physiology of Human Pregnancy and Lactation

Section XIII: Pediatric Physiology

55 Growth and Development

56 Systemic Physiology of Fetus, Neonate and Childhood

Section XIV: The Kidneys and the Body Fluids

57 The Kidney

Plate 1

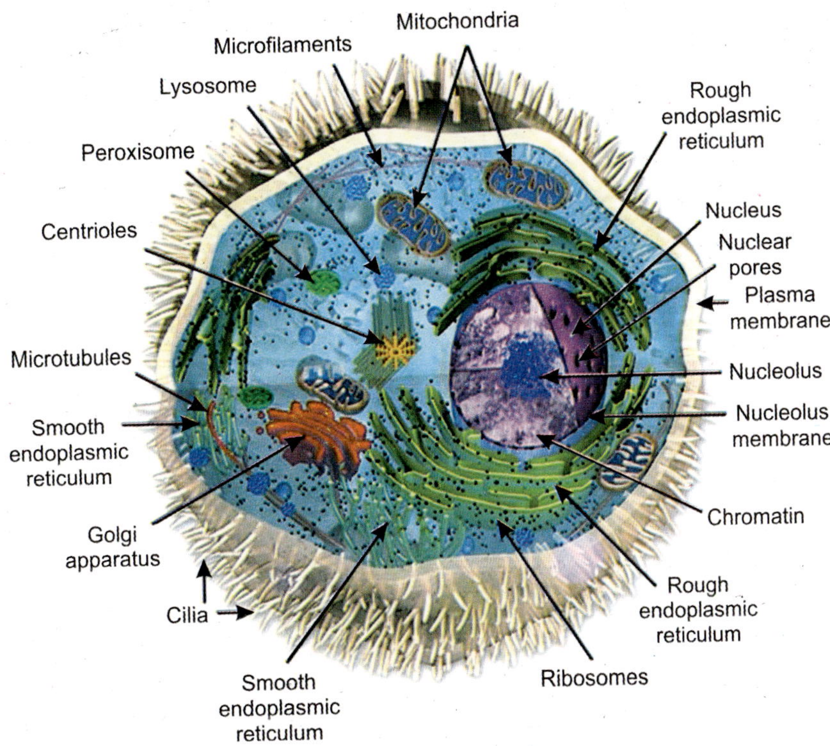

Fig. 1: Cell structure

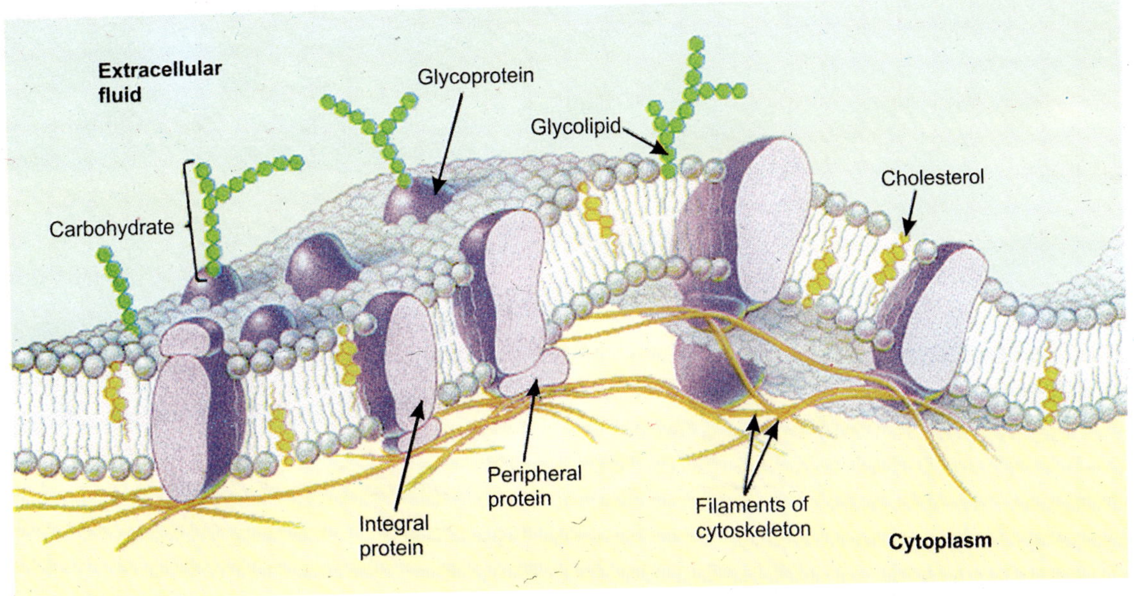

Fig. 2: Cell membrane

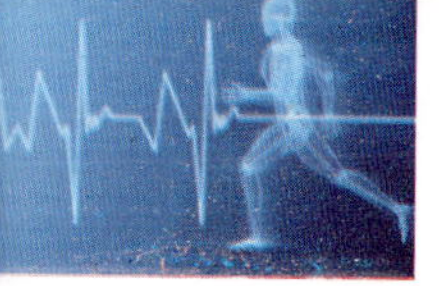

Plate 2

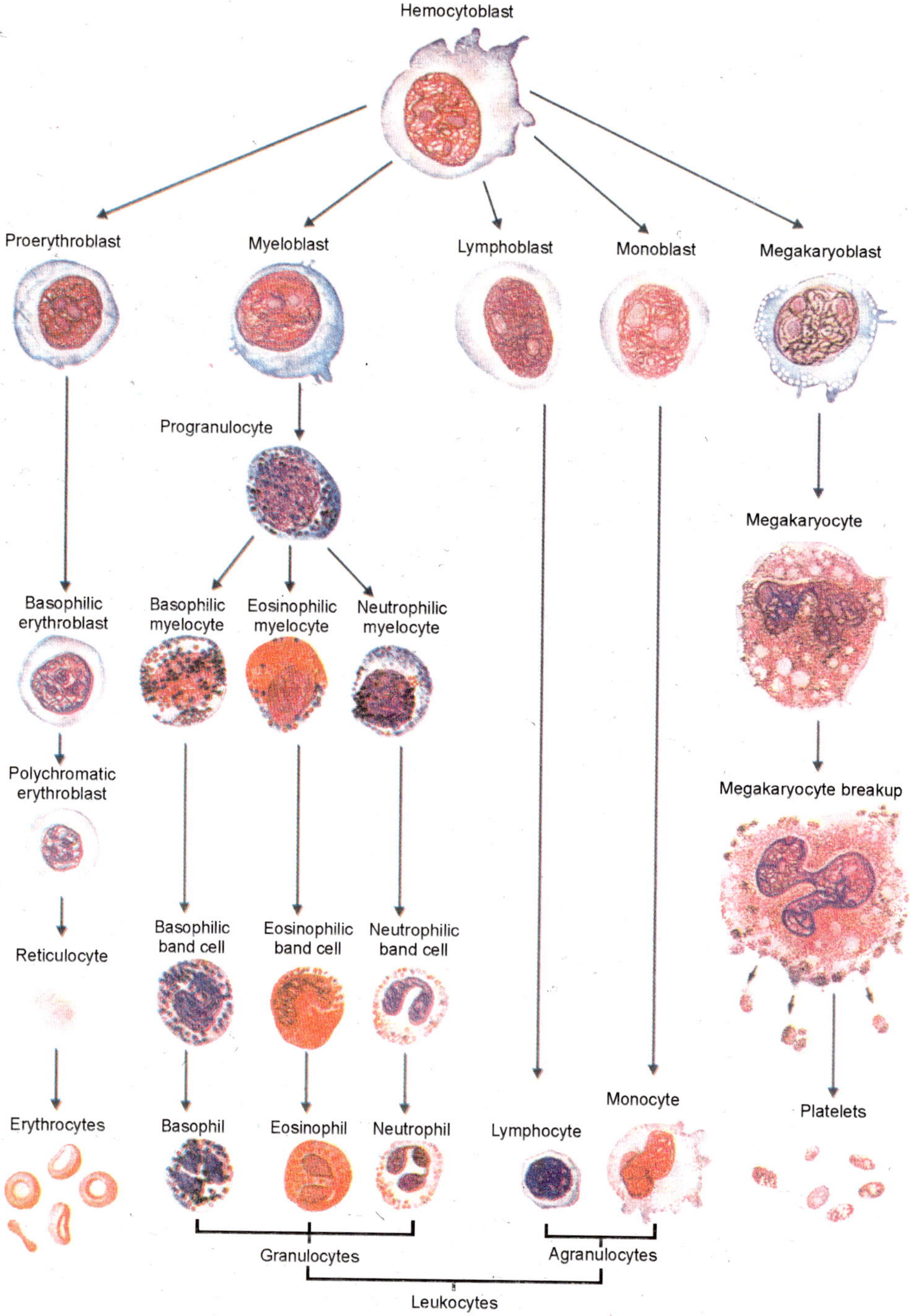

Fig. 3: Formation of blood cells

Plate 3

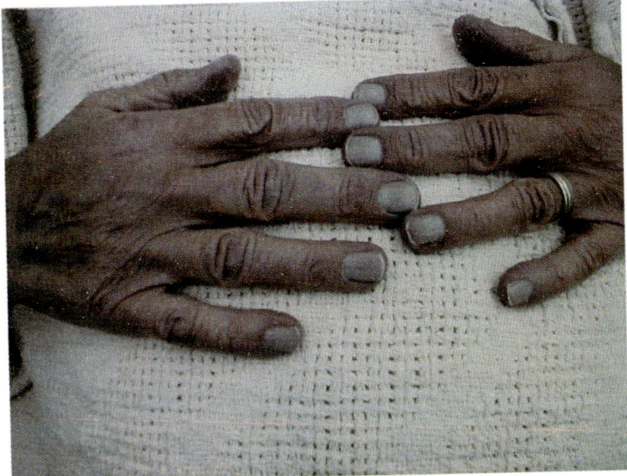

Fig. 4: Cyanosis

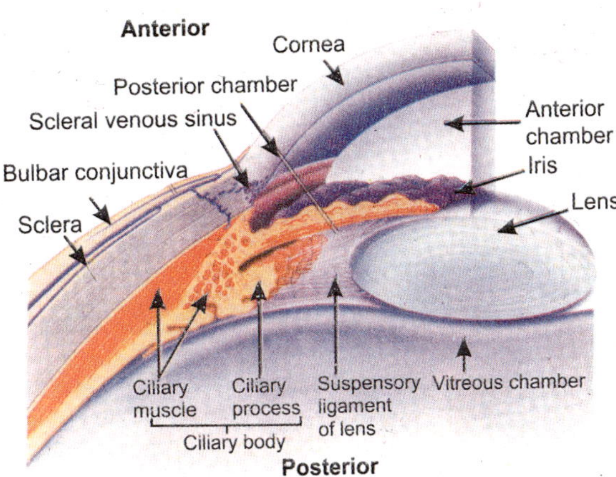

Fig. 5: Detailed structure of corneo-scleral junction

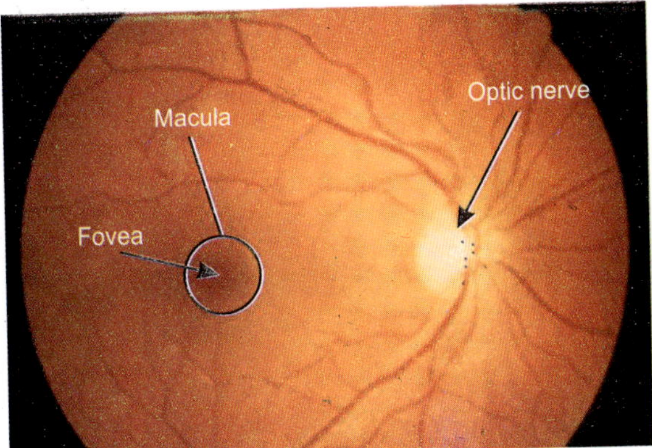

Fig. 6: Fundus (back) of the eye

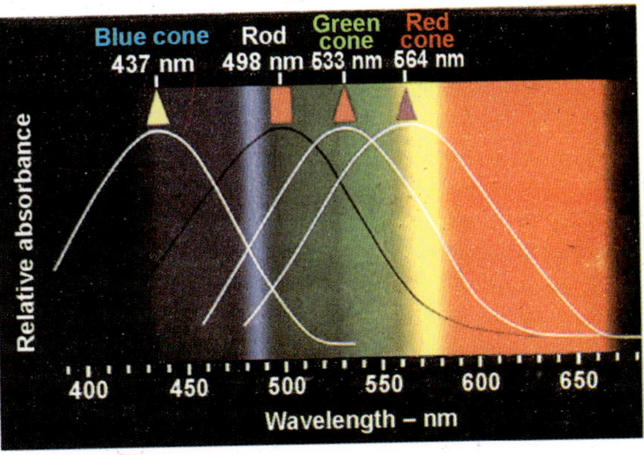

Fig. 7: Absorption spectrum of three types of cones

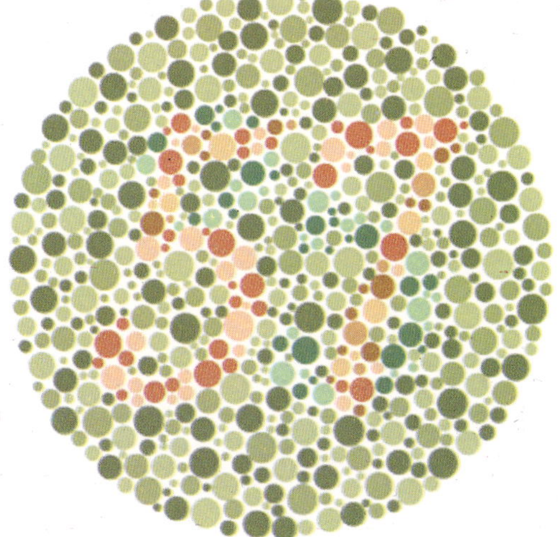

Fig. 8: Colour-blindness chart

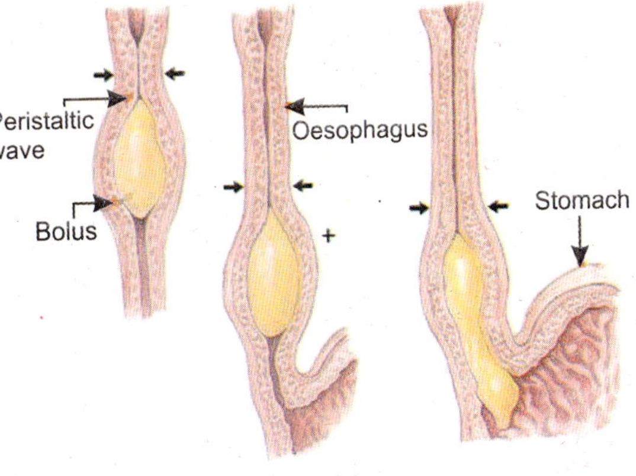

Fig. 9: Peristalsis

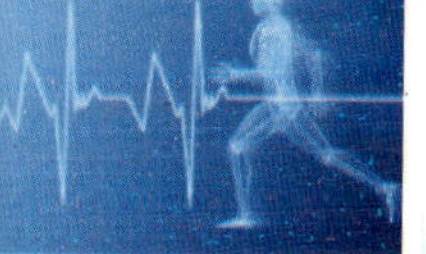

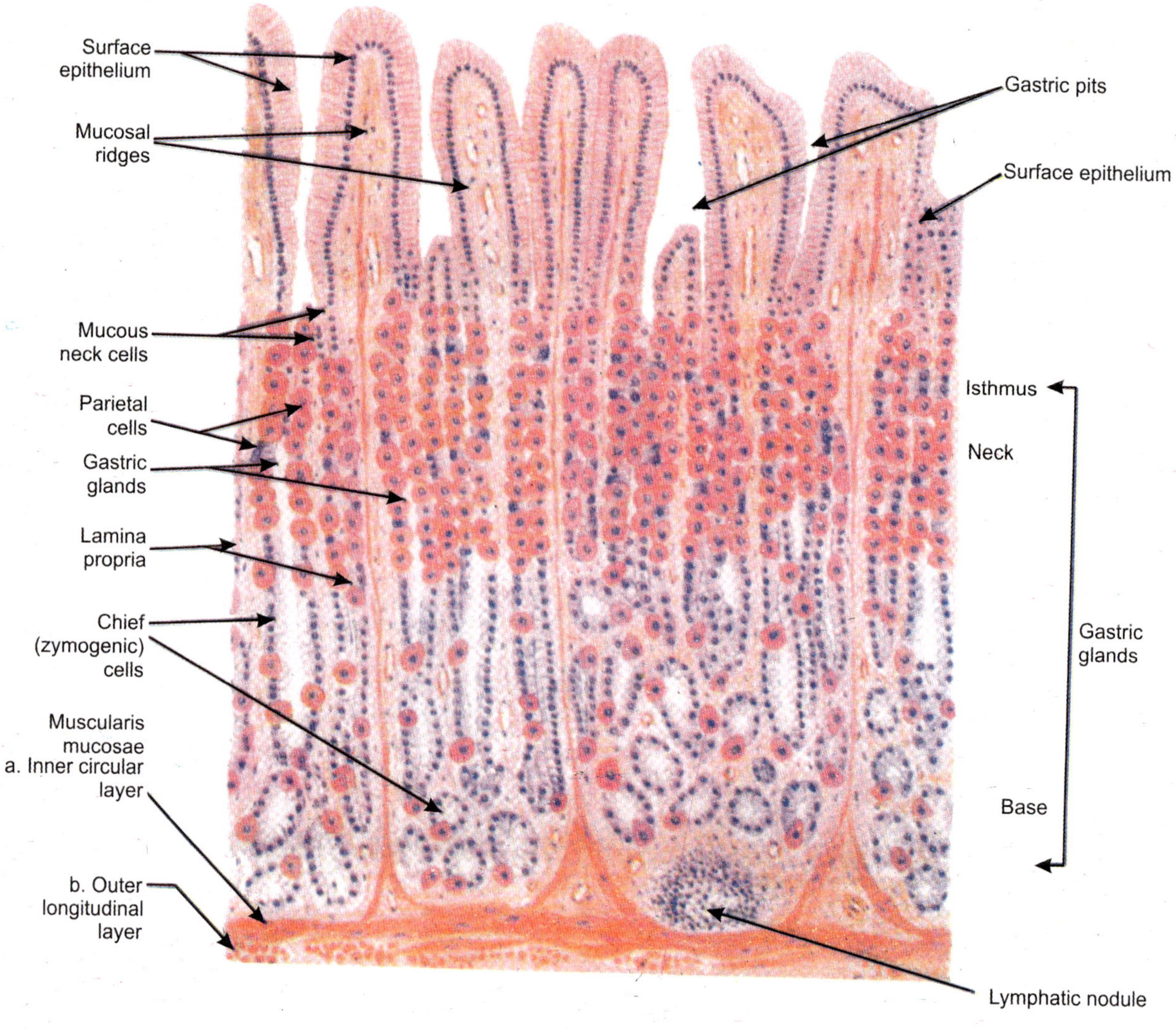

Plate 4

Surface epithelium
Mucosal ridges
Mucous neck cells
Parietal cells
Gastric glands
Lamina propria
Chief (zymogenic) cells
Muscularis mucosae
a. Inner circular layer
b. Outer longitudinal layer
Gastric pits
Surface epithelium
Isthmus
Neck
Gastric glands
Base
Lymphatic nodule

Fig. 10: Mucosa of body of stomach

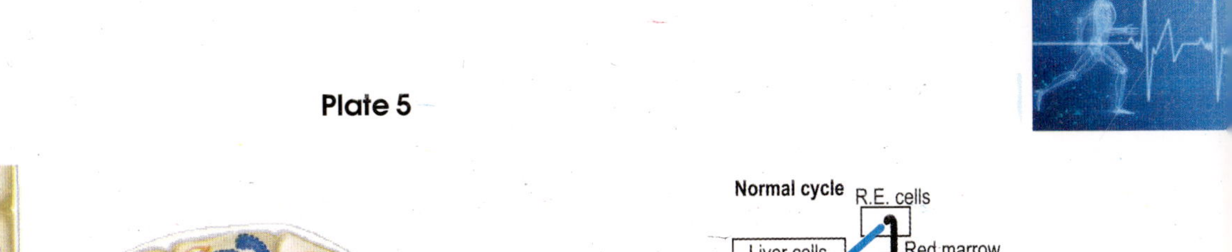

Plate 5

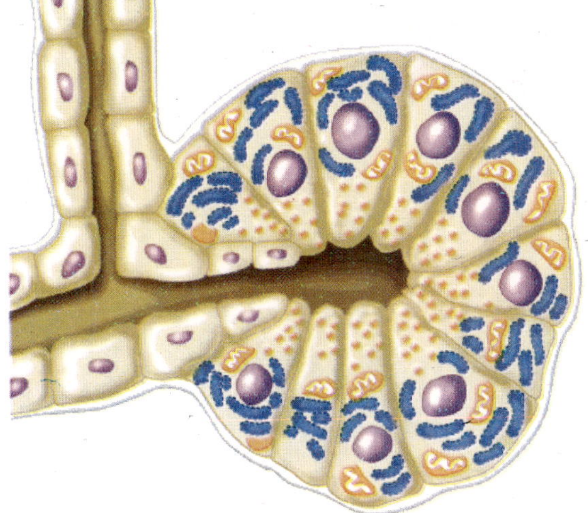

Fig. 11: Exocrine pancreas acinus

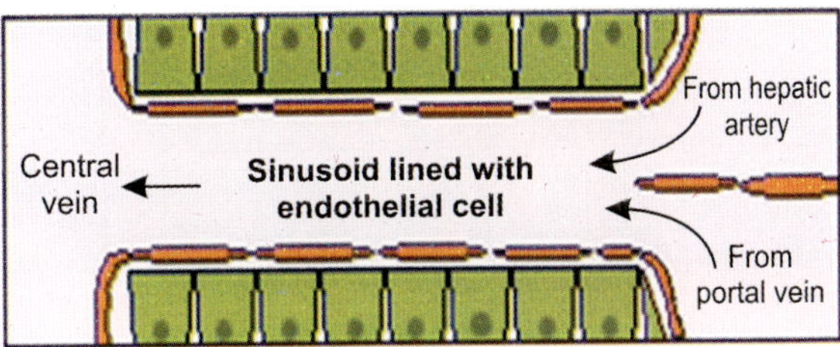

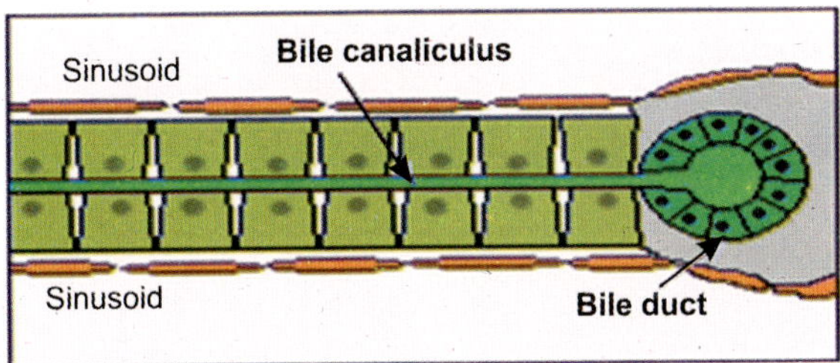

Fig. 12: A hepatic sinusoid and a bile canaliculus

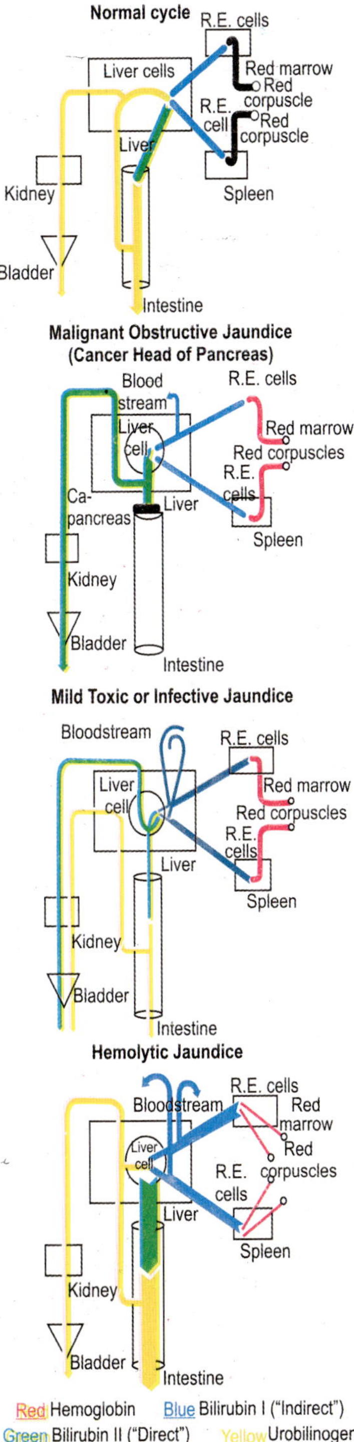

Fig. 13: Bile pigment metabolism in three types of jaundice

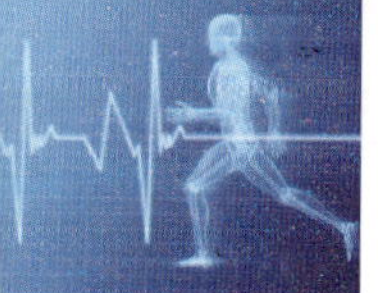

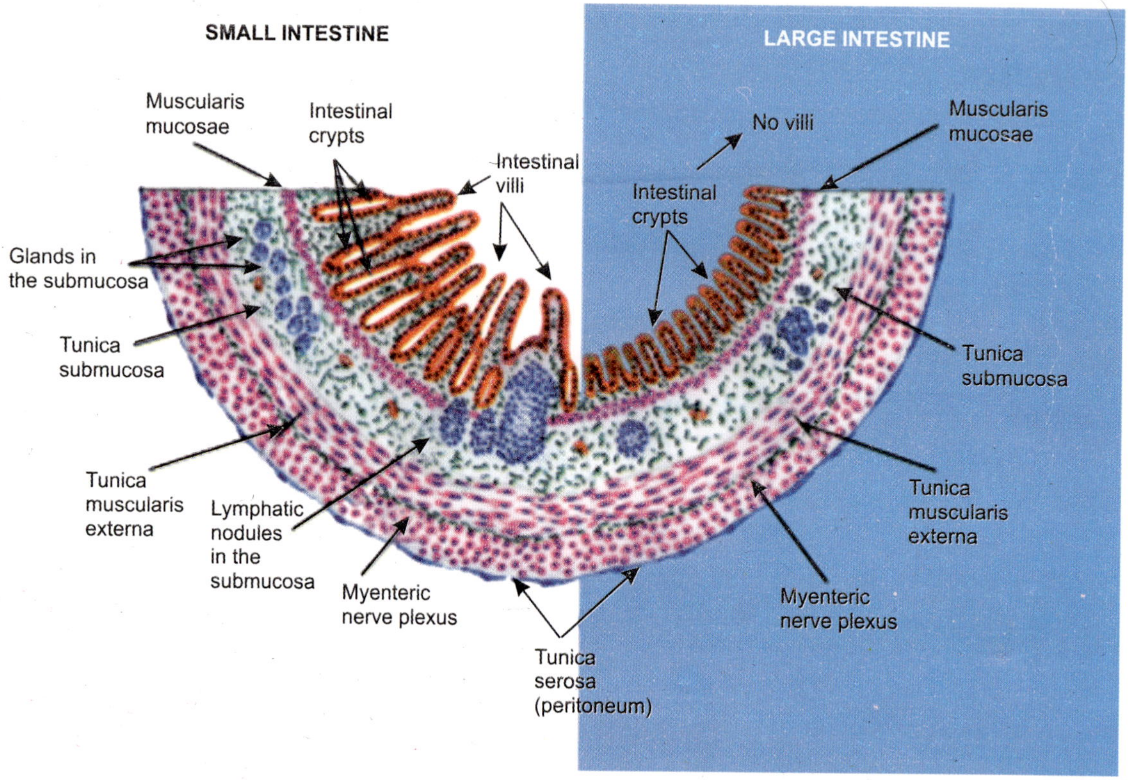

Plate 6

SMALL INTESTINE

LARGE INTESTINE

Muscularis mucosae

Intestinal crypts

Intestinal villi

No villi

Muscularis mucosae

Intestinal crypts

Glands in the submucosa

Tunica submucosa

Tunica submucosa

Tunica muscularis externa

Lymphatic nodules in the submucosa

Myenteric nerve plexus

Tunica muscularis externa

Myenteric nerve plexus

Tunica serosa (peritoneum)

Fig. 14: Mucosa of small and large intestines

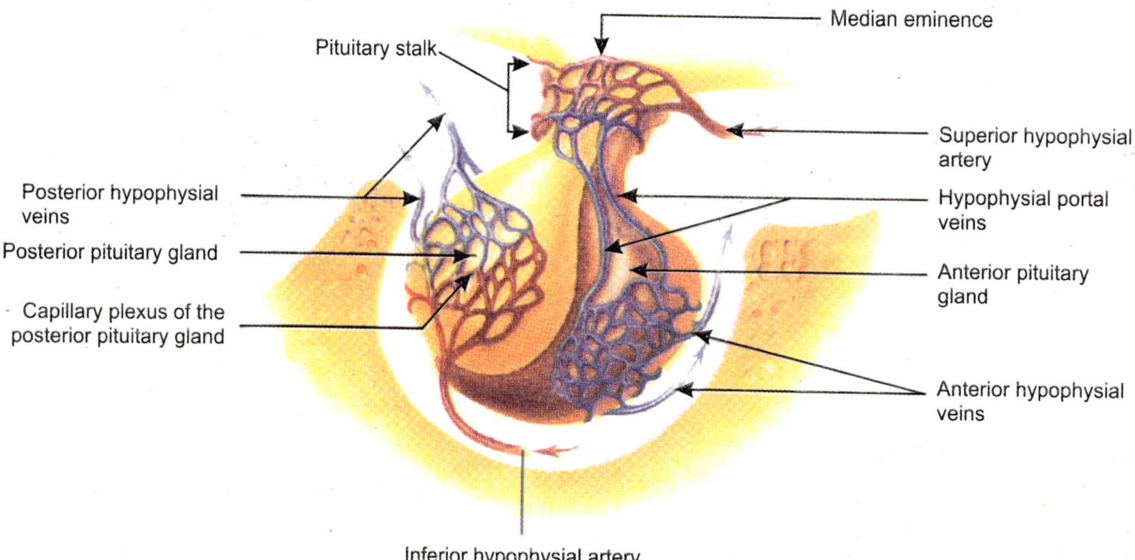

Fig. 15: Blood supply of pituitary gland

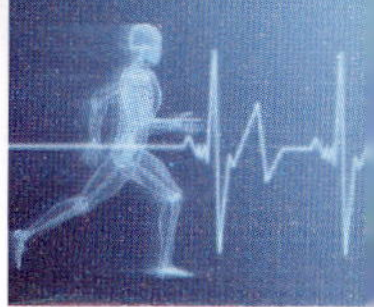

Plate 7

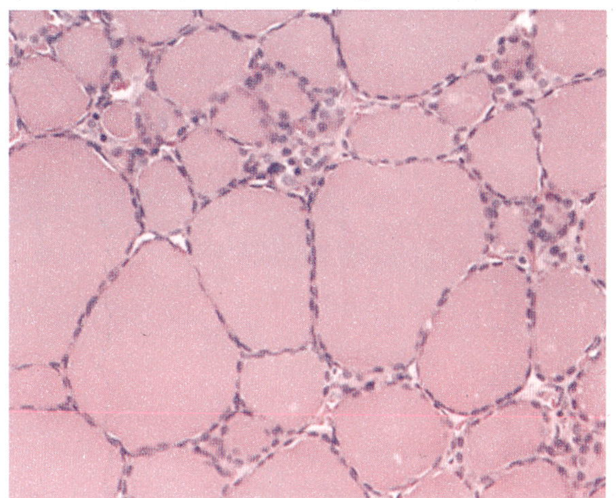

Fig. 16: Thyroid gland (histology)

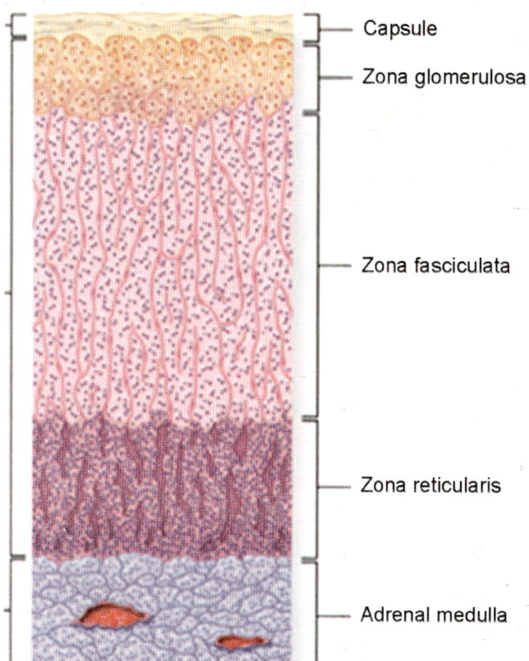

Fig. 17: Adrenal gland (histology)

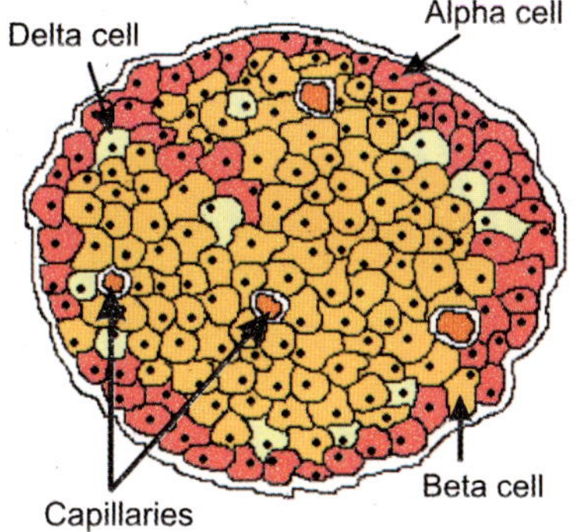

Fig. 18: Islet of Langerhans

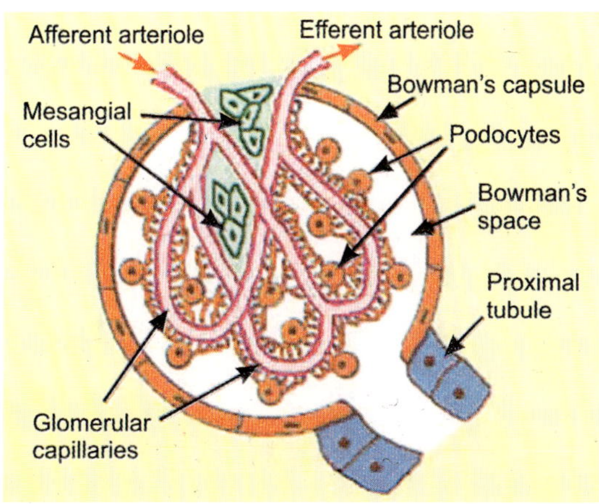

Fig. 19: Malpighian corpuscle

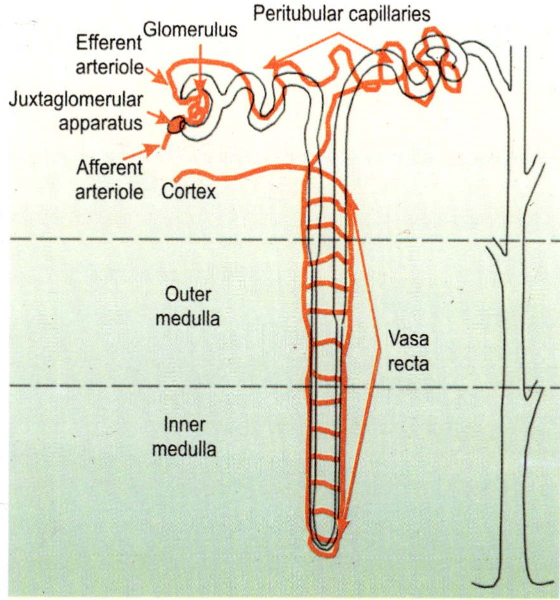

Fig. 20: Renal peritubular capillaries and vasa recta

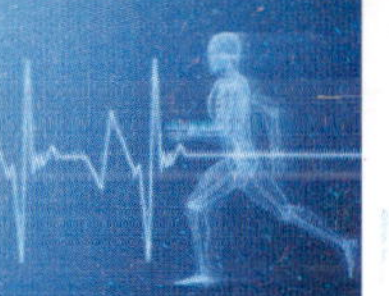

Plate 8

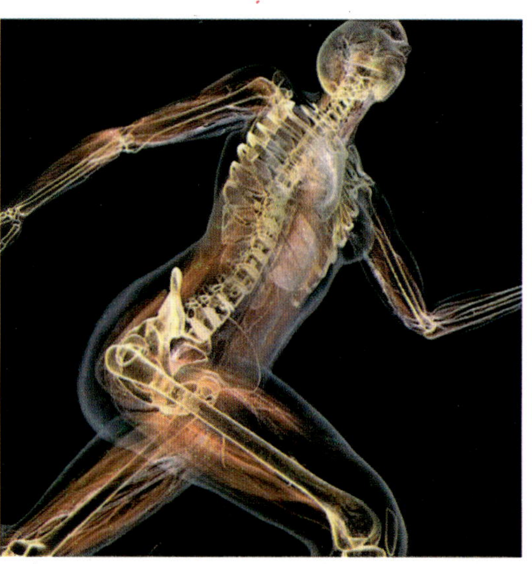

Section I

General Physiology

1 CHAPTER

The Cell

INTRODUCTION

The cells are functional units of living organisms. Some fundamental properties are common to almost all the cells, but in a multicellular organism, the cells are differentiated to perform a particular function more efficiently than others. For example, the muscle cell is specialized for the function of contraction, the intestinal mucosal cell for the absorption of food stuffs and so on. The aggregations of specialized cells constitute the tissues, the organs and organ systems. The science of human (or mammalian) physiology involves the study of interrelationships between different organs and organ systems necessary for the survival of the body as a whole.

Adaptation and *homeostasis* are the two fundamental features of life. Simple forms of life can survive over a wide range of temperature and can adapt themselves to the changes in the environment and to food stuffs available. Adaptation of man to environments varying from a desert to arctic conditions or adaptation of vision to varying degree of illumination (dark/light adaptation) are some of such examples. However, most of the physiological responses are directed towards preservation of constant physical and chemical internal environment (milieu interieur). The internal environment is constituted by the extracellular fluid which surrounds the tissue cells. The electrolyte concentration, osmotic pressure and temperature, etc. of the extracellular fluid must remain within the normal range, if the tissue cells are to function normally. Maintenance of a constant internal environment is called homeostasis. The subject of physiology is devoted to the mechanisms which help in homeostasis. Failure of homeostatic mechanism results in disturbed body function known as disease.

A common denominator of all physiological processes is their contribution to survival. But, for real understanding of the subject of physiology, and application of this knowledge in the diagnosis and treatment of a disease, the mechanism and not merely the purpose of each phenomenon must be clearly understood. The purpose of increased gastric secretion after ingestion of food is obvious even to a lay man, but only the scientific knowledge of the mechanism of gastric secretion can help in the diagnosis and treatment of gastric disorders. Therefore, while learning the subject of physiology, the student should try to understand the mechanism of a phenomenon and not teleology (explanation of events in terms of purpose).

THE CELL STRUCTURE (Colour Plate 1, Fig. 1)

Under ordinary light microscope, a cell is seen to consist to two basic components, namely, the cytoplasm and the nucleus. In a living cell, numerous granules, particles and long filaments can be seen in the cytoplasm, many of which oscillate back and forth, as if floating in the liquid medium (water). Electron microscopy reveals the complex nature of the cytoplasm and the nucleus. The functional morphology of the various components of human cells shall be briefly discussed. The cell is surrounded by a membranous covering called the cell membrane or the plasma membrane, which separates it from its extracellular environment. The cytoplasm is composed of a fluid matrix or cytosol in which several structures are dispersed. These structures can be classified into three groups, namely, (i) the organelles, (ii) the inclusions and (iii) "other components". The organelles are the permanent components of the cell. They have a limiting membrane and contain enzymes that participate in cellular metabolic activity, e.g. the endoplasmic reticulum, the mitochondria and Golgi apparatus, etc. The cytoplasmic inclusions generally are temporary components of certain cells. They consist of accumulated pigments, lipids, proteins or carbohydrates that may or may not be enclosed in a membrane. The "other components" or the cytoskeleton includes the microtubules, centriole and microfilaments. These structures are not enclosed in a membrane and do not participate directly in cellular metabolism. They act as supportive network within the cytoplasm.

The Cell Membrane (Colour Plate 1, Fig. 2)

The cell membrane is about 7.5 nm thick and hence can be seen only under the electron microscope. The cell membrane is primarily a lipid bilayer. Chemically, the lipid molecules are phospholipids and cholesterol. Each layer consists of lipid molecules with a shape of clothes-pin (Fig. 1.1).

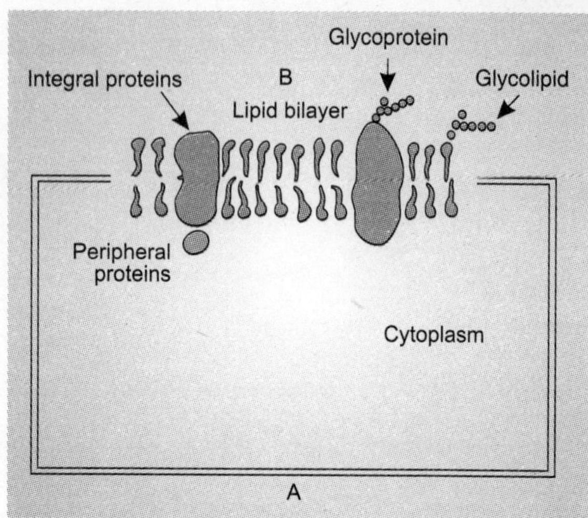

Fig. 1.1: The cell membrane. A : As seen under electron microscope. B : Fluid mosaic model of the cell membrane proposed by Singer and Nicolson.

The globular part of the molecule is hydrophilic (water soluble) and contains phosphate moiety of phospholipids or hydroxyl radical of cholesterol. The tails are hydrophobic (water insoluble); consisting of fatty acid or steroid radical of cholesterol. The lipid molecules are arranged in such a way that their non-polar hydrophobic ends are directed towards the centre of the membrane whereas their polar hydrophilic ends are directed outwards on either side of the membrane. The membrane lipid bilayer constitutes the major barrier to the permeability of water soluble molecules like ions and glucose. On the other hand, fat soluble substances like oxygen, fatty acids and alcohol can pass through the membrane with ease.

Proteins are also important molecular constituents of cell membrane and constitute nearly 50% of its weight. Two types of proteins have been recognized as constituents of the cell membrane, namely the integral proteins and the peripheral proteins. *Integral proteins* are large globular molecules distributed randomly among the lipid molecules of the membrane. They protrude out of the membrane on either side. Integral proteins act as channels for diffusion of water and water soluble substances across the cell membrane. These proteins have selective action and diffusion of some substances is preferred over others. Some of the integral protein molecules act as carrier proteins producing facilitated diffusion, while others act as receptor proteins for binding neurotransmitters and hormones. *Peripheral proteins* stud the inside or outside of the cell membrane (Fig. 1.1). These proteins modify the processes within the cell by acting as enzymes, receptors, antigens, etc.

The membrane carbohydrates occur in combination with proteins or lipids in the form of glycoproteins or glycolipids. The carbohydrate chains protrude out of the outer surface of the cell membrane (Fig. 1.1). The carbohydrate moieties act as receptor sites for binding certain hormones. Others may act as antigens. Many of these carbohydrate moieties are negatively charged and therefore influence the membrane permeability by repelling the negatively charged ions.

It should be remembered that the cell membrane is a fluid and not a solid partition. Portions of the membrane, especially the integral protein molecules, move from one point to another within the plane of the membrane.

The structure of other membranes within the cell, i.e. nuclear membrane and membranes of cytoplasmic organelles is basically similar to the cell membrane, i.e. made up of lipid bilayers. But, probably due to structural and chemical differences, each membrane has distinct receptor sites and permeability.

The Cytoplasm

The Cytoplasmic Organelles (Fig. 1.2)

1. The Mitochondria The mitochondria are spherical or cylindrical bodies having two lipid bilayer protein membranes. The inner mitochondrial membrane is folded in to form shelves or cristae. The cristae increase the internal surface area of the mitochondria. The inner cavity of a mitochondrion is filled with a gel-like matrix containing large quantities of dissolved enzymes of citric acid (Krebs') cycle and enzymes of fatty acid β-oxidation. The enzymes and other compounds involved in oxidative phosphorylation, (electron transport system) leading to generation of ATP are located on the inner mitochondrial membrane. The number of mitochondria varies in different types of cells depending on their energy requirements. One hepatocyte may contain as many as 2500 mitochondria. Within the cell, the mitochondria tend to accumulate in that part of cytoplasm where activity is more intense, e.g. at the base of the proximal tubular cell in the kidney or the apex of the ciliated epithelial cell of the respiratory mucosa.

2. The Endoplasmic Reticulum Endoplasmic reticulum is a network of membranous tubules and vesicles interconnected with each other. They are filled with a fluid called endoplasmic matrix, which is different from the cytosol. The vast

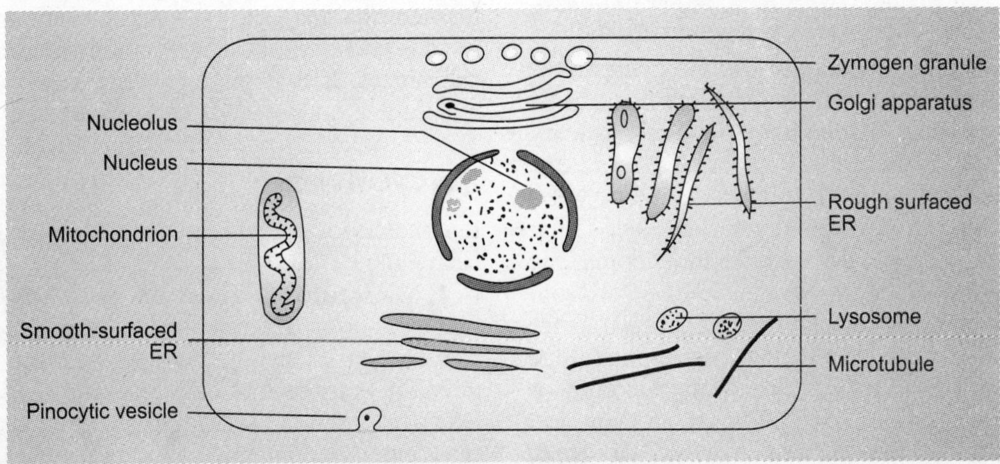

Fig. 1.2: Ultrastructure of a cell.

surface area of the reticulum and the attachment of many enzyme systems to the membrane provide machinery for: (a) synthesis of proteins, carbohydrates and lipids including steroid hormones and enzymes, (b) transport of the synthesized substances from one part of the cell to another.

Two types of endoplasmic reticulum can be recognized. They are called rough and smooth endoplasmic reticulum depending on the presence or absence of the ribosomes on their outer surface. The presence of ribosomes produces the rough or the granular appearance of the reticulum. Ribosomes are small electron-dense particles containing RNA. The abundance of rough endoplasmic reticulum is a characteristic feature of cells involved in protein synthesis, such as pancreatic acinar cells, neurons, plasma cells and fibroblasts, etc. The presence of ribosomes gives basophilic property to the cytoplasm when stained and viewed in light microscope.

3. Smooth (Agranular) Endoplasmic Reticulum The absence of attached ribosomes gives smooth appearance to the reticulum. This type of endoplasmic reticulum is associated with synthesis of a wide variety of substances. It is abundant in cells synthesizing steroid hormones (e.g. Leydig cells and cells of adrenal cortex) or in cells involved in conjugation and methylation reactions, e.g. liver cells. In the skeletal and cardiac muscle, smooth-surfaced endoplasmic reticulum is modified to form sarcoplasmic reticulum which is involved in the release and sequestration of calcium ions during muscular contraction.

4. The Golgi Apparatus The Golgi apparatus is usually composed of 4–6 flat smooth-surfaced vesicles stacked like dinner plates. It is very prominent in the cells involved in secretory processes. In such cells, it is positioned between the nucleus and the secretory surface. The Golgi apparatus is closely associated with endoplasmic reticulum. Small "transport vesicles" bud off from the ends of endoplasmic reticulum and transfer the synthesized product to the Golgi apparatus for further processing. The important function of Golgi apparatus consists of concentration and packaging of the secretory protein to form secretory vesicles or the lysosomes. Glycosylation of protein to form glycoproteins also takes place in the Golgi apparatus.

5. The Lysosomes The lysosomes are formed by the Golgi apparatus and appear as vesicles containing digestive enzymes. As many as 40 different enzymes have been identified in the lysosomes. These enzymes can digest proteins, carbohydrates, nucleic acids and lipids. Lysosomes are particularly abundant in cells involved in phagocytic activity, e.g. neutrophils, macrophages, etc. The membrane surrounding the lysosomes prevents the enclosed enzymes from acting on other cytoplasmic organelles. When bacteria are phagocytosed, the phagocytic vacuole fuses with the lysosomes and the bacterial digestion occurs within the phagolysosome. Besides destruction of the engulfed foreign bodies, the lysosomes are also concerned with turn over of the cytoplasmic organelles. The products of digestion produced by the lysosomal enzymes diffuse into the cytoplasm whereas the indigestible products are retained as residual bodies.

Cytoplasmic Inclusions

These are transitory components of the cytoplasm consisting of accumulated lipid droplets (e.g. adipose tissue, adrenal cortex and liver) or glycogen (e.g. liver, skeletal muscle) or proteins, (e.g. secretory granules). In some cells, pigments like melanin may be stored, e.g. epidermis, retina and basal ganglia. Lipofuscin is a yellowish brown pigment that increases in quantity with age. It is believed to represent accumulation of indigestible substances. It is commonly seen in the cardiac muscle and brain of the aged individuals.

The Cytoskeleton

It consists of microtubules, cilia and microfilaments.

1. Microtubules These are pipe-like or rod-like structures of variable length. Each tubule consists of 13 protofilaments running longitudinally in its wall. Microtubules are rigid bodies that give shape to the cells. They are also implicated in the intracellular transport. For example, axoplasmic transport in neurons and melanin dispersion or movement of secretory vesicles takes place through the microtubules.

The *centrioles* are two short cylindrical structures located near the nucleus. Microtubules in groups of three run longitudinally in the wall of the centriole. In the transverse section of a centriole, 9 such triplets can be seen around the circumference. The centrioles are concerned with the movement of chromosomes during cell division.

2. Cilia and Flagella These are motile processes extending from the surface of the cell. Their core is made up of microtubules. In a cilium or a flagellum, 9 pairs of microtubules are arranged around the circumference and a pair of tubules in the centre. In humans, only one type of cell contains a flagellum, i.e. the spermatozoa. True cilia are present in the cells of the respiratory mucosa, fallopian tubes, etc. The flagellum provides motility to the cell as a whole (sperm). On the other hand, cilia help in the movement of material overlying them, e.g. ovum in the fallopian tube or mucus laden with dust particles in the respiratory mucosa.

3. Microfilaments Most of the cells contain microfilaments made up of protein actin. The microfilaments are scattered in an unorganized network. They can be observed in the microvilli of the intestinal epithelium or associated with desmosomes. In the skeletal muscle, the presence of actin microfilaments is associated with the presence of another type of microfilaments, the thick, myosin microfilaments. The interaction of actin and myosin microfilaments is responsible for the shortening of the muscle.

The Nucleus

The nucleus controls all the cellular activities including reproduction of the cells. The control is mediated by the genes which are chemically made up of deoxyribonucleic acids (DNA).

The nucleus is surrounded by a double layered envelope called the nuclear membrane. The outer membrane is continuous with the endoplasmic reticulum. The space between the two nuclear membranes, called perinuclear cistern, is continuous with the lumen of the endoplasmic reticulum. The nuclear membrane is penetrated by a number of pores called the nuclear pores. Proteins with molecular weight as high as 44,000 can easily pass through these pores. The messenger RNA (mRNA) formed in the nucleus reaches the endoplasmic reticulum of the cytoplasm by passing through these pores.

The nucleus of most of the cells contains one or more nucleoli. Nucleoli are more prominent in growing cells or in cells actively synthesizing a protein. The nucleolus is rich in RNA. When a cell is not dividing, the nuclear matrix or the nucleoplasm shows dark staining chromatin material dispersed throughout the nucleus. Chemically, the chromatin material consists of DNA. It is during the cell division that the chromatin material becomes condensed and can be identified as 23 pairs of chromosomes, in all the cells, except an ovum or a spermatozoon which contain only 23 chromosomes (haploid number).

LINKAGE BETWEEN CELLS

In most of the tissues, the cells are separated from each other by interstitial spaces. However, the protective function of the epithelial tissue necessitates the presence of adhesions between the adjacent cells. The adhesions take the form of tight junctions, desmosomes and gap junctions

Tight Junctions They can be observed in the epithelia of the intestine, renal tubules and the gall-bladder. Near the apical margin, the two cell membranes fuse completely over a short distance (Fig. 1.3). Tight junctions help to bind the adjacent

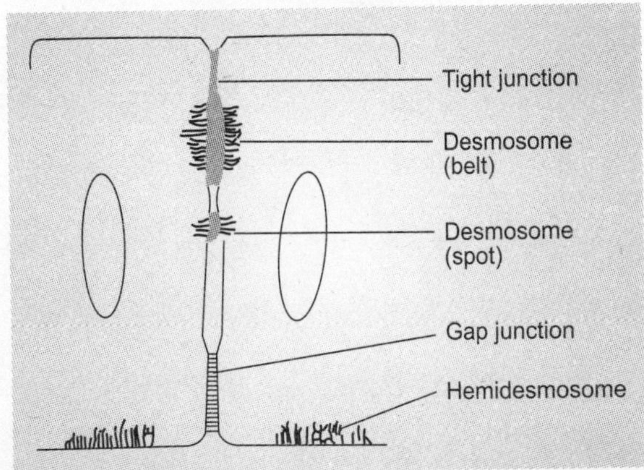

Fig. 1.3: Types of linkage between adjacent cells.

cells to each other. They also prevent movement of ions and other molecules across the intercellular spaces. Consequently, the absorption can be regulated by active or passive processes operating at the surface of cell membrane. However, the tight junctions are not completely impermeable. In some tissues, NaCl is allowed to pass through the tight junctions.

Desmosomes They occur as belt desmosomes, spot desmosomes and hemidesmosomes. These are characterised by local thickening of the adjacent cell membrane of the two epithelial cells. Attached to the thickened cell membrane are strong cytoplasmic fibrils which radiate out into the cytoplasm. Belt desmosomes are bands present below and parallel to the tight junctions. Spot desmosomes are small button-like points of attachment between the two membranes distributed randomly. Desmosomes act like spot-welds that strongly anchor one epithelial cell to the next. Hemidesmosomes are present at the basal border of the epithelial cells. They help to attach the epithelial cells firmly to the underlying connective tissue.

Gap Junctions They are intercellular connections that serve an entirely different function. Gap junctions are typically seen in cardiac and smooth muscle. They consist of proteinaceous tubes called *connexons* that allow ions to pass from one cell to the next without having to pass through the cell membrane (Fig. 1.4). Gap junctions act as areas with very low electrical resistance. Consequently, electrical impulses (action potentials) can easily spread from one cell to the next through the gap junctions. In the cardiac muscle, the gap junctions are present at the periphery of intercalated discs.

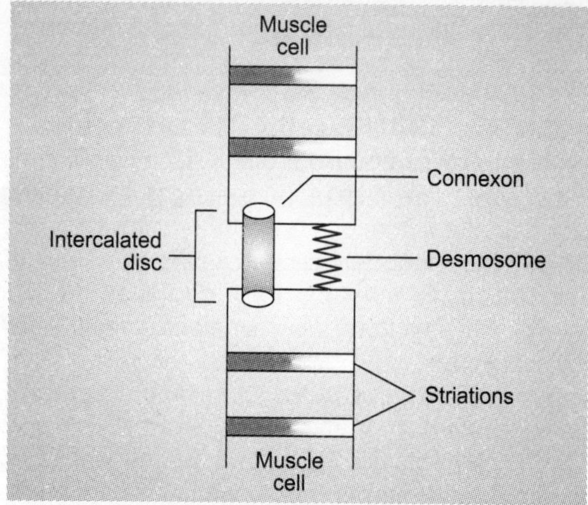

Fig. 1.4: Gap junction in cardiac muscle.

CHAPTER 2

Transport through the Cell Membranes

BODY FLUIDS

Water constitutes approximately 60% of total body weight. Thus, an adult weighing 70 kg contains 42 litres of water. Of these 42 litres, 28 litres are present inside the cells constituting the intracellular fluid volume. The remaining 14 litres of water are present outside the cells constituting the extracellular fluid volume. The extracellular fluid is mainly present as blood plasma (3.5 L) and interstitial fluid (10.5 L) (Fig. 2.1). Relatively small amount of fluid are present as cerebrospinal fluid and fluids in the eyeball and joints separated from the rest of the extracellular fluid and hence called transcellular fluid.

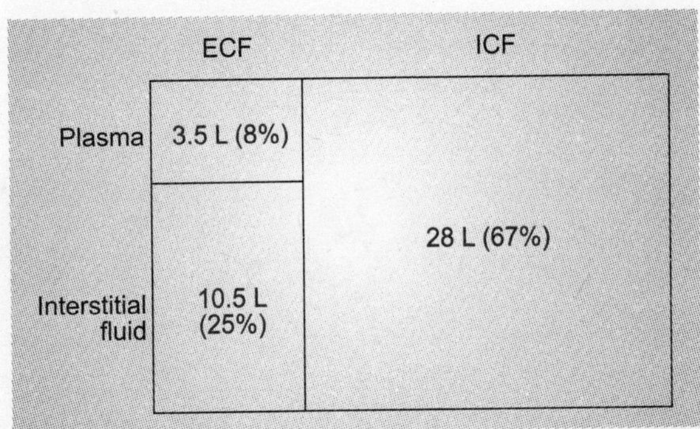

Fig. 2.1: Distribution of body water in various compartments.

Measurement of Body Fluid Volumes

The volume of any body fluid compartment, i.e. total body water, intracellular fluid (ICF), extracellular fluid (ECF), or plasma can be measured by dilution method.

Dilution Method Suppose 5 g of a marker (e.g. a dye) is added to a beaker containing unknown volume of water. After equilibrium, if the marker concentration in water is 1 g/100 ml, the volume of water in the beaker can be calculated as follows:

$$\text{Volume of water} = \frac{\text{Total amount of marker}}{\text{Conc. of marker in water}}$$

$$= \frac{5\text{ g}}{1\text{ g}/100\text{ ml}} = 500\text{ ml}$$

There are a few prerequisites for a substance to be a good marker for a particular body fluid compartment:

1. After injection, it should be confined to and evenly distributed throughout the compartment.
2. It should not be metabolized in the body.
3. It should be physiologically inert.
4. It should be non-toxic.
5. It should be easy to measure.

Some of the markers that have been used for this purpose are as follows.

Body fluid compartment	Marker
Total body water	Tritiated water
Extracellular fluid	Inulin, mannitol, sucrose
Plasma	Evans blue, ^{125}I albumin

There is no marker for ICF compartment. Its volume is calculated as the difference between total body water and ECF volume.

In practice, the measurement of various body fluid compartments is slightly more complicated, because some amount of the marker is excreted while it is being distributed through the body. Therefore the amount excreted also has to be estimated and appropriate correction made as follows:

$$\text{Body fluid volume} = \frac{\text{Total amount of marker injected} - \text{amount of marker excreted}}{\text{Concentration of marker after equilibrium}}$$

Composition of Extracellular and Intracellular Fluids

The composition of extracellular fluid (ECF) and intracellular fluid (ICF) is given in Table 2.1.

Table 2.1: Composition of ECF and ICF

	Extracellular fluid (mEq/L)	*Intracellular fluid (mEq/L)*
Na^+	142	14
K^+	5.5	150
Ca^{2+}	2.5	0.0001
Mg^{2+}	1.2	58
Cl^-	103	4
HCO_3^-	28	10
PO_4^{2-}	4	75
Protein	5 (2 g%)	40 (16 g%)

It may be noted that the extracellular fluid contains larger concentration of Na^+ and Cl^- but very little protein. Intracellular fluid contains large concentration of K^+, PO_4^{2-} and proteins. These differences are of great importance for the survival of the tissue. The forces that produce movement of substances from one compartment to another shall now be discussed.

TRANSPORT MECHANISMS

The transport mechanisms involved in the movement of substances across the cell membrane may be classified into three categories:

(a) Passive transport mechanisms which include diffusion and osmosis
(b) Active transport mechanisms
(c) "The third mechanism" which includes exo- and endo-cytosis involved in the transport of macromolecules.

DIFFUSION

Diffusion is the movement of molecules from one compartment to another due to random molecular movement. All the molecules including water molecules and dissolved particles are in constant random motion (except at absolute zero temperature). The velocity of movement increases with the increase in the temperature of the medium. Diffusion occurs in liquid as well as in gases. Due to random movements, the molecules strike against each other and bounce like rubber balls. Each collision alters the direction of the movement of molecules. The hypothetical path of molecules named A, B, C and D is shown in Fig. 2.2. Due to these collisions, molecule A moves but remains within ECF, molecule B moves but remains within ICF. In contrast, molecule C manages to enter the cell, i.e. into ICF, whereas molecule D leaves the cell to enter the ECF.

Although individual molecules move at very high velocity, the number of collisions they undergo

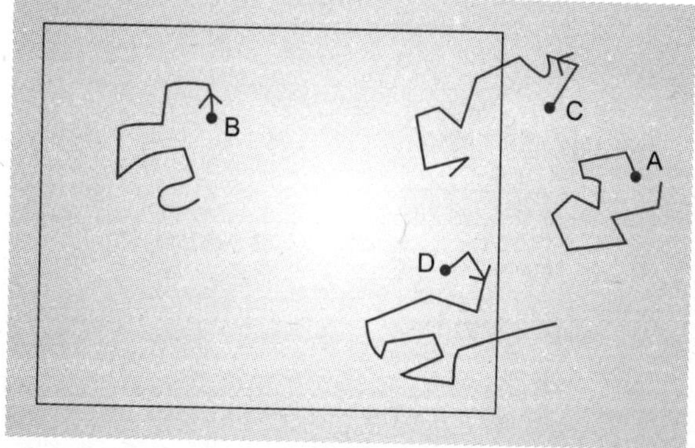

Fig. 2.2: Random movements of molecules causing diffusion.

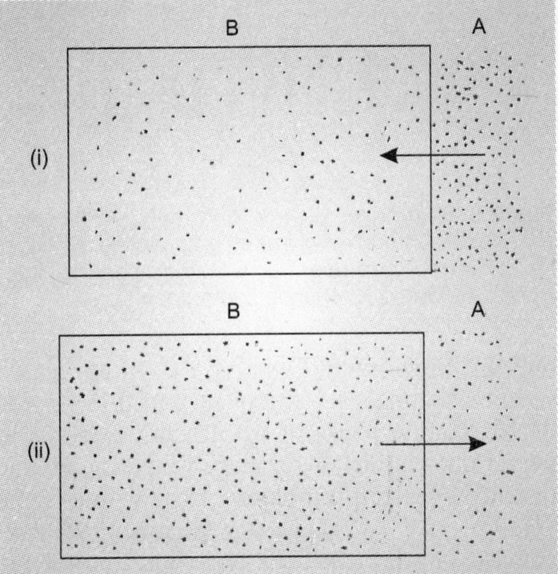

Fig. 2.3: Direction of net movement in diffusion is always down the gradient, i.e. from A to B in (*i*) and from B to A in (*ii*).

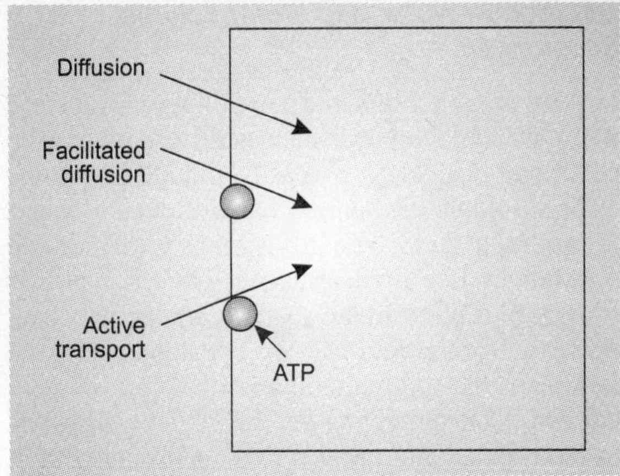

Fig. 2.4: Active transport can be uphill transport but simple diffusion or facilitated diffusion is always downhill.

prevents them from travelling very far. If the concentration of the solute molecules on the two sides of the cell membrane is similar, some molecules would enter the cell and a similar number is likely to leave it at any given moment, i.e. the net flux of the molecules is zero. Net movement of the solute molecules can occur only if concentration of molecules on one side of the membrane is greater than the concentration on the other side. In Fig. 2.3, the net movement is from fluid A to B in (i) and from B to A in (ii) because at any given time more solute molecules will pass from the fluid with higher molecule concentration to the area with lower molecule concentration. Diffusion always occurs down the gradient, i.e. from an area of high concentration to low concentration of the molecules. This phenomenon is called *simple diffusion.* In *carrier mediated diffusion*, though diffusion occurs down the gradient, it occurs with the help of a protein molecule located in the cell membrane called a carrier or a carrier protein (Fig. 2.4).

Simple Diffusion

As explained above, simple diffusion means diffusion of molecules or ions through a membrane without the help of any carrier protein. The rate of diffusion is proportionate to: (i) the difference in the concentration of the substance across the membrane (concentration gradient or chemical gradient), (ii) cross-sectional area of the membrane through which diffusion takes place, and (iii) inversely proportionate to the thickness of diffusion membrane. Electrical gradient causes diffusion of ions. Positively charged ions move towards an area with negative charge. Besides the physical factors mentioned above, diffusion across biological membranes is affected by permeability of the membrane to a particular substance, depending upon its lipid solubility, and specific and selective permeability of the membrane for different molecules. These factors shall now be discussed.

Diffusion of Lipid Soluble Substances

The extracellular and intracellular fluids are composed of water and water soluble substances. The lipid bilayer of the cell membrane forms a barrier for the diffusion of water soluble substances. However, lipids and lipid soluble substances like O_2, N_2, alcohol and steroids can diffuse across the membrane with great ease. Lipid solubility of a substance is therefore one of the determinants of the rate of diffusion across the biological membranes.

Diffusion of Water and Water Soluble Substances

In spite of the presence of lipid bilayer, water and many water soluble substances diffuse across the cell membrane relatively easily, though not as fast as lipid soluble substances. The diffusion of water is extremely rapid. The diffusion of water soluble substances like urea, glucose, Na^+, K^+, etc. is inversely proportionate to their molecular size. From these observations, it was postulated that the cell membrane contains pores of approximately 0.8 nm diameter. However, recent investigations have revealed that there are no such pores in the cell membrane. Instead, there are large *protein* molecules dispersed among the lipid molecules of the cell membrane which act as *channels* for the diffusion of water and water soluble substances. The size of the molecules or ions is not the only factor determining their diffusion through these protein channels. Selective permeability and "gating" of these channels further regulate the rate of diffusion.

1. Selective Permeability

There seem to be specific protein channels for different substances. Each allows only one type of ions to pass through. Protein channels for some substances like Na^+, Cl^-, K^+ and Ca^{2+} have been identified. Some of the ion channels are ungated i.e.always open. Sodium or potassium *leak channels* are examples of ungated ion channels. Most of the ion channels are gated.

2. Gating of Protein Channels

Gating of the protein channel means that the opening of the channel can be regulated by conformational change in the channel protein. A part of the protein molecule seems to act like a gate and close the opening. Lifting of the gate opens the channel (Fig. 2.5). Opening and closing of the gates may be controlled by three mechanisms.

1. Voltage Gating Some gates are opened or closed by a change in the electrical potentials across the cell membrane. Opening of voltage-gated sodium channels is largely responsible for the depolarization phase of the action potentials in nerve and muscle. A decrease in the membrane potential by approximately 15 mV opens the voltage-gated Na^+-channels. Opening of voltage-gated potassium channels is responsible for the repolarization phase of the action potentials in nerve and muscle (Chapter 20). Voltage-gated calcium channels have an important role in excitation-contraction coupling in the muscle. In the sino-atrial node of the heart, two types of calcium channels have been described: Transient (T-type) and long-lasting (L-type) depending on the duration for which the channels open (page 87).

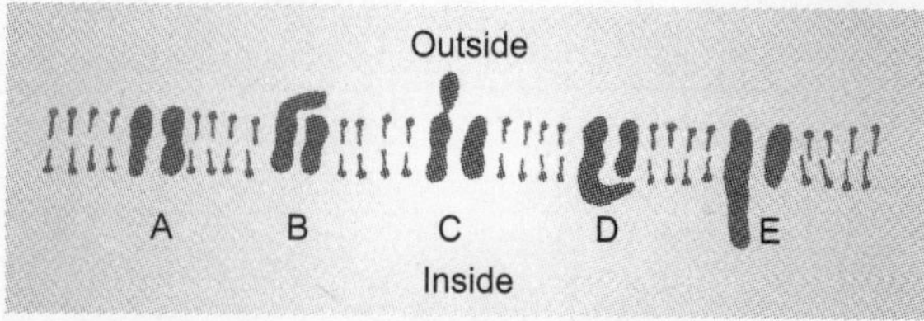

Fig. 2.5: Gating of protein channels. A. Ungated channel B. Gated Na^+-channel, gate closed. C. Gated Na^+-channel, gate open. D. Gated K^+-channel, gate closed. E. Gated K^+-channel, gate open.

2. Ligand Gating Some protein channels are opened by their binding with another molecule like a neurotransmitter or a hormone. For example, acetylcholine opens the Na^+-channels at the neuromuscular junction.

Aquaporins are water channels that help in the rapid transfer of water across the cell membranes. Like ion channels, aquaporins are made up of membrane protein. Most important ligand-gated aquaporins are found in the kidney. They are unique in the sense that the water channels are stored in the cytoplasm near the cell membrane. Presence of ADH in the blood leads to rapid translocation of aquaporins in the cell membrane and reabsorption of water from the collecting ducts (page 509).

3. Mechanically-gated Ion Channels Such channels open on exposure to a mechanical stress. The sensory receptors called mechanoreceptors contain mechanically-gated ion channels, e.g.

sensory receptors for touch, pressure, stretch, motion, and hearing. Opening of the ion channels in the receptors results in generation action potentials in the sensory nerve fibers arising from these receptors (page 271).

Certain drugs can block the ion channels in particular tissues. Sodium-channel blocker and calcium-channel blocker drugs have proved very useful in the treatment of cardiovascular disorders like angina pectoris and cardiac arrhythmias or for production of local anaesthesia. These actions shall be discussed at appropriate sections of the book.

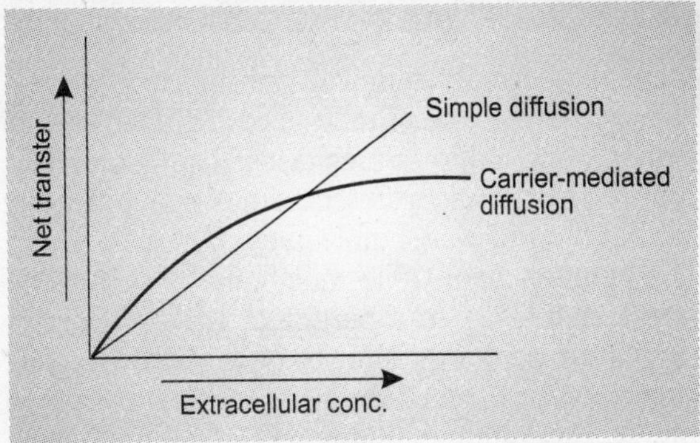

Fig. 2.6: Difference between simple diffusion and carrier-mediated diffusion: effect of saturation of the carrier.

Carrier-mediated Diffusion—Facilitated Diffusion

Diffusion of certain *large water soluble* molecules can occur only by facilitated diffusion, i.e. if helped by a protein molecule within the cell membrane. Glucose and amino acids are transported across the cell membrane by this method. Earlier, it was believed that the protein molecule acts like a shuttle between the outer and inner surfaces of the cell membrane. Now, it seems, there is no to and fro movement of the carrier protein. Molecules are transported merely by a configurational change in the protein molecule. The following characteristics of carrier-mediated diffusion differentiate it from simple diffusion.

Specificity The carrier proteins are highly specific for different molecules.

Saturation In simple diffusion, the net flux of molecules into the cell increases in direct proportion to the increase in concentration of the substance in the extracellular fluid, and it can increase to an unlimited extent. In contrast, in carrier-mediated transport, the flux into the cell increases in proportion to the increase in its concentration in the ECF only to a certain point, i.e. there is a limit beyond which further increase in the flux cannot occur (Fig. 2.6). When the maximum limit is reached, the carrier system is said to be saturated. A transport system is saturated when all the specific carrier sites on the cell membrane are occupied and the system operates at a maximum capacity.

Competition If two molecules, say (A) and (B), are transported by the same carrier, there is a competition between the two molecules for the transport. An increase in the concentration of molecule (A) may decrease the transport of molecule (B) and vice versa. No such competition occurs in simple diffusion.

Uniport and Cotransport

Some of the carrier proteins transport only one type of molecules. They are known as uniport carrier proteins. Others are called *cotransport proteins* when transfer of one substance is linked to the transport of another substance. For example, facilitated diffusion of glucose in the renal tubular cells in linked with the transport of sodium (*symport*). *Antiports* are transport proteins which exchange one substance for another, e.g. Na^+-K^+ exchange or Na^+-H^+ exchange in the renal tubules (Fig. 2.7).

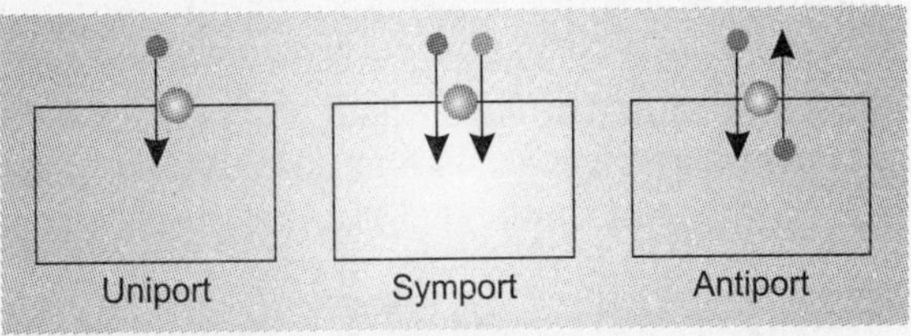

Fig. 2.7: Uniport, symport and antiport types of carrier proteins.

DIFFUSION OF WATER—THE OSMOSIS

Water is the most abundant substance to diffuse across the cell membrane. The diffusability of water is one million times faster than that of Na^+ ion. The term osmosis refers to the passive transfer or diffusion of water molecules. Osmosis occurs if a partially permeable membrane is permeable to water but not to a particular solute. The net diffusion of water occurs because of a concentration gradient of the water molecules against the cell membrane. Suppose the partially permeable membrane separates pure water from a solution of the solute, say glucose, or NaCl, to which the membrane is impermeable. In this case, the concentration of water molecules in pure water would be greater than that in which NaCl or glucose is also present. Consequently, water molecules diffuse from the side of higher concentration (pure water) to the side of lower concentration (glucose or NaCl solution). Osmosis will also occur if the membrane separates two solutions with different solute concentrations. The process of diffusion of solvent towards an area where there is higher concentration of solute is also called osmosis. Osmosis can be prevented by application of an appropriate degree of pressure on the side of higher solute concentration. The minimum pressure required to prevent diffusion of the solvent is called osmotic pressure (Fig. 2.8).

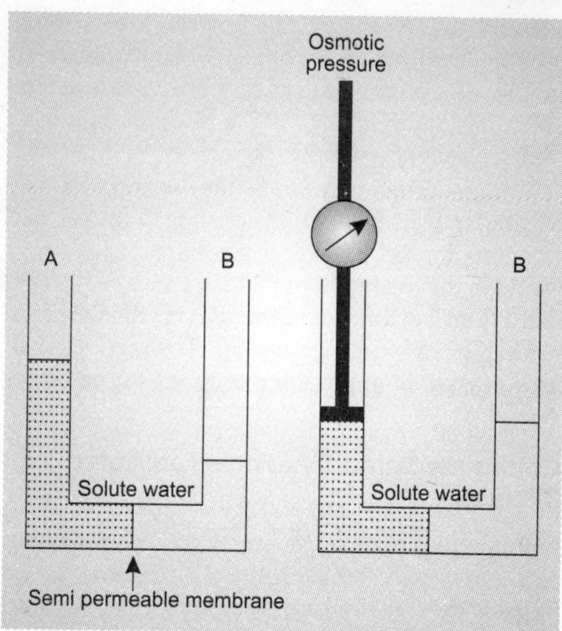

Fig. 2.8: Demonstration of osmotic pressure. Limb A contains solute solution whereas limb B contains pure water. Water enters by osmosis and increases the volume of limb A. The flow of water can be prevented by application of an appropriate pressure in side A, which is called the osmotic pressure.

Osmotic pressure depends on the number of particles rather than the type of particles present in the solution. In case of non-dissociated solutes, one gram molecular weight of any substance shall contain similar number of molecules and hence exert similar degree of osmotic pressure, i.e. equal to 22.4 atmospheres. In case of dissociated solutes, the osmotic pressure depends on the number of ions resulting from its dissociation. Thus, 180 g of glucose, i.e. 1 gram molecular weight exerts an osmotic pressure of 22.4 atmospheres. But one gram molecular weight of NaCl (58.5 g of NaCl) exerts an osmotic pressure of 44.8 atmospheres because NaCl completely dissociates into Na^+ and Cl^- ions.

The term osmole denotes the concentration of osmotically active particles in a given solution. One osmole equals the total number of particles in one gram molecular weight of the non-dissociable solutes per litre of water, or half of one gram molecular weight in case the solute dissociates completely into two ions. A complex fluid, like plasma, contains a variety of substances with varying degree of dissociation. In such cases, the osmolality can be determined more easily by an osmometer. This instrument is based on the principle of freezing point depression, which varies with the concentration of solute particles in a fluid. In case of physiological fluids, the term milliosmole (mOsm) is used. One milliosmole equals 0.001 Osm. Normal extracellular and intracellular fluids in the body have an osmolality of about 300 mOsm/kg (290 mOsm per kg to be exact).

Tonicity of Fluids

In clinical practice, the terms isotonic, hypotonic and hypertonic are commonly used. A fluid with an osmolality similar to that of plasma (290 mOsm/kg) is called *isotonic*. Red blood cells suspended in an isotonic fluid will neither shrink nor swell. A solution of 0.9% NaCl is isotonic with plasma. Any solution with osmolality greater than 290 mOsm/kg is called *hypertonic* and lower than this value is called *hypotonic*. A solution may be iso-osmotic with plasma but may not necessarily be isotonic, if the solute can penetrate the cell membrane more or less freely. For example, 0.9% NaCl is both iso-osmotic as well as isotonic but 5% glucose is iso-osmotic but hypotonic since glucose diffuses into the cell rapidly and metabolized.

In the plasma, of the total osmolality, 270 milli-osmoles are contributed by Na^+ and Cl^- and HCO_3^-. The remaining 20 mOsm are contributed by glucose and urea. Because of the large molecular weight and hence lesser number of particles, plasma proteins (70 g/L) contribute only 2 mOsm to the total plasma osmolality.

Total plasma osmolality may increase because of dehydration or increased blood glucose level (in severe diabetes mellitus) or urea (in uraemia). The consequent shrinkage of tissues may be disastrous. Decreased osmolality of plasma causes swelling of the tissues, e.g. due to excessive intravenous administration of 5% glucose.

Gibbs-Donnan Equilibrium

Diffusion of ions across a semipermeable membrane was studied by Gibbs. The theoretical calculations made by him were subsequently confirmed experimentally by Donnan.

In case the semipermeable membrane separates two solutions (a and b), one of which contains a non-diffusible anion z (side a), then the ions would distribute themselves in such a way that at equilibrium:

Side (a)	*Side (b)*
X_a^+	X_b^+
Y_a^-	Y_b^-
Z_a^-	

Semi-permeable membrane

(i) Each solution shall be electrically neutral, i.e.:

[Diffusible cation_a] = [Diffusible anion_a] + [Non-diffusible anion_a]

Or $[X_a^+] = [Y_a^-] + [Z_a^-]$

and

Diffusible cation_b = Diffusible anion_b

Or $[X_b^+] = [Y_b^-]$

(ii) The product of diffusible cations and anions on side (*a*) shall be equal to the product on side (*b*), i.e.:

[Diffusible cation 'a'] × [Diffusible anion 'a'] = [Diffusible cation 'b'] × [Diffusible anion 'b']

Or $[X_a^+] \times [Y_a^-] = [X_b^+] \times [Y_b^-]$

We might use arbitrary units to illustrate the point.

Side (a)	*Side (b)*
Diffusible cations = 16 units	Diffusible cations = 12 units
Diffusible anions = 9 units	Diffusible anions = 12 units
Non-diffusible anions = 7 units	
Equation (i) 16 = 9 + 7	12 = 12
Equation (ii) 16 × 9 = 144	12 × 144

The consequences of Gibbs-Donnan equilibrium are:

A. The concentration of diffusible cations is greater on the side containing non-diffusible anions (side a). On the other hand, the concentration of diffusible anions is greater on the other side, i.e. side (b).
B. The total concentration of diffusible ions on the side (a) is greater than on side (b).

The mammalian cells contain non-diffusible anions like proteins and organic phosphate where as K^+ and Cl^- are diffusible cation and anion respectively. The extracellular fluid contains K^+ and Cl^- as the diffusible cation and anion respectively. (The extracellular fluid is rich in Na^+ also, which is basically a diffusible cation, but the operation of Na^+-K^+ pump keeps the intracellular Na^+ concentrations very low).

Due to Gibbs-Donnan equilibrium:

1. Concentration of K^+ is greater in ICF than in ECF whereas concentration of Cl^- is greater in ECF than in ICF.
2. The higher concentration of K^+ in ICF generates the resting membrane potential.
3. Total concentration of ions is greater in the ICF than in ECF. Therefore, due to osmotic effect, the cells tend to imbibe water and swell up. This tendency is further accentuated by the higher concentration of Na^+ in the ECF because all the time, Na^+ (along with water) tends to enter the cells down the gradient but is prevented by the constant operation of Na^+-K^+ pump. If the pump fails, the cells gain sodium, lose potassium, imbibe water and swell up.

Ultrafiltration

So far, we have considered diffusion of solutes between ICF and ECF across the cell membrane. The extracellular fluid present in the blood vessels is separated from the ECF present in the interstitial spaces by the capillary endothelial cell membrane. Diffusion/osmosis occurs across the capillary membrane also. An additional factor is present at the capillary membrane, i.e. the capillary blood is under hydrostatic pressure. The pressure is 35 mmHg near the arteriolar end, and gradually declines to 12 mmHg near the venous end of the capillary.

The hydrostatic pressure causes ultrafiltration of all the constituents of plasma except proteins into the interstitial spaces. Filtration is the process in which a fluid passes through a membrane due to a difference in pressure on the two sides. Ordinary filter paper has very large pores. It holds back only large sized particulate matter. The capillary endothelium is a very fine filter. It allows filtration of water, electrolytes and other molecules with molecular weight less than 69,000 only. That is why; the term ultrafiltration is used to describe filtration across the capillary membrane.

Capillary wall is not permeable to plasma proteins, which therefore exerts an *oncotic pressure* (of 25 mmHg). The oncotic pressure opposes the movement of fluid out of the capillary walls. This factor (a) limits the outflow of fluid from the capillary near the arteriolar end and (b) causes the interstitial fluid to flow back into the capillary (by osmosis) near the venous end, where the oncotic pressure of proteins (25 mmHg) is greater than the hydrostatic pressure of blood (12 mmHg).

Biogenesis of Transmembrane Potential

In all the living cells, a difference of electric potential across the cell membrane can be demonstrated. This potential difference is called resting membrane potential or resting transmembrane potential or simply resting potential. The term resting potential indicates that the potential difference has been recorded when the cell was not undergoing any electrical change (action potential). It does not imply that the cell is metabolically quiescent. The transmembrane potential can be demonstrated by inserting a microelectrode into the cell and connecting it to a cathode ray oscilloscope (CRO) after suitable amplification (Fig. 2.9).

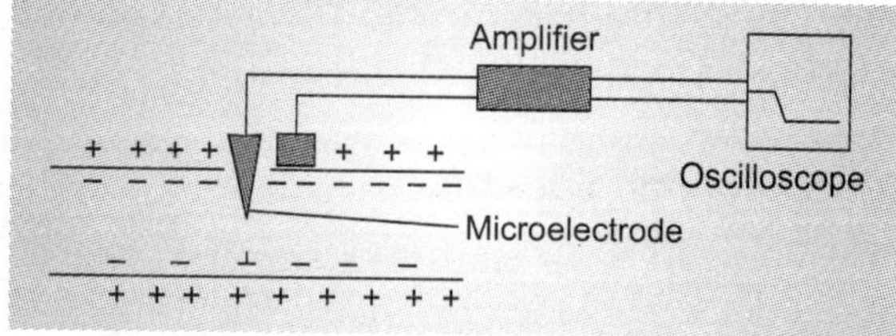

Fig. 2.9: Demonstration of transmembrane potential.

The interior of an excitable tissue cell, nerve or a muscle is 70 to 100 mV negative to the exterior. By convention, the transmembrane potential is written with a negative sign, i.e. the membrane potential inside the cell is taken as the resting membrane potential. For example, resting membrane potential of a nerve is described as –70 mV and that of a skeletal muscle cell as –90 mV.

Transmembrane potential is basically a diffusion potential, but Na^+-K^+ pump is of fundamental importance in maintaining the difference in the concentration of electrolytes between the intracellular fluid and the extracellular fluid.

1. The active transport mechanism, the Na-K ATPase pump keeps Na^+ out of the cell and pumps K^+ into the cell. Consequently, the concentration of intracellular K^+ is much higher (150 mEq/L) than that of the extracellular fluid (5 mEq/L).
2. The cell membrane is freely diffusible to K^+ ion.
3. The intracellular fluid contains non-diffusible anions in the form of proteins and organic phosphates.

Because of the large concentration gradient, positively charged K^+ diffuse out of the cells, but the non-diffusible negatively charged anions are left behind. Thus, a potential difference is created across the cell membrane with positively charged cations aligned just outside the membrane and negatively charged anions at the inner surface of the membrane. The electrical gradient so created puts a limit to the diffusion of K^+. At equilibrium, the potential difference is such that it effectively opposes any further diffusion due to chemical gradient. The degree of equilibrium potential for any diffusible ion is given by the *Nernest equation.*

$$\text{e.m.f. (millivolts)} = -61.5 \log \frac{\text{Conc. of diffusible ion inside } (C_i)}{\text{Conc. of diffusible ion outside } (C_o)}$$

For K^+, equilibrium potential E_K.

$$= -61.5 \log \frac{150}{5.5}$$

$$= -90 \text{ mV}$$

By similar calculation, the equilibrium potential for Cl^- is found to be – 70 mV.

The Na-K pump does not permit free diffusion of Na^+. If Na^+ could diffuse freely its equilibrium potential woule be

$$E\,Na_a^+ = -61.5 \log \frac{14}{142}$$

$$= +61 \text{ mV}$$

ACTIVE TRANSPORT

Active transport is also a carrier-mediated transport system with the difference that in this case, the transport of the molecules occurs faster than expected by facilitated diffusion. More importantly, active transport mechanism allows movement of substances *against an electrochemical gradient.* Such transport is also called *uphill transport* in contrast to only *downhill transport* possible with simple diffusion or facilitated diffusion (Fig. 2.4).

The movement of molecules against an electrochemical gradient involves expenditure of energy by the transport proteins. Thus, the transport proteins involved in active transport have ATPase activity incorporated into the protein molecule, which converts ATP to ADP.

Since carrier proteins are involved, specificity, saturation and competition are shown by active transport system as well. Na^+, K^+, H^+, Cl^-, I^- and several sugars, as well as, amino acids are transported by active transport mechanisms.

Sodium-Potassium ATPase (Na^+-K^+ Pump)

Sodium-potassium pump is responsible for maintaining the Na^+ and K^+ concentration differences across the cell membrane. Na^+-K^+ pump extrudes Na^+ out of the cell, and at the same time pumps K^+ into the cell. The Na^+-K^+ pump is a carrier protein which has three receptor sites for Na^+ on the portion of the protein protruding to the interior of the cell, and two receptor sites for K^+ on the portion projecting outside the cell. The inside portion of the receptor protein has ATPase activity. The ATPase activity is activated when three Na^+ and two K^+ bind to the receptor protein. The consequent release of energy from the ATP is believed to produce a conformational change in the carrier protein so that three Na^+ are extruded from the cell in exchange for two K^+ ions entering the cell. Both these ions are transported against their concentration gradients, since the intracellular fluid has high concentration of K^+, while extracellular fluid is rich in Na^+.

The Na^+-K^+ pump is an electrogenic pump since it produces a net movement of positive charge out of the cell. Thus, besides maintaining the ionic composition of the intracellular fluid, the Na^+-K^+ pump helps to maintain the electrochemical potential difference across the cell membrane. However, the sodium-potassium pump contributes

2

only – 4 millivolts to the total resting membrane potential of – 90 volts. It also helps to control the osmotic properties of the living cells.

The constant operation of Na^+-K^+ pump is responsible for about 30% of the energy utilization in most of the cells, and as high as 70% in case of neurons.

Secondary Active Transport

Transfer of many substances by active transport mechanism indirectly depends on the activity of Na^+-K^+ pump. This phenomenon is called secondary active transport. Glucose and amino acids are transported across the luminal membrane of the intestinal mucosal cells by secondary active transport. In the mucosal epithelial cell, the Na^+-K^+ pump operates at the basolateral border of the cell and maintains intracellular concentration of Na^+ very low. Luminal border of the cell contains cotransport transport proteins for facilitated diffusion of Na^+ as well as glucose. Since the intracellular Na^+ concentration is low, the facilitated diffusion of Na^+ is so powerful that glucose can be transported even when intracellular glucose concentration is higher than the intraluminal glucose concentration. In other words, downhill Na^+ transport leads to uphill glucose transport because both the molecules share a common transport system. Since glucose transport is secondary to the active Na^+-K^+ transport, it is named *secondary active transport* (Fig. 2.10).

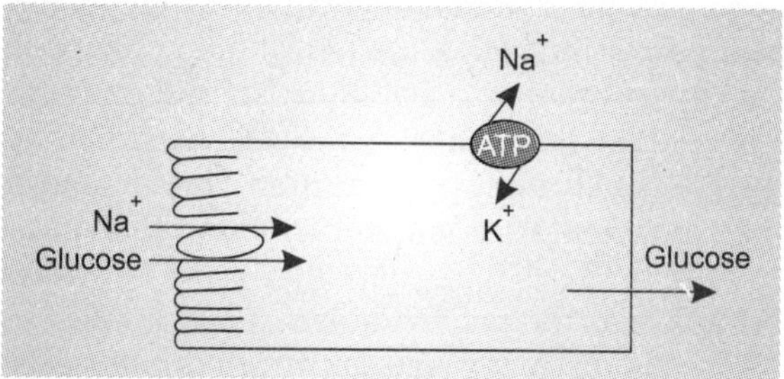

Fig. 2.10: Absorption of glucose in the small intestinal mucosa by secondary active transport.

Transport of amino acids in the intestine, or renal tubular cells is also by secondary active transport. Of course, different transport proteins are involved in this case. Secondary active transport proteins may act as antiport. For example, Na^+ is exchanged for K^+ or H^+ in the renal tubular cells or for calcium ion in the myocardial cells.

The Calcium Pump

The intracellular Ca^{2+}concentration is about 10,000 times less than that of extracellular fluid. Such low Ca^{2+} concentration is maintained by two calcium pumps. One of the calcium pumps extrudes Ca^{2+} out of the cell, whereas the other pumps cytoplasmic calcium into one or more of the cellular organelles like cytoplasmic reticulum of the muscle cells or mitochondria in all other cells. The carrier protein of both these Ca^{2+} pumps has ATPase activity. But the difference from the Na^+-K^+ pump is that the carrier protein binds Ca^{2+} rather than Na^+ and K^+.

TRANSPORT OF MACROMOLECULES—ENDOCYTOSIS AND EXOCYTOSIS

Macromolecules like large protein molecules cannot pass through the cell membrane by diffusion or active transport mechanism. They are transported into or out of the cells by a different mechanism, i.e. by endocytosis and exocytosis, respectively. When a large macromolecule comes in contact with the cell membrane, the membrane is invaginated to include the macromolecule as a vesicle. The vesicle is next pinched off to the interior of the cell and the cell membrane is restored (Fig. 2.11). This process, called endocytosis, may take the form of pinocytosis ("cell drinking") when the substances ingested are in solution or phagocytosis when a solid particle like a bacterium or a dead tissue, etc. is involved. Whereas pinocytosis occurs in most of the cells, phagocytosis occurs in a few cells like white blood cells and tissue macrophages.

There are two kinds of endocytosis:

1. *Constitutive endocytosis* is a non-specific continuous process.
2. *Receptor mediated endocytosis* is a more rapid and specific process. Specific

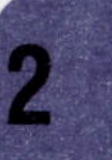

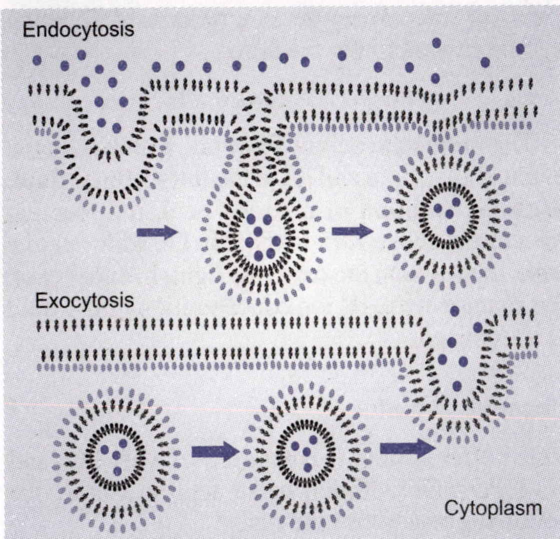

Fig. 2.11: Transport of macromolecules by endocytosis or exocytosis.

receptors are concentrated in small pits called coated pits. The inner surface of these pits is coated with dense material containing contractile filaments. Low density lipoproteins, insulin, etc. enter the cell by receptor-mediated endocytosis. Exocytosis is a reverse of endocytosis. This process is involved when secretory granules are extruded from the cell (Fig. 2.11).

Transport Across Epithelia

Epithelia are continuous sheets of cells covering the surfaces of the organs and lining the body cavities. In the GI tract, or in urinary tubules, substances are transferred from the lumen into the epithelial cell at its apical border, and then, from the basal border of the epithelial cell into the interstitium, and finally they are transported into blood capillaries. This, *transcellular pathway*, is the typical mode of transport. However, in certain epithelial cells it is not necessary for the substance to cross the whole length of the epithelial cells. Instead it may pass through the tight junctions, i.e., the point of tight adhesions between the two adjacent epithelial cells (*paracellular pathway*). In the epithelia of small intestine, proximal renal tubules and gallbladder most of sodium chloride passes through the paracellular pathway rather than traversing the entire length of the epithelial cells (Fig. 2.12).

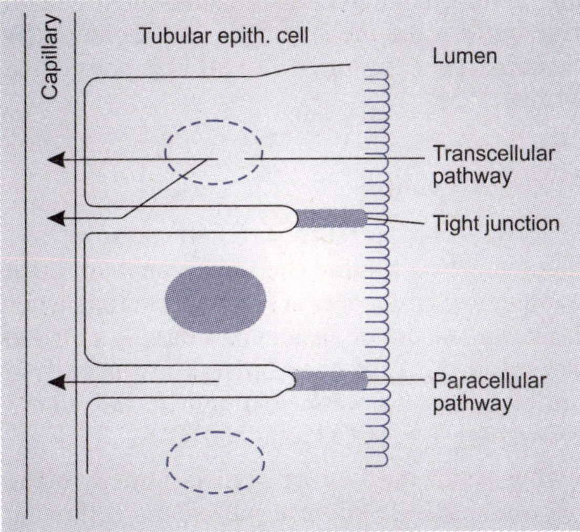

Fig. 2.12: Transport across epithelia.

HYDROGEN ION CONCENTRATION OF BLOOD

An acid is a substance that can contribute hydrogen ions (H^+) to a solution. A base is a substance that can combine with H^+ in a solution and remove it. Pure water undergoes extremely small degree of dissociation to yield H^+ and OH^- ions.

$$H_2O \rightleftarrows H^+ \text{ and } OH^-$$

The concentration of H^+ (or OH^-) in water is 10^{-7} mEq/L. Water is regarded as neutral. Acids are solution with H^+ concentration greater than 10^{-7} mEq/L (e.g. 10^{-6} or 10^{-5} mEq/L). Alkalies or bases are solutions with H^+ concentration less than 10^{-7} mEq/L (e.g. 10^{-8} or 10^{-9} mEq/L).

Expression of H^+ concentration in the body fluids as described above is cumbersome; hence a symbol pH came to be used.

$$pH = \log \frac{1}{[H^+]}$$

Thus, pH of pure water is written as 7. The pH of arterial blood is 7.4 (normal range 7.35–7.45).

2

A decrease in the pH value below 7.35 is known as acidosis, whereas an increase above 7.45 is known as alkalosis. Arterial blood pH values below 6.8 or above 8 are not compatible with life. In fact the arterial blood pH is maintained within very narrow range around 7.4 with the help of acid base buffers and the hydrogen ion secretion by the kidneys and the lungs. The pH of venous blood is about 7.35.

Acid-Base Buffers

Acid-base buffers are defined as solutions containing two or more chemical compounds that prevent marked changes in H^+ concentration, when moderate amount of an acid or a base is added to the solution. Acid-base buffers are usually a combination of a weak acid and its salt with a strong base, e.g. H_2CO_3 and $NaHCO_3$.

If a small amount of acid is added to the carbonic acid-bicarbonate buffer, the following reaction takes place:

$$HCl + NaHCO_3 \rightarrow H_2CO_3 + NaCl$$

Thus, strong acid HCl, an acid which undergoes complete dissociation and yields large number of H^+, has been converted to a weak acid (an acid which dissociates poorly to yield few H^+). Therefore in spite of addition of HCl, the H^+ concentration of the solution is only mildly increased. If a small amount of a strong base is added to the mixture, the following reaction takes place:

$$NaOH + H_2CO_3 \rightarrow NaHCO_3 + H_2O$$

Thus, a strong base has been converted into a weak base and the decrease in H^+ concentration is minimized.

Other Buffer Systems in the Body

Haemoglobin and Plasma Proteins

The plasma proteins in general, and haemoglobin in particular, constitute an important buffer system. Proteins are composed of amino acid chains. The terminal amino acids possess carboxyl (–COOH) and amino (NH_2) groups. At pH of 7.4, the carboxyl radicals ionize as a weak acid donating hydrogen ions to the medium.

$$\text{Protein} \rightleftarrows \text{Proteinate}^- + H^+$$

The proteinate anions form salt with Na^+ in the extracellular fluid and K^+ in the intracellular fluid. With the addition of a strong acid, the reaction mentioned above shift to the left. On addition of a base, the reaction moves to the right. In either case, the change in the H^+ ion concentration of the fluid is minimised.

Phosphate Buffer

This buffer system is composed of NaH_2PO_4 and Na_2HPO_4. On addition of an acid or a base, the following reactions take place:

$$Na_2HPO_4 + HCl \rightarrow NaH_2PO_4 + NaCl$$

$$NaH_2PO_4 + NaOH \rightarrow Na_2HPO_4 + H_2O$$

Ammonia Buffer

In the renal tubules, ammonia (NH_3) acts as an important buffer. It accepts H^+ to become NH_4 which is excreted in the urine.

Henderson-Hasselbalch Equation

Henderson–Hasselbalch equation gives the mathematical relationship between the ratio of concentrations of the acidic and basic elements of each buffer system on one hand and pH of the solution on the other.

$$pH = pK^1 + \log \frac{\text{base}}{\text{acid}}$$

K (or pK^1) is the ionization constant of the weak acid at a particular temperature, etc. From the equation, it is apparent that the pH will increase if the concentration of the base increases, or that of the acid decreases; pH shall decrease if the concentration of the base decreases, or that of the acid increases.

The efficiency of a buffer system is the best (i.e. the ability of the system to resist changes in pH is maximum) when pH of the solution is identical with that of the pK value of the buffer system. The pK value of the important buffers in the body is given in Table 2.2.

Table 2.2: pK value of buffer systems

Buffer systems	*pK[1]*
Carbonic acid bicarbonate	6.1
Phosphate buffer	6.8
Haemoglobin (histidine)	7.0

The pK[1] value of plasma proteins in general and haemoglobin in particular is closer to the pH of plasma. Moreover, their concentration in the blood (7.5 g% proteins and 15 g% Hb) makes them the most efficient buffers in the blood. Although the pK value of phosphate buffer is close to 7.4, but its poor concentration in the plasma (2–4 mg%) makes it most ineffective. However, intracellular fluids contain high concentration of phosphates as well as proteins. Hence, phosphate and proteins constitute important buffers in the intracellular fluids. Phosphates are also important urinary buffers because their concentration is markedly increased in the renal tubular fluid. The carbonic acid bicarbonate buffer is not so efficient because its pK value (6.1) is far removed from the pH of the plasma. The importance of carbonic acid bicarbonate buffer lies in the fact that both its components are subjected to regulation in the body: Carbonic acid concentration (CO_2) is regulated by the respiratory system, whereas the bicarbonate concentration is regulated by the kidneys.

Summary

Important buffers:

Blood	: Hemoglobin plasma proteins, bicarbonate
Interstitial fluid	: Bicarbonate
Intracellular fluid	: Proteins phosphates
Urine	: Phosphates ammonia

ISOHYDRIC PRINCIPLE

The three major buffer systems operating in vivo (proteins, particularly haemoglobin, bicarbonate-carbonic acid and phosphate) exert a mutual buffering action on each other. Any alteration in H^+ concentration will cause a corresponding shift in the base/acid ratio in each of the buffer pairs. This is called isohydric principle. The blood contains all the three buffers named above. But, it must be remembered that the *intracellular buffers (proteins and phosphates)* take care of over 50% of the excess acid load in metabolic acidosis and approximately 35% of the base load in metabolic alkalosis. In respiratory acidosis, or alkalosis, almost all the buffering is intracellular.

The chemical buffers of the cells and the extracellular fluid constitute the first line of defence against H^+ ion disturbances. Respiratory system constitutes the second line of defence and can partially compensate for metabolic acidosis or alkalosis. Ultimately, excess acid or alkali ingested or produced in the body is excreted by the kidney.

Section II

The Blood

CHAPTER 3

The Red Blood Cells and Blood Groups

The cardiovascular system contains about 5 litres of blood (about 7% of body weight). The blood is composed of specialized cells suspended in a fluid medium, the plasma. The unique fluid nature of this tissue is ideal for its function of transport of substances from one part of the body to another. The blood serves to provide nutrients and hormones to the tissues, and remove their waste products, etc. The function of blood is dependent upon the function of another organ system, the cardiovascular system. Adequate circulation of blood to every part of body is essential for the maintenance of millieu interieur.

The cellular elements of blood consist of three types of cells: the red blood cells (erythrocytes), the white blood cells (leucocytes) and the platelets (thrombocytes) (Fig. 3.1). The blood plasma is a solution of extraordinary complexity. It is a clear, slightly yellow liquid containing a large number of organic and inorganic substances dissolved in water. The plasma proteins constitute about 7.5% of the total weight of plasma. Another 1.5–2% of the solids present in plasma consist of inorganic constituents (like Na^+, K^+, Ca^{2+}, Mg^{2+}, Cl^-, HCO_3^-, PO_4^{2-} and SO_4^{2-}), organic

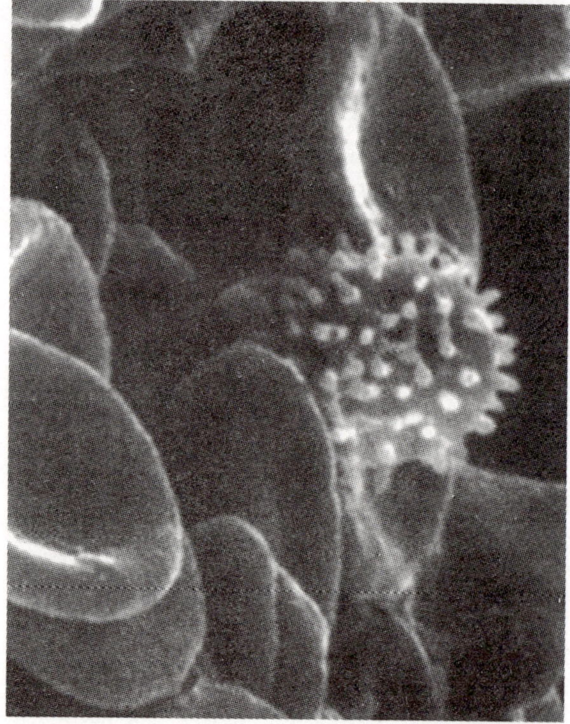

Fig. 3.1: Highly magnified view of red blood cells and a white blood cell.

constituents (like glucose, amino acids, lipids and cholesterol) (Table 3.1), vitamins, trace elements (like iron, copper, zinc), hormones and gases (like oxygen, carbon dioxide and nitrogen).

Table 3.1: Normal range of some important constituents of plasma

I. *Organic constituents (mg/dl)*	
Proteins	6000–8000 (6–8 g/dl)
Amino acids	30–50
Total lipids	400–600
Total cholesterol	150–200
Glucose	70–110
Urea	20–40
Uric acid	3.5–7.0 (males) 3.0–6.0 (females)
Creatinine	0.7–1.4
Bilirubin	0.2–1.0
II. *Inorganic constituents (mEq/L)*	
Sodium	136–145
Potassium	3.5–5.0
Calcium	2.1–2.5 (9–11 mg/dl)
Magnesium	0.7–0.9 (1.8–2.2 mg/dl)
Chloride	96–106
Bicarbonate	22–26
Phosphate	1.0–1.5 (2.5–4.5 mg/dl)

The fluidity of blood is maintained only as long as it circulates in the blood vessels. If experimentally removed from a vein and kept in a test tube, it becomes a solid mass within minutes by a process known as coagulation (or clotting) of blood. After about 30 minutes, the clot retracts to one side of test tube and a clear yellow fluid called *serum* is exuded out of the clot. If coagulation of the blood is prevented by the addition of a solid anticoagulant and centrifuged in a graduated tube called the haematocrit tube, the heavier red cells (sp. gravity 1.093) settle at the bottom of the tube leaving clear *plasma* (sp. gravity 1.026) above (Fig. 3.2). In this way, the percentage of total blood volume constituted by the red cells, known as the haematocrit, can be determined. Normal haematocrit is approximately 45% in males and 42% in females. White blood cells and platelets constitute only about 1% of the

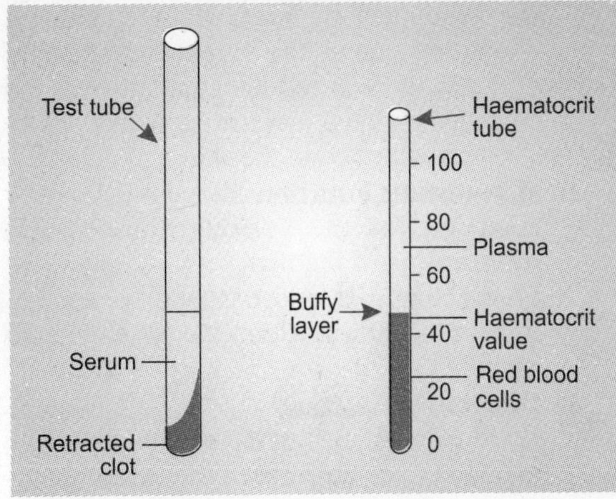

Fig. 3.2: Estimation of haematocrit (right side). Serum is obtained when the blood is allowed to clot (left side).

volume of blood, and are seen as a thin white layer called buffy coat on the top of the red cell mass in the haematocrit tube. The composition of the serum and the plasma is similar, except that in serum fibrinogen and a few other clotting factors have been removed during the process of clotting of blood. The high viscosity of blood as compared to that of water can chiefly be attributed to the presence of blood cells and plasma proteins. This property of blood has an intimate relation with haemodynamics of circulation.

FUNCTIONS OF BLOOD

1. **Transport Function** The primary function of the blood is transport of various substances from one part of the body to another:
   (a) Transport of nutrients like glucose, amino acids, fatty acids, vitamins, minerals (Fe, Cu, Co, Na, K, Ca) from the gastrointestinal tract to all the tissues.
   (b) Transport of gases. O_2 from the lungs to the tissues, and CO_2 from the tissues to the lungs.
   (c) Transport of hormones from the endocrine glands to the target tissues.
   (d) Transport of waste products of tissue metabolism like urea, uric acid, creatinine, bilirubin, etc. from the tissues to the sites of excretion, e.g. kidney or liver.

(e) Transport of heat. Heat is chiefly produced in the liver and skeletal muscle. It is redistributed all over the body to keep it warm in winter. Extra heat is lost from the skin.

2. **Homeostatic Function** Blood is essentially required for the various homeostatic mechanisms of the body, e.g. maintenance of glucose, pH and osmolality, etc. of extracellular fluid within the physiological range.

3. **Protective Function**
   (a) Protection against its own loss from the blood vessels by the presence of platelets and various coagulation factors.
   (b) Protection of the body against bacterial, viral and parasitic infections by the presence of white blood cells, specific immunoglobulins (antibodies) and complement proteins.

THE RED BLOOD CELLS (ERYTHROCYTES)

Each red blood cell (RBC) is a non-nucleated, biconcave disc with a mean diameter of approx. 7.5 μm and thickness of about 2 μm at the periphery and about 1 μm in the middle (Fig. 3.3). This shape of the red cell provides it with a large surface area: volume ratio which helps in an efficient gas diffusion throughout the interior of the cell. This shape also allows distortion during passage through narrow capillaries, and moderate swelling of the cell without stretching the cell membrane.

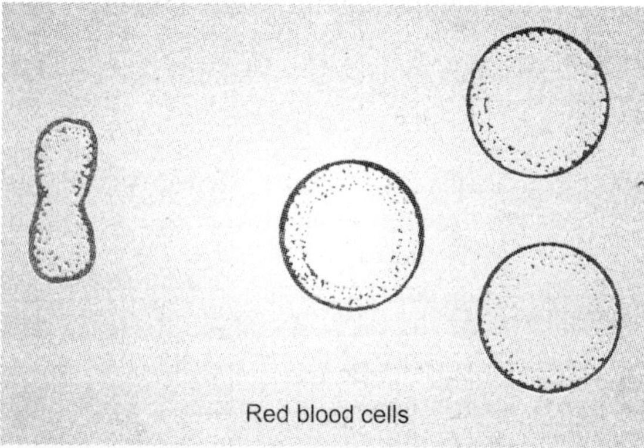

Fig. 3.3: Shape of red blood cells.

The red cell membrane is a typical lipid bilayer structure. It is freely permeable to water. A Na^+-K^+ ATPase pump keeps the intracellular Na^+ concentration low and K^+ concentration high. The energy for this active process is provided by ATP derived from glycolysis in the red cell. The red cell membrane contains certain specific glycoproteins which differ from person to person and form the basis of the blood groups.

Haemoglobin, an iron-containing red pigment is the most important constituent of the erythrocytes. It constitutes about 35% volume of the red cells.

Normal average red blood cell count is 5.5 million per μL of blood in adult males and 4.8 million per μL of blood in adult females (see Table 3.3). Deficiency of red blood cells and/or haemoglobin is called anaemia.

HAEMOGLOBIN

Haemoglobin (Hb), the most important red cell constituent, is a conjugated protein having a molecular weight of 64,400.

Haemoglobin A

This is the type of haemoglobin present in the red cells in the postnatal life. It consists of an iron-containing portion called the haem and a protein called the globin. Each haemoglobin molecule is made up of 4 subunits. Each subunit (mol. wt. 16,000) consists of iron-containing porphyrin. The iron atom in each subunit of haem is in ferrous form (Fe^{++}) and has a "bond" available for loose union with oxygen molecule (O_2) (Fig. 3.4). The globin part consists of 4 polypeptide chains two of which are known as alpha (α) chains (having 141 amino acids) and the other two, beta (ß) chains (having 146 amino acids). The α and ß chains differ from each other not only in the number but also in the sequence of the amino acids. Thus HbA is characterised by two α and two ß chains (HbA= α_2, β_2) (Fig. 3.5).

In adult males, mean Hb concentration of blood is 15.5 gm% (range 13 to 18 gm%). In adult females, the mean Hb conc. is 14 gm% (range 12 to 16 g%). At birth, the haemoglobin concentration

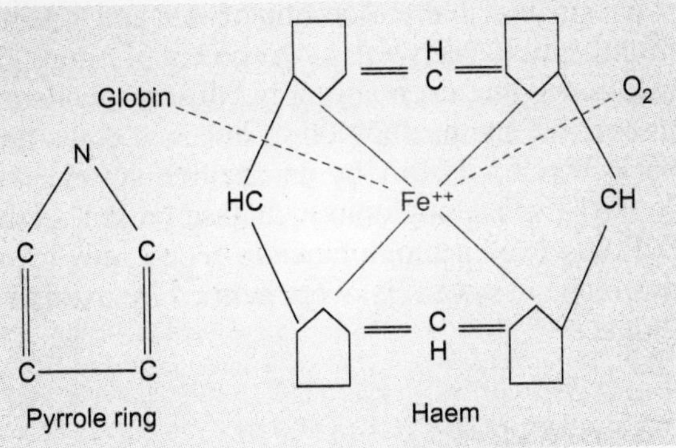

Fig. 3.4: Structure of haem.

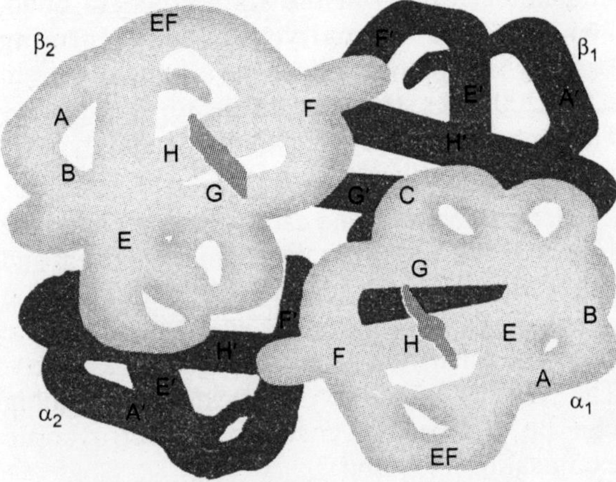

Fig. 3.5: Haemoglobin consists of 4 units of haem, each attached to one of the four polypeptide chains constituting globin.

of blood may be higher but it falls to about 10 gm% by the end of third month.

Functions

1. Haemoglobin molecules have an important property of forming a loose and reversible combination with O_2 to constitute oxygenated Hb (bright red in colour). One O_2 molecule is attached at the sixth covalent bond of each iron atom of the haemoglobin molecule. That means each Hb molecule can take up four molecules of oxygen. When fully saturated with O_2, each gram of Hb contains 1.34 ml of oxygen. Thus, each 100 ml of arterial blood contains approx. 20 ml of oxygen (15 × 1.34).

$$\underset{\text{Oxygenated haemoglobin}}{HbO_2} \rightleftharpoons \underset{\text{Deoxygenated haemoglobin (reduced Hb)}}{Hb} + O_2$$

In the tissues, oxygen molecules are released by the haemoglobin and deoxygenated Hb (dark red in colour) is formed. In this fashion, Hb serves the most important function of the transport of oxygen from the lungs to the tissues.

2. Haemoglobin is also involved in the transport of CO_2 from the tissues to the lungs. It must be stressed that CO_2 is transported by combination with amino acids of the globin part as shown below and not by combination with Fe^{++} atom.

$$\underset{\text{Haemoglobin}}{R{-}N{<}^{H}_{H}} + CO_2 \longrightarrow \underset{\text{Carbamino haemoglobin}}{R{-}N{<}^{H}_{COOH}}$$

Deoxygenated Hb forms carbamino compound more readily than oxygenated Hb. That is why venous blood becomes more suitable form of transport of CO_2 from tissues to the lungs.

3. Haemoglobin constitutes the most important acid-base buffer system of blood. Although the concentration of Hb is roughly twice the concentration of plasma proteins, Hb has 6 times the buffering capacity of plasma proteins.

Normally Hb remains within the red cells. In pathologic states, e.g. acute haemolytic disorders, Hb appears in plasma and may cause gross complications by increasing its viscosity and osmotic pressure. However, Hb circulating in the plasma is rapidly removed by tissue macrophages and by renal excretion as well.

Fetal Haemoglobin

During fetal life, the red blood cells contain a different type of Hb known as the fetal Hb (HbF). Structurally, HbF differs from HbA, i.e. it contains two α and two γ chains instead of two α and two β chains. The γ chains contain (like ß chains) 146 amino acids but 37 amino acids of γ chains are different from those of ß chains. As a result of this alteration, the affinity for oxygen is markedly increased, which helps in transport of O_2 during fetal life.

3 Fetal haemoglobin is normally replaced by haemoglobin A (HbA) soon after birth. This is achieved by replacement of gamma chains of globin molecule by ß chains. The exact mechanism of this switchover is not clear, but it is genetically determined. Due to a genetic defect, formation of ß chains may be inadequate, resulting in one type of thalassemias (see below).

Haemoglobin A_2

In normal adults, about 2.5% of haemoglobin has a different structure. This form contains 2 alpha (α) chains and 2 delta (δ) chains. This type is known as haemoglobin A_2. Delta chains also contain 146 amino acids but 10 amino acid residues are different from the ß chains. Presence of the small amount of HbA_2 in our blood has no physiological significance.

Haemoglobin A Derivatives

Glycosylated Haemoglobin (HbA_1)

A small percentage of haemoglobin A (< 7%) normally undergoes non-enzymatic attachment of glucose molecules to the terminal amino acid (valine) in each ß chain.The change called glycosylation (or glycation) of haemoglobin (HbA_1) does not produce any significant effect on the transport of gases. Three variants of HbA_1 can be isolated, namely, HbA_{1a}, HbA_{1b} and HbA_{1c}. Estimation of HbA_{1c} is of special interest in patients of diabetes mellitus. In patients with sustained hyperglycemia, 10–20% of total haemoglobin may be present as HbA_{1c} (Chapter 49).

Methaemoglobin

Methaemoglobin is a dark brown colored derivative of HbA. It is formed by conversion of Fe^{2+} (ferrous) atoms of haem molecules to Fe^{3+} (ferric) due to intake some certain oxidizing drugs. The ferric atoms cannot bind with oxygen. Hence, when a fairly large percent of HbA has been converted to methaemoglobin, the patient shows cyanosis (bluish discoloration of skin and mucous membranes) as well as hypoxia. It may be mentioned that even normally HbA has tendency to become methaemoglobin, but it is converted back to normal HbA by an enzyme system, the NADH-methaemoglobin reductase present in the red cells. Methaemoglobinemia occurs only when this enzyme system is overwhelmed by oxidizing drugs.

Carboxyhaemoglobin

Inhalation of carbon monoxide (CO) causes attachment of CO at the sixth covalent bond, (where O_2 is normally attached), forming carboxyhaemoglobin. Since the affinity of Fe^{2+} to CO is 200 times stronger than that for O_2, carboxy-Hb cannot take part in O_2 transport and hypoxia results. (For further details see Ch.19)

Methaemoglobin and carboxyhaemoglobin are formed by alterations in the haem component and can be reconverted to normal Hb by administration of reducing agents like methylene blue (or ascorbic acid) and inhalation of pure oxygen respectively. The presence of carboxy-Hb or methaemoglobin can be easily diagnosed by spectroscopic examination of blood.

Haemoglobinopathies

The red cells of certain individuals contain abnormal types of haemoglobin due to *genetically determined abnormalities* in the polypeptide chains of the globin component. These disorders include: thalassemia and sickle cell anemia.

Thalassemia

In this genetic disorder, there is a decrease or absence of α or ß chains of haemoglobin A. ß thalassemia is characterized by deficiency of ß chain synthesis, whereas α thalassemia is characterized by deficiency of α chain synthesis. Consequently, the red cells contain excess of the other type of globin chains. Such red cells have a shorter lifespan than the normal red cells and lead to severe anaemia.

Sickle Cell Anaemia

This type of haemoglobinopathy is caused by the presence of amino acid valine instead of glutamic acid at position 6 in the ß chain. Such haemoglobin is known as Hb S (haemoglobin S) because when it is deoxygenated, it becomes much less soluble making the red cells sickle-shaped (Fig. 3.6). Sickle-shaped cells are more prone to rapid destruction (haemolysis).

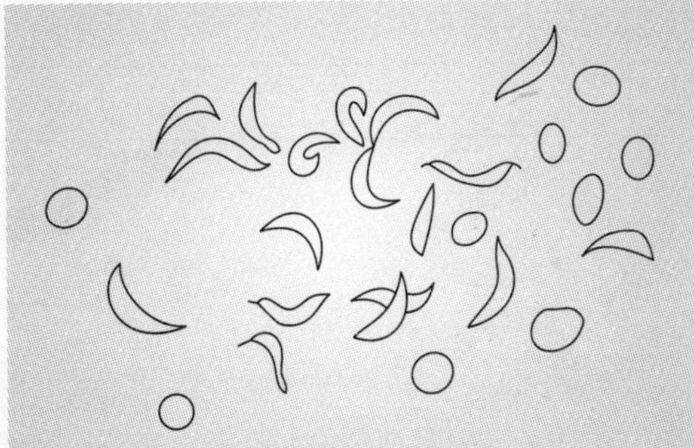

Fig. 3.6: Sickle cells.

Haemoglobin S is highly prevalent in black population of Africa. *Sickle cell anaemia* occurs only in those individuals who are homozygous for haemoglobin S gene, i.e. whose red cells contain only haemoglobin S. Children with sickle cell anaemia die young. *Sickle cell trait* is far more common. In certain areas, as much as 40% of the population have sickle cell trait. These individuals are heterozygous for haemoglobin S gene, i.e. their red cell contain haemoglobin S (50%) as well as haemoglobin A (50%). Persons with sickle cell trait do no suffer from excessive haemolysis of red cell. On the other hand, they are highly resistant to a very dangerous type of malaria (falciparum type) prevalent in those areas.

There are some other types of congenitally defective haemoglobins, e.g. Hb C, Hb E, Hb G, etc. Haemoglobinopathies can be diagnosed accurately by electrophoresis.

Haemopoiesis (Colour Plate 2, Fig. 3)

In the early fetal life, haemopoiesis (formation of blood cells) occurs intravascularly by proliferation of endothelial cells of the capillaries. Next, haemopoiesis occurs in the liver and spleen of the fetus. By the end of 4th month of fetal life, the bone marrow takes over the function of haemopoiesis. In children, blood formation occurs in the marrow cavities of most of the bones. The well marked cellularity gives red colour to the marrow when seen with a naked eye. Hence in children most of the marrow is red. Red marrow contains various developing stages of red cells, white cells and platelets as well as some adipose tissue and connective tissue cells. By 21 years age, the red bone marrow is limited to the axial skeleton (skull, vertebrae, ribs, sternum and pelvis) and the proximal ends of the femur and the humerus (Fig. 3.7). In the remaining parts of long bones, the marrow consists of adipose tissue and some blood capillaries. Such marrow is known as yellow bone marrow (Fig. 3.8). When the rate of formation of red cells (erythropoiesis) is to be markedly accelerated (e.g. after severe haemorrhage or in haemolytic anaemia), the yellow marrow is converted to red marrow. Thus yellow bone marrow acts as a reserve for increased blood formation in case of situations requiring rapid erythropoiesis.

The red marrow contains pluripotent stem cells (hemocytoblasts) which give rise to all types of blood cells. Various types of blood cells in different stages of development can be observed in a stained smear of red bone marrow obtained from iliac bone or sternum. A process of self-renewal without differentiation maintains stem cell population. Some of them migrate to other areas and produce lymphocytes. A process of commitment converts others into erythroid line of cells, myeloid line of cells or platelet forming cells. Certain humoral substances like erythropoietin, colony stimulating factors or thrombopoietin push the stem cells into the respective line of development. In the red bone marrow, normally, about 75% of cells are immature white cells and only about 25% cells are immature red cells. Thus normal myeloid: erythroid ratio is 3: 1, even though in the peripheral blood, the WBC: RBC ratio is 1: 600. This vast difference is related to the fact that the lifespan of red cells is far greater than that of the white blood cells. The development of white blood cells and platelets is discussed in Chapter 4 (page 50) and Chapter 5 (page 67) respectively.

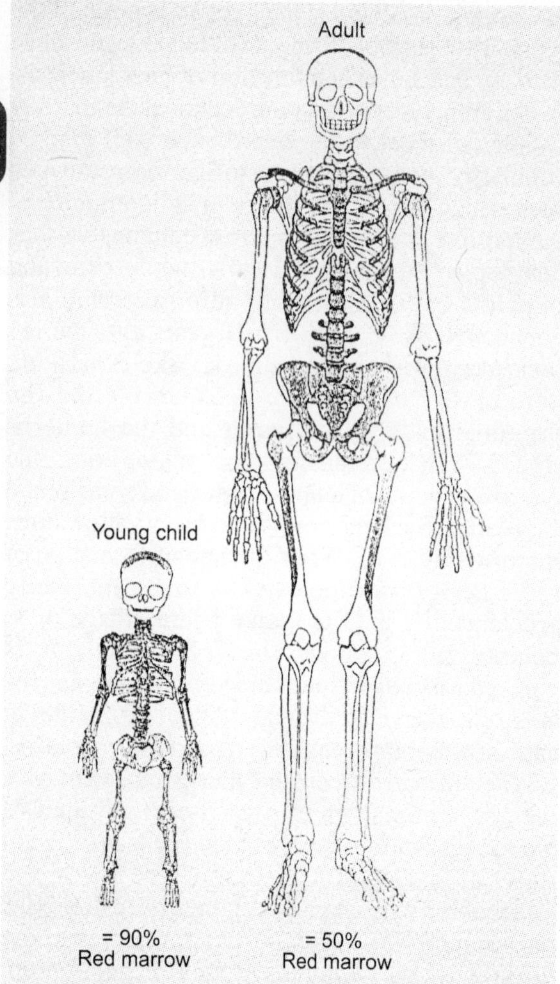

Fig. 3.7: Distribution of red bone marrow in a child and an adult.

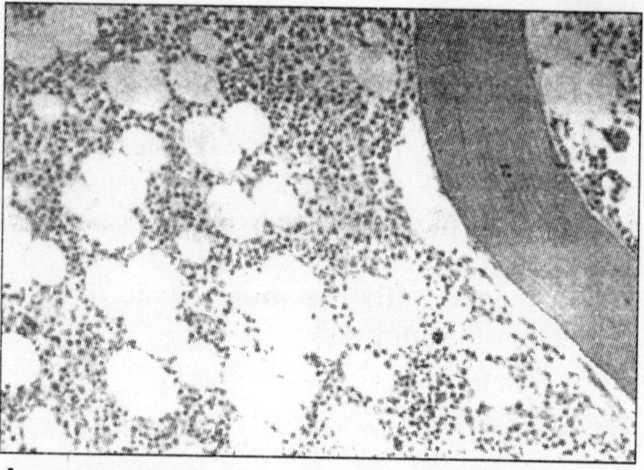

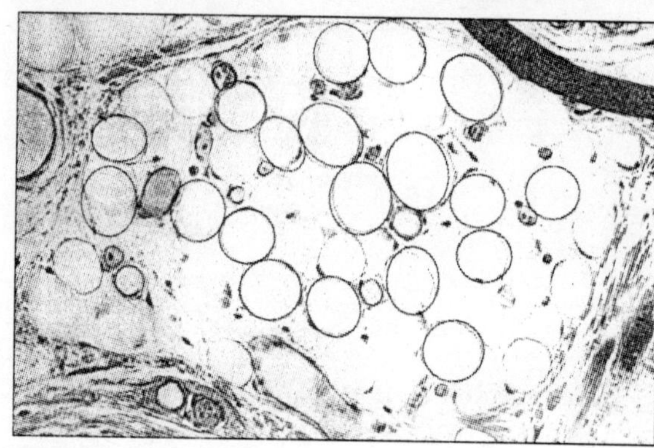

Fig. 3.8: Histological structure of red bone marrow (A) and yellow bone marrow (B).

Erythropoiesis

When the process of commitment pushes the stem cell into erythroid line of development (Fig. 3.9), the following stages can be differentiated.

1. **Proerythroblast (pronormoblast)** It is a large cell, 15–20 μm in diameter. The cytoplasm is deeply basophilic. A large central nucleus is seen to contain many nucleoli. The intense basophilia of the cytoplasm is due to the presence of abundant ribosomal RNA, indicating active protein synthesis.
2. **Basophilic (early) Normoblast** This cell has a diameter of about 12–16 μm. The cytoplasm is deeply basophilic. The nucleus is slightly condensed as compared to the previous stage, and the nucleoli are not seen. This stage shows active mitosis.
3. **Polychromatic (intermediate) Normoblast** This cell has a diameter of 12–14 μm. The nucleus is coarse and deeply basophilic. The most characteristic feature of this stage is the polychromatic cytoplasm since it contains basophilic RNA as well as small amount of acidophilic haemoglobin. Mitosis ceases at this stage.
4. **Orthochromatic (late) Normoblast** At this stage, the cell size is 7–10 μm. The cytoplasm is acidophilic due to accumu-

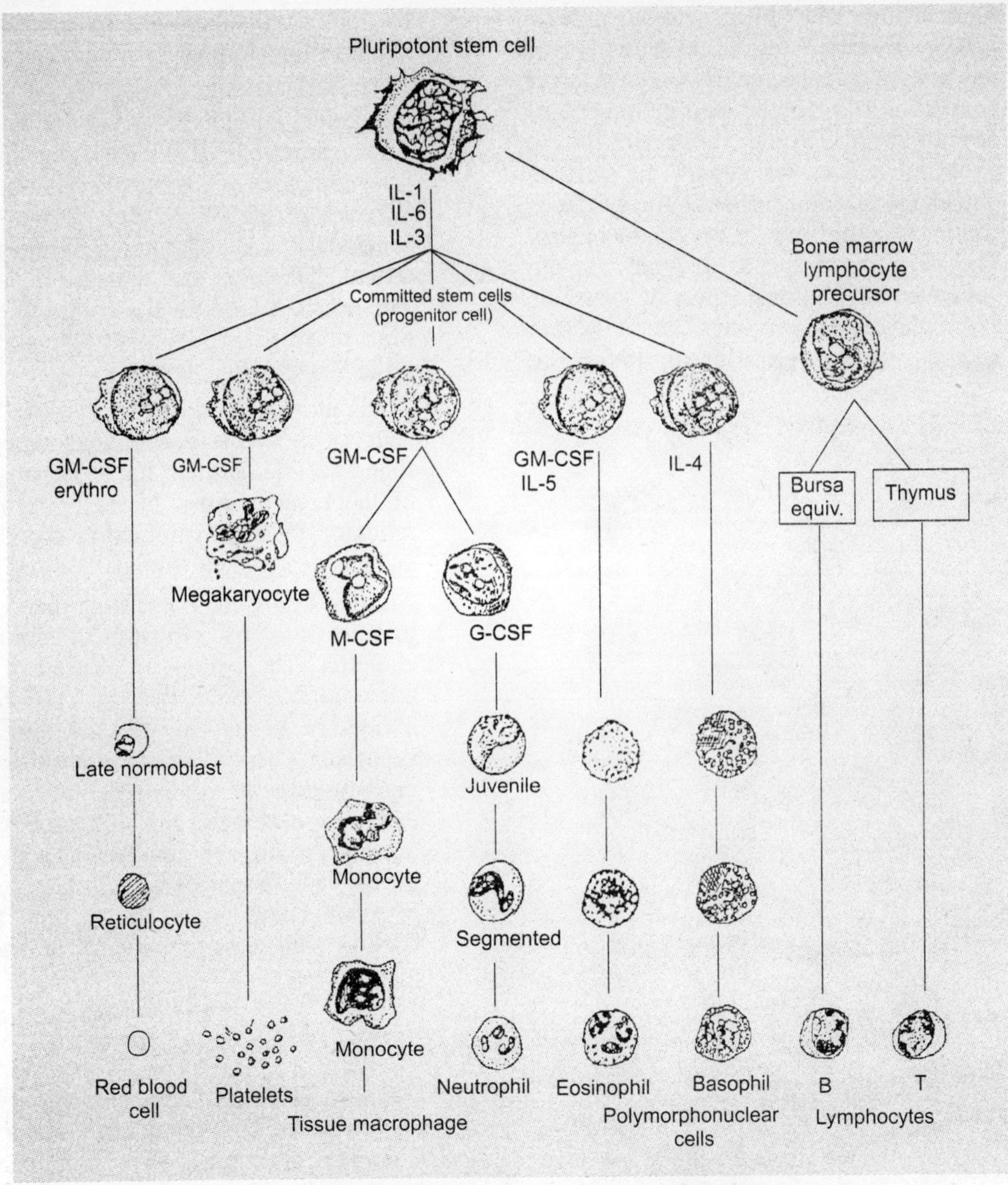

Fig. 3.9: Stages of development of various cells of the blood.

lation of haemoglobin. The nucleus is small with condensed chromatin taking a "cart-wheel appearance. Soon, it becomes pyknotic—uniform deeply stained. The pyknosis is a stage of degeneration of the nucleus, which breaks up and disappears either by lysis or by extrusion. With the destruction of the nucleus, a young red blood cell, reticulocyte is formed. Due to multiple mitosis, one proerythroblast gives rise to 8–32 reticulocytes.

5. **Reticulocyte** The young RBC is so called because on *vital staining* with cresyl blue, a network of basophilic material can be

seen in the acidophilic cytoplasm (Fig. 3.10A, B). The reticulum consists of remnants of cytoplasmic RNA seen in larger concentrations in the earlier stages of development. Since the reticulocyte contains a few ribosomes as well as mitochondria, some haemoglobin synthesis continues in this stage of development also. The reticulocyte spends 1–2 days in the bone marrow, and then enters its sinusoids to circulate in the peripheral blood. Within 1–2 days, the reticulocyte loses the basophilic reticulum and a mature red blood is said to be formed.

The normal range of reticulocyte count in the peripheral blood is 0.5–2.5% (average 1%) of the red blood cells. Reticulocyte count is a good index of the rate of erythropoiesis. When the rate of red cell formation is accelerated, e.g. following a haemorrhage, reticulocyte count may increase to 5–10%. The time required for the erythroid cell to mature from proerythroblast stage to reticulocyte is 5–7 days.

All the immature red and white blood cells, in various stages of development are found outside (around) the blood sinusoids of the bone marrow. Normally, only the reticulocytes and mature white blood cells and platelets are able to enter the circulation.

6. **Mature Red Cell** The mature red cell has lost its nucleus, ribosomes and mitochondria. The cytoplasm is packed with haemoglobin molecules, but the cell is incapable of any further haemoglobin synthesis. The cell depends on anaerobic glycolysis for its energy requirements. The enzymes necessary for this process are already synthesized and remain active for the normal life span of the cell. The absence of the nucleus allows the red cell to be packed with a larger amount of haemoglobin.

Rtc

A

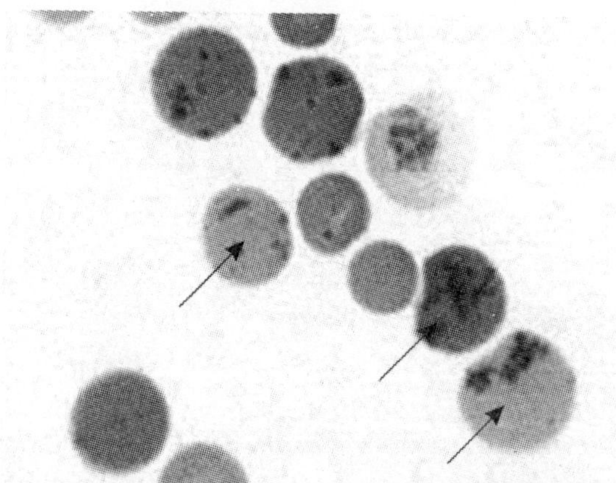

B

Fig. 3.10: Reticulocytes in a normal person (A) and in a patient of pernicious after administration of Vitamin B_{12} (B).

Biosynthesis of Haemoglobin

Haemoglobin is synthesized chiefly by the nucleated stages of developing red cells, a little by reticulocytes, and none at all by adult red cells. Haem is synthesized in the mitochondria from glycine, a non-essential amino acid, and succinyl coenzyme A, an intermediary of Kreb's cycle, and iron. The globin component of haemoglobin is synthesized in the ribosomes from amino acids.

Regulation of Erythropoiesis

Erythropoietin The rate of erythropoiesis is regulated by a glycoprotein (mol. wt. 34,000) called **erythropoietin**. Erythropoietin is chiefly formed in the kidneys by endothelial cells of peritubular capillaries in the renal cortex. Small amount (10–15%) of the circulating erythropoietin is synthesized in the liver. Liver is the main site of inactivation of erythropoietin. A certain basal level of this hormone is necessary for the normal rate of erythropoiesis. A decrease in the number of red cells (e.g. after haemorrhage or in haemolytic anaemia) and hypoxia are potent stimuli for the production of erythropoietin. That explains why polycythaemia (increased red cell count) is observed in hypoxic states such as in normal individuals residing at high altitude or in patients suffering from cardiopulmonary disorders. On the other hand, transfusion of blood in a normal person leads to a decrease in the rate of erythropoiesis till normal RBC count is restored. Anaemia is commonly seen in patients with chronic renal failure, which persists in spite of administration of anti-anaemic drugs, because the fundamental problem is deficient erythropoietin production.

Renal production erythropoietin is increased by testosterone. That explains higher RBC count in adult males than in females. Physiological concentrations of ACTH and adrenal cortical hormones stimulate the production of erythropoietin, but larger concentrations are inhibitory. Estrogens in moderate concentrations are inhibitory to erythropoietin production.

Erythropoietin exerts its chief effect on the stem cells, causing them to differentiate into proerythroblasts (erythroid series). The development of later stages of erythropoiesis, including haemoglobin synthesis, also seems to be promoted by erythropoietin. Now, erythropoietin is commercially available for the treatment of anaemia of chronic renal failure.

Nutrients required for Normal Erythropoiesis

Erythropoiesis involves a very rapid rate of cell division. Almost 1% of the total red cells are destroyed every day and an equal number of reticulocytes are released into the circulation. Haemoglobin has to be synthesized in each red cell. Amino acids, iron, vitamin B_{12}, folic acid, pyridoxine, copper, and several endocrines are not always available and their deficiency results in inadequate and/or defective erythropoiesis leading to various types of anaemias.

1. Iron Iron is an essential component of haemoglobin. About 50% of the total body iron is present in the red blood cells. Destruction of the aged red cells in the tissue macrophages results in the release of iron, which is transported to the bone marrow by the plasma protein transferrin and reutilized for haemoglobin synthesis. Thus, iron stores of the body are efficiently conserved and utilized. In males, less than 1 mg of iron is lost from the body every day, which is replenished by a normal diet. However, in females, there is a cyclic loss of iron in the menstrual blood and transfer of iron to the baby during pregnancy and lactation. As a result, average daily requirement of an adult female is twice that of an adult male. That is why; iron deficiency anaemia is fairly common in females. It may also be added here, that normally only about 10% of the dietary iron can be absorbed in the gut and very few food stuffs contain iron in appreciable amounts.

2. Proteins Essential amino acids are required for the synthesis of globin component of haemoglobin. That is why severe protein caloric malnutrition is associated with anaemia, even though iron deficiency may not be present. Dietary animal proteins, in general, are more effective than vegetable and cereal proteins in haemoglobin synthesis.

3. Vitamin B_{12} Vitamin B_{12} is required for DNA synthesis, and therefore, has a critical role in normal haemopoiesis. Deficiency of vitamin B_{12} is characterised by abnormal maturation of proliferating cells. The bone marrow becomes hyperplastic; spreading throughout the shaft of long bones. Even then, because of maturation defect the circulating red cell count is extremely low (about 2 million/c.mm). In the bone marrow, the erythroid series of red cells are megaloblasts, i.e. larger in size than the corresponding stages of normal erythropoiesis. The mature red cells ultimately released into circulation have an average diameter of 9.5 μm (macrocytes).

3

4. Folic Acid Folic acid deficiency also causes megaloblastic erythropoiesis and macrocytic anaemia, since folic acid is also required for DNA synthesis.

Interaction of folic acid and vitamin B_{12}:

Dietary folic acid appears in the plasma as methyltetrafolate (MeTHF).

In the tissues, the following reaction takes place:

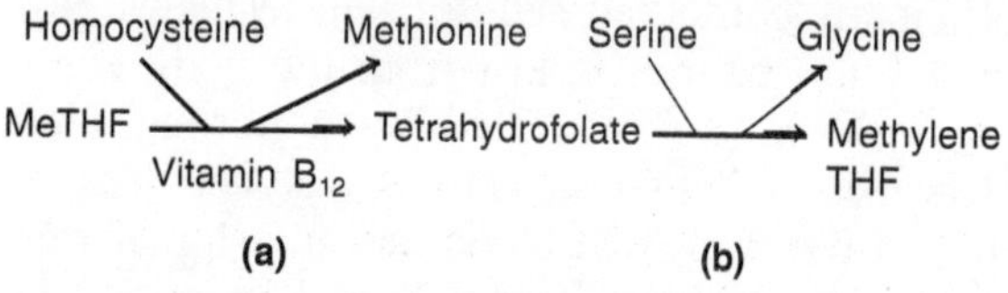

Methylene tetrahydrofolate (methyleneTHF) is essential for the synthesis of DNA. Vitamin B_{12} mediated reaction (a) generates amino acid methionine, which is required for the synthesis of myelin in the neurons. Thus deficiency of either vitamin B_{12} or folic acid causes megaloblastic anemia. Neurological problems are seen in vitamin B_{12} deficiency only.

5. Hormones Thyroxine, cortisol, growth hormone and androgens are involved in erythropoiesis in an indirect manner. Physiological plasma concentrations of these hormones are essential for the normal secretion of erythropoietin. Anaemia is commonly observed in patients suffering from deficiency of any of these endocrines (especially in hypothyroidism).

6. Others Copper, cobalt, pyridoxine (vitamin B_6), pantothenic acid and vitamin C also seem to be essential for normal erythropoiesis. However, their requirements are so small that in humans, anaemia can seldom be attributed to the deficiency of these substances. Ceruloplasmin, the copper-containing plasma protein acts as a ferroxidase and appears to be essential for transfer of iron from tissue macrophages to plasma transferrin. Cobalt is a component of vitamin B_{12}. Pantothenic acid and pyridoxine are required for synthesis of haem. Vitamin C is required for normal folic acid metabolism. It also helps in iron absorption by reducing dietary ferric (Fe^{3+}) ion to ferrous (Fe^{2+}) ion.

RED CELL METABOLISM

Glucose is the main source of energy in the red blood cells. Glucose enters the red cells by insulin-independent carrier-mediated facilitated diffusion using glucose transporter 1(GLUT 1). Since a mature RBC does not possess mitochondria, glucose can be metabolized only by the anaerobic Embden-Mayerhoff pathway. About 90% Of glucose is metabolized through the straight chained-reactions of this pathway (Fig. 3.11). The remaining 10% of glucose 6-phosphate passes via the *hexosemonophosphate (HMP) shunt* (shunt A, Fig. 3.11). An enzyme, glucose 6-phosphate dehydrogenase (G 6PD) is essential for entry of glucose into HMP shunt. The shunt pathway rejoins the Embden-Mayerhoff pathway. The metabolism via HMP does not yield any extra ATPs. The importance of glucose metabolism via this pathway lies in the fact that it generates reduced NADP (NADPH). Reduced NADP maintains high concentration of reduced glutathione in the red cells which is essential for maintaining the iron atoms of haemoglobin in ferrous state.

G6PD deficiency occurs as an X chromosome-linked genetic disorder. The patients develop haemolytic episodes when exposed to an oxidant stress like viral or bacterial infections or administration of certain drugs (aspirin, anti-malarials, and sulphonamides).

2, 3, diphosphoglycerate (2, 3 DPG) shunt (Shunt B, Fig. 3.11): In the straight chained glycolytic pathway, 1, 3 diphosphoglycerate (1, 3 DPG) is converted to 3, phosphoglycerate with the generation of 2 ATPs. An enzyme, diphosphoglycerate mutase converts 1, 3 DPG to 2, 3, DPG. Another enzyme diphosphoglycerate phosphatase causes reentry of 2, 3 DGP into glycolytic pathway as 3 phosphoglycerate. ATPs

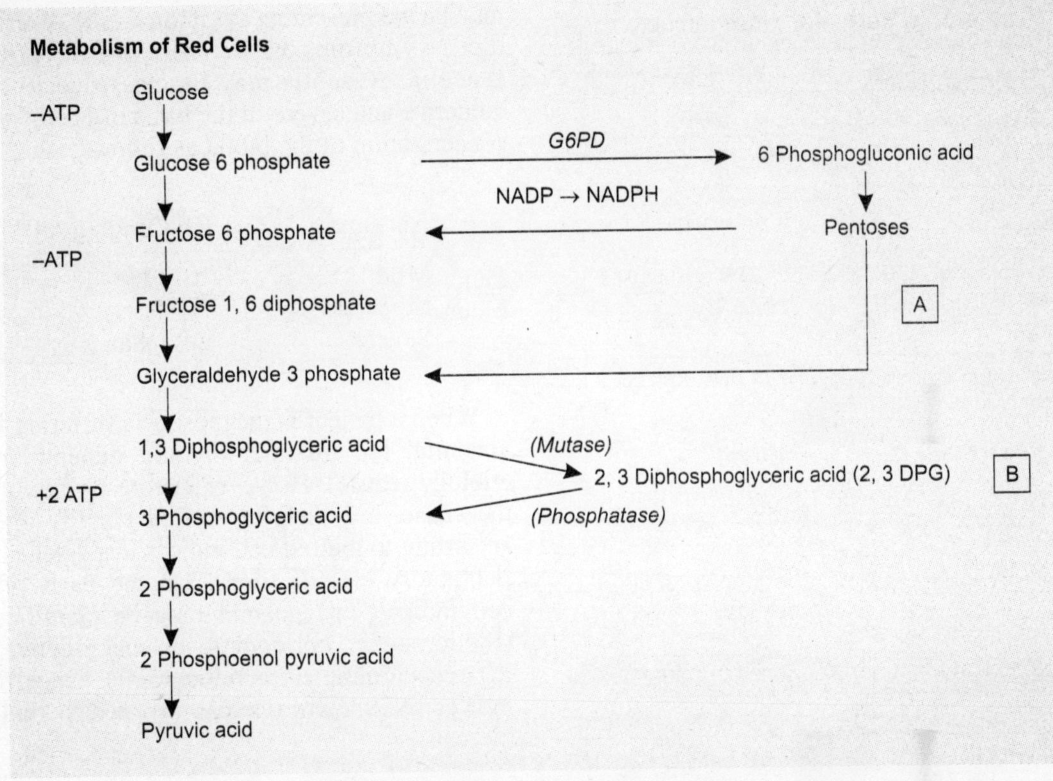

Fig. 3.11: Glucose metabolism in red cells.

are not generated if 1, 3, DPG enters 2, 3, DPG shunt. The importance of this shunt lies in the fact that it generates 2, 3 DPG. Over half of the phosphorus in the red cells is present as 2, 3 DGP. 2, 3 DPG reduces the affinity of haemoglobin for oxygen and hence its presence in the red cells is fundamentally essential for off-loading of oxygen from oxyhaemoglobin.

RED CELL INDICES

If the RBC count, haemoglobin concentration and haematocrit (PCV) value are known, certain indices (or absolute values) of the red cells of the person can be calculated. These absolute values are helpful in the *laboratory diagnosis of anaemia*. The method of calculation and normal range of each index is given below in Table 3.2.

On the basis of MCV, the red cells may be classified as macrocytes, normocytes and microcytes, i.e. those above, within and below the normal range respectively.

Red cells with MCHC below 32% or MCH below 26 pg are known as hypochromic cells and those with MCHC or MCH within the normal range are called normochromic. In a patient of anaemia, the knowledge of these indices is often useful in the detection of the cause of anaemia. Some important normal values in haematology are given in Table 3.3.

PATHOPHYSIOLOGY OF ANAEMIAS

Anaemia is defined as a condition in which the haemoglobin concentration is below the normal range, for the age and sex of the individual. In adults, the lower extreme of the normal range is taken as 13 g/dl in males and 12 g/dl in females (or haematocrit below 40% in males and 35% in females).

Table 3.2: Normal red cell indices

Index	*Normal range*	*Method of calculation*
1. Mean corpuscular volume (MCV)	80–100 μ^3	$\frac{\text{PCV} \times 10}{\text{RBC count (in million/mm}^3)}$
2. Mean corpuscular haemoglobin (MCH)	26–34 pg	$\frac{\text{Hb (g\%)} \times 10}{\text{RBC count (million/mm}^3)}$
3. Mean corpuscular haemoglobin conc. (MCHC)%	32–38%	$\frac{\text{HB (g\%)} \times 100}{\text{PCV \%}}$

For example, if in a patient, Hb conc. is 10 gm%, RBC count is 4 million/mm^3 and PCV is 40%, then

$$\text{MCV} = \frac{40 \times 10}{4} = 100\ \mu^3$$

$$\text{MCH} = \frac{10 \times 10}{4} = 25\ \text{pg}$$

$$\text{MCHC\%} = \frac{10 \times 100}{40} = 25\%$$

Table 3.3: Important normal values in haematology

	Men	*Women*
Haemoglobin, g%	13–18	12–16
Haematocrit, %	40–52	35–47
Red cell count, million/μL	4.4–5.9	3.8–5.2
White cell count, thousand/μL	4–11	80–100
Mean corpuscular volume, μ^3	4–11	80–100
Mean corpuscular Hb, pg	26–34	26–34
Mean corpuscular haemoglobin concentration, %	32–36	32–36
Platelet count, thousand/μL	150–440	150–440
Reticulocyte count, %	0.8–2.5	0.8–4.0
Erythrocyte sedimentation rate, mm 1st hour	0–10	0–20

Subnormal levels of haemoglobin decrease the oxygen carrying capacity of the blood leading to hypoxia. The function of tissues with high oxygen demand such as heart, brain and exercising muscles are most affected. The symptoms of anemia include tiredness, palpitation, easy fatiguability, generalized muscle weakness, lethargy, and headache. In older patients, angina pectoris, mental confusion, visual disturbances or intermittent claudications (pain in the skeletal muscles during exercise which disappears on rest) may be the presenting symptoms. The severity of these symptoms varies with the severity of anaemia. Anaemia may be classified as mild, moderate and severe in the basis of haemoglobin concentration of the blood as follows:

Anaemia	Hb Conc. (g /dl)
Mild	10–11.9
Moderate	7–9.9
Severe	Less than 7

When a patient is diagnosed as suffering from anaemia, the treatment would depend on its etiology (cause). However, before trying to find the cause, it is helpful to first classify anemia according to the red cell indices discussed above (laboratory classification). On the basis of red cell indices, an anaemia may be classified as (i) microcytic, normocytic or macrocytic, and (ii) hypochromic or normochromic. Once these indices are known, one can proceed to find out the cause.

ETIOLOGICAL CLASSIFICATION OF ANAEMIAS

1. Deficiency anaemias
2. Haemorrhagic anaemias
3. Haemolytic anaemias
4. Aplastic anaemias

Deficiency Anaemias

Iron Deficiency Anaemia Iron deficiency is probably the commonest cause of anaemia in the world. As explained above, it is more common in the females than in males. Iron deficiency results in the production of a smaller number of red cells, which are not only deficient in Hb (hypochromic), but also smaller in size (microcytic). Thus in iron deficiency, the MCH is below 26 pg, MCHC below 32% and MCV below 80 μ^3. Severe iron deficiency not only interferes with erythropoiesis but also with cell division in many other tissues. Severe iron deficiency is associated with not only severe anaemia, but also with disorders of tongue (atrophic glossitis), oesophagus (dysphagia) and nails (koilonychias, spoon-like nails). Iron deficiency can be easily treated by oral administration of Fe^{2+} salts.

Pernicious Anaemia Pernicious anaemia is caused by deficiency of vitamin B_{12} in the body. Although vitamin B_{12} content of the diet of these patients is usually normal, the vitamin is not absorbed in the gut. Normally, a glycoprotein (mol. wt. 45,000), known as intrinsic factor (IF), secreted by the gastric mucosa, helps in the absorption of vitamin B_{12} in the ileum. Atrophy of gastric mucosa results in the absence of intrinsic factor, leading to malabsorption of vitamin B_{12}. As discussed earlier, deficiency of vitamin B_{12} produces a megaloblastic bone marrow reaction and a very severe degree of anaemia. In the peripheral blood, the red cells are larger in size (macrocytes, MCV greater than 100 μ^3) but contain a normal concentration of haemoglobin (normochromic), i.e. vitamin B_{12} deficiency causes macrocytic normochromic type of anaemia. Blood smear shows another two characteristic features of red cells. Firstly, the cells show a wider variation in shape, i. e. all the red cells are not circular disks (poikilocytosis). Secondly, the cell size varies from 4 to 12 µm, average 9.5 µm (normal: variation 6.7 to 7.7 µm, average 7.5 µm) (anisocytosis).

Besides anaemia, deficiency of vitamin B_{12} is associated with peripheral neuropathy and degeneration of spinal cord. The disorder, if not treated, is invariably fatal. Recent evidence suggests that pernicious anaemia is an autoimmune disease. The auto-antibodies destroy both the parietal and chief cells of gastric mucosa (gastric atrophy).

Pernicious anaemia can be treated by regular administration of vitamin B_{12} by intramuscular route. Even after a single intramuscular injection of a large dose of vitamin B_{12}, the reticulocyte count in the peripheral blood may be as high as 40%, indicating an explosive increase in the rate of erythropoiesis (Fig. 3.10B).

Folic Acid Deficiency Anaemia Folic acid deficiency is fairly common during pregnancy. It produces macrocytic normochromic type of anaemia but there are no neurological problems.

Haemorrhagic Anaemias

Following an acute haemorrhage, anaemia is normochromic, normocytic type. But chronic blood loss, e.g. due to bleeding piles or excessive menstrual bleeding, leads to excessive loss of iron from the body. Hence such patients usually show hypochromic microcytic (iron deficiency) type of anaemia.

Haemolytic Anaemias

Lifespan of red cells may be shortened by congenital defects like thalassemia and sickle cell disease. Haemolytic anaemia may also be due to the presence of auto-antibodies in the plasma, which destroy the red cells (autoimmune haemolytic anaemia). Such anaemias are usually normocytic, normochromic type. To overcome excessive destruction of red cells, the rate of erythropoiesis in the bone marrow is increased. That is why patients with this type of anemia show high reticulocyte count (10–20%). Increased rate of red cell destruction also leads to excessive production of bilirubin. Therefore mild jaundice (haemolytic type) is another characteristic feature of haemolytic anaemia.

Aplastic Anaemias

Complete cessation of erythropoiesis is a very serious and often fatal complication of hypersensitivity reaction to certain drugs, e.g. chloramphenicol, sulfonamides, etc. Excessive irradiation and cytotoxic drugs used in the treatment of malignant disorders also depress the bone marrow. In most of such cases, besides very severe anaemia, severe leucopenia and thrombocytopenia are also present. Death may occur due to infection or severe blood loss. Bone marrow examination reveals presence of adipose tissue where red bone marrow is normally present, indicating cessation of haemopoiesis.

3

POLYCYTHAEMIA (ERYTHROCYTOSIS)

The term polycythaemia or erythrocytosis refers to higher than normal haemoglobin concentration (above 18g/dl in men or 16 g/dl in women) and/or higher than normal red cell count (above 6 million/uL in men or 5.5 million/uL in women). Polycythaemia may result from: (i) Increased red cell mass or (ii) Decreased plasma volume.

When elevated haemoglobin concentration/RBC count is solely due to contracted plasma volume, the condition is called *relative polycythaemia.* Polycythaemia due to actual increase in red cell mass because of hypoxia, leading to increased production of erythropoietin, is known as *secondary polycythaemia*. Polycythaemia vera (*primary polycythaemia*), a rare condition, is discussed below.

Secondary polycythaemia, due to hypoxia, may be seen in the following conditions:

(i) Physiological: in fetal life.
(ii) High altitude: in those residing at altitude of 10,000 feet or above.
(iii) Chronic pulmonary disorders interfering with O_2 uptake in the lungs.
(iv) Congenital heart disorders with shunting of venous blood to the left side of the heart.
(v) Heavy smoking leading to high concentration of carboxyhaemoglobin in the blood.

Polycythaemia Vera (Primary Polycythaemia)

It is a rare disorder in which there is uncontrolled over-production of mature red blood cells, white blood cells and platelets. The circulating blood cells (unlike in leukemia) are morphologically normal. It is basically a malignant disorder of bone marrow. In contrast to secondary polycythaemia, patients of polycythaemia vera have very low plasma erythropoietin levels (negative feedback effect on erythropoietin production).

OSMOTIC FRAGILITY OF RED CELLS

When the red blood cells are suspended in isotonic saline, their biconcave shape is maintained for many hours. In mildly hypotonic solutions, the osmotic difference causes movement of water into the cells, making them spherical in shape. In highly hypotonic solutions or distilled water, the cells swell up to such an extent that they burst (haemolysed). Younger red blood cells can tolerate slightly more hypotonicity than older red blood cells. That is why, if the red blood cells are placed in serial saline solutions with decreasing osmolality, the haemolysis usually begins in 0.48% saline, but all the cells are completely haemolysed in 0.32% saline solution. The red cells of venous blood are slightly more fragile than those of arterial blood, since the former contain larger number of osmotically active ions (Cl^-/HCO_3^-).

In a congenital disorder known as **congenital spherocytic anaemia**, the red cells formed in the bone marrow are spherical rather than biconcave. Hence, in serial saline solutions, such cells begin to haemolyse in 0.7% saline and haemolysis is complete in 0.45% saline solution. On the other hand, more flattened shape of red cells in sickle cell anaemia and thalassaemia makes them more resistant to hypo-osmolar solutions.

Congenital spherocytic anaemia (Hereditary spherocytosis) is primarily due to a genetic defect in the skeleton of the red cell membrane. Spectrin and ankyrin are two important proteins which maintain normal shape of the red cell membrane (Fig. 3.12). Genetic deficiency of either spectrin or ankyrin leads to reduced membrane stability

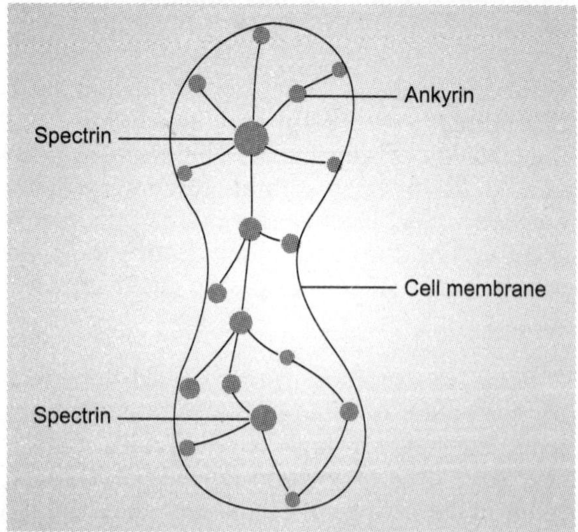

Fig. 3.12: Skeleton of a red cell consisting of protein—spectrin and ankyrin.

and spontaneous membrane loss. The resulting reduction in cell surface to volume ratio forces the red cells to assume smallest possible diameter for a given volume, namely, a sphere. Spherical shape makes the red cells less flexible. It cannot bend or twist as it passes through the capillaries, specially in the spleen, and hence destroyed. Thus haemolytic anaemia results.

ERYTHROCYTE SEDIMENTATION RATE

If the blood is mixed with an anticoagulant and allowed to stand in a narrow tube, the heavier red cells start settling down leaving clear plasma at the top (Fig. 3.13). The upper column of the red cells is read after 1 hour. The result is known as erythrocyte sedimentation rate (ESR). The normal range of ESR is 0–10 mm in males and 0–20 mm in females. In later months of pregnancy, an increase in ESR is physiological. In severe anaemia, ESR is increased, because the decrease in red cell number favours their sedimentation.

ESR is markedly increased in many pathological conditions like tuberculosis, rheumatoid arthritis and malignancy, etc. In such conditions, the increased ESR has a *non-specific diagnostic significance*. In chronic inflammatory disorders, like tuberculosis, serial estimation of ESR helps to assess the response of the patient to treatment. This is known as *prognostic value* of ESR. A progressive decrease in ESR indicates a good prognosis.

The red blood cells, in vitro, have a tendency to pile on the top of each other. The phenomenon is known as rouleaux formation. Rouleaux formation increases the mass/surface area ratio of the red cells (Fig. 3.14), and favours sedimentation.

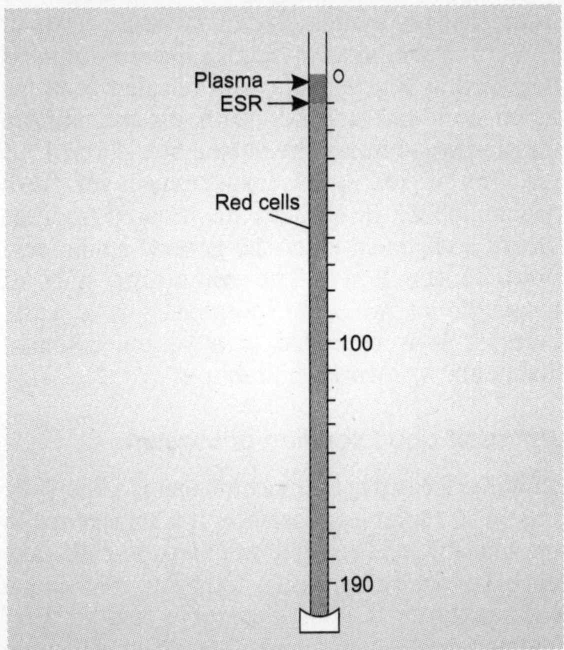

Fig. 3.13: Estimation of erythrocyte sedimentation rate in a Westergren tube.

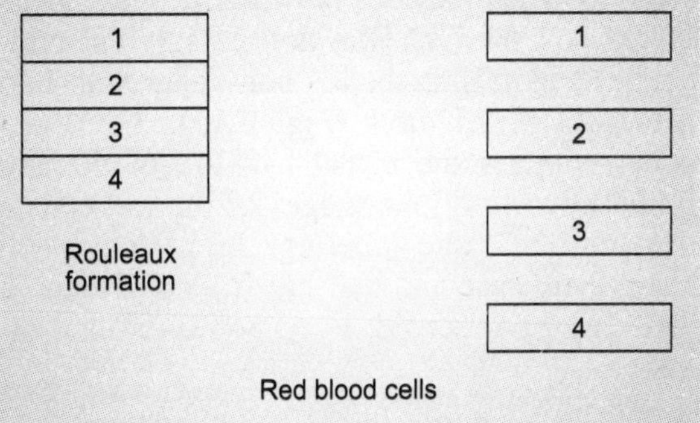

Fig. 3.14: Effect of rouleaux formation. The mass of the red cells remains same but the surface area decreases.

Increase in the plasma fibrinogen concentration favours rouleaux formation. Plasma fibrinogen level is increased in pregnancy as well as in pathological conditions mentioned above.

Some important causes of variations in ESR are given below:

ESR increased	*ESR decreased*
Anaemia	Polycythaemia
Old age	Spherocytosis
Infections	Hypofibrinogenemia
Inflammations	Extreme leucocytosis
Pregnancy	
Malignancy	

LIFESPAN OF RED BLOOD CELLS

Average lifespan of red blood cells is normally 120 days. It may be markedly reduced in patients with haemolytic anaemia. Many decades ago, the lifespan of red cells was determined by differential agglutination method. Nowadays, a more accurate method using radioactive chromium is used. In this method, small amount of the patient's blood is withdrawn, incubated with radioactive sodium chromate ($Na_2{}^{51}CrO_4$) and reinjected. The radioactive salt is strongly adsorbed on the treated red cells. Radioactivity of the blood sample withdrawn 10 minutes after reinjection gives baseline (100%) value. At regular intervals, blood samples are withdrawn and tested for radioactivity. The radioactivity of the blood gradually decreases due to disappearance of aged ^{51}Cr-tagged red cells. Residual radioactivity indicates the degree of red cell survival. The normal survival curve obtained by this method is non-linear with half-life ($t_{1/2}$) of 25 days (Fig. 3.15). The curve underestimates the actual half-life of 60 days (120/2) due to different ages of the red cells at the time of radio-labeling. In patients with haemolytic anaemia, half-life ($t_{1/2}$) of 5 days or less may be observed.

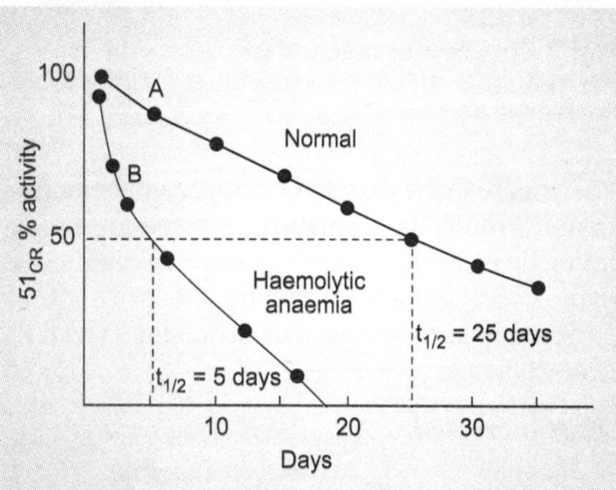

Fig. 3.15: Half-life ($T_{1/2}$) of red cells laden with radioactive chromium (^{51}Cr) in a normal person (A) and a patient of haemolytic anaemia (B).

DESTRUCTION OF RED BLOOD CELLS

By 120 days of age, the activity of cytoplasmic oxidative enzymes is decreased and hence the energy-deficient aged red cell is not able to maintain its normal shape and volume. Such deformed cells are removed from the blood by tissue macrophages present in the spleen, bone marrow, liver, lymph nodes, etc. Within a phagocyte, the aged cell is broken down and haemoglobin is degraded.

The aged red cells are mostly trapped by the tissue macrophages and destroyed. However, about 10% of the aged red cells undergo haemolysis while in circulation. Intravascular haemolysis releases haemoglobin into the plasma, from where it can be excreted in the urine. However under normal circumstances, free haemoglobin in the plasma binds with a plasma protein, haptoglobin and hence its renal excretion is prevented. The haptoglobin-haemoglobin complex is removed from the circulation by the tissue macrophages and degraded. In certain conditions, massive intravascular haemolysis may occur, e.g. some types of hemolytic anaemias or mis-matched blood transfusion. In such cases, the amount of haemoglobin released by intravascular haemolysis is far in excess of the binding capacity of plasma haptoglobin. In such circumstances, haemoglobin is excreted in the urine (haemoglobinuria).

Within the macrophages, haemoglobin is degraded as follows: The iron released from the haem component binds with plasma protein transferrin and transported to the iron stores. Thus the iron is reutilized for synthesis of fresh haemoglobin. The amino acids released from the globin component enter the general amino acid pool of the body. The remaining part of haemoglobin molecule, porphyrin, is a waste product. It is degraded to a yellow coloured compound known as bilirubin.

Transport and Excretion of Bilirubin

Bilirubin formed in the macrophages is a lipophilic (non-water soluble) substance. It is transported in the blood bound to albumin. Hepatic cells take up bilirubin by an active transport mechanism and conjugate it with glucuronic acid to form water soluble compounds known as bilirubin monoglucuronide and bilirubin diglucuronide (conjugated bilirubin). These compounds are excreted into the bile. In the large intestine, bacterial degradation converts these compounds to stercobilinogen (= urobilinogen). Some of the urobilinogen is absorbed into the portal blood to reach the systemic circulation. Being water soluble it is excreted into the urine by the kidneys (Fig. 3.16). The remaining stercobilinogen (40–280 mg/day) is excreted in the faeces. On exposure to air, stercobilinogen is oxidised to stercobilin which gives brown colour to the faeces.

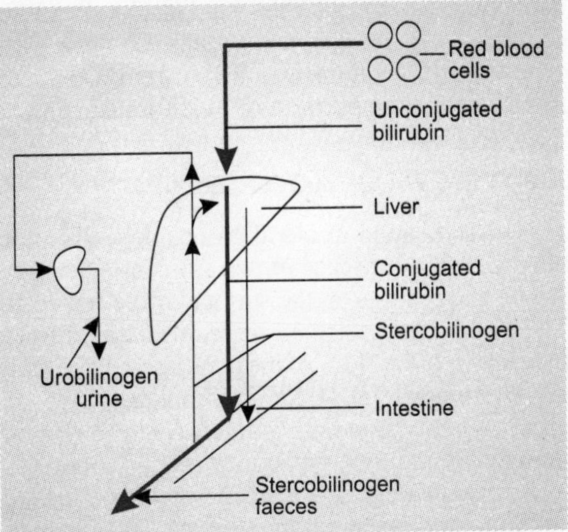

Fig. 3.16: Fate of bilirubin (formed in the tissue macrophages).

When urine is exposed to air, e.g. allowed to stand in a urine glass, urobilinogen is converted to urobilin and gives brown colour to the urine.

PATHOPHYSIOLOGY OF JAUNDICE

Presence of an excess of bilirubin in the plasma and tissue fluids causes yellow discolouration of the skin, conjunctivae and other tissues. The condition is called jaundice. The normal range of plasma bilirubin level is 0.2–1.0 mg%. Jaundice is clinically detectable when the plasma bilirubin level exceeds 2 mg%. Jaundice can occur due to a variety of causes. Broadly speaking it can be classified into 3 types: haemolytic jaundice, hepatic jaundice and post-hepatic jaundice.

Haemolytic Jaundice

It is caused by excessive haemolysis of red blood cells. Because of some congenital corpuscular defects (e.g. thalassaemia, sickle cell disease, congenital spherocytic anaemia) or presence of some haemolysins in the plasma, lifespan of the RBC may be shortened. If the rate of RBC production fails to keep pace with the rate of destruction, anaemia (haemolytic type) results. At the same time increased rate of red cell destruction increases the production of bilirubin. When its rate of bilirubin production exceeds the excretory capacity of the liver, bilirubin begins to accumulate in the blood.

Haemolytic jaundice is characterized by the presence of an excess of non-conjugated (lipid soluble) bilirubin in the plasma and absence of bilirubin in the urine (being non-water soluble, it cannot pass through the kidney filter). The urine and faeces contain an excess of urobilinogen and stercobilinogen respectively. Van den Bergh test is indirect positive (see below).

Hepatic Jaundice

It is most commonly produced by viral hepatitis. There is widespread swelling and destruction of the hepatocytes. Intrahepatic biliary obstruction causes regurgitation of conjugated bilirubin into the blood circulation. Therefore, blood contains an excess of conjugated bilirubin. Being water soluble, conjugated bilirubin appears in the urine giving it a dark brown colour. Since the bile cannot reach the intestine, stercobilinogen is absent in the faeces, leading to a pale, chalky colour of the stools. In such cases, unconjugated bilirubin may also accumulate in the blood since the injured hepatic cells have poor power of conjugation. Therefore, Van den Bergh test is biphasic positive (see below).

Post-Hepatic Jaundice

It is caused by obstruction in the extrahepatic biliary passages (e.g. by a stone in the common bile duct or carcinoma of the head of the pancreas). This type of jaundice is again due to regurgitation of conjugated bilirubin into the blood circulation.

Van den Bergh test, therefore, is direct positive (see below). Urine contains bilirubin, but stools and urine do not have stercobilinogen/urobilinigen. Due to absence of stercobilinogen, the stools are clay-colored, instead of normal yellowish-brown colour. Post-hepatic jaundice can be differentiated from the hepatic jaundice by the normal hepatocellular function in the former. The three types of jaundice have been compared in Table 3.4.

The Van den Bergh Test

This is a test to detect the presence of excess of bilirubin in the serum as well as to find out the type of bilirubin present. In this test, the diazo reagent (a mixture of sulphanilic acid, hydrochloric acid and sodium nitrite) is added to the serum. Conjugated bilirubin, if present in the serum, gives reddish violet colour whose maximum intensity reaches in 30 seconds. The result is called Van den Bergh direct positive. If no colour appears, alcohol is also added. Appearance of reddish violet colour indicates the presence of (lipid soluble) unconjugated bilirubin. This result is called indirect positive. If the serum contains both types of bilirubin, the reddish violet colour appearing at the first stage deepens further on addition of alcohol. The result is called biphasic positive. The concentration of bilirubin can be quantified if the intensity of colour is estimated in a photocolorimeter. In haemolytic jaundice, the Van den Bergh test is indirect positive. In post-hepatic jaundice, the test is direct positive. In hepatic jaundice, the test is biphasic positive.

BLOOD GROUPS

The cell membrane of human erythrocytes contains a variety of antigens called agglutinogens, depending upon which the human blood can be differentiated into different groups. Of these, two types A-B-O system and Rh system are more important for the purpose of blood transfusion.

A-B-O SYSTEM OF BLOOD GROUPS

This classification of blood groups depends upon the presence or absence of two antigens— antigen A and antigen B—on the surface of the red cells. The blood group is named according to the antigen present. In India, 40% of the population have antigen B (Blood group B), 20% have antigen A (Blood group A), 8% have both antigen A and B (Blood group AB) and 32% have none (Blood group O).

Antibodies against agglutinogens are called agglutinins. The agglutinin against A antigen is

Table 3.4: Comparison of the three types of jaundice

	Haemolytic (prehapatic) jaundice	*Hepatocellular (hepatic) jaundice*	*Obstructive (post-hepatic) jaundice*
Cause	Excessive haemolysis	Hepatocellular damage	Extrahepatic biliary obstruction
Total serum bilirubin	Increased	Increased	Increased
Serum unconjugated bilirubin	Increased	May increase	Normal
Serum conjugated bilirubin	Normal	Increased	Increased
Van den Bergh reaction	Indirect +	Biphasic +	Direct +
Faecal stercobilinogen	Increased	Decreased/ absent	Absent
Urinary urobilinogen	Increased	Decreased/ absent	Absent
Urinary bilirubin	Absent	Present	Present
Hepatocellular function	Normal	Disturbed	Normal
Serum alkaline phosphatase level	Normal	Mildly elevated	Markedly elevated

called α-agglutinin or anti-A agglutinin; agglutinin against B antigen is called ß-agglutinin or anti-B agglutinin. When plasma containing α-agglutinin is mixed with group A red cells, the cells undergo agglutination (clumping) and are subsequently haemolysed. Similarly ß-agglutinin causes clumping followed by haemolysis of group B red cells (Fig. 3.17). Chemically, the α- and ß-agglutinins are IgM type of immunoglobulins. Group AB cells undergo agglutination in the presence of either agglutinin. Group 'O' cells, do not contain any antigen, and hence cannot be clumped by either agglutinin.

The group specific antigens are present not only on the red cells but also in many other tissues like salivary glands, pancreas, kidney, liver, lungs and testis. The saliva, semen and amniotic fluid contain these group specific substances.

When a particular blood group antigen is present in the blood of a person, his plasma obviously would not contain the corresponding antibody, but surprisingly, it always contains the opposite antibody. This fact is known as *Landsteiner's law*. Thus, plasma of blood group A always contains β-agglutinin, that of blood group B always contains α-agglutinin, that of blood group O contains both α- and β-agglutinins. In a person with blood group AB, both the agglutinins are absent in the plasma. It needs to be reiterated that Landsteiner's law is applicable to A-B-O blood group system only.

The blood group of a person is genetically determined and antigens A and B are present during intrauterine life. On the other hand, agglutinins are absent at birth but they begin to appear by 10 days of age, to reach maximum concentration by 10 years of age. The mechanism of appearance of α- and β-agglutinins is not exactly clear. It seems antigens like A and B group substances are present in many foods and intestinal bacteria. Exposure of the newborn child to these antigens results in the development of agglutinins to the antigen recognized as non-self (e.g. not present in its own body).

Recently, chemical structure of blood group A, B and O substances have been identified (Fig. 3.18).

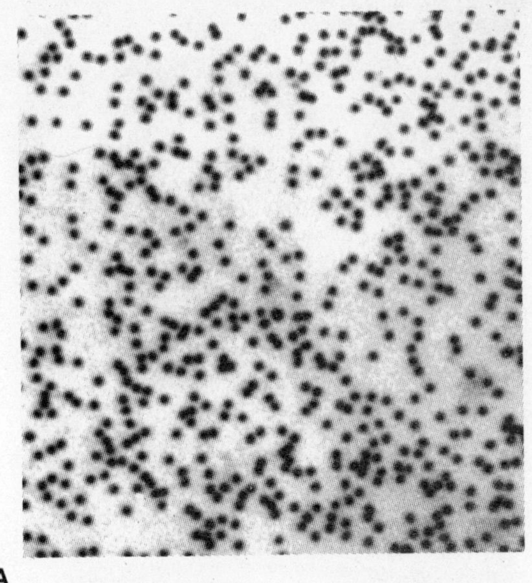

A

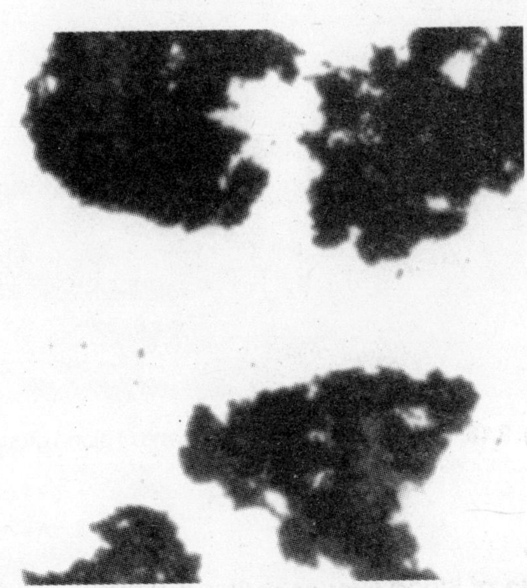

B

Fig. 3.17: (A) Normal red cells in saline solution. (B) Agglutination of red cells.

The blood group of a person can be determined by mixing a suspension of his red cells (in isotonic saline) with a drop each of α and β agglutinins separately. The blood group will be shown by the presence of agglutination with one, both or none of the agglutinins (Table 3.5).

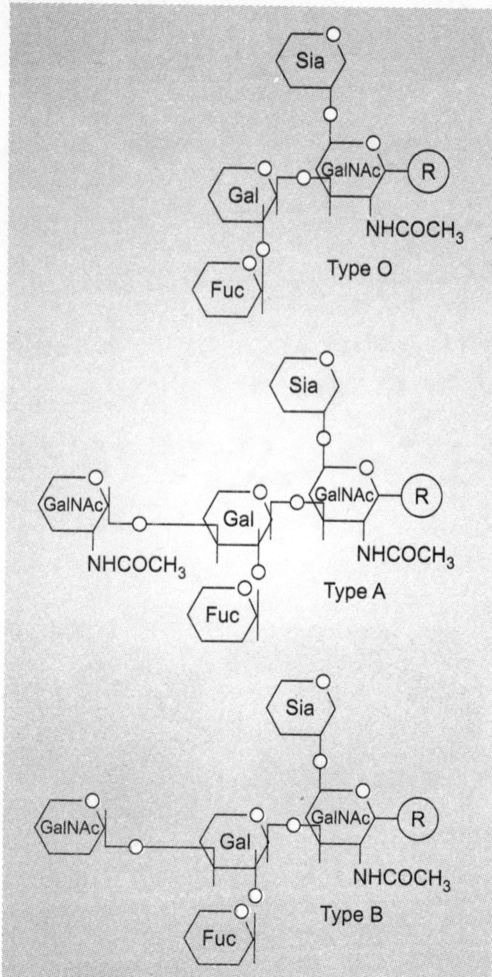

Fig. 3.18: Chemical structure of A, B and O blood group substances.

Role of Blood Groups in Blood Transfusion

When blood transfusion is given, the donated red cells are liable to agglutination and haemolysis if the recipient plasma contains the corresponding agglutinin. In other words, it is dangerous to transfuse A group blood to individuals with blood group B (whose plasma contains α-agglutinin). The compatibility/incompatibility of different blood group is given in Table 3.6. For this purpose, the possible reaction between donor's red cells and recipient's plasma is considered.

Table 3.5: Determination of blood group of an individual

Cells (blood group)	*α agglutinin (anti A)*	*β agglutinin (anti B)*
(i)	(ii)	(iii)
A	+	–
B	–	+
AB	+	+
O	–	–

+ Agglutination; – No agglutination

The agglutinins present in the donor's plasma are not considered since they are rendered ineffective by dilution in recipient's blood circulation.

From Table 3.6, it is obvious that it is safest when the donor's blood group is same as that of the recipient, i.e. patients with blood group A should be transfused with group A blood, and those with blood group B should be transfused with group B blood and so on. However, in emergency, group O blood can be transfused to a recipient with any other blood group, since these cells do not contain any agglutinogen. That is why persons with blood group O are sometimes called *universal donors*. However if the group O blood contains very strong concentration (titre) of α and β agglutinins, it may produce agglutination if transfused into a patient with blood group A, B, or AB. Persons with blood group AB are called *universal recipients* because they may be transfused with any blood group.

Table 3.6: Effect of injection of red cells of any group into a person with any group

Blood group of recipient	*Recipient's agglutinin*	*Blood group of donor*			
		A	*B*	*AB*	*O*
A	(β)	–	+	+	–
B	(α)	+	–	+	–
AB	(–)	–	–	–	–
O	(α β)	+	+	+	–

+ Agglutination; – No agglutination

Before transfusion, it is safest to *crossmatch* the two blood samples: (A) donor's red cells against recipient's serum, and (B) donor's serum against recipients red cells. This procedure ensures complete compatibility of donor's blood with the blood of the recipient.

INHERITANCE OF A AND B ANTIGENS

The blood group of a person is genetically determined by the two genes he/she receives: one from each parent. Genes A, B and O give rise to antigens A, B and non-antigenic O substance respectively. Genes A and B are codominant. Consequently, the genotype of persons with different blood groups may be as follows:

Blood group	*Geno type*
A	AA; AO
B	BB; BO
AB	AB
O	OO

Some cases of disputed paternity of a baby can be decided on the basis of this knowledge, e.g. if the child's blood group is O, whatever the blood group of the mother, a person with blood group AB cannot be the father. Or if the child's blood group is AB, whatever the blood group of the mother, a person with blood group O cannot be the father. The value of such a test is strengthened further when other blood group systems are also determined. Nowadays, a far more decisive test, the DNA test has rendered blood group testing for this purpose redundant.

Rh SYSTEM OF BLOOD GROUPS

Originally, this group system was known when red cells of rhesus monkey were injected into a rabbit. The rabbit's tissues reacted by forming antibodies against rhesus red cells. When such a rabbit's serum was tested against human red cells, agglutination occurred in about 90% of the cases, i.e. these persons' red cells contained antigen which reacted against antibody formed against rhesus red cells. Such persons are called Rh +ve. The remaining 10% are called Rh –ve.

There are 3 types of Rh antigens (C, D and E antigens) but D antigen is the commonest. Therefore, Rh +ve and Rh –ve individuals are also sometimes called D +ve and D –ve individuals.

An important difference between Rh system and ABO system of blood groups is that, in the former the anti-D agglutinins are not present naturally. In contrast, α or β antibodies are always present in the blood if the appropriate antigen is absent. Rh antibodies develop in:

(a) Rh –ve individuals who have been transfused with Rh +ve blood or
(b) Rh –ve women who give birth to an Rh +ve fetus. The first Rh +ve transfusion or the first Rh +ve baby usually does not produce any significant effect because the Rh antibodies develop slowly over several months. However in any subsequent Rh +ve transfusion or pregnancy with Rh +ve fetus, severe incompatibility reaction occurs. In Rh +ve re-transfusion, the results are like any other mismatched blood transfusion (see below). Pregnancy with Rh +ve fetus leads to haemolytic disease of the newborn. Unlike AB antigens, Rh antigens are not present in any other tissue or body fluid.

Haemolytic Disease of the Newborn

Erythroblastosis Fetalis

Although the fetal and maternal circulations do not mix, some of the fetal cells do enter the maternal circulation especially during delivery. If the fetus is Rh +ve and the mother in Rh –ve, the transfer of Rh +ve fetal red cells to the mother leads to development of Rh antibodies in the maternal tissues. Such antibodies are IgG type and hence can diffuse through placental membrane and destroy the Rh +ve fetal red cell. (The Rh –ve maternal red cells, however, are not effected.) As a result, severe anaemia occurs in the fetus and may cause death of the fetus in utero or soon after birth. If the death does not occur, the newborn child may be born with severe anaemia and jaundice. The jaundice commonly worsens in the neonatal period, because maternal Rh antibodies continue to destroy the newborn's red cells. In an effort to compensate for massive haemolysis, the bone marrow regenerative response is so intense that besides reticulocytes, even nucleated red cells (erythroblasts) can be seen in the peripheral blood. Hence, the disorder is also known as erythroblastosis fetalis. The haemolytic jaundice so produced may cause permanent motor or mental disability, because bilirubin may be deposited in the brain especially in the basal ganglia. This complication called *kernicterus* is likely to occur when plasma bilirubin level exceeds 18 mg%. Similar rise of plasma bilirubin level in adults does not cause kernicterus because of the development of the blood-brain barrier in infancy.

Incompatibility of ABO blood groups between the mother and the fetus is very common but there is seldom any complication, mainly because α or ß agglutinins (IgM type) cannot cross the placental barrier.

Blood Transfusion

Blood transfusion is a life-saving measure in patients suffering from severe haemorrhage. It is also often required during major surgical operations. In all such cases, it is advisable to transfuse fresh blood. However, for emergency purposes, blood is stored at 4°C in blood banks. Each unit of blood (420 ml) is mixed with 100 ml of 2% disodium hydrogen citrate and 20 ml of 15% dextrose (ACD. diluent). Acid citrate not only acts as an anticoagulant but also lowers the pH of the mixture. Glucose acts as a substrate for the metabolism of stored red cells. By liberating lactic acid, it also helps to lower the pH of the mixture. A fall in the pH helps the survival of red cells during storage. When stored in this way, the blood can be used up to 21–42 days.

Changes During Cold-Storage During cold-storage, low temperature reduces the metabolism of red blood cells leading to a decrease in the active transport mechanisms, especially the Na^+-K^+ pump. Consequently, there is a gradual increase in intracellular Na^+ and extracellular (plasma) K^+ concentrations. At the end of two weeks of storage, intracellular Na^+ concentration increases from normal 14 mEq/L to 30–40 mEq/L. As a result, the stored red cells imbibe more water and become spherocytes. Such cells may rupture in vitro in salt concentration as high as 0.8%. Plasma K^+ concentration of the stored blood may rise from 5 mEq/L to 20–30 mEq/L. There is a decrease in the intracellular ATP concentration also. However, when the stored blood is transfused, the red cells become normal in less than 48 hours with respect to Na^+ and K^+ content, volume, shape and saline fragility. *Due to their short lifespan, the granulocytes and platelets are practically absent in the stored blood.*

Exchange Transfusion is performed for the prevention or treatment of severe jaundice in the infants with erythroblastosis fetalis. The baby's Rh positive blood is withdrawn in small quantities and replaced by equal volume of ABO-compatible Rh negative blood. Rh negative red cells are not destroyed by the Rh antibodies circulating in the baby's blood and hence plasma bilirubin level falls. Of course, baby's bone marrow would again produce Rh positive red cells, but with in a few days, Rh antibodies disappear from the baby's circulation.

Dangers of Blood Transfusion

Blood transfusion should be given only when it is really indicated, since every transfusion carries certain risks:

1. Infections Transfusion of blood, especially if the donor is unknown, carries risk of transferring blood-borne infections like malaria, *viral hepatitis* or *AIDS.*

2. Hyperkalaemia Stored blood has high plasma K^+ concentration. It takes about 48 hours before potassium returns back to the red cells. Therefore, *massive* blood transfusion may produce severe hyperkalaemia which may be fatal.

3. Alkalosis Citrate present in the transfused blood is normally metabolized to bicarbonate in the liver and excreted in the urine. In patients with compromised kidney function, accumulation of bicarbonate may produce alkalosis.

4. Hypocalcaemia In patients with liver disease or in induced hypothermia, the metabolism of transfused citrate may be delayed. In such patients, massive blood transfusion may produce a decrease in plasma ionized calcium level. The risk of hypocalcaemia can be eliminated by simultaneous administration of calcium gluconate.

5. Circulatory Overload In patients with severe chronic anaemia, red cell mass is reduced but the total blood volume is normal. Transfusion of whole blood for the treatment of anaemia may produce circulatory overload especially when the cardiac function is compromised by the anaemia. Such patients should be treated by transfusion of packed red cells rather than whole blood.

6. Incompatibility Reaction: Mismatched Blood Transfusion Unless cross-matching has been done, every transfusion carries a risk of incompatibility reaction. Mismatching of blood leads to agglutination and subsequent haemolysis of the donor cells. The following types of clinical reactions may follow:

(a) **Inapparent Haemolysis** The injected blood cells may be destroyed within a few days without producing any other symptom.

(b) **Post-transfusional Jaundice** If the rate of haemolysis is rapid, the accumulation of unconjugated bilirubin in the blood may produce jaundice, which gradually disappears.

(c) **Severe Incompatibility Reaction** In some patients, severe incompatibility reaction may produce massive intravascular agglutination leading to obstruction of blood flow in vital organs and death within minutes. In others, agglutination followed by severe haemolysis releases large amount of haemoglobin in the plasma. The patient complains of severe pain in the back or elsewhere or tightness in the chest. These symptoms are attributed to blockade of capillaries by clumps of red cells. There is a marked decrease in the arterial blood pressure.

The arterial hypotension and blockade of glomerular capillaries produces severe reduction in glomerular filtration rate and oliguria. Haemoglobin released into plasma by haemolysis partly gets bound to plasma protein haptoglobin and removed by tissue macrophages. Remaining plasma haemoglobin is filtered by the renal glomeruli into renal tubules leading to haemoglobinuria. In the renal tubules, the filtered haemoglobin may be precipitated as acid haematin especially if the urine is acidic and GFR is low. The lumen of the renal tubules is thus blocked, leading to acute renal failure and death within 8–10 days.

Transfusion of Blood Products

Severe haemorrhage and exchange transfusion are the chief indications for transfusion of whole blood. In other conditions, only a specific product of blood should be transfused. For example, in chronic anaemia, packed red cells should be transfused rather than the whole blood. If bone marrow hypoplasia leads to severe thrombocytopenia, or neutropenia, platelet concentrate or granulocyte concentrate should be transfused. Indications for transfusion of whole blood and various blood products are summarized in Table 3.7.

Table 3.7: Indications for transfusion of whole blood and blood products

Blood product	*indications*
1. Whole blood	(i) Severe haemorrhage. (ii) Erythroblastosis fetalis (exchange transfusion).
2. Packed red cells	Severe chronic anaemia.
3. Platelet concentrate	Severe thrombocytopenia.
4. Granulocyte concentrate	Severe neutropenia.
5. Fresh frozen plasma	(i) Multiple coagulation factor deficiency. (ii) Immediate antidote to dicoumarol toxicity.
6. Albumin	(i) Chronic hypoproteinemia due to extensive burns or hepatic failure. (ii) Hypovolaemic shock.
7. Immune serum globulin	Congenital agammaglobulinemia.
8. Rh immune globulin	Immunization of Rh negative mother soon after delivery of Rh positive baby.
9. Factor VIII concentrate	Haemophilia A.
10. Factor IX concentrate	Haemophilia B.

3

Blood Donation

Effects on the donor Usually 250–450 ml of blood is donated at a time. This amount may be donated every 4–6 months without any ill effect, provided the donor's dietary intake of iron is adequate. The donor should not indulge in heavy work or exercise during the next few hours after a blood donation. Some donors may have transient fainting sensation after blood donation, but it disappears with rest and fluid intake.

Contraindications Following are the contraindications for donation of blood:

(a) Age below 18 years and above 65 years.

(b) Pregnancy.

(c) Anaemia, i.e. haemoglobin level below 13 gm% in males and 12 gm% in females.

(d) History of viral hepatitis, malaria and other infectious diseases. Nowadays particular care is taken to exclude AIDS.

CHAPTER 4

The White Blood Cells and Immunity

The white blood cells can be classified into three categories (Fig. 4.1):

1. Granulocytes
2. Lymphocytes
3. Monocytes.

1. Granulocytes (10–14 μm) are characterized by the presence of granules in the cytoplasm and a lobed nucleus. Using Leishman's stain, three types of granulocytes can be identified: Neutrophil with fine red-brown granules and 2–5 lobed nucleus; eosinophil with large red granules and a 2-lobed spectacle-shaped nucleus, and basophil with large purple-blue granules which mask a mildly indented nucleus.

2. Lymphocytes (Small lymphocytes, 6–10 μm; large lymphocytes, 10–14 μm diameter) are round cells with large round nucleus and scanty non-granular cytoplasm.

3. Monocytes (10–18 μm) are characterized by abundant agranular cytoplasm and a kidney-shaped or irregularly folded nucleus.

The normal total leucocytes count of blood is 4,000 to 11,000 leucocytes/cmm of blood. Of these, 50–70% are neutrophils, 1–4% eosinophils, 0–1% basophils, 20–40% lymphocytes and 2–8% monocytes (Table 4.1). Acting together, the white blood cells provide a powerful defence mechanism against bacterial, viral and parasitic infections.

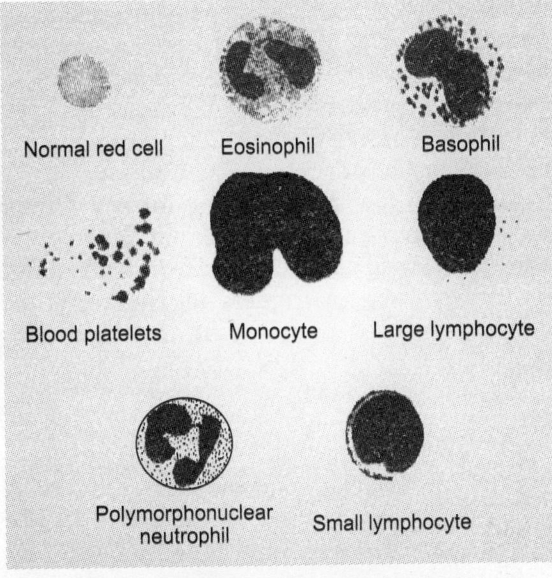

Fig. 4.1: Various types of blood cells.

FUNCTION OF POLYMORPHONUCLEAR NEUTROPHILS

The living neutrophil, when seen on a glass slide under a phase contrast microscope, shows active amoeboid movements. Its cytoplasm contains 50–200 dense granules (lysosomes) which contain proteolytic enzymes. The cell contains very little endoplasmic reticulum and a few mitochondria. The neutrophils perform their function outside the

4

Table 4.1: Normal values of the leucocytes

Cell	*Cells/cmm (Average)*	*Cells/cmm (Normal range)*	*Percentage of total leucocytes*
Total WBC	9000	4,000–11,000	–
Neutrophils	5400	3,000–6000	50–70
Eosinophils	275	150–300	1–4
Basophils	35	0–100	0–1
Lymphocytes	2750	1,500–4,000	20–40
Monocytes	540	400–600	2–8

blood vessels. In the tissue spaces, they actively seek out, engulf, and destroy the bacteria and other foreign proteins. These cells constitute the first line of defence against bacterial infections.

Average half-life of a neutrophil in *circulation* is only 6 hours. Some neutrophils are constantly migrating out of the blood capillaries. They squeeze through the gaps between the endothelial cells by a process called *diapedesis*. After migration into the tissues, neutrophils do not return back to the bloodstream. They survive in the tissues for a few days, looking for any foreign protein. Many neutrophils enter the lumen of the alimentary canal and the bronchi. Invasion of the tissues by bacteria triggers the inflammatory response which consists of the following (Fig. 4.2).

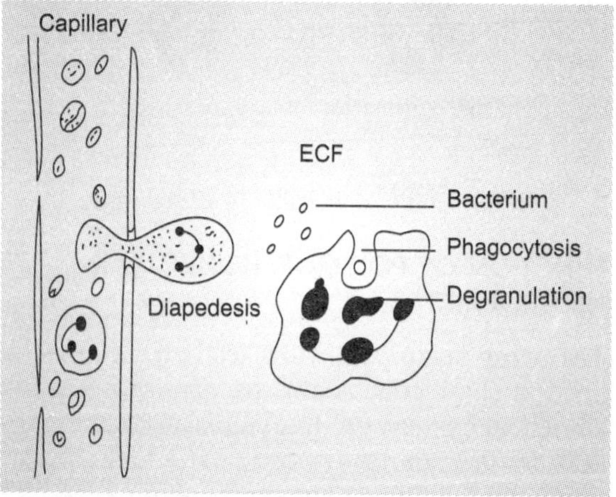

Fig. 4.2: Response of neutrophils to infection: Diapedesis, phagocytosis and degranulation.

1. Increased Rate of Diapedesis and Chemotaxis In case of infection, the rate of diapedesis in the involved tissue is dramatically increased because the bacterial products interact with plasma factor (called complements), to produce agents that attract the neutrophils to the infected area. This phenomenon is called *chemotaxis*.

2. Phagocytosis It is the next step. Not only bacteria but also other foreign proteins and necrotic tissues are phagocytosed by the neutrophils. This process is greatly helped by *opsonization* of the bacteria, i.e. specific antibodies (IgG) and complement proteins adhere to the bacterial membrane, making them 'attractive' to the phagocytes.

3. Degranulation occurs when bacterium enclosed in a phagocytic vesicle comes in contact with granules (lysosomes) of the neutrophils. By exocytosis, the neutrophil granules discharge their contents into the phagocytic vesicle to constitute phagolysosome. The lysosomal proteolytic enzymes digest the bacterium.

Degranulation is accompanied by activation of two enzymes present in the leucocyte granules, namely, NADPH oxidase and myeloperoxidase. Activation of NADPH oxidase is associated with a sharp increase in oxygen consumption in the neutrophil (*the respiratory burst*) leading to generation of highly toxic free radicals, superoxide (O_2^-) and hydrogen peroxide (H_2O_2). Myeloperoxidase catalyses the formation of toxic hypochlorous acid (HoCl). These toxic agents facilitate the bactericidal action of lysosomal enzymes. NADPH oxidase and myeloperoxidase are called oxygen-dependent bactericidal mechanisms. In addition, the granules contain a large number of bactericidal agents which do not require oxygen for their activity. These oxygen-independent bactericidal agents include lysosomal hydrolases, collagenases, elastases, proteinases, bactericidal permeability-increasing proteins, defensin, apolactoferrin, etc. Degranulation results in bacterial killing. However, some of the superficially placed granules discharge their contents into the extracellular fluid which results in some degree of tissue necrosis as well as other manifestations of inflammation (local vasodilatation, oedema, pain, etc.).

When a neutrophil engulfs a large number of bacteria, the strong proteolytic activity not only destroys the bacteria but also the neutrophil itself. Thus ultimately all the neutrophils in the inflamed area die and are subsequently removed by the monocyte macrophages. In more severe infection, pus is formed. It consists of necrotic tissue, dead neutrophils and dead macrophages.

Pools of Neutrophils

In normal persons 2–3 × 10^{10} neutrophils are circulating in the blood at any one time (*circulating pool*). An equal number of neutrophils are adherent to the endothelial cells of post-capillary venules (*marginated pool*). After heavy exercise, or injection of epinephrine, the blood granulocyte count is (moderately) increased because of a transfer of the cells from the marginated pool to circulating pool. Within a few hours after the onset of acute inflammation, the number of neutrophils in the peripheral blood increases 4–5 folds. This is due to mobilization of young granulocytes (band form) already formed and stored in the bone marrow (*storage pool*). A number of chemicals released from the inflamed tissue, collectively called *granulocyte-releasing* factors, are carried to the bone marrow causing the release of neutrophils from the storage pool into the systemic circulation. The *rate of production* of granulocytes is also increased by another group of chemicals collectively called colony *stimulating factor*, released from the inflamed tissues.

Eosinophils

The exact function of eosinophils is not clear. Eosinophils are weak phagocytes and do not seem to have any role in ordinary bacterial infections. However, their number is markedly increased in tissues with parasitic infections. The parasites are too big to be engulfed by eosinophils. Probably eosinophils attach themselves to the parasites and kill them by releasing toxic substances. The eosinophil granulocytes contain a large number of extremely potent toxins called major basic proteins (MBP). MBP is believed to be responsible for their antiparasitic activity.

Blood eosinophil count increases in various types of allergic disorders. Although normally blood contains only a few eosinophils (1–4% of total leucocytes), skin and submucosa of respiratory, gastrointestinal and genitourinary tracts contains a large number of eosinophils. In these tissues, during allergic reaction (in which mast cells are primarily involved) eosinophil number is markedly increased. Eosinophils seem to decrease the clinical manifestations of allergy by degrading the products of mast cells, especially histamine.

Basophils

Very few basophils circulate in the blood. Their exact function is not known. Mast cells, which histologically resemble the basophils, are present in large numbers outside the capillaries in many tissues. Mast cells and basophils seem to play an important role in allergic reactions. Immunoglobulin IgE attaches itself to the mast cells. When the specific antigen subsequently reacts with the antibody, the granules of mast cells release large amount of histamine, bradykinin, serotonin and heparin. These agents cause local vascular manifestations of allergy.

Monocyte-Macrophages

Like granulocytes, circulating monocytes also perform their function after migration into the tissues. Granulocytes arrive in the tissues fully prepared for their phagocytic function, but blood monocytes are not capable of phagocytosis as such. In the blood, monocytes have a half-life of about 70 hours. In the tissues, monocytes undergo further differentiation. Their size may increase up to 80 μm in diameter. An extremely large number of lysosomes and mitochondria develop in the cytoplasm. These cells are now called *macrophages*. A macrophage has a larger phagocytic power than a neutrophil. A macrophage may engulf as many as 100 bacteria as compared to 5–20 by a neutrophil. A macrophage may engulf a whole red blood cell or a malarial parasite which granulocytes cannot. Besides these, necrotic tissue and dead neutrophils are also removed by the macrophages. Like neutrophils, a few monocyte-

4

macrophages are always wandering through the tissues looking for any foreign protein or extraneous material. The lifespan of these tissue macrophages is several months. Macrophages accumulate in large numbers at the site of infection. The processes of chemotaxis, opsonization, formation of digestive vesicle and lysosomal digestion of the bacteria, etc. occur in macrophages as in the granulocytes. However, at the site of acute inflammation, granulocytes appear first. The macrophages appear a little later and constitute the second line of defence. Certain specific chemicals released from the inflamed area (colony stimulating factor) reach the bone marrow and increase the rate of production of monocytes.

Beside the phagocytic function described above, monocyte macrophages are also involved in the processing of antigen and modulation of lymphocytic activity during immune responses. Some of the macrophages constitute the fixed tissue macrophage system.

Tissue Macrophage System

As mentioned above, the blood monocytes migrate and differentiate into macrophages and wander through the tissues. Some of these macrophages become attached to the tissues and remain there for several months. This tissue macrophage system includes macrophages lining the sinusoids of the liver (Kupffer cells), spleen, bone marrow, lymph nodes, and in the lung parenchyma (alveolar macrophages), bone (osteoclast cells), brain (microglia) and skin (Langerhan's cells). The tissue macrophage system was earlier known as reticulo-endothelial system. The function of tissue macrophages is similar to that of mobile macrophages. They remove bacteria, viruses and necrotic material from the tissues and also from the circulating blood and lymph. If needed, in response to chemotaxis, fixed macrophages can lose their attachment and become mobile macrophages to reach the area of infection.

Functions of Monocyte Macrophages

(i) Phagocytosis of microorganisms (second line of defence), dead tissue cells, denatured connective tissue of matrix.

(ii) Antigen processing and modulation of lymphoid activity in immune responses.

(iii) Clearance from blood of senescent (aged) red blood cells, or invading micro-organisms is also a function of fixed tissue macrophages.

(iv) Release of interleukin-1 leading to increased production of erythrocytes, granulocytes, platelet and monocytes.

THE SPLEEN

Spleen is the largest lymphoid organ in the body. It constitutes an important defence system against antigens entering the circulation.

Human spleen is enclosed in a thick fibrous capsule. Unlike some animals such as cat and dog, the capsule of human spleen contains very few smooth muscle fibres. Hence, it is not capable of marked contraction.

With naked eye, the cut surface of the spleen is seen to contain white spots, in the background dark red tissue. These spots are called white pulp, whereas the dark red tissue is called the red pulp. The capsule extends into the spleen forming a sponge-like framework of thin septa. A finer network of reticular fibres, reticular cells and macrophages supports the lymphocytes and blood sinusoids. This finer network forms a filtering bed that filters out *abnormal* red cells, white cells and platelets passing through the red pulp.

In the white pulp, the reticular cells are arranged around a central artery. At intervals, large collections of lymphocytes constitute the lymph follicles, in which an artery (called the central artery) occupies an eccentric position. The lymph follicles chiefly contain B-lymphocytes. The red pulp consists of thin-walled blood sinusoids and splenic cords between them. The splenic cords consist of collections of lymphocytes in the fine network of reticular cells and fibres (Fig. 4.3).

The central artery gives off a number of penicillar arterioles. These open into large sinusoids from where the blood is drained into the venous channels. This pattern of circulation is called the closed circulation. According to another

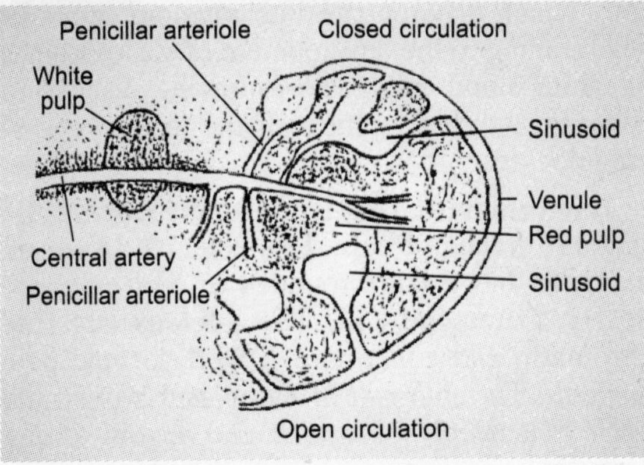

Fig. 4.3: Histological structure of the spleen illustrating the closed type and open type of circulation.

view, the spleen has an open circulation i.e. the penicillar arterioles open into the fine network of red pulp. Ultimately blood is drained into sinusoids and venous channels.

These two types of circulations are shown diagrammatically in Fig. 4.3. Whether splenic circulation is open or closed has not been settled as yet.

FUNCTIONS OF SPLEEN

1. Reservoir Function In some animals, the spleen serves as a reservoir for mobilization of red cells. In man, this function is not important because the splenic capsule cannot contract to any significant degree. However, spleen seems to serve as a storehouse for platelets. As much as 30% of the total circulating platelets may be present in the spleen adhering to the reticular cells in the red pulp or to the endothelial cells of the sinusoids.

2. Erythropoiesis During 2nd and 3rd month of fetal life, erythropoiesis occurs in the spleen. In postnatal life, erythropoiesis may occur in the spleen only if the entire bone marrow has been damaged.

3. Production of Lymphocytes The lymph follicles and the red pulp are active sites for the production of T and B lymphocytes.

4. Phagocytosis Aged erythrocytes or those damaged by the action of antibodies are removed by tissue mononuclear macrophages in different organs like spleen, bone marrow, liver, etc. Spleen seems to possess a special capability of trapping even mildly damaged erythrocytes. This ability has been attributed to the uniquely slow circulation of red cells among the splenic cords where red cells come in close contact with the splenic macrophages. Prolonged stasis of red cells causes haemoconcentration as well as fall of pH and sugar content of the blood. As a result, even mild damage to the red cells is exaggerated and phagocytosis follows. White blood cells and platelets are also treated similarly by the phagocytes. The ability to detect and destroy abnormal type of blood cells has been called *culling action* of spleen.

5. Iron Metabolism Although destruction of old and damaged red cells may occur in any of the tissue monocyte macrophage system of cells, spleen macrophages seem to have a special ability to recycle the liberated iron for synthesis of fresh haemoglobin in the bone marrow. Some other macrophages, e.g. in the lung parenchyma do not have this ability at all.

6. Antibody Production Spleen is one of the important sites of antibody production. After splenectomy, antibody production continues to occur in other lymphatic organs but the antibody response is delayed and the antibody titre does not rise as high as in normal individuals.

Effects of Splenectomy

Some types of anaemia are treated by splenectomy, e.g. congenital spherocytic anaemia. The removal of spleen produces the following effects:

1. Abnormal types of red cells appear in the circulation. The red cells tend to be thinner and have decreased osmotic fragility.
2. The total leucocyte count is moderately raised (10,000–15,000/μL).
3. There is moderate elevation of platelet count.
4. Infections tend to be more fulminating.

LYMPH NODES

Lymph nodes are kidney-shaped or ovoid structures varying in size from 1 mm to over 1 cm. They are more numerous at the axilla, groin, mediastinum and retroperitoneal region. The lymph nodes constitute a series of in-line filters. Lymph must pass through at least one lymph node before mixing with the bloodstream.

Trabeculae arising from the fibrous capsule of the node divide the parenchyma into sponge-like compartments. A network of reticular fibres, reticular cells and macrophages supports the lymphocytes of the parenchyma. Each lymph node has a cortex below the capsule and deeper medulla which reaches the surface at the hilum (Fig. 4.4). The cortex contains dense aggregates of lymphoid and reticular cells called lymphatic nodules. The medullary region consists of medullary cords comprised of dense lymphoid tissue and intervening medullary sinuses composed of loose lymphatic tissue. The afferent lymphatic vessels open into the convex surface of the node through a series of openings. Lymph percolates slowly through the cortex and medullary region and leaves through the efferent lymph vessels at the hilum. The lymph flow in the node is unidirectional due to the presence of valves in the afferent and efferent lymph vessels. Over 99% of the lymph passes through the lymph sinuses and only 1% penetrates the lymph nodules. However, it is in the nodules that bulk of antigenic material is processed and antibody production occurs.

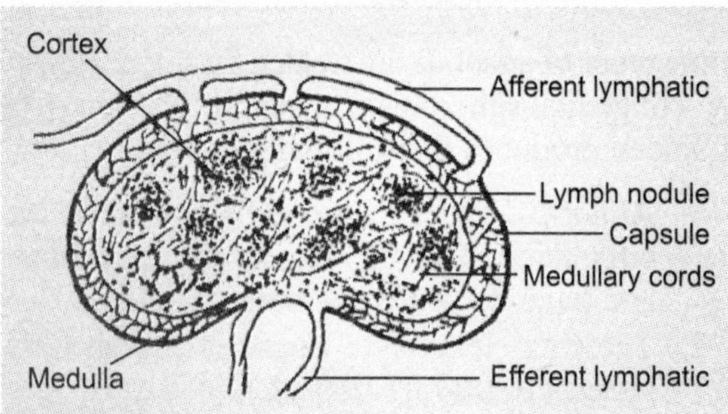

Fig. 4.4: Histological structure of a lymph node.

LEUCOPOIESIS

All the white blood cells develop from the haemopoietic stem cells present in the bone marrow (Fig. 3.9). A process of differentiation converts some of the stem cells to committed stem cells which differentiate into myeloid series of cells leading to the development of various types of white blood cells. The following discussion concerns the development of the three types of granulocytes.

1. Myeloblast This is the first recognizable stage of granulopoiesis. This cell, 10–18 μm in diameter, has a large rounded or oval nucleus, nearly filling the cell. The nucleus has fine chromatin and contains 2–5 well defined pale nucleoli. The thin rim of cytoplasm around the nucleus is deeply basophilic and devoid of any granules.

2. Promyelocyte At this stage, the cell is slightly larger than a myeloblast (12–18 μ diameter). The nucleus is large but chromatin is mildly condensed. The nucleoli are fewer than in the previous stage. The main feature which distinguishes it from the previous stage is the presence of a few azurophilic primary (non-specific) granules.

3. Myelocyte This stage is characterized by the appearance of specific (secondary) granules in the cytoplasm. Hence, neutrophilic, eosinophilic or basophilic myelocytes can be identified by the colour of specific granules. The primary granules persist but do not take up any stain (can be seen under E/M). In a melocyte, as compared to the previous stages, the cytoplasm is more extensive and less basophilic while the nucleus is smaller and more basophilic.

4. Metamyelocyte A metamyelocyte (10–18 μm diameter) is characterized by a clearly indented or horseshoe-shaped nucleus with dense or clumped chromatin. The cytoplasm contains still larger number of secondary granules. Primary granules though present cannot be seen since they do not take any stain, (but can be seen under E/M).

5. Band form This name is given to a juvenile granulocyte (10–14 μm diameter). At this stage, the nuclear chromatin is further condensed. The nucleus takes the shape of a band or a thin strip of uniform thickness.

6. Segmented Granulocytes A mature granulocyte (neutrophil, eosinophil, or basophil) is said to be formed when the indentation appears in the nuclear band to give it a lobed appearance. Mainly at this stage, the granulocytes enter the peripheral circulation, though some band forms may be seen normally. When the granulopoiesis is accelerated, many band forms can be seen in circulation. As a granulocyte, particularly a neutrophil, ages, the number of lobes increases. As a result, 4–5 lobes of the nucleus, connected by strands of nuclear material, may be seen in the aged neutrophil.

Granules of a Neutrophil

A mature neutrophil contains three types of cytoplasmic granules, which under E/M, are seen to be lysosomes. They are named as primary, secondary (specific) and tertiary granules. The primary granules appear at promyelocyte stage as azure-coloured cytoplasmic granules. They persist in all the subsequent stages, although they lose their staining property. The secondary granules appear in myelocyte stage and their number increases in the subsequent developmental stages. Secondary granules give specific staining reaction, based on which a myelocyte can be classified as a neutrophil, an eosinophil, or a basophil. In a mature neutrophil, the secondary and primary granules are present in the ratio of 2:1. Tertiary granules are few in number and appear only in band and subsequent development stage. Tertiary granules can be seen only under E/M. The three types of granules present in a mature neutrophil contain different types of bactericidal enzymes (Table 4.2).

Table 4.2: Enzymes present in the three types of granules in a mature neutrophil

Primary granules (azurophilic granules)	*Secondary granules (specific granules)*	*Tertiary granules*
Lysozyme	Lysozyme	Lysozyme
Myeloperoxidase	Collagenase	Gelatinase
Defensins	Apolactoferrin	
Elastase		
Proteinase 3		
Bactericidal permeability-increasing protein		

Development of Monocytes

Monoblasts are similar to myeloblasts but promonocytes are characterized by a round or mildly indented nucleus, and deeply basophilic cytoplasm containing a few azurophilic granules. Young circulating monocytes are identified by their kidney-shaped or folded nucleus and abundant grayish blue cytoplasm, which may contain a few azurophilic granules. As the monocyte matures, the granules, though present, cannot be stained.

The development of lymphocytes is discussed on page 53.

Regulation of Leucopoiesis

A number of glycoproteins regulate the production of white blood cells in the bone marrow. They are called *colony stimulating factors (CSF)*, because in tissue culture they cause a single stem cell to proliferate into a colony of a particular type of white blood cells, e.g. granulocyte colony stimulating factor (GCSF), macrophage colony stimulating factor (MCSF) and granulocyte-macrophage colony stimulating factor (GM-CSF). These factors are produced in the area of acute inflammation and transported to the bone marrow thorough blood circulation.

Like red blood cells, the development of white blood cells also requires vitamin B_{12} and folic acid. Deficiency of these vitamins results in leucopenia.

Pathophysiology

An increase in the number of total white blood cells in the periphral blood in known as *leucocytosis*. If the differential blood cell count confirms that leucocytosis is due to an absolute increase in the number of neutrophils, the term *granulocytosis* or more accurately, *neutrophilia* is used. In acute infections, like tonsillitis or acute appendicitis, total WBC count is between 15,000–40,000/cmm with 80–90% or more being neutrophils.

A total WBC count above 50,000/cmm should arouse the **suspicion** of cancerous growth of the myeloid tissue of the bone marrow (myeloid leukemia) or of lymphoid tissue (lymphoid leukemia). Besides very high white blood cell count (50,000–100,000/cmm), the most characteristic feature of leukemia is the presence of immature *blast cells* of myeloid or lymphoid series in the peripheral blood.

Reaction to certain drugs sometimes produces cessation of production of neutrophils (*agranulocytosis*). The *peripheral blood smears* show almost complete absence of granulocytes. In such cases, any severe infection may lead to death within a few days.

Causes of Neutrophilia (Neutrophilic leucocytosis)

I. Physiological
   (i) Exercise
   (ii) Pregnancy

II. Pathological
   (i) Acute infections, localized or generalized, e.g. abscess, tonsillitis, appendicitis, pneumonia.
   (ii) Non-infectious inflammations like myocardial infarction, burns and surgical operations.
   (iii) Acute haemorrhage.
   (iv) Acute haemolysis.

Causes of Neutropenia (Decreased Neutrophil Count)

(i) Certain infections, e.g. typhoid, viral influenza, viral hepatitis, malaria.
(ii) Overwhelming bacterial infections or septicemia.
(iii) Drug-induced bone marrow depression.
(iv) Vitamin B_{12} deficiency.

Causes of Eosinophilia

(i) Allergic disorders, e.g. bronchial asthma, hay fever.
(ii) Parasitic infections, e.g. intestinal parasites.

Causes of Eosinopenia

(i) Administration of ACTH or adrenal glucocorticoids.

Causes of Basophilia (Rare Condition)

(i) Some cases of chronic myeloid leukemia.
(ii) Polycythaemia vera.

Causes of Lymphocytosis

(i) Certain acute infections, e.g. viral hepatitis, infectious lymphocytosis, infectious mononucleosis.
(ii) Certain chronic infections, e.g. tuberculosis.

Causes of Lymphopenia

(i) Most acute infections.
(ii) Bone marrow depression due to drugs/radiation.
(iii) Corticosteroid therapy.

Causes of Monocytosis

(i) Certain bacterial infections, e.g. tuberculosis.
(ii) Viral infections.
(iii) Protozoal infections, e.g. malaria.

IMMUNITY

The human body is able to resist most of the foreign organisms that invade the body. This ability is known as immunity. Part of the resistance results from non-specific processes like:

A. Resistance of the skin to invasion by organisms.
B. Destruction of the ingested bacteria by gastric acid or gastrointestinal proteolytic enzymes.
C. Phagocytosis and killing of the bacteria by granulocytes and tissue macrophages, and natural killer (NK) lymphocytes.

This type of *non-specific innate* immunity, however, is not sufficient to give full protection against the invading organisms.

ACQUIRED IMMUNITY

Human body has an ability to develop an extremely powerful and specific immunity against invading agents like bacteria or viruses or their toxins. This is called *acquired immunity*. Lymphocytes are key constituents of this immune system. There are 2 types of acquired immunity, i.e. humoral immunity and cell-mediated immunity.

Humoral Immunity

It is due to the presence of circulating antibodies (immunoglobulins), which are capable of attacking the invading agent. Immunoglobulins are components of gamma-globulin fraction of plasma proteins. They are produced by lymphocytes after transformation into plasma cells. Immunoglobulins constitute the major defence system against bacterial infections.

Cell-Mediated Immunity (Cellular Immunity)

It is produced by activated lymphocytes that can directly attack intracellular pathogenic microorganisms like viruses and fungi as well as many bacteria. These cells are also involved in the removal of malignant cells and rejection of incompatible tissue grafts.

It would be obvious that lymphocytes play a key role in the production of acquired immunity. Lymphocytes can be broadly classified into two types namely T lymphocytes, which are involved in cellular immunity, and B lymphocytes, which are involved in humoral immunity. In the peripheral blood, T and B lymphocytes are present in the ratio of 80: 20, but cannot be differentiated from each other by usual microscopic methods.

DEVELOPMENT OF LYMPHOID TISSUE AND IMMUNE SYSTEM

The *peripheral lymphoid* tissue consists of: (i) The lymph nodes, distributed throughout the body, and (ii) special lymphoid tissue located in the spleen, tonsils and submucosal collection of lymphocytes in the gut (particularly in the terminal ileum), respiratory tract, the urinary tract and the bone marrow. It is obvious that lymphoid tissue is strategically located at each possible route of entry of invading organisms. The spleen and the bone marrow remove organisms that may enter the blood circulation. The lymph nodes remove organisms that may enter the lymphatics.

The lymphocyte precursors are formed in the bone marrow from pluripotent stem cells. From the bone marrow, lymphocyte precursors migrate to **central lymphoid tissues** like thymus *for preprocessing*. In the *thymus*, they undergo cell division and differentiation to form immunocompetent T lymphocytes which are released into circulation. Most of the processing of T lymphocytes occurs shortly before birth and for a few months after birth. In experimental animals, thymectomy abolishes cell-mediated immunity, if performed soon after birth, but has no effect if performed in an adult animal. However even in adult life, thymus seems to have a "supportive hormonal effect" on T cell function in the peripheral lymphoid tissues.

In birds, *bursa of Fabricius*, located near the cloaca, is the other central lymphoid tissue where the pre-processing of the lymphocyte precursors occurs to produce immuno-competent B lymphocytes. Bursectomy performed in fetal life leads to failure of development of humoral immunity after birth. In mammals, the equivalent central lymphoid tissue has not been identified but seems to be located in the fetal liver and bone marrow in postnatal life.

The T and B lymphocytes released from the central lymphoid tissues circulate in the blood. Within few hours, however, they are trapped ("seeded") in the areas of future peripheral lymphoid tissues named above. There, the T and B lymphocytes proliferate and further differentiate as a result of exposure to antigens. The lifespan of T lymphocytes may be 2–4 years. The B lymphocytes, however, have a lifespan of a few weeks only.

Specificity of T and B Lymphocytes

There are at least 1 million different types of B lymphocytes. Each is capable of activation by a specific antigen to differentiate into *plasma cells* and form a specific antibody against the antigen. Similarly, *there are at least 1 million* types of T lymphocytes, each capable of being activated by a specific antigen.

Once activated by an antigen, the T or B lymphocytes undergo a tremendous proliferation to produce a huge number of their duplicates.

Role of Macrophages in Immunity

Most invading organisms are first phagocytosed by macrophages which partially digest the bacteria and transfer the antigenic products to a lymphocyte having specific receptors for the antigen on the cell membrane.

4

The macrophages are also believed to secrete a hormone-like chemical messenger called interleukin 1 which promotes the growth and reproduction of specific activated lymphocytes.

Memory Cells

After exposure to an antigen, some of the T or B lymphocytes do not become effector cells. Instead, they remain as immunological memory cells for months and even years. On re-exposure to the similar antigen, these memory cells produce a quicker and much larger immunological response.

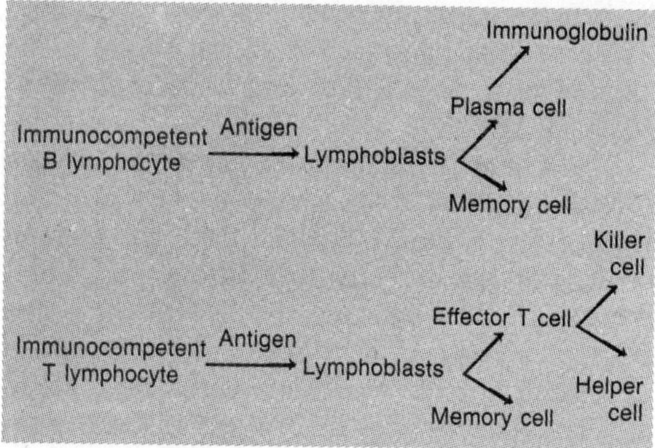

T Lymphocyte Function

There are three types of T lymphocytes; (i) cytotoxic T cells or killer cells, (ii) helper T cell and (iii) suppressor T cells.

i. Cytotoxic T Cells (T_C)

On coming in contact with specific antigen on the surface of an organism or a mutant cell, the T cell binds tightly to the organism, enlarges in size and releases cytotoxic substance (probably lysosomal enzymes) into the organism. The killer cell can attack several similar organisms one after another and kill them without suffering any harm to itself. Killer T cells particularly attack cells containing viruses or those with mutant genes (cancer cells). If a tissue is transplanted which is foreign to the body, it is rejected by the activity of a large number of killer cells collected at the site of transplant (incompatible graft rejection site).

ii. Helper T Cells

An antigen not only activates a specific type of cytotoxic T cells (T_C cells) but also helper T cells (T_H cells). Activated helper T cells secrete certain hormone-like chemical messengers, called cytokines or interleukins, which enhance the immune response of activated cytotoxic T cells (cellular immunity) as well as activated B lymphocytes (humoral immunity). Two subtypes of T_H cells have been identified. T_H1 cells secrete interleukin 2 which interacts with cytotoxic T cells, whereas T_H2 cells secrete interleukin-4 and -5 which interact with B lymphocytes. In the absence of cytokines from the helper T cells, the remainder of the immune system is almost paralyzed, as happens in patients suffering from AIDS. In this disorder, the human immunodeficiency virus (HIV) attacks and destroys helper T cells of the body.

iii. Suppressor T Cells

These cells can suppress the activity of the cytotoxic T cells and the helper T cells.

A major function of T cells is to recognize and destroy the cancer cells. Cell mutation occurs very frequently but such cells have surface antigen different from the normal cells. Hence, they are recognized as foreign cells by the circulating T cells and destroyed. Failure of this system seems to be one of the reasons for the multiplication of mutant cells resulting in the condition called cancer.

B Lymphocyte Function

On exposure to an antigen, specific B lymphocytes, located in one or more of the peripheral lymphoid tissues are activated. As a result, B lymphocytes are converted into lymphoblast-like cells. Some of these lymphoblast-like cells remain as such and are called memory cells. Others differentiate further into plasma blast cells which rapidly divide and form huge number of plasma cells. The plasma cells secrete immunoglobulins at a rapid rate. The immunoglobulins (antibodies) are carried to the general circulation via lymph. Each plasma cell continues to produce the specific antibody for several days or even weeks till it dies.

It would be obvious that whereas activated T lymphocytes can function in the blood or any other tissue, activated B lymphocytes differentiate into the plasma cells (which secrete antibodies) in the peripheral lymphoid tissues only.

The major differences between T and B lymphocytes tabulated below in Table 4.3.

Natural Killer Cells (NK Cells)

Most of the circulating *large lymphocytes* are activated B lymphocytes. Some of them, however, are natural killer cells (NK cells). NK cells are large lymphocytes containing a few azurophilic granules in their cytoplasm. These cells can engulf and destroy antigens (bacteria). However, unlike cytotoxic T cells, their action is non-specific, i.e. their activity does not require prior antigenic stimulation.

Interleukins (Cytokines)

Lymphocytes, macrophages and some other somatic cells secrete a variety of hormone-like chemical messengers that affect the immune response. The chemical messengers were initially called *lymphokines*. Nowadays, they are known as *cytokines* because, as mentioned above, they are produced by not only lymphocytes but also by other cells. Cytokines whose amino acid sequence is known are called *interleukins*. The list of some important interleukins with their principal source and chief effects is given in Table 4.4. The systemic effects of interleukin-1 have been listed separately (Table 4.5).

IMMUNOGLOBULINS

Immunoglobulins or antibodies are present in the gamma globulin fraction of the plasma proteins.

Table 4.4: Some important interleukins

Interleukins	*Cell source*	*Principal effects*
IL-1	Macrophages, other somatic cells	Costimulation of T cells, and B cells, systemic effects (Table 4.5)
IL-2	Activated T_H1 cell, T_C cells	Proliferation of activated T and B cells
IL-3	T lymphocytes	Growth of early haemopoietic progenitors.
IL-4	T_H2 cells, mast cells	B cell proliferation, Ig production, T_H2 cell and T_C cell proliferation and function. Eosinophil and mast cell growth and function.
IL-5	T_H2 cells, mast cells	Eosinophil growth and function

Table 4.3: Differences between T and B lymphocytes

	T lymphocytes	*B lymphocytes*
Origin	Bone marrow → Thymus → lymphoid tissue	Bone marrow → Bursa-equivalent → lymphoid tissue
Life span	Months to years	Less than one month.
Location		
Lymph nodes	Perifollicular	Germinal centre
Spleen	Perifollicular	Germinal centre
Payer's patches	Perifollicular	Central follicles
Number in blood	80%	20%
Function	(i) Cell-mediated immunity via Tc cells (ii) Immunoregulation of T and B lymphocytes via T_H cells	Humoral immunity via immunoglobulins

Table 4.5: Systemic effects of interleukin-1

A. CNS effects
Fever
Increased slow wave sleep
Increased secretion of CRH
Decreased appetite
B. Metabolic effects
Increased synthesis of hepatic proteins
Increased Na^+ excretion
Lactic acidosis
C. Haematological effects
Increased circulating neutrophils
Decreased circulating lymphocytes.
Increased secretion of colony-stimulating factors
Increased non-specific resistance
D. Vascular wall effects
Increased leucocyte adherence.
Increased prostaglandin synthesis.
Increased release of platelet-activating factor
Increased capillary permeability
Hypotension

Their molecular weight varies between 150,000 and 900,000 approximately. Immunoglobulins are composed of polypeptide chains. Most of the antibodies have two heavy chains and two light chains. Each light chain lies parallel to the terminal part of the heavy chain and linked by disulphide bridges (Fig. 4.5). The specificity of each antibody is due to a specific amino acid pattern of the terminal portions (variable portions) of both light and heavy chains. Antigen antibody binding occurs in this portion. In general, five classes of immunoglobulins are recognized. They have been called IgA, IgM, IgE, IgD, IgG.

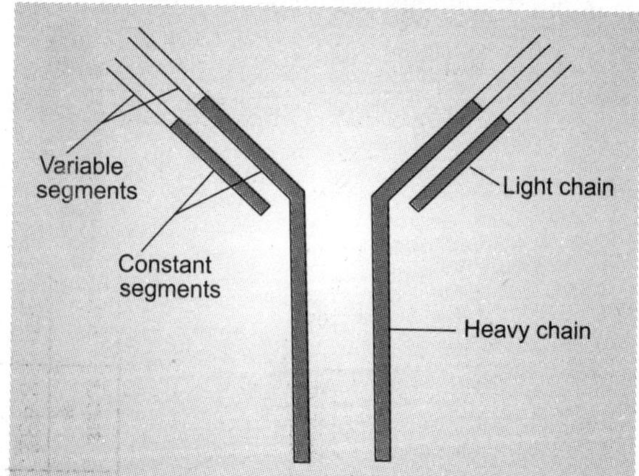

Fig. 4.5: Structure of an immunoglobulin molecule.

IgG is the most abundant immunoglobulin in the plasma. Its production is stimulated by bacterial or viral infections and by artificial immunization. These antibodies are distributed between blood and tissue fluids. They cross the placental barrier by active transport. IgG antibodies are found in the salivary, nasal and bronchial secretions and in the milk. They act by activation of complement system.

IgA are formed by the mucosal and submucosal aggregation of lymphoid tissue and passed on to the epithelial cells which secrete it by exocytosis. The presence of these immunoglobulins provides an effective defence mechanism in the mucosa of the alimentary canal, lungs, genitourinary tract and female reproductive tract. IgA act by producing lysis of the bacteria.

IgM have large molecular size and hence remains predominantly intravascular. IgM activate complement fixation, promote phagocytosis and particularly cause lysis of the bacteria.

IgE are the antibodies responsible for anaphylactic reaction. They get attached to the tissue cells, as well as, the mast cells. When an antigen comes in contact with antibody attached to the mast cells, the latter rupture and release histamine. In normal individuals, plasma IgE level is extremely low.

IgD is present on the surface of B lymphocytes which are destined to differentiate into antibody producing plasma cells. Plasma concentration of IgD is very low. Its exact function is not known. It is believed to help in antigen recognition (Table 4.6).

Mechanism of Action of Antibodies

An antibody may protect the body against an invading organism or its toxic products either by (A) *a direct action* or by (B) *activation of the complement system.*

A. Direct Action

The antibody may combine with the antigen and directly produce:

Table 4.6: Summary of properties and functions of immunoglobulins

	IgG	*IgA*	*IgM*	*IgD*	*IgE*
Molecular weight	150,000	170,000	900,000	180,000	200,000
Plasma conc.(mg/dl)	700–1500	250	100	3	0.03
Presence plasma/ECF	+	-	-	-	-
Presence intravascular	-	-	+	-	-
Presence secretions	-	+	-	-	-
Mast cell binding	-	-	-	-	+
Crossing placental barrier	+	-	-	-	-

(a) Agglutination of the bacteria (or the red blood cells) to form large clumps;
(b) *Precipitation* of the soluble toxins;
(c) *Neutralisation* of the toxins;
(d) *Lysis* of the bacteria.

B. Complement System

This is a more common mode of action of antibodies. The complement system consists of about 20 proteins present in the plasma and tissue fluids that are involved in the defence mechanism of the body. Of these, 11 are more well-known and are named C_1 through C_9, B and D (Fig. 4.6). The first named (C_1–C_9) belong to the classical pathway in which the proteins present as enzyme precursors are activated, one after another, as a cascade of sequential reactions (cf. clotting cascade). The series of reactions are set into motion by the activation of C_1 protein by an antigen-

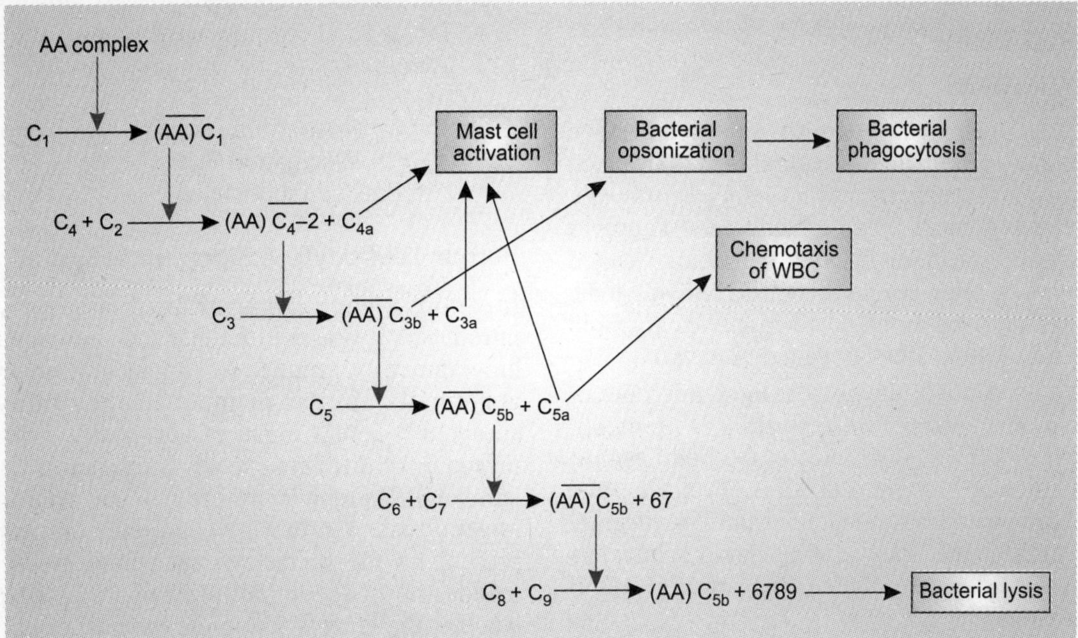

Fig. 4.6: Cascade of reactions in the activation of complements. A bar (—) over a figure means that the product has acquired enzymic property. Small letters (a) and (b) indicate that the parent complement has split into two components. AA = Antigen antibody complex. The biological responses of various activated products are indicated in rectangles.

antibody reaction. In the clotting cascade reactions, only the final activated product fibrin is the mediator of biological response. In contrast, in the complement system, many of the activated products along the cascade, not only activate the next step, but also produce some biological responses. The activated components of the complement system help in the defence mechanism against the invading organism by:

(i) **Opsonisation** Activated complement may make the bacteria tastier to the neutrophils and macrophages (opsonisation), e.g. activated C_3. They probably act as receptors to which macrophages can bind before phagocytosis (Fig. 4.6).
(ii) **Lysis** A combination of activated complements ($C_{5,\ 6,\ 7,\ 8,\ 9}$) together have a direct effect of rupturing the cell membrane of the bacteria.
(iii) **Agglutination** of the bacteria.
(iv) **Neutralization** of the viruses.
(v) **Chemotaxis** The activated complement attracts large number of neutrophils and macrophages to the site of infection.

VACCINATION

The immunological responses described above occur during the course of natural infections. Such type of *active immunity* may be induced artificially by injecting small doses of *weakened microbes* (live polio vaccine) or modified toxins called toxoids (e.g. tetanus toxoid), or harmless antigenic material derived from killed microbes (typhoid vaccine). The process is called *vaccination.*

The exposure of the body to these microbes or their products results in activation of immunological processes which protect the body against the particular bacterium or virus. Typically, two doses are given at a short interval and subsequently booster doses are repeated at regular long intervals to maintain a high level of immunological protection (Fig. 4.7).

Passive immunity can be induced by a direct transfer of antibodies formed in another person or an animal. For example, γ-globulins are transferred from the mother to the fetus across the placenta and in breast milk. Specific antibodies or pooled globulins are sometimes given to produce immediate protection against infections like tetanus or viral hepatitis. However, passive immunization gives protection only for a short period.

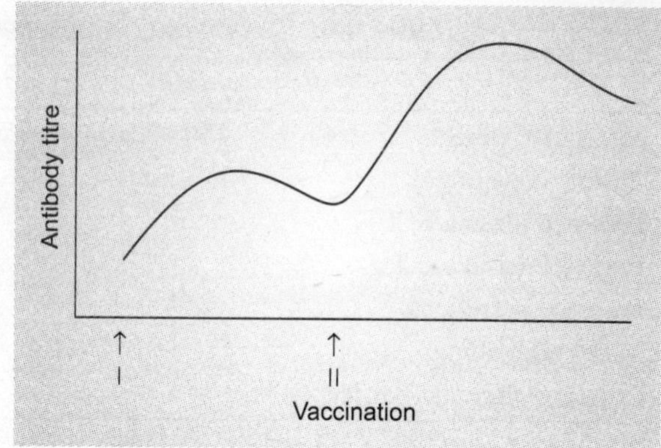

Fig. 4.7: Effect of first and second dose of a vaccine on the antibody titre.

Summary

Types of Immunity
1. Innate (non-specific, weak)
2. Acquired (specific, strong)
   (i) Active (long-lived)
      (a) Natural infections
      (b) Vaccination
   (ii) Passive (short-lived)

Human Leucocyte Antigen (HLA) System

In 1960s, when organ transplantation was introduced, it was realized that each individual is biochemically unique. An organ grafted from genetically similar member of the family is accepted, whereas organ of genetically different person or of different species is rejected. A large number of T lymphocytes can be found at the graft rejection site. Certain glycoproteins (antigens), present on the surface of each nucleated cell, decide the histocompatibility of the graft, i.e. whether the graft is foreign to the host or not. In humans, these antigens were initially discovered in the leucocytes and were therefore called human leucocyte antigens. But actually these antigens are present on the surface of all nucleated cells.

Now, a physiological role of HLA has been discovered. A T lymphocyte can recognize and attack a foreign protein e.g. a virus or a bacterium, only when the latter is associated with HLA molecule. A macrophage (antigen presenting cell, APC) engulfs a bacterium or a virus, processes it by removing some amino acid segments and presents it on the surface of the macrophage enclosed in HLA molecule (Fig. 4.8).

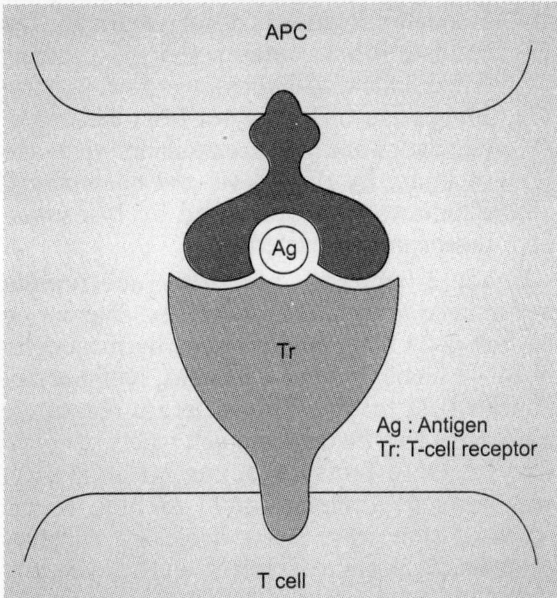

Fig. 4.8: Physiological role of human leucocyte antigen (HLA).

HLA antigens are encoded by a cluster of genes known as major histocompatibility complex (MHC). In humans, the genes of MHC are located on chromosome 6.

Pathophysiology

1. Allergy Normally, an immune response is beneficial to the body, since it eliminates or neutralizes foreign antigens. However, in some individuals, due to a genetic variation, exposure to certain specific antigens produces a harmful response in the form of severe inflammatory reaction and tissue damage. The condition is called allergy. The antigens which produce allergic responses are called allergens. In such individuals, exposure to an allergen produces large amount of antibodies IgE (besides the usual IgG and IgM). IgE gets attached to mast cells and basophils in a particular tissue, e.g. skin, bronchi, etc. When the allergen enters the body again, the antigen-antibody (allergen-IgE) reaction causes rupture of the basophils and mast cells leading to release of a number of chemical substances like histamine, heparin, a protease, a platelet activating factor, an eosinophil chemotactic substance, a neutrophil chemotactic substance, etc. These substances cause dilatation of blood vessels, increased capillary permeability, tissue damage, smooth muscle contraction and attraction of neutrophils and eosinophils to the involved tissues. The result may be (a) **urticaria** when allergen-IgE reaction occurs in the skin; (b) **hay fever** (nasal allergy) when it occurs in the nasal mucosa; or (c) **asthma** (bronchial spasm) when it occurs in the bronchioles of the lungs. (d) **Anaphylaxis** is a particularly dangerous form of allergic reaction to injection of certain drugs like penicillin or even insect stings. Widespread allergen-IgE reaction occurs within blood vessel as well as tissues immediately outside the capillaries. Release of large amount of histamine and other agents named above causes widespread peripheral vasodilatation, increased capillary permeability and loss of plasma proteins from the circulation. Unless treated immediately, the patient dies of circulatory shock. Severe bronchospasm may cause death by suffocation.

2. Autoimmune Diseases The immunological apparatus is geared to detect antigens that are foreign to the body. The immuno-competent cells of the body can recognise the difference between body's own antigens and those of foreign agent and react only against the latter. Frequently, because of various factors like interaction with drugs, genetic mutation, or infection by closely related microbes, the immunological apparatus may fail to differentiate between "self" and "non-self". In other words, the immunological apparatus starts forming antibodies against one's own tissues and destroy them. Such disorders are grouped as autoimmune diseases.

For example, in rheumatic fever, the antibodies act against connective tissue especially in heart and joints. In one type of acute *glomerular nephritis*, the antibodies act against the basement membrane of renal glomeruli. In *myasthenia gravis*, antibodies attack the acetylcholine receptor proteins at the neuromuscular junction.

Following is the list of some of the diseases produced by an autoimmune disorder.

1. Adult hypothyroidism
2. Graves' disease
3. Idiopathic Addison's disease
4. Autoimmune atrophic gastritis (pernicious anaemia).
5. Insulin dependent diabetes mellitus
6. Ulcerative colitis
7. Autoimmune hemolytic anaemia
8. Autoimmune hepatitis
9. Autoimmune thrombocytopenia
10. Myasthenia gravis
11. Membranous glomerulonephritis
12. Rheumatic heart disease
13. Rheumatoid arthritis
14. Systemic lupus erythematosis
15. Scleroderma

3. Acquired Immunodeficiency Syndrome (AIDS) It is a sexually transmitted disease. It is caused by a virus called human immunodeficiency virus (HIV). Infection by this virus causes severe deficiency of helper-T lymphocytes leading to failure of cellular immunity as well as humoral immunity. The immunity is decreased to the extent that even non-pathogenic organisms invade the body. Bacterial infections and cancer are the usual terminal events.

4. Inflammation Inflammation is a complex tissue reaction provoked by cellular injury. It involves reactions in blood vessels, blood cells and tissue cells. The sequence of changes usually leads to healing (repair). The causes of inflammation include:

(a) Infections by bacteria.
(b) Allergic reactions including autoimmune disorders.
(c) Trauma: Mechanical or thermal.

The clinical signs of inflammation include local redness, swelling, heat, pain and loss of function (to a variable degree).

Acute Inflammation It has three major pathophysiologic components:

1. Alterations in vascular calibre that lead to increased blood flow (which causes local redness and rise of local temperature).
2. Structural changes in microvasculature that permit the plasma proteins to leave the circulation (cause of local swelling). The exudate often contains 4–5 g% proteins (albumin and globulins).
3. Emigration of leucocytes from the microcirculation and their accumulation at the site of injury by diapedesis and chemotaxis. Phagocytosis is followed by lysosomal destruction of bacteria.

In acute bacterial infections, neutrophils predominate in the inflammatory exudate during the first 6–24 hours and replaced by monocytes by 24–48 hours. In viral infections, lymphocytes may be first to arrive. In allergic reactions, eosinophils may be the chief cell type.

Systemic effects of acute inflammation (mediated by interleukin-1) include fever, increased slow wave sleep, decreased appetite, increased degradation of proteins and hypotension.

Chronic Inflammatory Process It is characterized by infiltration with macrophages, lymphocytes and plasma cells, extensive tissue destruction and proliferation of fibroblast cells.

When tissue damage is extensive, or when fibrin exudate is abundant, healing is accompanied by formation of collagen fibrous tissue called scar.

Chemical Mediators of Inflammation A large number of chemical mediators originating from the plasma or cells at the site of injury are involved in the genesis of inflammatory response (Table 4.7).

5. Histamine The main sources of histamine in the body are the mast cells, blood basophils and platelets. Histamine is also present in gastric mucosa and in histaminergic neurons of CNS. In all these cells, histamine is produced by decarboxylation of amino acid histidine (Fig. 4.9).

Table 4.7: Chemical mediators of acute inflammation

	Mediator	Source
1. *Cellular*		
(a) *Preformed mediators*	Histamine	Mast cells, basophils and platelets
	Serotonin	Platelets
	Lysosomal enzymes	Neutrophils Macrophages
(b) *Newly synthesized mediators*	Prostaglandins	All leucocytes
	Leucotriens	All leucocytes
	Interleukin-1	Macrophages
2. *Plasma*	Bradykinin	—
	Coagulation/ fibrinolysin factors	—
	Activated complements	—

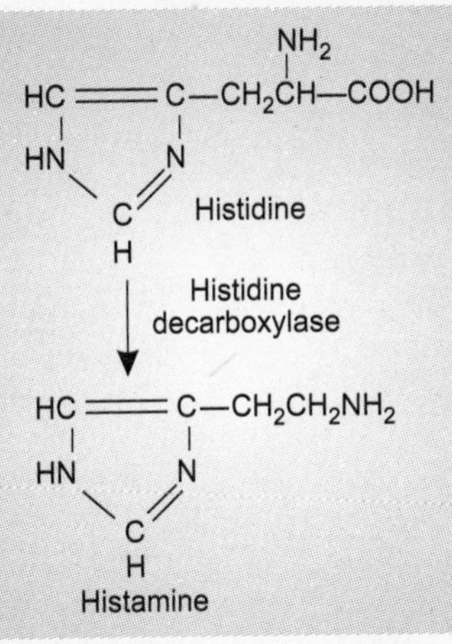

Histidine

Histidine decarboxylase

Histamine

Fig. 4.9: Synthesis of histamine.

Mast cells are widely distributed in the tissues. They are present just adjacent to the blood vessels. A number of stimuli cause rupture of mast cells leading to release of histamine, e.g. physical or thermal injury, allergic (IgE-mediated) reactions, leucotriens and substance P. In humans, histamine causes dilation of arterioles and precapillary sphincters and increased vascular permeability. Severe fall of blood pressure may occur when large amount of histamine is produced, e.g. during anaphylactic shock. Histamine also causes contraction of smooth muscle of bronchioles and intestine. In the stomach, histamine is a powerful stimulant of hydrochloric acid secretion.

Besides the role in gastric secretion, mast cell histamine seems to serve as an immediate mechanism for onset of acute inflammatory response. In pathological conditions, it causes allergic reactions, e.g. urticaria, allergic rhinitis, asthma, or anaphylaxis.

Two types of histamine receptors are known. H_1 receptors mediate most of the vascular and smooth muscle responses. H_2 receptors are involved in gastric secretion. Drugs which block H_1 receptors (e.g. promethazine) are useful in the treatment of allergic disorders. H_2 blockers (e.g. cemetidine) are useful in the treatment of gastric hyperacidity and peptic ulcer.

6. Tissue Transplantation A transplant of a tissue or organ from one part of the body to another part of the body of the same person is called an *autograft*; from one identical twin to another, an *isograft*; from one animal to another animal of same species or from one human being to another, an *allograft;* from a lower animal to a human or from animal of one species to an animal of another species, a *xenograft*.

In autograft, since all the tissues have exactly similar HLA, there is no rejection. For example, in treatment of extensive burns, skin from a healthy area of the patient is grafted on the burnt areas. In isograft also, grafted tissue has virtually similar HLA and hence accepted by the host. On the other hand, because of dissimilarity of HLA, allografts are usually rejected. The T lymphocyte system is responsible for the rejection of the transplanted tissue. Large number of T_C cells can be seen at the site of graft rejection. Therefore, if an organ like kidney is to be transplanted, it is essential to find a donor with maximum HLA similarity. The best success in tissue antigen matching can be expected between close relatives, e.g. siblings or between a parent and child. Since some degree of antigenic dissimilarity always exists in a case of allograft, it is likely to be rejected unless T cell function is suppressed in

4

the recipient. Some of the therapeutic agents for this purpose (immunosuppression) are as follows:

(a) Glucocorticoids: inhibit the growth of all lymphoid tissues.
(b) Drugs like azathioprine: have toxic effects on lymphoid tissue.
(c) Antilymphoid globulin.
(d) Cyclosporine: It has a specific inhibitory effect on the proliferation of T cells. It has proved most valuable because it does not suppress other aspects of immune system.

Immuno-suppressed individuals are liable to suffer from massive bacterial or viral infections. In addition, the incidence of cancer is several times greater in such individuals. Skin, kidney, cornea, heart, liver, glandular tissue and bone marrow can be transplanted. Of these, transplantation of skin, cornea and kidney have been most successful.

CHAPTER 5

The Plasma Proteins and Haemostasis

PLASMA PROTEINS

The total plasma protein concentration of blood is approximately 7.5 g% (range 6.4–8.3 g%). More than 100 types of plasma proteins have been identified by different techniques. Original classification of plasma proteins was based on their precipitation by salts. On this basis, plasma proteins are classified as albumin (4.8 g%), globulins (2.3 g%), and fibrinogen (0.3 g%). By electrophoresis techniques (Fig. 5.1), globulins can be further separated into a number of fractions namely α-1, α-2, ß, and γ globulins. The relative shapes and molecular weights of the plasma proteins are given in Fig. 5.2.

Functions

Plasma proteins have such a large number of functions that they cannot be discussed in detail at one place. Some of the important functions are briefly described below.

1. Osmotic Pressure The capillary walls are impermeable to plasma proteins. Consequently, the proteins exert an oncotic pressure of about 25 mmHg across the capillary wall. This constitutes one of the Starling forces responsible for the regulation of filtration and reabsorption of tissue fluids in the capillaries.

Osmotic pressure is determined by the number of solute particles in the solution. Therefore, albumin makes more important contribution to the oncotic pressure than the globulins because: (i) The total concentration of albumin in the plasma is almost twice that of globulins, (ii) Due to smaller molecular weight, albumin contains greater number of particles than globulins per gram weight.

2. Buffer Action Plasma proteins contain –COOH and $–NH_2$ radicals which act as weak acids and bases respectively. Therefore, plasma proteins act as buffers and prevent marked variation in plasma pH. On the whole, plasma proteins contribute about 15% of the total buffering capacity of the blood.

3. Viscosity of Blood Viscosity of blood is an important factor in the maintenance of vascular peripheral resistance and hence the blood pressure. Plasma proteins and blood cells contribute about 50% each to the total viscosity of blood.

4. Coagulation Plasma contains a large number of proteins called clotting factors, which are involved in the clotting mechanism of the blood.

5. Fibrinolytic System Plasminogen, plasminogen activator and inhibitor are the plasma proteins concerned with slow dissolution of the clot after the injured wall of the blood vessel has been repaired.

5

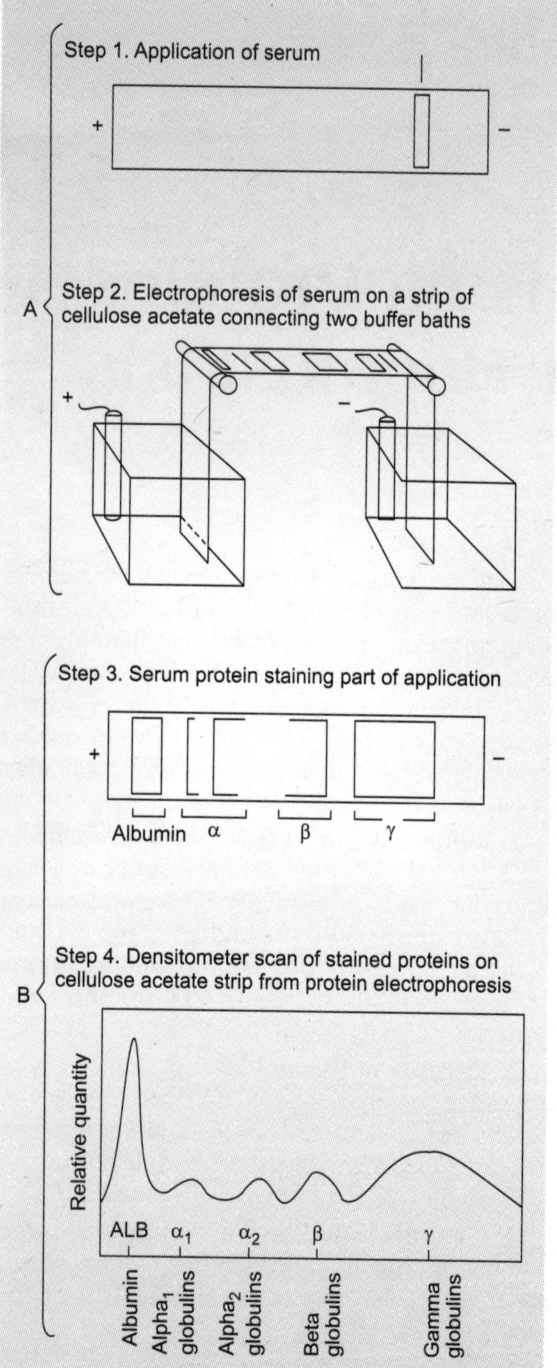

Fig. 5.1: An electrophoresis specimen application and chamber (A). This type of equipment is used to separate proteins for identification and quantification. The serum protein electrophoresis pattern is presented here (B).

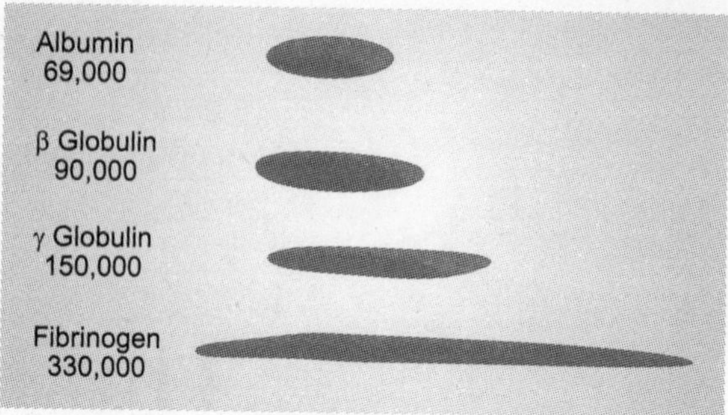

Fig. 5.2: Molecular weights and shapes of different types of plasma proteins.

6. Defence Mechanisms (Immunity) Immunoglobulins and complement system are the plasma proteins concerned with the body defence mechanisms.

7. Carrier Proteins Many plasma proteins act as carriers of metals, hormones, lipids and even drugs. The binding of hormones, metals and drugs with the plasma protein limits their free diffusion into the ECF, and hence limits their biological activity. The protein bound substances serve as a reservoir from which small amounts of these substances are gradually released. The protein binding also prevents their quick excretion in the urine.

The transport of water-insoluble lipids in blood would be a serious problem. In combination with plasma proteins, which are amphiphilic, the lipid protein complex can be transported in the aqueous medium of the plasma. The names and the functions of some of the important plasma proteins are discussed in greater detail below and summarized in Table 5.1.

1. Albumin This is the major constituent of plasma proteins (3–5 g/dl). Human albumin has molecular weight of 69,000. Albumin is exclusively synthesized in the liver. About 12 g of albumin is produced per day, which represents approximately 25% of total hepatic protein synthesis. The important functions of albumin include:

(i) Major contribution to oncotic pressure of plasma.

(ii) Major contribution to buffering action of plasma.

(iii) Nutritive function: In nutritional deprivation, plasma albumin is catabolised to

Table 5.1: Names and functions of some of the plasma proteins

Protein	*Mol. wt.*	*Major functions*
Albumin	69,000	Osmotic effect, buffering, nutritive and transport (free fatty acids, bilirubin, steroid hormones, calcium, copper, many drugs).
Pre-albumin	61,000	Transport of thyroxine, vitamin A.
Alpha-1-globulins		
α_1 antitrypsin	54,000	Inhibition of trypsin.
α_1 lipoprotein	–	Transport of cholesterol, phospholipids
Retinol binding protein	21,000	Transport of vitamin A.
Thyroxine binding globulin	58,000	Transport of thyroid hormones
Transcortin	52,000	Transport of adrenal glucocorticoids
Alpha-2 globulins		
Haptoglobin	90,000	Binds with plasma free haemoglobin and prevents its renal excretion.
Prothrombin	68,000	Participates in blood coagulation.
Ceruloplasmin	150,000	Binds with copper, oxidation of Fe^{++} to Fe^{+++}
Beta globulins		
β lipoprotein	–	Transport of triglycerides and cholesterol
Transferrin	76,000	Transport of iron
Plasminogen	140,000	Forms plasmin: involved in fibrinolysis
Gamma globulins	–	Function as antibodies
Fibrinogen	340,000	Participates in coagulation

help in the synthesis of more important tissue proteins.

(iv) Transport of a large number of substances (Table 5.1).

2. Alpha-Antitrypsin (α-antiproteinase) It is a glycoprotein. It is the major constituent of α-1 globulin. Its plasma concentration is 200 mg/dl. It inhibits the activity of proteolytic enzymes such as trypsin, elastase, etc. During inflammatory response to a bacterial infection, degranulation in an activated leucocyte releases proteolytic enzymes into the phagosomes. Some of these proteolytic enzymes leak into the extracellular spaces where they are likely to produce tissue destruction. Normally, the leaked extracellular enzymes are destroyed by α-antitrypsin present in the plasma and body fluids. Deficiency of α-antitrypsin may be a congenital defect. A more common cause is cigarette smoke, which predisposes the individual to emphysema.

3. Alpha-2 Macroglobulin It is a high molecular weight (800,000) plasma protein. It is the major constituent of α-2 globulin fraction of plasma proteins. It has antiprotease activity and serves as an important natural anticoagulant in the plasma.

4. Ceruloplasmin It is a copper-containing α-2 globulin (mol.wt 150,000). About 90 % of plasma copper is bound to ceruloplasmin. This binding is tight and its copper is not available to the tissues. About 10% of plasma copper, transported loosely bound to albumin, is available for tissue metabolism. Thus, the important function of plasma ceruloplasmin is not as a transport carrier for copper but to act as ferroxidase, i.e. it converts ferrous iron absorbed from the intestinal epithelial cells into blood to ferric state for combination with plasma protein transferrin.

5. Haptoglobin It is a component of α-2-globulin fraction. Its function is to bind any free haemoglobin present in the plasma as a result of intravascular haemolysis, and prevent its urinary excretion. Hb-haptoglobin complex is rapidly removed from the blood by mononuclear macrophage system.

6. Transferrin It is a glycoprotein, a component of ß–globulin fraction of plasma proteins. It is a transporter of iron in blood circulation.

7. Fibrinogen It shall be discussed later in this Chapter

8. Immunoglobulins They have been discussed in Chapter 4.

ORIGIN AND CATABOLISM OF PLASMA PROTEINS

Immunoglobulins, present in the γ-globulin fraction of the plasma proteins, are manufactured by B lymphocytes-plasma cells. Albumin and most of the other plasma proteins including fibrinogen are manufactured in the liver. The factors regulating the rate of synthesis of plasma proteins in the liver are poorly understood.

Different plasma proteins are degraded at different rates. Intravascular half-life of albumin and IgG is approximately 20 days as compared to 4 days of fibrinogen and haptoglobin, and only few hours of factor VII and factor VIII clotting proteins.

Hypoproteinemia may result from severe malnutrition, or chronic liver disease (leading to decreased protein synthesis) or nephrosis (leading to increased urinary protein loss). The consequent decrease in plasma protein oncotic pressure commonly produces oedema. Congenital absence of certain plasma proteins (agammaglobulinemia or afibrinogenaemia) is rare.

THE PLATELETS (THROMBOCYTES)

The platelets are small, (2–4 μm), non-nucleated, colourless, spherical or oval cells. In blood smears stained with Leishman's stain, a platelet shows faint bluish cytoplasm containing reddish purple granules. Electron microscopy reveals Golgi apparatus, endoplasmic reticulum, a few mitochondria, microtubules, microvesicles, and granules in the cytoplasm (Fig. 5.3).

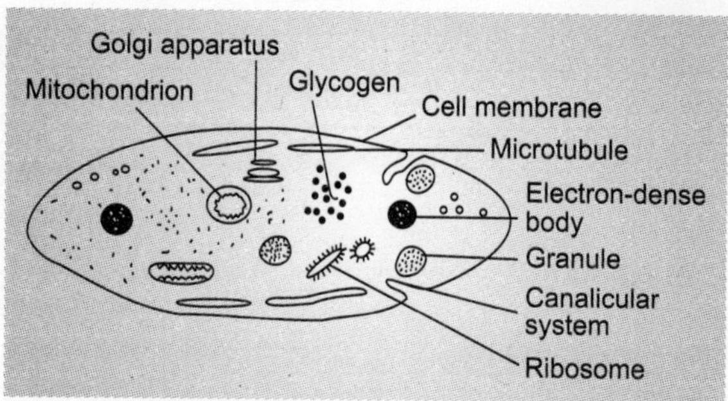

Fig. 5.3: Ultrastructure of a platelet.

Chemically, platelets have been shown to contain numerous oxidative enzymes, contractile proteins, (the actin and the myosin), ATP, ADP, histamine, 5-hydroxy tryptamine (5-HT) and prostaglandin synthesizing system. Clot promoting phospholipids are found in the granules and in the cell membrane. Platelets also contain fibrin-stabilizing factor (factor XIII), von Willebrand factor (vWF) and platelet-derived growth factor.

The normal platelet count ranges from 150,000 to 440,000/mm^3.

FUNCTIONS

1. Primary Haemostasis Platelets perform a crucial role in the arrest of bleeding (haemostasis) after injury to a blood vessel. At the site of injury, the platelets are exposed to sub-endothelial extracellular matrix, particularly collagen fibres. This initiates the haemostatic reaction in which the platelets undergo the following three important changes:

(a) **Adhesion and Shape-Change** The platelets assume an irregular star shape (Fig. 5.4) and adhere tightly to collagen. vWF is necessary for such adhesions by serving as a molecular bridge between the two.

(b) **Secretion** The release of the contents of platelet granules occurs next. Platelets contain two types of granules. *Alpha granules* contain fibrinogen and platelet derived growth factors (PDGF). The other types of granules are *electron dense bodies* which contain ADP, ATP, ionized calcium, histamine, serotonin and epinephrine. ADP is a potent mediator of platelet aggregation.

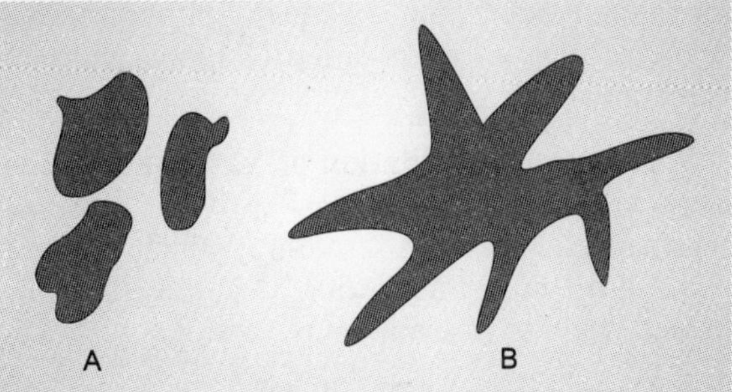

Fig. 5.4: (A) Normal circulating disc-shaped platelets. (B) An activated platelet.

Ca^{++} helps in coagulation. The release of the granule contents activates a phospholipid complex on the platelet surface. This complex is an important component of the intrinsic pathway of blood clotting. In addition, thromboxane A2 is synthesized by the activated platelets.

(c) **Platelet Aggregation** It closely follows platelet adhesion and secretion. It is induced by ADP and thromboxane A2. As a result, a ball of aggregated platelets called *platelet plug* is formed, which can plug small leaks in the endothelial lining. Release of serotonin from the platelets produces local vasoconstriction. The platelet plug formation occurs within minutes of injury and constitutes primary haemostasis. The clotting of blood constitutes secondary haemostasis.

2. Blood Clotting If the vascular injury is severe, platelet plug formation is not able to control the leakage of blood out of the vessels. In that case, a number of plasma factors come into action and cause clotting of the shed blood. The blood clot forms a more efficient and durable bung at the injured site. The platelets play an important role in this process by releasing a phospholipid called platelet factor-3. Platelets are also responsible for retraction of the clot.

3. Phagocytosis Certain viruses and antigen-antibody complexes are phagocytosed by platelets.

4. Storage and Transport Platelets contain stores of 5-HT and histamine, which are released by disintegration of the platelets. 5-HT is synthesized by the argentaffin cells of the gastrointestinal mucosa and released into blood circulation. The chemical is taken up by platelets and stored.

Thrombopoiesis

The platelets are produced in the bone marrow. The stem cells committed to form platelets differentiate into *megakaryoblasts*. A megakaryoblast is a moderately large cell (15–20 μm) with an irregularly oval nucleus, and a small amount of deeply basophilic cytoplasm. It matures into a **megakaryocyte**. A megakaryocyte is a large (35–160 μm) cell containing multilobulated nucleus and plenty of cytoplasm containing reddish purple granules. The megakaryocyte extends cytoplasmic pseudopodia through the endothelial lining of sinusoids of the bone marrow. The pseudopods fragment and circulate in the blood as platelets.

The lifespan of platelets is about 8–12 days. They are destroyed mainly in the spleen.

The humoral agents called *thrombopoietin* and *megakaryocytic-colony stimulating activity* (Meg CSA) seems to regulate the thrombopoiesis. The factors stimulating the synthesis and release of these agents are not yet known.

Thrombocytopenia or deficiency of platelets in the blood is a common accompaniment of agranulocytosis and aplastic anaemia. Deficiency of all the formed elements of blood may occur due to bone marrow depression by allergic reactions, irradiations or intake of certain drugs like chloramphenicol and anticancer drugs. Thrombocytopenia can occur independently also. Whatever the cause, low platelet count results in purpura (thrombocytopenic purpura).

HAEMOSTASIS AND BLOOD COAGULATION

When a blood vessel is injured, a number of mechanisms operate to minimize and ultimately arrest bleeding. Haemostatic mechanisms are successful in controlling the bleeding from small vessels like arterioles, capillaries and veins. Venous bleeding is especially less dangerous because of lower venous pressure and collapsible vessel wall. In contrast, bleeding from large arteries requires immediate surgical intervention or at least tourniquet, otherwise it can be fatal. Haemostatic events may be summarised as the following five overlapping steps:

1. Initial constriction of injured blood vessel.
2. Formation of a platelet plug.
3. Humoral facilitation of vasoconstriction.
4. Coagulation of blood.
5. Ultimate fibrous tissue growth into the blood clot permanently sealing the breach in the vessel wall. The clot is finally removed by proteolytic enzymes (fibrinolysis).

1. Initial Constriction of the Injured Blood Vessel The immediate response of a bleeding vessel is constriction of the vessel wall, over several centimeters in both the directions from the site of injury. The degree of spasm is proportionate to the degree of trauma to the blood vessel. The vasoconstriction may be intense enough to stop the bleeding from small vessels. The vasoconstriction is caused by a direct effect of injury on the vascular smooth muscle. The initial vasoconstriction is transient but is maintained for several minutes or even hours by humoral facilitation (Step 3).

2. Formation of Platelet Plug When the platelets come in contact with the damaged endothelial lining of the blood vessel and particularly with the collagen fibres exposed in the blood vessel wall, a series of changes occur in the platelets. The platelets begin to swell up and assume an irregular shape. A number of processes protrude from their surface and become very sticky. Consequently, the platelets stick to the collagen fibres and secrete large quantities of ADP and a prostaglandin, **thromboxane-A**, which activates other platelets in the blood, making them sticky as well. The activated sticky platelets tend to aggregate and form a platelet plug which may close the opening in the vascular wall. In day to day life, numerous small leaks tend to occur in the capillaries but are immediately dealt with by the platelet plugs. Because the platelet plug is basically soft, it is not able to stop bleeding from a large leak in the blood vessels. In that case also, activated platelets play an equally important role in the process of coagulation of blood and clot retraction.

3. Humoral Facilitation of Vasoconstriction Activated platelets release powerful vasoconstrictors, including serotonin, which produce secondary vasoconstriction that may last for several minutes or even hours.

4. Coagulation of Blood This is the most important step in the process of haemostasis. This is shown by the fact that any congenital or acquired defect in the mechanism of coagulation always results in severe bleeding even after minor injuries. However, the role of the first three steps should not be under-estimated. They not only help in minimizing the blood loss but also facilitate the clotting process. In this process, a soluble plasma protein fibrinogen is converted into a gel-like insoluble protein fibrin. Fibrin is laid down as highly adhesive long threads in the form of a network. These fibrin threads not only stick to one another but also to the adjacent vascular wall forming an efficient plug in the vascular opening. Erythrocytes, leucocytes and platelets are also entrapped in the fibrin threads. Within minutes, the clot contracts, making the clot a very firm bung which stops bleeding from the injured vessel permanently (Fig. 5.5).

The phenomenon of blood clotting including clot contraction (or retraction in vitro) can be best observed by pouring 10 ml of blood in a glass tube and observing it for next 35–45 minutes in a water bath at 37°C. Within 5–10 minutes, the fluid blood solidifies by the process of clotting. About 30 minutes later, the clot retracts to one side of the tube leaving light yellowish *serum* on the top (Fig. 3.2). [Plasma is obtained when blood mixed with an anticoagulant is centrifuged.]

MECHANISM OF COAGULATION

A large number of substances, mostly proteins, are present in the blood and tissue fluids which are involved in the process of coagulation. These substances have been called clotting factors and are given Roman numerals (Table 5.2).

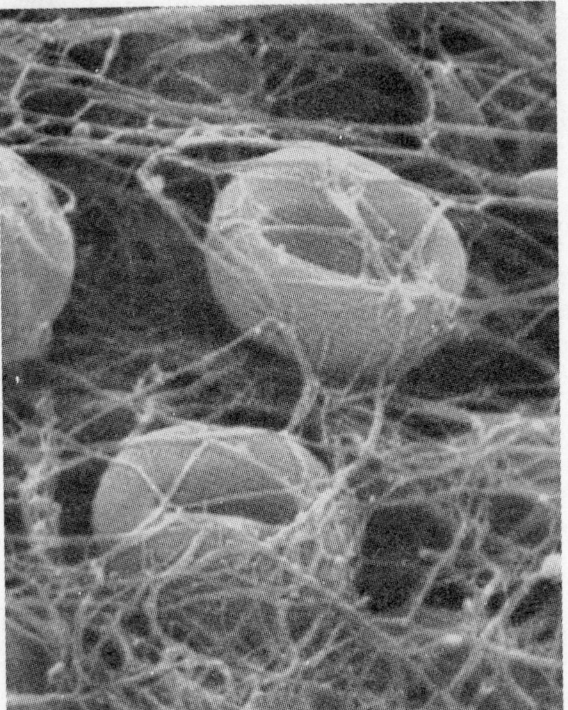

Fig. 5.5: Magnified view of fibrin threads in a blood clot.

Table 5.2: List of clotting factors and their synonyms

Clotting factor	*Synonym*
I	Fibrinogen
II	Prothrombin
III	Tissue thromboplastin
IV	Calcium
V	Labile factor
VII	Stable factor
VIII	Antihaemophilic factor-A (antihaemophilic globulin, AHF)
IX	Christmas factor (antihaemophilic factor B)
X	Stuart-Power factor
XI	Plasma thromboplastin antecendent (PTA) (antihaemophilic factor C)
XII	Hageman factor
XIII	Fibrin stabilizing factor

Basically, the mechanism of clotting involves three essential steps:

1. Generation of *prothrombin activator*: initiated by vascular injury.
2. Prothrombin activator converts the plasma protein prothrombin to a proteolytic enzyme, *thrombin.*
3. Thrombin converts soluble protein fibrinogen into thread-like and sticky *insoluble protein called fibrin.* Fibrin is laid as a meshwork which entangles the red cells, the white cells and platelets, and forms a solid mass (Fig. 5.5).

STEP 1: Generation of Prothrombin Activator

In spite of the presence of all the clotting factors in the blood, the blood does not clot spontaneously, unless a vessel wall has been injured. This is due to the fact that normally all the factors are present in an inactive form and therefore, prothrombin activator is absent from the blood. Moreover, the blood contains small amounts of naturally occurring anticoagulants. In short, *clotting occurs only when the blood contains prothrombin activator*.

Prothrombin activator is formed by a cascade of reactions in which activation of one factor leads to activation of the next clotting factor. This sequence of changes can occur in two pathways, the *extrinsic pathway, and the intrinsic pathway*, each ultimately leading to the generation of prothrombin activator. Both pathways are activated when a blood vessel is injured and bleeding has occurred. The reactions of extrinsic system are initiated by a factor called tissue-thromboplastin *released by the injured tissues around the vessel wall.* The intrinsic system is initiated by activation of factor XII, *present in the plasma itself*, by the vascular injury.

The Extrinsic Pathway

In the extrinsic pathway (Fig. 5.6), the injured tissue releases several substances which are together known as *tissue thromboplastin* (or tissue factor or factor III). They include phospholipids from the cell membrane and a glycoprotein. The tissue factor combines with factor VII. Next, tissue factor—factor VII complex, in the presence of Ca^{2+} activates factor X to factor X_a. The steps subsequent to the activation of factor X are common to extrinsic and intrinsic pathways.

The Intrinsic Pathway (Fig. 5.6)

Exposure of blood to the collagen fibres underlying the vascular endothelium (or electronegatively charged wettable surface such as glass, in vitro) activates plasma factor XII and initiates the intrinsic pathway of blood clotting, as well as, activates the platelets. Activated factor XII [XII_a] activates factor XI to XI_a. Factor XI_a in turn activates factor IX to IX_a.

Activation of Factor X

Factor IX_a, in the presence of factor VIII_a, platelet-phospholipids released by activated platelets, and ionic calcium, convert factor X to X_a.

As mentioned above, factor X is activated by tissue factor—factor VII complex in the extrinsic pathway, as well as by factor IX_a along with factor VIII_a and platelet phospholipids in the intrinsic pathway. Serious bleeding occurs in patients who lack factor VIII (haemophilia A) or factor IX (haemophilia-B, Christmas disease) (involving intrinsic pathway) only or in those who lack factor VII only (involved in extrinsic pathway). This shows that activation of factor X by both the pathways is essential for normal clotting.

Formation of Prothrombin Activator

In the presence of platelet phospholipid, Ca^{2+} and factor V_a, *factor X_a acts as prothrombin activator,* i.e. it catalyses the conversion of prothrombin to thrombin.

STEP 2: Formation of Thrombin

Prothrombin is a plasma protein (α-2 globulin) with a molecular weight of 72,000. Its normal

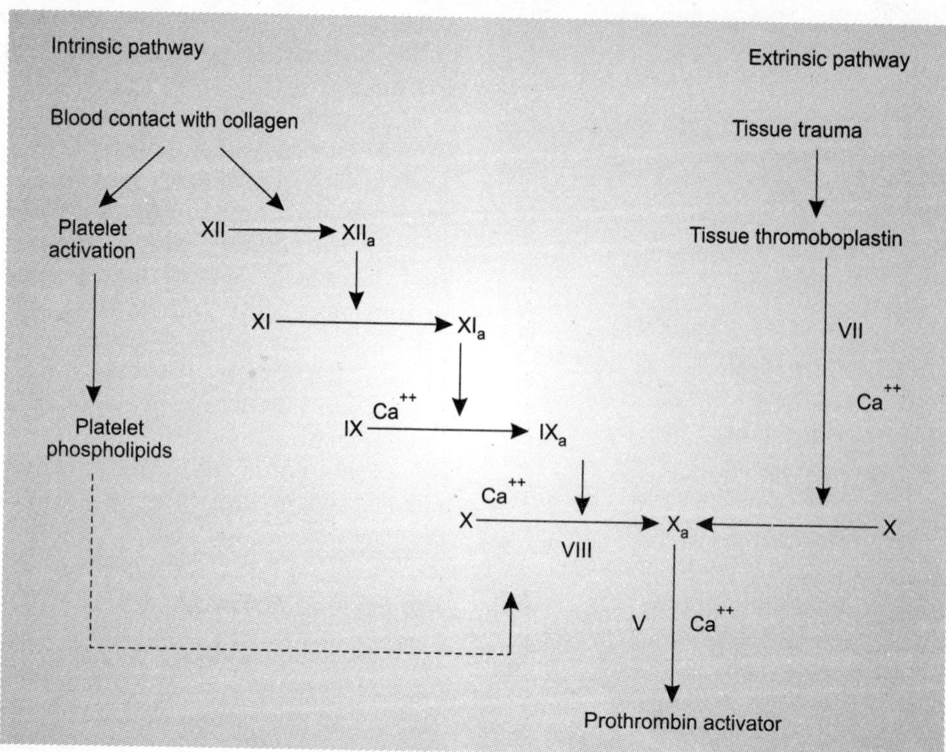

Fig. 5.6: The extrinsic and intrinsic pathways of coagulation leading to generation of prothrombin activator.

plasma concentration is about 15 mg%. It is synthesized in the liver in the presence of vitamin K. (Hepatic synthesis of factor VII, IX and X is also dependent on the presence of vitamin K). The prothrombin activator acts as a proteolytic enzyme, and splits prothrombin into a number of smaller compounds, one of which is thrombin with a molecular weight 33,700. Ca^{2+} is essential for this step.

$$\text{Prothrombin} \xrightarrow[\text{Ca}^{++}]{\text{Prothrombin activator}} \text{Thrombin}$$

STEP 3: Formation of Fibrin Threads

$$\text{Fibrinogen} \xrightarrow[\text{Monomer}]{\text{Thrombin}} \text{Fibrin} \xrightarrow[\text{Polymerization}]{\text{Factor XIII a, Ca}^{2}} \text{Fibrin threads}$$

Fibrinogen is a plasma protein with a molecular weight of 3,40,000. Its normal plasma concentration is about 0.3 g%. Fibrinogen is synthesized in the liver.

Thrombin, acting as a proteolytic enzyme removes four low molecular weight peptides from each molecule of fibrinogen to form a fibrin monomer. Fibrin monomers tend to polymerise spontaneously. But the process is catalysed by another plasma factor called fibrin stabilizing factor (activated factor XIII). Thrombin activates factor XIII also. In the presence of Ca^{2+}, factor XIIIa causes formation of covalent cross-linkages between fibrin threads. Thus, a dense meshwork of fibrin threads is formed, which traps the remaining components of plasma as well as the blood cells to form a solid mass called the blood clot. The blood clot becomes adherent to the injured vascular walls, plugging it permanently.

CLOT RETRACTION (CONTRACTION)

Within a few minutes of its formation, the clot begins to contract and expel most of its fluid content, known as serum. Within the next 30–60 minutes, the clot becomes one-third of its original size. Platelets are essential for clot contraction (retraction). They adhere to the fibrin threads and send out pseudopodia. The pseudopodia then contract, pulling the fibrin threads closer to each other and squeezing out the serum. The contraction of pseudopodia is produced by the contractile proteins actin and myosin present in the platelets. In patients with thrombocytopenia, the clotting mechanism is normal but clot retraction is very poor. Clot retraction is an in vitro phenomenon. Clot contraction occurs in vivo.

Importance of Ca^{2+} In Clotting

Except for the first two steps in the intrinsic pathway, Ca^{2+} acts as a cofactor in all the steps of coagulation. Therefore, coagulation of blood can be prevented in vitro (e.g. for storage in the blood bank or for separation of plasma) by removal of Ca^{2+}. The use of oxalates or citrates as in vitro anticoagulants is based on this principle. In vivo, the degree of hypocalcaemia (e.g. due to deficiency of vitamin D or hypoparathyroidism) compatible with life does not cause bleeding disorders.

von Willebrand Factor (vWF). It is a high molecular weight glycoprotein present in the plasma and in platelets. It is synthesized by the endothelial cells (sources of plasma vWF) and megakaryocytes (source of platelet vWF). In the plasma, vWF serves as a carrier protein for the transport of clotting factor VIII. Hence, it is essential for the normal clotting process. It is also essential for primary hemostasis since it helps the adhesion of platelets to injured endothelial cells.

NATURAL ANTICLOTTING MECHANISMS

Normally, the flowing blood does not clot in the blood vessels. Even after injury to a blood vessel, the clot is limited to the area of bleeding and does not extend inside the vessel. Obviously, some mechanisms operate in the circulation which prevent intravascular clotting. Some of the known anticlotting mechanisms are as follows:

1. *Smoothness of normal intact endothelial linings* is one of the most important factors. The intrinsic or extrinsic clotting pathways cannot be initiated as long as the endothelium is not injured.
2. *Heparin* is a powerful anticoagulant but its concentration in the normal circulation is so low that its independent physiological

role is doubtful. However, the circulating heparin may supplement the activity of antithrombin-III.

3. *Antithrombin-III* is probably the most important anticoagulant in the normal circulation. It is an α-globulin. It inhibits thrombin, factor X_a and IX_a. Its activity is markedly enhanced by combination with heparin.
4. Protein C is another natural anticoagulant present in the plasma. As such, it is inactive. It is activated by exposure to thrombin formed during clotting. Thrombin interacts with an endothelial modulator to activate protein C. Activated protein C inhibits factors V_a and VII_a.
5. Some of the activated intermediates of the process of coagulation enter the circulation but are quickly removed by the macrophages in the liver and elsewhere.
6. The fast velocity of blood flow in larger blood vessels in itself prevents coagulation. Slowing of blood flow is one of the important contributory factors in genesis of intravascular blood clotting (thrombosis).

FIBRINOLYTIC SYSTEM

Following a vascular injury and clot formation, the discontinuity of the vessel wall is gradually repaired by proliferation of adjacent fibroblasts, smooth muscle cells and endothelial cells. The clot, no more required, is gradually dissolved by degradation of fibrin into small soluble fragments called fibrin-degradation products (FDPs). The phenomenon, called *fibrinolysis*, is a normal secondary response in haemostasis. The dissolution of clot occurs by the action of a proteolytic enzyme, plasmin, activated in the clot. Normal plasma contains a protein plasminogen (mol.wt 92,000) synthesized in the liver. Cleavage of a single peptide bond converts plasminogen into an active proteolytic enzyme called plasmin. The cleavage of plasminogen into plasmin can occur under the effect of (i) thrombin, or (ii) plasminogen activator. When a clot is formed, plasminogen is also incorporated in it. Thrombin formed during the process of clotting slowly begins to convert plasminogen into plasmin. Moreover, the deposition of fibrin within the vessel wall gives rise to stimuli which trigger the release of plasminogen activator from the endothelial cells (Fig. 5.7). Plasmin system plays a role not only in (i) dissolution of a blood clot but also in (ii) tissue remodeling in inflammation, (iii) ovulation and (iv) mechanisms by which tumour cells invade a tissue.

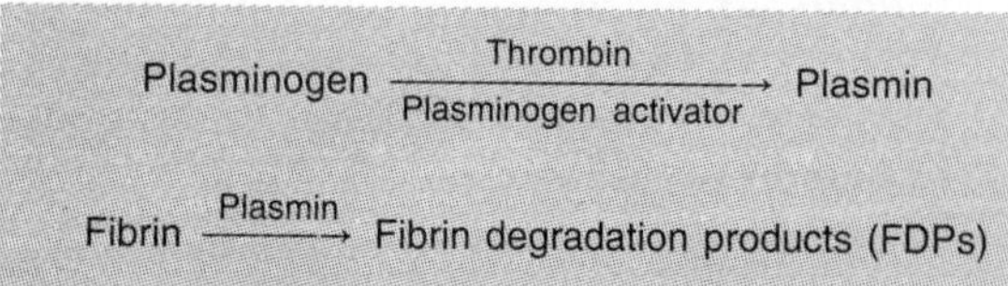

Fig. 5.7: The fibrinolytic system.

PATHOPHYSIOLOGY OF HAEMOSTASIS

Bleeding Disorders

1. Haemophilia Haemophilia is a congenital bleeding disorder. A relatively minor trauma like falling on the knees, or tooth extraction is sufficient to start prolonged bleeding, which may last for days or even weeks (Fig. 5.8). Most commonly, there is congenital deficiency of factor VIII. The condition is called (haemophilia-A or classical haemophilia). In a few cases, factor IX is deficient (haemophilia B or Christmas disease). The disorder is transmitted as X-chromosome linked recessive trait. That is why; it occurs almost exclusively in the males. Females act as carriers and transmit the disease to 50% of their male offspring, and transmit the carrier state to 50% of the female offspring. The only effective therapy is intravenous injection of the deficient clotting factor. On investigation, the clotting time is found to be prolonged but the bleeding time is normal.

2. Acquired Clotting Disorders The synthesis of prothrombin and clotting factors VII, IX and X in the liver is vitamin K dependent. Severe liver disease or deficiency of vitamin K may cause deficiency of these clotting factors leading to severe and prolonged bleeding after a minor trauma. Deficiency of fat soluble vitamin K is typically caused by intestinal malabsorption

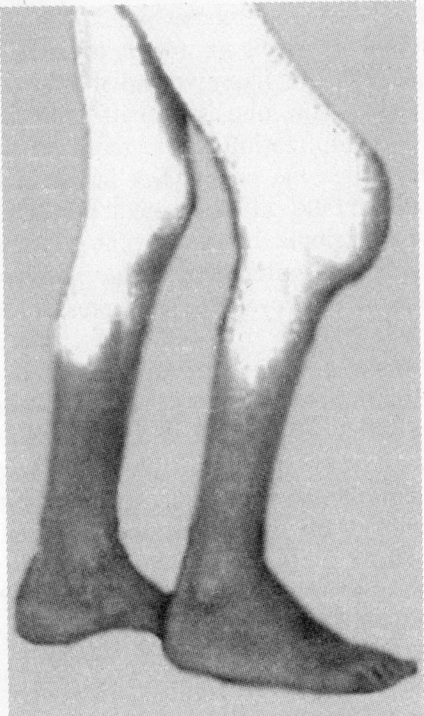

Fig. 5.8: A patient of haemophilia.

disorders. It is characterized by prolonged clotting time and normal bleeding time.

3. von Willebrand Disease It is a fairly common bleeding disorder. It is caused by a congenital deficiency of von Willebrand factor. It is characterized by long history of easy bruisability, and bleeding from mucous membranes. It is often detected when bleeding does not stop after a surgical procedure like tooth extraction or tonsillectomy. On investigation, characteristic features include prolonged bleeding time, normal platelet count and deficiency of factor VIII in the plasma.

4. Purpura This bleeding disorder is characterised by easy *bruisability* and spontaneous multiple haemorrhages under the skin and mucous membranes. At an early stage, the patient may present with numerous red spots of the size of pinhead on the skin and mucous membranes (*petechial haemorrhages*). Purpura is most commonly due to thrombocytopenia (Fig. 5.9). The platelet count in the blood is usually less than 50,000/mm^3.

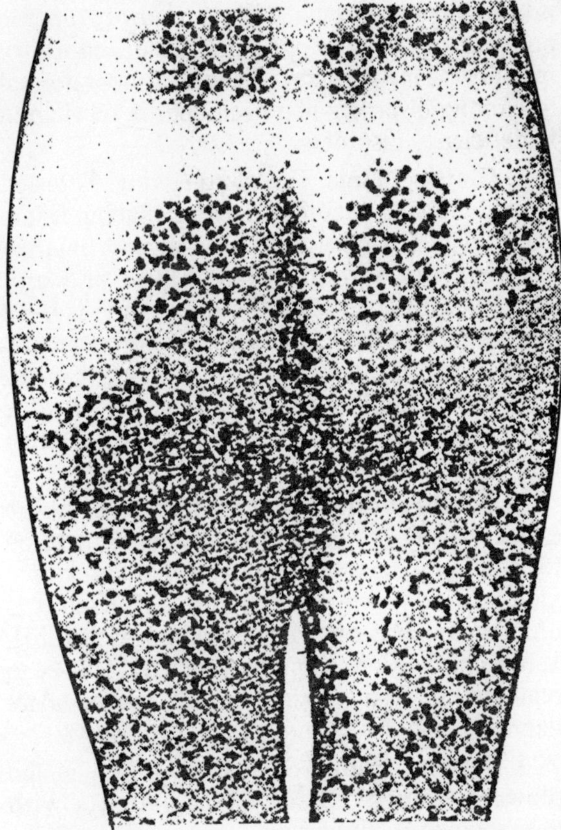

Fig. 5.9: A patient with thrombocytopaenic purpura.

In senile purpura, or purpura due to deficiency of vitamin C, the platelet count is normal. The spontaneous bleeding is due to increased capillary fragility.

LABORATORY INVESTIGATIONS IN BLEEDING DISORDERS

A battery of tests is usually required to diagnose the exact cause of a bleeding disorder. The principle of some of these tests is described below.

1. The Bleeding Time The bleeding time is determined by measuring the time required for bleeding to stop from an incised small subcutaneous vessel, e.g. in the ear lobe, or fingertip. Normally, the bleeding ceases in 2–6 minutes. The bleeding time investigates the early stages of haemostasis, e.g. vasoconstriction and platelet plug formation. Therefore, the bleeding time is prolonged in patients with thrombocytopenic purpura or in those with increased capillary fragility (senile purpura). Bleeding time is normal in clotting disorders like haemophilia or vitamin K deficiency disorders.

5

2. Clotting Time The clotting time is tested by withdrawing venous blood and placing it in a small glass test-tube at 37°C. The time interval between the withdrawal of blood and clot formation is noted. Normal clotting time is 6–12 minutes. It is prolonged in patients with congenital or acquired disorders of coagulation, e.g. haemophilia-A, haemophilia-B or bleeding disorders due to deficiency of vitamin K. In purpura, clotting time is normal.

3. Prothrombin Time In this test, tissue extract is added to the plasma and the time taken for clotting reflects the adequacy of other *clotting factors* involved in the *extrinsic pathway*. It is prolonged in patients with deficiency of factor II, V, VII and X. More commonly, this test is used to regulate the dose schedule of oral anticoagulant like dicoumarol.

4. Platelet Count Severe reduction in the platelet count is observed in patients with thrombocytopenic purpura.

5. Tourniquet Test Blood pressure cuff is tied on the arm and inflated to a pressure midway between systolic and diastolic pressures for 5 minutes. The forearm is observed for evidence of petechial spots. The test is positive in patients with purpura due to thrombocytopenia or increased capillary fragility.

6. Deficiency of Specific Clotting Factor, e.g. Factor VIII, or IX or VII, etc. It can be detected precisely by using *thromboplastin generation test*. Such investigations are important for appropriate therapy in cases of haemophilia.

Thrombosis

Physiologically, clotting of blood occurs only extravascularly, after a vessel has been injured and bleeding has occurred. Pathologically, clotting may occur within an intact blood vessel. The process of intravascular clotting is known as *thrombosis*, and the blood clot so formed is known as a *thrombus*. Thrombosis within the coronary or cerebral arteries is a common cause of serious medical problems like myocardial infarction and hemiplegia. Thrombosis in calf-veins is more often a complication after major surgery or delivery when the patient lies in the bed for a few days and the calf veins are compressed. Two factors contribute to the thrombus formation: (i) Roughened endothelial surface of a vessel, e.g. due to atherosclerosis, or pressure on the veins; (ii) Slowing of blood flow.

A thrombus, once formed, has a tendency to extend and block the blood vessel. In addition, the thrombus may get detached from its original site, circulate as small fragments called *emboli* and block a blood vessel at a distant site. For example, pulmonary artery may be blocked by an embolus arising from a calf-vein (pulmonary embolism). A cerebral artery may be blocked by an embolus arising from a carotid artery (cerebral embolism).

Extension of a thrombus can be prevented by administration of anticoagulants like heparin and dicoumarol. But these agents cannot dissolve a clot once formed. In early stages of coronary thrombosis, the clot can be removed surgically (coronary angioplasty) or medically by intravenous administration of a fibrinolytic enzyme of bacterial origin, called *streptokinase*. The therapy is ineffective against an old thrombus.

ANTICOAGULANTS

Anticoagulants are the agents that can be used to delay or prevent coagulation of blood. They can be classified into: (1) in vitro and (2) in vivo anticoagulants depending on whether they are used in the laboratory or can be administered to a patient respectively.

1. In Vitro Anticoagulants

These anticoagulants are used to prevent clotting of blood in the laboratory, e.g. to store blood in a blood bank, obtain plasma or packed red cells or estimation of ESR, etc. The commonly used in vitro anticoagulants are:

(i) Sodium citrate
(ii) Ammonium and potassium oxalate

(iii) Ethylene diamine tetraactate (EDTA). Agents (i) to (iii) act by removing Ca^{++} from the blood.

(iv) Heparin. It is effective in vitro also though it is mainly used in vivo.

2. In vivo Anticoagulants

These agents are used to decrease the coagulability of blood so as to prevent the extension of an already formed clot, e.g. in patients of coronary thrombosis or deep vein thrombosis, etc. In vivo anticoagulants include heparin and dicoumarols.

Heparin

Heparin is a powerful anticoagulant. It is administered intravenously, since it is ineffective orally. Its action begins within a few minutes and lasts for several hours. Heparin acts by inhibiting thrombin, factor X_a, and IX_a. It is administered in patients who are at risk of thrombosis.

Chemically, heparin is a polysaccharide containing many sulphate groups. It is related to chondroitin. It is normally secreted by the mast cells present in many tissues like the lungs, liver and intestinal mucosa. It was initially isolated from the liver, hence the name. Commercially, it is obtained from the lungs of the ox or intestinal mucosa of the pig.

Besides, acting as an anticoagulant, heparin has another physiological role. It releases a lipoprotein lipase from the endothelial cells which hydrolyses the chylomicrons and lipoproteins.

Toludine blue and protamine can neutralize the anticoagulant action of heparin. These chemicals (drugs) are used as antidote if over-dosage of heparin leads to a bleeding disorder.

Dicoumarol

This drug has chemical structure similar to vitamin K. Therefore, it acts as vitamin-K-antagonist in the liver, and elsewhere, by the phenomenon of *substrate competition*. As a result, the synthesis of vitamin-K-dependent clotting factors like prothrombin (factor-II), factor VII, IX and X is depressed. Due to its mode of action, dicoumarol can act as anticoagulant *in vivo* only. Dicoumarol is administered in patients who are at risk of a thrombotic disorder. Dicoumarol is more conveniently administered than heparin since it is effective orally. However, onset of its action is delayed. Hence, initially heparin is given intravenously for immediate results. Dicoumarol is administered simultaneously and after a couple of days heparin is withdrawn but oral anticoagulant is continued. The dose schedule of dicoumarol is so adjusted that the coagulability of blood is depressed but not to the extent that spontaneous bleeding occurs. Estimation of prothrombin time at regular intervals is essential during dicoumarol therapy.

Section III

The Heart

CHAPTER 6

The Physiology of Cardiac Muscle

INTRODUCTION

The cardiovascular system constitutes a transportation system that delivers to all the tissues materials necessary for their normal functions (e.g. O_2, nutrients, hormones, etc.), as well as, removes the waste products produced by cellular metabolism (e.g. CO_2, uric acid, urea, etc.). A number of defence systems against infection (e.g. leucocytes, immunoglobulins, etc.) also circulate in the bloodstream. Moreover, the cardiovascular system helps to regulate the body temperature by transporting heat, generated by metabolic processes to the areas where it can be dissipated.

The cardiovascular system consists of a pump, the heart, and a series of distributing and collecting tubes, i.e. arteries and veins respectively and extensive system of extremely thin vessels, the capillaries. The most important function of blood vessels, i.e. the rapid exchange of materials between the blood and extracellular fluid bathing the tissue cells, is served by the capillaries.

FUNCTIONAL ANATOMY OF THE HEART

The human heart consists of four chambers, the two atria (right and left) and two ventricles (right and left). The atria are receiving chambers, whereas the ventricles are ejecting chambers. An interatrial septum separates the two atria, whereas an interventricular septum separates the two ventricles. The right atrium receives blood from the great veins (superior and inferior vena cava) and pumps it into the right ventricle. The right ventricle pumps blood into the ***pulmonary circulation***. Four pulmonary veins bring blood from the pulmonary circulation into the left atrium, which pumps blood into left ventricle. The left ventricle pumps blood into the aorta and thereby into the ***systemic circulation***, all over the body. All the venous blood reaches right atrium through superior and inferior vena cava. In this way, the two cardiac pumps, the right and the left heart, work in series (Fig. 6.1).

The wall of each chamber of the heart consists of:

(i) Epicardium, the visceral layer of serous pericardium.
(ii) Myocardium, the thick middle layer composed of cardiac muscle fibres.
(iii) Endocardium, the innermost layer formed by the endothelial cells and subendothelial connective tissue.

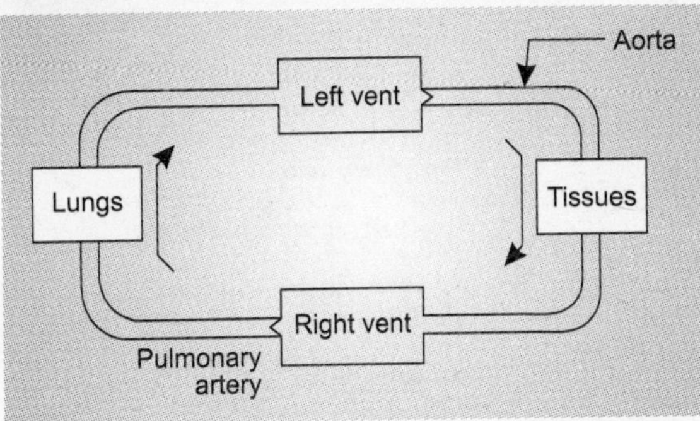

Fig. 6.1: Interrelation between the systemic and pulmonary circulations.

Pericardial cavity is the potential space between the parietal and visceral layers of serous pericardium. It normally contains a thin film of fluid that enables the heart to contract and relax in a frictionless environment.

Fibrous Skeleton of the Heart

The fibrous skeleton of the heart consists of a complex framework of dense collagen fibres forming four fibrous rings. The atrial and ventricular muscle fibres have their origin and insertion in the fibrous skeleton of the heart. The atrial muscle fibres are attached to the superior surface of the fibrous skeleton, whereas the ventricular muscle fibres are attached to the inferior surface. The functions of the fibrous skeleton include:

(i) To keep the orifices of AV and semilunar valves patent.
(ii) Protection of the orifices of AV and semilunar valves against over-distension when a large volume of blood flows through them.
(iii) Provide attachment for the leaflets or cusps of the cardiac valves.
(iv) Provide attachment to the atrial muscle on the superior surface and the ventricular muscle on the inferior surface of the fibrous skeleton.
(v) Form an electrical insulation between the atria and the ventricles. As a result, the atria and the ventricles are excited and contract independent of each other.

Of the four cardiac chambers of the heart, walls of the left ventricle and interventricular septum are thickest (about 10 mm). The thickness of the right ventricular wall is about one-third of left ventricular wall. The walls of the two atria are still thinner (< 2 mm). The thickness of cardiac chamber may be correlated with the peak pressure generated in each chamber (Table 7.1).

Ventricular Muscle

The muscle bundles of the ventricular wall wind spirally around the ventricular chambers. Three distinct layers of the myocardial fibres can be identified. The fibres run in a clockwise direction in the outer layer, horizontally in the middle layer, and counter clockwise in the innermost layer. As a result of this arrangement, blood is virtually wrung out of the heart during the ventricular contraction. The heart rotates to the right so that the apex is pushed in close approximation to the chest wall in the region of the left 5th intercostals space, which can be palpated as "apex beat."

The AV Valves

The atrioventricular orifices are large oval-shaped apertures between an atrium and the respective ventricle. The right AV orifice can admit tips of three fingers, whereas the left AV orifice can admit tips of two fingers. The right AV orifice is guarded by the tricuspid valve (it has three cusps), whereas left AV orifice is guarded by the mitral valve (also called bicuspid valve, since it consists of two cusps). The AV valves allow the blood to flow in one direction only, i.e. from the atria to the ventricles. During ventricular contraction, the tendency of blood to flow back to the respective atria is prevented by the closure of the valve (Fig. 6.2).

The papillary muscles are conical muscular projections arising from the ventricular walls. From their apices, arise tendinous cords (cordae tendineae) which are attached to the border and inferior surfaces of the cusps of AV valves. During ventricular contraction, the papillary muscles also contract and help to

(i) Draw the cusps of AV valves together so as to close the AV orifice and prevent regurgitation of blood back into the atria; and

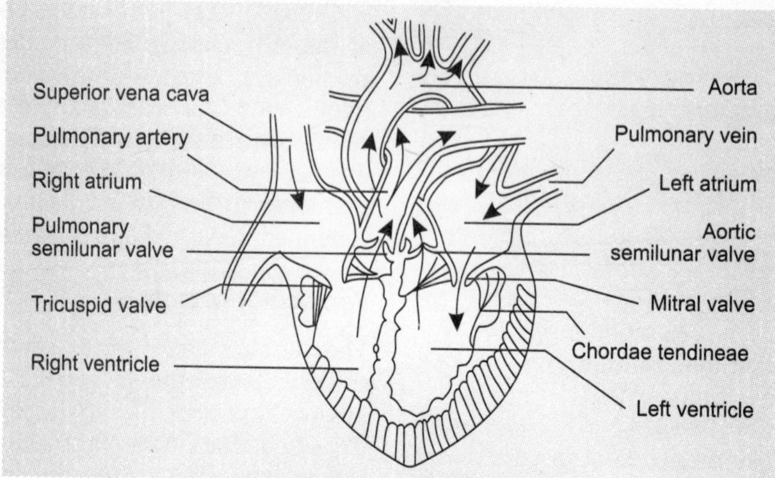

Fig. 6.2: Internal structure of the heart.

(ii) Prevent the membranous cusps from prolapsing into the atria. During atrial contraction, blood passes through the AV orifice, pushing the cusps of AV valve aside like a curtain.

The Semilunar Valves

The aortic and pulmonary orifices are rounded apertures, smaller than the respective AV orifices. They are guarded by the aortic and pulmonary valves, respectively. These valves are also known as the semilunar valves since each consists of three half-moon-shaped cusps. These cusps allow the blood to flow from the ventricle to the respective arterial trunk (aorta or pulmonary artery) during ventricular contraction by getting aside to the wall. When the ventricles relax, the tendency of the blood to flow back into the ventricles is prevented by the three cusps, which by opening like pockets, close the orifice (Fig. 6.2).

The Cardiac Muscle

Cardiac muscle fibres are striated like skeletal muscle fibres but the most characteristic histological feature of the cardiac muscle is a syncytium-like appearance. (A syncytium is a multinucleated mass of cytoplasm which is not divided by end-membranes into individual cells.) Cardiac muscle fibres seem to divide and reunite with the adjacent muscle fibres. Early histologists described the cardiac muscle as an anatomical syncytium. Subsequently, electron microscopic studies have revealed that the dense partitions seen at regular intervals under light microscopy, and called *intercalated discs* (Fig. 6.3), are actually end membranes that separate one muscle cell from another. Intercalated discs are desmosomes which provide a strong union between the adjacent cardiac muscle cells.

At the outer border of the intercalated disc, the adjacent cell membranes contain proteineous tunnels called connexons or *gap junctions*

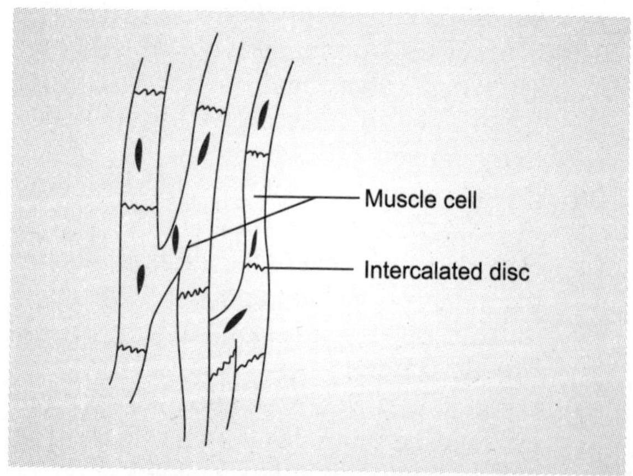

Fig. 6.3: Structure of cardiac muscle.

(Fig. 1.4). Electrical resistance in these gap junctions is 400 times less than in other parts of the cell membrane. Electrical impulse arising in one muscle fibre spreads to the next muscle fibre through these gap junctions. In this way, the cardiac impulse spreads throughout the muscle mass quickly, resulting in a coordinated contraction of the whole tissue. Therefore, the cardiac muscle behaves as a *functional syncytium*, although anatomically it is not so.

The cardiac muscle cell contains actin and myosin filaments, the sarcotubular system and other organelles seen in the skeletal muscle. The mitochondrial content of cardiac muscle is much larger than that of the skeletal muscle.

ELECTROPHYSIOLOGY OF MYOCARDIUM

The description which follows pertains to electrical properties of the cardiac muscle fibres of the ventricles and the atria.

Resting Membrane Potential (RMP)

The resting membrane potential of the cardiac muscle is –90 mV, i.e. interior of the cardiac muscle cell is 90 mV negative with respect to its surface. The ionic basis of RMP in the cardiac muscle is same as in other excitable tissues like nerve or skeletal muscle: selective permeability of cell membrane to different ions and operation of electrogenic Na^+—K^+ pump at the cell membrane (Ch. 20).

Cardiac Action Potential

Action Potential When an excitable tissue is stimulated, there is a transient reversal of a transmembrane potential of the tissue, i.e. the inner surface of the cell membrane becomes positive (+ 20 to 35 mV) with respect to the outer surface. This change from – 90 mV (– 70 mV in case of nerve) to + 20 to 35 mV in the transmembrane potential is called *depolarization*. Soon, the transmembrane potential is restored to normal (i.e. – 90 or – 70 mV). This change is called *repolarization*. The sudden change in the transmembrane potential is called an *action potential* and it consists of two phases: a phase of depolarization followed by a phase of repolarization. (The action potential of a nerve fibre and its ionic basis is given in Chapter 20. The reader is advised to go through that discussion before reading further in this chapter). After this general discussion on an action potential, cardiac action potential shall be discussed in detail.

The Cardiac Action Potential The cardiac action potential is shown in Fig. 6.4. It consists of a phase of depolarization (phase 0) and a phase of repolarization (consisting of phases 1, 2 and 3) followed by a phase 4 in which resting membrane potential is maintained steady.

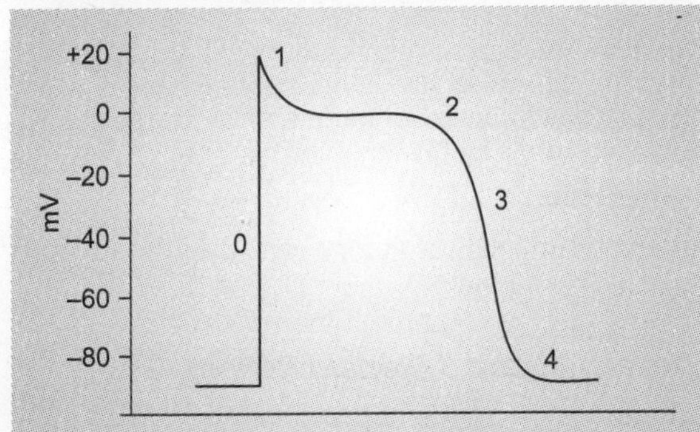

Fig. 6.4: Phases of cardiac action potential: 0, depolarization; 1. initial rapid repolarization; 2. plateau phase, 3. late rapid repolarization; 4. baseline.

Phase 0 (Depolarization)

This phase is recorded as a rapid upstroke. The membrane potential changes from the resting value of – 90 mV to + 20 mV, within 2 ms only. The rapid depolarization is caused by opening of voltage gated Na^+ channels. Consequently, the positively charged sodium ions enter the cardiac muscle cell following concentration and electrical gradients (Na^+ conc: 142 mEq/L outside and 14 mEq/L inside and membrane potential – 90 mV inside) (Fig. 6.5).

The voltage-gated Na^+ channels in the myocardium have two gates: an *outer gate* that *opens* at the beginning of depolarization and an *inner gate* that *closes* soon after the opening of the outer gate. The inner gate remains closed till the cell membrane is repolarized back to – 80 mV. Prolonged closure of the inner gate is responsible

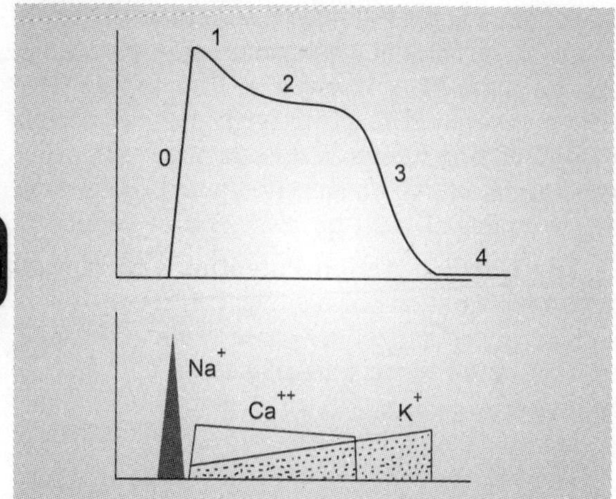

Fig. 6.5: Ionic conductance during cardiac action potential. Increased Na^+ conductance-phase 0, Ca^{++} conductance in phase 2 and gradually increasing K^+ conductance during phases 2 and 3.

for the prolonged refractory period in the cardiac muscle (see below).

Phases 1, 2 and 3 (Repolarization)

In the cardiac muscle, the repolarization, recorded as a down stroke, is a slow process. It is completed in 200–300 ms. It can be divided into phases 1, 2 and 3.

Phase 1 This is a brief initial phase of rapid repolarization, in which the membrane potential changes from + 20 mV to – 10 mV. It has been variously attributed to: (i) closure of Na^+ channels or (ii) brief opening of voltage-gated K^+ channels.

Phase 2 The brief phase 1 is followed by a prolonged *plateau phase* which takes about 200 ms. In this phase, the membrane potential is held relatively steady. Phase 2 gives the characteristic shape to the cardiac action potential. The plateau phase is because of: (i) opening of voltage-gated Ca^{++} channels leading to increased Ca^{++} permeability and (ii) simultaneous opening of voltage-gated K^+ channels (Fig. 6.5). Thus, the Ca^{++} influx balances the effect of K^+ efflux and hence the membrane potential remains steady.

The transfer of Ca^{++} into the cell during phase 2 has an implication in the excitation-contraction coupling in the cardiac muscle (see below).

Phase 3 This is a phase of relatively rapid repolarization. In this phase, the membrane potential reverts back to – 90 mV over a short period. This phase is caused by: (i) inactivation of Ca^{++} channels and (ii) opening of voltage gated K^+ channels (Fig. 6.5). Consequently, positively charged potassium ions leave the cell and restore the membrane potential of RMP value.

Phase 4 In this phase, the membrane potential is maintained steady at the resting value (–90 mV). Thus, this phase is recorded as a flat baseline.

During this phase the energy dependent Na^+-K^+ ATPase pump is activated. Therefore, extra Na^+ which entered the cell during depolarization are extruded. At the same time, K^+ which left the cell during repolarization are taken back. Calcium ions, which entered the cell during plateau phase, are also extruded by a Na^+-Ca^{++} pump.

In the pacemaker tissues (SA node and AV node), the shape of the action potential is characteristically different. It shall be discussed in detail later in this chapter.

Refractory Period

The cardiac muscle does not respond to another stimulus for about 200 ms after the beginning of an action potential. This duration is called *absolute refractory period* (Fig. 6.6). It is related to the closure of inner gate of Na^+ channels soon after

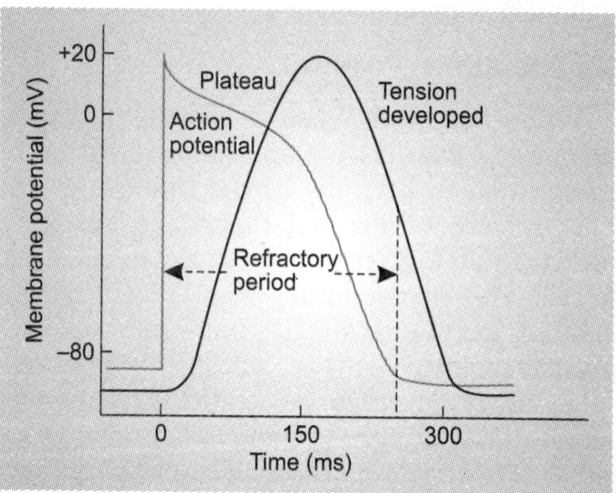

Fig. 6.6: Refractory period in the myocardium and its relation to myocardial contraction (tension).

the beginning of an action potential. The gate remain closed till the membrane potential is repolarized back to about – 80 mV (lower part of phase 3 of the action potential). During this period, any Na^+ influx (essential for the next depolarization) is not possible. During the subsequent 50 ms approximately, the cardiac muscle is said to be in *relative refractory period* (Fig. 6.6). During this period, only a stronger than normal stimulus can excite the cell membrane. Relative refractory period is because of the opened K^+ channels (a repolarizing force). Hence, a stronger depolarizing stimulus is required to initiate depolarization during this period.

All or None Law

As in nerve and skeletal muscle, the action potential of a cardiac muscle follows all or none law. If stimuli of gradually increasing strength are applied to a strip of cardiac muscle, it would be seen that weak stimuli (called subthreshold stimuli) fail to produce an action potential. Stimulus of a particular strength (known as threshold strength) produces an action potential. Application of stronger stimuli (called supra-threshold stimuli) does not produce any further increase in the extent (height) of the action potential. All action potentials are of same extent (from – 90 mV to + 20 mV). This property is called *all or none law*. It is due to the fact that whenever voltage-gated Na^+ channels open, they open fully and the degree of Na^+ influx is similar irrespective of the fact that a stimulus is of threshold strength or supra-threshold strength. All or none law holds true provided Na^+ concentration of ECF and other environmental conditions do not change.

Automaticity and Rhythmicity

These two important properties seen in the cardiac muscle are not seen in a nerve fibre or skeletal muscle. The myocardial tissue, even if cut into small pieces, has the property of contracting automatically and rhythmically (periodically). Activation of the cardiac muscle by a neural stimulus is not essential. The properties of automaticity and rhythmicity are due to the presence of *pacemaker tissue* (specialized conduction tissue) within the myocardium. The pacemaker tissue and its activity are discussed in detail later in this chapter.

Conductivity

The action potential, once generated, is conducted by the cardiac muscle from one region of the heart to another. The conduction velocity of the action potentials in the cardiac muscle is rather slow (0.2–1 m/s). The specialized conduction tissue of the heart has greater conduction velocity (1–4 m/s).

MECHANICAL PROPERTIES OF MYOCARDIUM

The Contractile Response

Development of an action potential (an electrical response) in any muscle results in a brief contraction followed by relaxation once again. In the cardiac muscle fibre, the mechanical response (contraction) begins just after the depolarization of the muscle and lasts for about 300 ms. Thus, the time courses of electrical (250 ms) and mechanical responses of the cardiac muscle are almost same (Fig. 6.6). This is in contrast to the *skeletal muscle* where the duration of the action potential (refractory period) is short and the mechanical response begins a few milliseconds *after the end of repolarization* and lasts approximately 100 ms (Fig. 6.7). Therefore in skeletal muscle, repetitive stimulation results in summations of contractions (sustained contraction: tetanus, Chapter 21). From the comparison of the time courses of the electrical and mechanical events in the cardiac muscle (Fig. 6.6), it would be apparent that, the cardiac muscle is refractory to any stimulation during the contraction phase (systole). Thus, unlike skeletal muscle, the cardiac muscle cannot be tetanized. This property of the cardiac muscle is physiologically very useful because the heart has to function as a pump. It must relax, get filled up with blood and then contract to pump out the blood. A tetanized heart (a state of continued contraction) would be useless as a pump.

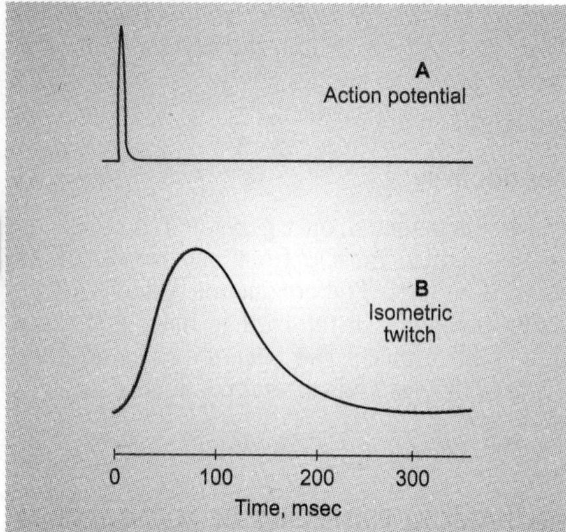

Fig. 6.7: The time course of action potential (A) and the mechanical response (B) in skeletal muscle.

All or None Law

In an isolated muscle fibre, whether skeletal or cardiac, the mechanical response follows the all or none law. It means that a stimulus of sub-threshold strength does not produce any contraction whereas all stimuli of threshold and supra-threshold strength produce a similar degree of contraction. If a *bundle of skeletal muscle fibres* is stimulated, it does not follow all or none law because adjacent muscle fibres are insulated from each other by sarcolemma. Therefore, a threshold stimulus may activate a few muscle fibres only. With increase in strength of stimuli more and more, muscle fibres are activated and made to contract. On the other hand, even a *bundle of cardiac muscle fibres* follows all or none law. With a subthreshold stimulus, the cardiac muscle bundle does not contract at all. With threshold and supra-threshold stimuli, the cardiac muscle bundle contracts to the same extent. The all or none response of the cardiac muscle contraction is due to the presence of gap junctions (at the periphery of intercalated discs) between the adjacent muscle cells. Consequently, excitation of one cardiac muscle cell results in excitation of all the muscle cells. Therefore, *cardiac muscle mass always contracts as a whole.* The all or none mechanical response of the heart is a physiological necessity. To act as a pump effectively, all the muscle fibres of the atria (or ventricles) must contract simultaneously.

The gradation of skeletal muscle power can be achieved by recruitment of progressively greater number of motor units. This mechanism cannot work in the cardiac muscle. In stead, gradation of cardiac muscle power is achieved by increasing the sympathetic discharge to the heart, through the inotropic effect of norepinephrine.

Length-Tension Relationship

By stimulating a papillary muscle, isometric tension can be recorded at varying degrees of initial (resting) length. Like skeletal muscle, within physiological limits of stretch, cardiac muscle also shows an increase in the isometric tension with the increase in the initial length (Fig. 6.8). This property forms the basis of the *Starling's law of the heart* which is applicable to skeletal muscle as well and can be explained on the basis of sliding filaments theory (Chapter 21).

At any given length, the tension produced in the cardiac muscle can be increased by addition of norepinephrine in the bathing fluid. This effect of catecholamines on the cardiac muscle is known

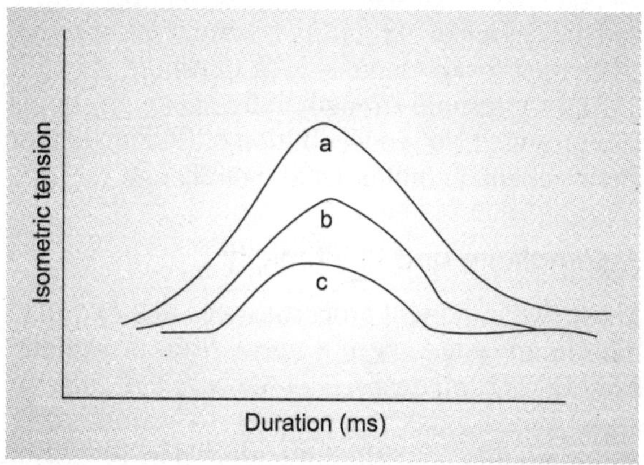

Fig. 6.8: Length-tension relation in cardiac muscle. Gradual stretch of cardiac muscle (c, b, a) causes progressively increasing tension (force).

as *positive inotropic effect* (Fig. 6.9). *Under the effect of norepinephrine, the cardiac muscle contracts more forcibly as well as with greater velocity.*

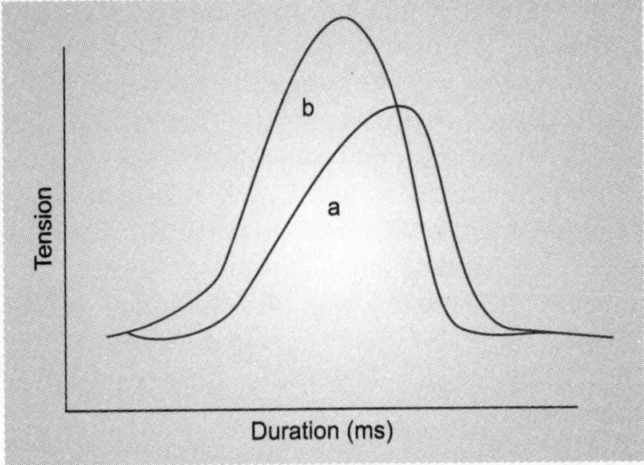

Fig. 6.9: Positive inotropic effect. Curves a and b obtained with similar stretch (length) of the cardiac muscle but curve b obtained after addition of norepinephrine to the bathing fluid.

Excitation-Contraction Coupling

The process of excitation-contraction coupling in the cardiac muscle is basically similar to that in the skeletal muscle, except for some differences which have important clinical implications.

As the action potential passes over the cardiac muscle, it passes into the interior of the cells through T-tubules. The T-tubules in the cardiac muscle are much larger than those in the skeletal muscle. As the T-tubules undergo an action potential, (unlike in skeletal muscle) fairly large amount of Ca^{++} diffuse into the sarcoplasm from the ECF (in the lumen) of the T-tubules. This influx of Ca^{++} occurs during the plateau phase of the action potential. In addition, the action potential causes release of Ca^{++} from the terminal cisterns. Since Ca^{++} are transferred directly from the ECF in the T-tubules, the strength of contraction of the cardiac muscle depends to a greater extent on the concentration of Ca^{++} in the ECF. In contrast, Ca^{++} concentration in ECF has no significant effect on the strength of contraction of the skeletal muscle. Calcium ions bind with troponin-C and result in sliding of myosin filaments over actin filaments leading to shortening of the muscle. (For details of shortening mechanism, see Chapter 21).

During diastole, Ca^{++} are extruded out of the cardiac muscle fibre by a carrier system operating at the sarcolemma in which two Na^+ are exchanged for each Ca^{++} extruded (Fig. 6.10). The rate of Ca^{++} transport depends on the gradient of Na^+ created by Na^+-K^+ ATPase. A cardiotonic drug, digitalis, inhibits Na^+-K^+ ATPase, thereby increasing intracellular Na^+ concentration in the cardiac muscle. The resulting decrease in Na^+ gradient diminishes the rate of Ca^{2+} extrusion. As a result, intracellular Ca^{++} concentration increases. This explains the increased cardiac contractility observed on administration of digitalis in patients with congestive heart failure.

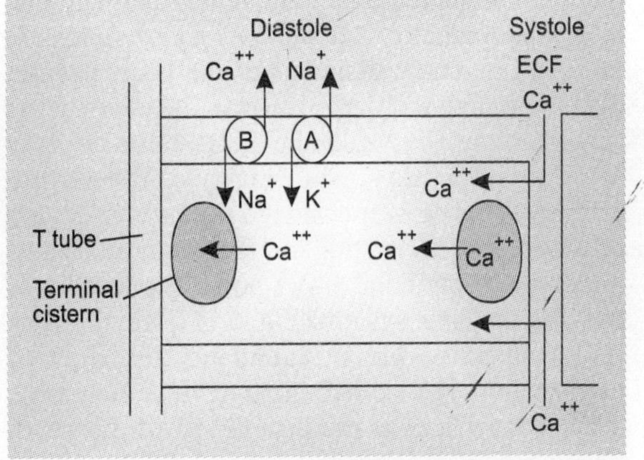

Fig. 6.10: During cardiac systole Ca^{++} diffuses into the sarcoplasm from the T-tubes as well as terminal cisterns. During diastole, Ca^{++} is transported back into (i) terminal cisterns and (ii) ECF. Transport into ECF by a Na^+-Ca^{++} pump (B) is driven by low intracellular Na^+ concentration (created by Na^+-K^+ ATPase pump (A).

Cardiac Muscle Metabolism

The cardiac muscle is characterized by higher myoglobin content and more numerous mitochondria than in the skeletal muscle. It also has more abundant blood supply. All these features are indicative of high metabolic rate in the cardiac muscle. The metabolic processes are almost completely *aerobic* and cardiac muscle cannot undergo O_2 debt (cf. skeletal muscle). That is why even brief ischemia in the myocardium produces necrosis (infarction).

Oxidation of *free fatty acids* accounts for 60% of the cardiac energy requirements. About 35% of its energy requirement is met with by the *carbohydrates* and the rest by amino acids and ketone bodies.

SPECIALIZED EXCITATORY AND CONDUCTION TISSUES OF THE HEART

The heart is innervated by both the sympathetic, as well as the parasympathetic nerves. The autonomic nerves regulate the frequency at which the heart beats, and the vigour (force) of each beat. Changes in the discharge rate of autonomic nerves to the heart help to adjust the cardiac function appropriate to the various stressful states the body is subjected to. However, the heart has unique properties of *automaticity* and *rhythmicity*, i.e. even if totally denervated; the heart has not only the capacity to initiate its own beat (automaticity) but also the heart beats at very regular intervals (rhythmicity). These two properties reside in specialized *pacemaker tissues of the heart,* consisting of the sinoatrial (SA) node, atrioventricular (AV) node, the bundle of His and Purkinje system (Fig. 6.11). Rhythmicity of the heart is due to automatic discharge of cardiac impulses at regular intervals. Normally, the SA node acts as the *pacemaker* of the heart, i.e. its impulse discharge determines the rate at which the heart beats. The cardiac impulses generated in the SA node spread to the atrial muscle, and little later, through the bundle of His and Purkinje tissue, to the ventricles. The pacemaker tissues other than the SA node normally act as conductive tissues only, even though they have the capacity to generate impulses on their own. The reason why normally they do not do so is that the intrinsic rhythmicity of the SA node (*sinus rhythm, 60–80 minute*) is far greater than the intrinsic rhythmicity of other pacemaker tissues. Therefore, other pacemaker tissues receive an impulse arising from SA node before they can generate their own impulse. Only in abnormal conditions cardiac impulse may arise from AV node at the frequency of *40–60/minute (nodal rhythm)* or even from Purkinje fibres, at the frequency of *15–40/minute (idioventricular rhythm).*

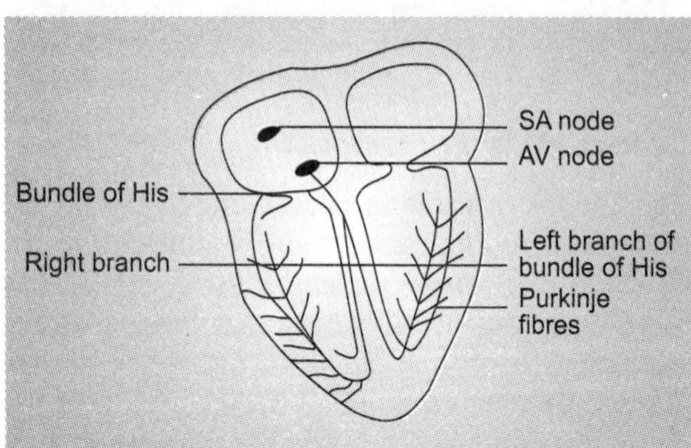

Fig. 6.11: Conduction system of the heart.

Sinoatrial (SA) Node

The sinoatrial node is a small strip of specialized cardiac muscle tissue, measuring 25 × 2 mm, located in the right atrial wall immediately anterior and lateral to the opening of the superior vena cava. The muscle fibres of SA node are 3–5 μm in diameter in contrast to 15–20 μm diameter of the surrounding atrial muscle fibres. Located in the centre of SA node are still smaller modified cardiac muscle cells called the *stellate cells* or *P cells*. P cells are believed to be the real pacemaker cells. The SA node also contains parasympathetic autonomic ganglia and postganglionic sympathetic and parasympathetic fibres. The pacemaker activity of P cells is modulated by the activity of autonomic nerve fibres.

Internodal Pathways

These are three bundles of Purkinje type fibres which connect SA node with AV node. The bundles are called the anterior, middle and posterior *internodal tracts*. The cardiac impulse initiated at SA node reaches the AV node via conduction through atrial muscle (conduction velocity 0.8 metre/S) and through faster conducting internodal tracts (conduction velocity 2 metre/S). However, it may be mentioned that even the existence of the internodal pathway is controversial.

Atrioventricular (AV) Node

The atrioventricular node is situated subendocardially in contrast to the subepicardial location of the SA node. The AV node, measuring 20 × 3 mm, is located in the wall of right atrium at the right posterior portion of the interatrial septum. It consists of specialized muscle fibres resembling those of the SA node, including the P cells. The AV node is connected to the bundle of His through modified cardiac muscle cells called the transitional cells.

The bundle of His is the only electrical link between the atrial muscle mass and the ventricular muscle mass. Therefore, the AV node acts as an electrical gate. Cardiac impulse arising from the SA node spreads all over the atrial muscle mass but has to pass through the AV node before transmission to the ventricular muscle mass. At the AV node, there is always a delay of about 200 mS before the impulse is transmitted to the bundle of His. The physiological significance of AV nodal delay is discussed later in this chapter.

Another important property of AV node is that it is not capable of transmitting impulses at a very rapid rare. If pathologically, the atria start firing impulses at a rate faster than 200/min, the AV node allows only some of these to pass into the ventricles, i.e. the ventricles are not allowed to beat at very rapid rates. This is physiologically useful since very high rates of ventricular contraction make it ineffective as a pump.

The His-Purkinje System

The Purkinje system consists of bundle of His and its branches. It contains muscle fibres with diameter of 70–80 μm. Thus, these fibres are even larger than the typical ventricular muscle fibres. The Purkinje tissue cells are richer in glycogen and have more sarcoplasm than the typical cardiac muscle cell. These fibres are striated but do not have distinct cell boundaries. Their conduction velocity is 4 m/S as compared to 1.0 m/S in the typical myocardial fibre. The faster conduction velocity helps to spread the wave of excitation rapidly over the two ventricles, so that the two contract simultaneously.

The bundle of His begins from the AV node, passes through the fibrous AV ring into the top of interventricular septum. Almost immediately it divides into the right and left bundle branches, which supply the right and the left ventricles, respectively. The left bundle branch further divides into anterior and posterior fascicles. The anterior branch is thinner of the two and supplies the anterior wall of the left ventricle. The thicker posterior branch supplies the posterolateral wall of the left ventricle. The right branch and the two fascicles of the left branch run subendocardially on the respective sides of the septum. At the apex of the heart, these fibres divide further into a large number finer branches that spread into the subendocardial region of the respective ventricles.

INNERVATION OF THE HEART

The parasympathetic (cholinergic) fibres to the SA node are supplied mainly by the right vagus nerve and to the AV node by the left vagus nerve. This may be correlated with the fact that, developmentally, the SA node and the AV node are right-sided and left-sided structures, respectively. The parasympathetic fibres innervate SA node, AV node and the atrial muscle but do not innervate the ventricular musculature. Stimulation of the vagus produces decreased heart rate and decreased force of atrial contraction. The cardiac output is decreased only moderately because of decrease in the heart rate.

The sympathetic (noradrenergic) fibres innervate all parts of the heart, i.e. SA node, AV node, His-Purkinje tissue and atrial as well as ventricular musculature. Stimulation of sympathetic fibres to the heart produces increased heart rate (positive chronotropic effect) as well as increased force of contraction of the atria and the ventricles (positive inotropic effect) (Table 6.1). As a result, the output of the heart is markedly increased.

THE ORIGIN AND SPREAD OF CARDIAC IMPULSE

The Origin

As mentioned above, the properties of automaticity and rhythmicity reside in pacemaker tissues of the

Table 6.1: Summary of the effects of autonomic nerves on the heart

	Parasympathetic stimulation	*Sympathetic stimulation*
Heart rate	Decreased	Increased
Force of contraction		
Atrial	Decreased	Increased
Ventricular	No effect	Increased
AV delay	Prolonged	Shortened
Conduction in		
His-Purkinje tissue	Slower	Faster
Refractory period	Prolonged	Shortened

6

heart. The basis for this specialized function lies in the electrical properties of the pacemaker tissue. It may be recapitulated that the resting membrane potential of a typical atrial or ventricular muscle fibre is approximately –90 mV. The action potential recorded from the atrial or the ventricular muscle consists of phases of rapid depolarization (phase 0), rapid repolarization (phase 1), plateau (phase 2), late rapid repolarization (phase 3) and baseline (phase 4) (Fig. 6.12).

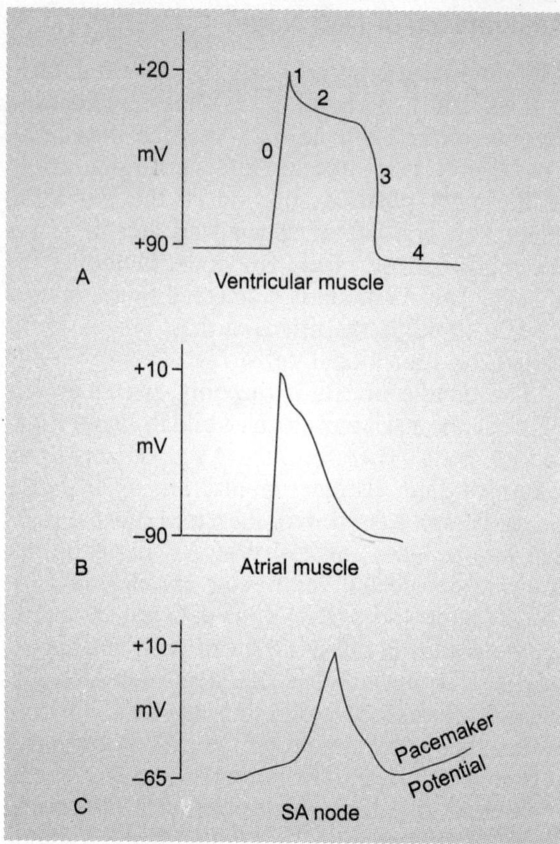

Fig. 6.12: Action potentials recorded from ventricular muscles (A), atrial muscle (B) and SA node (C).

Pacemaker Potential (Prepotential)

A typical transmembrane action potential recorded from a mammalian SA node is shown in Fig. 6.12. As compared to atrial or ventricular transmembrane potential, the *resting membrane potential* of SA nodal fibres is less: approximately *–65 mV*. Moreover, the depolarization (*phase 0*) has much *slower velocity*; rapid repolarization and the plateau (*phases 1 and 2*) *are absent* and the late rapid repolarization (*phase 3*) *is more gradual. The most prominent difference, however, lies in phase 4*. In the atrial (or ventricular) muscle action potentials, there is a constant transmembrane potential between the two adjacent action potentials. In contrast, in the nodal tissues, the phase 4 shows *slow depolarization called pacemaker potential* (or *prepotential*). Pacemaker potential is the name given to the slow and gradual depolarization recorded between two action potentials. The slow depolarization proceeds at a steady rate until the "firing level" (about –40 mV) is attained; and then the next action potential is fired.

Pacemaker potentials can be normally recorded from SA node and AV node only, but under abnormal conditions, the bundle of His or other parts of the Purkinje system can develop pacemaker potentials, e.g. when the ventricle is electrically isolated from the atria (complete heart block).

Atrial and ventricular muscle cells may also develop pacemaker potentials under pathological conditions.

Ionic Basis of SA Nodal Rhythmicity

Study of ionic conductance in the SA node in relation to the action potential reveals that, in general, the nodal muscle fibres are quite leaky to sodium ions. As a result, the resting membrane potential of the SA node is less negative than that of the adjacent atrial muscle fibres. The prepotential or the gradual depolarization immediately after the end of an action potential is caused by a slow increase in Ca^{++} permeability through *T (for transient) Ca^{++} channels.* When the firing level is reached, opening of *L (for long lasting) Ca^{++} channels* cause the upstroke (depolarization). The down stroke (repolarization) is produced by an increase in K^{+} permeability. Thus, changes in Na^{+} permeability do not play a significant role in the production of action potential in nodal tissues.

Effect of Autonomic Nerves on Pacemaker Potential

Changes in the heart rate can occur due to a change in the resting membrane potential and/or a change in the slope of the pacemaker potential. The parasympathetic stimulation (acetylcholine) decreases the heart rate by producing: (a) slight hyperpolarization of the SA node and (b) reducing the slope of pacemaker potential. Consequently, for each action potential more time is required to reach the firing level (Fig. 6.13). Very strong stimulation of the vagus nerve may abolish the spontaneous discharge of the SA node for some time. On the other hand, sympathetic stimulation (norepinephrine) increases the heart rate by increasing the slope of prepotential (Fig. 6.13).

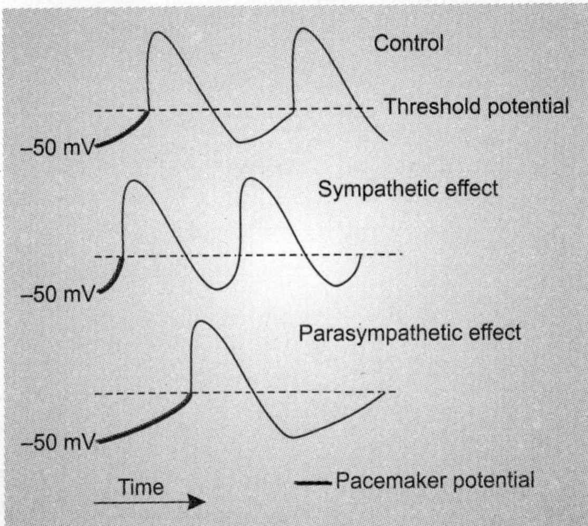

Fig. 6.13: Effect of stimulation of autonomic nerves on the slope of pacemaker potential.

The effects of acetylcholine and norepinephrine on the prepotential are mediated through changes in K^{+} and Ca^{++} permeability in the nodal tissue.

Acetylcholine increases K^{+} permeability and slows the opening of Ca^{++} channels, whereas norepinephrine facilitates the opening of L-Ca^{++} channels in the nodal tissue. Norepinephrine also increases Ca^{++} permeability of the myocardium, thereby increasing the force of each contraction.

The frequency of spontaneous discharge in the SA node is influenced by temperature of blood in the right atrium. This at least partly explains the increase in heart rate (tachycardia) associated with fever.

Spread of Cardiac Impulse

The Atrial Spread

The cardiac impulse (action potential) generated in the SA node spreads radially throughout the myocardium of the two atria simultaneously (like ripples in a pond) and eventually reaches the AV node. Atrial depolarization is completed in approximately 0.1 S and is followed by atrial contraction.

Three special bundles that contain Purkinje type of fibres constitute the internodal pathways between the SA and AV nodes. These pathways conduct the cardiac impulse to the AV node more rapidly, i.e. approximately 0.04 S after its origin in the SA node.

Nodal Delay

In the AV node, the cardiac impulse is delayed for about 200 mS, before it spreads to the ventricles via the bundle of His. Nodal delay serves a very useful function. It ensures that the two atria complete their contraction and empty themselves, well before the ventricles begin to contract. Mild vagal stimulation decreases the excitability of AV node and therefore increases the duration of nodal delay. Strong vagal stimulation may partially or completely block all the impulses coming from SA node. Conversely, sympathetic stimulation decreases the nodal delay.

Ventricular Conduction

The His-Purkinje system has high conduction velocity, 1–4 m/S. Therefore once the impulse reaches the bundle of His, it rapidly spreads throughout the two ventricles within 0.08–0.1 S. The interventricular septum is first to be depolarized. Its left side is initially depolarized and the wave of depolarization spreads towards the right side of the septum. As the impulse reaches the apex of the heart, it returns along the subendocardial region of the two ventricles to the AV groove. In the meantime, it spreads throughout the ventricular wall from the subendocardial to the epicardial surface. The last parts of the ventricles to be depolarized are the posterobasal portions of the left ventricle and pulmonary conus region of the right ventricle. The sequence of spread of cardiac impulse described above is responsible for the pattern of PQR and S waves observed in electrocardiogram (ECG).

7 CHAPTER The Heart as a Pump

THE CARDIAC CYCLE

As mentioned in the previous chapter, periodically a cardiac impulse originates in the SA node and spreads first into the atrial and then into the ventricular myocardium. The depolarization of the atria results in a brief atrial contraction (*atrial systole*). Subsequent ventricular depolarization results in ventricular contraction (*ventricular systole*). Each contraction is followed by a period of relaxation known as diastole (*atrial or ventricular diastole* (Fig. 7.1). When the terms *cardiac systole* and *cardiac diastole* are used, they refer to ventricular systole and diastole only. The period from the beginning of one cardiac contraction to the beginning of next cardiac contraction is known as a *cardiac cycle*. At normal heart rate (75/min), the duration of each cardiac cycle is 0.8 S.

$$\left[\frac{60\text{ S}}{75} = 0.8\text{ S}\right]$$

PRESSURE AND VOLUME CHANGES DURING A CARDIAC CYCLE

Atrial Systole (Duration 0.1 S)

Before the atrial systole begins, the mitral and tricuspid valves (AV valves) located between the atria and ventricles are open and most of the atrial blood has already been transferred passively into the ventricles. Atrial systole contributes only about 30% of the ventricular filling. However, when the heart rate is fast, and consequently, the duration of ventricular diastole is shortened, atrial systole contributes a higher percentage of ventricular filling. Even though there are no valves at the opening of the vena cavae and the pulmonary veins into the atria, the regurgitation of blood into the veins is prevented by narrowing of the venous orifices due to contraction of the atrial muscle. Atrial systole lasts only 0.1 S. For the remaining 0.7 S of the cardiac cycle, the atria remain in diastole.

Ventricular Systole (Duration 0.3 S)

Ventricular systole begins just after the end of atrial systole. As the ventricular systole begins, the intraventricular pressure begins to rise, leading to an abrupt closure of the AV valves. The intraventricular pressure continues to increase, but ejection of blood into the aorta or the pulmonary artery does not occur, since the semilunar valves are still closed. This period between the beginning of ventricular systole and opening of semilunar valves, lasting about 0.05 S, is known as *isovolumic (isometric) contraction phase*. It is only when the intraventricular pressure exceeds the pressure in the aorta and the pulmonary artery

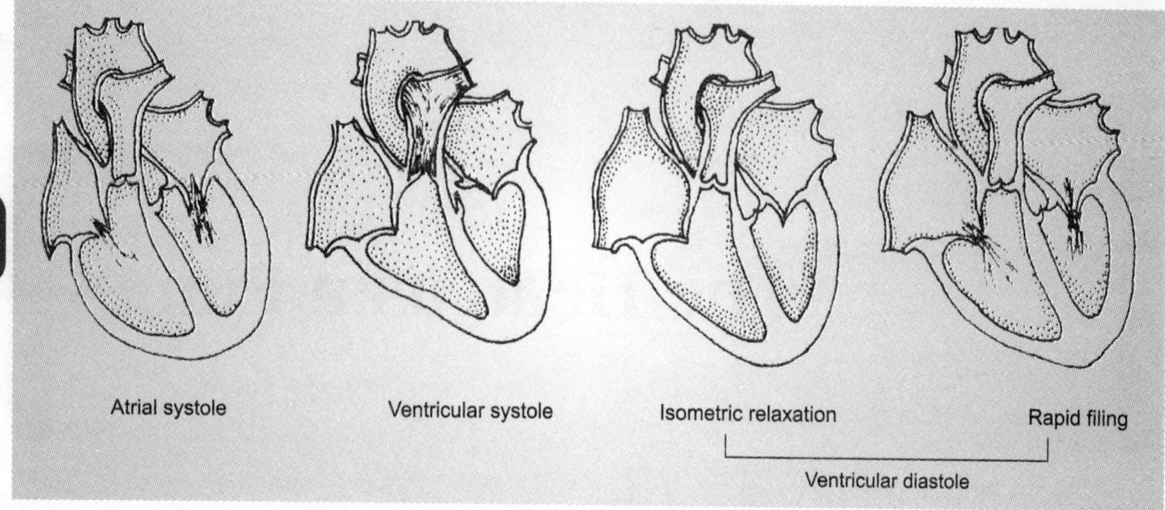

Fig. 7.1: Phases of the cardiac cycle.

(80 and 10 mmHg, respectively) that the semilunar valves open and ventricular ejection begins. The ejection of blood is rapid at first (*rapid ejection phase*), but slows down during the later part of ventricular systole (*slow ejection phase*) (Fig. 7.2). Intraventricular pressure reaches highest level during the rapid ejection phase. Peak intraventricular pressure is about 120 mmHg in the left ventricle and 25 mmHg in the right ventricle (Table 7.1) The amount of blood ejected out of each ventricle in each systole (*stroke volume*) at rest is about 70 ml and another 50 ml of blood are left in each ventricle at the end of systole (*end systolic volume*). In other words, of the 120 ml of blood present in each ventricle at the end of diastole (*end diastolic volume*), only 70 ml are ejected during each systole. Therefore at rest, the *ejection fraction* (percentage of ventricular blood ejected with each stroke) is about 60% [70/120 × 100]. During exercise (or stimulation of sympathetic nerves), greater ejection fraction is observed.

Table 7.1: Pressure values (mmHg) in various cardiac chambers during the cardiac cycle

Chamber	*Peak pressure in systole*	*Minimum pressure in diastole*
Left ventricle	120	5
Right ventricle	25	1
Left atrium	15	5–8
Right atrium	5	0

Ventricular Diastole (Duration 0.5 S)

As the ventricles begin to relax, there is a steep fall in the intraventricular pressure. The pressure gradients between the ventricles and the aorta (or the pulmonary artery) are reversed. Consequently, the blood tends to regurgitate back into the ventricles. This is prevented by the closure of semilunar valves almost immediately after the end of ventricular systole. The intraventricular pressure continues to decrease till it falls below the atrial pressure (0–5 mmHg) and then the AV valves open. The interval between the closure of semilunar valves and the opening of AV valves is known as *isovolumic (isometric) relaxation phase*.

Throughout the ventricular systole, the atria are being filled with blood from the great veins (or pulmonary veins). When the AV valves open, blood rushes from the atria into the ventricles (even though the atria are still in diastole). Ventricular filling is rapid at first (*rapid filling phase*), but slows down during the later part of ventricular diastole (*slow filling phase or diastasis*). The next cardiac cycle begins with the onset of next atrial systole.

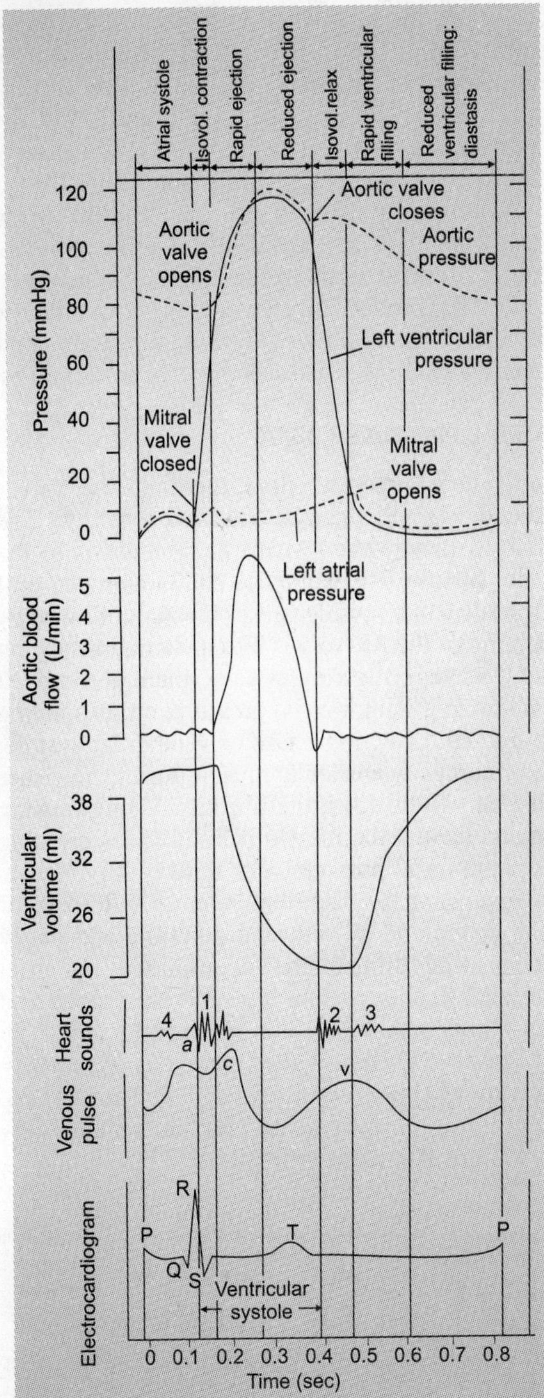

Fig. 7.2: Left atrial, aortic and left ventricular pressure pulses correlated in time with aortic flow, ventricular volume, heart sounds, venous pulse, and the electrocardiogram for a complete cardiac cycle.

Volume Changes during Cardiac Cycle (Fig. 7.2)

At the end of atrial systole, the ventricular volume increases to a maximum of approximately 120 ml. The ventricular volume remains unchanged during the isovolumic (isometric) contraction phase. The ventricular volume decreases quickly during the rapid ejection phase, but the rate of decline slows down during the reduced ejection phase. During the ejection phases, the ventricular volume decreases by about 70 ml so that approximately 50 ml of blood is left behind in each ventricle.

Ventricular volume remains unchanged during the isovolumic (isometric) relaxation phase. When the AV valves open, the passive transfer of blood causes a rapid increase in ventricular volume initially (rapid filling phase), but there may be no increase during the phase of diastasis. At the end of diastasis phase, each ventricle contains approximately 90 ml of blood. Approximately 30 ml of blood are added to the ventricular volume by the atrial systole.

Pressure Volume Relationship Loop

The pressure volume relationship has been determined by cardiac catheterization. It is depicted in Fig. 7.3. The importance of pressure volume loop shall become apparent during the discussion on congestive heart failure (Fig. 14.4).

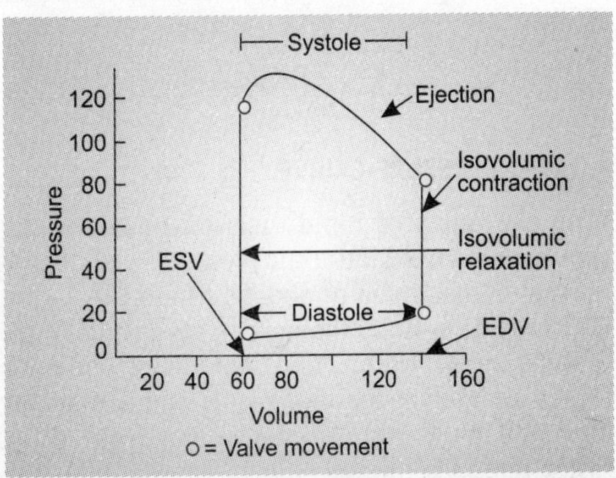

Fig. 7.3: Pressure volume loop in a cardiac cycle.

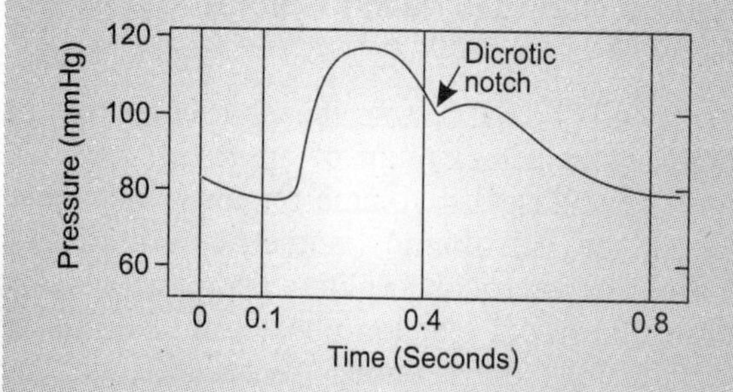

Fig. 7.4: Aortic pressure curve.

VARIATIONS IN DURATION OF SYSTOLE AND DIASTOLE

An increase in heart rate reduces the duration of systole as well as diastole. The durations of cardiac (ventricular) systole are 0.3 sec and 0.16 sec at heart rates of 75/min and 200/min, respectively. More significant, however, is the still greater reduction in the duration of ventricular diastole from 0.5 sec. to 0.14 sec. (Table 7.2). As mentioned above, most of the ventricular filling occurs during diastole. At very fast heart rates, the ventricular filling may be compromised to such an extent that the output of heart decreases.

Table 7.2: Effect of heart rate on the duration of cardiac systole and diastole

H.R.	*Duration (Seconds)*		
	Cardiac cycle	*Systole*	*Diastole*
75/min	0.8	0.3	0.5
200/min	0.3	0.16	0.14

AORTIC PRESSURE CURVE (Fig. 7.4)

With the onset of rapid ejection phase of the ventricular systole, the aortic pressure rises steeply to reach a maximum of about 120 mmHg. In the later part of systole, the aortic pressure declines to some extent. The ejection of blood into the aorta causes a stretch on the aortic walls, and also makes the blood in the entire arterial system to move at a faster rate. The decrease in the aortic pressure, starting in the later part of ventricular systole, continues throughout the ventricular diastole, to reach a minimum of about 80 mmHg during the isometric contraction phase of the next cardiac cycle. The elastic recoil of the aorta and the resistance of arterioles help to maintain relatively high aortic pressure during diastole.

A notch (also called incisura) is recorded in the early part of down stroke of the aortic pressure curve. It corresponds to the closure of the aortic valves. It is produced by the sudden backward flow of aortic blood followed by the immediate cessation of backflow due to closure of the aortic valves.

ATRIAL PRESSURE CURVE

In the atrial pressure curve, three positive waves named; a, c and v can be observed (Fig. 7.5). The first positive wave (a-wave) corresponds to the atrial systole. The isometric contraction phase of the ventricular systole causes closure followed by bulging of the AV valves into the atria, producing the c-wave. Following c-wave, there is a sudden decline in the intra-atrial pressure, corresponding to the rapid ejection phase of ventricular systole. Shortening of ventricular muscle during this phase suddenly pulls down the fibrous AV ring causing enlargement of the atrial lumen and thus decreasing the intra-atrial pressure. The third positive wave, v-wave, is partly due to the release of fibrous AV ring at the end of ventricular systole and partly due to atrial filling by the venous blood. The atrial pressure declines when the AV valves open and the blood rushes into the ventricles.

The atria are thin-walled chambers. When they contract, the AV valves are already open. Therefore, the intra-atrial pressure remains low even during atrial systole (Table 7.1).

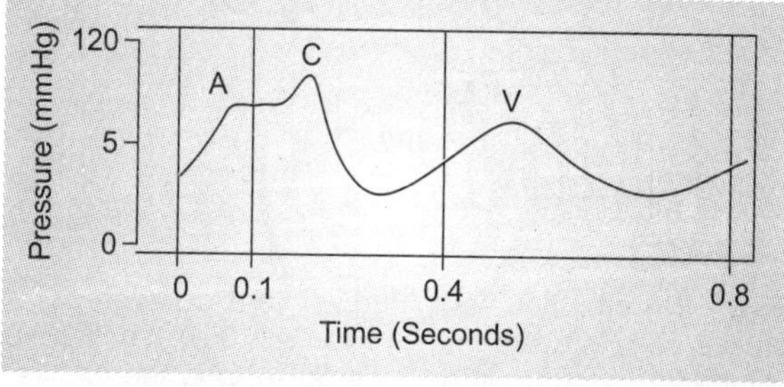

Fig. 7.5: Atrial pressure curve.

Jugular Venous Pulse

Changes in the right atrial pressure result in corresponding waves form in the right internal and external jugular veins, because they are in direct communication with the right atrium. Therefore, changes in the right atrium can be predicted by merely observing the pattern of pulsations in the jugular veins. Study of right internal jugular vein pulsations is more reliable than observation on the external vein because: (i) external jugular vein contains venous valves which interfere with the conduction of pressure pulses from the right atrium, and (ii) external jugular vein passes through more facial planes than the internal jugular vein. Therefore, it is more likely to be affected by extrinsic compression from other structures in the neck and thorax.

Jugular venous pulse tracing shows three positive waves, namely 'a', 'c' and 'v' and two negative waves named 'x' and 'y'. The 'c' wave is so small that its presence cannot be appreciated by visual examination (Fig. 7.6).

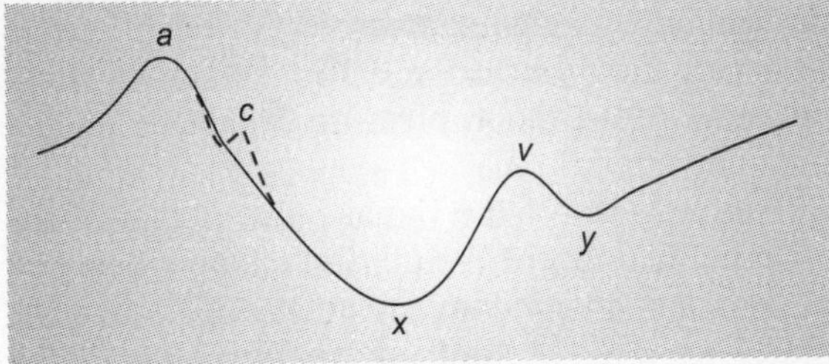

Fig. 7.6: Jugular venous pulse.

The 'a' wave is most prominent of the three positive waves. It is caused by atrial systole due to an abrupt stoppage of blood flow from superior vena cava into the right atrium. Decline in the 'a' wave follows the end of atrial systole. The small 'c' wave is caused by an increase in right atrial pressure due to bulging of the tricuspid valve into the right atrium during the isovolumic contraction phase. The negative 'x' wave represents the fall in right atrial pressure caused by descent of fibrous AV ring during the rapid ejection phase, leading to an enlargement of the atrium. The third positive 'v' represents the rise in right atrial pressure due to: (i) inflow of blood into the right atrium, when the tricuspid valve is closed, and (ii) relaxation of fibrous AV ring at the end of ventricular systole. The negative 'y' wave represents the decline in right atrial pressure following opening of the tricuspid valve.

Prominent 'a' waves are caused by:

(a) Right atrial hypertrophy due to tricuspid stenosis or pulmonary hypertension. In such cases, the right atrial pressure rises more markedly during systole since the atrium contracts against a narrowed valve or non-compliant ventricle, respectively.
(b) Cannon waves: In cases with complete heart block (discussed in the next chapter), there is complete dissociation between atrial and ventricular contractions. So, occasionally, atria contract when the AV valves are closed because of simultaneous ventricular contraction. All the force of right atrial contraction is transmitted back into the great veins, producing *giant 'a' waves (cannon waves)*. The cannon waves are interspersed in normal 'a' waves. 'a' wave is absent in cases with atrial fibrillation.

Prominent 'c' waves or *giant 'c' waves* are seen in cases with tricuspid valve incompetence due to regurgitation of blood into the right atrium during ventricular systole.

Cardiac Catheterization

The pressure and volume changes in various chambers of the heart have been investigated by cardiac catheterization (Fig. 7.7). The technique involves insertion of a long and flexible catheter into a *vein* at the elbow. Under fluoroscopic control, it is pushed up through the various venous channels into the right atrium, right ventricle and the pulmonary artery. By using pressure and volume sensors at the catheter tip, measurements can be made in the right heart. Blood samples can be withdrawn from each chamber of the right heart and pulmonary artery and analyzed for its oxygen content. The procedure described above is known as *right heart catheterization*. The procedure is absolutely safe and routinely used in cardiology departments.

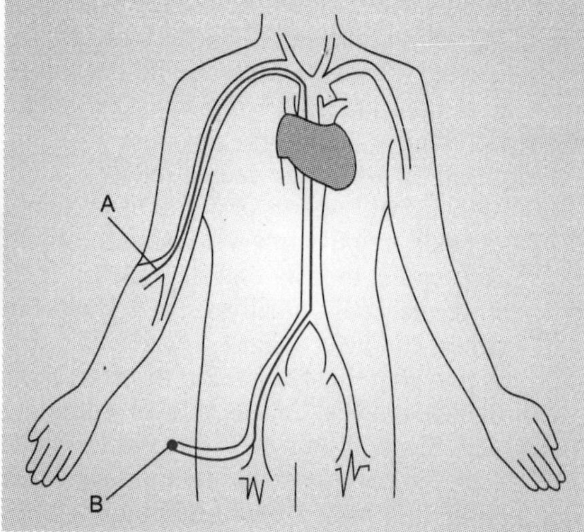

Fig. 7.7: Path of cardiac catheter. **A.** Catheter inserted through a blood vessel in the arm, **B.** Catheter inserted through a blood vessel in the groin.

Left heart catheterization involves insertion of a catheter in a *femoral artery* and pushing it up under fluoroscopic control till it reaches the left ventricle and then the left atrium.

Indications for Cardiac Catheterization

(i) Measurement of pressure and volume in various chambers of the heart and great vessels.

(ii) By taking blood samples, oxygen concentration of blood in various chambers of the heart and great vessels can be known. Pressure and oxygen concentration values are useful in the diagnosis of various types of congenital heart defects like atrial septal defect, ventricular septal defect, patent ductus arteriosus, etc.

(iii) Cardiac catheterization is required for estimation of cardiac output by Fick principle.

(iv) By releasing radio-contrast media, cardiac catheterization can be used to visualize the cardiac chambers.

(v) Coronary arteriography: Patency of the coronary artery and its major branches can be tested by releasing contrast media in the coronary artery through left heart catheterization.

(vi) Coronary angioplasty: Dilatation of a narrowed segment of coronary artery can be achieved by inflating a balloon at the tip of the catheter inserted in the coronary artery.

(vii) Balloon valvuloplasty: A narrowed cardiac valve may be dilated using a balloon tipped catheter.

Arterial Pulse

As mentioned before, ejection of blood into the aorta during systole stretches the wall of the ascending aorta. The stretch of the aorta sets up a pressure wave that travels with a velocity considerably faster than the velocity of blood flow. In young adults, the pressure pulse travels at a velocity of 4 m/S in the aorta; 8 m/S in large arteries; 16 m/S in small arteries. The velocity of arterial pulse is inversely related to the amount of elastic fibres in the arterial wall. The velocity increases with age due to a gradual decrease in the elasticity of the arterial tree.

The strength (volume) of the arterial pulse is determined by the pulse pressure, i.e. the difference between the systolic and the diastolic blood pressure. Mean blood pressure cannot be judged from the arterial pulse.

Examination of the radial pulse is one of the essential features of the clinical examination of a patient. It is a very convenient way of finding out the heart rate. In addition, the strength of the arterial pulse reflects the stroke volume of the heart. The radial pulse is fast and strong after exercise, indicating an increase in the rate and stroke volume of the heart. In hypovolemic shock, the pulse is fast but weak (thin and thready). Besides the radial artery, the arterial pulse can be palpated from many other superficial arteries, e.g. common carotid, brachial, femoral, dorsalis pedis. Clinically, the radial pulse is examined for the following features:

1. Rate of pulse.
2. Rhythm of pulse.
3. Volume of pulse.
4. Character of pulse.
5. Presence of any delay in femoral pulse compared to radial pulse.

1. Rate of Pulse Pulse rate in beats per minute is counted. Normally, the pulse rate reflects the heart rate (except in cases with pulse deficit: see below). Pulse rate is increased in conditions associated with tachycardia, e.g. exercise, emotional excitement, fever, thyrotoxicosis, haemorrhage, etc. It is also increased in abnormalities of cardiac rhythm like atrial tachycardia, flutter or fibrillation or ventricular tachycardia. Low pulse rate is seen in athletes (physiological bradycardia), raised intracranial pressure, complete heart block, myxoedema, jaundice, sick sinus syndrome, etc.

Pulse Deficit In atrial fibrillation, the pulse rate counted at the wrist is lower than the heart rate counted by auscultation at the apex beat. The difference between the two is known as pulse deficit (see atrial fibrillation, Chapter 8).

2. Rhythm of the Pulse Normally, the rhythm of the pulse is regular, i.e. it appears at regular intervals. An abnormal rhythm may be: (i) completely irregular, i.e. there is no rhythm at all, or (ii) irregularly irregular, i.e. otherwise regular rhythm is occasionally interrupted by an irregular beat. In atrial fibrillation, the pulse is completely irregular. Irregularly irregular rhythm is seen in patients with premature heart beats (extra-systoles) (see Chapter 8).

3. Volume of the Pulse The pulse volume is a rough guide to the pulse pressure (systolic blood pressure minus diastolic blood pressure) or stroke volume of the heart and vascular compliance. Pulse volume is high during exercise because of increased stroke volume. In old age, pulse volume is high even though stroke volume is normal. It is because of loss of elasticity (decreased compliance) of aorta and large arteries (Chapter 10).

4. Character of the Pulse The character of the pulse can be understood better if, at first, the graphic record of the radial (arterial) pulse is discussed (Fig. 7.8). Normally, arterial pulse tracing shows a rapid upstroke (an ascending limb) to a summit followed by a somewhat less rapid downstroke. A notch called dicrotic notch is present in the upper region of the downstroke followed by a secondary dicrotic wave. The arterial wave pattern basically follows the aortic pressure wave pattern. The rise and fall of the radial pulse can be appreciated by palpation of the radial artery at the wrist. The pulse may show the following variations in its character.

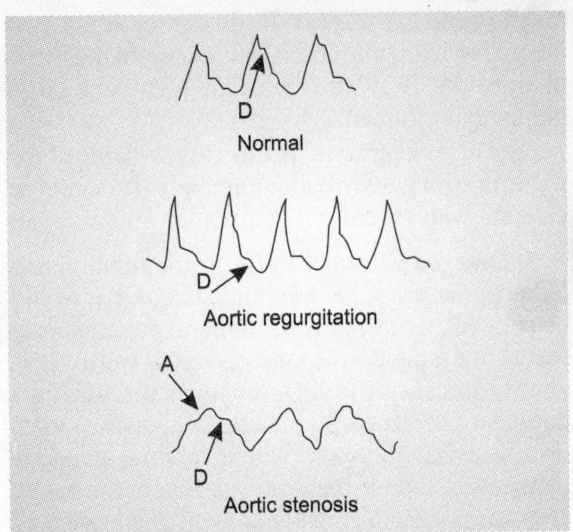

Fig. 7.8: Arterial pressure curve in a normal individual, a patient of aortic regurgitation, and a patient of aortic stenosis. (D) = dicrotic notch. A = anacrotic notch.

(a) *Slow rising pulse* (*anacrotic pulse*): It is seen in patients with aortic valve stenosis. In this case, volume of the pulse is low and the upstroke is as slow as the downstroke. A notch called anacrotic notch may be recorded in the upper region of the upstroke (Fig. 7.8).

(b) *Collapsing pulse (water hammer pulse)* It is a high volume pulse with rapid upstroke and an equally rapid (collapsing) downstroke. It is seen in patients with aortic valve regurgitation (Fig. 7.8). During systole, the ejection of a large volume of blood produces the large upstroke. The rapid downstroke of the pulse is caused by regurgitation of blood from the aorta into the left ventricle through the incompetent aortic valve during the diastole. The regurgitated blood is added to the blood coming from the right ventricle. Therefore, a larger than normal volume of blood is ejected during each ventricular systole.

(c) *Bisferiens pulse* It is a combination of low rising pulse with a collapsing downstroke. It is seen in patients suffering from both aortic valve stenosis as well as incompetence.

(d) *Pulsus paradoxus* In this case, volume of the pulse shows marked decrease during each inspiration. It is an important sign of a large pericardial effusion.

(e) *Pulsus alternans* In this case, volume of the pulse is strong and weak alternately. It occurs in patients with severe left ventricular failure.

5. Delayed Femoral Pulse If the femoral and radial pulses are palpated simultaneously, it would be noticed that normally the femoral pulse appears earlier than the corresponding radial pulse. It is simply because the difference in the distance between the ascending aorta (where the pulse originates) and the site where femoral artery is palpated is shorter than the site where the radial artery is palpated. In patients with coarctation of the aorta (a congenital narrowing of the aorta in the area where the ductus arteriosus joins the aorta), the transmission of pulse to the femoral artery is delayed by the obstruction in the narrowed segment. Therefore in such cases, with each heart beat, the femoral pulse appears later than the radial pulse.

Heart Sounds and Murmurs

Four sounds are produced during each cardiac cycle. The first two can normally be heard through a stethoscope. With suitable amplification, all the four sounds can be recorded graphically. The record is known as a *phonocardiogram* (Fig. 7.9).

First Heart Sound (S_1)

It is relatively prolonged (0.15 S) and low pitched (frequency 25–45 Hz) sound. It is produced by the closure of *AV valves* at *the beginning of ventricular systole.* Though both the AV valves contribute to the production of S_1, the main contribution is by mitral valve, since higher pressure generates in the left ventricle makes it snap shut.

Second Heart Sound (S_2)

This heart sound is shorter in duration (0.12 S) and high pitched (50 Hz) than the S_1. It is produced by closure of the *semilunar valves* (chiefly aortic valve) at the *end of ventricular systole*. Phone-

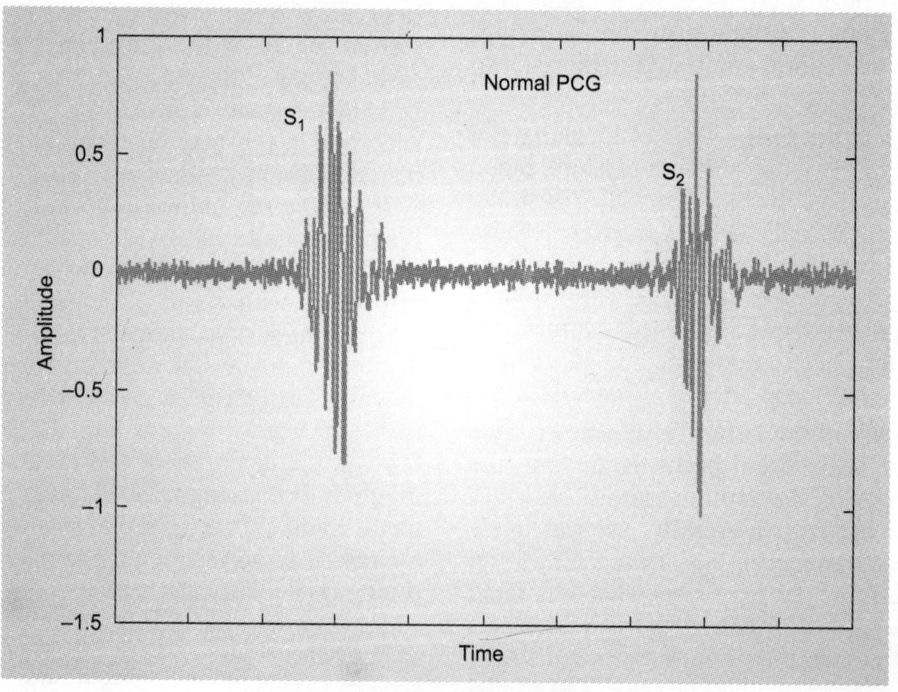

Fig. 7.9: A phonocardiogram.

tically, the first two heart sounds are described as *lubb* and *dup* respectively.

Third Heart Sound (S_3)

This heart sound coincides with the rapid filling phase of the ventricular diastole when tensing of chordae tendineae occurs because of rapid expansion of the ventricles. This soft low pitched sound can be heard with the stethoscope in children and some young adults only. When heard in a middle-aged or older patient, S_3 indicates a disease, e.g. congestive heart failure or mitral or tricuspid regurgitation.

Fourth Heart Sound (S_4)

The fourth heart sound consists of a few vibrations *recorded* during the atrial systole in a phonocardiogram. It is not heard by a stethoscope in normal individuals. When heard, it indicates a vigorously contracting atrium against a stiffened non-compliant ventricle.

Factors Affecting Intensity of First Heart Sound (S_1)

1. Velocity of AV Valve Closure It is the most important factor. At fast heart rate, S_1 is louder than normal.

2. Integrity of AV Valve A diseased AV valve may not close completely, resulting in decreased intensity of S_1, e.g. in mitral or tricuspid regurgitation.

3. Mobility of AV Valve If the mitral valve is calcified and relatively fixed, S_1 is attenuated (decreased intensity).

4. Status of Ventricular Contraction In patients with severe anaemia, anxiety or pregnancy, S_1 is usually louder than normal because of stronger ventricular wall contraction. On the other hand, weak myocardial contraction produces attenuated S_1, e.g. in patients with acute myocardial infarction, myxoedema or cardiac myopathy.

5. Transmission Characteristics of Thoracic Cavity Obesity, emphysema, pericardial effusion would decrease the intensity of all heart sounds because these conditions interfere with the transmission of heart sounds from the heart to the stethoscope.

Factors Affecting Intensity of Second Heart Sound (S_2)

1. Pressure in the Aorta or Pulmonary Artery S_2 is found to be of louder intensity in systemic or pulmonary hypertension. In these conditions, the retrograde flow of blood in the arterial trunks at the beginning of ventricular diastole strikes with greater force against the closed semilunar valves.

2. Same as factor 5 above.

AUSCULTATORY AREAS OF PRECORDIUM

Normal heart sounds, as well as, murmurs due to defect of different valves, are conducted in particular directions and are best heard over specific areas of the chest. These areas are known as the auscultatory areas (Fig. 7.10). An auscultatory area is not located directly over the anatomic position of the particular valve.

(i) The *mitral area* corresponds to the apex beat.
(ii) The *tricuspid area* lies just to the left of lower sternum.
(iii) The *aortic area* is at the right of sternum in the second intercostal space.
(iv) The *pulmonary* area is at the left of sternum in the second intercostals space.

Murmurs

Auscultation of the first two heart sounds is an important part of the clinical examination of a patient since they indicate the beginning and the end of ventricular systole, respectively. Many valvular defects of the heart can be diagnosed accurately by careful auscultation, since these defects produce abnormal heart sounds called 'murmurs'.

A murmur is defined as a relatively prolonged series of *audible vibrations heard between the heart sounds*. Murmurs may vary in intensity (loudness), frequency (pitch) and duration. Any murmur heard between first (S_1) and the second heart sound (S_2) is called a systolic murmur. A murmur heard between S_2 and S_1 is known as a diastolic murmur.

Murmurs are basically produced by turbulence in the blood as it flows through a cardiac valve or a narrowed blood vessel. Turbulence in blood flow arises when the blood flow velocity becomes

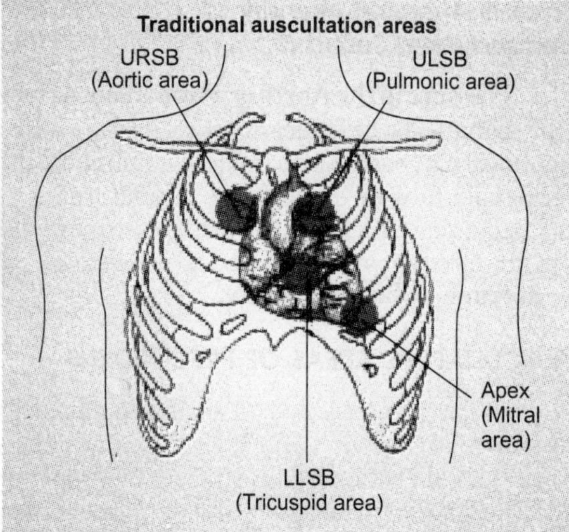

Fig. 7.10: Auscultatory areas. URSB upper right sternal border. ULSB upper left sternal border. LLSB lower left sternal border.

critically high. In the heart, it may happen because of four reasons:

(i) High blood flow rate across a normal valve, e.g. in patients with hyperdynamic circulation due to severe anaemia or hyperthyroidism.

(ii) Blood flow across a partial obstruction, e.g. stenosed aortic or mitral valve.

(iii) Regurgitant blood flow across an incompetent valve, e.g. incompetent aortic or mitral valve.

(iv) Shunting of blood from a high pressure chamber to a low pressure chamber of the heart across an abnormal opening, e.g. atrial septal defect, ventricular septal defect or patent ductus arteriosus.

SYSTOLIC MURMURS

Systolic murmur would be produced when turbulence in blood flow occurs during systole of cardiac cycle; e.g. blood flow through the stenotic (narrowed) aortic valve, or regurgitation of blood from the left ventricle into left atrium due to mitral valve incompetence. Although both these abnormalities produce systolic murmurs (Fig. 7.11), the disorders can be differentiated because.

(i) Systolic murmur of aortic stenosis would be best heard at the right second intercostals space near the sternum (aortic area), whereas that due to mitral regurgitation would be best heard over the apex of the heart (mitral area).

(ii) The murmur due to mitral regurgitation (MR) shall be heard throughout systole (pansystolic murmur), because the left

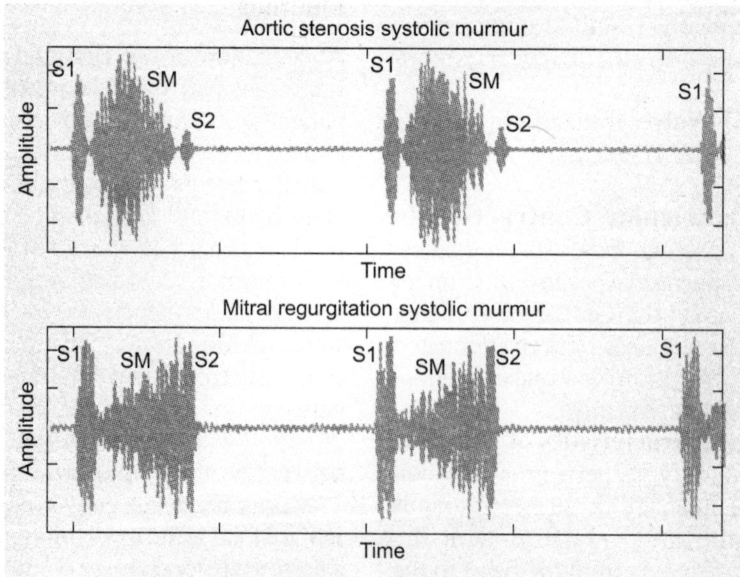

Fig. 7.11: Systolic murmurs.

ventricular pressure exceeds left atrial pressure throughout systole. So, the blood regurgitates throughout systole. In aortic stenosis, it would be heard in the middle of systole (midsystolic murmur), since there is no blood flow during the initial isovolumic contraction phase and blood flow slows down in the last part of systole (slow ejection phase).

In ventricular septal defect (VSD), the left ventricular pressure is greater than right ventricular pressure throughout systole. Therefore, abnormal blood flow from left to the right ventricle would continue throughout systole. In other words, a pansystolic murmur would be produced. There is no confusion with MR because in VSD, the murmur is best heard at the left sternal edge.

Diastolic Murmurs

Diastolic murmur shall be produced by a turbulence in blood flow occurring during diastolic phase of cardiac cycle (Fig. 7.12). It could be due to regurgitation of blood from the aorta into the left ventricle due to an incompetent aortic valve (aortic regurgitation or aortic valve incompetence).

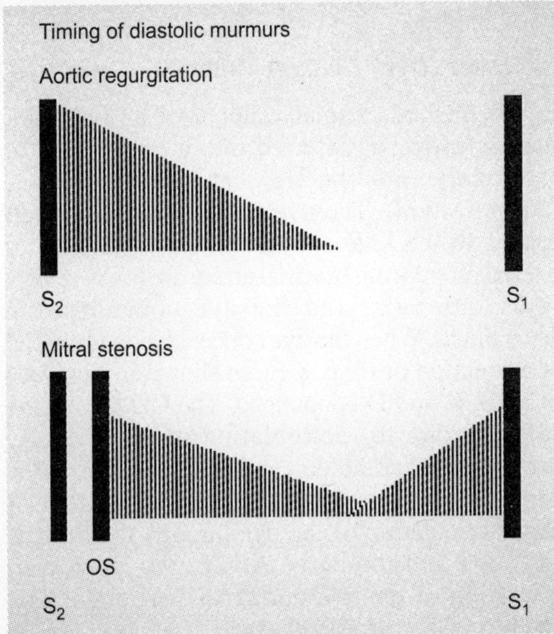

Fig. 7.12: Diastolic murmurs: (a) Early diastolic murmur. (b) mid-diastolic murmur.

Such a diastolic murmur would be best heard over the aortic area, but in early diastole only (early diastolic murmur).

Diastolic murmur, best heard over the mitral area, is due to stenosis of the mitral valve (mitral stenosis). The narrow valve interferes with the flow of blood from the left atrium to the left ventricle during the rapid filling phase of ventricular diastole. Therefore, the murmur due to mitral valve stenosis shall begin to be heard during middle of diastole only (mid-diastolic murmur).

Detailed discussion of various types of cardiac murmurs is beyond the scope of this book. Some examples have been cited above to illustrate the importance of the knowledge of events in the cardiac cycle in diagnosis of some of the cardiac disorders.

CARDIAC OUTPUT

Cardiac output is the quantity of blood pumped by the left ventricle into the aorta each minute. In adults, the average cardiac output is about 5 litres/min.

The cardiac output in females is approximately 10% less than in males of the same body size.

Cardiac output is related to the body surface area. Therefore, it may be described in terms of *Cardiac Index*. The cardiac index is defined as the cardiac output per minute per square metre of body surface area. Average cardiac index is about 3.2 L/min/m^2 of BSA. The cardiac output is sometimes described in terms of *stroke volume (or stroke output)* instead of minute output defined above. Stroke volume is the amount of blood pumped out of either of the two ventricles per beat. Normal stroke volume is approximately 70 ml. Therefore:

$$\begin{aligned}\text{Cardiac output} &= \text{Stroke volume (ml)} \times \text{Heart rate (per min.)}\\ &= 70 \times 75 = 5250 \text{ ml}\\ &\cong 5 \text{ L per minute}\end{aligned}$$

Since, the stroke output of the two ventricles is similar, it would be obvious that the cardiac output of the right ventricle is equal to that of the left ventricle.

MEASUREMENT OF CARDIAC OUTPUT

In animals, the cardiac output may be directly measured by placing an electromagnetic or ultrasonic flow meter over the aorta. Indirect methods used to measure the cardiac output in humans are described below.

7

Fick Principle Method

Fick principle is an important concept which can be used to calculate the cardiac output or the blood flow rate in many other organs (e.g. the liver, kidney).

Fick principle states that the amount of any substance taken up or excreted by an organ per minute (x) must be equal to the rate of blood flow per minute (Q) multiplied by the difference between the concentration of the substance before (C_1) and after (C_2) passing through the organ.

$$X = Q \times (C_1 - C_2)$$

$$\therefore \quad Q = \frac{X}{C_1 - C_2}$$

By measuring the amount of O_2 taken up by the blood from the lungs and the O_2 concentration difference between the pulmonary artery (PAO_2) and the pulmonary vein (PVO_2), the amount of blood flow through the lungs per minute can be calculated (Fig. 7.13).

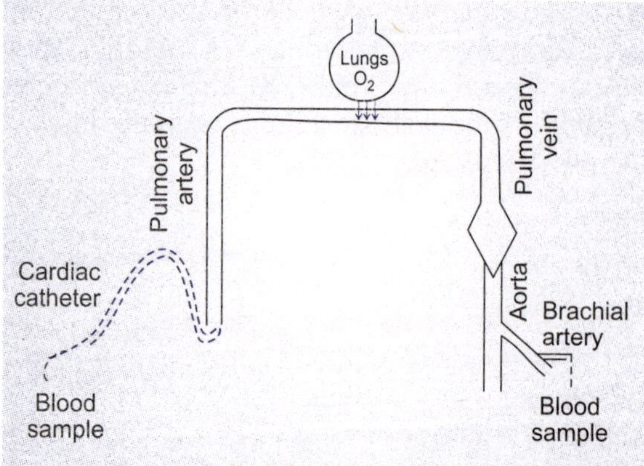

Fig. 7.13: Estimation of cardiac output by Fick principle.

It may be remembered that:

Right ventricular output = Pulmonary blood flow/mt
= Left ventricular output

$$\therefore \quad \text{Cardiac output} = \frac{O_2 \text{ consumption (uptake) per minute}}{PVO_2 - PAO_2}$$

In actual practice, the O_2 uptake from the lungs is known by using a spirometer. A sample of blood is obtained from the pulmonary artery by cardiac catheterization. Because of practical difficulties, blood sample from a pulmonary vein cannot be obtained. However, the blood sample from any peripheral artery (e.g. brachial artery) can be used since the oxygen content of all the major arteries is almost similar to that of pulmonary veins. A typical set of values for the calculation of cardiac output is given below:

O_2 uptake = 250 ml/min

O_2 content of venous (Pulmonary arterial) blood = 14 ml/100 ml

O_2 content of arterial (Brachial arterial) blood = 19 ml/100ml

$$\therefore \text{Cardiac output} = \frac{250}{19 - 14} = \frac{250}{5 \text{ ml}/100} = \frac{250 \times 100}{5}$$

$$= 5 \text{ L per minute}$$

Indicator (Dye) Dilution Method

In this method, a small amount of an indicator, such as a dye, is injected into a large vein (or preferably into the right atrium by cardiac catheterization). The dye passes through the left heart into the arterial system. Serial samples of arterial blood from brachial artery are taken at very short intervals, and the dye concentration determined. When the dye concentration is plotted as a function of time, a curve shown in Fig. 7.14 as A, B, C and D is obtained. The CD part of the curve is due to recirculation of the dye. By extrapolation of the descending limb (BC) of the curve to the time scale (BCE), the duration of single circulation of the dye through the heart is known. From the curve ABCE, the mean concentration of the dye during its first circulation can be calculated as follows:

The area under the triangle ABE is represented as a rectangle, with same area but with base of the

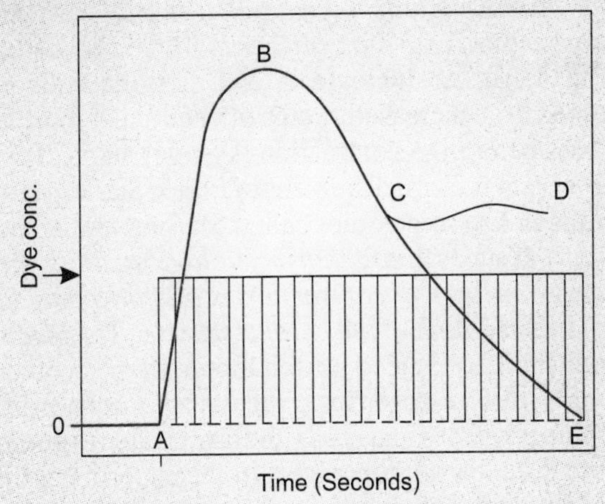

Fig. 7.14: Estimation of cardiac output by indicator dye dilution method. The arrow points at the calculated mean dye concentration.

rectangle as AE, which represents the duration of 1st circulation of the dye.

From these values, the cardiac output can be calculated as follows:

$$\underset{\text{(in 1/min)}}{\text{Cardiac output}} = \frac{\text{Dye injected in mg} \times 60}{\underset{\text{(mg/1)}}{\text{Mean dye conc.}} \times \underset{\text{(in second)}}{\text{Duration of 1st circulation}}}$$

The nature of the dye should be such that it stays in circulation for the duration of the test, and has no toxic or haemodynamic effects.

In recent years, *thermodilution method* has become more popular. In this method, cold saline is injected into the right atrium through one side of a double-lumened catheter and the temperature change in the blood of the pulmonary artery is recorded through a thermister placed at the tip of the catheter. The temperature change is inversely proportionate to the amount of blood flow through the pulmonary artery, i.e. we determine the extent to which cold saline is diluted by the blood. Since cold is dissipated in the tissues, the problem of recirculation does not occur. Moreover, brachial arterial puncture is not required in this method.

Echocardiography

It is one of the most widely used test for the diagnosis of cardiovascular disease. Its most important feature is that it is non-invasive and has no risk or side effect. In this method, pulses of ultrasonic waves at a frequency of 2.25 MHz are emitted from a transducer that also functions as a receiver to detect sound waves reflected from various parts of the heart (Fig. 7.15).

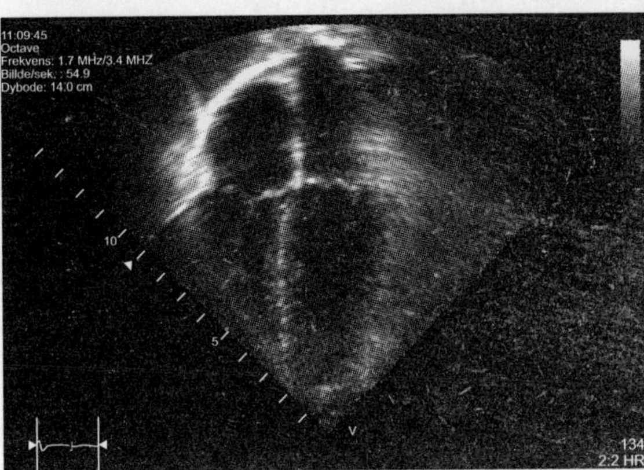

Fig. 7.15: An echocardiogram.

Echocardiography can be used to detect the following:

- Size and shape of the heart.
- Thickness of the various chambers of the heart.
- Condition of the valves.
- Congenital cardiac defects
- Cardiac output : Easiest and safest method.
- Ejection fraction
- Ischemic necrosis

Causes of Increased Cardiac Output

(A) *Physiological*

- Exercise (CO increases up to 25–35 L/min)
- Pregnancy
- High environmental temperature
- Anxiety (50–100%.)
- After food intake (30%.)

(B) *Pathological*

- Severe anaemia
- Hyperthyroidism

- Beriberi (vitamin B_1 deficiency)
- Arteriovenous fistula
- Polycythaemia

Causes of Decreased Output

(A) *Physiological*

- Change from supine to standing posture (20–30%.)

(B) *Pathological*

- Congestive heart failure
- Haemorrhage
- Burns
- Extensive surgery
- Dehydration
- Myocardial infarction
- Cardiac arrhythmias
- Toxic myocarditis
- Anaphylactic shock

REGULATION OF CARDIAC OUTPUT

Cardiac output can change from a resting value of 5 L/min to more than 25 L/min during exercise. Increase in cardiac output could be because of an increase in one or both of the two variables that determine the cardiac output, i.e. heart rate and stroke volume, (since CO = HR × SV). Under physiological conditions, the cardiac output may increase because of a change in *intrinsic regulation* (change within the heart) or a change in *extrinsic regulation* (a change in the neural input to the heart. The importance of intrinsic regulation can be experimentally shown by studying the cardiac output in a dog after complete denervation. If such a dog is made to run, the increase in cardiac output is almost similar to that in a normal dog undergoing similar exercise.

Intrinsic Regulation of Cardiac Output (Frank-Starling Mechanism)

This phenomenon was shown by two physiologists Otto Frank and Earnest Starling. Using a denervated heart, they found that *within physiological limits, the stroke volume increased linearly with an increase in end-diastolic volume of the heart* (Fig. 7.16). An increase in end diastolic volume results in an increased stretch of ventricular muscle fibres before the contraction (systole) starts. This observation formed the basis of Frank-Starling law of the heart (some times called Starling law of the heart). It states that *within physiological limits, the energy or force of contraction is proportionate to the initial length of the cardiac muscle* (The law is applicable to skeletal muscle fibres also). In other words, due to an intrinsic regulatory mechanism, within physiological limits, the heart is able to pump out all the blood it receives. In the experiment on denervated dog mentioned above, the exercise increased venous return to the heart. Thus, in each diastole, there was greater ventricular filling and therefore the ventricular muscle fibres underwent greater stretch. Therefore, the ventricles pumped out greater amount of blood with each systole. In other words, the *increase in cardiac output was because of an increase in stroke volume of the heart*, (because the heart rate cannot increase significantly during exercise after denervation of the heart).

The molecular basis of the Frank-Starling law is the sarcomere geometry (Fig. 21.10). When a muscle is optimally stretched, there is formation

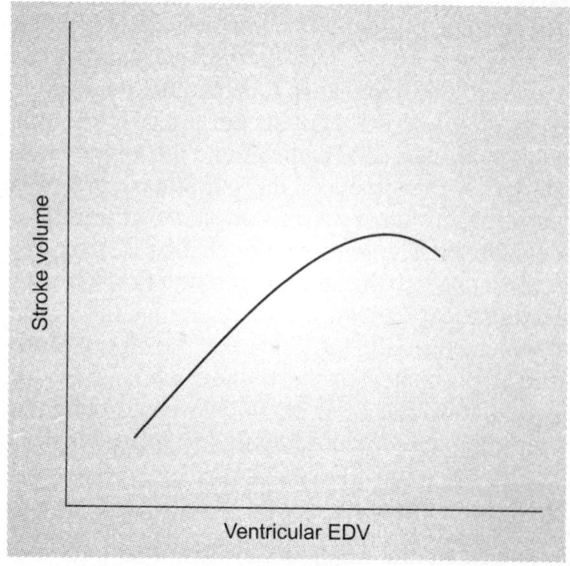

Fig. 7.16: Frank-Starling curve.

of largest number of cross-bridges between the actin and myosin filaments and hence maximum tension is developed during contraction. When the muscle is under-stretched or over-stretched, the cross-bridges formed are lesser and hence tension developed is less. (See Chapter 21 for details of this length tension relationship).

Extrinsic Regulation of Cardiac Output

Both the heart rate and stroke volume of the heart can be altered by an *extrinsic mechanism.* Increased sympathetic discharge to the heart increases the heart rate (chronotropic effect) as well as the stroke volume (force of ventricular contraction, inotropic effect). Thus the cardiac out put is increased proportionate to the increase in sympathetic discharge. Increase discharge in parasympathetic nerves to the heart decreases the cardiac output by decreasing mainly the heart rate.

In the extrinsic regulation, the increase in stroke volume is by a mechanism different from the intrinsic mechanism. In the extrinsic mechanism, the increase in stroke volume is achieved by better emptying as shown be a *decrease in end-systolic volume of the heart.* Under the effect of catecholamines, the cardiac muscle contracts more forcibly. Thus at the end of each systole, only about 30 ml of blood may be left in each ventricle in stead of the usual 50 ml (see cardiac cycle discussed above).

Even under the effect of extrinsic regulation, the intrinsic regulation, the fundamental property of cardiac muscle, persists (Fig. 7.17). In other words, the heart can utilize both the intrinsic as well as extrinsic mechanism simultaneously. Epinephrine and norepinephrine released from adrenal medulla and circulating in the blood can also activate the extrinsic mechanism and increase the cardiac output.

INTEGRATED CONTROL OF CARDIAC OUTPUT

In the previous section, the intrinsic and extrinsic mechanisms regulating the cardiac output have been described. Their relative role in the production of increased cardiac output in exercising animals/ humans is a matter of debate.

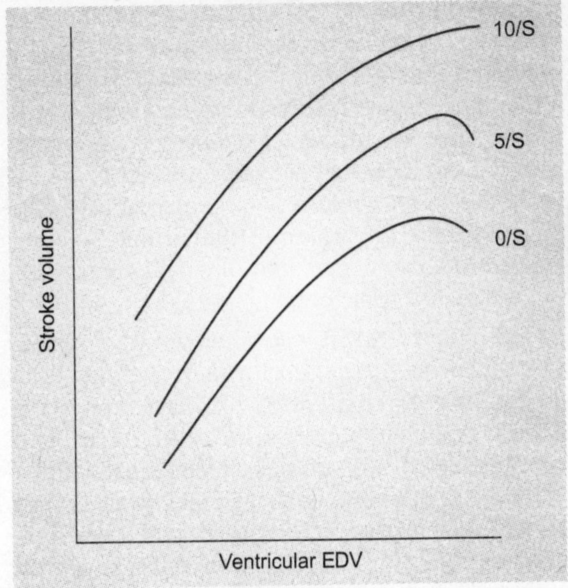

Fig. 7.17: Family of Frank-Starling curves at various rates of sympathetic stimulation.

Some authors attribute the increased cardiac output in mild and moderate exercise to an increase in venous return. According to them, the increased venous return increases the cardiac output by Frank-Starling mechanism alone. Sympathetic stimulation increases the cardiac output only when the exercise is severe enough to require cardiac output greater than 15 L/min (in humans). There is no doubt that the venous return is increased in exercise. In a closed circulation, the cardiac output and venous return have to be equal; the heart cannot pump out more blood than it receives for any length of time (except transiently). The only question is: do we observe an increase in end-diastolic volume of the heart during exercise (because the prerequisite for Frank-Starling mechanism is the change in end-diastolic volume)?

Actual measurements of end-diastolic and end-systolic volumes in exercising animals and humans have revealed no change or even a decrease in the end-diastolic volume in mild to moderate exercise. At the same time, there is evidence of increased sympathetic discharge to the heart (i.e. decrease end-systolic volume and tachycardia). It is apparent that the increased venous return, produced by skeletal vasodilatation, muscle pump action and increased respiration, is tackled by improved pumping ability of the heart. Therefore, it may be inferred that the pumping ability of the heart is increased by greater sympathetic discharge in mild and moderate exercise. In severe exercise, when the venous return is large enough to raise the end-diastolic volume, the Frank-Starling mechanism also comes into play and contributes to very high cardiac output.

The Frank-Starling mechanism is a fundamental intrinsic regulator, which operates even during resting conditions, by maintaining the precise balance between the outputs of two ventricles. The two ventricles eject equal amount of blood per stroke, even though they work against widely different peripheral resistance (i.e. right ventricle against 15 mmHg, left ventricle against 100 mmHg). Any discrepancy between the outputs of the two ventricles, if maintained for some time, would be disastrous. Moreover in patients with transplanted heart, the Frank-Starling mechanism is practically the only mechanism regulating the cardiac output.

Factors Affecting Myocardial Contractility

"Contractility is the inherent capacity of the myocardium to contract independently of changes in the preload or afterload. It remains an essential core concept to separate the effects of a primary change in loading conditions from an intrinsic change in the force of contraction. It is a basic property of cardiac muscle and is strictly linked to the activation quantity of actin myosin transverse bridges in the myocardial fibers, and to the velocity of cross-bridge activation at the systole onset.

Increased contractility, is reflected in higher myocardial fiber shortening velocity, with a more highly developed tension peak and a steeper pressure rise, when preload, afterload, and heart rate are constant: in the cytosol, calcium release is more and faster from SR with a higher cytosol calcium concentration in systole: more troponin is activated from higher levels of calcium with more actin-myosin cross-bridges, and ultimately myocardial fiber contraction is more forceful and faster.

Decreased contractility is reflected in lower myocardial fiber shortening velocity, with a lower tension peak and a blunted pressure rise, when preload, after load, and heart rate are constant: in the cytosol, calcium release is less and slower from SR with a lower cytosol calcium concentration in systole: less troponin is activated from lower levels of calcium with less actin-myosin cross-bridges, and ultimately myocardial fiber contraction is less forceful and slower.

Cardiac Contractility is Increased by

(i) Increased sympathetic neural discharge to the heart.
(ii) Circulating catecholamines
(iii) Digitalis
(iv) Dopamine

Cardiac Contractility is Decreased by

(i) Increased parasympathetic discharge to the heart
(ii) Loss of myocardium (myocardial infarction)
(iii) Congestive heart failure (Fig. 7.18)
(iv) Acidosis
(v) Hypoxia
(vi) Hypercapnoea

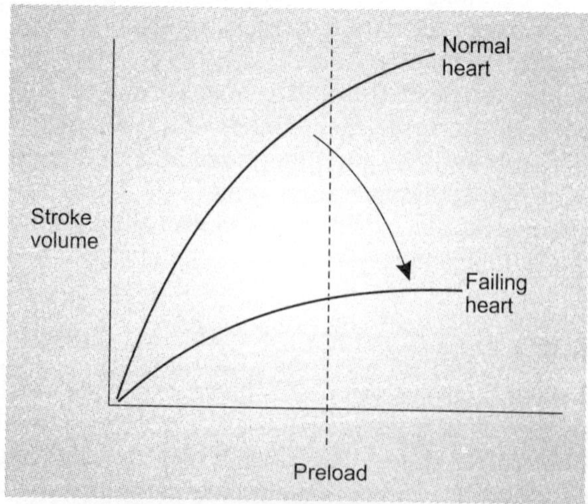

Fig. 7.18: Decrease in myocardial contractility.

(vii) Many pharmacological agents like verapamil.

Cardiac Preload and Afterload

Skeletal muscle or cardiac papillary muscle may be experimentally stimulated and made to lift a load. The load may act on the muscle before the contraction has started. This is called preloaded condition or simply preload (Fig. 7.19 A). If the load attached to the muscle is made to rest on a platform, it would act on the muscle only when the muscle begins to contract. This condition is called afterloaded condition or simply "afterload".

A muscle consists of: (i) contractile element (CE) namely actin and myosin filaments, and (ii) series-elastic (SE) element, namely, tendon. During preloaded condition, the load stretches the muscle (both CE and SE). On stimulation, the muscle contracts forcibly and lifts the weight (starling mechanism). In the afterloaded condition, there is no initial stretch on the muscle. On stimulation, initial contraction of CE merely leads to generation of tension in SE (isometric contraction). Only when the tension generated is greater than the load, shortening of the muscle occurs and the load is lifted. In either case, the load has been lifted but by increasing initial length, preload produce greater shortening than afterload (Fig. 7.19A and B).

In vivo, the diastolic filling of the left ventricle acts as preload whereas blood pressure (peripheral resistance) acts as afterload. As explained under intrinsic regulation of cardiac output, an increase in preload or afterload can be tackled by a normal heart by production of greater force of contraction (Starling mechanism). However, in a damaged heart, an excessive preload or afterload may precipitate congestive heart failure. Excessive blood volume would increase venous return to the heart and hence increase preload. Venular dilatation increases the size of venous reservoir and therefore, decreases the venous return (preload). An increase in peripheral resistance or aortic stenosis are examples of increased afterload. Modern treatment of angina pectoris or congestive heart failure involves medications to decrease the preload, afterload or both.

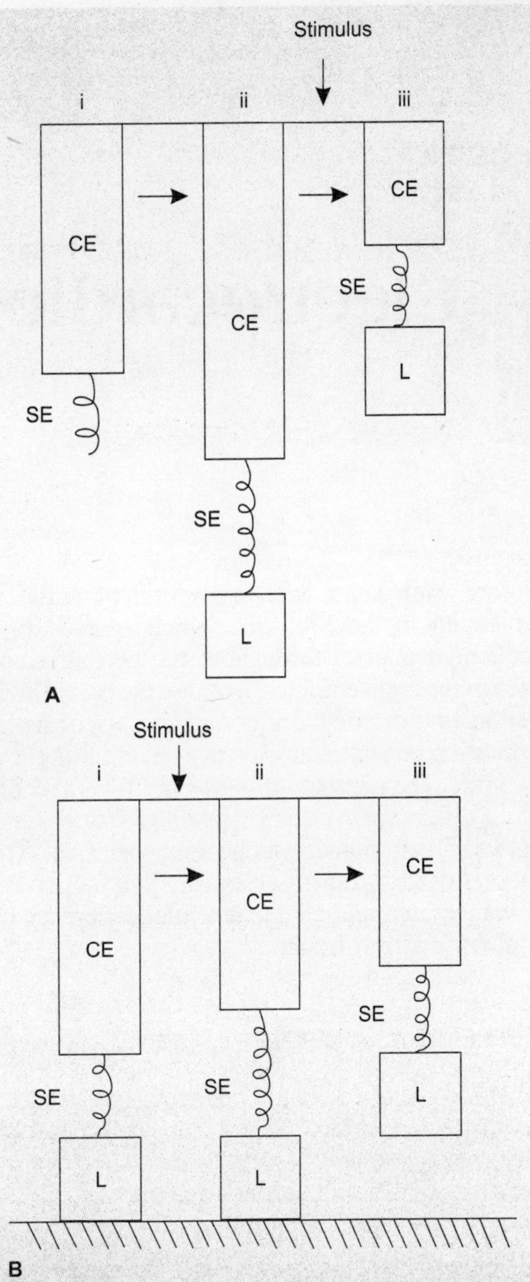

Fig. 7.19: Muscle contraction with a "preload" (A) and "afterload" (B). (Ai) Muscle unloaded. (Aii) "Pre-load" stretches CE and SE. (Aiii) Stimulation causes shortening of muscle and load is lifted. (Bi) "Afterload" does not stretch the muscle. (Bii) Stimulation causes partial contraction of CE and tension in SE but no shortening of muscle. (Biii) Further contraction of CE lifts the load off the platform (shortening of muscle).

CHAPTER 8

Electrocardiography

Before each heart beat, an action potential is generated in the SA node which spreads in a sequential manner throughout the two atria and then in the two ventricles. Because the body fluids act as a volume conductor, the myocardial excitation generates an electrical field throughout the body. The *electrocardiogram* (*ECG*) is a record of the difference in electrical potentials (or voltage) between two points on the body surface. The electrocardiograph, essentially a sensitive galvanometer, records the potential difference on a moving strip of paper.

THE HEART AS A DIPOLE

As the wave of excitation begins to spread in the heart, the depolarized surface of the cells becomes electronegative with respect to the region not yet depolarized. Thus the excited and the non-excited parts of the heart constitute a dipole or a two terminal battery, in which the excited part forms a negative pole and the non-excited part, the positive pole (Fig. 8.1). This phenomenon generates an electric field throughout the body fluids. The dipole spreads in a fixed direction. Therefore, depending on the position of the recording electrodes, the potential difference may produce a positive or a negative deflection. The galvanometer (electrocardiograph) is so adjusted that when the recording electrode faces the excitation front (positive side of the dipole) an upward deflection is recorded.

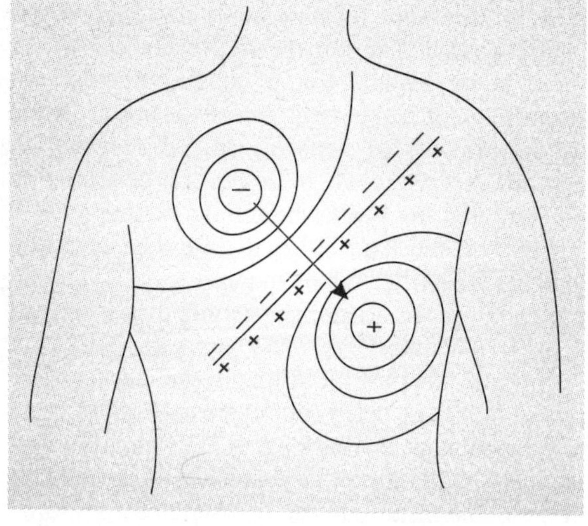

Fig. 8.1: The heart as a dipole.

As a result of sequential spread of the excitation front in the atria, the interventricular septum, the two ventricular walls (Fig. 8.2), and finally the repolarization of the myocardium, a series of positive and negative waves are generated. These positive and negative waves designated P, Q, R, S and T waves can be recorded with each heart beat (Fig. 8.3).

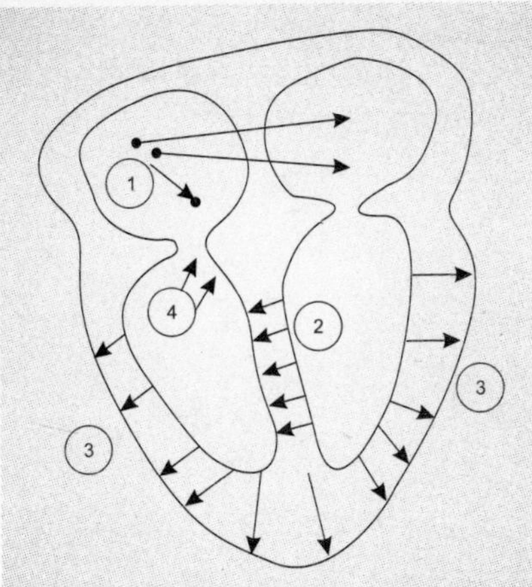

Fig. 8.2: Stages of sequential depolarization of the heart. 1. atria, 2. interventricular septum, 3. the two ventricular walls and finally, 4. the pulmonary conus region of the right ventricle.

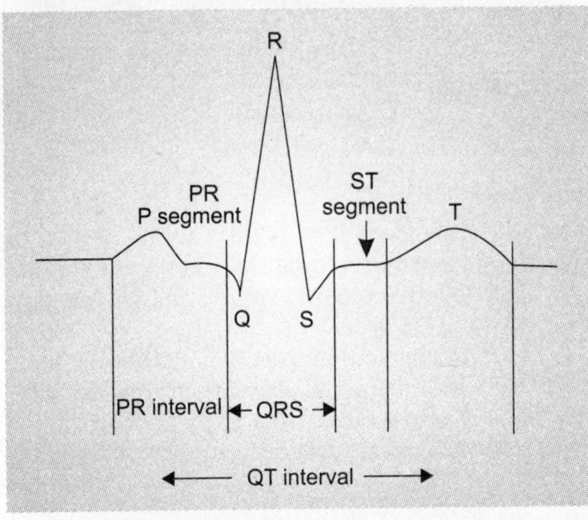

Fig. 8.3: Normal electrocardiogram.

ELECTROCARDIOGRAPHIC LEADS

An electrocardiogram is recorded by picking up potentials from two parts of the body. The two sites selected for this purpose constitute the electrocardiographic *lead*. Usually ECG is recorded using three bipolar (standard) limb leads, three unipolar limb leads and six unipolar chest leads.

Bipolar (Standard) Limb Leads

In bipolar recording, potential difference between two active electrodes placed on two limbs is recorded. It makes no difference whether the electrodes are placed in proximal or distal parts of the extremities, but for convenience they are placed near the wrists and ankles. Three electrodes are used, one each on the left arm, the right arm and the left leg. An electrode placed on the right leg is connected to an electrical ground to minimize electrical interference (Fig. 8.4). The standard bipolar limb leads are designated by Roman numerals.

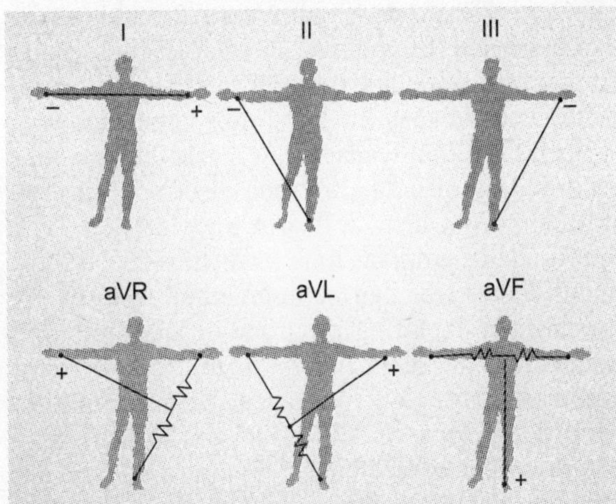

Fig. 8.4: Arrangement of electrodes in standard (bipolar) and unipolar limb leads.

Table 8.1 shows the position of the electrodes and their connection to the electrocardiograph in each of the three bipolar limb leads.

For example, in lead I, the electrode on the left arm is connected to the positive terminal and that

Table 8.1: Position of electrodes and their connection to the electrocardiograph in bipolar limb leads

Lead	*Positive terminal*	*Negative terminal*
I	Left arm (LA)	Right arm (RA)
II	Left leg (LL)	Right arm (RA)
III	Left leg (LL)	Left arm (LA)

on the right arm is connected to the negative terminal of the galvanometer (electrocardiograph).

Unipolar Leads

In unipolar leads, one *exploring* (active) *electrode* is placed over a limb (unipolar limb lead) or over the chest (unipolar chest lead) and connected to the positive terminal of the electrocardiograph. An *indifferent electrode,* kept at approximately zero potential by connecting electrodes placed at RA, LA and LL through a resistance, is connected to the negative terminal. By this arrangement, the instrument records the potential at the site of exploring electrode, since the potential at the indifferent electrode remains 'zero' throughout the cardiac cycle. In contrast, in each of the bipolar limb leads, the instrument records potential difference between the two limbs connected.

Unipolar limb leads VR, VL and VF are thus recorded by placing exploring electrode, turn by turn, on right arm, left arm and left leg. The amplitude of unipolar limb leads thus recorded is small. Their size can be augmented by 50% by placing the exploring electrode on one limb and connecting the *other two limbs* to the indifferent electrode through a resistance. For example, to record *augmented VR* (*aVR*) lead, exploring electrode is placed on the right arm while the left arm and left leg are connected to the indifferent electrode. For recording lead aVL, exploring electrode is placed on the left arm whereas right arm and left leg are connected to the indifferent electrode. In this way, augmented limb leads aVR, aVL and aVF are recorded (Fig. 8.4).

The position of the exploring electrode in unipolar limb leads and unipolar chest leads (precordial leads) is shown in Table 8.2. The unipolar leads are designated by the letter 'V'. Position of exploring electrodes in unipolar chest leads is as shown in Fig. 8.5.

The configuration of a typical electrocardiographic pattern observed in a bipolar limb lead is shown in Fig. 8.3 and shall be described in detail a little later. The configurations of ECG records in unipolar limb and unipolar chest leads are shown in Fig. 8.6. It would be apparent that the P, Q, R, S and T waves occur in all the leads simultaneously but with different shape and the polarity due to differences in the orientation of each lead with respect to the heart. The description of the pattern of record in different unipolar electrocardiographic leads is beyond the scope of this book.

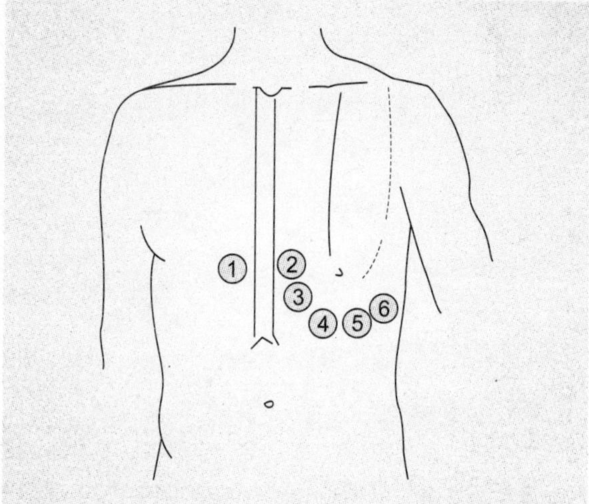

Fig. 8.5: Position of exploring electrodes in unipolar chest leads.

Table 8.2: Position of exploring electrodes in unipolar limb leads and unipolar chest leads

	Position of exploring electrode
Unipolar limb leads	
aVR	RA
aVL	LA
aVF	LL (F foot)
Unipolar chest leads (Fig. 8.5)	
V_1	Right fourth intercostal space at sternal margin
V_2	Left fourth intercostal space at sternal margin
V_3	Midway between V_2 and V_4
V_4	Left fifth intercostal space at midclavicular line
V_5	Left fifth intercostal space at anterior axillary line
V_6	Left fifth intercostal space at midaxillary line

CALIBRATION OF TIME AND VOLTAGE

The electrocardiogram is recorded on a special heat-sensitive graph paper having 1mm and 5 mm squares. The paper moves at a constant speed of 25 mm/S. On horizontal axis, therefore, each millimetre represents 0.04 sec. (1/25 S). The

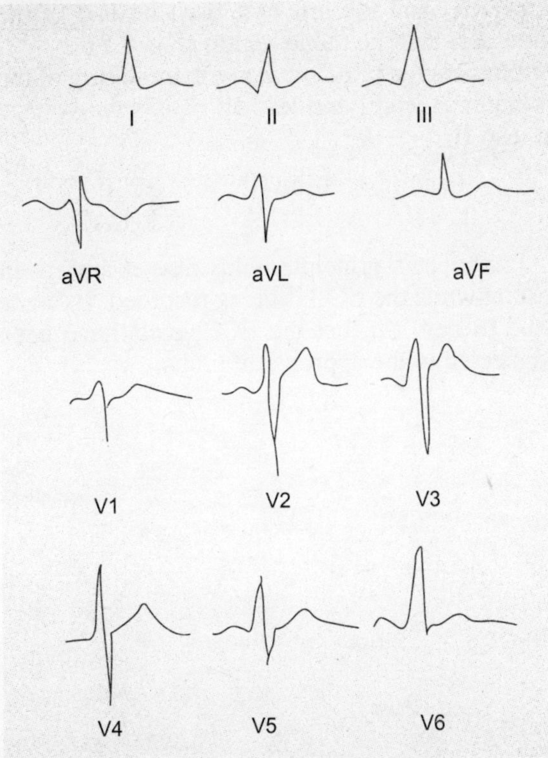

Fig. 8.6: Configurations of ECG records in bipolar limb leads (I, II, III), unipolar limb leads (aVR, aVL, aVF) and unipolar chest leads (V1-V6).

sensitivity of the electrocardiograph is adjusted in such a way that an impulse of 1 mV causes a vertical deflection of 10 mm. On vertical axis, therefore, each millimetre represents 0.1 mV potential (Fig. 8.7).

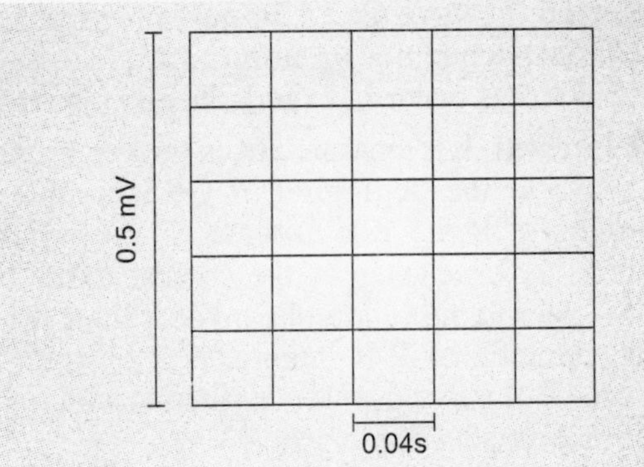

Fig. 8.7: Calibration of time and voltage in ECG.

Normal ECG (In a Bipolar Limb Lead)

The P wave The P wave is produced by atrial depolarization. It is an upright (positive) and rounded deflection. Normally, the duration of P wave is not more than 0.1 S and its height not more than 2.5 mm. In pathological conditions, P wave may be larger, bifid, and prolonged (e.g. in left atrial hypertrophy due to mitral stenosis). P wave could also be tall (5 mm) and peaked with normal duration, e.g. in right atrial hypertrophy (due to tricuspid stenosis). P wave may be inverted if (ectopic) cardiac impulses arise from a source other than the SA node (in atrial extrasystoles).

The QRS Complex The P wave is followed by a short isoelectric *P-R segment,* and then a QRS complex is recorded. The QRS complex represents ventricular depolarization. Q wave may be normally absent. When present, it is defined as the first downward deflection in the QRS complex, which precedes the R wave. R wave is the first upward (positive) deflection of the QRS complex. S wave is defined as the first downward deflection after the R wave. The normal duration of QRS complex ranges from 0.08 to 0.12 S. The normal depth of Q wave is less than 2 mm. Deep Q wave (along with the presence of other electrocardiographic signs described later) is an important sign of myocardial infarction. The R wave is usually a tall upward deflection, but its amplitude varies in different individuals. The taller R waves are seen in ventricular hypertrophy. Low voltage QRS complex (when the sum of Q, R, S waves in each of lead I, II, and III measures less than 5 mm) is seen in hypothyroidism or pericardial effusion. An R wave taller than 13 mm in lead I indicates left ventricular hypertrophy. Similarly, a tall R wave in lead III occurs in right ventricular hypertrophy. The duration of QRS complex is prolonged in bundle branch block.

The T Wave An isoelectric period called S-T segment follows the QRS complex. It gradually merges into the T wave. The T wave represents the ventricular repolarization. It is an upright (positive) dome-shaped deflection. Its height is usually between 2–5 mm and duration approximately 0.27 S.

Inverted T wave is an important sign of myocardial ischaemia or infarction. Tall and peaked T waves occur in hyperkalaemia.

PR Interval It is measured from the beginning of P wave to the beginning of QRS complex (beginning of R wave if Q wave is absent). It represents the time taken by the impulse to travel from SA node to the ventricular myocardium. The normal duration of P-R interval is 0.12–0.2 S. Prolonged P-R interval is seen in patients with first degree A-V conduction block.

QT Interval This interval is measured from the beginning of Q wave to the end of T wave. It represents ventricular depolarization and ventricular repolarization. The normal QT interval is up to 0.4 S. Prolonged QT interval is seen in patients with hypocalcaemia.

The duration of different electrocardiographic waves and intervals is summarized in Table 8.3. The wave due to atrial repolarization is not seen because the atria are repolarized when ventricles are being depolarized. The small wave caused by atrial repolarization is submerged in much larger QRS complex.

Table 8.3: Duration of electrocardiographic waves and intervals

	Duration (S)	*Cause*
P wave	0.1	Atrial depolarization
QRS complex	0.08–0.12	Ventricular depolarization
T wave	0.27	Ventricular repolarization
PR interval	0.12–0.2	Atrial and AV bundle conduction
QT interval	0.4	Ventricular depolarization + repolarization

Vector Analysis

The three standard bipolar limb leads are based on the assumption of the electrophysiologist, Einthoven, that the body is like an electrically homogeneous plate in which the right and left shoulders and the pubic region form the corners of an equilateral triangle with the heart in its centre (*Einthoven's hypothesis*). For convenience, the electrodes are connected to the left arm (LA), right arm (RA) and the left foot (LF) instead of the shoulders and the pubic region (Fig. 8.8).

Einthoven's principle states that the sum of the voltages in lead I and lead III equals the voltage in lead II.

Lead I	+	Lead III	=	Lead II
(LA-RA)		(LL-LA)		(LL-RA)

Einthoven's principle holds true at any given instant while the ECG is being recorded. It can be used to confirm that the ECG leads have been connected to the appropriate limbs.

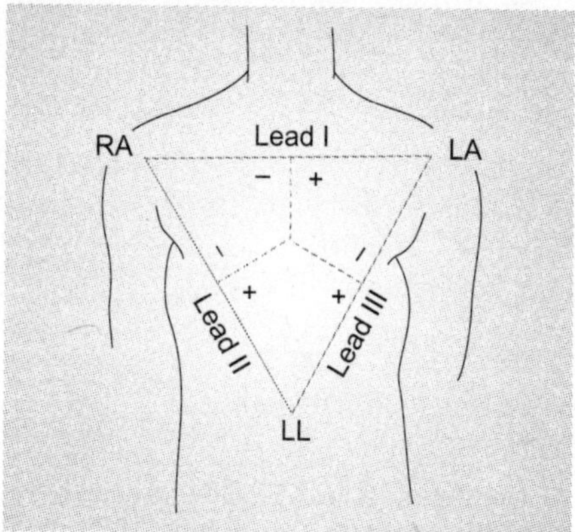

Fig. 8.8: Einthoven's triangle.

Vector During each cardiac cycle, the cardiac current flows in a particular direction at a given instant. A vector is an arrow that points in the direction of the current flow and the arrow points in the positive direction. By convention, the length of the arrow is drawn in proportion to the voltage generated by the current flow. The direction of the vector is denoted in terms of degrees. Fig. 8.9 shows the magnitude and the direction of vectors of eight successive instants in a normal QRS complex (ventricular depolarization). It is recorded on an oscilloscope and the result is recorded as a loop called *vectorcardiogram*. The loop will be similar to the one obtained by joining the positive ends of all the vectors. In different individuals, the shape of the loop may vary due to a change in the position of the heart in the thorax or due to hypertrophy of one of the ventricles. For practical purposes, the vectorcardiogram is not commonly

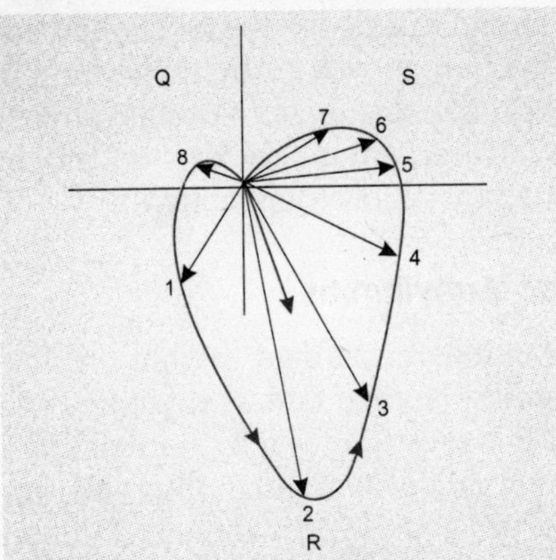

Fig. 8.9: Vector cardiographic loop. The thick arrow indicates the mean electrical axis.

used. Instead, mean electrical axis of the ventricles (QRS complex) is calculated from the magnitude of QRS waves in the three standard limb leads.

Mean Electrical Axis

The three sides of Einthoven triangle are redrawn so that they intersect each other at 60° angle (triaxial system). In lead I, the algebraic sum of positive wave (R) and negative waves (Q and S) is calculated in millimetres and the result is plotted on lead I axis at appropriate + or – point (Fig. 8.10).

Similarly, the algebraic sum of QRS waves in lead III is calculated and plotted on lead III axis at appropriate point. From these two points on lead I and lead III axes, perpendiculars are drawn. The point where the two perpendiculars intersect is connected to the point of intersection of the three axes. The result represents the average direction and magnitude of the QRS vector during the entire ventricular depolarization. Hence, it is called the *mean electrical axis* (*MEA*). The result is read from the horizontal axis, lead I (positive side).

The mean electrical axis in normal individuals is + 60°. It means during most of duration of ventricular depolarization, the current flows from the base of the ventricles to the apex. The normal range of MEA varies from – 20° to + 100°. Left axis deviation is said to be present when the MEA is less than – 20°. It is caused by left ventricular hypertrophy, e.g. in essential hypertension. Right axis deviation is said to be present when MEA is

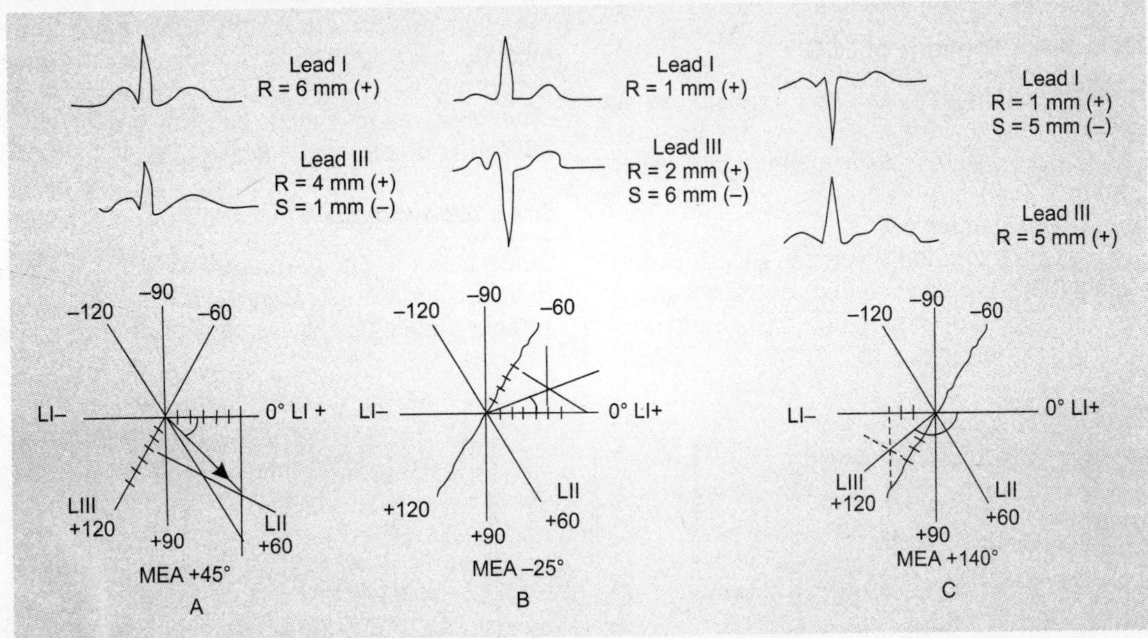

Fig. 8.10: Triaxial system of vector analysis for calculation of mean electrical axis. A. Normal; B. Left axis deviation; C. Right axis deviation.

greater than + 100°. It is caused by right ventricular hypertrophy, e.g. in pulmonary stenosis. Left or right axis deviations can also occur physiologically by changes in the position of the heart. Left axis deviation is seen in obese persons, when the abdominal fat pushes the diaphragm and keeps the heart in more horizontal position. Right axis deviation is normally seen in tall, lanky individuals, when the heart occupies a more vertical position.

Relation of ECG to the Cardiac Cycle

Using a polygraph, mechanical events in the heart like ventricular pressure curve, phonocardiogram and the electrical events, i.e. ECG can be recorded simultaneously. Fig. 7.2 illustrates such a record. It would be seen that P wave representing atrial depolarization occurs just before the onset of atrial systole. (An electrical event always precedes the mechanical event). QRS complex representing ventricular depolarization is recorded just before the beginning of ventricular systole. The T wave representing ventricular repolarization begins just before the end of ventricular systole and extends to the ventricular diastole.

Clinical Applications of ECG

An electrocardiogram can help to diagnose not only a number of cardiac disorders but also quite a few other systemic abnormalities like hyperkalaemia (tall T waves), or hypocalcaemia (prolonged QT interval).

Among the cardiac disorders, electrocardiography is the only method to diagnose accurately the various types of arrhythmias. ECG is also very useful in the diagnosis of myocardial ischaemia and infarction as well as the hypertrophy of the various cardiac chambers. (Nowadays hypertrophy of the cardiac chambers can be more easily diagnosed by echocardiography.)

Cardiac Arrhythmias

Abnormalities of cardiac rhythm are known as arrhythmias. Normal (sinus) rhythm is shown by normal P waves followed by normal QRS and T waves recorded at regular intervals, at a rate between 60 and 100 per minute. Following are some of the more important abnormalities of cardiac rhythm.

Sinus Arrhythmia

During deep breathing in adults or even during quiet breathing in children, the heart rate is faster during inspiration than during expiration. This phenomenon, called sinus arrhythmia, is seen on an ECG as slightly shorter R-R intervals recorded during inspiration than those recorded during expiration (Fig. 31.11). Sinus arrhythmia is believed to be due to irradiation of impulses from the inspiratory centre to the vagal centre in the medulla. It is a normal physiological phenomenon, which has no clinical significance. Its absence, often observed in diabetic patients, is taken as an indication of autonomic neuropathy.

Sinus Tachycardia

Sinus tachycardia is diagnosed when *normal PQRST* complexes are recorded at a rate faster than 100 per minute (Fig. 8.11). Sinus tachycardia is a

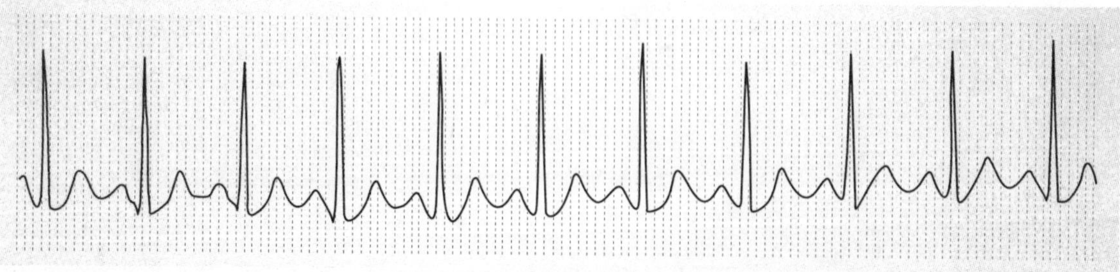

Fig. 8.11: Sinus tachycardia.

normal physiological response to excitement and anger. It is also seen during exercise, fever, haemorrhage, or administration of catecholamines, caffeine or atropine.

Sinus Bradycardia

Sinus bradycardia occurs when the SA node discharges impulses at a rate slower than 60 per minute. Except the rate, there is no abnormality in PQRST complexes. It is seen physiologically in trained athletes (Fig. 8.12). It may be due to administration of drugs like digitalis or β-blockers. Pathologically, conditions associated with sinus bradycardia include myxoedema, obstructive jaundice (as an effect of bile salts on SA node), uraemia and increased intracranial pressure.

When the above mentioned causes have been excluded, bradycardia is presumed to due to a functional defect in the SA node leading to lower rate of impulse generation. The condition, called *sick sinus syndrome*, is usually due to degenerative changes in the SA node (Fig. 8.13). Bradycardia may be severe enough to cause dizziness or attacks of syncope. Sick sinus syndrome is treated by insertion of an artificial pacemaker in the heart.

Heart Block

This term actually means a block in the conduction of impulses in the conduction tissue of the heart, i.e. AV node, His bundle or its branches. Inflammation or ischaemic damage in these tissues may lead to one of the following types of heart block:

(a) *First degree (1°) heart block* In this case, there is prolongation of PR interval beyond 0.2 seconds (Fig. 8.14). It indicates only mild damage to the conduction tissue.

(b) *Second degree (2°) heart block* More severe damage to the conduction tissue produces second degree heart block. Second degree heart block may be 2:1 block or 3:1 block, i.e. one QRS follows every 2 or 3 P waves (Fig. 8.15). The remaining impulses arising from SA node are dropped in the conduction tissue.

(c) *Complete heart block (3rd degree block)* It is said to be present when the conduction from the atria to the ventricles is completely interrupted. As a result, the atria and the ventricles beat at their own independent rhythms. The atria contract at the usual

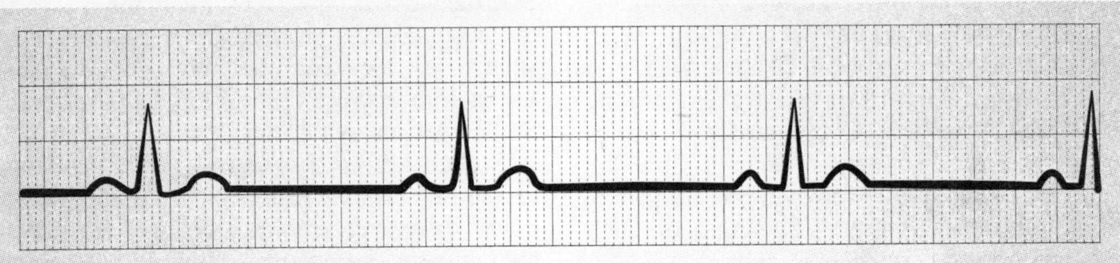

Fig. 8.12: Sinus bradycardia.

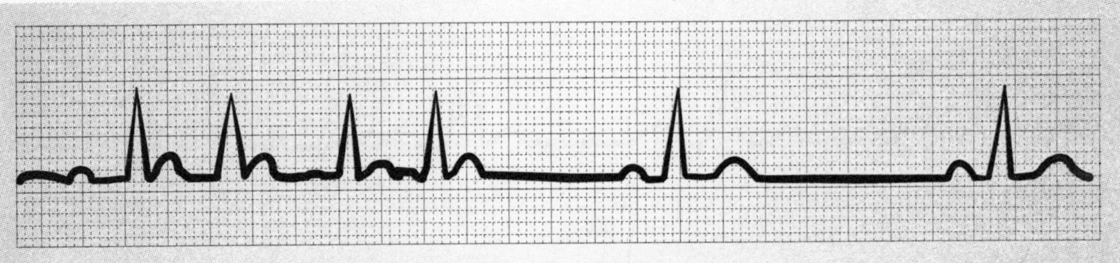

Fig. 8.13: Sick sinus syndrome. A brief tachycardia is followed by slow sinus node discharge.

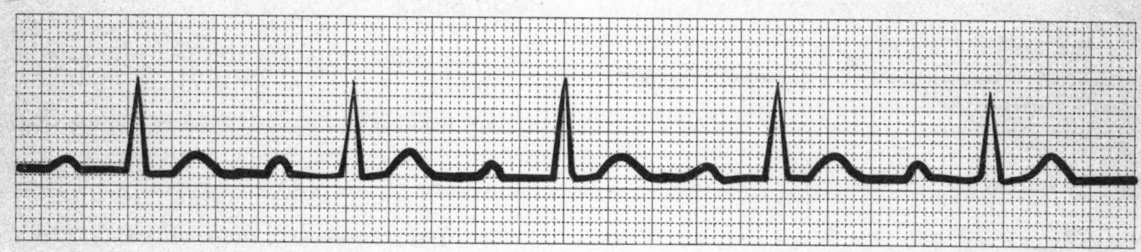

Fig. 8.14: First degree heart block. The PR interval is prolonged.

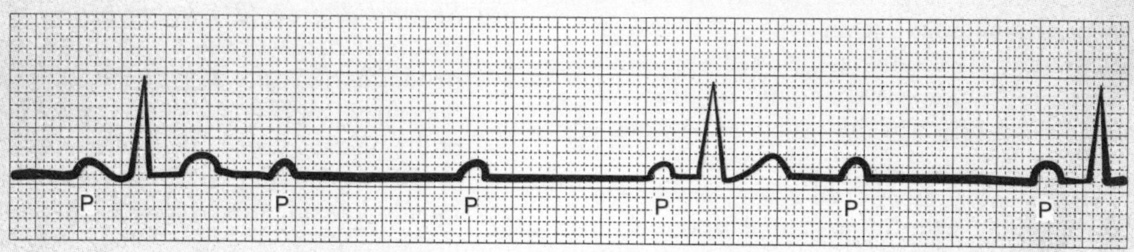

Fig. 8.15: Second degree 3:1 heart block.

rate of 70–80/min. The ventricles beat at a much lower rate of 15–40/min (*idioventricular rhythm)*, since the ventricular pacemaker is located in the Purkinje system having much lower intrinsic rhythmicity. Electrocardiogram of a patient with complete heart block is characterized by a complete dissociation of P waves from the QRS complexes. Consequently, P waves may precede, merge with or follow the QRS complexes. Moreover, the frequency of P waves is higher than that of QRS complexes (Fig. 8.16).

If the complete heart block is at AV node (*AV nodal block*), the remaining nodal tissue or adjacent His bundle becomes the pacemaker and the ventricles beat at the rate of about 40/min.In case the block is *infranodal, i.e.* in the His bundle, the pacemaker is situated more peripherally. In such cases, the ventricles may beat at a rate as low as 15/min. Such cases are likely to suffer from Stokes-Adams syndrome.

Stokes-Adams Syndrome When the damage to the AV bundle results in third degree heart block, there is commonly a delay of few seconds to a minute, before the idioventricular rhythm

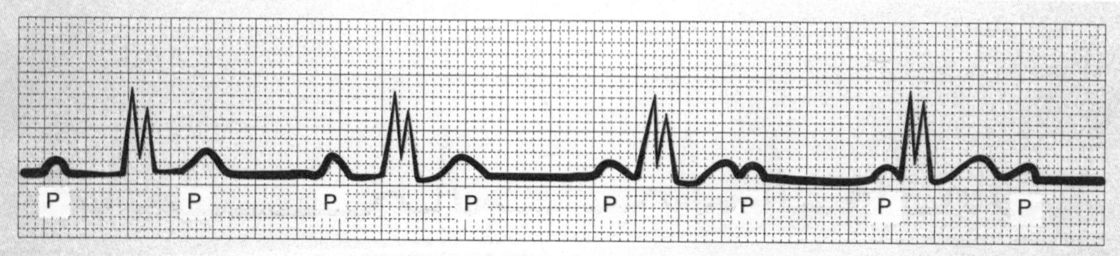

Fig. 8.16: Complete heart block. P waves and QRS complexes are independent of each other. Wide and split R wave indicates bundle branch also exists.

sets in. During this period of *asystole*, blood is not ejected from the heart and cerebral ischaemia results in dizziness and fainting or even convulsions. The condition is called Stokes-Adams syndrome. In patients who suffer from repeated attacks of Stokes-Adams syndrome, artificial pacemaker is usually inserted in the chest wall. It is an electronic device which stimulates the heart at the regular (normal) rate of 70–80 per minute (Fig. 8.17).

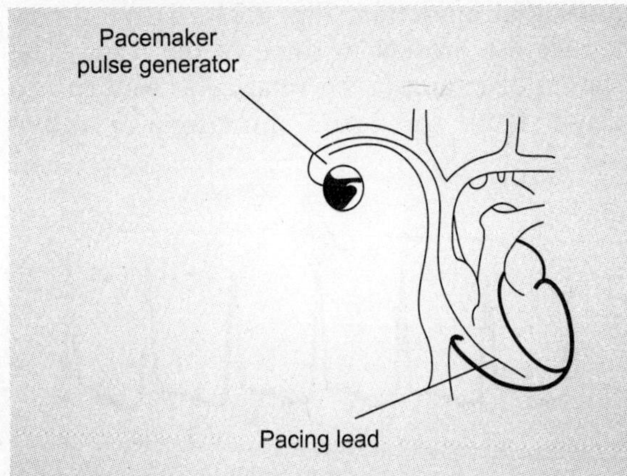

Fig. 8.17: Principle of artificial pacemaker.

Bundle Branch Block

Blockade of conduction may occur in either of the two branches of the bundle of His. In such patients, the electrical impulse travels down the unblocked branch first to depolarize the corresponding ventricle before spreading to the ventricle of the blocked side. Consequently, the QRS complex is prolonged in duration and abnormal in shape (Fig. 8.16).

Ectopic Foci of Excitation

(a) Premature Beats (Extrasystoles) SA node is the normal pacemaker of the heart. In pathological conditions, Purkinje tissue or even atrial and ventricular musculature may start discharging impulses spontaneously. Since the ectopic impulse reaches the ventricles earlier than the next impulse arising from the SA node, it results in a premature heart beat or an extrasystole (Fig. 8.18). A premature heart beat is usually followed by a prolonged diastole, called the *compensatory pause*. The reason for the compensatory pause lies in the fact that the subsequent impulse arising from the SA node finds the ventricle in absolute refractory period because of premature contraction. Since the premature beat is immediately followed by absence of a normally expected beat, the term premature is more appropriate than the term extra systole. An *atrial premature beat* is characterized by an abnormal shaped or inverted P wave, followed by a normal QRS complex. A *ventricular premature beat* is characterized by a widened and deformed QRS complex without any preceding P wave (since the impulse arises from an abnormal source in the ventricle itself).

An occasional atrial premature beat is not pathological. It commonly occurs during anxiety states or after excessive consumption of tea or coffee. Ventricular premature beats should be considered potentially serious.

(b) Tachycardia In *atrial paroxysmal tachycardia*, attacks of high heart rate occur, because suddenly an ectopic focus in the atria starts discharging impulses at the rate of about 150–200/min. Abnormal looking P waves followed by

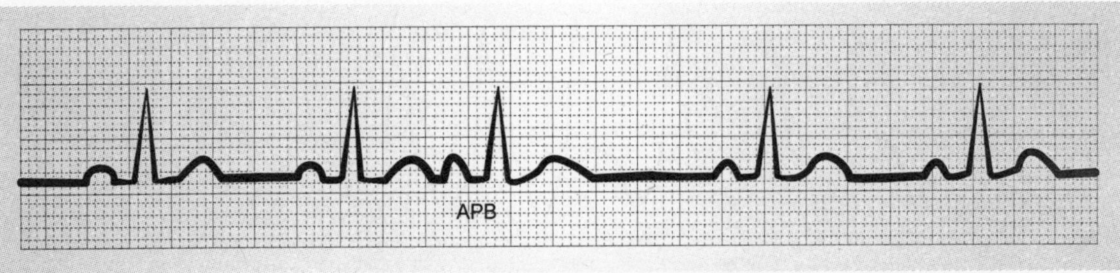

Fig. 8.18: Atrial premature beat (APB).

normal QRS complexes are characteristic feature of atrial tachycardia (Fig. 8.19). In *atrial fibrillation*, the atria are excited at the rate of 300–500/min, due to the origin of impulses from multiple foci in the atrial muscle. The AV node cannot conduct impulses at such a fast rate and hence, blocks the conduction of impulses irregularly. Consequently, the ventricles contract irregularly at a rate of about 80–160/min. In the ECG, the P waves appear as very small F waves which are irregular in time and amplitude (Fig. 8.20).

Ventricular paroxysmal tachycardia (Fig. 8.21) and *ventricular fibrillation* (Fig. 8.22) are serious complications. The latter is almost immediately fatal, because the quivering ventricles are ineffective as a pump. The onset of ventricular fibrillation is the most frequent cause of death in patients with myocardial infarction.

Myocardial Infarction

Probably the most common use of electrocardiography is in the diagnosis of myocardial infarction (ischaemic necrosis of a part of myocardium).

Elevation of ST segment, T wave inversion and a deep Q wave are cardinal ECG features of myocardial infarction (Fig. 8.23). These abnormalities are present in some of the leads. The location of infarct in the ventricular wall can be known from the leads showing the above

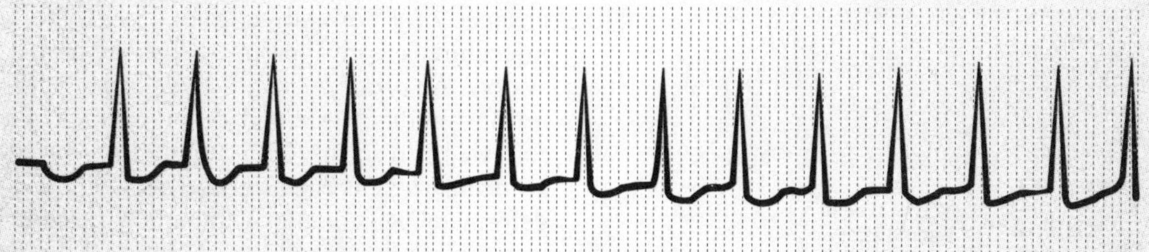

Fig. 8.19: Paroxysmal supraventricular tachycardia.

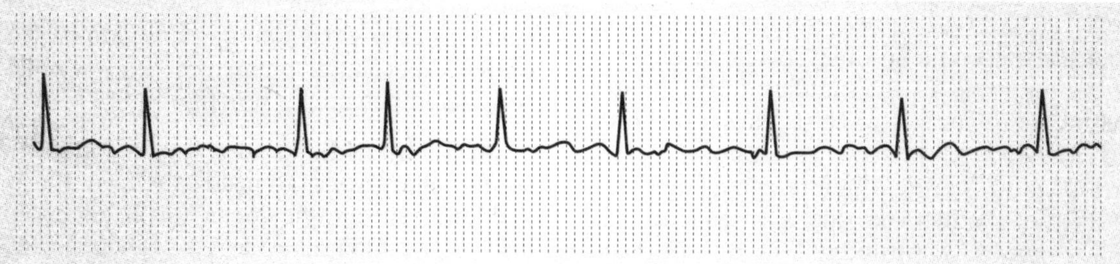

Fig. 8.20: Atrial fibrillation.

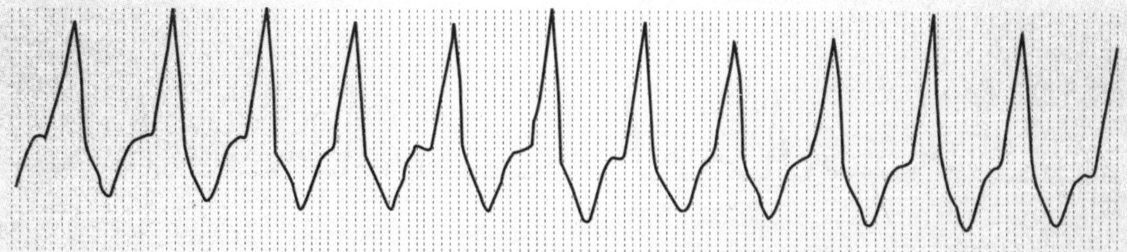

Fig. 8.21: Ventricular tachycardia.

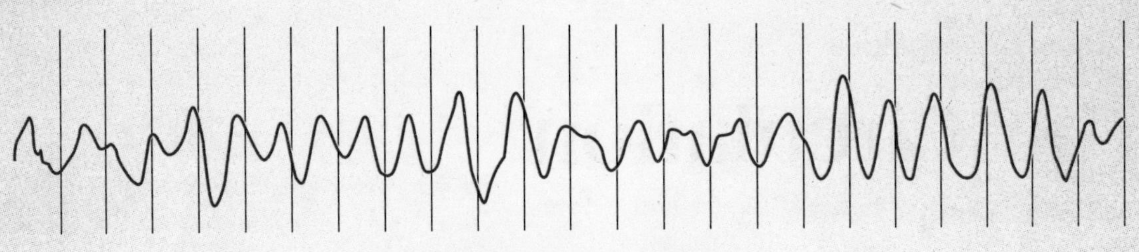

Fig. 8.22: Ventricular fibrillation.

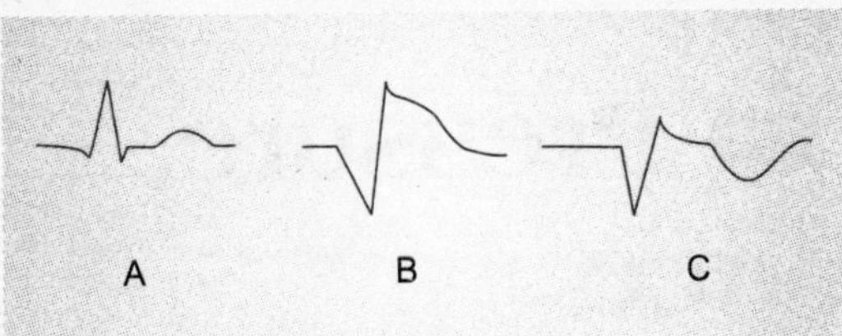

Fig. 8.23: Myocardial infarction: evolutionary changes in ECG. (A) Normal (B) A few hours after infarction—a prominent Q wave and elevated ST segment. (C) A few days later—Q wave persists, ST segment returns to baseline, T wave deeply inverted.

mentioned features, e.g. in lead I, aVL and V_5 and V_6 in case anterolateral infarction, in lead II, III, and aVF in case of an inferior wall infarct.

Myocardial Hypertrophy

Hypertrophy of the left ventricle occurs in patients with hypertension or aortic valve stenosis. In such patients, the ECG is characterized by tall R wave in lead I, aVL, V_5 and V_6 (left axis deviation). Hypertrophy of the right ventricle occurs in patients with some congenital heart diseases or in pulmonary valve stenosis. In such patients, ECG is characterized by tall R waves in lead III, a VR, V_1 and V_2 (right axis deviation).

Exercise ECG Test

In this test, the patient is asked to perform exercise of gradually increasing severity on a treadmill (Fig. 8.24), or a bicycle ergograph. An ECG is recorded continuously throughout the test. Following are the electrocardiographic manifestations of myocardial ischaemia relative to the increased myocardial oxygen demand of exercise:

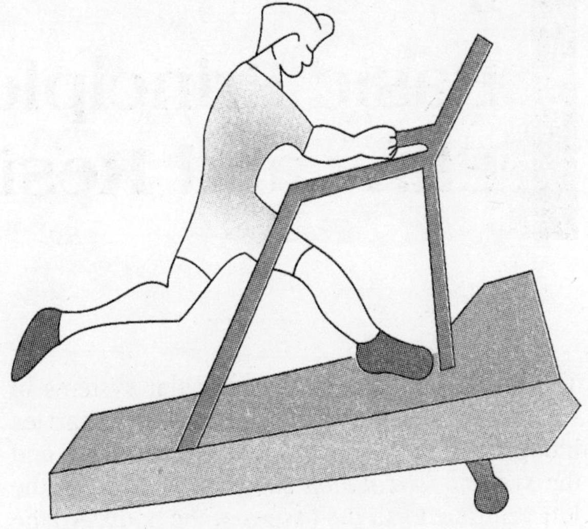

Fig. 8.24: A treadmill.

- ST segment elevation
- ST segment depression
- An increase in R wave amplitude
- Appearance of bundle branch block
- Appearance of multifocal ventricular premature beats

Following are some of the important indications for this test.

(i) Evaluation of a patient with symptoms of angina but normal ECG at rest.
(ii) Screening of asymptomatic patients who have one or more of risk factors for coronary artery disease, e.g. family history of myocardial infarction, diabetes mellitus, myxoedema, familial hypercholesterolaemia, etc.
(iii) Assessment of severity of coronary artery disease.

Section IV

The Circulation

CHAPTER 9

Basic Principles of Pressure, Flow and Resistance

The blood circulates in two vascular systems in succession; the *pulmonary circulation* carries blood from the right ventricle to the lungs, and the *systemic circulation* supplies blood from the left ventricle to all the tissues of the body. All the output of the right ventricle (5 L/min) flows through the lungs. On the other hand, the output of the left ventricle (5 L/min) flows through different *circuits in parallel*, e.g. to the brain, to the kidneys, to the limbs, etc. (Fig. 9.1). This arrangement of systemic circulation permits wide variations in the regional distribution of blood flow.

The vascular system includes not only the arteries, arterioles, capillaries and veins of systemic and pulmonary circulations but also *lymph vessels*. Lymphatics begin in extracellular spaces as small thin-walled capillaries, closed at one end, called the lymph capillaries. The lymph capillaries converge into larger lymphatic vessels, which ultimately drain into great veins near the heart. The lymphatic vessels contain a fluid called the lymph.

The flow of blood through the vessels is governed by certain basic principles of haemodynamics with some modifications imposed by the properties of blood and the vascular system.

BASIC PRINCIPLES OF PRESSURE, FLOW AND RESISTANCE

Poiseuille's Law

Fluid flows (F) through a tube in response to difference in pressure between the two ends of the tube, i.e. pressure gradient $(P_1 - P_2)/(\Delta P)$ and does not depend upon the absolute pressure values (Fig. 9.2).

$$F \propto P_1 - P_2\ (\Delta P) \qquad \text{...(i)}$$

The rate of flow also depends upon the resistance (R), against which fluid will flow through the tube.

$$F \propto \frac{1}{R} \qquad \text{...(ii)}$$

Higher the resistance, lesser would be the rate of flow. Resistance is the impediment to the flow of a fluid in a tube.

Poiseuille (a French physiologist) determined in detail the factors governing the rate of flow in a

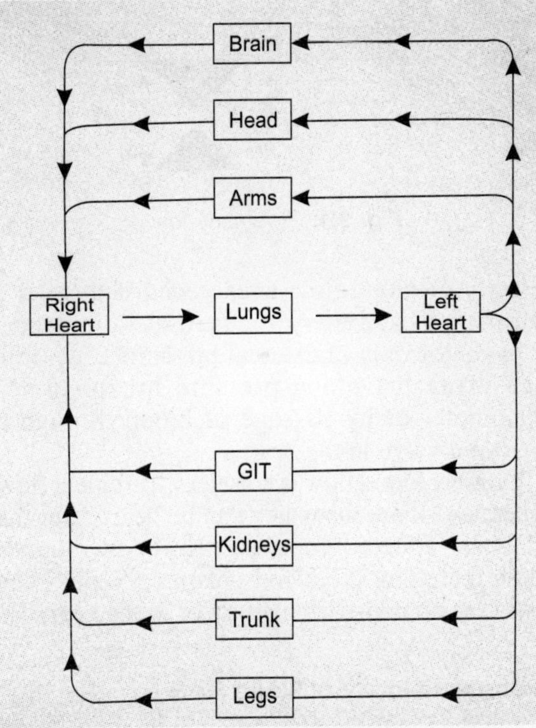

Fig. 9.1: The circulation.

Fig. 9.2: Pressure gradient ($P_1 - P_2$) rather than absolute pressure determines the flow in a tube.

rigid tube. He showed that, the resistance to flow is directly proportionate to the length of the tube (L) and viscosity of the fluid (n) and is inversely proportionate to the radius (r) of the tube. The relation is shown by the equation given below:

$$R = \frac{8\,nL}{\pi\, r^4} \quad \text{...(iii)}$$

If we consider the equations (i), (ii) and (iii) together, we get an equation known as the Poiseuille's law

$$Q = \frac{\Delta P\, \pi\, r^4}{8\,nL}$$

where Q stands for the rate of flow of fluid in a rigid tube.

Vascular Length and Vascular Resistance

As mentioned above, three factors determine the degree of resistance to flow of a fluid in a tube, namely the length and the radius of the tube and the viscosity of the fluid. In the body, since the length of blood vessels remains constant it is not a factor in the regulation of vascular resistance.

9

Vascular Radius and Resistance

As shown in equation (iii) above, the resistance to flow is inversely proportionate to the fourth power of the radius (r^4) of the vessel. In other words, even a small change in the calibre of blood vessel produces a marked change in the blood flow as shown below.

Pressure gradient	*Diameter of vessel*	*Flow rate*
ΔP = 100 mmHg	1 mm	1 ml/min
ΔP = 100 mmHg	2 mm	16 ml/min
ΔP = 100 mmHg	4 mm	256 ml/min

Arterioles are the chief site of vascular resistance because of small bore (30 μm diameter) and the presence of large amount of smooth muscle fibres in their wall. The lumen of the arterioles can be altered by the action of vasomotor nerves as well as many humoral factors. Consequently, the arterioles constitute a regulatory mechanism for variations in the regional blood flow. Capillaries are also an important site of vascular resistance but the resistance is not subjected to regulation because of absence of smooth muscle in capillary wall.

Viscosity and Resistance

In the blood, viscosity depends on the haematocrit as well as the plasma protein concentration. In vitro, even a moderate increase in haematocrit causes a marked increase in the viscosity of blood. In small vessels like arterioles and capillaries (the chief sites of vascular resistance), the effect of mild or moderate change in haematocrit on the viscosity of blood is not very significant. However, marked alterations in haematocrit, e.g. severe polycythaemia and severe anaemia do produce a significant increase or decrease in the vascular resistance, respectively. In addition, abnormalities in the shape of the RBCs (congenital spherocytosis) or abnormally high immunoglobulin levels also produce a clinically significant increase in the viscosity of blood, leading to an increase in peripheral resistance and therefore in cardiac workload.

When the temperature of the blood is lowered, its viscosity increases. This may be one of the factors aggravating tissue damage in cold injuries (frost bite).

Laminar and Turbulent Flow

The blood flow in a blood vessel is normally *laminar*. The fluid flowing through a blood vessel may be considered to be consisting of a series of thin layers slipping over each other (Fig. 9.3). An extremely thin layer immediately in contact with the vessel wall almost does not move. The next layer has some velocity, and the subsequent inner layers have gradually increasing velocities, the core of the bloodstream having the maximum velocity.

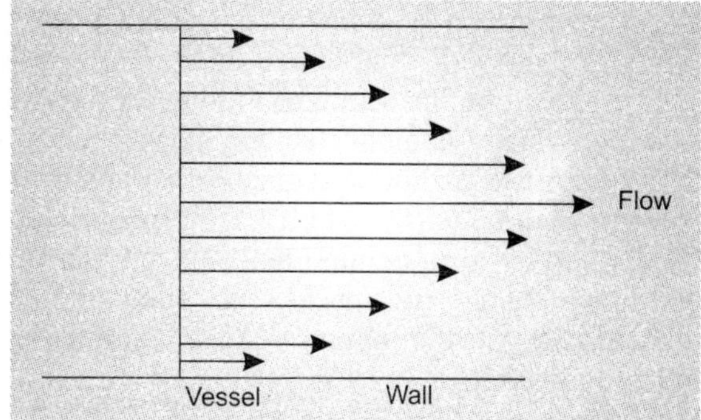

Fig. 9.3: Laminar flow. The core of the bloodstream has greatest flow rate.

When the velocity of flow exceeds a certain limit, called the *critical velocity*, the flow becomes *turbulent*, instead of being laminar. In turbulent flow, the fluid particles move in irregular and constantly varying paths (Fig. 9.4). Critical velocity of blood flow is exceeded if there is a constriction of an artery by atherosclerotic plaque, or by application of external pressure, e.g. while measuring the blood pressure by sphygmomanometer or by passage of blood through a narrowed valve in the heart.

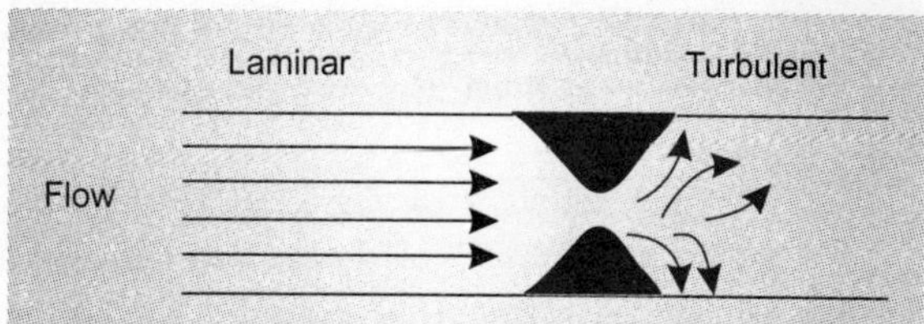

Fig. 9.4: Turbulent flow.

Laminar blood flow is noiseless. Turbulent flow generates vibrations which can be heard over the artery by a stethoscope, e.g. Korotkow sounds while recording the blood pressure, or murmurs heard over a constricted artery or in the heart.

Average Velocity of Blood Flow

The rate of blood flow is measured as the amount of blood flowing per unit time (e.g. cubic centimetre/sec). Velocity of blood is the displacement of blood per unit time (e.g. centimetre/sec). The relation between the flow and velocity is as follows :

$$V = \frac{Q}{A}$$

V = Velocity
Q = Quantity of blood
A = Area of cross-section of the vessel

If the quantity of blood flow remains constant, and the cross-sectional area increases, the velocity of blood flow decreases. Total cross-sectional area of the capillaries is 1000 times the cross-sectional area of aorta. Accordingly, the velocity of blood flow in capillaries is approximately 1 mm/S, as compared to mean velocity of 40 cm/S in the aorta. Extremely slow velocity of blood flow in the capillaries is useful in the transcapillary exchange of tissue fluids and gases. The total cross-sectional area of the various types of blood vessels in the systemic circulation is compared as follows.

Type of vessel	*Lumen diameter*	*Cross-sectional area (cm²)*
Aorta	2.5 cm	4.5
Artery	0.4 cm	20
Capillary	5 μm	4500
Vein	0.5 cm	40
Vena cava	3.0 cm	18

Circulation Time

If a substance is injected into one segment of the circulation and its presence can be detected at another point, the circulation time between two points can be estimated. For example, the interval between the injection of bile salts in the vein of an arm, and the appearance of bitter taste of the bile salts, gives the *arm to tongue circulation time* (average normal: 15 S). Similarly *arm to lung circulation time* can be estimated by noting the interval between the injection of a bolus of ether into the vein of an arm, and the appearance of coughing produced by its arrival in the lungs (average normal: 6 S). Nowadays, circulation time is hardly ever estimated in clinical medicine, but it is educative to know that a dye injected into the vein of a foot reaches the other foot, after circulation through the heart, within 30 S.

Critical Closing Pressure

In a rigid tube, there is a linear relationship between the pressure and flow (Fig. 9.5) and flow ceases only if the pressure is zero. On the other hand, in a blood vessel, blood flow may cease even when the mean blood pressure is 20 mmHg or even higher. The pressure value at which the flow ceases is called critical closing pressure. The blood flow ceases because certain intraluminal pressure is required to push the RBCs (with average diameter of 7.5 μm) through the capillaries (with average diameter of 5 μm). Moreover, a certain amount of tissue pressure is exerted over the blood vessels. Blood vessels would remain patent only if the intraluminal pressure is greater than the tissue pressure.

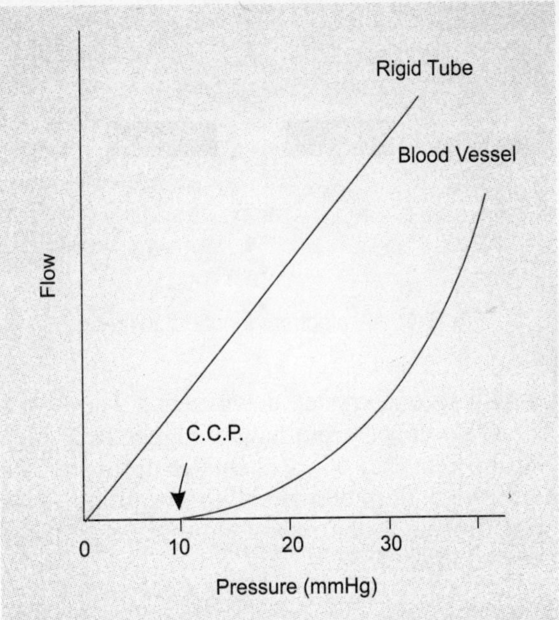

Fig. 9.5: Relation of pressure and flow in a rigid tube and a blood vessel (CCP—critical closing pressure).

Measurement of Blood Flow

Blood flow in some of the organs like the lungs, heart and the brain can be measured using Fick principle. Renal blood flow is determined by estimation of PAH clearance. Blood flow through a vessel (artery or vein) can be known using a flow meter. Nowadays, electromagnetic and Doppler flow meters are commonly used in the diagnosis of vascular diseases to locate the site of obstructions/occlusion.

Electromagnetic Flow Meters This instrument is based on the principle that when a blood vessel is placed between the poles of a strong magnet, a voltage is generated as the blood flows through the magnetic field. The magnitude of voltage is proportionate to the volume of flow (Fig. 9.6).

Ultrasonic (Doppler) Flow Meter This instrument is based on the principle of 'Doppler effect'. When a minute piezoelectric crystal is used to send ultrasonic waves diagonally across a blood vessel, some of the waves are reflected from the RBCs and WBCs. The reflected waves are picked

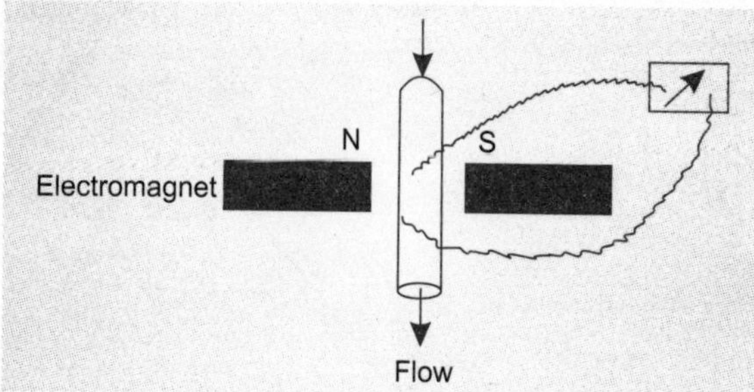

Fig. 9.6: An electromagnetic flowmeter.

up by a second crystal, downstream. The waves picked up downstream have a higher frequency than the frequency of waves emitted upstream. The difference between the two frequencies is proportionate to the rate of flow because of the Doppler effect (Fig. 9.7).

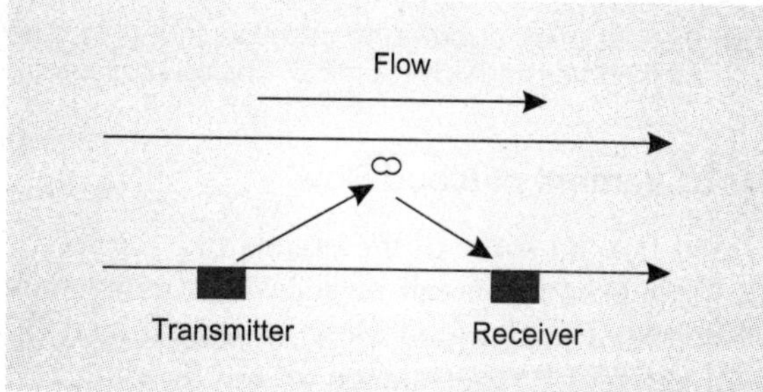

Fig. 9.7: An ultrasonic (Doppler) flowmeter.

Venous Occlusion Plethysmography In the absence of flow meters described above, the flow to a limb may be measured by a simple (but crude) method known as venous occlusion plethysmography. A limb (say a forearm) is enclosed in a watertight chamber (the plethysmograph) connected to a volume recorder. Venous drainage from the limb is occluded for a few seconds by inflating the sphygmomanometer cuff to 60 mmHg. The increase in the volume of the limb reflects the arterial blood flow to the limb during that period (Fig. 9.8).

Law of Laplace

This law describes the relation between the distending pressure (P) and the tension (T) on the

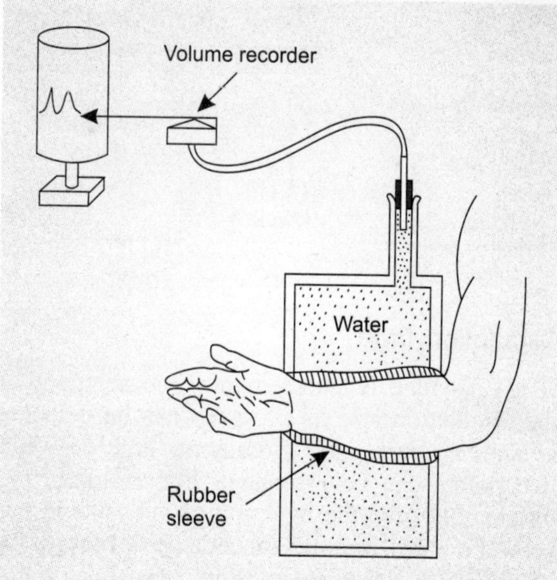

Fig. 9.8: Estimation of blood flow to the forelimb by venous occlusion plethysmography.

wall of a distensible (elastic) cylinder. According to Laplace, the distending pressure in a distensible hollow object is equal at equilibrium to the tension in the wall divided by two principal radii of the curvature of the object (r_1 and r_2).

$$P = T\left(\frac{1}{r_1} + \frac{1}{r_2}\right)$$

In a sphere $r_1 = r_2$ therefore $P = \frac{2T}{r}$

This equation is applicable to the alveoli of the lungs. In a blood vessel since one of the radii is indefinite, the equation would be :

$$P = \frac{T}{r}$$

The equation shows that smaller the size of the vessel, lesser would be the tension in the wall of the vessel necessary to balance the distending pressure. In the human aorta, with mean blood pressure of 100 mmHg, the tension on the walls is 170,000 dynes/cm. The tension in the walls of a blood capillary is 10,000 times less (approximately 16 dynes/cm) even though the capillary blood pressure is one-fourth of the aortic pressure. This explains why the thin-walled capillaries do not rupture, in spite of fairly high distending pressure.

BLOOD PRESSURE

Blood pressure means the force exerted by the blood column against a unit area of the vessel wall. It is usually measured in millimetres of mercury (mmHg). The term blood pressure is used without any further qualification to denote *arterial blood pressure*. When describing pressure in other types of blood vessels, the type of vessel is also mentioned, e.g. capillary pressure, venous pressure, etc.

The arterial blood pressure varies with the phases of cardiac cycle (Fig. 9.9). It rises to a peak value, in the systolic phase, and the peak value is known as the *systolic blood pressure* (about 120 mmHg). The arterial blood pressure falls gradually to reach a minimum value in the diastolic phase. The lowest value is known as the *diastolic blood pressure* (about 80 mmHg). The difference between systolic and diastolic blood pressure values is called the *pulse pressure.* The normal range of systolic blood pressure is from 100 to 140 mmHg. Normal diastolic blood pressure ranges from 60–90 mmHg. Conventionally, systolic BP and diastolic BP are denoted as numerator and denominator respectively, e.g. B.P. of a normal individual is written as 120/80 mmHg. When blood pressure values are above 140 mmHg systolic and/or above 90 mmHg diastolic, the condition is known as *hypertension*. When the blood pressure value is below the normal range the condition is known as *hypotension*.

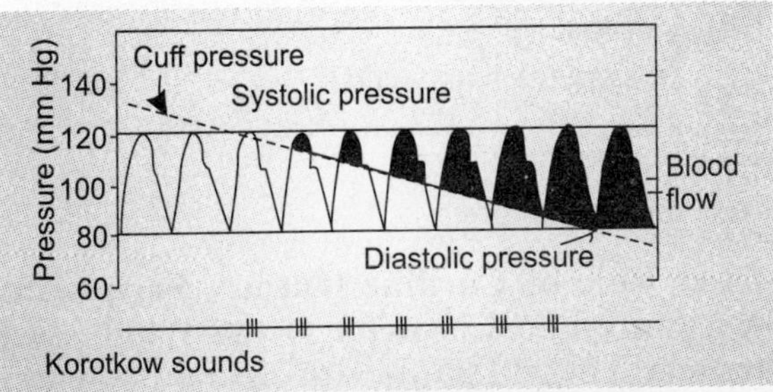

Fig. 9.9: Systolic and diastolic variations in blood pressure. Manner of production of Korotkow sounds.

Mean Arterial Pressure It is the average arterial blood pressure throughout the cardiac cycle. Mean blood pressure is not equal to the algebraic mean of the systolic and diastolic blood pressure, i.e it is not equal to

$$\frac{\text{Systolic BP + Diastolic BP}}{2}$$

because the duration of the cardiac systole is shorter than the duration of diastole. Mean arterial blood pressure is roughly equal to:

$$\text{Diastolic BP} + \frac{1}{3}\text{ Pulse pressure}$$

For example, if systolic BP is 120 mmHg and diastolic BP 80 mmHg, the mean blood pressure would be

$$80 + \frac{1}{3} \times 40 = 93 \text{ mmHg}$$

$$(\text{and not } \frac{100 + 80}{2} = 100 \text{ mmHg})$$

METHODS FOR MEASUREMENT OF BLOOD PRESSURE

1. Direct Method In experimental animals, a cannula or a 'T'-tube is inserted into an artery and connected to a strain-gauge transducer.

2. Indirect Methods In clinical practice, arterial blood pressure is measured using a sphygmomanometer and a stethoscope. The sphygmomanometer consists of an inflatable rubber cuff attached to a mercury manometer. The cuff is wrapped around the arm and the pressure in the cuff is rapidly raised to a value well above the expected systolic pressure. The pressure is then gradually lowered while the chest-piece of the stethoscope is placed over the brachial artery at the elbow (Fig. 9.10). At a certain level, soft tapping sounds, corresponding to the heart-beat are heard through the stethoscope. As the pressure is further lowered, the sounds at first become louder, and then suddenly muffled and finally disappear. These sounds are known as Korotkow sounds. The level at which the sounds begin to be heard is the systolic blood pressure of the individual. The level at which the sounds

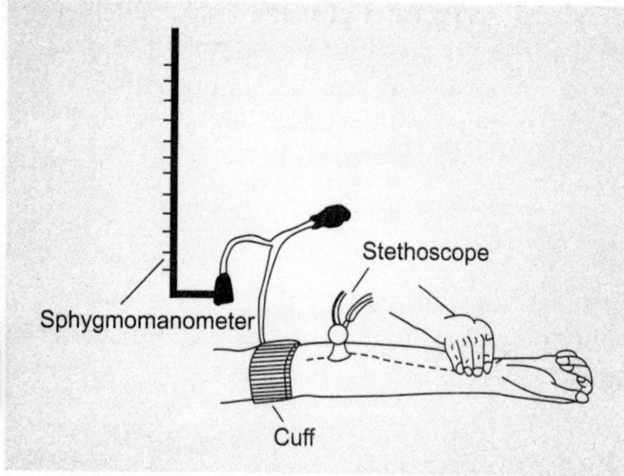

Fig. 9.10: Record of BP by auscultatory method.

disappear is the diastolic pressure (Fig. 9.9). In some clinical situations, the level at which the sounds become muffled is taken as diastolic blood pressure (because in conditions like hyperthyroidism and aortic valve insufficiency, the sounds continue to be heard even when the pressure in the cuff is very low).

Korotkow Sounds

With careful auscultation, the following phases of Korotkow sounds can be differentiated:

Phase I: Synchronous with each heart beat, faint tapping sounds begin to be heard. Their intensity increases for about 10–15 mmHg fall in pressure.

Phase II: Softer bruit during the next 15 mmHg fall in pressure.

Phase III: Sounds become louder and clearer for about 15 mmHg fall in pressure.

Phase IV: Sounds become muffled for next 4–6 mmHg fall in pressure.

Phase V: Sounds disappear.

Korotkow sounds are produced by turbulent flow of blood in the brachial artery. With cuff-pressure higher than the systolic blood pressure, the blood flow in the brachial artery completely ceases and no sounds are heard. When the cuff-pressure is just below the systolic pressure, blood trickles down the artery at the peak of each systole. As long as the cuff pressure is above the diastolic blood pressure, the blood flow in the brachial artery remains intermittent and hence turbulent, producing a sound with each systole. When the cuff pressure falls below the diastolic blood pressure, the blood flow becomes continuous and laminar and hence the sounds are no more produced.

While recording blood pressure in very obese individuals a cuff of greater width must be used for accurate results. In infants, the cuff size is proportionately smaller.

Auscultatory Gap

In some of *the hypertensive* subjects, the phase II Korotkow sounds are not heard. That is, after the initial phase I, there are no sounds during the next 20–40 mmHg fall of pressure. And then phase III to V Korotkow sounds are heard. The phenomenon is called auscultatory gap. The exact mechanism of auscultatory gap is not clear. However, it has an important clinical implication. While recording blood pressure of a hypertensive patient, if the cuff pressure is not adequately elevated in the beginning, the phase III Korotkow sounds may be mistaken for phase I sound and therefore a false low systolic pressure would be recorded. The error can be avoided if *in all cases*, a rough idea of systolic blood pressure is initially obtained by *the palpatory method.* Then, while recording blood pressure by *auscultatory method,* the pressure in the cuff is raised well above the systolic pressure obtained by the palpatory method.

Determinants of Arterial Blood Pressure

Following are the important determinants of arterial blood pressure:

1. Cardiac output.
2. Peripheral resistance.
3. Elasticity of the aorta and large arteries (windkessel vessels).
4. Blood volume.

(A) Role of Cardiac Output, Peripheral Resistance and Elasticity of the Windkessel Vessels These factors are of fundamental importance in the creation of arterial pressure. To exert pressure on the vessel wall, first of all, blood needs to be pumped into the arterial system. To be under pressure, the amount of blood entering the arterial system has to be slightly greater than the amount leaving it. Such a situation is created by pumping of blood by the heart into the aorta with each beat and the resistance exerted by the arterioles in its exit out of the arterial system. The importance of these two factors is shown by the equation:

$$\text{Blood pressure} = \text{Cardiac output} \times \text{peripheral resistance}$$
$$= \text{CO} \times \text{PR}$$

Since ejection of blood occurs during ventricular systole (0.3 seconds), the arterial pressure is likely to fall to very low levels during diastole (0.5 seconds). The maintenance of fairly high pressure during diastole (80 mmHg) is achieved by elasticity of the aorta and its immediate branches (windkessel vessels) and the action of arterioles. The heart ejects about 70 ml of blood during each systole. As a result, the aortic pressure rises to a peak value of approximately 120 mmHg and stretches the elastic wall of the aorta and its immediate branches. During diastole, the arterial pressure begins to decline, but does not fall below approximately 80 mmHg because of: (a) elastic recoil of the windkessel (elastic) vessels and (b) resistance offered to the outflow of blood by the arterioles. Elasticity of the windkessel vessels prevents the excessive rise of blood pressure during ventricular systole. The recoil of the elastic fibres helps to maintain fairly high pressure during diastole, when there is no ejection of blood from the heart into the arterial system (c.f. pressure in the left ventricle falls to near zero in diastole) (Fig. 9.11).

In old age, there is a gradual decrease in the elasticity of the windkessel vessels (due to age-related degeneration of the elastic fibres). As a result, the normal cardiac output produces a greater rise in systolic blood pressure, but the diastolic pressure declines to a value lower than normal. In a normal healthy individual aged about 70 years, typical blood pressure reading is 160/70 mmHg. The condition is known as *systolic hypertension.*

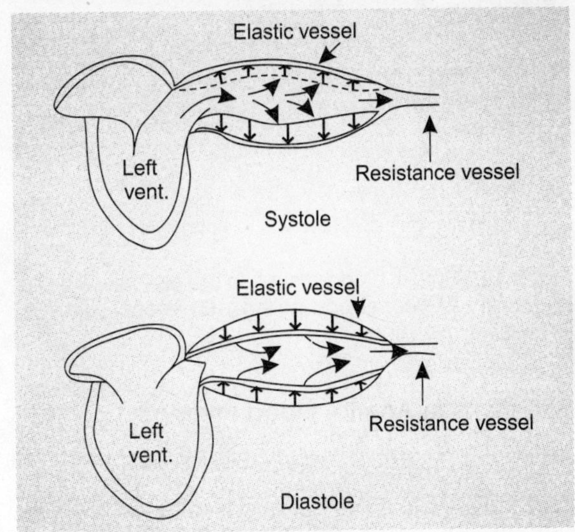

Fig. 9.11: Role of elastic vessels and arterioles in maintaining arterial pressure and flow during diastole of the heart.

(B) Role of Blood Volume/ECF Volume The blood volume is an important determinant of arterial blood pressure. To exert pressure on the vessel wall, the blood content of the vessel should be slightly more than its capacity (Fig. 9.12). If extracellular fluid volume is increased or decreased, the blood pressure changes accordingly by the following sequence of events.

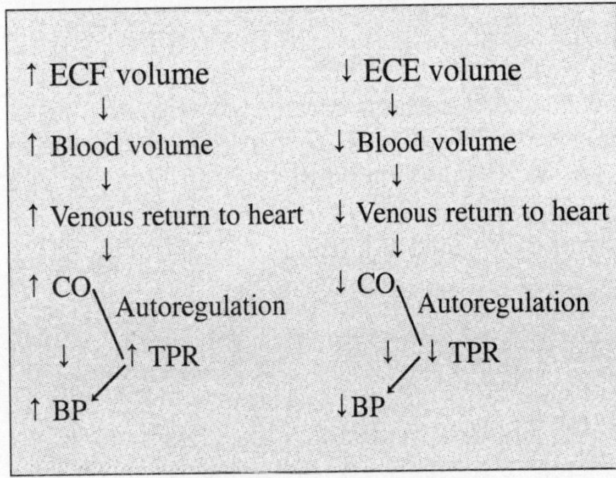

A decreased blood volume is an important cause of a fall in blood pressure, e.g. due to haemorrhage, dehydration or burns, etc.

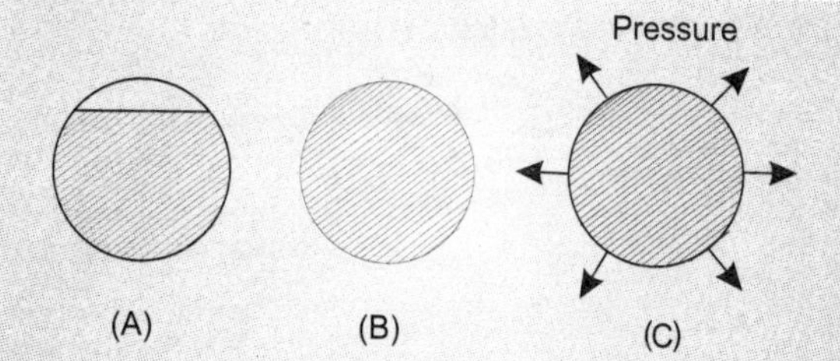

Fig. 9.12: Role of blood volume in the genesis of blood pressure (A) vessel underfilled, (B) vessel just full, (C) vessel overfilled.

Variations in Arterial Blood Pressure

(Factors affecting arterial blood pressure)

Since BP = CO × PR, variations in blood pressure can occur because of a change in cardiac output (CO), peripheral resistance (PR) or both.

In general, changes in CO produce relatively more effect on the systolic blood pressure whereas changes in peripheral resistance produce relatively more effect on the diastolic blood pressure. The peripheral resistance primarily depends on the calibre of arterioles. Only occasionally changes in viscosity of blood may be the cause of altered PR, e.g. anaemia or polycythaemia. Various factors which may produce a variation in arterial blood pressure are discussed below.

1. Age Both systolic and diastolic blood pressure values tend to increase with age (Fig. 9.13). Since the cardiac output does not increase with age, increased blood pressure is primarily because of increased peripheral resistance. After the age of 60 years, there is a sharper increase in systolic BP but diastolic BP tends to decrease. The condition is called systolic hypertension. This change is related to a decrease in elasticity of the aorta and its large branches.

2. Sex During the reproductive age of the female (from puberty to menopause), the blood pressure tends to be 5–10 mmHg lower than in males of the corresponding age. The lower BP is related to the presence of female sex hormones (oestrogens and progesterone). After menopause when the plasma levels of these sex hormones falls to very low levels, the difference in BP between males and females disappears (Fig. 9.13).

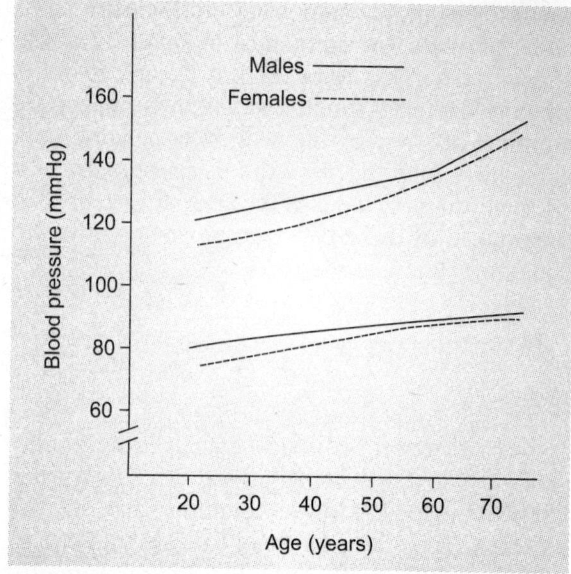

Fig. 9.13: Effect of age and sex on arterial blood pressure.

3. Body Built In obese subjects, the recorded blood pressure tends to be higher than in lean individuals of similar age and sex. The higher value of BP is partly because of a procedural artifact. The manometer records pressure in the cuff wrapped around the upper arm whereas Krotokoff sounds depend on the pressure exerted over the brachial artery lying deep in the tissues. In obese individuals, the communication of pressure from the cuff to the artery is poor, i.e. pressure exerted on the artery is lower than pressure recorded in the manometer. In addition, there is evidence that in obese subjects, BP is actually higher than in lean individuals and the difference may be evident even in obese children.

4. Weather In hot weather, BP is lower than in cold weather. Hot weather results in extensive cutaneous vasodilatation leading to low peripheral resistance. In contrast, exposure to cold weather produces cutaneous vasoconstriction leading to increased peripheral vascular resistance.

5. Sleep During sleep, blood pressure is 10–20 mmHg lower than in day time.

6. Exercise During exercise, the cardiac output is increased in proportion to the severity of exercise. On the other hand, peripheral resistance is increased in some vessels (cutaneous, splanchnic area) and decreased in others (coronary, skeletal vessels). Hence, during exercise, systolic BP is always increased in proportion to the severity of exercise. Diastolic BP may be slightly elevated, slightly lowered or there may be no change. Mean blood pressure is usually elevated.

7. Emotions During emotional excitement, e.g. rage, anxiety, emotional stress, sexual excitement, etc., both systolic and diastolic BP increase, particularity the former (Fig. 9.14).

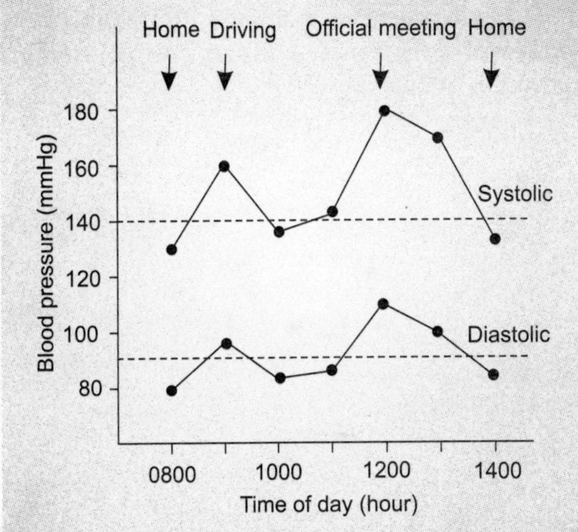

Fig. 9.14: Effect of emotional stress (driving in a rush hour, stormy official meeting) on the arterial blood pressure of a normotensive ("normal") individual.

In some individuals, high BP is recorded in the doctor's clinic. But, when the same individual is re-examined at his/her home, the BP recorded is found to be normal. This condition, called *white coat hypertension*, is an example of the effect of emotions on BP. Patients with white coat hypertension may ultimately develop real hypertension in later life.

8. Gravity Blood pressure should be recorded with the subject in recumbent position and the sphygmomanometer placed at the level of the heart. In this position, all the large arteries have similar blood pressure. In standing posture, the blood pressure recorded in the dorsalis pedis artery is approximately 80 mmHg greater than in measured in supine position. For example, say the blood pressure recorded in *supine position* is 120/80 mmHg in the brachial artery. It would be similar in dorsalis pedis artery as well. If measured in *standing position*, the pressure recorded in the dorsalis pedis artery is likely to be approximately 200/160 mmHg. The higher blood pressure in the arteries of the lower limbs in standing posture is because of the hydrostatic (gravitational) effect the column of blood from the heart to the level of recording. For every centimetre below the level of heart, the blood pressure increases by 0.77 mmHg. For similar reasons, in standing posture, the blood pressure in the cranial arteries would be *lower* by 20–35 mmHg (Fig. 9.15).

9. Change of Posture A change from supine to standing posture results in a transient fall in BP due to decreased venous return leading to decreased cardiac output. However, within a few seconds,

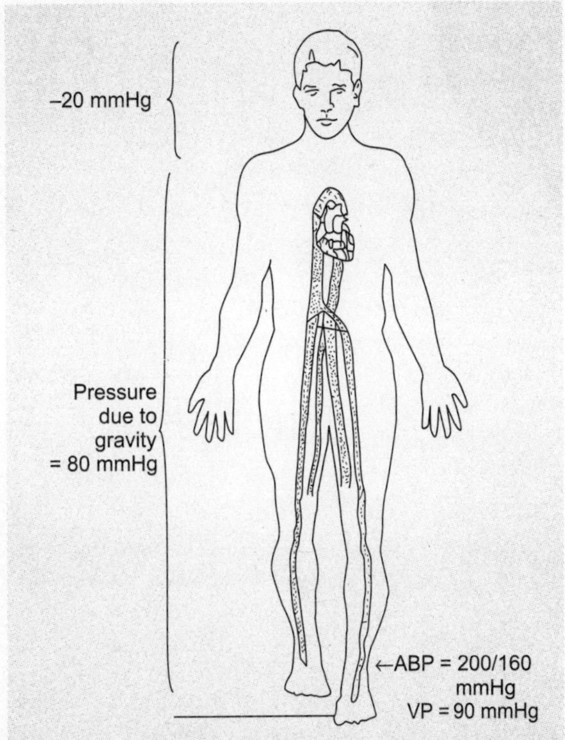

Fig. 9.15: Effect of gravity (standing posture) on arterial and venous pressure.

9

baroreceptor-mediated reflexes bring the BP back to normal primarily by increasing the peripheral vascular resistance (for further details see Ch. 14).

10. Blood Volume As discussed earlier, blood volume is an important determinant of BP. That is why BP falls in cases with decreased blood volume, e.g. haemorrhage, burns, dehydration, etc.

9

11. Pregnancy In later months of pregnancy, blood volume is increased by about 30%. However, instead of the expected increase, the BP remains normal or may even decrease by 5–10 mmHg. This is related to the high plasma progesterone level in pregnancy. Progesterone decreases peripheral resistance by its action on vascular smooth muscle.

12. Food Intake During digestion and absorption of food, there is a moderate (about 30%) increase in cardiac output. However, BP does not increase because of simultaneous vasodilatation (decreased PR) in the blood vessels of gastrointestinal system.

13. Anaemia/Polycythaemia Red blood cells make an important contribution to the viscosity of blood, which in turn, influences peripheral vascular resistance. Therefore, in severe anaemia, BP is low because of decreased PR. On the other hand, polycythaemia tends to produce hypertension by increasing PR.

Pressure and Flow in Different Segments of Circulatory System

10 CHAPTER

THE ARTERIAL SYSTEM

The arterial vessels comprise: (a) the large *elastic vessels* or windkessel vessels such as aorta and its immediate branches (windkessel; a German word meaning elastic reservoir), (b) large muscular *distributing arteries* such as radial, ulnar, popliteal arteries, etc. and (c) the small arteries and arterioles also known as the *resistance vessels*. The function of the large arteries is to transport blood under high pressure to the tissues. The arterioles, the small lumened final branches of the arterial system have strong muscular walls. They act as control valves to regulate the amount of blood released into the capillaries. In addition, the arterioles and the large elastic vessels act together to convert the periodic ejection of blood from the heart to a steady continuous flow in the tissue capillaries.

The average velocity of blood flow in the aorta is about 40 cm/s. During systole, the peak velocity of blood flow in the aorta may reach up to 120 cm/s.

As mentioned earlier, the resistance to flow varies inversely with the fourth power of the radius of the vessel. In the aorta, and the large arteries up to 3 mm diameter, there is very little resistance to flow and the arterial pressure remains practically unchanged. Even in small arteries, mean blood pressure may be as high as 85 mmHg.

THE ARTERIOLES

Each arteriole is only a few millimetre long and has an average diameter of 30 μm. Each arteriole branches many a time and supplies about 10–100 capillaries. The most characteristic feature of an arteriole is its thick muscular wall having profuse vasomotor (sympathetic) innervation. Because of their small lumen, the arterioles are the major sites of the peripheral resistance. The arterial pressure drops by about 50 mmHg as the blood passes through a few millimetre long arterioles (Fig. 10.1).

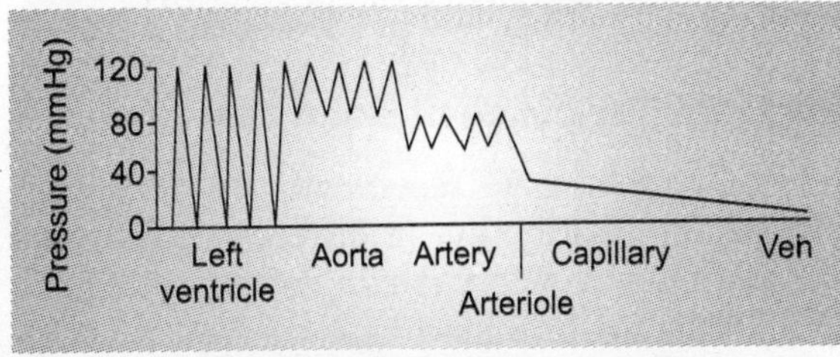

Fig. 10.1: Blood pressure in the left ventricle and in different segments of the systemic vessels.

More important is the fact that the smooth muscle in the wall of arterioles responds to changes in the sympathetic discharge. Since resistance = $1/(\text{radius})^4$, even a small change in the lumen of arterioles produces a marked change in the peripheral resistance. Because of their large bulk, the skeletal muscles and the abdominal viscera (splanchnic area) contain large number of arterioles and together constitute the major site of *total peripheral resistance.*

The arteriolar smooth muscle responds not only to the variations in the *sympathetic neural discharge* but also to the *products of local metabolism.* By these two mechanisms, the regional blood flow can be controlled in such a way that it is almost exactly proportionate to the metabolic requirement of the tissues in any situation. For example, during muscular exercise, strong sympathetic discharge causes constriction of the arterioles in the splanchnic area (where the blood is not immediately required). At the same time, local metabolites like adenosine, CO_2, H^+ and lactic acid cause marked arteriolar dilation in the blood vessels of the skeletal muscle and the myocardium. Consequently, the blood flow is temporarily diverted from the abdominal viscera to the skeletal muscles and the heart to meet the latter's markedly elevated metabolic demand.

Another effect of arteriolar resistance is that, beyond the arterioles the blood flow becomes non-pulsatile (Fig. 10.1). The pressure pulse is an important feature of the arterial tree but is absent in capillaries and veins. Pulsations of blood flow are well marked in the aorta as shown by the variations in the velocity of flow in different phases of cardiac cycle. In the capillaries and veins, the blood flow is steady and non-pulsatile.

Regional Distribution of Blood Flow

At rest, about 5 L of blood enter the aorta each minute. Its distribution in different organs and tissues under rest and maximum vasodilatation (VD) is shown in Table 10.1.

In terms of tissue weight, the liver, the heart and the brain have very high resting blood flow rate reflecting very high metabolic demand. The kidneys have extremely high blood flow per 100 gm weight, but it is related to the excretory function rather than to the metabolic requirement of the renal tissue. Figure 10.2 shows the blood flow in different tissues at rest and after maximal vasodilatation.

Table 10.1: Regional distribution of cardiac output

Organ	*Blood flow*			
	Per organ (ml/min)		*Per 100 g tissue (ml/min)*	
	Rest	*Max. V.D.*	*Rest*	*Max. V.D.*
Heart	250	1200	80	400
Brain	750	2100	55	150
Skeletal muscle	750	20000	4	70
Kidney	1200	1400	400	450
Skin	500	3500	15	150

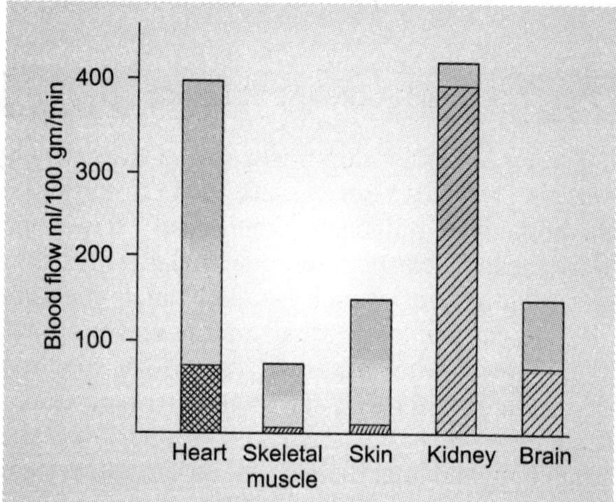

Fig. 10.2: Blood flow in different organs at rest (shaded areas) and at maximum vasodilatation (unshaded areas).

THE CAPILLARY CIRCULATION

This is the most important segment of the circulatory system. The exchange of materials between the blood and the tissue fluid takes place only in the capillaries. The activity of all the remaining segments of the cardiovascular system is regulated so as to ensure capillary exchange adequate for the metabolic requirement of tissues.

Architecture of Micro-Circulation

From the arterioles, blood reaches the venules through two routes. A direct short route is the *metarteriole*, or the *thoroughfare vessel*. Secondly, the blood may traverse the true capillaries, the endothelial tubes devoid of any perivascular smooth muscle, interposed between the proximal and the distal portions of the metarteriole (Fig. 10.3). The proximal end of the capillary is surrounded by one or two smooth muscle cells which constitute the *precapillary sphincter*. When the precapillary sphincters are closed, the true capillaries are excluded from the active circulation and the blood flows through the thoroughfare vessels only. In many tissues, like skeletal muscle, where metabolic activity may vary markedly between rest and heavy exercise, the number of true capillaries is approximately 10-times the number of thoroughfare channels. In such tissues, only one or two capillaries are open at rest. The tissue fluid and gas exchange in the distal segments of metarterioles and one or two open capillaries are sufficient to meet the metabolic requirement of the resting muscle. During exercise, when the metabolic demand is enormously increased, the blood supply to the muscle is markedly increased by the opening up of all the precapillary sphincters as well as by dilatation of the arterioles and the metarterioles. On the other hand, in tissues like the mesentery, where metabolic activity does not vary, there are only few capillaries for each metarteriole. *Precapillary sphincters, and metarterioles,* unlike the arterioles, have *very little sympathetic innervation.* Their muscle fibres are controlled almost entirely by local metabolites like CO_2, pH, etc.

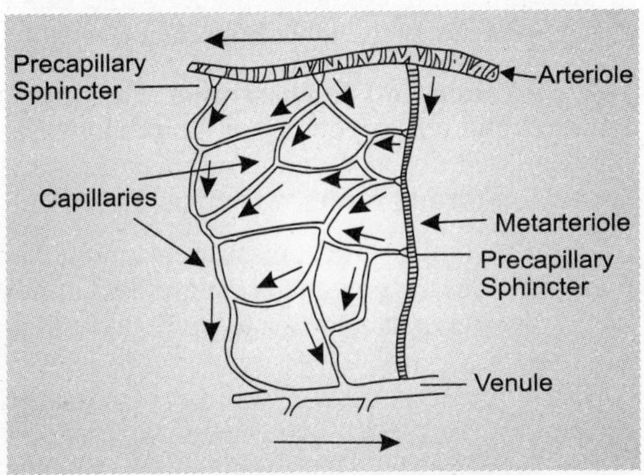

Fig. 10.3: The microcirculation.

Arteriovenous anastomoses (AV anastomoses) are short vessels with thick muscle coat, connecting arterioles with venules, bypassing the metarterioles and capillaries. These vessels are abundantly innervated by vasomotor sympathetic fibres. Such vessels are specially found in the skin of the fingers, toes and ear lobes. The cutaneous AV anastomoses play an important role in the regulation of body temperature.

10

Types of Capillaries

The capillaries have an average diameter of 5 μm. The capillary wall consists of a single layer of endothelial cells. Under electron microscope, three different types of capillaries may be identified, i.e. continuous, fenestrated and discontinuous type (Fig. 10.4).

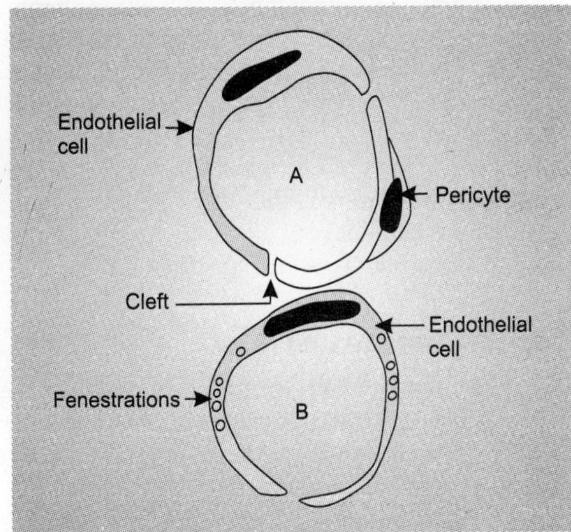

Fig. 10.4: Structure of a capillary; continuous type (A) and fenestrated type (B).

(a) Continuous Type This is the most common type of capillaries. They are found in the skeletal muscle, adipose tissue, connective tissue and pulmonary circulation. The capillary wall is a continuous membrane of endothelial cells, about 1 μm thick except at the site of the nucleus. Actually, the endothelial cells forming the capillary walls are not continuous with each other. A small cleft of 10 nm size always separates the two adjacent endothelial cells. It is believed that most of the water soluble ions and molecules pass across the capillary through these clefts (or *slit-pores*).

(b) Fenestrated Type These capillaries are named so because of large intracellular gaps, 20–100 nm in diameter, found in the cytoplasm of the endothelial cells. Such capillaries are found in the endocrine glands, intestinal villi and renal gromeruli. The fenestrations permit the passage of relatively large molecules and make the capillary porous.

(c) Discontinuous Type In this type of capillary, the wall is interrupted at intervals by large intercellular gaps (600–3000 nm in diameter) through which even formed-elements of blood can pass freely. Such capillaries are found in the bone marrow and sinusoids of the liver and spleen.

Capillaries and postcapillary venules have certain cells called *pericytes* outside the endothelial cells. These cells have long processes that wrap around the vessels. Pericytes are contractile. They also release a wide variety of vasoactive substances. Their physiological function seems to be regulation of flow of fluids through the junction between the endothelial cells, particularly in the presence of inflammation (Fig. 10.4).

Capillary Pressure and Flow

Because of many variations, it is difficult to describe a generalized picture of capillary pressure and flow. In the *nailbed*, the average capillary pressure is about 25 mmHg, but it varies over the length of the capillary. The capillary blood pressure is approximately 35 mmHg at the arteriolar end, and about 10 mmHg at the venular end. Average capillary pressure is less than 10 mmHg in the *pulmonary capillaries* and *hepatic sinusoids*. The velocity of blood flow in the capillary is extremely slow (less than 1 mm/S). The transit time of blood between the arteriolar end to the venular end of an average sized capillary is 1–2 seconds.

Transcapillary Exchange

In the tissues, the spaces between the cells are collectively called the *interstitium*. It consists of a fluid called the interstitial fluid trapped between extremely fine proteoglycon filaments (98% hyaluronic acid and 2% protein) forming a sort of gel known as the *tissue gel*. Gases, nutrients and cellular waste products diffuse through the tissue gel very freely.

Adequate capillary blood flow is essential for the survival of the tissues. Capillary blood brings oxygen, electrolytes and nutrients to the tissues and removes the waste products of cellular metabolism. The exchange of these substances between the capillary blood and the interstitial fluid occurs across the thin membrane formed by the endothelial cells. *Diffusion*, as well as, *filtration-reabsorption* constitute the chief mechanisms of transcapillary exchange. *Pinocytosis* does not contribute to the transcapillary exchange to any significant degree but it provides an active transport mechanism for the macromolecules like the gamma globulins which cannot reach the tissue spaces by diffusion or filtration.

1. Diffusion This is by far the most important means of transcapillary exchange of materials between the plasma and the interstitial fluid. Lipid soluble substances like O_2 and CO_2 diffuse most freely. Water and water soluble (lipid-insoluble) micromolecules like Na^+, Cl^-, K^+, glucose, urea, etc. diffuse almost freely through the intracellular and intercellular pores in the capillary membrane. Broadly speaking, the pore size is such that all substances with molecular weight less than 69,000 can diffuse freely. The capillaries are impermeable to albumin (molecular wt. 69,000) and other plasma proteins with higher molecular weight.

2. Filtration and Reabsorption The rate of filtration and absorption at any point along the capillary wall depends on the balance of forces, known as **Starling forces**, which include:

(i) The hydrostatic pressure gradient, i.e. hydrostatic pressure in the capillary minus the hydrostatic pressure in the interstitial space.
(ii) Oncotic pressure gradient across the capillary wall, i.e. colloidal osmotic pressure of the plasma minus the colloidal osmotic pressure of the interstitial fluid.

(iii) Capillary permeability. Capillary filtration coefficient is proportionate to the permeability of the capillary and surface area available for filtration. The interstitial osmotic pressure (Π_i) is practically zero. The interstitial hydrostatic pressure (P_i) is about –2 mmHg in subcutaneous tissue, but positive in the liver and the kidneys, and as high as +6 mmHg in the brain.

$$\text{Fluid movement} = K\,[P_c - P_i] - [\Pi_c - \Pi_i]$$
$$= K\,[P_c - \Pi_i] - [P_i - \Pi_c]$$

where
- K = Capillary filtration coefficient
- P_c = Capillary hydrostatic pressure
- Π_i = Interstitial osmotic pressure
- P_i = Interstitial hydrostatic pressure
- Π_c = Capillary osmotic pressure

At Arteriolar End

The forces that tend to cause movement of fluid out of the capillary at the arteriolar end are:

(i) Capillary hydrostatic pressure = 35 mmHg
(ii) Negative interstitial hydrostatic pressure = –2 mmHg

Total outward force

$$P_c - P_i = [35 - (-2)] = 37 \text{ mmHg}$$

Forces that tend to move the fluid inward is plasma protein osmotic pressure (Π_c) which is 25 mmHg since ($\Pi_i = 0$).

Net filtering force

$$[P_c - P_i] - [\Pi_c] = 37 - 25 = 12 \text{ mmHg}$$

At Venous End of Capillary

Outward forces are i. $P_c = 10$ mmHg
ii. $P_i = -2$ mmHg

Total outward force $= [P_c - P_i] = [10 - (-2)] = 12$ mmHg

Inward force $= \Pi_c = 25$ mmHg

Net inward force $= [P_c - P_i] - [P_c]$
$= 12 - 25 = -13$ mmHg

The example given above refers to the position at the extreme ends of the capillary. Over the length of the capillary, the hydrostatic pressure gradually decreases. Therefore, the filtration is maximum at the arteriolar end of the capillary and gradually declines to zero near the middle of the capillary. From here, the inward forces become dominant and reabsorptive process starts to reach its maximum at the venular end (Fig.10.5).

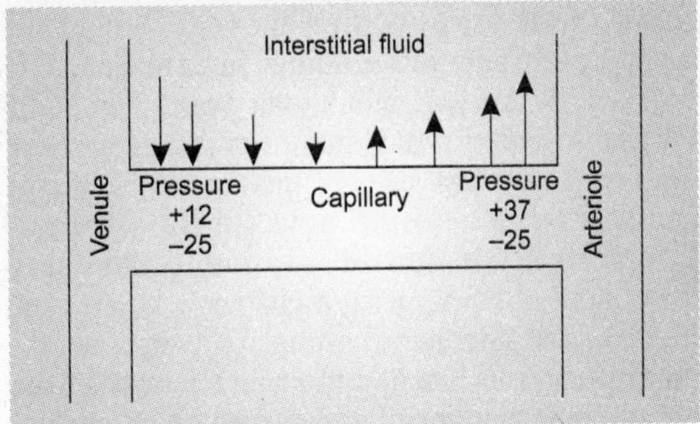

Fig. 10.5: Filtration and reabsorption in a capillary due to interplay of Starling's forces.

The description given above may not apply to all the capillaries. For example, under normal circumstances, due to low hydrostatic pressure, filtration does not occur at all in the pulmonary capillaries.

Leaving aside the glomerular capillary filtration, approximately 14 ml of fluid is transferred per minute from the capillaries to the interstitial spaces of the body. Of this, about 90% of fluid is reabsorbed back to the capillaries and the rest is returned to the circulation via the *lymphatics*. The filtered fluid contains all the constituents of the plasma except proteins.

Although capillaries are said to be impermeable to plasma proteins, a small amount of albumin does pass out of the capillary membrane. Practically whole of it is returned to the circulation through the lymphatics.

THE LYMPHATIC CIRCULATION

Lymphatic capillaries are present in all the tissues except the brain and the cartilage. They are closely associated with the blood capillaries. The lymphatic system constitutes an accessory route for the removal of interstitial fluid. More important is the drainage of proteins and other large particulate matter present in the interstitial spaces. The lymphatic capillaries begin in the interstitial spaces as thin-walled capillaries closed at one end.

They join together to form larger lymphatic vessels which ultimately form two large lymphatic vessels, known as the thoracic duct and the right lymphatic duct. The thoracic duct brings lymph from the whole of the lower part of the body, left upper limb, the left sides of the thorax, head and neck. It drains into the left subclavian vein. The right lymphatic duct drains lymph from the right upper limb, and the right sides of the thorax, head and neck. It opens into the right subclavian vein. Lymph nodes are situated at various points along the course of the larger lymphatics, e.g. axillary, inguinal and abdominal groups of lymph nodes. Foreign proteins like bacteria which may enter the lymphatics are trapped and destroyed by macrophages in the lymph nodes and thus prevented from dissemination throughout the body.

The lymphatic capillary network in the tissues is as extensive as the network of blood capillaries. The diameter of the lymphatic capillaries varies widely. Like blood capillaries, the lymphatics are lined by a single layer of endothelial cells. Edges of the endothelial cells overlap in such a way that they form minute flap-valves. Fluid and even larger particulate matter in the interstitial space can push the valve open and flow into the capillary but once inside, the fluid cannot go out of the capillary since the tendency to back flow closes the flap-valve (Fig. 10.6).

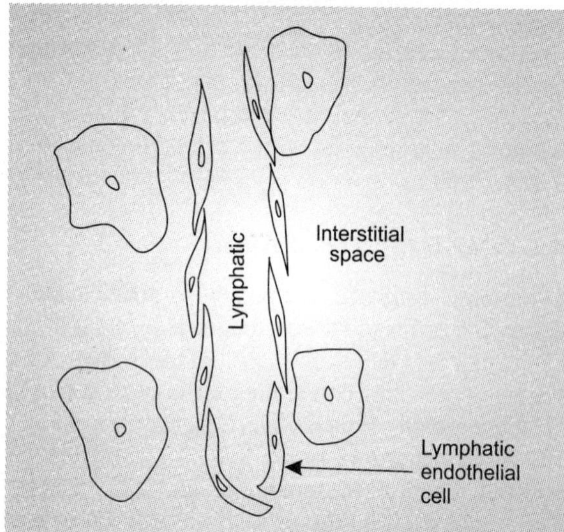

Fig. 10.6: Structure of a lymph capillary.

Formation of Lymph

About 90% of the fluid filtered out of the blood capillaries is reabsorbed back into them at the venous end. The remaining fluid enters the lymphatic vessels to constitute the lymph. Therefore, the lymph has the same composition as the interstitial fluid except that it is richer in proteins. This would be apparent because all the protein content of the filtered fluid is drained into lymphatics along with only 10% of the filtered fluid. Moreover, the protein content of lymph formed in the liver is approximately 6 gm% and that of the intestine is 3–5 gm%. Since more than half of the lymph is derived from the liver and intestines, the thoracic duct lymph has protein concentration of 3–5 gm%.

The lymphatic system also provides a route of absorption of long-chained fatty acids and cholesterol from the intestine (in the form of chylomicrons).

As the lymph passes through the lymph nodes, it picks up the lymphocytes and the gammaglobulins formed in the nodes.

The formation of lymph is very slow, and only 2–4 L of lymph are drained into the great veins every day. The rate of formation of lymph is somewhat accelerated by regional venous obstruction (leading to decreased absorption of tissue fluids into blood capillaries), or by arteriolar dilatation (leading to increased tissue fluid formation).

Factors Affecting Flow of Lymph

Large lymphatic vessels contain valves which allow one way flow of the lymph. Contraction of the skeletal muscles, and the negative intrathoracic pressure increase the rate of flow of lymph. The suction effect of high velocity of blood flow in the veins, where the lymphatics terminate, and the rhythmic contraction of the walls of the large lymphatic ducts are the two other factors promoting the flow of lymph.

Oedema

Oedema is the term applied to an excessive accumulation of fluid in the tissue spaces. It is due to an abnormality in the mechanism of transcapillary exchange, i.e. the outflow and inflow are not perfectly in balance. From the discussion of the Starling forces, it would be obvious that the following factors would tend to increase the volume of interstitial fluid.

1. Increased Capillary Hydrostatic Pressure It can occur in venous obstruction, congestive heart failure *(cardiac oedema)*, or local inflammation *(inflammatory oedema)*. In the inflammatory oedema, the bacterial toxins produce arteriolar vasodilatation as well as increased capillary permeability.

2. Decreased Plasma Protein Osmotic Pressure Oedema occurs when the plasma albumin concentration falls below 2.5 gm% (normal 4.5 gm%). Severe malnutrition (decreased protein synthesis), and certain renal diseases (increased excretion of proteins) are important causes of *nutritional oedema* and *renal oedema* respectively.

3. Chronic Lymphatic Obstruction Chronic obstruction of the lymphatic vessels by scars, or by parasites (e.g. filariasis), or operative removal of lymph nodes (e.g. in treatment in cancer), causes interference with the drainage of proteins from the tissue spaces. Therefore, protein-rich fluid accumulates in the tissue spaces causing a special type of oedema called *lymphoedema*. Lymphoedema differs from all other types of oedema mentioned above in having higher protein concentration of the oedema fluid. In filariasis, the gross oedema gives elephant-like appearance to the lower limbs (elephantiasis). Application of pressure by thumb on the skin overlying a bone (say just above the medial malleolus) leaves a small depression in all other types of oedema (pitting oedema) (Fig. 10.7) but not in lymphoedema (non-pitting oedema.)

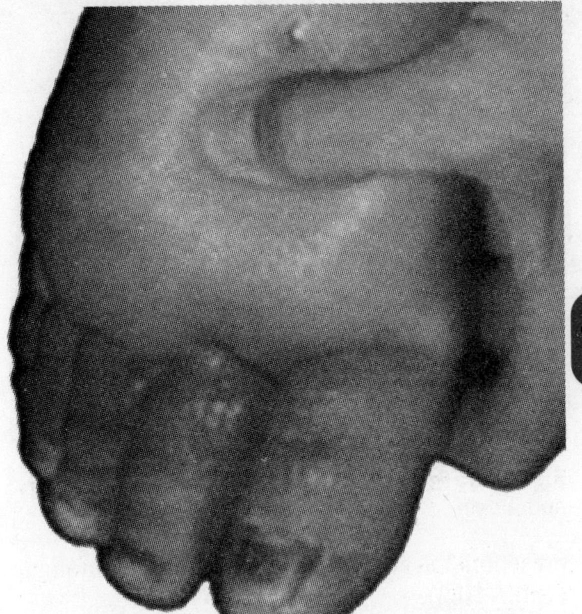

Fig. 10.7: Pitting oedema.

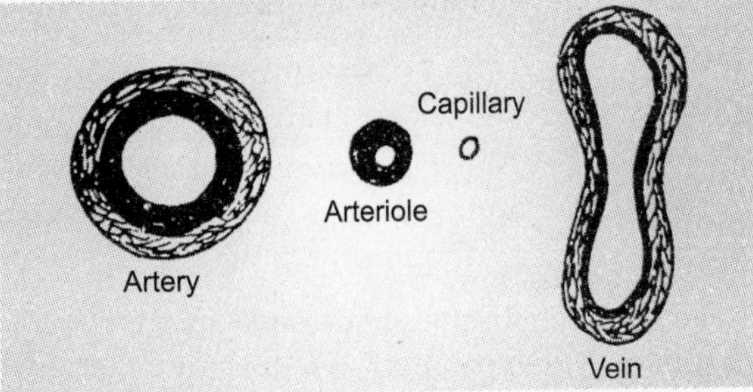

Fig. 10.8: Structural differences between an artery and a vein.

THE VENOUS CIRCULATION

As compared to arteries, at equivalent levels in the vascular tree, veins have more numerous tributaries, thinner walls, larger lumen, lesser smooth muscle and greater distensibility (Fig. 10.8). The venules, though larger in lumen and thinner than the arterioles, can to some extent alter the post-capillary resistance by responding to various neural and chemical stimuli. Most of the veins, however, act as low resistance conduits and capacitance vessels.

Besides *distensibility*, *collapsibility* is another characteristic feature of the veins. When their blood content decreases, the veins assume an elliptical profile. As the venous blood content increases, they assume more and more circular profile to accommodate progressively greater amount of blood per unit length. Further increase in the volume of blood is accommodated by distension of the walls without any significant increase in the venous pressure (Fig. 10.9). Due to this property, veins are called the *capacitance vessels*. About 60% of the total blood volume is

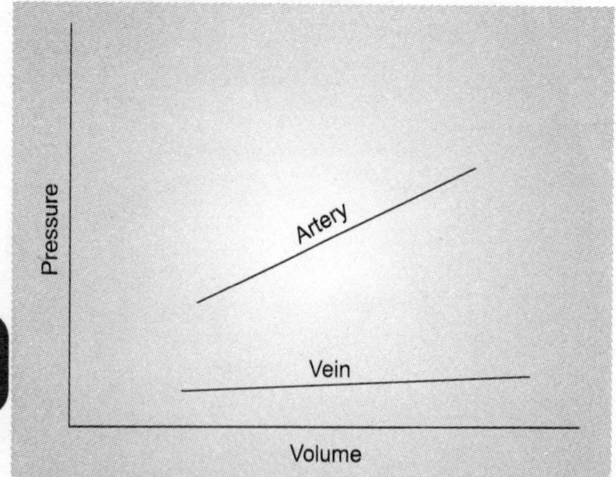

Fig. 10.9: Pressure-volume relationship in an artery and a vein.

present in the systemic veins at any given moment (Table 10.2).

Table 10.2: Distribution of blood volume in different portions of the circulatory system

Heart	7%	Venules and small veins	25%
Large arteries	8%	Large veins	39%
Small arteries	5%	Pulmonary vessels	9%
Arterioles	2%	Capillaries	5%

The smooth muscle in the walls of the veins is supplied by sympathetic vasoconstrictor nerves. Increased discharge in these nerves produces contraction of the smooth muscle but the result of venous and venular constriction is a decrease in their capacity leading to increased venous return to the heart. There is no significant increase in the venous resistance. After blood loss from an external or internal injury, reflex increase in sympathetic discharge decreases the capacity of the veins. Since the veins contain over 60% of the total blood volume, the decrease in the capacity of the veins helps to maintain the cardiac output by maintaining normal venous return in spite of blood loss.

Venous Pressure and Flow

Hydrostatic pressure in the venules is approximately 10 mmHg. As the veins approach the heart, there is a gradual decrease in the venous pressure. In the great veins near the heart (the central), venous pressure is approximately 5 mmHg. In the right atrium, during its diastole, the pressure is nearly zero.

In standing posture, the effect of gravity modifies the venous pressure. At the level of the feet, the effect of gravity results in an increase of venous pressure by approximately 80 mmHg. For similar reason, the pressure in the veins above the heart is decreased in proportion to the distance from the heart (Fig. 9.15). In the neck veins, when the pressure falls to zero, the veins collapse. But in the skull, the dural sinuses cannot collapse because of the tough non-collapsible nature of dura mater and hence, sub-atmospheric pressure develops in the dural sinuses in sitting or standing posture of the body. Certain neurosurgical procedures are performed with the patient in semi-recumbent position. During such procedures, any accidental opening of dural sinuses results in suction of air into the sinus (air embolism).

The velocity of blood flow in the veins increases with increase in the size of the vein. In inferior vena cava, the average velocity of blood flow is 10 cm/sec.

Air Embolism This dangerous complication may occur due to accidental opening of dural sinuses (vide supra) or in Caisson's disease (Ch. 19). Some times as little as 5 ml of air may be lethal. When a bolus of air enters a vein, it is transported by blood to the heart where it fills the cardiac chambers. It is not propelled out of the heart by cardiac contractions because of its easy compressibility. Absence of outflow of blood proves fatal within minutes. Small bubbles of air can be swept across the heart but they ultimately lodge in the small arteries and block the blood flow. It may result in serious tissue damage in the vital organs like the brain which may be fatal.

Factors Affecting Venous Return

The pressure gradient between the venules (10 mmHg) and the right atrium (O mmHg) is rather small. Venous blood is returned to the heart even though, in some blood vessels, the blood flow has to occur against gravity, e.g. in veins of lower limb and abdomen. A number of factors are involved in the mechanism of the return of venous blood to the heart.

1. *Pumping action of the heart* This is the most fundamental factor responsible for the flow of blood in the veins. The pumping action of the heart creates a pressure head of about 100 mmHg in the arterial system, which gradually decreases to about 10 mmHg in the venules. There is no venous return when the heart stops beating. This force driving the blood in the veins is known as *vis a tergo* (force from behind).

2. *Suction of venous blood by the heart* During rapid ejection phase of cardiac cycle, the intra-atrial pressure becomes negative. The negative pressure acts as a suction force for the blood in superior and inferior vena cavae. This action is called "vis a fronte" (*force from front*).

3. *Thoracic pump* The intrathoracic pressure varies between – 5 cm H_2O in expiration and –10 cm H_2O in inspiration. The negative intrathoracic pressure acts as a suction force and promotes the venous return from the extrathoracic segments to the intrathoracic segments of the great veins. During artificial respiration, positive pressure breathing may interfere with the venous return to the heart.

4. *Intrabdominal pressure* During inspiration, the intra-abdominal pressure rises because of the descent of diaphragm. Therefore, there is greater flow of venous blood from the abdominal veins towards the thorax.

5. *Gravity* The force of gravity promotes venous return from the head and neck towards the heart. In the veins below the level of the heart, gravity tends to interfere with the venous return. Despite the pull of gravity, venous return occurs in these vessels because of factors 1, 2, 3 and 6 discussed here.

6. *Muscle pump* Veins in the limbs have venous valves which allow the blood to flow in one direction only, i.e. from the periphery towards the heart (Fig. 10.10). When a person is standing quietly, the valves in the veins of the lower limb are open and there is a slow continuous flow of blood in the veins towards the heart. As the lower limbs move, the muscular contraction squeezes the veins present in between them. As a result, venous blood is propelled towards the heart. Retrograde movement of blood is prevented by the venous valves. This role of skeletal muscle contraction on the venous blood flow is known as *muscle pump action*.

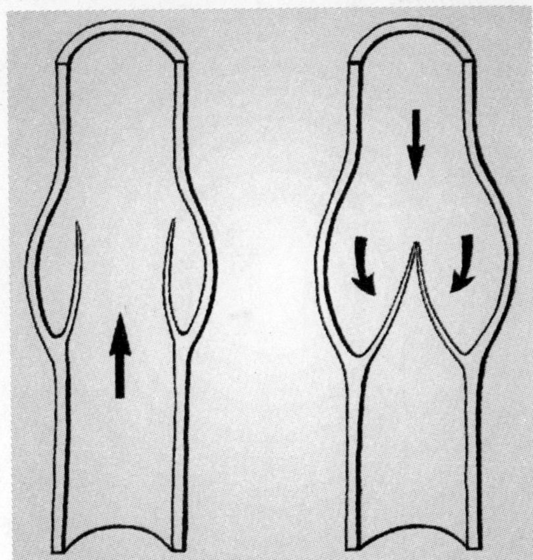

Fig. 10.10: Action of venous valves.

7. *Role of venous valves on venous pressure* Besides promoting the venous return by the muscle-pump action described above, rhythmic muscular contractions help to lower the venous pressure in the veins of the lower limb. During quiet standing, the continuous flow of blood in the veins of lower limb produces a column of blood extending from the heart to the feet producing a pressure of nearly 90 mmHg in the veins at the level of the feet. During walking, the pressure is reduced to about 20 mmHg. The rhythmic muscular contractions break up the column of venous blood into smaller segments by closure of the venous valves. As a result, the gravitational effect on the veins at the ankle is exerted by a column of blood up to the nearest closed venous valve, instead of the column of blood extending up to the heart (Fig. 10.11).

Certain persons like nurses, or traffic policemen have to keep standing for long hours every day. Excessive venous pressure stretches the veins of

10

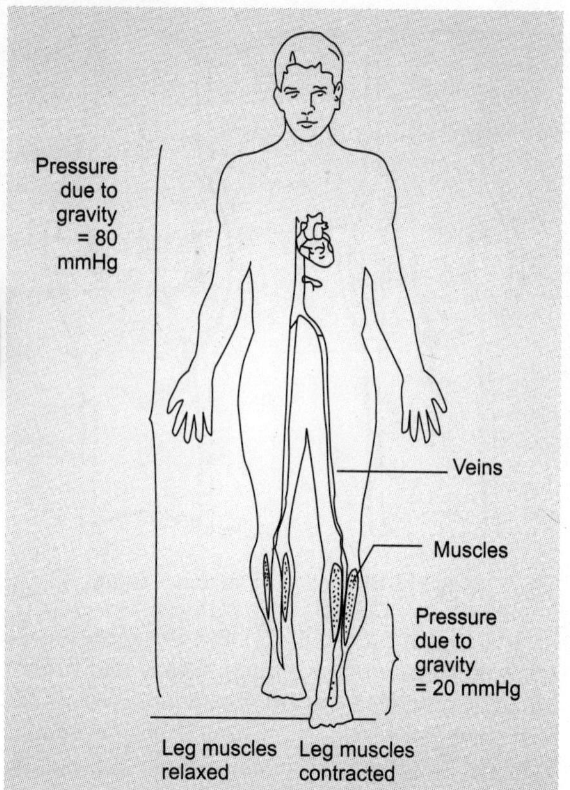

Fig. 10.11: Role of muscle pump action and venous valves. Contraction of the muscles causes closure of the venous valves and reduction of hydrostatic pressure in the veins of the feet.

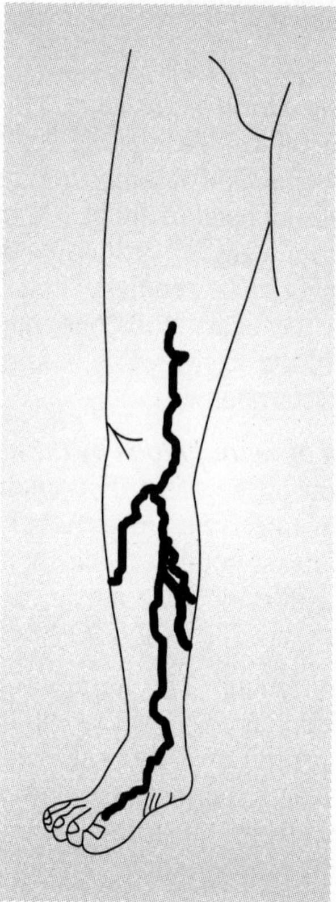

Fig. 10.12: Varicose veins.

the leg to such an extent that their diameter increases. The venous valves, therefore, become incompetent. As a result, veins of the lower limbs become large, bulbous, and tortuous. Such veins are called varicose veins (Fig. 10.12).

8. *Blood volume* An increase in blood volume increases the venous return and vice versa.

9. *Sympathetic discharge* An increase in sympathetic discharge to the veins increases the venous tone, i.e. lowers their capacitance. Hence, venous blood is displaced towards the heart.

10. *Right atrial pressure* An increase in right atrial pressure interferes with the venous return, e.g. in congestive heart failure.

11 CHAPTER

Regulation of Systemic Arterial Blood Pressure

Adequate blood flow through the vital organs like the brain and the heart must be maintained all the time. The brain is irreversibly damaged within three minutes of ischaemia. In contrast, many other tissues such as the skin, skeletal muscle or the GI tract can tolerate reduction of the blood flow for a longer duration. The excretory function of the kidney is also critically dependent on normal arterial blood pressure (which provides driving force for the glomerular filtration). It would be obvious that the maintenance of blood pressure within the physiological range is of fundamental importance for the survival of an individual. Besides this, the circulatory system is subjected to various types of stress which may vary from simple change of posture (from supine to upright) to severe haemorrhage. For such eventualities, multiple cardiovascular regulatory systems have been evolved in the mammals. Of these, the *neural regulatory mechanism* is most important, since it responds within a few seconds. Later in the chapter, some *slow-reacting mechanisms* shall be discussed. These slow mechanisms provide a second line of defence against a disturbance in blood pressure.

NEURAL CARDIOVASCULAR REGULATORY MECHANISMS

Neural cardiovascular regulatory mechanisms consist of a medullary cardiovascular centre commonly called the vasomotor centre (VMC) and its afferent and efferent connections.

MEDULLARY CARDIOVASCULAR CENTRE (Vasomotor Centre)

The primary cardiovascular regulatory centre is located in the medulla oblongata of the brainstem. It consists of a bilateral group of neurons situated in the reticular formation, at the floor of the fourth ventricle. These neurons control the blood pressure by changing the vascular tone, as well as, the cardiac output. This group of neurons exerts a predominantly excitatory effect on the thoraco-lumbar sympathetic neurons innervating the heart and the blood vessels.

In the initial experimental studies, the effect of stimulation of this area was recorded on blood pressure only. Therefore, it was assumed that this area mainly affects the arteriolar tone and the term *vasomotor centre (VMC)* was used for these neurons. However, subsequently it was revealed that the increase in the BP was not only because of increased vascular tone but also because of increased sympathetic discharge to heart leading to increased cardiac output. Therefore, although the term *medullary cardiovascular centre* is more appropriate, this area is still widely known as vasomotor centre.

11

Further studies revealed that whereas stimulation of rostral and lateral region of the VMC predominantly increases the heart rate and BP, stimulation of the most medial and caudal region of the same area results in bradycardia and a fall in BP. The terms *pressor area* and *depressor area*, have been applied to the two components of VMC. Pressor area exerts an excitatory influence on the thoracolumbar sympathetic neurons supplying the heart and the blood vessels (chiefly arterioles and venules). The depressor area, when activated (by certain reflex mechanisms), exerts an inhibitory influence on thoracolumbar sympathetic neurons. The depressor area also increases the parasympathetic (vagal) discharge to the heart (Fig. 11.1).

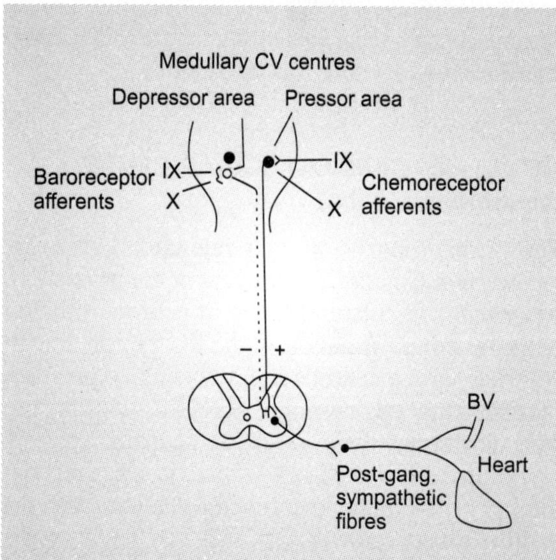

Fig. 11.1: Pathways for neural regulation of the heart and the blood vessels.

The neurons of the pressor area of the VMC have an inherent tonic discharge leading to a steady discharge in the vasomotor nerves supplying the blood vessels. This can be experimentally demonstrated by producing a transverse section in the lower cervical region of the spinal cord. The blood pressure of the animal immediately falls to about 40 mmHg. After a few days, the spinal sympathetic neurons resume some tonic activity and the blood pressure rises to some extent. However, there is no regulation of blood pressure under stressful conditions because of the lack of connection of the thoracolumbar sympathetic neurons with medullary VMC.

Factors Affecting the VMC (Fig. 11.2)

Higher Centres of the Brain

The influence of the cerebral cortex on the BP is well known. Tachycardia and hypertension during emotional stress or sexual excitement, or bradycardia and fainting during sudden emotional shock are examples of the influence of the limbic system on the medullary VMC.

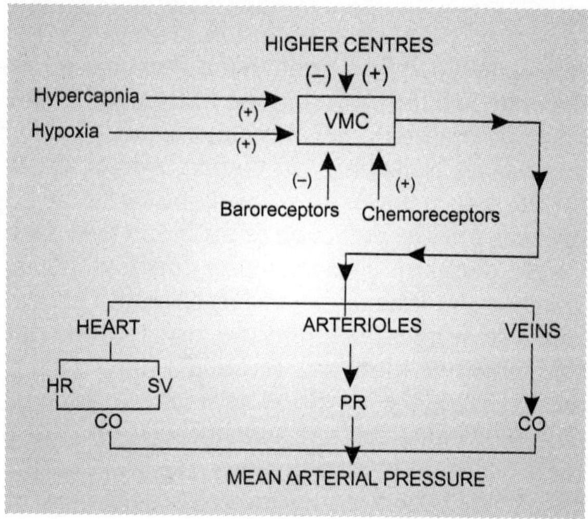

Fig. 11.2: Neural vasomotor control.

In normotensive individuals, arterial blood pressure may show moderate to marked increase while driving an automobile in heavy traffic or during a stormy official meeting, which subsequently returns to normal (Fig. 11.3). These are examples of the effect of emotional stress on blood pressure.

The hypothalamus serves to integrate many somatic and autonomic responses, e.g. for temperature regulation, or for defence reactions. The cardiovascular elements of these responses are brought about by the hypothalamus through its connection with the VMC.

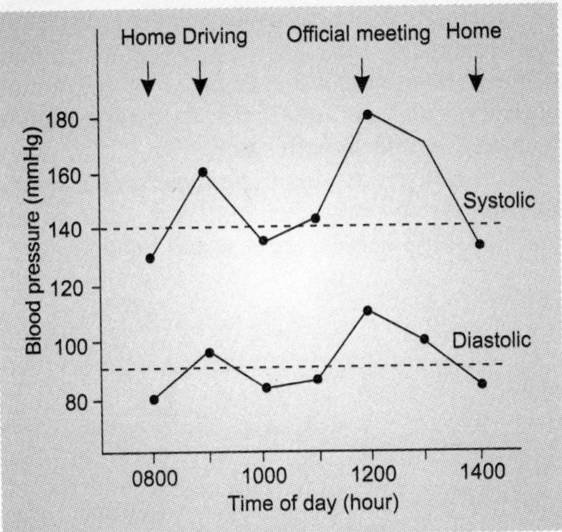

Fig. 11.3: Effect of emotional stress (driving in a rush hour; stormy official meeting) on the arterial blood pressure of a normotensive ("normal") individual.

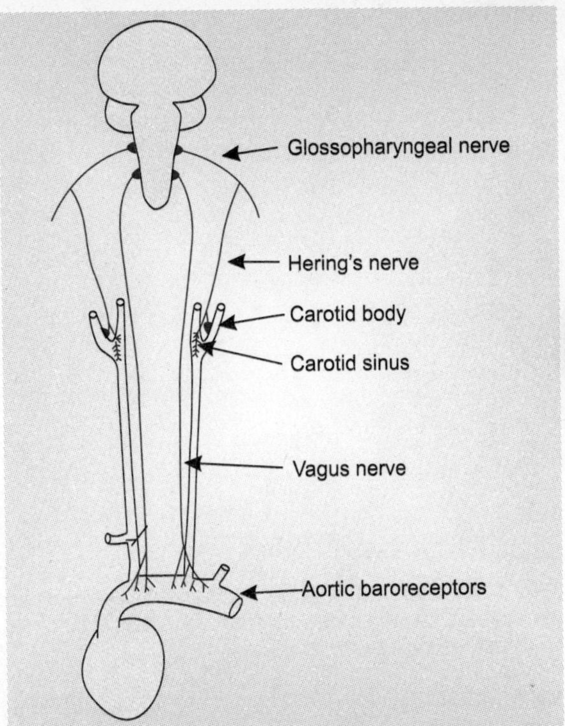

Fig. 11.4: The sino-aortic baroreceptors.

Baroreceptor Afferents

Baroreceptors are stretch receptors (mechanoreceptors) located in the wall of the heart and certain segments of the blood vessels. They respond to changes in the BP. Of these, the arterial baroreceptors are concerned with very rapid control of the arterial BP. Cardiopulmonary baroreceptors, to be described subsequently, are concerned with the regulation of central venous pressure (CVP) blood volume.

(a) Arterial Baroreceptors At its origin from the common carotid artery, the internal carotid artery shows a small dilatation, called the *carotid sinus*. The wall of the artery is thinnest at this site and the tunica adventitia contains a large number of highly branched, coiled and inter-twined naked nerve endings of myelinated nerve fibres (Fig. 11.4). These nerve-endings are highly sensitive to distortion or stretch produced by pressure within the artery. These afferent fibres along with the afferents from the carotid body form the *sinus nerve*, a branch of 9th cranial nerve. Similar stretch receptors are located in the tunica adventitia of the arch of aorta. The afferent nerve fibres, along with those from the aortic body, form the *aortic nerve*, a branch of 10th cranial nerve.

The baroreceptor afferents from the carotid sinus and the arch of aorta are often collectively called the *buffer nerves*, because they act to prevent any rise or fall in the arterial blood pressure.

(i) *Pattern of discharge* The baroreceptors do not respond to perfusion pressure below 60 mmHg. Above this pressure, the discharge rate increases with increase in perfusion pressure, but the response is non-linear. Baroreceptors are most sensitive to pressure changes around the normal mean arterial pressure of the species, i.e. in humans even a small change in blood pressure around the mean pressure of 100 mmHg produces marked changes in the baroreceptor discharge rate. Beyond 200 mmHg pressure, there is no further increase in the rate of the discharge in the baroreceptors (Fig. 11.5).

(ii) *Effect of changes in baroreceptor discharge* Increased discharge in baroreceptors *inhibits* tonic discharge of the medullary *VMC* to the heart and blood vessels and also *increases* the *vagal discharge* to the heart. Consequently, there is

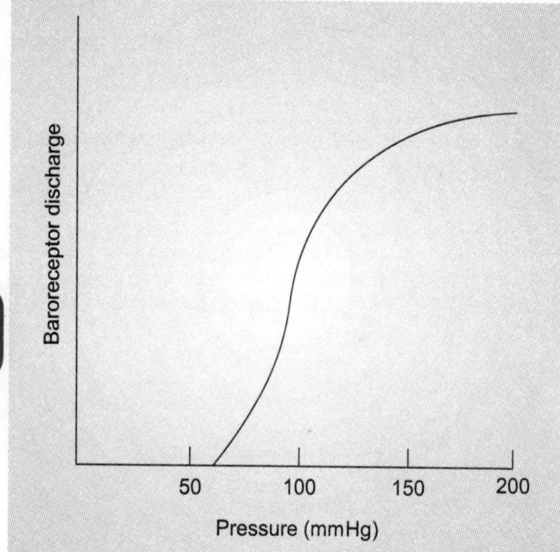

Fig. 11.5: Effect of change in perfusion pressure in an isolated carotid sinus on (baroreceptor) discharge in the sinus nerve.

vasodilatation (decreased peripheral resistance), venodilatation, bradycardia and decreased cardiac output. As a result of all these changes, *the blood pressure falls* (Fig. 11.6).

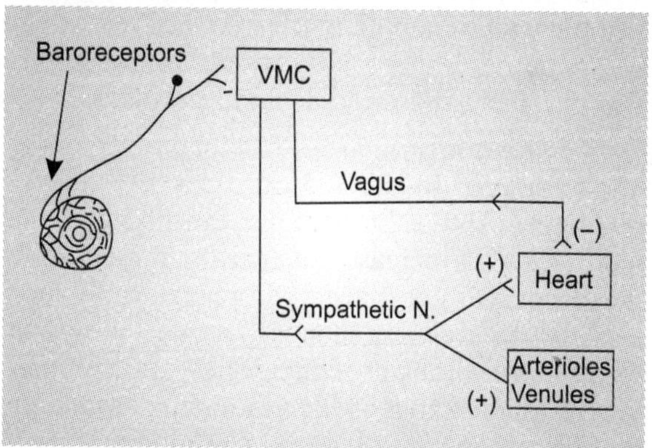

Fig. 11.6: Relation between baroreceptors, VMC and the heart and blood vessels.

A decrease in the baroreceptor discharge produces the reverse effects, i.e. increased activity of VMC leading to vasoconstriction (increased peripheral resistance), venoconstriction (decreased venous pooling and thus increased venous return), increase in heart rate and cardiac output. As a result of all these changes, the *blood pressure increases*.

Experimentally, arterial baroreceptor discharge can be markedly reduced by: (a) bilateral clamping of the common carotid arteries, or by (b) cutting both the sinus nerves. It results in a moderate tachycardia and hypertension (Fig. 11.7). More marked tachycardia and hypertension (BP = 300/200 mmHg) occurs when both, the sinus nerves and the aortic nerves, are resected bilaterally.

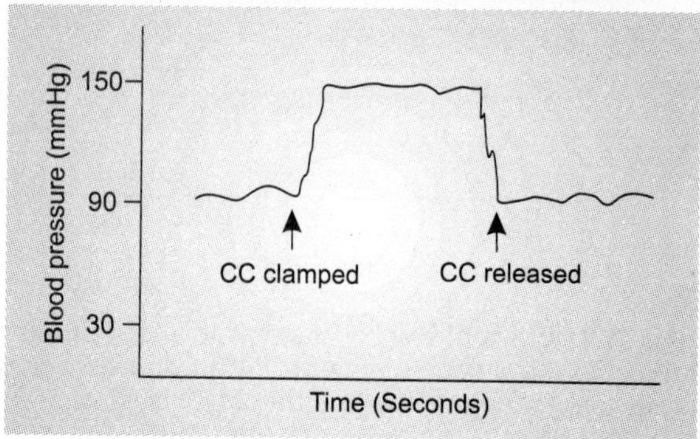

Fig. 11.7: Effect of clamping common carotid artery.

(iii) *Function of arterial baroreceptors* The normal BP is the result of a tonic discharge in the sympathetic fibres to the arterioles and venules, initiated from the VMC. The tonic discharge of the VMC is constantly under slight inhibitory effect of the arterial baroreceptors. The constant vagal (parasympathetic) discharge to the heart (vagal tone) is also reflex in nature and depends on steady baroreceptor discharge. Thus, the baroreceptors and the sinus-aortic nerves constitute the afferent limbs of a reflex arc in which the VMC acts as the centre and the sympathetic and vagus constitute the efferent limbs (Fig. 11.8).

This reflex arc acts as a feedback mechanism which maintains the BP and the HR at a steady normal level. Any rise in BP results in greater impulse discharge in the buffer nerves. The resultant inhibition of VMC decreases the CO as well as the PR. As a result, BP falls to near normal

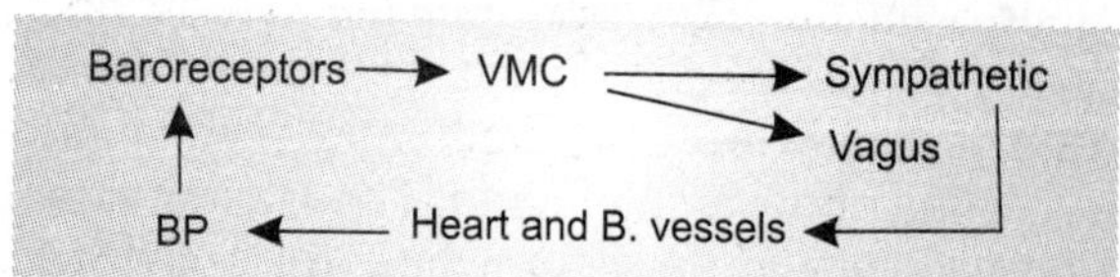

Fig. 11.8: Feedback control of BP.

level (Fig. 11.9A). Any drop in the systemic arterial BP decreases the inhibitory discharge of the buffer nerves on the VMC causing compensatory increase in CO, PR and hence BP is restored to near normal (Fig. 11.9B).

(iv) *Resetting of 'barostat'* As explained above, the baroreceptors maintain the B. P. within a normal narrow range. In that case, one may ask, how a person can ever become hypertensive? The answer is that the baroreceptors respond to short term deviations in the arterial BP If the BP of a person is chronically elevated, there is resetting of the baroreceptor reflex mechanism and the receptors try to maintain the BP at the newly elevated level rather than the previous normal level.

(b) Other Baroreceptors

(i) *Atrial baroreceptors* Two types of stretch receptors are present in the subendocardial region of the atria, specially the left atrium. Atrial stretch receptors seem to monitor the central venous pressure and act as *volume receptors*. Their stimulation by hypervolaemia results in increased secretion of *atrial natriuretic peptide (ANP)* from the atrial myocytes and *inhibition of ADH secretion* from the posterior pituitary gland.

Bainbridge reflex Rapid infusion of intravenous saline (or blood) in anaesthetised animals produces tachycardia, if initially the heart rate is low. This effect is known as the Bainbridge reflex. It seems to be the effect of stimulation of atrial baroreceptors. The physiological significance of the reflex is not clear.

(ii) *Left ventricular baroreceptors* In experimental animals, the distension of the left ventricle has been shown to produce bradycardia and hypotension. However, distension required to produce these effects is so high that no physiological significance can be attached to these

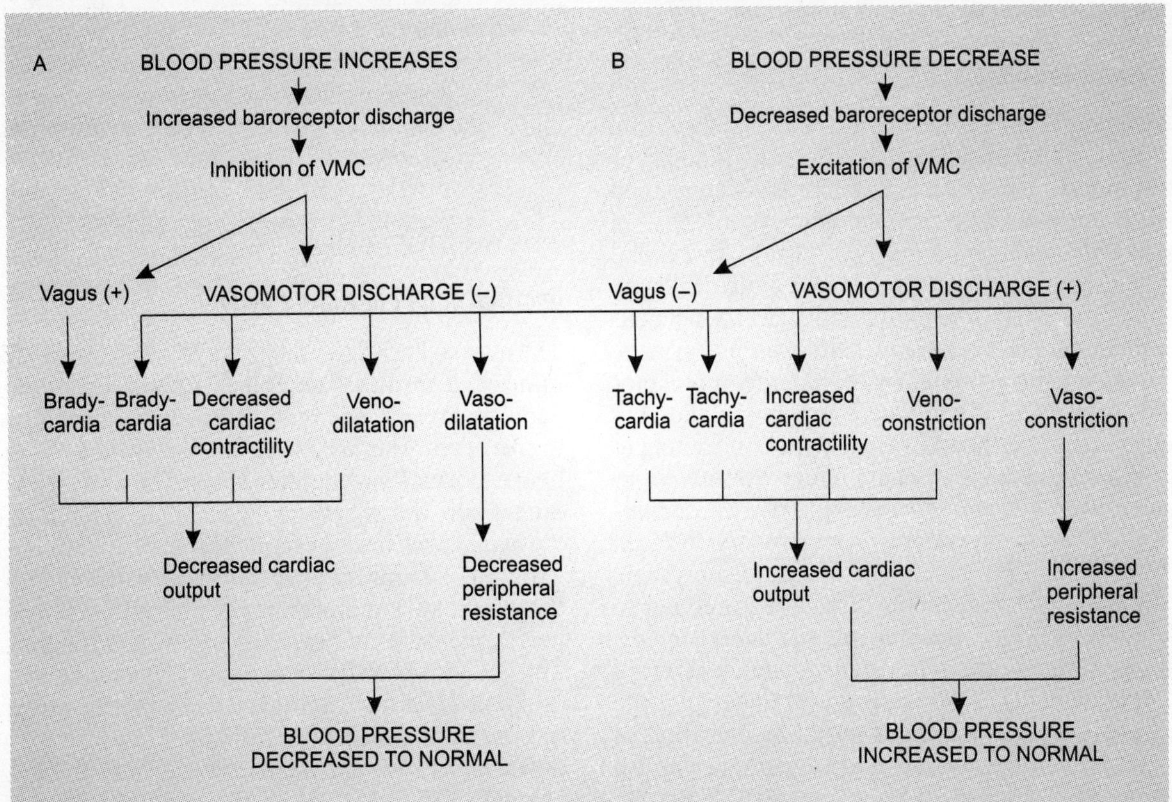

Fig. 11.9: Blood pressure regulation by baroreceptor mechanism.

receptors. Injection of certain drugs like varatridine or nicotine into the left coronary artery also produces hypotension and bradycardia (but the injection of the drugs in the right coronary artery is ineffective). The response is called *coronary chemo-reflex* or *Bezold-Jarisch reflex*. The response is abolished by bilateral vagotomy. Bezold-Jarisch reflex is probably produced by the chemical stimulation of left ventricular stretch receptors. It has been speculated that the persistent hypotension in some patients of myocardial infarction may be due to the stimulation of ventricular stretch receptors by substances released from the necrotic cardiac tissue.

(iii) *Pulmonary arterial baroreceptors* The walls of pulmonary arterial trunk contain baroreceptors in the tunica adventitia. These baroreceptors act as low pressure volume receptors, like the atrial baroreceptors. They are stimulated by volume overload and result in inhibition of ADH secretion as well as increased secretion of atrial natriuretic hormone.

Chemoreceptors

Chemoreceptors in the *carotid body* and the *aortic body* respond to changes in pO_2, pCO_2, and pH of the blood. These receptors are primarily concerned with the regulation of pulmonary ventilation. In physiological conditions, i.e. a healthy individual breathing normal air, there is very little discharge from the chemoreceptors and there is no contribution to the regulation of cardiovascular system. However, in hypoxia, increased chemoreceptor discharge, not only produces hyperventilation but also causes peripheral vasoconstriction leading to a rise in arterial BP. Thus, unlike *the inhibitory action of arterial baroreceptors, the chemoreceptors have an excitatory action on the VMC*. In hypotension produced by severe haemorrhage, increased chemoreceptor discharge may help to elevate BP. This protective role of chemoreceptors in severe hypotension can be demonstrated experimentally. Bilateral section of sinus and aortic nerves in normal animals produces elevation of BP. In severe hypotensive animals, similar surgical procedure produces further fall in BP. Since, in such animals, the baroreceptor discharge is already absent, the section of sinus and aortic nerves abolishes the chemoreceptor drive as well. The further fall in BP indicates that the chemoreceptors were contributing to the maintenance of BP to some extent.

Direct Actions on VMC

(i) Arterial hypoxia (low pO_2) and hypercapnia (elevated pCO_2) stimulate the VMC directly. Peripherally, increased arterial pCO_2 has inhibitory action on the vascular smooth muscle. Therefore, in case of CO_2, the peripheral and central effects cancel each other and only severe rise of arterial pCO_2 causes a mild increase in BP.

(ii) An increase in the intracranial pressure interferes with the cerebral circulation resulting in ischemia of the brain including the VMC. The resulting local hypoxia and hypercapnia stimulate the VMC causing a rise in the systemic arterial BP. This reflex, called the *Cushing reflex*, tends to restore the cerebral blood flow by increasing the arterial pressure. The resulting increase in the BP causes reflex bradycardia via arterial baroreceptors. Thus, bradycardia is an important clinical feature of raised intracranial pressure (Fig. 11.10).

REGULATION OF HEART RATE

The normal heart rate (range 60–90/min, mean 75/min.) is a result of combined effects of strong parasympathetic and mild sympathetic discharge to the heart. The SA node, the pacemaker of the heart, normally generates impulses at a much higher rate. It is shown by the fact that, in humans, the *denervated* heart beats at the rate of about 110–120/min. Administration of atropine (which blocks the effect of parasympathetic discharge to the heart), elevates the heart rate to a similar degree. The constant discharge in the vagus nerve is known as the *vagal tone*. The vagal tone is a reflex effect of constant baroreceptor discharge.

Variations in the heart rate can occur by a change in the vagal discharge and/or change in sympathetic discharge. In trained athletes, the

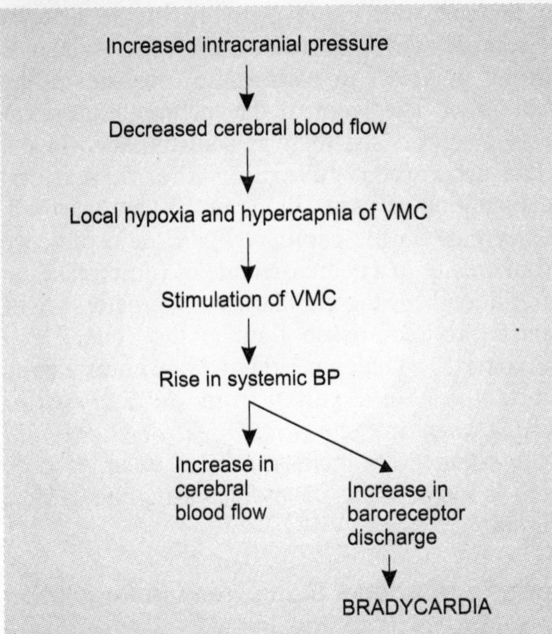

Fig. 11.10: Effect of increased intracranial pressure on the heart rate and BP.

resting heart rate is around 60/min, because the athletic training increases the vagal tone. In maximal athletic activity (or exercise on a treadmill) the heart rate may increase to a value as high as 180–200/min.

During deep breathing in adults or even quiet breathing in young children, the heart rate is faster during inspiration than during expiration. This phenomenon called *sinus arrhythmia* is due to irradiation of inhibitory impulses from the inspiratory centre to the vagal nucleus in the medulla (Fig. 31.11).

The stimuli which increase or decrease the heart rate are given in Table 11.1. Except fever, thyroid hormones and catecholamines, which act locally on the SA node, all other factors affect the heart rate through medullary cardiovascular regulatory centres (VMC).

It may be reiterated that stimuli which increase the heart rate also increase the blood pressure, whereas those causing bradycardia decrease the blood pressure. An exception to this general rule is the bradycardia and hypertension produced by Cushing's reflex.

Table 11.1: Factors affecting the heart rate

Causes of tachycardia	*Causes of bradycardia*
1. Excitement and anger	1. Athletic training
2. Painful stimuli (Somatic)	2. Fear and grief
3. Exercise	3. Rise in intracranial pressure
4. Epinephrine and nor-epinephrine	4. Visceral or trigeminal pain
5. Hyperthyroidism	5. Complete heart block with idioventricular rhythm
6. Fever	6. Myxoedema
7. Bainbridge reflex	
8. Hypotension due to haemorrhage or dehydration	

NON-NEURAL REGULATORY MECHANISMS

The neural regulatory mechanisms discussed above provide a very rapid means of BP regulation. The neural mechanisms can counteract both a rise and a fall of BP. In contrast, the regulatory mechanisms described below are not only relatively slow to act but also are mainly effective against a fall of blood pressure only.

When the BP remains low for more than a few minutes (in spite of neural regulation), certain hormonal and fluid shift mechanisms are activated, which supplement the neural mechanism for restoration of BP to normal.

HORMONAL MECHANISMS

1. Vasopressin Vasopressin, also known as antidiuretic hormone (ADH), is secreted from the posterior pituitary. It is primarily concerned with the regulation of body water. When present in physiological concentration in the blood, the antidiuretic action is prominent. Fall of BP due to haemorrhage or hypovolemia due to dehydration causes release of larger amounts of ADH from the posterior pituitary. At higher plasma concentrations of the hormone, the *vasopressor action* becomes quite significant, which, along with the antidiuretic action, helps to restore the blood volume as well as the BP. The vasopressor action increases the arteriolar resistance, whereas the antidiuretic action improves the blood volume (Chapter 46).

2. Renin-angiotensin Vasoconstrictor Mechanism The renin-angiotensin system is described in detail elsewhere but summarised in Fig. 11.11.

11

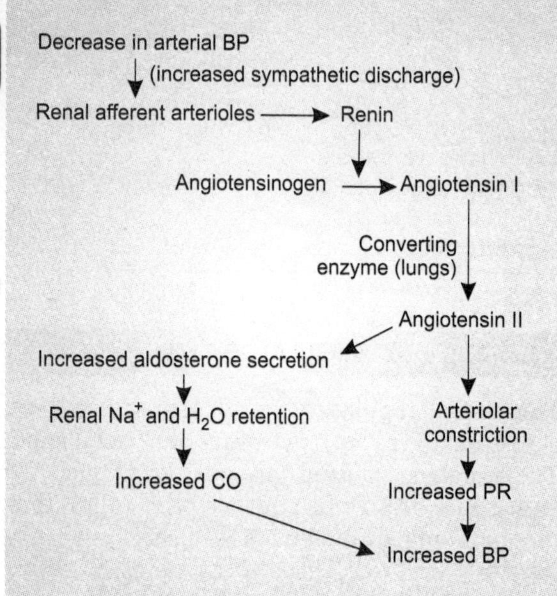

Fig. 11.11: The renin-angiotensin mechanism.

Angiotensin-II is the most potent vasoconstrictor known. It causes arteriolar constriction to increase the peripheral resistance. In addition, angiotensin-II acts on the adrenal cortex to increase the secretion of aldosterone. Aldosterone causes retention of Na^+ and H_2O by acting on renal tubules. Thus, plasma volume, cardiac output and PR are all increased and BP is restored to normal. Renin-angiotensin system takes at least 20 minutes to be fully operative, but it makes a significant contribution to the recovery of BP after severe haemorrhage.

CAPILLARY FLUID SHIFT MECHANISM

Reflex arteriolar vasoconstriction is one of the important neural responses to a fall in blood pressure, e.g., in a patient suffering from haemorrhagic hypotension. This response tends to increase the blood pressure in the arterial system. However, increased arteriolar resistance results in a fall in hydrostatic pressure in the capillaries. Therefore, if the increased arteriolar resistance persists, there is a disturbance in the Starling forces governing the formation-reabsorption of tissue fluids in the capillary bed. A decrease in the capillary hydrostatic pressure would result in a decreased rate of filtration at the arterial ends of the capillaries and greater rate of reabsorption of tissue fluid at the venous end (Chapter 10). Over a period of a few hours a large amount of fluid shifts from the *interstitial compartment* into the *vascular extracellular fluid compartment*. The increase in blood volume would help to increase the BP by increasing the cardiac output.

Long-Term Arterial Blood Pressure Regulation

Earlier in this chapter, the neural regulation of blood pressure has been discussed. It is the most rapidly acting mechanism. Some slow acting short-term regulatory mechanisms like the role of vasopressor hormones and fluid shift mechanisms have also been discussed. However, when the blood pressure change is slow; over a period of many days, the neural mechanism loses almost all of its ability to react to the change. Therefore, there has to be a long-term regulatory mechanism which maintains the arterial blood pressure in the normal range, week-after-week and month-after-month. The kidneys play a dominant role in this long-term regulation of blood pressure.

In the discussion on the arterial blood pressure, the importance of blood volume as one of the important determinants was highlighted. The long-term regulation of blood pressure is achieved by changes in the blood volume (or ECF volume). The kidneys have an ability to regulate the ECF volume by regulation of salt (NaCl) and water excretion. In addition, the renin-angiotensin-aldosterone system helps in the regulation of salt and water excretion by the kidneys. In an experiment on dogs, all the neural mechanisms were blocked and then about 500 ml of blood was transfused. There was an almost instantaneous increase in cardiac output as well as arterial blood pressure to almost double the initial value. The increase in blood pressure was followed by many fold increase in urinary output. Over a period of one hour, the blood pressure became normal once again.

In normal individuals, any persistent increase in arterial blood pressure leads to increased urinary salt and water excretion resulting in a decrease in ECF volume and arterial blood pressure. Any persistent decrease in arterial blood pressure leads to decreased urinary salt and water excretion. The resultant increase in ECF volume restores the blood pressure to normal. A failure of this long term regulatory mechanism is responsible for the disorder known as essential hypertension (Chapter 14).

CHAPTER 12

Regulation of Blood Flow in the Tissues

There is a great variation in the degree of blood flow in different organs. In most of the organs, the blood flow is related to its rate of metabolism—greater the metabolic rate of the organ, greater is the blood flow.

Further blood flow to an organ may have to be temporarily curtailed so as to divert more blood to a metabolically active organ. From this discussion, it would be obvious that blood flow is to be regulated at the tissue level. Blood flow to an organ can be increased by arteriolar dilatation (vasodilatation) and curtailed by arteriolar constriction (vasoconstriction). Broadly speaking, the caliber of the arterioles can be affected by two groups of mechanisms:

1. Neural mechanisms
2. Humoral mechanisms

NEURAL MECHANISMS

Neural Vasoconstriction

All the blood vessels, whatever their size, receive noradrenergic sympathetic innervation. The density of sympathetic innervation (also known as vasomotor innervation) varies in different circulations. Veins receive smaller number of sympathetic fibres than the corresponding arteries. Small arteries and arterioles of the skin, skeletal muscles and the abdominal viscera receive far greater sympathetic innervation than those in the brain and myocardium.

Under resting conditions, a mild adrenergic discharge (1–3 impulses / sec) maintains the blood vessels in a state of mild tonic contraction. Basal vascular tone is rather low in cerebral, pulmonary and coronary vessels, but strong in skeletal muscle vascular beds.

Increased vasomotor discharge causes contraction of vascular smooth muscle of the blood vessel. Contraction of smooth muscle produces practically no haemodynamic effects in the *large blood vessels* such as the aorta, large arteries or vena cavae. Widespread vasomotor discharge in the *venules and larger veins* reduces their capacity leading to displacement of a large volume of blood to the arterial circulation. Most important effect of increased vasomotor discharge occurs in the *resistance vessels (arterioles)*. By regulating the caliber of the arterioles, variations in the vasomotor discharge regulate the regional blood flow. Strong vasomotor discharge, e.g.10 impulses/sec can produce severe reduction in blood flow in certain circulations such as skeletal muscle, cutaneous and splanchnic area.

Neural Vasodilatation

(i) Decreased Adrenergic Discharge A decrease in adrenergic vasomotor discharge produces dilatation in most of the blood vessels. However, the consequent increase in blood flow is well marked only in a few vessels like AV anastomoses, where resting vasomotor discharge is high. In most of the tissues, local (humoral) factors are far more important means of vasodilatation and increased blood flow.

(ii) Sympathetic Vasodilators Besides the *sympathetic adrenergic vasoconstrictor fibres*, the blood vessels of the skeletal muscle are also supplied by a separate system of *cholinergic sympathetic fibres*. Increased discharge in these nerve fibres causes vasodilatation in the skeletal muscle.

Sympathetic vasodilator system originates in the cerebral cortex. The neurons relay in the hypothalamus and mesencephalon (mid-brain) but (unlike sympathetic vasoconstrictors) have no connection with medullary vasomotor centres. These fibres terminate around the lateral horn cells in the thoracolumbar region of the spinal cord. The preganglionic neurons of this system follow the usual sympathetic pathways but the postganglionic fibres are cholinergic in nature (Fig. 12.1).

The functional significance of this system is not yet clear. Sympathetic vasodilator fibres seem to increase the blood flow in thoroughfare channels, just before the start of exercise. At this stage, the cardiac output is increased due to emotional factors. Increased discharge in the sympathetic vasodilator fibres, occurring at this time, lowers the peripheral resistance and prevents undue rise of blood pressure.

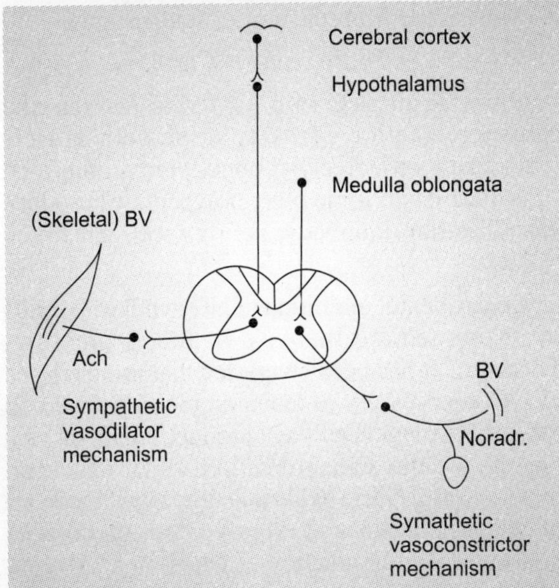

Fig. 12.1: Pathways of sympathetic vasodilator system (on the left) as compared to sympathetic vasoconstrictor system (on the right).

(iii) Parasympathetic Vasodilators Vasodilatation because of increased discharge in parasympathetic nerve fibres occurs in the *external genitalia only*. Vasodilatation produced by parasympathetic stimulation in the gastrointestinal exocrine glands is not truly a neural vasodilatation (see below).

(iv) Axon Reflex (See Chapter 13).

HUMORAL MECHANISMS

Local Metabolites

Certain products of tissue metabolism act as highly potent vasodilators. A decrease in the partial pressure of O_2 (pO_2), and decrease in pH or increase in pCO_2, or increase in local temperature act as vasodilators by producing relaxation of the smooth muscle of the arterioles and the precapillary sphincters. Local accumulation of K^+, lactate, or adenosine also causes vasodilatation in these vessels.

The vasodilatation produced by these metabolites is far more pronounced than that produced by decreased adrenergic (neural vasoconstrictor) discharge. For example, abolition of vasomotor adrenergic discharge increases the blood flow in skeletal muscles from 2 ml /100 gm /min to 4 ml/ 100 gm/min only, but during exercise the local metabolites increase the skeletal blood flow up to 70 ml/100 gm/min.

Another advantage of the control of tissue blood flow by local metabolites is that the blood flow can be exactly matched to the metabolic requirements. In the myocardium, adenosine (derived from ATP) or low pO_2 seem to be the chief regulator of blood flow. Increased pCO_2 is the most potent dilator of cerebral vessels. In the skeletal muscle, accumulation of K^+, or lactate, as a result of metabolic activity, seems to regulate the blood flow during exercise.

12

Bradykinin

In certain tissues like sweat glands, salivary glands and intestine, the exocrine secretion is accompanied by the release of a proteolytic enzyme called kallikrein into the extracellular fluid. Kallikrein acts on kininogen, (an α-2 globulin) present in the tissue fluids, to produce a polypeptide called bradykinin (Fig. 12.2). Bradykinin is a powerful vasodilator and it increases capillary permeability as well. Bradykinin, thus, increases the blood flow when these tissues are actively secreting their products.

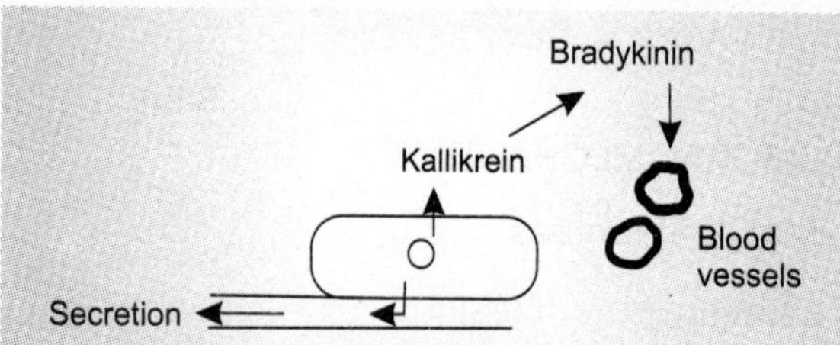

Fig. 12.2: Mechanism of production of bradykinin during secretory activity of an exocrine gland.

Circulating Vasoactive Substances

Epinephrine and norepinephrine (released from the adrenal medulla during generalized sympathetic response to stress) act on α and β adrenergic receptors present in the walls of blood vessels. Circulating *norepinephrine* produces vasoconstriction but the effect is much weaker than that produced by norepinephrine released from adrenergic nerve endings. Circulating *epinephrine* dilates the skeletal vessels through β-receptors.

Vasopressin and *angiotensin-II* act as generalized vasoconstrictors. These polypeptide hormones play a significant role in the maintenance of blood pressure after severe blood loss or in severe dehydration.

Histamine is probably not involved in physiological regulation of tissue blood flow. It is released by the mast cells as a tissue response to injury. It is a powerful vasodilator and it increases the capillary permeability as well.

Histamine seems to be one of the many chemical mediators of vascular response to inflammation.

Role of Endothelial Cells The endothelial cells collectively constitute an important organ. They release many growth factors as well as many vasoactive substances. The growth factors play a key role in vascular development (angiogenesis). The vasoactive substances produced by the endothelial cells include prostaglandins, nitric oxide and endothelins.

(a) Prostaglandins In many physiological and pathological conditions, tissue blood flow seems to be regulated by prostaglandins produced locally. Some of the prostaglandins are vasoconstrictors, but most of them act as local vasodilators. Change from supine to standing posture results in wide spread vasoconstriction as shown by a net increase in total peripheral resistance. However, renal blood flow and GFR do not decrease due to simultaneous production of renal prostaglandins. In acute inflammations, prostaglandins are one of the chemical mediators producing local vasodilatation.

(b) Nitric Oxide Different stimuli may act on the endothelial cells to produce *endothelium-derived relaxing factors* (EDRF), a substance that is now known to be *nitric oxide* (NO). Nitric oxide is synthesized from the amino acid arginine.

Arginine → Nitric oxide + Citrulline

Nitric oxide acts in a paracrine fashion and causes relaxation of vascular smooth muscle (vasodilatation). Acetylcholine, bradykinin, VIP, substance P and some other polypeptides produce vasodilatation indirectly, i.e. by local generation of NO.

Experimental inhibition of NO synthesis results in an immediate increase in blood pressure. Therefore, it has been suggested that tonic release of NO is necessary to maintain blood pressure in the normal range. Deficient production of NO may be one of the causative factors in essential hypertension. Nitric oxide is an important mediator of vasodilatation and engorgement of corpora cavernosa during erection of penis.

(c) Endothelins Endothelin-1 is a 21-amino acid polypeptide produced by endothelial cells. It is the most potent vasoconstrictor known as yet. Endothelin 1 is produced by endothelial cells and secreted towards tunica media, where it acts in a paracrine fashion on the vascular smooth muscle. Its presence in very low concentrations in the plasma is probably due to an overflow from the endothelial cells; it does not have endocrine mode of action. The release of endothelin 1 is increased by angiotensin II, catecholamines and inhibited by prostaglandins and NO. Thus, endothelin seems to be primarily a local paracrine regulator of vascular tone. In the kidney, endothelin-2 produces mesangial cells-mediated increase in renal vascular resistance and a decrease in glomerular filtration rate. An endothelin seems to be involved in the closure of ductus arteriosus at birth. Factors affecting the caliber of arterioles have been summarized in Table 12.1.

REACTIVE HYPERAEMIA

If the arterial supply to a limb is stopped for a few seconds, (e.g. by raising the pressure in the sphygmomanometer cuff above the systolic blood pressure (>160 mmHg), and then restored, the skin becomes markedly red indicating the *cutaneous hyperaemia*. The increased blood flow in the underlying muscles can also be demonstrated by plethysmography. The degree and the duration of hyperaemia varies with the duration of initial arterial occlusion (Fig. 12.3). This phenomenon, called *reactive hyperaemia* is due to accumulation of vasodilator products of hypoxic tissue metabolism during the period of arterial occlusion. On release of occlusion, blood flow remains above the basal level till the local metabolites are washed away/destroyed.

Table 12.1: Summary of factors affecting caliber of arterioles

	Vasoconstriction	*Vasodilatation*
Neural factors	(i) Increased discharge in noradrenergic vasomotor nerves	(i) Decreased discharge in noradrenergic vasomotor nerves (ii) Activation of cholinergic sympathetic vasodilator discharge(skeletal muscle) (iii) Increased parasympathetic discharge to external genital vessels. (iv) Axon reflex (in inflammation)
Local factors	(i) Decreased local temperature (ii) Autoregulation (iii) Endothelin I (iv) Thromboxane A2 (v) Serotonin	(i) Increased local temperature (ii) Increased tissue pCO_2 (iii) Decreased tissue pO_2 (iv) Increased tissue adenosine (v) Increased tissue K^+ (vi) Increased tissue lactate (vii) Decreased local pH (viii) Autoregulation (ix) Nitrous oxide (x) Kinins (xi) Prostaglandin PGE2
Circulating hormones	(i) Epinephrine (except in skeletal muscle and liver (ii) Norepinephrine (iii) Vasopressin (iv) Angiotensin II	(i) Epinephrine (in skeletal muscle and liver) (ii) Substance P (iii) Histamine (iv) ANP (v) VIP

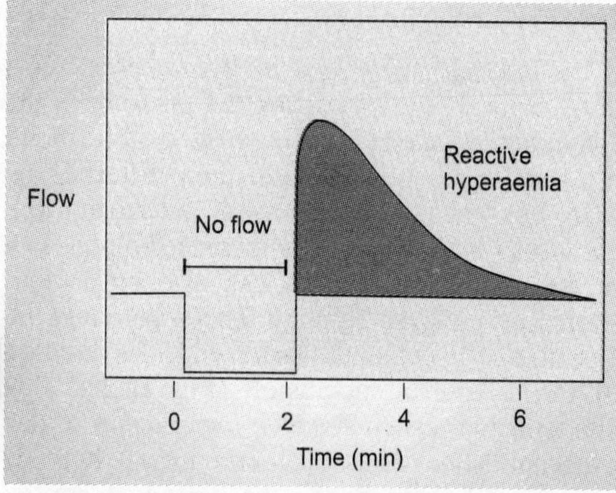

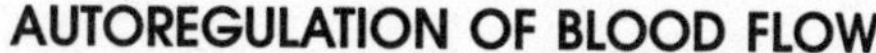

Fig. 12.3: Reactive hyperaemia.

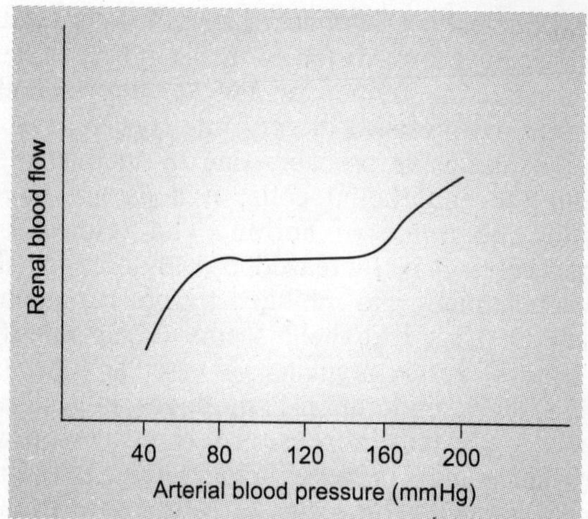

Fig. 12.4: Autoregulation of blood flow in the renal blood vessels.

AUTOREGULATION OF BLOOD FLOW

Since, flow = pressure/resistance, increase in the perfusion pressure (arterial blood pressure) is expected to produce an increase in the flow of blood to the tissues. Actually, in most of the tissues, notably *the kidney, the heart, the brain, skeletal muscle and liver,* blood flow remains relatively constant between mean arterial pressures of 70 to 150 mmHg. The maintenance of blood flow at near normal level in spite of marked changes in the arterial pressure is called autoregulation of blood flow (Fig. 12.4).

The intrinsic mechanism responsible for autoregulation is not known. It can be observed even after denervation of an organ. According to the *myogenic theory,* the vascular smooth muscle responds to increased stretch by increasing its tension. In other words, an increased perfusion pressure is accompanied by a proportionate decrease in the calibre of the arterioles, leading to an increased vascular resistance. Consequently, the flow of blood remains constant.

According to the *metabolic theory*, a sudden increase in the perfusion pressure initially increases the blood flow, but this causes excessive removal of the local vasodilator metabolites. The consequent increase in the vascular resistance restores the blood flow to normal.

13

CHAPTER

Regional Circulations

CORONARY CIRCULATION

FUNCTIONAL ANATOMY

In man, there are two coronary arteries, the right and the left coronary arteries, which originate from the sinuses of Valsalva, just above the aortic valve leaflets. In approximately 90% of human subjects, the right coronary artery is "dominant", i.e. larger than the left coronary artery and supplies blood to a major part of the heart. It supplies blood to the right atrium, right ventricle, posterior wall of the left ventricle and the vital SA node and the AV node. The left coronary artery supplies blood to the left atrium, the interventricular septum and anterior and lateral walls of the left ventricle.

Each coronary artery divides progressively into smaller branches which spread on the surface of the heart. These branches give off tiny arterioles which penetrate the myocardium at right angles. The coronary arteries are basically end-arteries; there are no anastomoses between the two coronary arteries. That is why; thrombosis of one coronary artery is invariably followed by ischaemia or infarction of the part of myocardium supplied by the blocked artery.

The heart has a huge demand for oxygen since it is continuously active; pumping blood all over the body. Moreover, the myocardium is dependent purely on aerobic metabolism of the substrates (glucose and FFA). That is why myocardium has far greater capillary density (2500 capillaries/ square mm) than skeletal muscle (400 capillaries/ square mm).

Most of the venous blood from the myocardium is drained by the coronary sinus and anterior cardiac veins into the right atrium. A small amount of venous blood (less than 10%) is drained by deep venous channels (thebesian veins) directly into the cardiac chambers.

CORONARY BLOOD FLOW

Coronary blood flow, at rest, is about 250 ml per minute (5% of total CO). Because of high metabolic rate of the myocardium, even at rest, 70–80% of the oxygen is extracted from each unit the arterial blood (cf. 25% oxygen extraction in the body taken as a whole). During exercise, the increased oxygen demand of the myocardium is met with by almost total extraction of O_2 from the coronary arterial blood and by manifold increase in the rate of coronary blood flow.

Although the perfusion pressure (aortic pressure) is greater during ventricular systole, most of the coronary blood flow (over 70% of total) occurs during the ventricular diastolic phase (Fig. 13.1A). The difference in the amount of coronary blood flow during cardiac systole and diastole is not merely because of longer duration of diastole. In exercise, when the duration of diastole may be equal to or even shorter than systole, most of the coronary blood flow still occurs during diastole (Fig. 13.1B). Extramural pressure on the coronary arteries is the determining factor. In the left ventricle, the tension developed in the myocardium is so high that it has throttling effect on the branches of coronary vessels penetrating through them. During some moments of the isometric contraction phase, the coronary blood flow to the left ventricle practically ceases. In diastole, the absence of extramural compression permits free flow of blood.

In the right ventricle, the pattern of blood flow is basically similar, with a difference that the reduction in blood flow during systole is not so drastic. The difference is related to the degree of tension developed in the two ventricles during systole. From this discussion, it is easy to understand why the *subendocardial region* of the left ventricle (which develops maximum tension during systole) is particularly prone to ischaemia and is the most common site of myocardial infarction.

In severe tachycardia, the duration of diastole is drastically curtailed. This tends to reduce the coronary blood flow, but due to local metabolic regulation, the blood flow to the myocardium is not seriously affected.

Regulation of Coronary Blood Flow

1. Aortic Pressure The aortic pressure is the driving force for the coronary perfusion. Therefore, coronary blood flow may be expected to vary with changes in the blood pressure. However, over a fairly wide range of arterial BP, the coronary blood flow remains practically constant. The phenomenon is called autoregulation of coronary blood flow.

The coronary autoregulation fails when *mean* blood pressure falls below 70 mmHg, and the coronary perfusion is seriously impaired.

2. Autonomic Control Coronary vessels are supplied with noradrenergic sympathetic fibres. In the intact animal, stimulation of sympathetic fibres to the heart produces coronary vasodi-

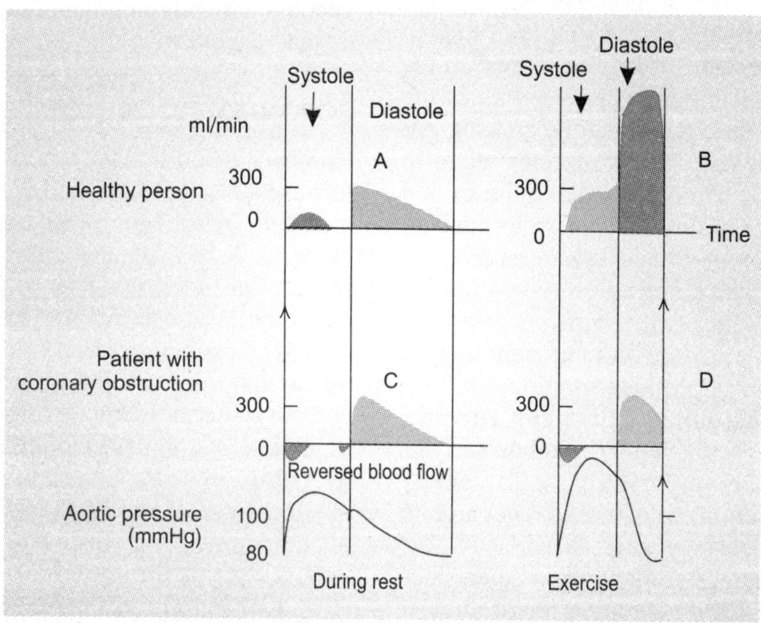

Fig. 13.1: Effect of different phases of the cardiac cycle on the blood flow in the left coronary artery, and on the aortic pressure; at rest and during exercise.

latation. This is an indirect effect of simultaneous increase in the myocardial activity and the resultant excessive production of local vasodilator metabolites. Experimentally, when the positive inotropic and chronotropic adrenergic effects on the myocardium are blocked by prior administration of a β-adrenergic blocker, sympathetic stimulation produces a weak coronary vasoconstriction.

3. Local Metabolites Coronary blood flow can be shown to increase in proportion to the increase in cardiac out put or cardiac work. A direct and almost linear correlation can be observed between the coronary blood flow and the myocardial O_2 consumption (Fig. 13.2). How the O_2 consumption regulates the coronary vascular resistance is not exactly clear. A decrease in the tissue pO_2 could act on the arterioles directly or it may act through an increase in the concentration of adenosine (a powerful vasodilator product formed by degradation of ATP).

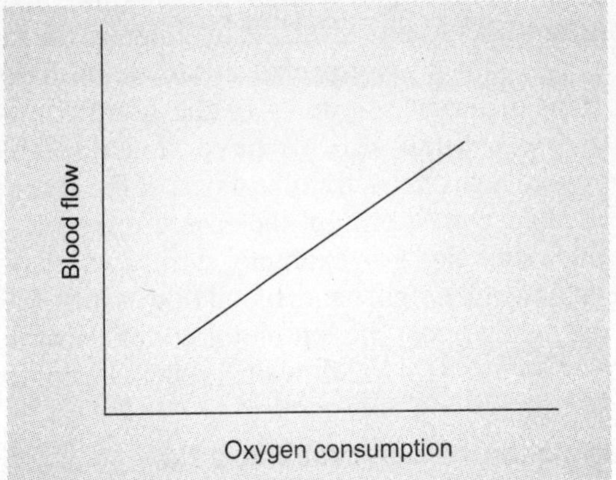

Fig. 13.2: Relation between coronary blood flow and myocardial oxygen consumption.

CORONARY ARTERY DISEASE

Angina Pectoris

Atherosclerotic changes in one or more branches of the coronary artery may reduce the lumen to such an extent that, in times of increased demands like exercise, the blood flow to the myocardium fails to increase in proportion to the metabolic requirement (Fig. 13.1C and D). The consequent accumulation of anoxic metabolites like lactic acid or some other products (e.g. kinins) stimulates the pain nerve endings in the myocardium. The pain is usually felt beneath the upper sternum and often referred to the left shoulder, left arm or left side of the neck. This condition is called *angina pectoris*. The pain of angina pectoris characteristically occurs during exercise and subsides on taking rest.

An acute attack of angina pectoris is treated by sublingual administration of a vasodilator, glyceryl trinitrate. Being a smooth muscle-relaxant, it causes arteriolar dilatation (decreased peripheral resistance, afterload) and venular dilatation (decreased preload). Thus, by decreasing the cardiac workload, it decreases the O_2 demand of the myocardium. In normal individuals, it dilates coronary vessels also but this action is probably unimportant in patients with angina in whom the coronary vessels are hardened by atherosclerosis.

In patients with frequent attacks of angina, oxygen demand of the heart can be limited by regular administration of a calcium channel blocker which reduces afterload by producing arteriolar dilatation. Regular administration of a β-blocker is also helpful since it limits the increase in the rate and force of cardiac contraction (oxygen demand) associated with exercise or anxiety.

Myocardial Infarction

A branch of a coronary artery may be completely occluded by thrombus formation over an atherosclerotic plaque. Depending upon the size of the vessel occluded, part of the ventricular myocardium undergoes ischemic necrosis (infarction). The condition is called myocardial infarction. It may occur in patients who previously suffered from angina pectoris or may occur without any previous warning.

Pain is the most important symptom of myocardial infarction. It occurs in same sites as angina pain but it is far more severe and lasts longer. In addition, breathlessness, pallor, sweating and syncope are commonly observed. These are signs of cardiogenic shock leading to activation of reflex sympathetic activity.

Myocardial infarction results in typical electrocardiographic changes in some of the ECG leads, depending upon the part of the ventricle affected.

Certain enzymes, normally present within the myocardial cells, leak into the circulation from the infarcted tissue. Elevated serum levels of these enzymes are important additional evidence of myocardial infarction. The enzymes most commonly estimated are creatine kinase and lactate dehydrogenase and cardiac troponins T and I.

Myocardial infarction is one of the leading causes of death in India and other countries. Daily administration of a small dose of aspirin is believed to be helpful in the prevention of coronary thrombosis since it has anti-platelet-aggregation action. The therapy is particularly useful in individuals who have predisposing factors for myocardial infarction, e.g. hypertension, hyperlipidemia, heavy smoking, diabetes mellitus or family history of myocardial infarction.

Aortic Coronary Bypass Coronary arteriography may reveal areas of atherosclerotic narrowing. Such cases can be treated by anastomosing a small vein graft between the aorta and the coronary artery more peripheral to the obstruction. This operation, called *aortic coronary bypass,* brings dramatic relief to patients with severe angina. Nowadays, coronary angioplasty is a preferred procedure when the atherosclerotic blockage is small and is confined to one artery. In this operation, by left heart catheterization, a tiny balloon is inserted and inflated at the site of arterial obstruction. A small metal coil called *stent* is left permanently to prevent the artery from narrowing at that site in future.

CEREBRAL CIRCULATION

Four arteries, the two internal carotids and two vertebral arteries supply blood to the brain. The two vertebral arteries unite to form the basilar artery, which along with the two internal carotid arteries form the *circle of Willis* at the base of the brain (Fig. 13.3). Six large arteries arising from the circle of Willis supply blood to the cerebrum. The two alternative sources of arterial blood (internal carotid and vertebral) and their anastomosis to form a circle of arteries seems to be an ideal mechanism to assure adequate cerebral blood flow even if one of the four arteries is completely blocked. However, in older subjects, the widespread atherosclerotic changes make the anastomosis practically nonfunctional, and occlusion of one of the arteries often produces cerebral ischaemia and infarction. The anatomical peculiarities of cerebral capillaries and their role in the blood-brain barrier are discussed in Chapter 30.

CEREBRAL BLOOD FLOW

The average cerebral blood flow is 750 ml/min. This is equivalent to blood flow of 50–55 ml/100 gm of brain per min. In other words, the cerebral blood flow is as high as in actively contracting skeletal muscle. This may be correlated with the total consumption of 45 ml of O_2/min by the brain, which is 20% of the total O_2 consumption of the whole body at rest. The O_2 consumption of the grey matter (3.3 ml/100 gm/min) is far greater than that of the white matter (0.2 ml/100 gm/min).

Total cerebral blood flow remains fairly constant and is not affected by intense mental activity. Using highly specialized technique, blood flow in different segments of the brain can be estimated. Such studies have revealed that increased neuronal activity in a part of the brain is associated with a prompt increase in blood flow in that segment. For example, during voluntary clenching of the right hand, blood flow is increased in the hand area of the left motor cortex. Reading a book increases blood flow in the occipital cortex.

Regulation of Cerebral Blood Flow

1. Arterial Blood Pressure Cerebral blood flow shows an autoregulation, i.e. it is not affected over a fairly wide variation in arterial blood pressure.

Only when the mean arterial blood pressure falls below 65 mmHg, the cerebral circulation is seriously affected. The mechanism of autoregulation of cerebral circulation is believed to be chiefly metabolic in nature.

2. Autonomic Nerves The cerebral blood vessels are supplied with vasoconstrictor sympathetic nerve fibres. However, their role in the regulation of cerebral blood flow is not exactly

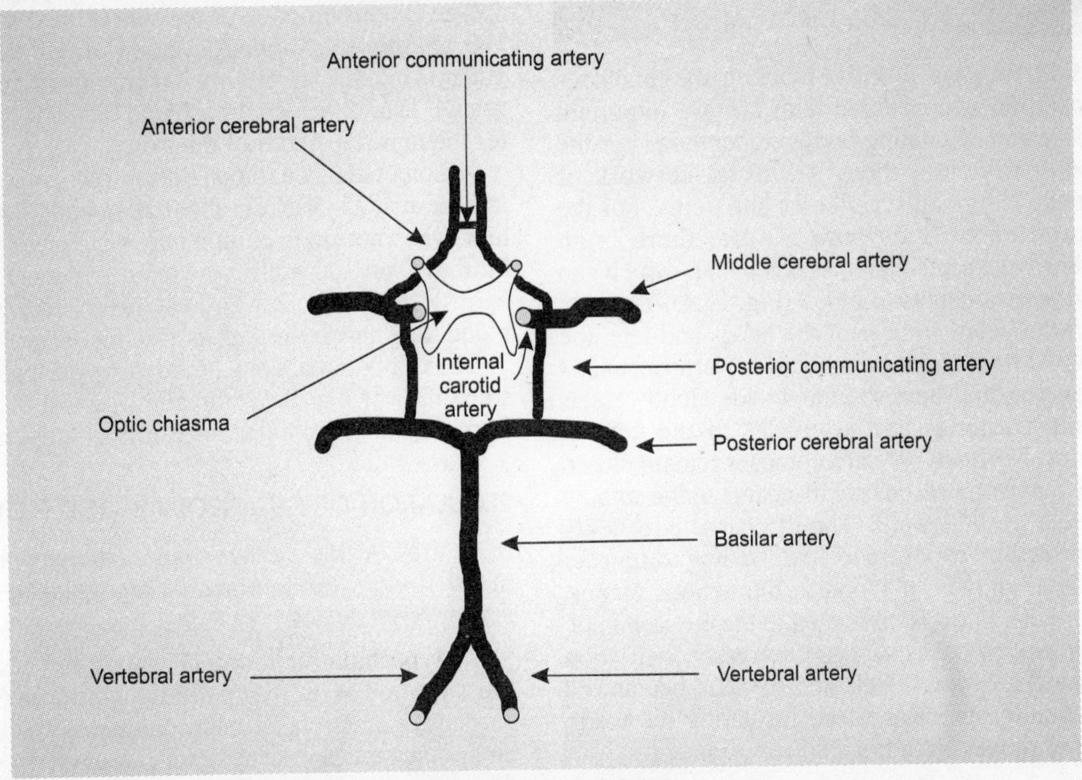

Fig.13.3: Circle of Willis.

clear. Increased sympathetic discharge during severe exercise increases systemic blood pressure to a fairly high level. At that time, neural vasoconstrictor discharge in large and medium sized cerebral arteries may prevent the transmission of high blood pressure to the smaller cerebral vessels. In this way, the risk of cereberal haemorrhage may be prevented.

3. Metabolic Factors *Carbon dioxide* is a very potent vasodilator in the cerebral resistance vessels. There is a linear relationship between the arterial pCO_2 and the cerebral blood flow over a fairly wide range of pCO_2. A decrease in the arterial pCO_2 by vigorous voluntary hyperventilation lowers the arterial pCO_2 to such an extent (15–20 mmHg; normal 40 mmHg) that extreme cerebral vasoconstriction occurs. It causes blurring of vision (due to retinal vasoconstriction) and dizziness (due to oxygen lack in the cerebral cortex). CO_2 acts by formation of carbonic acid and subsequent dissociation to form H^+ ion.

Low pO_2 is another factor causing cerebral vasodilatation. High pO_2 causes mild vasoconstriction. Hyperbaric O_2 therapy (inhalation of O_2 under more than one atmospheric pressure) causes marked cerebral vasoconstriction. This is a useful protective action because high cerebral tissue pO_2 is toxic. It causes a disruption of neuronal metabolism leading to convulsions, coma and even death.

4. Intracranial Pressure Acute rise of intracranial pressure would tend to interfere with the cerebral blood flow by causing extramural compression. However, there is a compensatory increase in the perfusion pressure, due to a reflex increase in the systemic arterial blood pressure. Increased intracranial pressure causes bulbar asphyxia leading to a direct stimulation of VMC and increased vasomotor discharge to the systemic resistance vessels (*Cushing reflex*, Chapter 11). Therefore, cerebral blood flow may remain normal despite a fairly large increase in intracranial pressure.

CUTANEOUS CIRCULATION

Besides the usual nutritive function, the cutaneous circulation is concerned with a more important function of regulating body temperature. For the former function, there is a usual network of arteries, arterioles, capillaries and veins. For the regulation of body temperature, there is an extensive subcutaneous venous plexus which can hold large amounts of blood (Fig. 13.4). The skin over the volar surfaces of the hands and feet, the lips, the nose and the ears contains *arteriovenous anastomoses*. These short and wide blood vessels connect arteries and arterioles to the venous plexus. Normally, AV anastomoses remain closed due to a strong vasomotor discharge to the smooth muscle in their walls. The discharge is reflexly abolished by exposure to heat, leading to transfer of large amount of blood to the venous plexus, from where heat is dissipated to the environment. Exposure to cold causes reflex vasoconstriction in the cutaneous vessels and the skin becomes a practically bloodless sheet, insulating the warm deeper tissues from the cold environment.

CUTANEOUS BLOOD FLOW

The cutaneous blood flow varies with the temperature of the environment or the rate of metabolic activity of the body and not with any change in the nutritive needs of the skin itself.

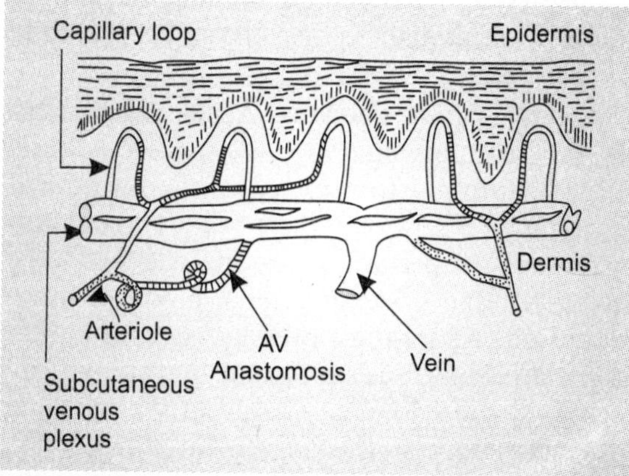

Fig. 13.4: Microcirculation of the subcutaneous region.

The O_2 consumption of the skin is only 0.3 ml/100 gm/min (cf. O_2 consumption of 3.3 ml/100 gm/ min in brain and 9.7 ml/100 gm/min in cardiac tissue). Therefore, very little blood flow is required for the nutritive needs of the skin.

Average cutaneous blood flow in a person resting in a room at 25–30°C, is about 10–15 ml/100 gm/min. On exposure to cold, it may be reduced to as little as 1 ml/100 gm/min without any metabolic harm to the skin. During heat stress, cutaneous blood flow may be as high as 150 ml/100 gm/min.

Thus, total cutaneous blood flow during heat stress may be over 3 L/min, allowing loss of heat from the skin by conduction and evaporation.

REGULATION OF CUTANEOUS BLOOD FLOW

In contrast to most other tissues, the cutaneous blood flow is predominantly regulated by the *neural mechanisms*.

1. Hypothalamic Control Cutaneous vessels are supplied with sympathetic noradrenergic vasoconstrictor fibres. Under conditions of rest and environmental thermal neutrality (28–30°C), these fibres have a mild tonic discharge. During exposure to heat stress, reflex decrease in the neural discharge results in vasodilatation and increased cutaneous blood flow. In the skin of the hands, feet, and the face, the reflex opening of AV anastomosis causes a marked increase in cutaneous blood flow.

Exposure to cold causes widespread cutaneous vasoconstriction. The reflex increase or decrease in the sympathetic discharge for thermoregulation is mediated through the temperature regulating centres of the hypothalamus.

2. Bradykinin In other parts of the skin, where AV anastomoses are not present, removal of sympathetic tonic discharge cannot increase the cutaneous blood flow to a significant extent. In these parts, massive increase in blood flow occurs only during sweating. Although, sweating is the result of cholinergic sympathetic discharge to the sweat glands, cutaneous vasodilatation is not produced by acetylcholine. Instead, bradykinin produced as a result of the secretory activity of the sweat glands acts as a powerful vasodilator (Chapter 12).

3. Baroreceptor-mediated Reflexes Cutaneous vessels participate in the baroreceptor-mediated reflexes. In times of circulatory stress, like exercise or haemorrhage, considerable cutaneous vasoconstriction and occurs.

4. Cortical Control Emotions affect the cutaneous circulation. The expressions "being pale with fear" or "blushing" refer to blanching and dilatation in the cutaneous vessels of the face respectively. They are produced through cortico-hypothalamic-VMC pathway.

Cold Vasodilatation

Exposure to cold normally produces cutaneous vasoconstriction. However, prolonged and severe vasoconstriction may lead to tissue damage known as *frost-bite*. This painful condition is characterized by cutaneous *vasodilatation* following a prolonged exposure to cold. This response is basically meant to prevent further tissue damage by increasing the cutaneous blood flow, in spite of continued exposure to cold. Severe frost bite can lead to permanent tissue damage in the parts of the body affected. This phenomenon is largely due to the axon reflex (see below) operating on the AV anastomoses in the affected tissues. Low skin temperature also causes the release of histamine and plasma kinins which stimulate the pain-nerve endings. In a different context, cold vasodilatation is the cause of ruddy cheeks seen in fair complexioned individuals on a cold day. It is a harmless, actually likable, physiological response.

The Triple Response (Cutaneous Vascular Response to Injury)

Cutaneous trauma, even as simple as stroking the skin with a fine pencil point, brings out a series of responses known as the triple response. It consists of: (i) the red reaction, (ii) the flare and (iii) the wheal.

The red reaction appears in about 10 seconds and is limited to the area of injury. It is followed in a few minutes by a diffusedly spreading and irregularly outlined reddening called the flare. If the stroke stimulus is strong enough, a swelling or a localized oedema, known as the wheal, develops within the area of the flare.

The *red reaction* is due to the dilatation of the precapillary sphincters in the injured area. The *flare* is due to dilatation of the arterioles and precapillary sphincters. An arteriole supplies blood to the capillaries in an irregularly outlined area. That explains the irregular outline of the flare. The *wheal* is due to increased capillary permeability leading to local oedema.

The triple response is produced by histamine and/or some polypeptides released from the damaged skin. These substances dilate the precapillary sphincters and cause the red reaction by a direct action. Local anaesthetization of the skin abolished the flare and the wheal formation but not the red reaction, indicating that the former two phenomena are mediated through nerves. However, blockade of the concerned afferent fibres, away from the site of injury, does not abolish the response. For example, blockade of the ulnar nerve at the elbow, when the skin is injured in the forearm does not abolish the triple response. It shows that, although the flare and wheal are nerve-mediated phenomena, unlike a typical reflex, they do not depend upon the connections with the central nervous system.

It is believed that the flare is produced by the *axon reflex*. As the pain receptors are stimulated by histamine (or some other polypeptide), the impulses are conducted orthodromically in the pain afferents to produce the sensation of pain. However, close to the site of injury the impulses are also conducted antidromically, in some branches of the sensory fibres which terminate around the adjacent arterioles and cause their dilatation. It is believed that the *substance P* released from these nerve endings acts as a strong vasodilator (Fig. 13.5). It causes flare and also produces extravasation of fluid (wheal).

THE SPLANCHNIC CIRCULATION

The combined vascular beds of the *liver, spleen and the gastrointestinal tract* are known as the splanchnic circulation. The liver receives about 1500 ml of blood/min. Of this about 25% comes

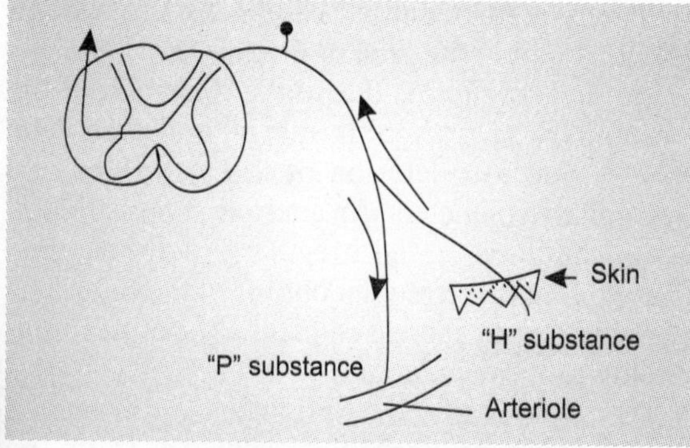

Fig. 13.5: The axon reflex arc.

13

from the hepatic artery and the remaining 75% from the portal vein, which in turn drains blood from the gut, the pancreas and the spleen.

Regulation of Gastrointestinal Blood Flow

About 80% of the portal blood is derived from the abdominal parts of the alimentary canal and the rest from the pancreas and the spleen. In the gastrointestinal tract, most of the arterial blood is supplied to the mucosa to help the intestinal secretory activity and reabsorptive processes.

Neural Regulation Splanchnic blood vessels are supplied with noradrenergic sympathetic fibres. Mild tonic discharge in these fibres maintains moderate vascular resistance in the splanchnic blood vessels. Removal of sympathetic discharge increases the intestinal blood flow by about 25% only. Splanchnic vasomotor nerves participate in the baroreceptor-mediated reflexes.

Humoral Regulation During increased activity of the gut, i.e. after food intake, the increase in the gastrointestinal blood flow is well marked (functional hyperaemia). However, since the digestive and reabsorptive processes proceed in different parts of the alimentary canal in a sequential manner, the overall increase in the gastrointestinal blood flow during the digestive period is only modest, i.e. about 50% above the level in post-absorptive period. The exact mechanism of increased blood flow is not known. The gastrointestinal hormones like VIP, gastrin, secretin, CCK, etc. released during digestion cause mucosal vasodilatation. Bradykinin also seems to be generated during the secretory processes and causes local vasodilatation.

Regulation of Hepatic Blood Flow

Total hepatic blood flow rate (100 ml/100 gm/ min) is rather high. Even the arterial blood supply to the liver (25–30 ml/100 gm/min) is quite high and reflects the high metabolic activity of the organ. Hepatic *arterial blood flow is autoregulated* by the local vasodilator metabolites. The portal blood flow, however, is not autoregulated and increases during the digestive period.

The entire splanchnic vascular system contains about 20% of the total blood volume. The liver alone contains about 300–400 ml of blood in its sinusoids. An increase in the right atrial pressure causes expansion of the liver, which may accommodate as much as 1 litre of blood. On the other hand, increased sympathetic discharge, e.g. during haemorrhage, may cause constriction of the intrahepatic portal vessels, leading to a marked reduction in the capacity of the hepatic blood reservoir.

PULMONARY CIRCULATION

As compared to the systemic circulation, pulmonary circulation is a low pressure, low resistance system. The thickness of the right ventricular wall and pulmonary artery is approximately one-third of the thickness of left ventricular wall and aorta, respectively. The pulmonary vessels, in general, have thinner and more distensible walls than the systemic vessels. The pulmonary arterioles have very little smooth muscle in their walls. The pulmonary capillaries are larger in diameter than systemic capillaries and have multiple anastomoses. As a result, each alveolus seems to be enclosed in a basket of capillaries.

Pressure and Flow

During each cardiac cycle, the right ventricular pressure reaches a peak value of about 25 mmHg in systole (cf. 120 mmHg in the left ventricle) and falls to 0–1 mmHg in diastole (cf. 5 mmHg in the left ventricle).

In the pulmonary artery, the average systolic and diastolic pressure values are 25/8 mmHg (cf. 120/80 mmHg in aorta). Mean pulmonary arterial pressure is 15 mmHg. Since the mean left atrial pressure is about 8 mmHg, the pressure gradient in the pulmonary system is only 7 mmHg (pressure gradient is 100 mmHg in the systemic circulation).

Mean pulmonary capillary pressure is approximately 10 mmHg. Since this pressure value is far below the oncotic pressure of plasma proteins (25 mmHg), there is hardly any formation of interstitial fluid. Thus, the alveoli remain free of any fluid. In patients with left ventricular congestive heart failure (due to hypertension or aortic valvular disease), the pulmonary venous and capillary pressures rise, leading the pulmonary oedema. Presence of fluid in the interstitial spaces and the alveoli causes severe interference with the gaseous exchange in the lungs. The resultant hypoxia may be rapidly fatal.

Effect of Gravity

Like systemic blood vessels, gravity affects the pulmonary vessels also but the effect is more marked in the latter. In normal adults in supine posture, pulmonary mean arterial pressure is the same all over the lung. However, in erect posture, as compared to the pressure at the heart level, the mean arterial pressure is greater by 8 mmHg at the base of the lungs and less by 15 mmHg at the apex of the lungs. Consequently, the capillary pressure and blood flow at the apex of the lungs may be near zero. (*Zone I : area of zero blood flow*). In the middle of the lungs, i.e. at the heart level, the mean pulmonary arterial pressure is 15 mmHg, but it varies from 25 mmHg in the systolic phase to 8 mmHg in the diastolic phase. Since minimum left atrium pressure is about 5 mmHg, there is practically very little gradient between the pulmonary artery and the left atrium during later part of diastole, when the pulmonary blood flow practically ceases (*Zone II: area of intermittent blood flow*). At the base of the lung, pulmonary arterial pressure is 33/16 mmHg and adequate pressure gradient allows continuous and well-marked blood flow throughout the cardiac cycle (*Zone III: area of continuous blood flow*).

Zone I is absent is normal individuals. However, if intra-alveolar pressure is increased (as occurs while blowing into musical instruments), the arterial pressure cannot overcome the external compression on the pulmonary capillaries and hence Zone I becomes a significant upper part of the lungs.

It must be reiterated that all the discussion on the three pulmonary zones given above refers to the erect posture. In supine position, all the parts of the lung are uniformly perfused.

Pulmonary Blood Volume

The pulmonary vessels contain around 450 ml of blood, i.e. about 9% of the total blood volume. The pulmonary vessels act as capacitance vessels and their blood content can vary from 200 to 900 ml. In physiological conditions like standing, increased vasomotor discharge decreases the capacity of pulmonary vessels, and the extra blood is shifted to the systemic circulation. In this way, there is partial compensation of blood pooled in the leg veins due to gravity. Thus, the pulmonary vessels act as a reservoir of blood. This phenomenon becomes still more important in pathological conditions like haemorrhage.

Mean transit time in the pulmonary circulation from pulmonary valves to the left atrium is about 4 seconds. A red cell traverses a pulmonary capillary in approximately 0.75 sec at rest; and 0.3 sec during exercise. Even in this brief duration, adequate gaseous exchange between the red cells and the alveolar air can occur.

Regulation of Pulmonary Blood Flow

Neural Control

Pulmonary vessels are innervated by sympathetic vasoconstrictor fibres. Pulmonary vessels participate in the vasomotor reflexes e.g. baroreceptor stimulation produces reflex dilatation of pulmonary vessels, whereas chemoreceptor stimulation causes pulmonary vasoconstriction. However, the effect of vasodilatation or vasoconstriction is more on the capacity rather than the resistance of the pulmonary vessels.

The pulmonary trunk and its two major branches contain baroreceptors in the tunica adventitia. An increase in the pulmonary arterial pressure produces reflex bradycardia and systemic hypotension.

On the whole, the neural control on the pulmonary circulation is not very strong, since all the cardiac output has to pass through the pulmonary circulation. Mostly, pulmonary vessels act as passive distensible tubes that enlarge with increasing luminal blood volume and become narrow with the decrease in blood volume.

Chemical Control

Local hypoxia induces pulmonary vasoconstriction. This is a local and direct action, since it can be demonstrated in isolated (denervated) perfused lungs. Increased *tissue* pCO_2 or *acidosis* also causes pulmonary vasoconstriction. The effects of pCO_2 or acidosis on pulmonary vessels are just opposite to those in the systemic vessels where these stimuli produce vasodilatation.

Obstruction of a bronchus or a bronchiole results in hypoventilation of the alveoli in the corresponding parts of the lung. The consequent *local tissue* oxygen deficiency and accumulation of CO_2 causes vasoconstriction in the involved segment. As a result, the blood is diverted to the capillaries around the normally ventilated alveoli. In this way, the local chemical control of the pulmonary vessels helps to maintain uniformity of ventilation: perfusion ratio in all the segments of the lungs.

14 CHAPTER

Cardiovascular Homeostasis in Health and Disease

EFFECT OF POSTURE ON CARDIOVASCULAR HAEMODYNAMICS

A change from supine to erect posture produces complex haemodynamic changes, which tend to reduce the cardiac output and arterial blood pressure. This is shown by the fact that sudden passive tilting of a normal individual on a tilt table, in head-up position, often leads to a transient loss of consciousness (syncope) due to a severe fall of blood pressure. But, normally when we change the posture by active movements of the limbs, prompt baroreceptor-mediated neural compensatory reactions prevent any significant fall of blood pressure.

In the standing posture, the pressure due to the column of blood in the arteries and veins is added to the intravascular pressure recorded in supine position (Chapters 9 and 10). In normal adults, the blood pressure at the level of the feet in both arteries and veins is increased by approximately 80 mmHg. Thus the mean arterial and venous pressures at the level of the feet are 170 mmHg and 90 mmHg respectively as compared to 90 mmHg and 10 mmHg in the supine position. As such, the pressure gradient between the arteries and the veins is not disturbed and the flow of blood is not affected. The increased intraluminal pressure has no significant effect on the thick-walled arteries. The effect of gravity on the thin-walled and distensible veins is far more important. Under high intraluminal pressure, the veins normally partially collapsed, open up and even get distended. In this way, the veins of the lower limbs may accommodate as much as 500 ml of extra blood. This change is called *venous pooling*. Venous pooling of blood results in a decrease in the venous return to the heart. The resulting decrease in cardiac output leads to a fall in blood pressure. However, within seconds, the arterial baroreceptor-mediated *compensatory mechanisms*, discussed below, set in and restore the blood pressure to normal.

1. An increase in heart rate (by 5–10 beats/min) and force of cardiac contraction.
2. Arteriolar constriction in cutaneous, splanchnic and renal circulations leading to increased total peripheral resistance.
3. Venoconstriction leading to a mild decrease in capacity of the veins including those of the lower limbs.
4. Decreased capacity of pulmonary and splanchnic blood reservoir. The central venous pool is decreased by approximately 400 ml.
5. Increased secretion of renin and aldosterone.

In spite of the compensatory reactions mentioned above, the stroke volume and cardiac output in standing posture are approximately 25%

less than those in supine posture. However, an approximate 25% increase in the total peripheral resistance restores the blood pressure to the level observed in the supine posture.

In some individuals, especially after prolonged illness, the blood volume is decreased and the compensatory mechanisms described above are slow to develop. These patients complain of transient blurring of vision, dizziness or even fainting on sudden standing. Similar symptoms occur in patients with diabetic autonomic neuropathy or in those receiving sympatholytic drugs. The condition is known as *orthostatic (or postural) hypotension*. It is diagnosed by recording BP in supine and standing postures. A decrease of systolic BP by 30 mmHg or more on standing from supine posture is diagnostic.

EFFECTS OF SEVERE GRAVITATIONAL FORCES

The effect of gravity on the circulatory system has been discussed above. In elevators, aircrafts and space flights, the effect of gravity may be multiplied many folds. The force acts on all the tissues of the body but the mobile circulatory system is most affected. The force acting on the body as a result of acceleration is expressed in 'g' units.

When the *acceleration* of a rocket exceeds 5 'g', the pressure in the veins in the lower limbs would be over 450 mmHg. The consequent passive dilatation of veins of the lower limbs retains so much blood that the venous return and therefore, cardiac output is markedly reduced. The astronaut feels *black out* of vision and unconsciousness follows. During *deceleration*, the effect of negative 'g' results in accumulation of blood in the head and neck leading to intense congestion of the eyes, and mental confusion (*red-out*). These effects are seen when the gravitational force acts in the direction of head to feet. The effects of acceleratory forces are minimised if they act on chest to back direction rather than in head to feet direction. Due to this reason, during take off, the astronauts are positioned in such a way that the force of gravity acts in chest to back direction.

Further protection against the effect of gravitational forces is obtained by using anti-'g' suits. These consist of double-walled pressure suits which compress the abdomen and the legs with a force proportionate to the increase in the positive 'g'. Thus, the venous pooling and the consequent risk of black out is minimised.

Effects of Zero Gravity The effects of acceleratory forces are important during the launch and reentry of the spacecraft. The continued flight of a spacecraft lasting weeks and even months brings about the problem of weightlessness or *zero gravity*. Due to the absence of normal gravitational stress, the movements of limbs become effort-free. In fact, the astronauts float about inside the spacecraft, and need to cling to a hand hold for any propulsive movement. The absence of gravity causes absence of hydrostatic pressure of the blood. There is decrease in *blood volume* including *total red cell mass*, loss of *muscle mass*, and the demineralization of the *bones*. The circulating *T lymphocytes* also decrease in number.

CIRCULATORY SHOCK

Circulatory shock is a clinical syndrome which occurs when the cardiac output is inadequate to maintain the normal tissue nutrition and O_2 supply.

It is characterised by *tachycardia, decreased pulse pressure, (rapid and thready pulse); pale, cool, and moist skin; rapid breathing; intense thirst, and oliguria. Blood pressure* may be normal initially, but as the condition worsens, it falls. The patient is often *restless and apprehensive*.

Broadly speaking, circulatory shock may be classified into three types : (i) cardiogenic shock, (ii) hypovolemic shock, (iii) low resistance shock.

1. **Cardiogenic Shock** This type of shock is characterized by decreased CO, primarily due to cardiac disorders like myocardial infarction, toxic myocarditis and cardiac arrhythmias.
2. **Hypovolemic Shock** It is characterised by decreased CO due to a reduction in blood volume, e.g. in dehydration, haemorrhage, burns, trauma, etc.
3. **Low Resistance Shock** It is produced by severe vasodilatation in the face of normal CO, e.g. septic shock, or anaphylactic shock. Because of its more common occurrence,

the haemorrhagic shock shall be described in detail.

Haemorrhagic Shock

About 10% of the total blood volume may be lost without any ill-effect. Acute blood loss more than 10% leads to a significant decrease in the CO and B.P. Blood loss greater than 30% of the total blood volume is fatal unless treated immediately. Decreased blood volume, due to loss of blood (or any other cause of hypovolemia mentioned above) produces the following changes:

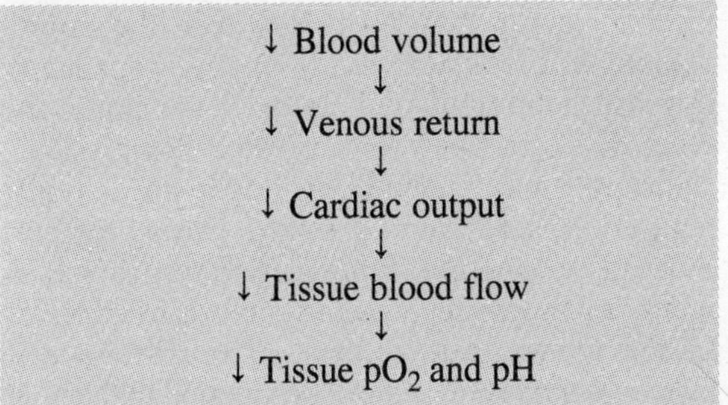

The loss of blood sets into motion certain rapid compensatory mechanisms which, in the face of reduced cardiac output, try to maintain normal blood flow to the vital organs. If the patient survives, long-term compensatory mechanisms restore the plasma proteins and red cell mass to normal in 4 to 8 weeks.

Compensatory Mechanisms

1. Neural Mechanism Even when the blood pressure has not fallen, the decrease in pulse pressure is sufficient to decrease the impulse discharge from the arterial baroreceptors. As a result, there is a generalized increase in the sympathetic vasomotor discharge to the heart, the arterioles and the veins. The net effect of all these reactions is improvement in cardiac output, an increase in total peripheral resistance and maintenance of BP, in spite of diminished blood volume (Fig. 14.1). Vasoconstriction is more marked in the cutaneous, splanchnic, renal and skeletal muscle vessels. The coronary and cerebral vessels do not participate in the generalized vasoconstriction. In fact, all the compensatory mechanisms are geared to maintain blood pressure at such a level that the blood flow to the vital organs like heart and brain is not affected. However, blood flow to the vital organs is provided at the cost of many other tissues of the body, e.g. skin, abdominal viscera, kidney and skeletal muscles, etc. The compensatory mechanisms discussed above account for most of the symptoms and signs observed in patients with circulatory shock.

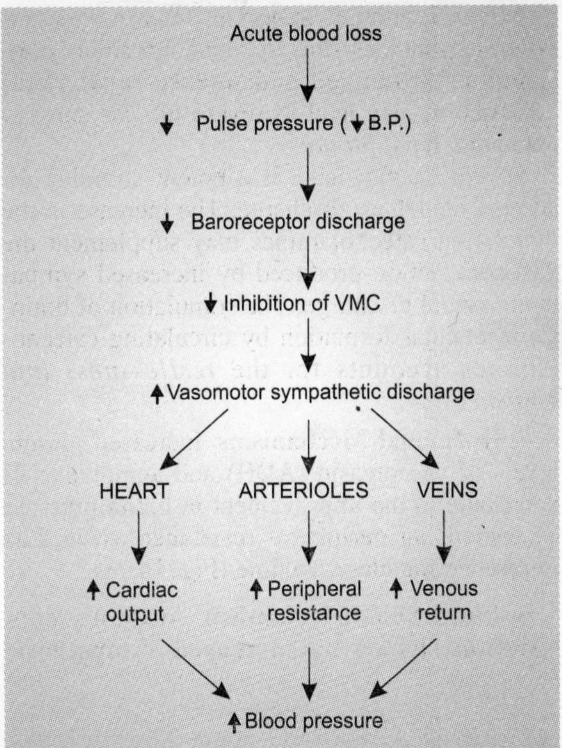

Fig. 14.1: Rapid (neural) compensatory mechanism in hypovolemic shock.

Decreased blood flow to the skin and sweating (due to increased sympathetic discharge) is responsible for the *pale, cool and moist skin*. The skin may have *cyanotic tinge* because of increased O_2 extraction from the blood.

Tachycardia and *fall in pulse pressure* produce the *thin and thready pulse*, a characteristic feature of hypovolemic shock. *Increased rate and force of respiration* is due to greater sino-aortic chemoreceptor discharge.

Oliguria, another important feature of hypovolemic shock is due to renal arteriolar constriction. Prolonged and intense renal vasoconstriction may lead to severe tubular damage and *acute renal failure.*

Severe haemorrhage is a potent stimulus for adrenal medullary discharge. The increase in the circulating catecholamines may supplement the vasoconstriction produced by increased sympathetic neural discharge. The stimulation of brainstem reticular formation by circulating catecholamines accounts for the *restlessness and apprehension.*

2. Hormonal Mechanisms Increased plasma levels of vasopressin (ADH) and angiotensin-II contribute to the improvement in blood pressure by increasing peripheral resistance as well as improving the blood volume (Fig. 14.2).

3. Fluid Shift Mechanism Arteriolar constriction caused by increased sympathetic discharge produces a drop in the capillary pressure. Hence, fluid moves into the capillaries along most of its course. The shift of fluid from the interstitial compartment into the circulation helps to improve the circulating blood volume. The decrease in the volume of ECF causes cellular dehydration, which accounts for the *intense thirst* felt by the victims of circulatory shock. The thirst may also be due to action of angiotensin-II on subfornical organ, a specialized receptor area in the hypothalamus.

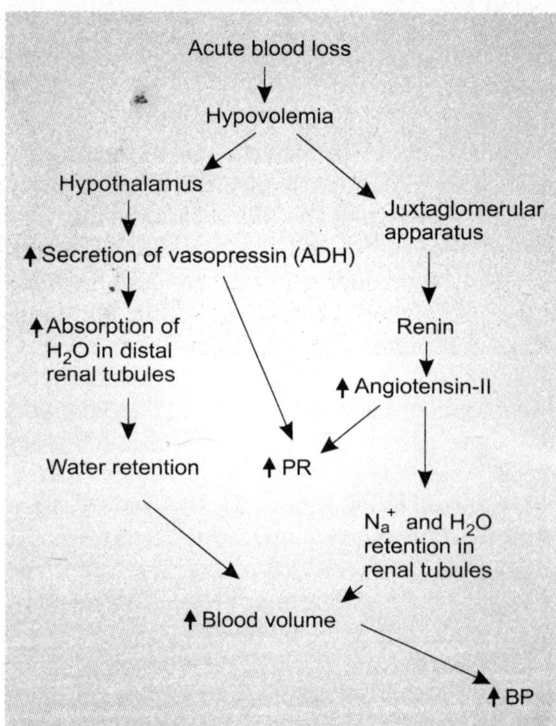

Fig. 14.2: Hormonal compensatory mechanisms in hypovolemic shock.

4. Long-Term Compensatory Mechanisms After a moderate haemorrhage, the plasma volume is restored by the hormonal and fluid shift mechanisms in 2–3 days. However, the improvement in blood volume is merely because of increase in the amount of plasma water along with electrolyte content. The plasma protein concentration and haematocrit values are actually reduced (due to haemodilution). During the next 3–4 days, plasma protein concentration is improved by greater protein synthesis by the liver. In the mean time, release of erythropoietin increases the rate of red cell production in the bone marrow. The red cell mass is restored to normal in 4–8 weeks. The treatment of circulatory shock should consist of correcting the cause, e.g. replacement of the fluid lost, i.e. blood (in haemorrhagic shock) or plasma (in burns), or saline (in dehydration).

Irreversible Shock

In the treatment of hypovolemic shock, administration of vasoconstrictor drugs (e.g. norepinephrine) is not recommended because it may lead to a condition called irreversible shock. Even otherwise, an untreated severe hypovolemic shock may deteriorate to a stage when no treatment is effective. Prolonged and sustained vasoconstriction in the renal, splanchnic and skeletal muscle vessels may give rise to certain changes in the microcirculation, due to which the cardiac output remains depressed, even if the blood volume is subsequently restored to normal. The condition is called irreversible shock and eventually the patient dies.

A number of factors seem to lead a patient in shock to the irreversible stage:

(a) A severe fall of blood pressure may cause cerebral ischaemia and failure of medullary cardiovascular centres. It may also cause myocardial ischaemia and cardiac depression.

(b) Hypoxic damage to the tissues in the splanchnic area, because of intense and prolonged vasoconstriction, is another important contributory factor.

The hypoxic local metabolites (lactacidosis) cause failure of the arteriolar and precapillary sphincters to respond to the vasomotor discharge.

(c) Severe vasoconstriction causes a breakdown of normal protective mucosal barrier in the gut leading to the entry of intestinal bacteria into the portal circulation. Simultaneous deterioration of hepatic function permits bacterial toxins to reach the systemic circulation. The endotoxins cause failure of arteriolar and precapillary sphincter function. At this stage, no amount of treatment can restore the circulatory function to normal.

HYPERTENSION

Hypertension is defined as being present when the arterial blood pressure of an individual *persistently* exceeds 140/90 mmHg. In nearly 10% of the cases, the cause of hypertension can be established. Such cases are said to suffer from *secondary hypertension*. The rest 90% of cases, in whom no apparent cause can be found, are said to suffer from *essential hypertension*.

Secondary hypertension may be caused by:

1. Renal Diseases Secondary hypertension is most commonly due to renal diseases like chronic nephritis, chronic pyelonephritis or renal artery stenosis. In many cases of renal hypertension, increased secretion of renin-angiotensin-II or aldosterone can be demonstrated.

2. Pheochromocytoma In this case, a norepinephrine-secreting tumour of the adrenal medulla causes hypertension.

3. Primary Hyperaldosteronism A tumour of zona glomerulosa of adrenal cortex secretes excessive amount of aldosterone leading to excessive salt and water retention and hypertension.

4. Coarctation of the Aorta This condition is associated with hypertension in the arteries above the constriction in the aorta, and hypotension below. Since the constriction of the aorta is commonly above the origin of renal arteries, the decreased renal blood flow causes excessive secretion of renin and angiotensin-II as well.

Many of the cases with secondary hypertension can be cured by surgical removal of the cause.

14

Essential Hypertension

In patients with essential hypertension, the cardiac output and the viscosity of blood are normal. Hence, increased arteriolar resistance is the basic cause of increased blood pressure. Hypertrophy of the tunica media of the arterioles can usually be demonstrated. The etiology of the hypertrophy of the smooth muscle is not clear.

According to *one hypothesis*, the essential hypertension is primarily due to a genetic defect leading to reduced renal excretion of sodium. As a result, there is an increase in extracellular fluid volume and cardiac output. The autoregulatory mechanisms produce vasoconstriction in the resistance vessels so as to prevent tissue overperfusion.

Another hypothesis proposes vasoconstriction as the primary defect. It is believed to be due to a genetically induced defect in Na^+/Ca^{++} transport in the vascular smooth muscle. This results in an increase in intracellular Ca^{++} leading to contraction of smooth muscle. Thus, there is an increased sensitivity of resistance vessels to physiological stimuli. Vasoconstriction may also be caused by a genetically induced increase in secretion of vasoconstrictor agents like renin, catecholamines and endothelins.

Important environmental factors implicated in the causation of hypertension include *stress, obesity, smoking, inactivity and heavy consumption of salt.*

Elevated blood pressure not only imposes higher work-load on the heart, but also predisposes the patient to coronary thrombosis, cerebral thrombosis, cerebral haemorrhage and renal failure. High intraluminal pressure can damage the endothelial lining specially when there is underlying atherosclerosis. The damaged endothelium initiates thrombus formation which may itself occlude the vessel or it may get loose and transported by circulation to block an artery at a distant site (embolism).

Treatment

14

The principles of treatment of essential hypertension include: (a) measures to decrease body sodium and (b) measures to decrease peripheral resistance.

(a) Body sodium can be decreased by: (i) decreasing salt intake and (ii) by increasing urinary excretion of sodium chloride by administration of a saluretic (a diuretic drug which increases urinary NaCl excretion).

(b) Peripheral resistance can be decreased by use of one or more of the following vasodilator agents:
   (i) Calcium channel blockers produce relaxation of arteriolar smooth muscle.
   (ii) Angiotensin converting enzyme (ACE) inhibitors decrease the level of angiotensin II and aldosterone in the plasma.
   (iii) β-blockers inhibit β-receptor activity in the heart, kidney and CNS, leading to a reduction in cardiac output, plasma renin-angiotensin-II as well as a decrease in generalized sympathetic discharge.

HEART FAILURE

Heart failure is said to be present when the cardiac output is not adequate to meet the needs of the body. More commonly, there is an absolute decline in the cardiac output (*low output heart failure*), e.g. in hypertension, myocardial infarction, or valvular defects. In some disorders, the cardiac output may be above normal, but still it is inadequate relative to the increased needs of the body (*high output heart failure*), e.g. in thyrotoxicosis. The manifestations of heart failure may vary from sudden death (e.g. ventricular fibrillation); shock like state (cardiogenic shock) to chronic congestive heart failure.

Chronic Congestive Heart Failure

This disorder is characterized by the presence of *cardiac enlargement*, *oedema* (prominent over the ankles or the sacrum), *hepatic enlargement*, *dyspnoea*, distended neck veins *(raised JVP)*, *weakness* and *exercise intolerance*. Weakness and exercise intolerance are due to inadequacy of the cardiac output (*forward failure*). Other symptoms and signs are the result of increased venous pressure and congestion (*backward failure*).

Patients in early stages of heart failure have merely exercise intolerance as shown by shortness of breath and early fatigue. Later on, as the cardiac output decreases further, full-fledged picture of congestive heart failure emerges.

The basic defect in low output congestive heart failure is decreased contractility of the myocardium, i.e. it works on a lower level of Starling's curve (Fig. 14.3). The compensatory mechanisms involve *increased sympathetic discharge* to the heart and the Starling mechanism, i.e. the heart operates at a *greater end diastolic volume* (Fig. 14.4).

The increased sympathetic discharge sets up certain complex reactions (Fig. 14.5) which lead

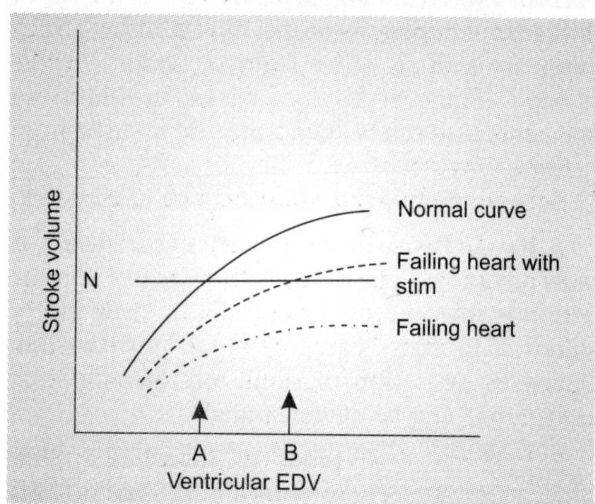

Fig. 14.3: Effect of sympathetic stimulation on a failing heart. Normal stroke volume (N) is achieved at greater EDV (B) than normal (A).

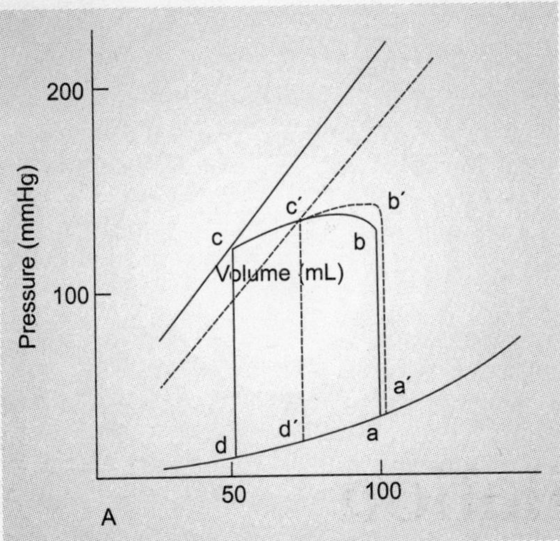

Fig. 14.4: Pressure volume loops: solid lines normal; dotted lines in congestive heart failure. In CHF, the loop operates at a higher end-diastolic volume.

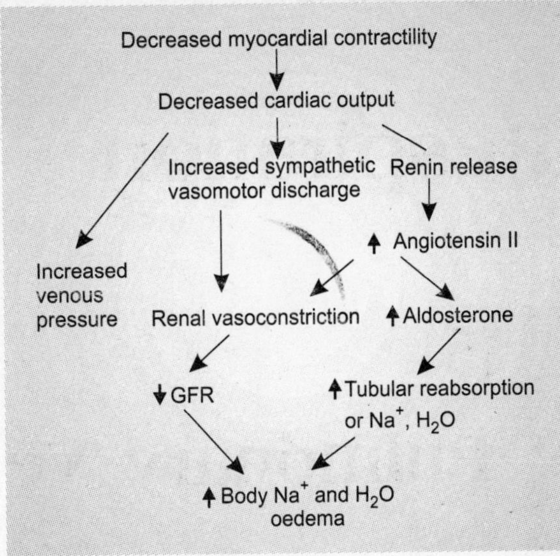

Fig. 14.5: Mechanism of fluid and water retention in chronic congestive heart failure.

to Na^+ and H_2O retention and expansion of ECF volume. The increased ECF volume causes increase in venous return and end-diastolic volume.

Elevated capillary and venous pressure causes oedema, pulmonary congestion and pulmonary oedema. Ultimately, the compensatory mechanisms stretch the heart to such an extent that the stroke volume actually decreases and the downhill course of the disease begins.

In the treatment of congestive heart failure, the primary aim is to lower the preload on the heart by administration of a saluretic which decreases the blood volume. Further, the afterload can also be decreased by administration of vasodilator drugs like ACE inhibitors.

The contractility (force of contraction) of the heart can be improved by administration of digoxin. The mechanism of action of this drug has been discussed earlier (Chapter 6). In brief, digoxin inhibits the activity of Na^+-K^+ ATPase in the cardiac muscle. The consequent increase in Ca^{++} in the myocytes improves myocardial contractility.

Section V

Respiration

CHAPTER 15

Pulmonary Ventilation

In most of the chemical reactions involved in the production of energy, oxygen is consumed and carbon dioxide is produced. An adult body consumes about 250 ml of O_2 and produces about 200 ml of CO_2 per minute. The respiratory system is concerned with the supply of O_2 to the tissues and removal of CO_2. Many steps are involved in this process:

(i) The lungs are the organs of gas exchange between the blood and external environment (atmosphere). The process of moving air from the environment into and out of the lungs is known as *ventilation*.

(ii) The next step involves diffusion of gases (O_2 and CO_2) across the alveolar membrane (*pulmonary diffusion*).

(iii) The blood circulation transports the gases between the lungs and the tissues (*transport of gases*).

(iv) Finally, the tissues utilize O_2 and produce CO2. The last step, which may be called *tissue respiration*, or internal respiration is out of the scope of this book. A standard textbook of biochemistry may be consulted for this purpose.

FUNCTIONAL ANATOMY

Conducting Air Passages

In order to reach the lungs, air has to pass through a series of air passages, such as the nose (or the mouth), pharynx, larynx, trachea, bronchi and bronchioles. The bronchi and bronchioles are a series of highly branched hollow tubes which become smaller and more numerous at each branching.

Between trachea and the alveoli, the air passages divide 23 times. The conducting zones constitute the first 16 divisions (Fig. 15.1). The next 7 divisions involve areas like respiratory bronchioles, alveolar ducts and alveolar sacs, where the gas exchange occurs. The multiple divisions greatly increase the cross-section area of the airways, and therefore, the velocity of air flow in the small airways declines to very low values. The conducting passages, though not taking part in gas exchange, serve many important functions.

Functions of Conducting Air Passages

1. The respiratory passages humidify the inhaled air. Dry air is harmful for the ciliary function in the respiratory passages.

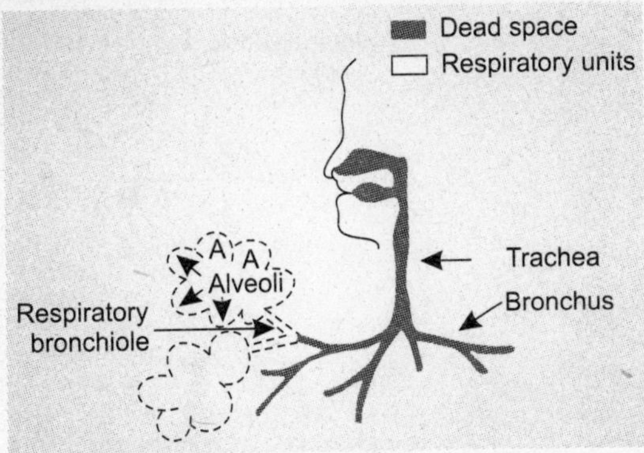

Fig. 15.1: The respiratory passages.

2. The inhaled air is warmed/cooled to the body temperature by the time it reaches the alveoli.
3. The mucous membrane of the trachea, bronchi and bronchioles is characterized by the presence of mucous glands and cilia. The cilia beat rhythmically towards the pharynx. The dust particles in the inhaled air are often coated with bacteria. As the air passes through the highly branched bronchial tree, it repeatedly comes in contact with the layer of mucus on the luminal surface of the respiratory passages. The dust particles and the bacteria are caught in the mucus and moved up to the pharynx by the cilia and swallowed. This "ciliary escalator" is an important defence system against air-borne organisms (Fig. 15.2). Cigarette-smoke paralyses the ciliary function. That explains the higher incidence of respiratory infections in smokers than in non-smokers.

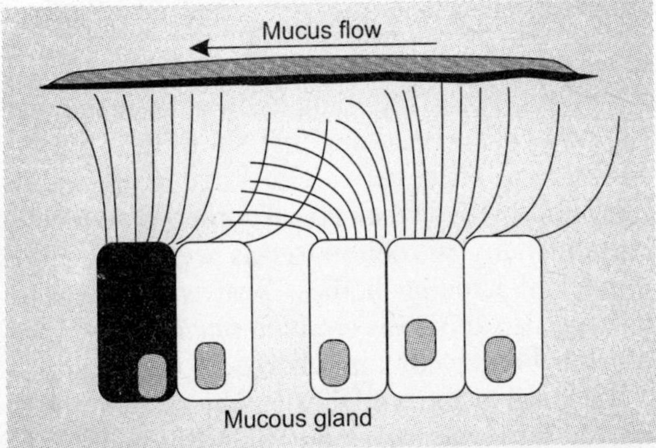

Fig. 15.2: The ciliary escalator in the respiratory mucosa.

4. The secretion of immunoglobulin-A (Ig A) in the bronchial secretions is an additional protection against respiratory infections.
5. Tonsils and adenoids are large collections of immunologically active lymphoid tissue in the pharynx. They provide an important defence mechanism against the ingested and inhaled microorganisms.
6. The rings of cartilage in the walls of bronchi and bronchioles do not allow them to collapse. The smooth muscle fibres in their walls can alter the size of their lumen, and thereby vary the airway resistance. The terminal bronchioles lack the cartilage but have abundant smooth muscle. Hence, pathological contraction of smooth muscle can obliterate their lumen.

   The respiratory smooth muscle is richly innervated by cholinergic parasympathetic nerve fibres. Their stimulation causes mild to moderate bronchial constriction. Though not innervated by sympathetic fibres, the bronchial smooth muscle fibres contain β_2-adrenergic receptors. Therefore, they respond to circulating epinephrine and inhaled or injected sympathomimetic drugs resulting in bronchodilation. Histamine is a potent bronchoconstrictor. During allergic reactions, it is released by the mast cells present in the bronchial mucosa.

   The *function of bronchial smooth muscle* is still a matter of debate. It may have a protective role against inhaled irritants. In allergic conditions, its contraction produces bronchospasm and difficulty in breathing (bronchial asthma) which can be relieved by the administration of sympathomimetic drugs.
7. Cough reflex: The laryngeal, tracheal and bronchial mucous membranes contain vagal afferent terminals which act as irritant receptors. Stimulation of these receptors by chemical or mechanical stimuli (excessive mucus, inadvertently inhaled food stuff, etc.)

produces a bout of coughing, which helps in expulsion of the foreign material.

THE RESPIRATORY PARENCHYMA

The exchange of gases between the blood and the air in the lungs occurs in the terminal region of the air passages. Each respiratory unit consists of a respiratory bronchiole which opens into a number of alveolar ducts. Each alveolar duct opens into a number of sac-like alveoli (Fig. 15.3). The two lungs contain about 300 million alveoli. Each alveolus has diameter of about 0.2 mm. The walls of the respiratory units are extremely thin and contain an extremely extensive network of capillaries (Fig. 15.4). The total area of the alveolar walls in contact with the capillaries in the two lungs is about 70 m^2.

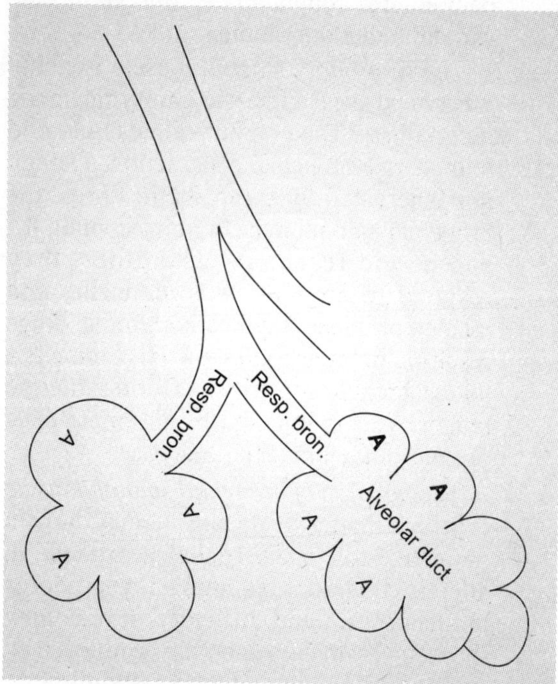

Fig. 15.3: The respiratory units; A-alveolus.

The alveoli are lined by two types of epithelial cells. Type-I cells, very thin flat cells with many cytoplasmic extensions, constitute approximately 95% of the surface area of the alveoli (Fig. 15.5). These cells contain only a few cytoplasmic organelles. Type-II cells, though similar in number as type I cells, constitute only 5% of the alveolar surface area. These cells are cuboidal in shape with many microvilli on their apical border. Type II cells contain many mitochondria as well as a large number of lamellar bodies. That is why type II cells are also known as *granular pneumocytes*. The lamellar bodies contain whorls of phospholipids synthesized by the type II cells. The phospholipids are an important element of pulmonary surfactant—the surface tension lowering agent present on the surface of alveolar epithelium.

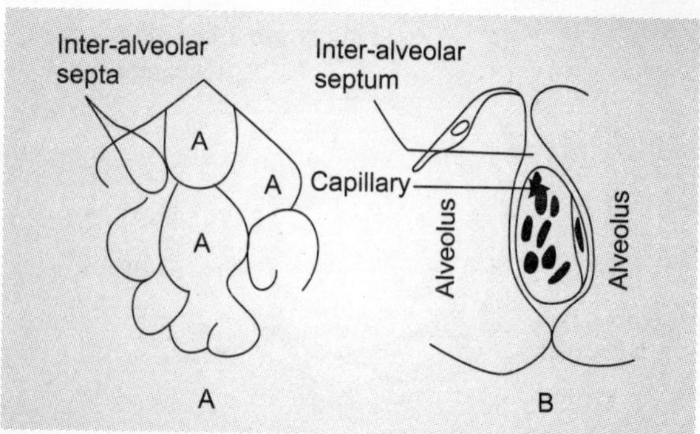

Fig. 15.4: (A) Structure of pulmonary parenchyma under ordinary microscope. (B) Highly magnified view of an inter-alveolus septum.

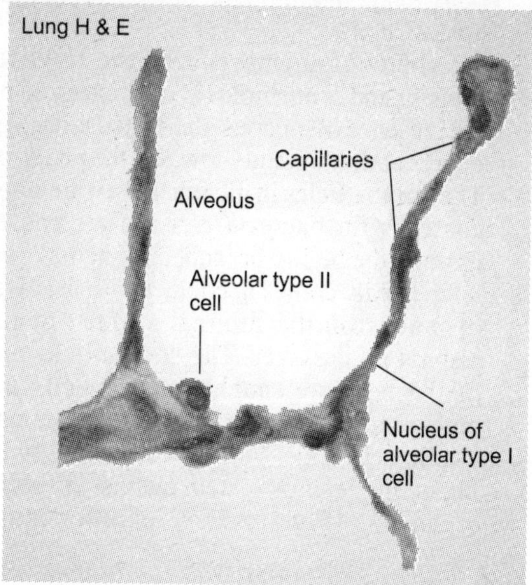

Fig. 15.5: The alveolar epithelial cells.

Besides blood capillaries, the alveolar walls contain a few elastic and collagen connective tissue fibres, a few mast cells and tissue macrophages called *pulmonary alveolar macrophages* (PAMs).

THE RESPIRATORY MEMBRANE

The respiratory membrane is the name given to the tissues which separate the capillary blood from the alveolar air. It consists of the following layers (Fig. 15.6):

1. A layer of fluid lining the alveolus (the fluid contains pulmonary surfactant).
2. A single layer of alveolar epithelial cells.
3. Basement membrane of the alveolar epithelial cells.
4. A very thin interstitial space between the epithelial and the endothelial cells.
5. Basement membrane of capillary endothelial cells.
6. A single layer of capillary endothelial cells.

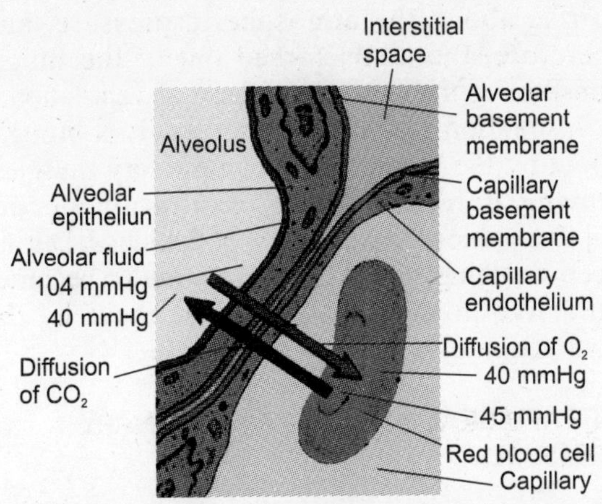

Fig. 15.6: The respiratory membrane.

All the layers mentioned above, together constitute a membrane not more than 0.2–1 μm thick. Hence, under normal circumstances, gases can diffuse across the respiratory membrane with great ease. Pathologically, the thickness of the respiratory membrane may increase due to exudation of fluid from the capillaries (pulmonary oedema). Under these conditions, the diffusion of gases, particularly O_2, is seriously hampered.

Non-Respiratory Functions of the Lungs

Besides the function of gas exchange and related function of surfactant synthesis, many other important non-respiratory functions are performed by the lungs:

(a) Metabolic Functions The pulmonary vessels have a large surface area of endothelial cells. These cells serve many metabolic functions. A converting enzyme called *angiotensin converting enzyme* (ACE) is present on the surface of the pulmonary endothelial cells which converts angiotensin-I to angiotensin-II. Many naturally occurring substances such as acetylcholine, serotonin, bradykinin, norepinephrine and prostaglandins (E & F type) are *taken up and destroyed* by the endothelial cells. Many of these products are released from the damaged tissues or from breakdown of platelets during the clotting of blood. By this action of the lungs, the rest of the body is protected from the possible adverse effects of these products. On the other hand, many substances such as epinephrine, vasopressin and other general hormones and prostaglandin A pass through the lungs without any change to produce their effects in the systemic circulation (Table 15.1). Many hormones act on the lungs. Corticosteroids promote maturation of type II epithelial cell of the fetal lungs which secrete surfactant. Thyroxine also seems to be required for the maturation process.

(b) Filtration Function The pulmonary capillaries act as an effective filter. These vessels trap and prevent microemboli such as fibrin clots, gas bubbles, or fat globules from reaching the systemic circulation.

(c) Reservoir Function Normally the pulmonary circulation contains approximately 450 ml of blood. The pulmonary vessels act as capacitance vessels and their capacity may vary from 200 to 900 ml (see Chapter13).

(d) Role in Defence The role of *ciliary escalator system* and *immunoglobulin A* present in the bronchial secretions has been discussed earlier. In addition, the lungs contain *pulmonary alveolar macrophages* which constitute an important defence mechanism of the body. Like

Table 15.1: Summary of metabolic functions of the lungs

Cleared by lungs:
Bradykinin
Norepinephrine
Serotonin
Prostaglandins E and F
Activated by lungs:
Angiotensin I
Released by lungs:
Prostaglandins
Histamine
Kallikreins
Slow-reacting substances of anaphylaxis
Unaffected by lungs:
Angiotensin II
Epinephrine
Vasopressin
Prostaglandin A

other fixed tissue macrophages, these cells are actively phagocytic. They ingest bacteria and small dust particles which escape the ciliary escalator system and reach the alveoli. Like other macrophages, alveolar macrophages are also involved in the processing of inhaled bacterial antigens and their transfer to immuno-competent cells. They also secrete chemotactic substances that attract granulocytes to the lungs, as well as chemicals that stimulate granulocyte and monocyte production in the bone marrow.

(e) Water Balance Lungs play a role in the water balance of the body. Respiratory water loss is due to the difference between the water vapour content of the inspired air and the expired air. About 400 ml of water is lost per day from the pulmonary epithelium. During hot and dry weather, there is still greater water loss from the respiratory passages. Factors that increase pulmonary ventilation (physical work, acidosis, etc.) also increase respiratory water loss.

Animals like dogs do not have sweat glands. They use respiratory system to regulate their body temperature. In hot weather, their breathing becomes more rapid and shallow (panting). Water vapourization from the upper respiratory passages causes substantial heat loss (as well as water loss).

It may seem surprising but large amount of water is lost from the respiratory passages in very cold climate also. Cold air contains very little water vapour even when fully humidified. Inspired cold air becomes warm and gets loaded with water vapour from the respiratory passages, which is lost in expiration. Therefore, mountain climbers and polar explorers run the risk of dehydration even when surrounded by frozen water all around.

PULMONARY VENTILATION

Pulmonary ventilation, i.e. movement of atmospheric air into and out of the lungs, is brought about by changes in the size of the thoracic cavity.

Expansion of the thoracic cage leads to a fall in the intrapulmonary pressure below the atmospheric air pressure. Due to the pressure gradient, the atmospheric air flows into the lungs, constituting the inspiratory phase of ventilation. Subsequently, the decrease in the size of the thoracic cage causes the intrapulmonary pressure to rise above the atmospheric pressure, and therefore, the air is forced out of the lungs, constituting the expiratory phase of ventilation.

Inspiration is an active process. It is brought about by the contraction of inspiratory muscles. During quiet breathing, expiration occurs passively due to elastic recoil of the lungs. During deep breathing, however, even expiration becomes an active process; it is brought about by the contraction of expiratory muscles.

INTRAPLEURAL AND INTRAPULMONARY PRESSURES

The lungs have a continuous tendency to collapse. This is called the *recoil tendency of the lungs*. It is caused by: (i) the presence of many elastic fibres in the alveolar walls which are under constant stretch in the inflated lungs; (ii) Surface tension of the fluid lining the alveoli due to which the alveoli tend to become progressively smaller and collapse.

The recoil tendency of the lungs is opposed by the recoil tendency of the thoracic cage. As a result, even when the inspiratory muscles are not contracting, the thoracic cage along with the parietal layer of the pleura tends to expand

(Fig. 15.7). In other words, the parietal and the visceral layers of the pleura tend to separate out in opposite directions, producing a subatmospheric intrapleural pressure. All these facts can be easily demonstrated by inserting an injection needle into a pleural cavity of an experimental animal (Fig. 15.8). Immediately, the lung collapses and the thoracic cage becomes bigger than on the normal side.

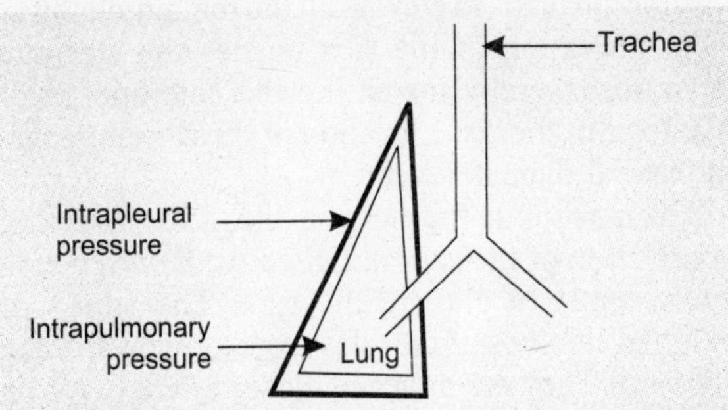

Fig. 15.7: The intrapleural and intrapulmonary pressure.

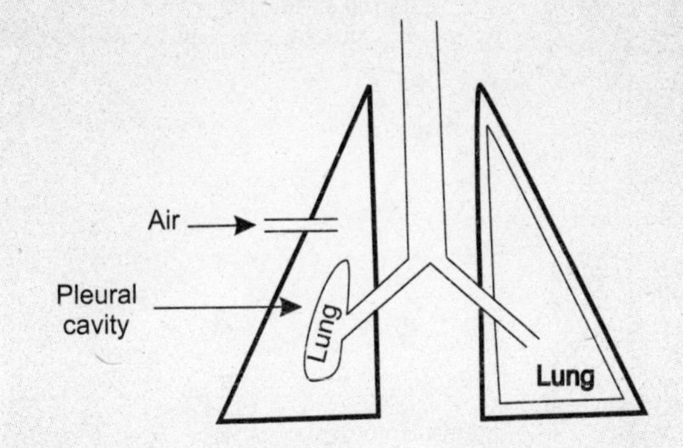

Fig. 15.8: Effect of absence of negative intrapleural pressure on the expansion of the left lung.

When the inspiratory muscles are relaxed, intrapleural pressure is approximately –3 mmHg. (3 mmHg below atmospheric pressure or 757 mmHg). During inspiration, contraction of the inspiratory muscles expands the chest wall and the intrapleural pressure becomes still lower (about –6 mmHg). Consequently, the lungs expand further, the intrapulmonary pressure becomes subatmospheric and inspiration occurs. Expiration occurs when the inspiratory muscles relax and the intrapleural pressure rises to –3 mmHg once again, and the lungs are allowed to recoil to a smaller volume. The increase in the intrapulmonary pressure above the atmospheric pressure forces the air out of the lungs (Fig. 15.9). The degree of inflation and deflation of the lungs varies with the extent of changes in the intrapleural pressure.

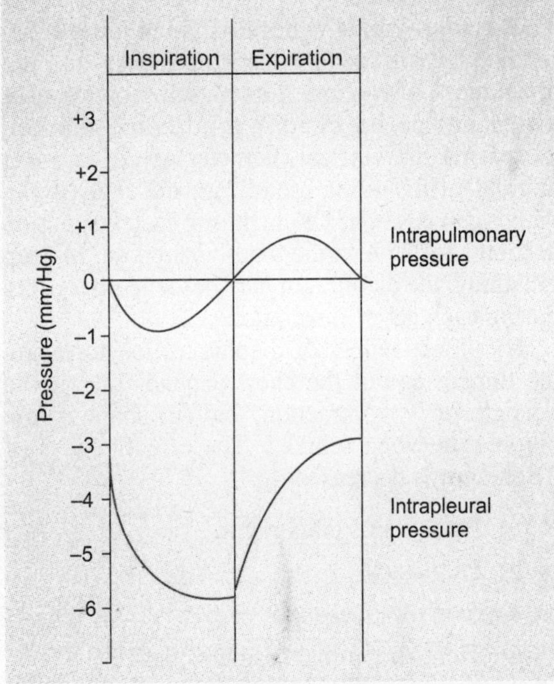

Fig. 15.9: The intrapleural and intrapulmonary pressures in the two phases of respiration.

During quiet breathing, the intrapleural pressure varies between –3 and –6 mmHg. During very forceful inspiratory effort, it may be as low as –100 mmHg. During forceful expiratory effort, the intrapleural pressure may even become positive.

During quiet breathing, the intrapulmonary pressure varies between –1 mmHg (during inspiration) and +1 mmHg (during expiration). During forceful inspiratory effort against closed glottis (Muller's manoeuvre), the intrapulmonary pressure may be as low as –80 mmHg. Forceful expiration against closed glottis (Valsalva's manoeuvre) may produce intrapulmonary pressure of as much as +100 mmHg.

MECHANISM OF VENTILATION

Inspiration

Enlargement of the thoracic cavity during inspiration is caused by contraction of the diaphragm and the external intercostal muscles.

Role of Diaphragm

The diaphragm is a dome-shaped, musculotendinous partition between the thorax and the abdomen. Contraction of its muscle fibres causes a descent of its central tendinous portion, increasing the vertical diameter of the thoracic cage. During quiet breathing, descent of the diaphragm by about 1.5 cm during each inspiration accounts for 75% of the total inspired air. In deep breathing, the diaphragm may descend up to 7 cm during each act of inspiration.

The effectiveness of diaphragm in increasing the dimensions of the chest depends on: (i) the strength of its contraction, and (ii) shape of the diaphragm when relaxed. The effectiveness of diaphragm is decreased by:

(a) Paralysis of diaphragm,

(b) Pregnancy,

(c) Extreme obesity,

(d) Tight abdominal garments, and

(e) Emphysema: In this disorder, the lungs are permanently over-inflated. Even during expiration, the diaphragm is flat, not dome-shaped. Hence, contraction of diaphragm during inspiration does not effectively increase the vertical diameter of the thoracic cage.

The nerve supply (phrenic nerve) to the diaphragm arises from cervical cord segments 3, 4 and 5, whereas the intercostals muscles are supplied by motor nerves from the corresponding thoracic spinal cord segments. That is why a spinal cord injury *above C 5* is immediately fatal because all the respiratory muscles are paralysed. On the other hand, a patient with spinal cord injury below *C 5* can breathe almost normally because of the intact function of diaphragm.

Role of Intercostal Muscles

From pivot-like joints with the vertebrae, the *ribs slope obliquely downwards and forwards.* The intercostal muscles are attached to the adjacent ribs. Thus, when they contract, they may be expected to pull the upper rib downward and the lower rib upward. However, the first rib is relatively fixed in position. Therefore, contraction of the external intercostal muscles during inspiration tends to elevate all the remaining lower ribs. Elevation of the ribs pushes the sternum outwards, thereby increasing the anteroposterior diameter of thorax. Elevation of the ribs increases the lateral diameter also.

Even without the help of the fixed first rib, contraction of the *external intercostal muscles,* as such, tends to elevate the ribs. The fibres of external intercostal muscles slope downward and forward. They are attached closer to the pivot on the upper ribs than on the lower ribs (Fig. 15.10).

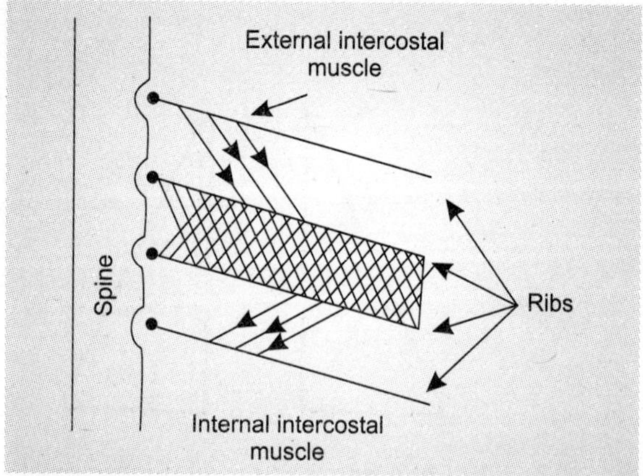

Fig. 15.10: Effect of the attachment of intercostal muscles on the mechanical advantage. Contraction of external intercostal muscles favours elevation of ribs whereas contraction of internal intercostal muscles favours the opposite.

As the force arm of the lower rib is longer as compared to that of the upper rib, the lever system operates in such a way that, because of the mechanical advantage, contraction of external intercostal muscle fibres would pull the lower rib upward rather than pull the upper rib downward.

(The reverse is true for the action of *internal intercostal muscles*. They slope downward and backward, therefore creating a longer force-arm for the upper rib. Hence, their contraction tends to pull all the ribs downwards).

Accessory Muscles of Inspiration

The *scalene* muscles attached to the first two ribs and *sternocleidomastoids* attached to the top of the sternum are called the accessory muscles of inspiration. Their action is to elevate the thoracic cage. They are so-called because they do not contract during quiet breathing. They contract vigorously during deep breathing such as during exercise. Visible contraction of these muscles in a patient indicates a difficulty in the breathing process (respiratory distress).

Expiration

In quiet breathing, expiration is a passive process. The volume of the thorax is decreased by relaxation of the diaphragm and external intercostal muscles. In deep breathing, however, the expiration becomes an active process. A number of expiratory muscles, like *internal intercostal* and *abdominal muscles,* are involved in active expiratory process. Contraction of abdominal muscles (rectus, transversalis, oblique): (i) increases the intra-abdominal pressure which pushes the diaphragm upwards: (ii) pulls the ribs downward and medially: (iii) fixes the lower ribs.

Consequently, contraction of the internal intercostal muscles lowers the ribs.

In addition, as explained above, the insertion of internal intercostal muscles on the adjacent ribs is such that their contraction pulls the ribs downwards.

Besides their role in deep breathing, the expiratory muscles are involved in other forced expiratory efforts, e.g. in coughing, vomiting, defaecation and Valsalva manoeuvre, etc.

Role of Laryngeal Muscles The abductor muscles of the larynx contract during inspiration, pulling the vocal cords apart. Contraction of the adductor muscles of the larynx is a part of deglutition reflex.

LUNG VOLUMES AND CAPACITIES

The term lung volume refers to one of the four primary, non-overlapping subdivisions of total lung capacity. Each capacity refers to two or more primary lung volumes. Lung subdivisions are measured from resting position at the end of spontaneous expiration. Most of the lung volumes and capacities can be easily estimated by a water-filled spirometer attached to a kymograph (Fig. 15.11).

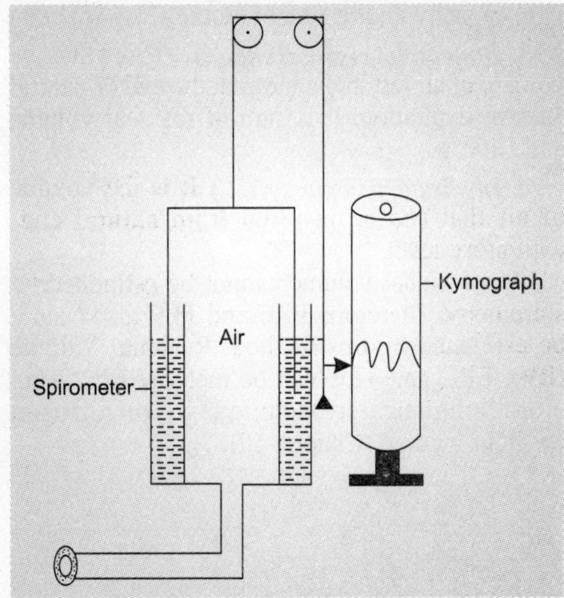

Fig. 15.11: A water-filled spirometer.

Static Ventilatory Function

Pulmonary Volumes

1. ***Tidal volume (VT)*** It is the volume of air that enters or leaves the lungs at each natural respiratory effort at rest.

2. ***Inspiratory reserve volume (IRV)*** It is the volume of air that can be inhaled by a maximum inspiratory effort over and above the inspired tidal volume.

3. ***Expiratory reserve volume (ERV)*** It is the volume of air that can be exhaled by the maximum expiratory effort after the end of natural (passive) expiration.

4. *Residual volume (RV)* It is the volume of air that remains in the lungs after maximum expiratory effort.

Pulmonary Capacities

1. *Vital capacity (VC)* It is the volume of air that can be expelled by the most vigorous expiratory effort after the deepest possible inspiration. It is equal to the sum of VT, IRV and ERV (Fig. 15.12).

2. *Total lung capacity (TLC)* It is the sum of vital capacity and residual volume (Fig. 15.12).

15

3. *Functional residual capacity (FRC)* It is the volume of air left in the lungs at the end of natural passive expiration. It is sum of residual volume and ERV.

4. *Inspiratory capacity (IC)* It is the volume of air that can be inspired from natural end-expiratory level.

The residual volume cannot be estimated by spirometry. Therefore, FRC and TLC also cannot be estimated by this method. Residual Volume (RV), FRC and TLC can be measured by using more sophisticated techniques like nitrogen washout method (Chapter 19).

The normal values of various pulmonary volumes and capacities in an adult male are given in Table 15.2. In an adult female, the values are 20% lower.

Table 15.2: Normal values of various volumes and capacities

Pulmonary volume/capacity	*Volume*
TV	0.5 L
IRV	3.0 L
ERV	1.0 L
RV	1.2 L
TLC	5.7 L
VC	4.6 L
FRC	2.2 L
MVV	125 L /min

FACTORS AFFECTING VITAL CAPACITY

Vital capacity varies with the size and muscular development of the subject. In adults, it is approximately 2.6 L/m^2 BSA in males and 2.1 L/m^2 BSA in females. Average vital capacity in adult males and females is 4.6 L and 3.5 L, respectively. Vital capacity is increased by athletic training. Vital capacity is decreased in (i) neuromuscular disorders

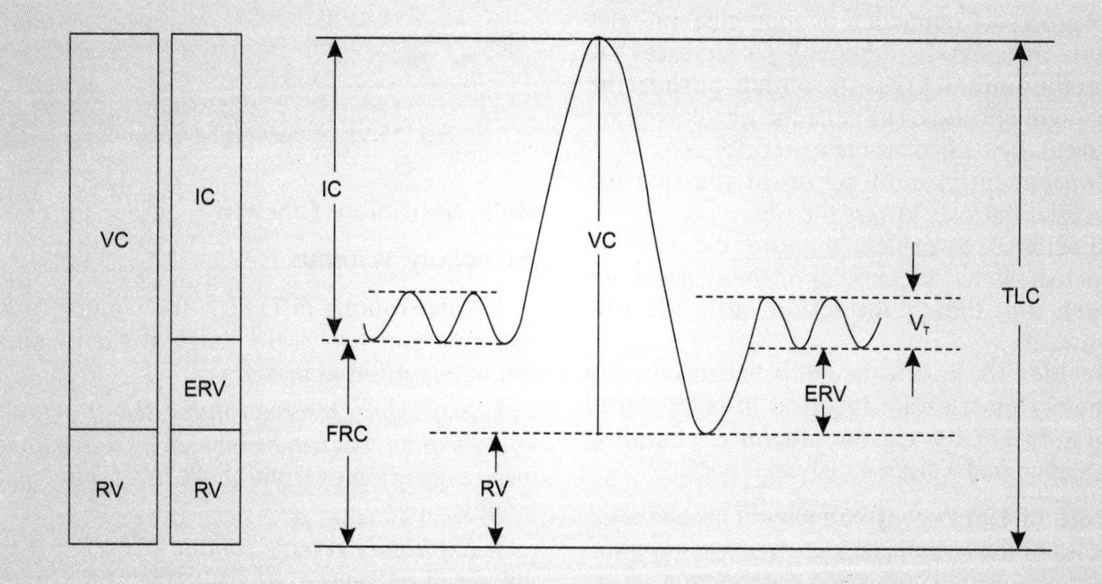

Fig. 15.12: Lung volumes. VC = vital capacity, RV = residual volume; IC = inspiratory capacity; ERV = expiratory reserve volume; FRC = functional residual capacity; V_T = tidal volume.

like poliomyelitis; (ii) pulmonary airways obstructive disorders like bronchial asthma; and (iii) restrictive pulmonary diseases like pulmonary fibrosis. Vital capacity is greater in standing posture than in supine because of decreased pulmonary blood volume in the former position.

Dynamic Ventilatory Function

Maximum Ventilatory Volume

Pulmonary ventilation is a dynamic process. It can be calculated if tidal volume as well as the rate of breathing per minute is known. At rest, the tidal volume is approximately 500 ml and the breathing rate is about 12/min. Hence, at rest, the rate of pulmonary ventilation is 6 L/min (12 × 0.5 L).

The greatest rate of pulmonary ventilation (125L/min) is called the maximum breathing capacity (MBC) or maximum ventilatory volume (MMV).

Timed Vital Capacity

Forced expiratory volume in the first second (FEV_1 %) is the fraction of total vital capacity that can be expired in the first second of the expiratory effort (Fig. 15.13). In early stages of obstructive lung disorders, FEV_1 is more affected than the vital capacity.

During exercise, the pulmonary ventilation increases in proportion to the severity of exercise. It may be 10 times the pulmonary ventilation at rest. The increase in pulmonary ventilation is because of:

(a) Increase in the rate of breathing. It may increase up to 50 breaths/minute.
(b) Increase in the depth of breathing. The tidal volume encroaches on the IRV, and ERV specially the IRV. However, the maximum depth of breathing remains usually less than 50% of the vital capacity (Fig. 15.14).

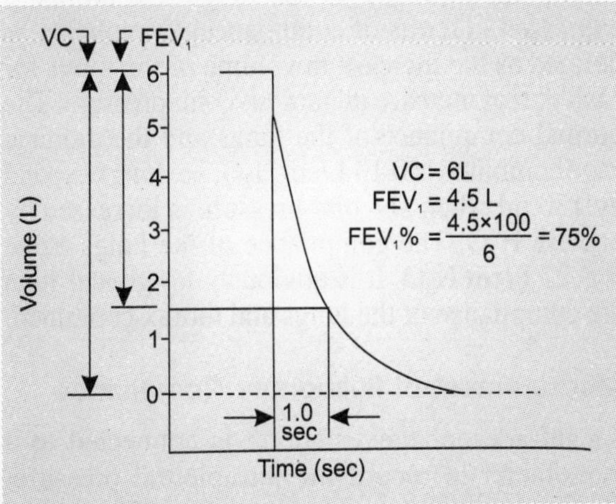

Fig. 15.13: Calculation of FEV_1 %.

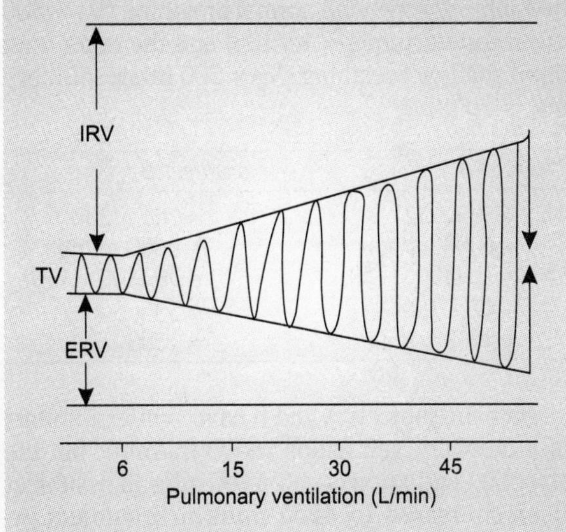

Fig. 15.14: Mechanism of increase in the depth. of breathing (by encroachment of IRV and ERV, more so on the former).

ALVEOLAR VENTILATION vs. PULMONARY VENTILATION

The respiratory passages where the gaseous exchange does not occur is called the dead space (Fig. 15.1). It is equal to approximately 150 ml. Thus, when tidal volume of 500 ml leaves the lungs, the last 150 ml of expiratory alveolar air remains in the conducting passages. Therefore, of 500 ml of air entering the lungs during next inspiration, 150 ml is not fresh atmospheric air but only the alveolar air left behind earlier. Only 350 ml of fresh atmospheric air reach the alveoli during each inspiration and mix with the alveolar air.

Rate of Alveolar Ventilation

Alveolar ventilation is the volume of fresh air which ventilates the gas-exchange areas of the lungs each minute. It is equal to the respiratory rate multiplied by the volume of air entering the alveoli with each breath.

$$V_A = \text{Respiratory rate} \times (V_T - V_D)$$

where V_A = Alveolar ventilation
V_T = Tidal volume
V_D = Dead space volume.

The importance of alveolar ventilation can be understood if we calculate alveolar ventilation of two subjects, one with normal breathing (V_T = 500 ml; respiratory rate = 12/min) and the other with rapid shallow breathing (V_T = 200 ml; respiratory rate = 30/min).

15

Subject A	*Subject B*
V_p = 500 × 12	V_P = 200 × 30
= 6000 ml/min	= 6000 ml/min
V_A = 12 (500 – 150)	V_A = 30 (200 – 150)
= 12 × 350	= 30 × 50
= 4200 ml/min	= 1500 ml/min

Both the subjects A and B have similar amounts of pulmonary ventilation (6000 ml/min); but the alveolar ventilation is only 1500 ml/min in subject B as compared to 4200 ml/min in subject A. Consequently, subject B would suffer from hypoxia and hypercapnia.

Anatomic and Physiologic Dead Space

As mentioned above, the volume of respiratory conducting passages above the level of respiratory bronchioles is called the *anatomic dead space*, because this volume of air does not participate in gas exchange. *Physiologic dead space* includes anatomic dead space plus the volume of air present in the alveoli where gas exchange does not occur because of insufficient blood supply. Hence, practically these alveoli must also be considered a dead space (Fig. 15.15). Normally, the number of such alveoli is very small and physiologic dead space nearly equals the anatomic dead space. However, in certain respiratory disorders, physiologic dead space may be as much as ten times the anatomic dead space. Obviously, such patients would have very little effective alveolar ventilation, which results in respiratory distress.

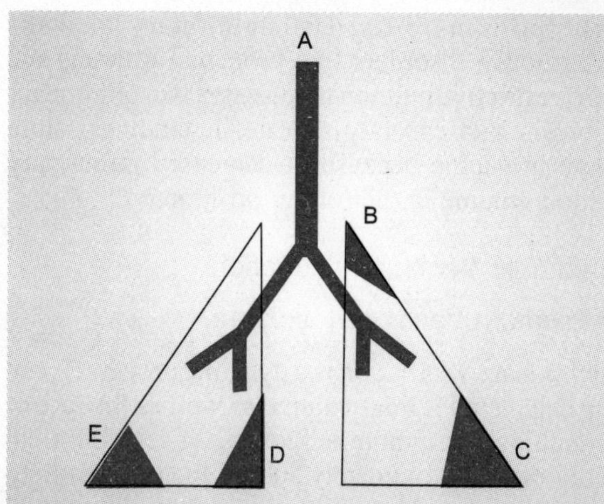

Fig. 15.15: Anatomic dead space (A). Physiological dead space includes (A) plus non-perfused areas of the lungs (B + C + D + E).

Expansibility of the Lungs and the Thoracic Cage

Both the lungs and the thoracic cage are visco-elastic structures. Elastic properties of the lungs are partly because of the presence of elastic connective tissue fibres in the parenchyma, and partly because of the surface tension of the fluid lining the alveoli. The elastic property of the thoracic cage is because of the elastic nature of the ribs, muscles and tendons. The major part of the energy is spent by the respiratory muscles in stretching the elastic structures of the lungs and thorax.

The expansibility of the lungs and thorax is expressed in terms of compliance. Compliance is defined as the increase in volume of the lungs for each unit of increase in intra-alveolar pressure. The normal compliance of the lungs and the thoracic cage combined is 0.13 L/cm H_2O, i.e. lungs expand by 130 ml when alveolar pressure is increased by one cm H_2O. The compliance of the lungs alone is 0.22 L/cm H_2O. It is obviously far greater than the compliance of the lungs and thorax combined.

Measurement of Pulmonary Compliance

An intraoesophageal balloon is connected to a manometer to record the intrapleural pressure. (The two pressures are almost similar). The subject inspires air from a spirometer in steps of 100 ml, and each time the intrapleural pressure is recorded. Similarly, intrapleural pressure is recorded during stepwise expiration. The relationship of changes in lung volume to changes intrapleural pressure ($\Delta V/\Delta P$) is plotted (Fig. 15.16). The curve which the lungs follow during inflation is different from that during deflation. This behaviour is known as *hysteresis*. The lung volume at any given pressure is greater during expiration than during inspiration. This is due to the viscous properties of the lungs. The volume midway between the two loops (dashed line in Fig. 15.16) gives the average compliance of the lungs.

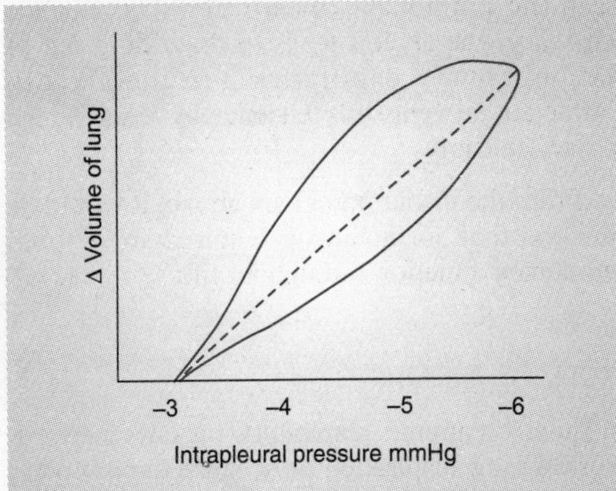

Fig. 15.16: Changes in intrapleural pressure in relation to lung volume change during quiet respiration. The dotted line represents the pulmonary compliance.

Pulmonary compliance is decreased by pulmonary fibrosis (pathologic replacement of elastic fibres by collagen fibres). Congestion or oedema of the lung also decreases pulmonary compliance. Compliance of the thoracic cage is reduced by deformities of spine or thoracic cage like kyphoscoliosis.

SURFACE TENSION

Besides the elastic fibres, surface tension of the fluid lining the alveoli is another very important factor affecting the pulmonary compliance. This can be demonstrated by recording the compliance of an isolated lung of an animal by distending it with air and then with saline (Fig. 15.17). The

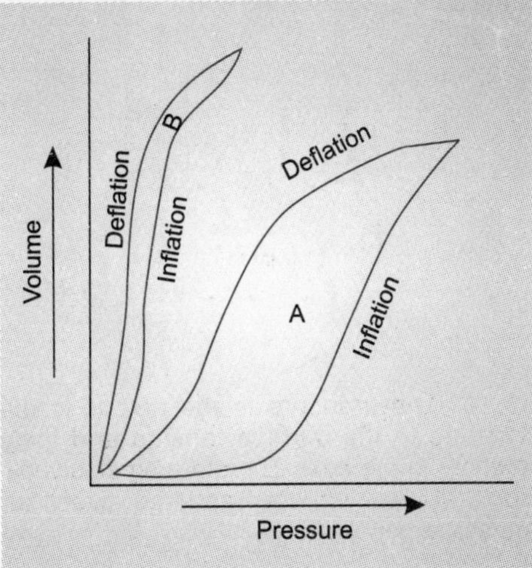

Fig. 15.17: Pressure volume relationship of an isolated lung filled with air (A) and with saline (B). Saline-filled lung has far greater compliance due to absence of surface tension at water-air interface (in the air-filled lung).

compliance of the saline-filled lungs is far greater (and hysteresis much smaller) than of air-filled lung. The difference is due to the fact that saline-filling abolishes the surface tension forces, and the compliance of such a lung depends only on the elastic fibres of the lungs.

The air in each alveolus is separated from the alveolar walls by a thin film of fluid. The alveoli are practically air-filled bubbles lined with water. At the air-water interface, the attractive forces between the water molecules cause the air bubbles to squeeze. This force called *surface tension* makes the alveolus to act like a small elastic balloon with constant tendency to collapse and resist further stretching. Much of the inspiratory effort is spent in overcoming this force. According to the law of Laplace, in spherical structures like alveoli, the pressure generated equals two times the (surface) tension, divided by the radius. $P = 2T/r$ (Fig. 15.18). So smaller alveoli with small radius tend to generate greater pressure, and hence empty into larger alveoli. Therefore, surface tension tends to produce collapse of the alveoli.

The surface tension of pure water is so high that every inspiration would require an exhausting muscular effort. However, the presence of a

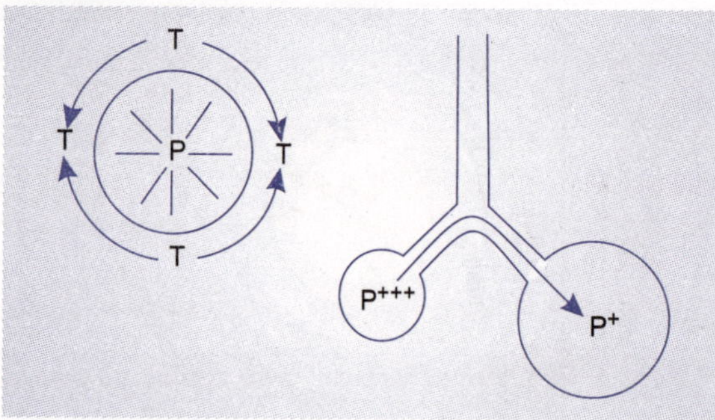

Fig. 15.18: The pressure in the alveoli is directly proportionate to the surface tension and inversely proportionate to the radii. Therefore small alveoli tend to become still smaller whereas large alveoli tend to become still larger.

phospholipoprotein complex called *pulmonary surfactant* in the fluid lining the alveoli reduces the surface tension to about one-fourth. As mentioned earlier, pulmonary surfactant is secreted by type-II alveolar epithelial cells, and it mixes with the water molecules on the alveolar surfaces.

In the absence of surfactant, the expansion of the lungs becomes extremely difficult. Such a problem occurs in some of the newborn babies. Premature babies are more liable to suffer from this disorder, called respiratory distress syndrome of the newborn, because the synthesis of surfactant starts only late in fetal life. The disorder is characterised by failure of expansion of many parts of the lungs at birth. Even those alveoli which expand have a tendency to collapse. As a result, the newborn baby suffers from respiratory distress and hypoxia. Hypoxia may be so severe as to cause cerebral damage, which may be irreversible. The condition is known as *infant respiratory distress syndrome* (IRDS).

The lamellar inclusions seen in type-II alveolar epithelial cells contain the material that is secreted as surfactant by exocytosis. The size and number of inclusions are increased by thyroxine. Glucocorticoids are involved in the maturation of surfactant. There is an increase in the concentrations of cortisol in fetal and maternal blood near term. Respiratory distress syndrome is also more common in infants with low plasma thyroxine level.

Surfactant not only increases the pulmonary compliance but also helps to maintain the equality of alveolar size. If an alveolus tends to become smaller, the concentration of surfactant per unit surface increases, causing further decrease in surface tension. Therefore, the alveolus enlarges.

Similarly, any tendency of an alveolus to enlarge would lead to smaller surfactant concentration per unit surface; hence greater surface tension. Therefore, the alveolus diminishes in size. In this way, pulmonary surfactant prevents any deviation from the normal size of the alveoli.

Another function of pulmonary surfactant is to keep the pulmonary alveoli dry. The surface tension of the alveoli tends to draw fluid out of the pulmonary capillaries into the alveoli. Surfactant prevents this tendency by reducing the surface tension.

From the discussion given above, it would be obvious that surfactant is required for normal pulmonary function throughout life.

WORK OF BREATHING

In quiet breathing, respiratory muscles perform work during inspiration only, since expiration is a passive process. Quiet expiration is produced by the elastic recoil of the lungs. The work of inspiration consists of energy required to overcome: (i) elastic resistance (65%), (ii) viscous resistance (7%), and (iii) airways resistance (28%). Factor (i) has been discussed above in detail. Viscous resistance is the resistance offered by the tissues as they slide over each other during stretch. Airway resistance is discussed below.

During normal quiet respiration, the energy cost of breathing accounts for only 2–3% of the total energy expenditure of the body. Pulmonary diseases which decrease pulmonary compliance, or thoracic cage compliance, or increase airway resistance, may increase the work of breathing to such an extent that breathing becomes an exhaustive work, consuming as much energy that the total energy expenditure of the body increases by over 33%.

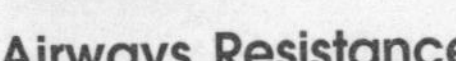

Airways Resistance

Resistance in the airways (Raw) is basically determined by same factors that govern the resistance in the blood vessels:

$$R_{aw} = \frac{8\ nL}{\pi r^4}$$

Airways resistance is directly proportionate to the viscosity of the air (*n*) and length of the airways (*L*). It is inversely proportionate to the fourth power of airways radius. In normal circumstances, length of the airways is almost constant and the viscosity of air does not change. Therefore, the major factor determining the airways resistance is the radius of the airway tubes. The term 4 denotes that a small change in the radius of the tube causes a large change in the airway resistance.

The pattern of flow of a fluid is another important factor that determines the resistance. Resistance is low when the flow is laminar but increases sharply when the flow is turbulent. The transition from laminar flow to turbulent flow pattern is a function of linear flow velocity. Linear flow velocity is large in trachea and up to medium sized bronchi (> 2 mm diameter). It is very low in bronchi smaller than 2 mm diameter because their number and consequently their total cross-section area is very large (cf. blood flow velocity in the aorta and capillaries). Therefore, even during quiet breathing air flow is turbulent in the upper respiratory passages (nose and pharynx), trachea and large bronchi, but laminar in bronchi smaller than 2 mm diameter. Hence, R_{aw} chiefly resides in upper airways (50%) and in trachea and bronchi > 2 mm diameter (40%). Bronchi smaller than 2 mm diameter offer very little resistance (10%).

Upper Airways Resistance

Upper respiratory airways resistance is not subjected to any physiological variation except that it can be markedly reduced by mouth breathing. During exercise, rapid air flow further increases the turbulence of air. This would tend to markedly increase the upper airways resistance. However, it does not happen because, by some unknown mechanism, we shift to mouth breathing during exercise.

An increase in the upper airways resistance may occur in pathological conditions like nasal congestion, deviation of nasal septum or enlarged adenoids. In such conditions also, mouth breathing is common.

Lower Airways Resistance

Physiological control of airways resistance chiefly lies in *medium-sized bronchi (2–4 mm diameter)*. Their walls not only contain supporting cartilage but also large amount of smooth muscle. Muscle contraction can substantially reduce the airways radius. The diameter of these bronchi, and therefore the airways resistance, may be altered by the following factors: (1) Bronchomotor muscle tone; (2) Radial traction by lung parenchyma; (3) Transmural pressure; and (4) Mucus secretions.

1. Bronchomotor Muscle Tone Changes in the bronchomotor muscle tone are the most important regulator of the diameter of medium-sized bronchi. The smooth muscle is innervated by cholinergic parasympathetic (vagal) nerve fibres. Increased parasympathetic discharge causes contraction of bronchial smooth muscle. In normal individuals, injection of atropine sulphate reduces the airway resistance by about 30%. This indicates a mild tonic discharge in the vagal fibres. It is doubtful whether bronchial smooth muscle is innervated by noradrenergic sympathetic nerve fibres.

The bronchial tone seems to be regulated purely by changes in parasympathetic neural discharge. However, bronchial smooth muscle cells respond to the circulating catecholamines and produce bronchodilation.

The following factors affect the bronchial smooth muscle tone and thereby bronchial diameter:

(i) *Irritant receptors* The mucosa of the lower respiratory passages contains certain irritant receptors. These are stimulated by mechanical or chemical irritants such as dust particles or irritant gases leading to reflex bronchoconstriction. Vagus nerve contains both the afferent and the efferent fibres for the reflex. The biological significance of this reflex in decreasing the amount of inhaled irritant material is obvious.

(ii) *Stretch receptors* Walls of the bronchi and bronchioles contain stretch receptors. Their stimulation by stretching of pulmonary parenchyma (e.g. over inflation of the lungs during deep breathing) results in reflex bronchodilation. This vagally-mediated reflex helps to increase the airflow in proportion to the increased capacity of pulmonary alveoli.

(iii) *Carbon dioxide* High CO_2 concentration causes relaxation of the bronchial smooth muscle leading to bronchodilation. Conversely, low CO_2 concentration produces bronchoconstriction. If any part of the lung tends to over-ventilate, the local tissue pCO_2 falls. The resulting bronchoconstriction increases the airway resistance and therefore ventilation of the part of the lung is restored to normal.

(iv) *Local hormones* In allergic asthma, a large number of local hormones such as histamine, prostaglandins, leukotriens, kinins, etc. are released, all of which produce varying degree of bronchoconstriction.

(v) *Circulating catecholamines* Circulating epinephrine produces bronchodilation by acting on β-2 adrenergic receptors present on the bronchial smooth muscle. Specific β-2 stimulating drugs like salbutamol are still more effective bronchodilators, and hence used in the treatment of bronchial asthma.

2. Radial Traction by Lung Parenchyma Bronchi and bronchioles are surrounded by the lung parenchyma, whose constant pull helps to keep the airways open. This supportive action is called the radial traction. As lung volume increases, so does the radial traction. Low lung volume tends to decrease the radial traction causing closure of some of the small airways and an increase in airways resistance. Diseases such as emphysema, which cause parenchymal destruction, cause loss of radial traction. As a result, the small airways collapse during expiration. Therefore in emphysema, in spite of increased pulmonary compliance, work of breathing is markedly increased due to increased airways resistance, especially during expiration (Fig. 15.19).

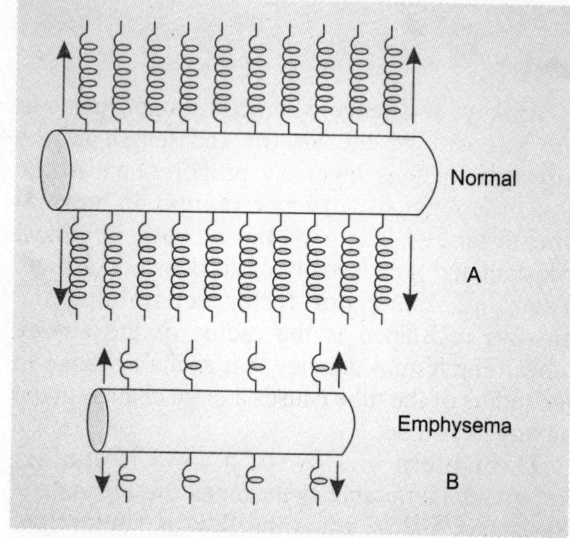

Fig. 15.19: (A) Radial traction keeps the normal airways open. (B) Effect of loss of radial traction on airway lumen.

3. Transmural Pressure During inspiration, intrapleural pressure is negative with respect to intrapulmonary pressure and that keeps the airways open. Similar situation remains during tidal expiration. However, during forced expiration, intrapleural pressure becomes strongly positive and that may cause dynamic airways collapse. Dynamic airway collapse causes expiratory flow limitation, i.e. beyond a limit increased expiratory efforts do not produce further increase in flow. The problem is worsened in emphysema.

4. Mucus Secretion The presence of excessive mucus or any other material in the lumen of the respiratory passages increases the airway resistance. Cigarette smoking or respiratory infections enhance the secretion of submucosal mucous glands and goblet cells of the respiratory passages.

16

CHAPTER

Pulmonary Diffusion

Pulmonary ventilation brings fresh environmental air into the alveoli. The next step in the external respiration consists of diffusion of O_2 from the alveolar air into the pulmonary capillary blood and diffusion of CO_2 in the opposite direction. Diffusion of gases occurs at tissue level also. Therefore, to understand these processes clearly, it would be advisable to recapitulate some of the physical laws that govern the behaviour of gases.

Gas Pressure

The molecules of a gas have kinetic energy and hence they are in continuous random motion. They bounce against each other or against the walls of the container. It would be obvious that greater the concentration of the molecules of the gas, the greater would be the force exerted by the molecules against the container at any given time. Therefore, *the pressure of a gas is directly proportionate to its concentration.*

Boyle's Law

At a constant temperature, the pressure (P) of a given mass of gas is inversely proportionate to its volume (V).

$$P \propto = 1/V$$

$$PV = \text{constant}$$

$$P_1V_1 = P_2V_2 \text{ (when temp. is constant)}$$

Charles' Law

At a constant pressure, the volume of gas is proportionate to its absolute temperature (T).

$$V \propto T \text{ (when pressure is constant)}$$

$$\text{or} \quad \frac{V}{T} = \text{constant}$$

$$\text{or} \quad \frac{V_1}{T_1} = \frac{V_2}{T_2}$$

$$\text{or} \quad \frac{V_1}{V_2} = \frac{T_1}{T_2} \text{ (when pressure is constant)}$$

Dalton's Law of Partial Pressures

When a mixture of gases is present in a container, each gas exerts a pressure according to its own concentration, independent of the concentration of other gases present in the mixture. In other words, each gas behaves as if it was present alone. The pressure of each gas in a mixture of gases is known as its *partial pressure* or *tension*. It is represented by the symbol 'p'. For example, environmental air is a mixture of 21% O_2 and 79% N_2. Therefore, the partial pressure of O_2 (pO_2) in the environmental air, at sea level (barometric pressure 760 mmHg), would be 21/ 100 × 760 = 160 mmHg. Similarly, partial pressure of N_2 (pN_2) in the environmental air, at sea level, would be 79/100 × 760 = 600 mmHg.

Total Pressure = $pO_2 + pN_2$ = 760 mmHg.

Partial Pressure of Gases in Water and Tissues

When a gas under pressure comes in contact with H_2O, some of the gas molecules move into water and get dissolved in it. As more and more molecules become dissolved, they diffuse all over the liquid medium and some of them start bouncing out of the aqueous phase into the gaseous phase. Ultimately, equilibrium is reached when the number of gas molecules entering the aqueous phase equals the number of molecules leaving it.

In this state of equilibrium, the partial pressure of the gas in aqueous phase is equal to the partial pressure of the gas in gaseous phase.

Henry's Law

The volume of a gas dissolved in a liquid is proportionate to its partial pressure and the solubility coefficient of the gas.

As compared to O_2, the solubility coefficient of CO_2 is 20 times greater whereas that of N_2 is one-half.

$$\text{Concentration of dissolved gas} = \text{Partial pressure of the gas} \times \text{Solubility coefficient of the gas}$$

Water Vapour Pressure

The inhaled air is humidified by the water vapours from the conducting passages. By the time it reaches the alveoli, it is saturated with water vapour. In the alveolar air, besides O_2 and N_2, water vapour also exerts its partial pressure. Vapour pressure of water is dependent on its temperature. In the alveoli (temperature 37°C), the water vapour pressure is 47 mmHg.

PHYSICAL LAWS GOVERNING RATE OF DIFFUSION OF A GAS ACROSS A MEMBRANE

1. **Gas Pressure Difference** This is the basic factor which promotes diffusion of a gas. Net diffusion of a gas always occurs from an area of high pressure to an area of low pressure. The rate of diffusion (D) is proportional to the difference in the pressure (ΔP) across the membrane (**D** $\propto \Delta P$).
2. **Solubility Coefficient (S)** of the gas ($D \propto S$).
3. **Cross-Section Area (A)** of the membrane ($D \propto A$).
4. **Distance (d)** through which the gas must diffuse ($D \propto 1/d$).
5. **Molecular Weight (MW)** of the gas $D \propto 1/\sqrt{MW}$).
6. **Temperature (t)** of the fluid ($D \propto t$).

Since, the body temperature remains fairly constant, the last factor is usually not considered. Therefore, in the lungs, or the tissues, the factors affecting the rate of diffusion of a given gas may be given by the following single formula.

$$D \propto \frac{\Delta P \times A \times S}{d \times \sqrt{MW}}$$

Now, the application of these factors in the pulmonary gas exchange shall be discussed.

PULMONARY DIFFUSION OF GASES

1. Pressure Gradient (ΔP) In the pulmonary alveoli, the respiratory membrane separates the gases (O_2 and CO_2) present in the alveolar air in gaseous phase from dissolved gases present in the blood of pulmonary capillaries. Oxygen diffuses from the alveolar air to the alveolar capillary blood because partial pressure (pO_2) of the alveolar air (100 mmHg) is far greater than that of alveolar capillary blood (40 mmHg), giving a pressure gradient of 60 mmHg. Carbon dioxide diffuses from the alveolar capillary blood to the alveolar air because pCO_2 of the alveolar capillary blood (46 mmHg) is greater than that of alveolar air (40 mmHg). In case of CO_2, the ΔP is merely 6 mmHg, but CO_2 transfer across the alveolar membrane is very efficient because it has 20 times greater diffusion coefficient than oxygen.

Diffusion of oxygen across the alveolar membrane is affected by a decrease in pO_2 of alveolar air in many conditions such as breathing at high altitude or hypoventilation because of narcotic poisoning, bronchial asthma or drowning, etc.

2. Cross-Sectional Area of Respiratory Membrane (A) It has been estimated that the total cross-sectional area of respiratory membrane is approximately 70 m^2 at rest. It is still greater during exercise because of the opening of a large number of previously dormant pulmonary capillaries. The total amount of blood in the pulmonary capillaries at any given moment is 60–140 ml, which spreads over a surface area of 70 m^2. That explains the extremely efficient gas exchange across the respiratory membrane. In pathological conditions, the surface area of the respiratory membrane may be decreased due to:

(i) Destruction of alveolar tissues as in the disorder called emphysema.
(ii) Surgical resection of a lung or a large lobe of a lung. When the total surface area of the respiratory membrane is decreased to about one-third of normal, the diffusion of gases (especially oxygen) is seriously affected.

3. Thickness of Respiratory Membrane (d) The thickness of respiratory membrane is normally very small (less than 1 μm). In many pathological conditions, respiratory membrane may become two or three times thicker. The result is a substantial interference in the gas exchange, particularly of oxygen. The thickness of respiratory membrane may be increased because of:

(i) Presence of oedema fluid in the alveolar interstitial tissue, or
(ii) Fibrosis of the interstitial tissue of the interalveolar septa (interstitial pulmonary fibrosis).

4. Solubility Coefficient and Molecular Weight of Gases The rate of diffusion of a gas varies directly with its solubility coefficient (S) and inversely with square root of its molecular weight. The molecular weight of CO_2 is 44 as compared to 32 in case of oxygen. But solubility coefficient of CO_2 is 24 times greater than that of oxygen. Therefore, in spite of having higher molecular weight, CO_2 diffuses 20 times faster than oxygen. That is why, in most of the respiratory disorders, pulmonary diffusion of O_2 is more severely affected than that of CO_2. Solubility coefficient and molecular weight of a gas are important factors governing its rate of diffusion into the liquid medium.

Diffusion Capacity of Lungs (Transfer Factor)

The overall ability of the respiratory membrane to transfer a gas between the alveolar air and the pulmonary blood is expressed in terms of diffusion capacity or transfer factor. Diffusion capacity is defined as a volume of a gas that diffuses through the respiratory membrane each minute for a pressure difference of one millimetre mercury. In young adult males, the diffusion capacity for O_2 under resting conditions is about 25 ml/min/mmHg. Mean oxygen pressure difference across the respiratory membrane under quiet breathing is about 11 mmHg. Therefore, at rest approximately 250 ml (25 × 11) of O_2 diffuses through the respiratory membrane per minute. During strenuous exercise, the diffusion capacity of O_2 may increase up to 90 ml/min/mmHg due to increase in the surface area of the respiratory membrane.

Diffusion capacity for CO_2 has never been measured because of technical difficulties. Carbon dioxide diffuses across the respiratory membrane so rapidly that the difference between the average pCO_2 of the capillary blood and pCO_2 of the alveolar air is less than 1 mmHg. Such a small difference cannot be detected by any available technique. However, from the knowledge of solubility coefficient of CO_2, diffusion capacity for CO_2 is believed to be about 400–450 ml/min/mmHg under resting condition and 1200–1300 ml/min/mmHg during strenuous exercise.

Due to a vast difference in the diffusion capacities for O_2 and CO_2, damage to the respiratory membrane may produce serious impairment of diffusion of O_2 while that of CO_2 may remain normal.

Effect of Ventilation-Perfusion Ratio on Pulmonary Gas Exchange

(The student is advised to pursue this topic after he/she is familiar with Chapter 17 of this book).

The resting alveolar ventilation of 4.2 L/min and pulmonary blood flow of 5 L/min give an overall ventilation-perfusion ratio of 0.84 (4.2 L/

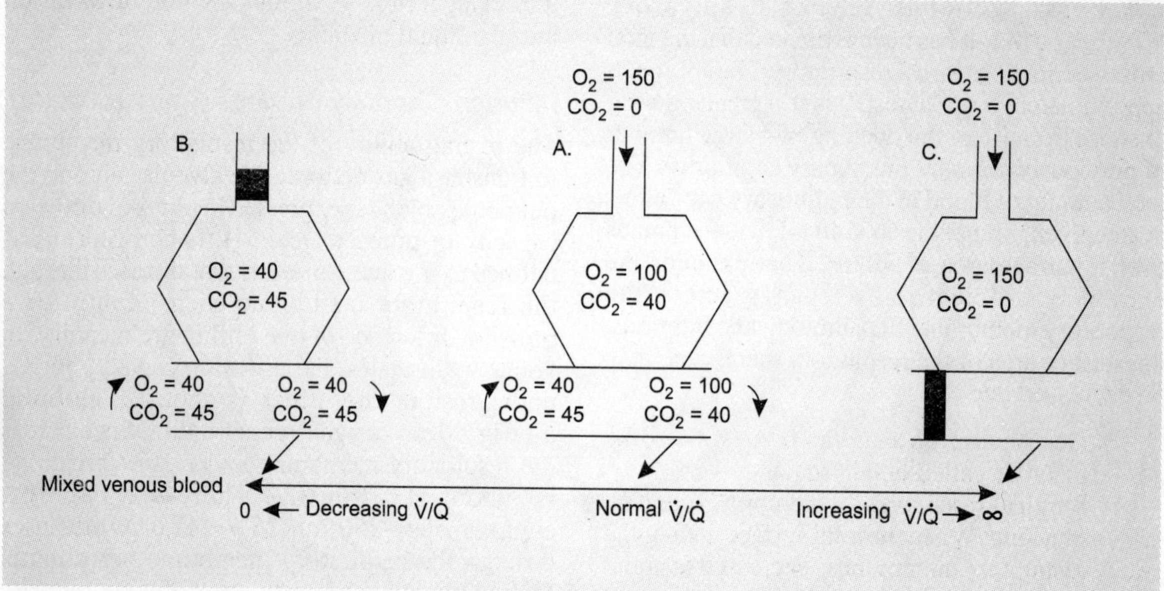

Fig. 16.1: Effect of changes in ventilation-perfusion ratio on gas exchange in the lungs (values are given in mmHg).

5 L = 0.84). Although there are some regional differences in the ventilation-perfusion ratio, on the whole, the amount of ventilation of the alveoli perfectly matches the amount of blood flow around it. Thus, optimum conditions are produced for gas exchange (Fig. 16.1A). In pathological states, the ventilation-perfusion ratio may become below or above normal.

Physiological Shunts

This term is used when ventilation perfusion ratio is below normal. Such a situation occurs when ventilation of a part of the lung is not adequate enough for the amount of blood flowing through it. Consequently, a certain fraction of the venous blood passes through the area without oxygenation. It seems as if some venous blood has been shunted to the arterial side without oxygenation, and hence the term physiological shunt (Fig. 16.1B). In many respiratory disorders like emphysema and pneumonia, physiological shunts constitute an important cause of fall in the arterial pO_2 (hypoxia) and sometimes may lead to even rise in arterial pCO_2 (hypercapnia).

Physiological Dead Space

In certain lung disorders, blood flow to part of a lung is blocked. Hence, ventilation-perfusion ratio in this region becomes abnormally high. Such alveoli do not take part in gas exchange and therefore constitute a physiological dead space (Fig.16.1C). A large increase in physiological dead space results in severe hypoxia as well as hypercapnia.

CHAPTER 17

Transport of Gases

Oxygen and carbon dioxide are transported to and from the tissues by the circulating blood. The exchange of gases across the alveolar membrane occurs because of a difference in their concentrations on the two sides. Similarly, in the tissues, the difference in the concentrations (and hence the pressure gradient) between the blood and the tissue cells causes its diffusion into or out of the cell. In this chapter, the mechanism of transport of gases in the blood shall be discussed.

COMPOSITION OF ATMOSPHERIC AIR AND ALVEOLAR AIR

The atmospheric air contains approximately 21% O_2, 79% N_2 and almost negligible (0.04%) CO_2. The composition of alveolar air is quite different from the inspired (atmospheric air) or the air expired from the lungs (Table 17.1). The marked differences between the composition of alveolar air and the atmospheric air are because of several factors:

(i) Oxygen is constantly removed from the alveolar air.
(ii) Carbon dioxide is added to the alveolar air.
(iii) Only a small amount of fresh air (350 ml) is added to the alveolar air (2.2 L) during each inspiration.
(iv) Atmospheric air is humidified by upper respiratory passages before it enters the alveoli.

Table 17.1: Composition of atmospheric air, alveolar air and expired air

	Atmospheric air		*Alveolar air*		*Expired air*	
	%	PP mmHg	%	PP mmHg	%	PP mmHg
O_2	20.84	159.0	13.6	104	15.7	120
CO_2	0.04	0.3	5.3	40	3.6	27
Nitrogen	78.62	597.0	74.9	569	74.5	566
H_2O (Vapour)	0.50	3.7	6.2	47	6.2	47
	100%	760.0	100%	760	100%	760

During quiet breathing (*eupnoea*), the composition of alveolar air does not change significantly during inspiration and expiration. This fact would look less surprising if it is realized that in each inspiration, only 350 ml of fresh air enters the alveoli and mixes with a much larger volume of alveolar air present at the end of tidal expiration (functional residual capacity: 2.2 L). The stability of alveolar air composition in eupnoea prevents extreme variations in the partial pressures of oxygen and carbon dioxide in the blood and tissue fluids. For example, voluntary hyperventilation can raise the alveolar pO_2 up to 150 mmHg. At the same time, alveolar air pCO_2 may fall to an extent that breathing stops for a few seconds.

17

Expired Air

The expired air is a mixture of dead space air (150 ml) and alveolar air (350 ml). Therefore, its composition is between that of humidified atmospheric air and the alveolar air, but nearer to the latter. If a person expires into a narrow 1 metre long tube, the dead space air would be first to be expired followed by the alveolar air. The pure alveolar air sample can be collected from the side tube situated close to the mouthpiece (Fig. 17.1).

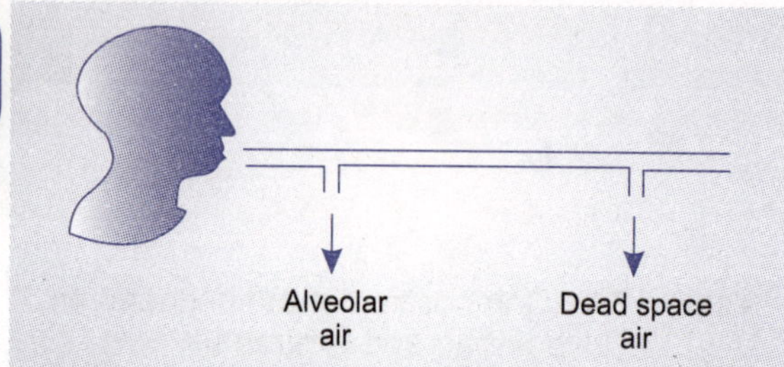

Fig. 17.1: A simple method to obtain a sample of alveolar air.

OXYGEN TRANSPORT IN BLOOD

Transport of oxygen is one of the most important functions of the blood. It is dependent primarily on the presence of haemoglobin in the red blood cells.

Oxygen Uptake in the Lungs

The venous blood entering the pulmonary capillaries has pO_2 value of 40 mmHg, because large amount of O_2 has been extracted by the tissues. The pO_2 of the alveolar air is 104 mmHg. Due to the pressure gradient, oxygen diffuses rapidly from the alveolar air to the pulmonary capillary blood. Equilibrium is attained even before the blood reaches midpoint of the capillary length (Fig. 17.2).

By the time, the blood reaches the aorta, however, pO_2 falls to about 100 mmHg. The mild decrease in oxygen content and pO_2 of the arterialized blood is because of the addition of small amount of *venous blood* from physiological shunts and the besian vessels to the *oxygenated blood* in the left ventricle.

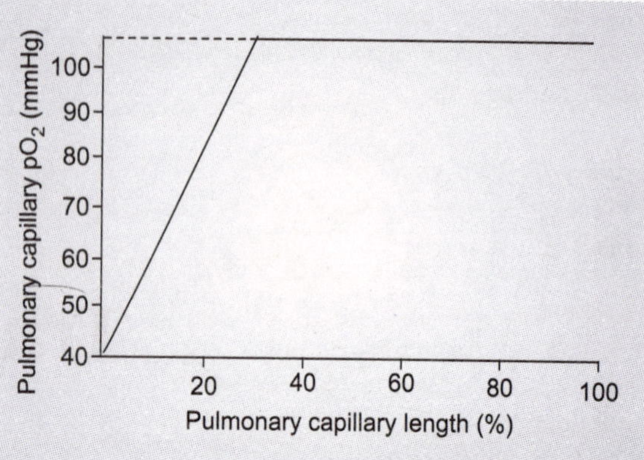

Fig. 17.2: The diffusion of gases across the alveolar membrane is so rapid that the pulmonary capillary blood becomes fully saturated with oxygen even before the blood has traversed half of the capillary length.

The solubility of O_2 in water (plasma) is so little that at pO_2 value of 100 mmHg, only 0.3 ml of O_2 is dissolved in 100 ml of blood. This amount is the *physically dissolved component* of the O_2 content of blood. The major mechanism of O_2 uptake and transport in the blood is in chemical *combination with haemoglobin* (Hb). In this form, nearly 20 ml of O_2 is transported per 100 ml of blood.

Role of Haemoglobin in Oxygen Transport

Haemoglobin molecules of the red blood cells have the unique property of forming loose and reversible combination with O_2 molecules. One O_2 molecule can be attached at the 6th covalent bond of ferrous (Fe^{2+}) atom in each of the four subunits of haemoglobin molecule.

$$\underset{\text{(Deoxygenated Hb)}}{Hb + O_2} \underset{\text{Tissues}}{\overset{\text{Lungs}}{\rightleftharpoons}} \underset{\text{(Oxygenated Hb)}}{HbO_2}$$

The amount of O_2 taken up by haemoglobin depends on the pO_2 value of the blood. At pO_2 of 100 mmHg, Hb can be fully (100%) saturated with O_2 and each gram of Hb can combine with 1.34 ml of O_2. Taking average normal Hb concentration to be 15 gm%, the ***oxygen carrying capacity*** of blood is **20 ml/100 ml** of blood (15 × 1.34).

Oxygen Delivery in the Tissues

As the arterial blood reaches the tissues, it is exposed to the interstitial fluid with pO_2 of about 40 mmHg. Due to the pressure gradient, O_2 diffuses out of the plasma into the interstitial fluid and consequently, the pO_2 of the plasma falls to 40 mmHg. At pO_2 of 40 mmHg, Hb can have a maximum O_2 saturation of 75% (see oxygen-haemoglobin dissociation curve, vide infra). In other words, each 100 ml of blood can hold only about 15 ml of O_2 (15 × 1.34 × 75/100) and the remaining 5 ml is released to diffuse into the tissues.

Thus, each 100 ml of arterial blood carries 20 ml of O_2 to the tissues where 5 ml of O_2 is given off and becomes "venous blood". The venous blood (deoxygenated blood) reaches the lungs to be arterialized once again. At rest, *coefficient of oxygen utilization* (i.e. O_2 uptake by the tissues/ O_2 content of the arterial blood) is about 25% (5 / 20 × 100). During heavy muscular exercise, the venous blood leaves the skeletal muscles with O_2-content less than 4 ml per 100 ml of blood. Under such circumstances, the coefficient of O_2-utilization may increase to about 80%.

Rate of Total O_2 Transport

Under resting condition, each 100 ml of blood gives off 5 ml of O_2 to the tissues. Therefore, with normal cardiac output of 5 L/min, 250 ml of O_2 (5/100 × 5000) is delivered to the tissues per minute. During heavy exercise, nearly 4000 ml of O_2 can be transported from the lungs to the tissues per minute. Delivery of such a massive amount of O_2 is achieved by: (a) more than 3-fold increase in the coefficient of O_2 utilization; and (b) by 5–6-fold increase in the cardiac output.

Oxygen-Haemoglobin Dissociation Curve

The relation between pO_2 and the degree of O_2 saturation of Hb can be demonstrated by plotting an O_2-Hb dissociation curve. Such a curve can be obtained by exposing a known amount of blood (Hb) to air with varying oxygen content (varying pO_2). The oxygen content of blood at each pO_2 value is analysed. Haemoglobin is said to be 100% saturated if its O_2 content is 1.34 ml/gm of Hb. If the O_2 content is 0.67 ml /gm Hb, it is said to be 50% saturated. The O_2-Hb dissociation curve is obtained by plotting pO_2 values on the X-axis and Hb % saturation on the Y-axis.

The normal O_2-Hb dissociation curve is shown in Fig. 17.3. The curve is *sigmoid-shaped.* The upper part of the curve is flat. At pO_2 values of 100 mmHg or above, Hb is 100% saturated. More important is the fact that even when pO_2 value falls to 60 mmHg, Hb saturation is still 90%. This property of Hb ensures fairly high uptake of O_2 by blood even when alveolar pO_2 is moderately decreased, e.g. because of high altitude or a pathological decrease in alveolar ventilation. *This part of the curve is related to the process of O_2 uptake in the lungs.*

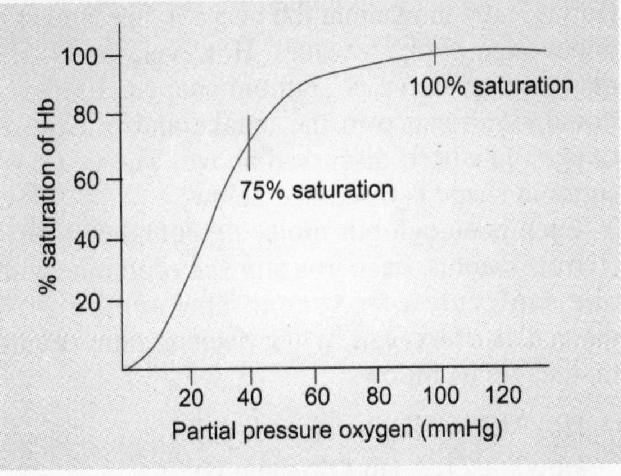

Fig. 17.3: The oxygen-haemoglobin dissociation curve.

The middle and lower parts of the O_2-Hb dissociation curve are concerned with O_2 delivery in the tissues. At pO_2 value of 40 mmHg, Hb is 75% saturated with O_2 (Figs. 17.3, 17.4). Thus, each 100 ml of blood can hold only 15 ml of O_2 as compared to 20 ml at pO_2 of 100 mmHg. At values of pO_2 lower than 40 mmHg, still larger volumes

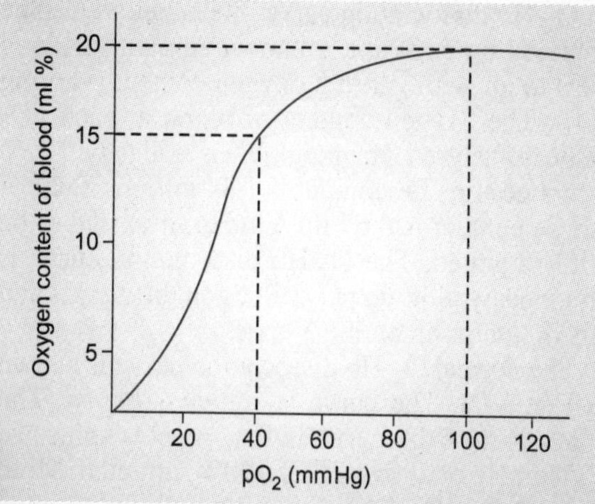

17

Fig. 17.4: The relation between pO_2 and oxygen content of the blood.

of O_2 would be off-loaded and become available to the tissues (e.g. during heavy exercise).

Cause of Sigmoid Shape of the Oxygen–Haemoglobin Dissociation Curve Study of the carbon dioxide-haemoglobin dissociation curve (Fig. 17.10) shows that the curve is linear over a wide range of pCO_2 values. However, the O_2-Hb dissociation curve is sigmoid-shaped. Its functional significance in the uptake and release of oxygen has been discussed above. The cause of sigmoid shape is discussed below:

Each haemoglobin molecule contains 4 Fe^{++} (ferrous) atoms. Each iron atom can combine with one molecule of oxygen. The uptake of 4 molecules of oxygen by the haemoglobin occurs in 4 stages as follows:

$Hb_4 + O_2 = Hb\ O_2$ (stage I)
$Hb_4O_2 + O_2 = Hb_4O_4$ (stage II)
$Hb_4O_4 + O_2 = Hb_4O_6$ (stage III)
$Hb_4O_6 + O_2 = Hb_4O_8$ (Stage IV)

Combination of the first haem (iron) atom with oxygen (stage I) increases the affinity of second haem (iron) atom for oxygen. Thus as the oxygen uptake of haemoglobin molecule increases, there is a progressive increase in affinity for oxygen, so that the oxygen uptake in stage 4 is easiest and most quick.

Factors Affecting O_2-Hb Dissociation Curve

Effect of pCO_2 and pH

The description of O_2-Hb dissociation curve given above holds true if the blood has pCO_2 value of 40 mmHg and a pH of 7.4 (as seen in the normal arterial blood). An increase in the pCO_2 of blood shifts the curve to the right. The phenomenon is called **Bohr effect** (Fig. 17.5). The result of shift of the curve to the right is that at a given value of pO_2, Hb saturation with O_2 is diminished, thus more of O_2 is off-loaded. As the arterial blood reaches the tissues, it is exposed to not only low pO_2 (40 mmHg) but also higher pCO_2 (46 mmHg). Due to Bohr effect, for a given decrease in pO_2, larger volume of O_2 is shed off (about 2% more).

A decrease in the pH of blood, as occurs in the tissues, also shifts the O_2-Hb dissociation to the right. This phenomenon is also known as the Bohr effect (Fig. 17.5).

Effect of Temperature

An increase in the temperature of blood also shifts the O_2-Hb dissociation curve to the right (Fig. 17.6). During muscular exercise, the higher tissue temperature (in the skeletal muscle) along with lowered pO_2, increased pCO_2 and decreased pH facilitate the delivery of larger amounts of O_2 to the actively contracting muscle.

P50 of Haemoglobin As discussed above, the oxygen-haemoglobin dissociation curve is shifted to the right by an increase in pCO_2, a decrease in pH or an increase in temperature of blood. The net effect is an increased off-loading of oxygen from the haemoglobin. This property can be expressed in another way: by describing **P50** of haemoglobin. This term is used to describe the value of pO_2 at which haemoglobin is 50% saturated with oxygen. It is an expression of the affinity of haemoglobin for oxygen. **P50** is derived from an oxygen-Hb dissociation curve (Fig. 17.5A). At pCO_2 of 40 mmHg, pH 7.4 and temperature 37°C (arterial blood), **P50** is 26 mmHg. An increase in the value of **P50** indicates decreased affinity of haemoglobin (greater off-loading of oxygen (Fig. 17.7).

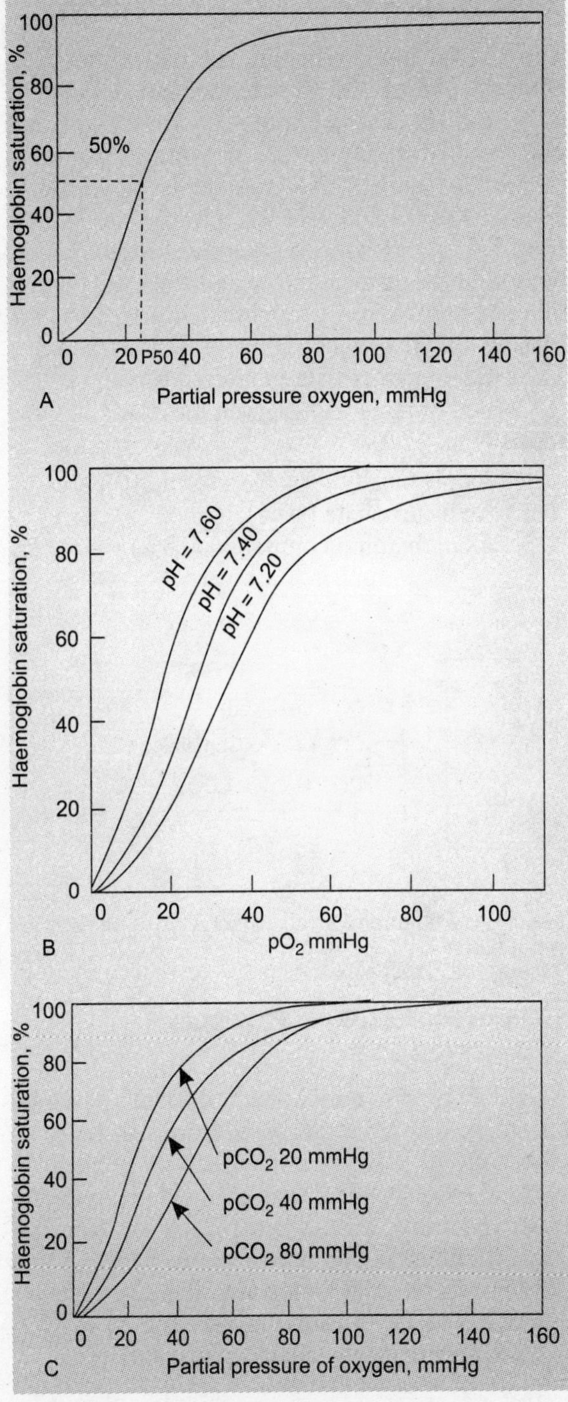

Fig. 17.5: (A) Typical adult oxyhaemoglobin dissociation curve. (B) and (C) Effects of arterial pH and pCO_2 on oxyhemoglobin dissociation curve.

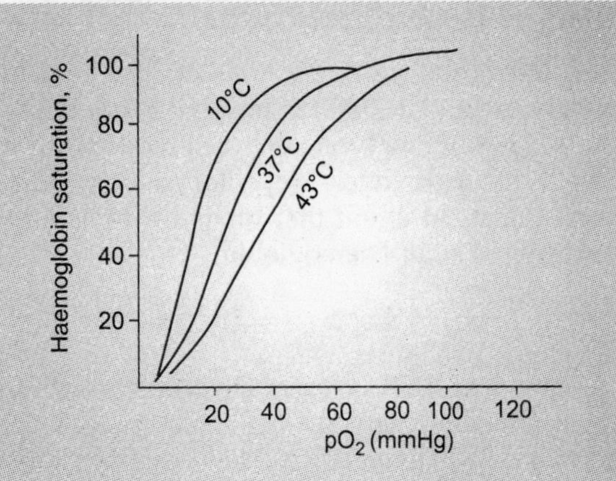

Fig. 17.6: Effect of a change in the temperature of blood on the oxygen-haemoglobin dissociation curve.

Conditions causing an increase in **P50:**

(i) An increase in pCO_2.

(ii) A decrease in pH.

(iii) An increase in temperature.

(iv) Increase in 2,3 DPG concentration because of:
Anaemia
High altitude
Chronic hypoxia
Exercise.

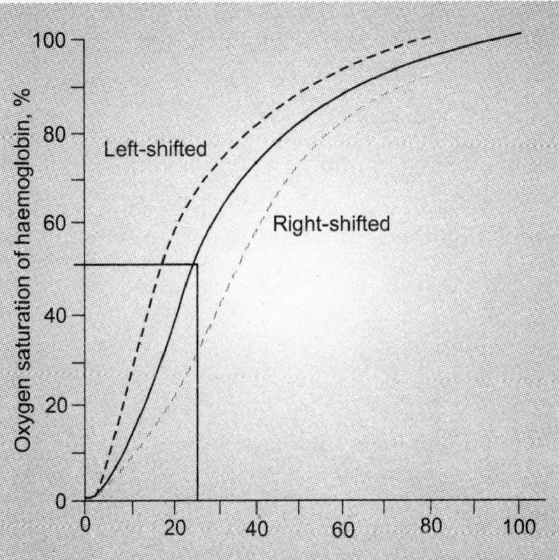

Fig. 17.7: Calculation of P**50**.

Effect of Diphosphoglycerate

The red blood cells are rich in 2, 3-diphosphoglycerate (2,3-DPG) (Chapter 3). It is formed from 1, 3-phosphoglyceraldehyde produced during glycolysis via Embden-Meyerhof pathway. It is a highly charged anion that binds to β-chains of oxygenated adult haemoglobin.

$$HbO_2 + 2,3\text{-DPG} \rightarrow Hb\text{–}2,3\text{-DPG} + O_2$$

Thus, 2,3-DPG decreases the affinity of Hb for O_2 resulting in greater off-loading of oxygen. The normal O_2-Hb dissociation curve described above is obtained only in the presence of normal concentration of 2–3 DPG. An increase in the concentration of 2, 3-DPG occurs in anaemia, or in those exposed to chronic hypoxia due to high altitude, or those suffering from certain pulmonary disorders. As a result, in all such people, the O_2 off-loading in the tissues is improved.

The O_2-Hb dissociation curve of fetal-Hb (HbF) is different from that of adult-Hb (HbA), since it is shifted far to the left (Fig. 17.8). The greater affinity of fetal-Hb for O_2 is due to the fact that fetal Hb contains two α chains and two γ-(gamma) chains and the gamma chains have very little affinity for 2,3-DPG. This property of fetal-Hb helps it to take up normal volumes of O_2 even though fetal blood is exposed to rather low pO_2 values of the maternal blood in the placenta.

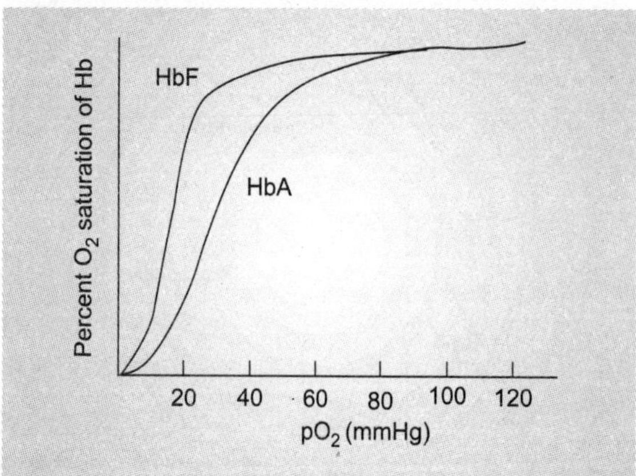

Fig. 17.8: Oxygen dissociation curves of HbA and HbF.

CARBON DIOXIDE TRANSPORT IN BLOOD

The arterial blood reaching the tissues has CO_2 content of 48 ml/100 ml of blood, and pCO_2 value of 40 mmHg. Diffusion of CO_2 from the tissue cells raises pCO_2 value of venous blood to 46 mmHg, and its CO_2 content is increased to 52 ml/100 ml of blood. The pH of blood drops from 7.4 to 7.35. Due to chloride shift, explained below, chloride content of red cells in venous blood is significantly greater than in arterial blood. Plasma HCO_3^- concentration of venous blood is 1–2 mEq/L greater than in arterial blood.

Carbon dioxide is present in the blood in three forms (Fig. 17.9) :

1. As physically dissolved form (10%),
2. As bicarbonate (80%), and
3. As carbamino compound (10%).

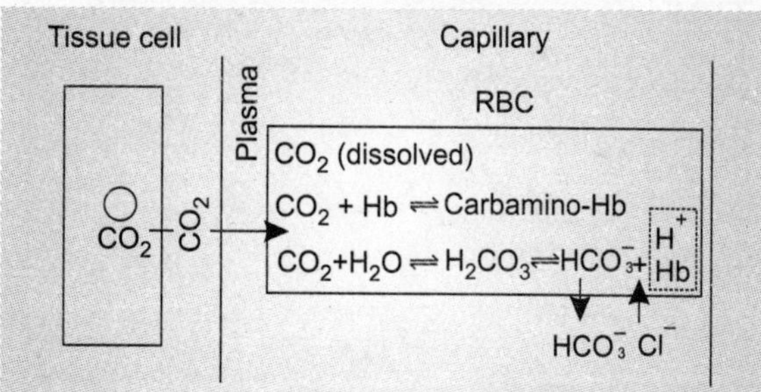

Fig. 17.9: The three forms in which CO_2 is transported in the blood.

1. Transport of CO_2 in Physically Dissolved Form

At pCO_2 of 46 mmHg, each 100 ml of blood contains approximately 5.2 ml of CO_2 in physically dissolved form. This is in contrast to only 0.3 ml of O_2 per 100 ml of blood in physically dissolved from, even when pO_2 is 100 mmHg. The difference is because of the fact that CO_2 is 20 times more soluble in water than O_2. Thus, as compared to O_2, a much larger volume of CO_2 is transported in physically dissolved form.

2. Transport of CO_2 as Bicarbonate

Diffusion of CO_2 from the tissues to the red blood cells brings about a very important chemical reaction. The red cells contain an enzyme called *carbonic anhydrase*, which accelerates the hydration of CO_2 to carbonic acid, by about 5000 folds. Thus, on entering the blood, CO_2 is instantaneously converted to carbonic acid in the red cells. Carbonic acid further dissociates into bicarbonate and hydrogen ions.

$$CO_2 + H_2O \underset{\text{Lungs}}{\overset{\text{Tissues}}{\rightleftharpoons}} H_2CO_3 \rightleftharpoons H^+ + HCO_3^-$$

Hydrogen ion is buffered primarily by the simultaneous deoxygenation of Hb because it binds more hydrogen than oxyhaemoglobin. This is because the deoxyhaemoglobin is a weaker acid than oxy-Hb.

The increase in bicarbonate concentration in the red cells leads to its diffusion into plasma down the concentration gradient. In order to maintain the electrical neutrality, chloride ions diffuse into the red cells. In this way, about 70% of bicarbonate ions formed in the red cells are transferred to plasma in exchange for chloride ions. This phenomenon, called **'chloride shift'**, is essential for the transport of CO_2 as bicarbonate. It occurs very rapidly.

Uptake of carbon dioxide by the red blood cells results in an increase in its bicarbonate/chloride ion content. In other words, the red cells of the venous blood contain a larger number of osmotically active particles than in the arterial blood. Consequently, the venous red cells imbibe more water and become relatively less biconcave. This explains a significantly greater osmotic fragility of red cells of venous blood as compared to the arterial blood. This also explains a greater value of PCV by about 3% for venous blood as compared to that of arterial sample.

3. Transport of CO_2 as Carbamino Compound

Carbon dioxide combines with amino groups (–NH_2) of haemoglobin to form carbamino compound.

$$\underset{\text{(Hb)}}{R{-}NH_2 + CO_2} \underset{\text{Lungs}}{\overset{\text{Tissue}}{\rightleftharpoons}} \underset{\text{(Carbamino Hb)}}{R{-}NH{-}COOH}$$

The deoxygenated haemoglobin has greater capacity to form carbamino compound than the oxygenated-Hb. Thus, in the tissue when Hb is deoxygenated the reaction given above shifts to the right. In the lungs, the oxygenation of Hb shifts the above reaction in the opposite direction. By this method, about 10% of CO_2 produced in the tissues is transported to the lungs.

In the lungs, the venous blood is exposed to the alveolar air with pCO_2 of 40 mmHg. Diffusion of CO_2 from the capillary blood to alveolar air decreases the pCO_2 of the blood to 40 mmHg. Therefore, CO_2 is evolved not only from the physically dissolved state but also from the chemical form, i.e. bicarbonate, (due to reversal of reaction catalysed by carbonic anhydrase and chloride shift as shown in the reaction above) and carbamino form.

Haldane Effect

The fact that deoxygenation of Hb increases its ability to carry CO_2 as bicarbonate and carbamino form is known as the Haldane effect. It may be remembered that in the tissues the Bohr's effect operates on the O_2 transport. Thus, Haldane effect and Bohr effect complement each other. In the tissues addition of CO_2 to the blood facilitates unloading of O_2 by Bohr effect. In turn, O_2 unloading favours uptake of CO_2 by Haldane effect.

Carbon Dioxide Dissociation Curve

The relationship between pCO_2 and total CO_2 content of blood is shown in Fig. 17.10. It can be observed that the relationship between the two is linear over wider range of pCO_2 than in case of O_2-Hb dissociation curve (Fig. 17.3). The ability of deoxygenated Hb to hold larger volume of CO_2, as compared to oxygenated Hb, is also obvious.

It needs to be stressed that, unlike pO_2, pCO_2 values of arterial and venous blood vary within a narrow range of 40–46 mmHg, whereas pO_2 values vary from 100 to 40 mmHg or even less.

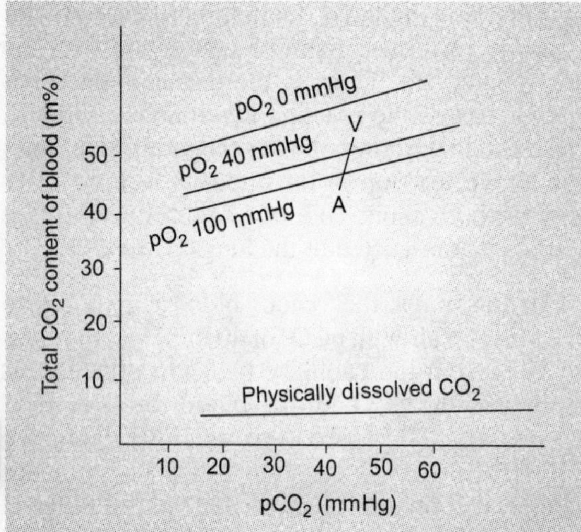

Fig. 17.10: The relation between pCO_2 and the total CO_2 content of blood. Physiologically the curve operates between the arterial (A) and venous (V) points.

Large variations in pCO_2 are not allowed to occur because of the profound effect on acid-base balance. The full range of CO_2 dissociation curve shown in Fig. 17.10 is an experimental phenomenon and does not operate in the body. Physiologically the curve operates only within 'AV' range.

Rate of Total CO_2 Transport

At rest, about 200 ml of CO_2 are transported from the tissues to the lungs per minute. In severe exercise, as much as 4 L of CO_2 may be transported per minute. Because of greater solubility and transport in different forms, the transport of such large volumes of CO_2 occurs without any difficulty. The conversion of most of the CO_2 into bicarbonate prevents any significant change in the pH of blood, even when such large volumes of CO_2 enter the circulation.

CHAPTER 18

Regulation of Respiration

The control of respiration needs to be considered under two headings: (i) The mechanism of rhythmic breathing, i.e. genesis of alternate inspiration and expiration and other *neural respiratory mechanisms*, and (ii) regulation of the minute ventilation that is under *chemical control*.

NEURAL CONTROL OF RESPIRATION

Neural Generation of Rhythmic Breathing

The rhythmicity of breathing is dependent on the cyclic neural discharge to the inspiratory muscles via phrenic nerve supplying the diaphragm and intercostals nerves supplying the external intercostal muscles. Inspiration is initiated by increased impulse discharge in these neurons. As the rate of impulse discharge increases, progressively more number of motor units are recruited leading to an expansion of the thoracic cage. Then, suddenly, all the inspiratory neurons stop firing, ending the contraction of inspiratory muscles. Expiration follows passively because of elastic recoil of the lungs. Neural discharge to the expiratory muscles occurs only during forced expiration.

The neural discharge in the spinal nerves supplying the muscles of respiration is under the control of certain neurons whose cell bodies are located in the brainstem. Their axons descend in the spinal cord and synapse with the cell bodies of neurons constituting the phrenic and intercostals nerves. The absolute dependence of respiratory muscles on the bulbar control can be experimentally demonstrated by making a transection in the spinal cord at the level of C_2 or C_5 segments. A transection at C_2 results in immediate cessation of respiration. A transection at C_5 results in paralysis of intercostals muscles but movements of the diaphragm continue.

The term *respiratory centre* is used to describe a widely scattered group of neurons located bilaterally in the medulla oblongata and pons.

Medullary Respiratory Centres

Medullary respiratory centres (Fig. 18.1) consist of: (i) a dorsal group of respiratory neurons, that contains inspiratory neurons *(I-neurons)* only; and (ii) a ventral group of respiratory neurons that contains both inspiratory neurons *(I-neurons)* and expiratory neurons *(E-neurons)*.

The **dorsal group** of respiratory neurons is located in the nucleus of the tractus solitarius. Tractus solitarius receives afferent signals from peripheral chemoreceptors and from various receptors in the lungs through IX and X cranial nerves. The basic rhythm of respiration is generated in the dorsal group of respiratory neurons called *I-neurons*. These inspiratory neurons fire periodically, i.e. they fire impulses for about 2–3 seconds after which the impulse

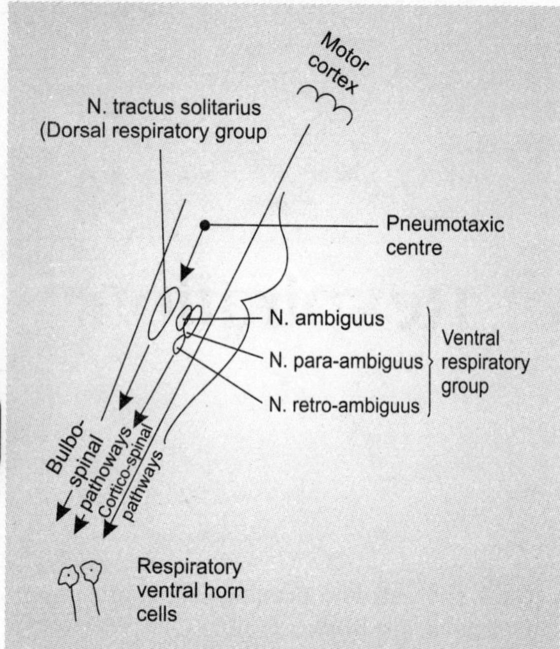

Fig. 18.1: The neural regulatory centres of respiration.

discharge abruptly ceases for about 3 seconds and then the next cycle begins (Fig. 18.2). Further, when the I-neurons fire, the frequency of impulse discharge gradually increases to maximum before coming to an abrupt end. This pattern of discharge has been called *ramp signals*.

The rate and depth of breathing are regulated by two factors: (i) The rate of increase of ramp

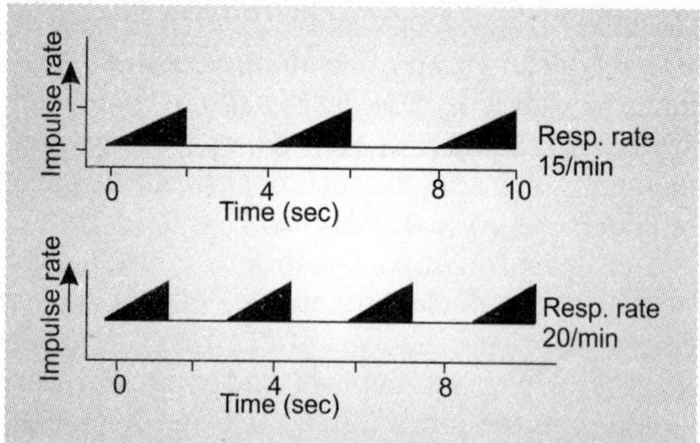

Fig. 18.2: The ramp signals in the medullary inspiratory neurons. The impulse discharge rate gadually increases and then comes to an end abruptly. A more rapid increase in the rate of discharge produces increased rate of respiration.

signals. During hyperventilation, the ramp increases rapidly which causes stronger inspiratory effort. (ii) Control of timing of point at which the ramp ceases. When it ceases early; the rate of respiration increases. However, it needs to be stressed that the basic cause of rhythmicity of discharge in the I-neurons of the dorsal group remains to be explained.

Recently pacemaker cells for respiration have been identified in the medulla oblongata. These cells, known as *Pre-Botzinger complex,* consist of a small group of synaptically coupled pacemaker cells situated close to the dorsal group of respiratory neurons. These pacemaker cells discharge impulses automatically and rhythmically even in a brain slice in vitro. Experimental destruction of pre-Botzinger complex abolishes rhythmic respiration whereas destruction of dorsal group of neurons does not.

The **ventral group** of neurons is located about 5 mm anterior and lateral to the dorsal group. Like the dorsal group, the ventral group of neurons is also present in the entire length of medulla oblongata. The ventral group of neurons consists of both *I- and E- neurons*. Both types of neurons fire only during deep breathing.

The Pneumotaxic Centre (The Pontine Respiratory Centre)

The pneumotaxic centre is located bilaterally in the upper pons. These neurons have an inhibitory influence on the dorsal respiratory group of neurons. The pneumotaxic centre is believed to regulate the switching-off point of the ramp signals, thereby regulating the rate of breathing. Strong pneumotaxic discharge may cut down the inspiratory phase to 0.5 second only. As a result, the breathing rate increases to 30–40/min. Conversely, weak pneumotaxic discharge increases the duration of ramp signals to as long as 5 seconds. As a result, breathing rate may slow down to 5–6 breaths per minute.

Role of Vagal Afferents

Stretching of the lungs during inspiration initiates afferent discharge in the vagus nerve that has an inhibitory influence on the medullary dorsal group of respiratory neurons. That can be proved by the observation that bilateral vagotomy in experimental animals results in an increase in depth of breathing. The effect is more prominent when bilateral vagotomy is performed along with a section at the upper border of medulla (to eliminate the role of pneumotaxic centre). The animal develops *apneustic breathing*—prolonged inspiratory spasms alternating with brief expiratory movements.

In brief, both vagal afferents and pontine pneumotaxic centre regulate the switch-off point of ramp signals, thereby regulating the rate and depth of breathing.

Other Neural Influences on Respiration

1. Higher Centres: Pain and emotional stimuli influence the rate and depth of breathing. It indicates the presence of afferents from the limbic system to the medullary respiratory neurons.

Voluntary Control Normally, breathing is not a conscious effort and goes on automatically. However, both inspiratory and expiratory muscles can be controlled voluntarily, at least for a short period. Breathing may be stopped voluntarily, but after about 50–70 seconds (breath-holding time), the chemical drive overrides the voluntary inhibition and breathing is resumed involuntarily. Similarly, one may overbreathe voluntarily for short periods.

The voluntary control of respiration is mediated by a pathway which originates from the neocortex, bypasses the medullary respiratory centres to project directly on the spinal respiratory neurons (Fig. 18.1).

2. Hering Breuer Reflexes In experimental animals, sustained inflation of the lungs, e.g. by occlusion of the trachea at the end of an inspiration results in prolonged expiration. This response is known as *Hering Breuer inflation reflex.* On the other hand, prolonged deflation of the lungs, e.g. by occlusion of the trachea at the end of an expiration results in a prolonged inspiratory contraction. This response is known as *Hering Breuer deflation reflex*. Hering Breuer reflexes are initiated by slowly adapting stretch receptors located in the smooth muscle of the respiratory airways. The impulses are carried to the medullary respiratory centers through thickly myelinated fibres in the vagus nerve.

Once upon a time, Hering Breuer reflexes were considered to play an important role in the regulation of the rate and depth of breathing. Recent evidence indicates that Hering Breuer reflexes are mostly inactive in human adults unless the tidal volume exceeds 1 L, e.g. during exercise. These reflexes seem to have more important role in the regulation of the rate and depth of breathing in new born infants.

3. Irritant Receptors Mucosa of the respiratory tract contains rapidly adapting receptors which respond to noxious gases, cigarette smoke, inhaled dust, cold air, etc. and therefore called irritant receptors. These receptors seem to be located below as well as between epithelial cells of the respiratory passages. The impulses are carried by myelinated fibres in the vagus nerve. Stimulation of such receptors in the trachea and large bronchi results in cough, bronchial constriction and increased mucus secretion. Irritant receptors are believed to play a role in the genesis of bronchial asthma.

Coughing It is a protective reflex. The reflex is initiated by irritation of the trachea and bronchi. The afferent impulses reach the medulla via vagus nerve and produce the following sequence of events: After a deep inspiratory effort, the glottis is closed. Contraction of abdominal muscles causes a marked rise in the intra-abdominal pressure (up to 100 mmHg). Then, suddenly the glottis opens and the air is expelled out explosively. Air velocity of several hundred kilometres per hour may be achieved in the upper respiratory passages. Consequently, the irritant foreign matter like dust particles or bronchial mucus are expelled out. Excessive production of mucus in the upper respiratory passages as a result of infection or allergy is most common cause of chronic cough.

Sneezing is also a reflex expiratory phenomenon produced by the irritation of nasal mucosa.

4. Juxtacapillary Receptors (J-receptors) These receptors are nerve endings of nonmyelinated (type-C) afferent fibres found in the vagus nerve. The receptors are named after their location in close proximity to the pulmonary capillaries in the alveolar walls. These receptors seem to be activated by engorgement of the alveolar capillaries and result in rapid shallow breathing. Physiological role of J-receptors has not been discovered so far. The dyspnoea (the uncomfortable or unpleasant sensation associated with hyperventilation) in left heart failure, interstitial lung disease, pneumonia or pulmonary microembolism has been attributed to the stimulation of J-receptors. In all these disorders, pulmonary congestion is the common patho-physiological feature.

5. Afferents from Proprioceptors Proprioceptive afferent impulses from the muscles and joints stimulate the inspiratory neurons. The increased pulmonary ventilation during muscular exercise can be partly attributed to the afferent impulses from the proprioceptors.

6. Visceral Reflexes Contraction of respiratory muscles is an important component of visceral reflexes like deglutition, vomiting and defaecation. These observations indicate the close connection between the respiratory centres and the medullary centres of vomiting, deglutition and defaecation, etc.

7. Role of Muscle Spindles Like all skeletal muscles, the respiratory muscles, especially the intercostals, contain numerous muscle spindles. These sensory receptors help to coordinate breathing during changes in posture or during speech. They also help to maintain normal tidal volume when breathing is impeded by an increase in airways resistance or a decrease in pulmonary compliance. The conscious proprioceptive impulses from the muscle spindles may be involved in the sensation of breathlessness during exertion or hypoxic cardiorespiratory disorders.

8. Pain and Temperature Acute pain produces a short period of apnoea followed by hyperventilation. Hyperventilation is a usual accompaniment of fever also. In fever, hyperventilation may help to promote heat loss from upper respiratory passages but it may produce respiratory alkalosis as well.

CHEMICAL CONTROL OF RESPIRATION

The chemical control of breathing is concerned with the regulation of pulmonary ventilation appropriate to the metabolic requirements. Tissue metabolism involves utilization of oxygen and release of CO_2. The latter, in turn, increases hydrogen ion concentration of the blood. Accordingly, certain chemoreceptors present in the body respond to changes in pO_2, pCO_2 and pH of the blood. Breathing is stimulated by a decrease in pO_2 or an increase in pCO_2 or H^+ concentration. The chemoreceptors are able to maintain the arterial pCO_2 and pH within a more narrow normal range than they can maintain the arterial pO_2.

Medullary (Central) Chemoreceptors

These chemoreceptors are believed to be located a few microns below the surface of medulla oblongata, ventral to the origin of IX and X cranial nerves (Fig. 18.3). The concept of central chemoreceptors and regulation of pulmonary ventilation by them is based on a number of experimental evidences, even though these receptors have not yet been histologically identified.

The central chemoreceptors monitor *H^+ concentration* of *cerebrospinal fluid* and interstitial fluid of the brain. Carbon dioxide penetrates the blood-brain barrier and blood-CSF barrier freely but H^+ and HCO_3^- penetrate these barriers slowly.

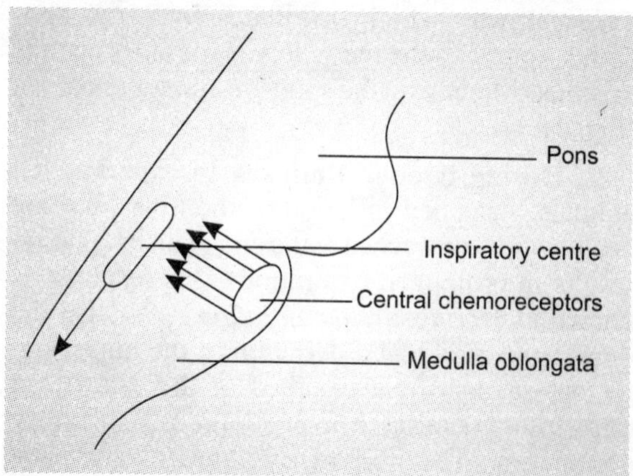

Fig. 18.3: The central chemoreceptors.

Central chemoreceptors are most sensitive to changes in arterial pCO_2 and less so to arterial pH. Even mild increase in arterial pCO_2 causes stimulation of medullary respiratory centres leading to increased pulmonary ventilation. These receptors do not respond to mild or moderate decrease in pO_2. Severe hypoxia, if present, depresses CNS including respiratory centres.

Peripheral Chemoreceptors (The Carotid and Aortic Bodies)

The carotid body is located on either side near the bifurcation of common carotid artery (Fig. 18.4). Two or more aortic bodies are located in the arch of the aorta. Each carotid (or aortic) body consists of islands of cells surrounded by large sinusoidal capillaries. Unmyelinated nerve endings are closely applied to the epithelial cells called type-I or glomus cells. Type-II cells, which are probably glial cells, are also closely applied to the type-I cells (Fig. 18.5). On leaving the carotid or the aortic body, the nerve fibres acquire the myelin sheath. Afferent fibres from the carotid body join the sinus nerve, a branch of IX cranial nerve. Those from the aortic body join the aortic nerve, branch of X cranial nerve. Peripheral chemoreceptors are stimulated by a decrease in arterial pO_2 (hypoxia), an increase in H^+ concentration or an increase in pCO_2 of the arterial blood.

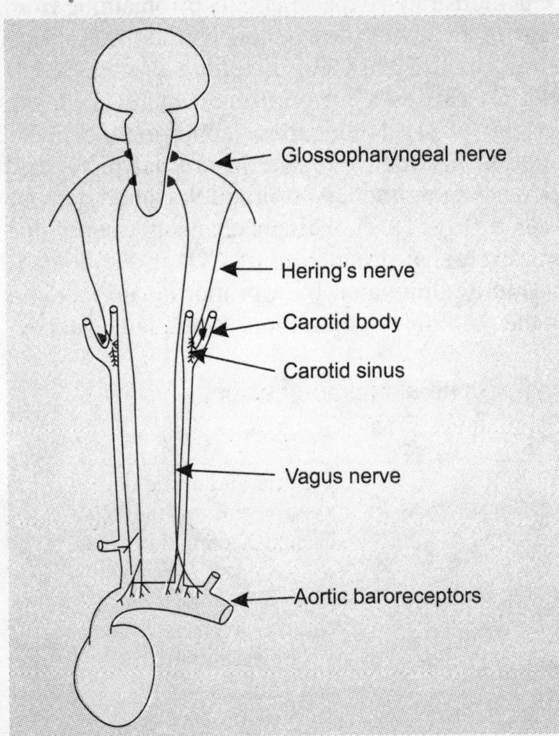

Fig. 18.4: Location of the carotid body.

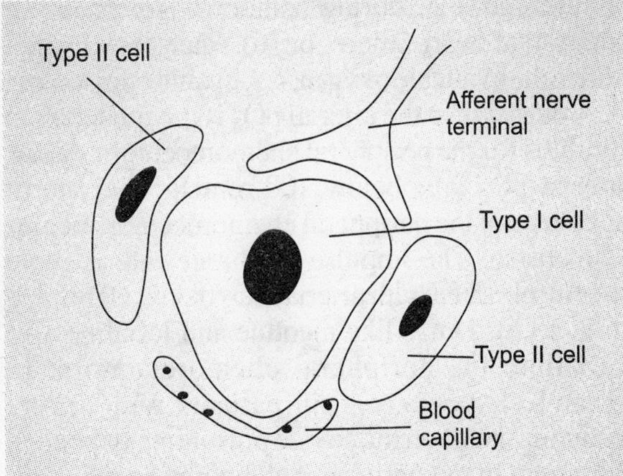

Fig. 18.5: Histological structure of the carotid body.

Mechanism of Hypoxic Stimulation

The type I cells resemble the adrenal medullary chromaffin cells, i.e. their cytoplasm contains numerous dense core granules containing dopamine, a catecholamine. These cells have oxygen-sensitive K^+ channels whose conductance is reduced in proportion to the degree of hypoxemia around them. The sequence of events is believed to be as follows: hypoxia → decreased K^+ efflux → cellular depolarization → Ca^{++} influx → action potential → dopamine release → excitation of afferent nerve endings.

Each carotid body weighs about 2 mg and its blood flow rate is 0.04 ml/min. Thus, the calculated rate of blood flow in the carotid body is 200 ml/100 gm tissue/min. Due to this enormous blood flow rate, the arteriovenous pO_2 difference in the carotid body is negligible, even though its metabolic rate is fairly high. As a result, pO_2 value of the chemoreceptor tissue practically remains similar to that of arterial pO_2.

Peripheral chemoreceptors are also stimulated, (i) when blood, (oxygen) supply to the carotid body is curtailed, e.g. during haemorrhagic shock or congestive heart failure, or (ii) when they cannot utilize the available oxygen, e.g. cyanide poisoning.

A decrease in the arterial pO_2 is the most potent stimulus for the peripheral chemoreceptors. As the arterial pO_2 falls below 100 mmHg, the rate of discharge in the peripheral chemoreceptors begins to increase. The impulse discharge rate is more steeply elevated with arterial pO_2 below 60 mmHg (Fig. 18.6). Drugs like nicotine and lobuline also stimulate the peripheral chemoreceptors. In anaemic hypoxia, e.g. in patients with severe anaemia or carbon monoxide poisoning, the rate of discharge in the peripheral chemoreceptors is not increased because the arterial pO_2 remains normal.

18

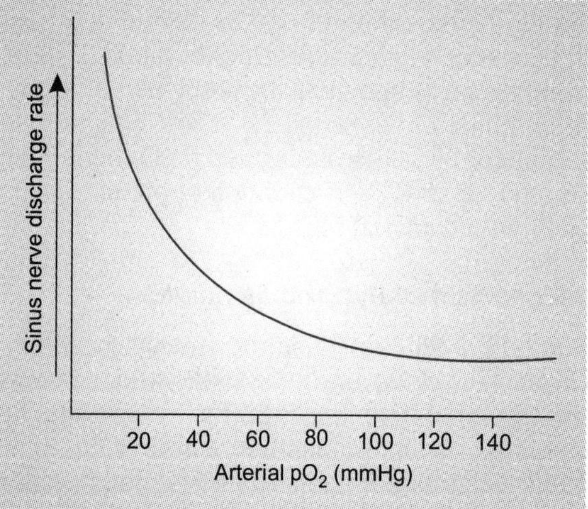

Fig. 18.6: The relation between arterial pO_2 and the impulse discharge rate in the sinus nerve (peripheral chemoreceptors).

An increase in the H^+ concentration of the blood also stimulates the peripheral chemoreceptors. This is in contrast to the central chemoreceptors where the blood-brain barrier and blood-CSF barrier are relatively impermeable to H^+ of the blood. The central chemoreceptors are very sensitive to changes in pH of CSF produced by an increase in its CO_2 content. Changes in the arterial pH due to causes other than increase in pCO_2 (metabolic acidosis or alkalosis) affect the peripheral chemoreceptors only because H^+ can penetrate their glomus cells with ease.

Peripheral chemoreceptors respond to changes in the arterial pCO_2 but their sensitivity to CO_2 is far less than that of the central chemoreceptors. The central and peripheral chemoreceptors have been compared in Table 18.1.

EFFECT OF CARBON DIOXIDE ON PULMONARY VENTILATION

Any increase in arterial pCO_2 causes a prompt increase in the pulmonary ventilation. This can be demonstrated experimentally by breathing from bags of air with different concentrations (varying from 5 to 10%) of CO_2. Breathing air with excess of CO_2 causes a proportionate increase in the arterial pCO_2. Under these conditions, a linear relation between increase in arterial pCO_2 and increase in pulmonary ventilation can be demonstrated (Fig. 18.7). This mechanism assures that any excessive production of CO_2 in the body is promptly eliminated by a proportionate increase in the pulmonary ventilation. As explained above,

Table 18.1: Comparison of central and peripheral chemoreceptors

	Central chemoreceptors	*Peripheral chemoreceptors*
Location	Medullary surface	Carotid and aortic bodies
Structure	Not known	Type I (chromaffin cells)
Afferent pathways to respiratory centres	?	IX and X cranial nerves
Respond to	pH of CSF	Arterial pO_2, pH, pCO_2
Max sensitivity to	Arterial pCO_2	Arterial hypoxia
Response on stimulation	Hyperventilation	1. Hyperventilation 2. Tachycardia 3. Vasoconstriction 4. Increased BP

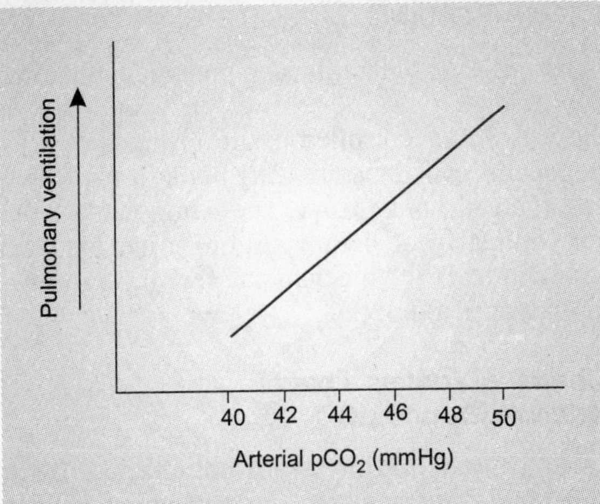

Fig. 18.7: The relation between arterial pCO_2 and pulmonary ventilation.

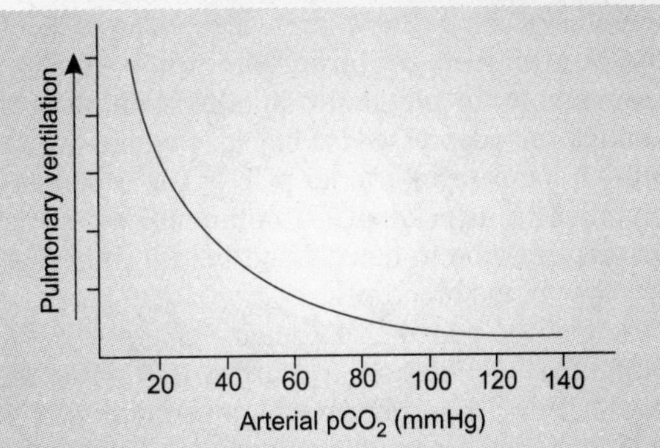

Fig. 18.8: The relation between arterial pO_2 and pulmonary ventilation.

CO_2 stimulates pulmonary ventilation chiefly through the stimulation of central chemoreceptors.

Carbon Dioxide Narcosis

Mild to moderate increase in arterial pCO_2 stimulates respiration. On the other hand, increase in arterial pCO_2 above 50 mmHg (normal arterial pCO_2 40 mmHg) depresses the central chemoreceptors and the respiratory centres. Depending on the degree of hypercapnoea (increase in arterial pCO_2), headache, confusion, convulsions and finally coma and death may occur. This condition, called CO_2-narcosis may occur in patients with emphysema (respiratory failure) or due to accidental inhalation of CO_2 (in breweries or refrigeration plants).

EFFECT OF HYPOXIA ON PULMONARY VENTILATION

Hypoxia stimulates respiration. However, if a person is made to breathe air with decreasing concentrations of O_2, it would be found that pulmonary ventilation increases only when arterial pO_2 falls below 60 mmHg (Fig. 18.8).This would look very strange because peripheral chemoreceptors begin to discharge at a higher rate even when the arterial pO_2 is just below 100 mmHg (Fig. 18.6). In other words, between arterial pO_2 of 100 to 60 mmHg, pulmonary ventilation does not increase, in spite of increased discharge in the peripheral chemoreceptors. There are two reasons for this phenomenon:

(i) Between pO_2 100–60 mmHg, the hypoxic drive does tend to increase pulmonary ventilation but it results in a decrease in the arterial pCO_2 which inhibits the respiratory drive.

(ii) Due to hypoxia, the arterial blood contains a greater percentage of Hb in the deoxygenated form. Since deoxygenated Hb is a weaker acid than oxy-Hb, hypoxia results in a mild decrease in H^+ concentration of the blood. Therefore, this factor also tends to nullify the hypoxic drive on pulmonary ventilation. At pO_2 values below 60 mmHg, the stimulation of peripheral chemoreceptors is so strong that it overrides the inhibitory effects of decreased arterial pCO_2 and H^+ concentration.

The reasons given above can be experimentally proved by holding the pCO_2 constant at 40 mmHg and decreasing arterial pO_2 simultaneously. Under these conditions, hyperventilation is observed even at pO_2 between 100–60 mmHg.

EFFECT OF ARTERIAL pH ON PULMONARY VENTILATION

Pulmonary ventilation is markedly increased in metabolic acidosis (e.g. ketoacidosis in diabetes

18

mellitus) leading to a decrease in the arterial pCO_2 by elimination of larger amounts of CO_2. Conversely, in metabolic alkalosis pulmonary ventilation is depressed leading to retention of CO_2 and an increase in arterial pCO_2. The secondary changes in arterial pCO_2 compensate for the primary metabolic defects and help to minimise changes in the blood pH.

It may be added that primary changes in the pulmonary ventilation also affect the pH of the blood. Primary pulmonary hypoventilation, e.g. due to narcotic poisoning, leads to elevation of arterial pCO_2 and acidosis (respiratory acidosis). Primary hyperventilation, e.g. voluntary hyperventilation causes a decrease in the arterial pCO_2 and alkalosis (respiratory alkalosis).

18

Interaction of pO_2, pCO_2 and pH

As mentioned above, each of hypoxia, increased pCO_2 and acidosis individually cause an increase in the pulmonary ventilation. In many physiological or clinical situations, more than one factor may be present. Under such conditions, the effects of H^+ concentration and CO_2 are additive. On the other hand, hypoxia and hypercapnoea interact to produce a much greater response than expected from the additive effects of the two stimuli (Fig. 18.9).

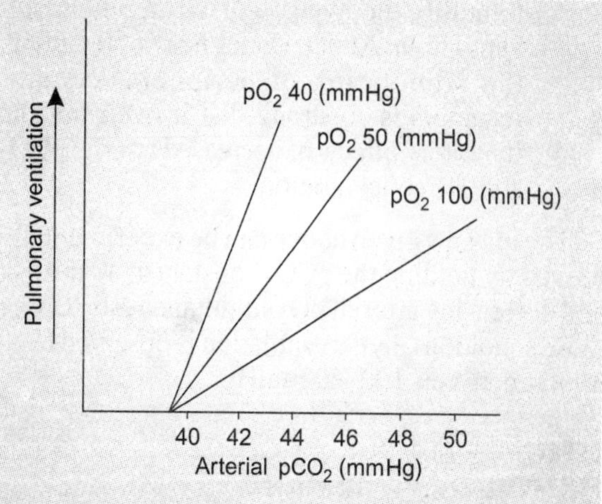

Fig. 18.9: The effect of interaction of arterial pCO_2 and pO_2 on pulmonary ventilation.

BREATH-HOLDING

A person can voluntarily stop breathing, but after approximately 50–70 seconds, in young adults, there is an uncontrolled desire to breathe. This moment is called the *breaking point.* It marks the end of breath holding time. The factors responsible for limitation of breath holding time include: (a) chemical, (b) mechanical/neural, (c) motivation, and (d) training.

Chemical Factors: Role of Arterial pO_2 and pCO_2

During the period of breath holding, the body continues to use oxygen and produce carbon dioxide. Therefore, there is a gradual decrease in (alveolar) arterial pO_2, as well as, an increase in (alveolar) arterial pCO_2. Breaking point is reached when arterial pO_2 decreases to approximately 50 mmHg and arterial pCO_2 increases to 55 mmHg. The combination of hypoxia and hypercapnoea makes the respiratory drive so powerful that the breath cannot be held any longer. The following observations support the chemical mechanism for the breaking point:

(i) Breath-holding time can be prolonged by 15–20 seconds by initial hyperventilation with room air, which lowers the arterial pCO_2 to about 15–20 mmHg (CO_2 wash out), and arterial pO_2 is elevated to approximately 150 mmHg. Therefore, breath-holding can be continued for a longer duration till arterial pCO_2 and pO_2 change to the level critical for the end of breath-holding.

(ii) Initial hyperventilation with pure oxygen can prolong the breath-holding time up to 5 minutes.

Mechanical /Neural Factors

Besides the chemical factors discussed above, some mechanical/neural factors also seem to be involved in limiting the duration of breath holding. This view is supported by the following observations:

(i) At the breaking point, if the subject is allowed to take a few breaths with an air mixture low in oxygen and high in CO_2 content, the person can hold the breath for about 20 seconds more. Inhalation of such a gas mixture could not have improved the arterial pO_2 or pCO_2 values. This experiment suggests that proprioceptive impulses from respiratory muscles may contribute to the end of breath-holding.

(ii) The unpleasant sensation associated with breath holding can be abolished by a temporary blockade of IX and X cranial nerves, which carry afferent impulses from the lungs.

At rest, our body consumes 250 ml of O_2 and produces only 200 ml of CO_2 per minute. Thus during breath holding, there is a gradual decrease in the lung volume, whereas the thoracic cage size is held constant by voluntary inhibitory control over the respiratory muscles. This discrepancy seems to set up pulmonary afferent impulses which result in an urge in the respiratory muscles to start rhythmic breathing.

Motivation and training can prolong the breath-holding time, since the subject learns to temporarily ignore the urge to start breathing at the breaking point.

EFFECTS OF HYPERVENTILATION

Severe Voluntary Hyperventilation

The effects of severe hyperventilation illustrate the role of arterial pCO_2 and pO_2 in the regulation of respiration. A person is asked to breathe, as rapidly and as deeply as he can, for one to two minutes, and then told to stop the voluntary effort. In most of the individuals, the end of hyperventilation is followed by a prolonged period of hypoventilation. In some individuals, complete cessation of breathing (apnoea) for 1–2 minutes may occur.

In few others, *periodic breathing,* i.e. alternate phases of apnoea and breathing may occur for some time, before normal breathing is restored. Examination of the composition of the alveolar air shows that after the bout of hyperventilation, alveolar (arterial) pO_2 is as high as 150 mmHg and pCO_2 as low as 15 mmHg. Apnoea is caused by the lack of CO_2 because it does not occur if the person hyperventilates a gas mixture containing 5% CO_2 and 20% O_2. During the phase of apnoea, the body metabolism causes a gradual decline in the arterial pO_2 and an increase in arterial pCO_2. When the arterial pCO_2 reaches the threshold value (38 mmHg), normal breathing is resumed. If the hypoxic stimulus becomes stronger before the pCO_2 has reached the threshold value, periodic breathing may result : a few breaths eliminate the hypoxic stimulus, breathing stops till pO_2 falls to the critical level and the cycle is repeated for a few times (Fig. 18.10). Soon, however, arterial pCO_2 level returns to normal and normal breathing pattern is restored.

18

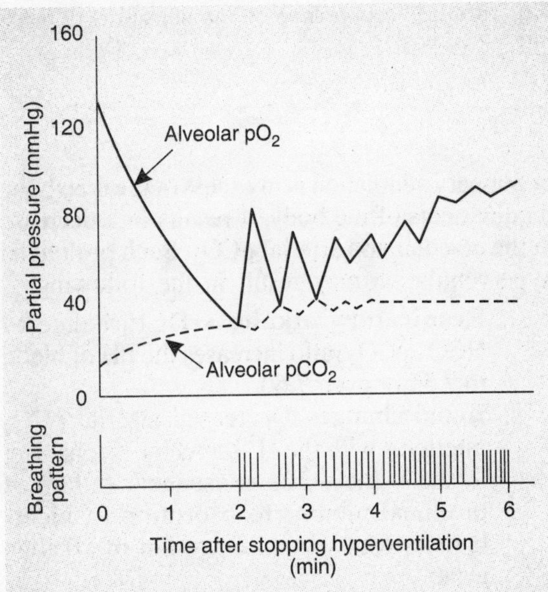

Fig. 18.10: Effect of hyperventilation on arterial pO_2, pCO_2 and respiration.

Periodic breathing when observed in a patient is called Cheyne–Stokes respiration. It may be observed in some patients of congestive heart failure and uraemia.

Moderate Degree of Hyperventilation

Two to five-fold increase in pulmonary ventilation may be maintained voluntarily for longer periods. It may also occur in residents of high altitude or clinically hypoxic patients. Since, the

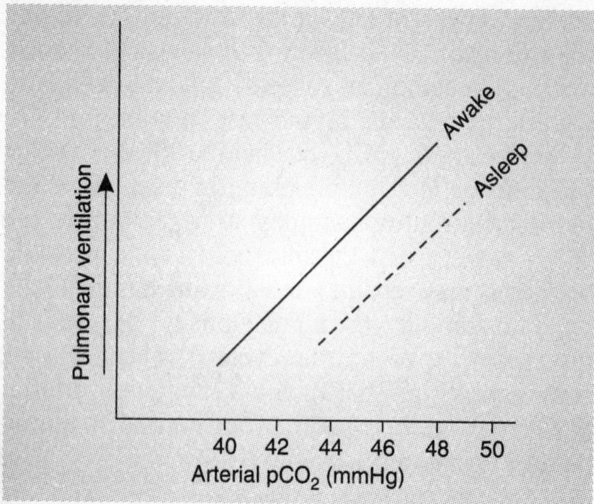

Fig. 18.11: Effect of sleep on the sensitivity of respiratory neurons.

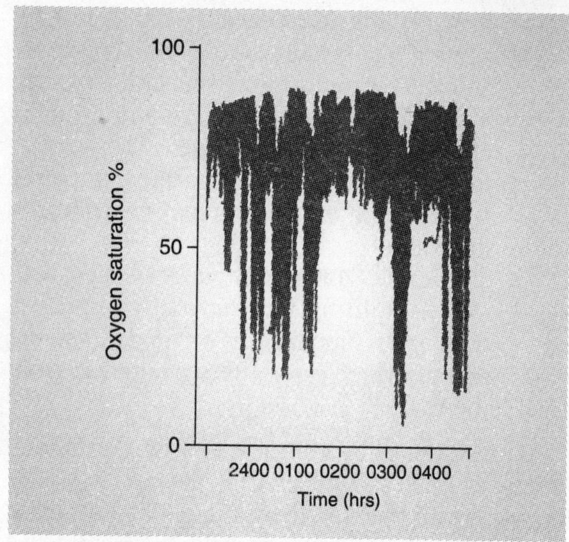

Fig. 18.12: Sleep apnoea syndrome: overnight oxygen saturation trace.

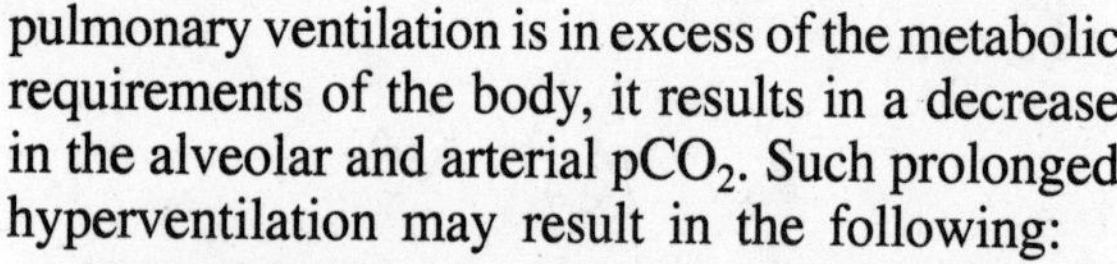

pulmonary ventilation is in excess of the metabolic requirements of the body, it results in a decrease in the alveolar and arterial pCO_2. Such prolonged hyperventilation may result in the following:

i. **Respiratory alkalosis** Disturbance of HCO_3^-/pCO_2 ratio increases the pH of blood to 7.55 or even 7.60.
ii. **Renal changes** Decreased arterial pCO_2 interferes with the H^+ secretory mechanism in the kidney. The consequent failure of proximal tubular reabsorption of bicarbonate results in an excretion of alkaline urine.
iii. **Neurological changes** Respiratory alkalosis produces symptoms of hypocalcaemic tetany, i.e. numbness and tingling in the extremities, carpo-pedal spasms, etc. Cerebral symptoms include dizziness and light headedness. Consciousness may be dulled or even lost. The cerebral symptoms are due to vasoconstriction of the cerebral vessels induced by low arterial pCO_2.
iv. **Cardiovascular changes** The cardiac output is moderately increased. It could be due to muscular effort involved in the production of hyperventilation.

Sleep Apnoea Syndrome

During sleep, the sensitivity of respiratory neurons to arterial pCO_2 seems to decrease (Fig. 18.11). Therefore, brief periods of apnoea (10 S duration) often occur during sleep. When the episodes of sleep apnoea are more prolonged (30–90 S) and frequent, the condition is called sleep apnoea syndrome.

Two types of sleep apnoea syndrome have been recognized. In the less common central (neurogenic) type, episodes of apnoea are due to lack of central neurogenic drive because of poor sensitivity of respiratory neurons to CO_2. The other, *obstructive (peripheral) type* is more common. It is usually observed in obese males who have persistent loud snoring. The exact cause of apnoea is not known. It seems, excessive relaxation of pharyngeal muscles during REM sleep obstructs the oropharynx. The sleep is repeatedly disturbed because each episode of apnoea leads to suffocation and arousal.

These patients suffer from hypoxia (Fig. 18.12), hypercapnoea, polycythaemia and even intellectual deterioration (due to repeated hypoxic episodes).

CHAPTER 19

Respiratory Adjustments in Health and Disease

HYPOXIA

Hypoxia means deficiency of oxygen in the tissues. Hypoxia may be classified into the following four categories: hypoxic hypoxia, anaemic hypoxia, stagnant hypoxia and histotoxic hypoxia.

Hypoxic Hypoxia

This is the commonest type of hypoxia seen in clinical practice. In this type of hypoxia, pO_2 *of the arterial blood is reduced*. As a result, oxygen content of the arterial blood is reduced as well. Hypoxic hypoxia is further characterized by *cyanosis*, hyperventilation and dyspnoea even at rest. Hypoxic hypoxia may be due to:

(a) Pulmonary Disorders *Decreased pulmonary ventilation* because of narcotic poisoning, bronchial obstruction, drowning, etc. leads to decreased entry of air into the lungs, causing a fall in alveolar pO_2. As a result there is a decrease in arterial pO_2 as well as arterial oxygen content. In *pulmonary oedema*, thickening of the alveolar membrane causes a decrease in arterial pO_2 (even though alveolar pO_2 is normal) because of an interference with the diffusion of O_2. Bronchial constriction (bronchial asthma), emphysema and pneumonia are the commonest causes of hypoxic hypoxia in clinical practice.

(b) Congenital Heart Disease In certain congenital heart disorders, the right-to-left shunt transfers deoxygenated (venous) blood to the left side of the heart. As a result, pO_2 of the arterial blood falls significantly.

(c) High Altitude Physiologically, pO_2 of the arterial blood may be reduced in residents at high altitude (over 3000 metres).

Anaemic Hypoxia

In this case, *arterial* pO_2 *is normal but oxygen content of arterial blood is reduced* because of non-availability of haemoglobin for transport of oxygen. Anaemic hypoxia may be due to:

(i) **Severe Anaemia**

(ii) **Altered Haemoglobin** Total haemoglobin content of the blood may be normal, but if a large percentage is in altered form, e.g. as carboxyhaemoglobin or methaemoglobin, the patient shall show signs of anaemic hypoxia.

Hyperventilation or dyspnoea are absent at rest in patients suffering from anaemic hypoxia because arterial pO_2 is normal and therefore peripheral chemoreceptors are not stimulated.

Stagnant Hypoxia

This type of hypoxia occurs in specific organs or regions of the body due to slowing of circulation, e.g. in congestive heart failure or circulatory shock. In the arterial blood, pO_2 and oxygen content are normal. However, the volume of blood flow in the tissues per minute is reduced. The venous blood contains larger amount of deoxygenated haemoglobin, because of greater O_2 extraction due to slowing of blood flow. *Cyanosis* is a prominent feature of this type of hypoxia.

Histotoxic Hypoxia

19

Cyanide poisoning is the best example of this type of hypoxia. The poison interferes with tissue oxidation by paralysing the enzyme cytochrome oxidase. Thus, the tissue metabolism suffers even when pO_2 and oxygen content of the arterial blood, as well as, the volume of blood flow per minute to the tissues are all normal. The four types of hypoxia have been compared in Table 19.1.

Effects of Generalized Hypoxia

Localized Hypoxia It occurs most commonly due to localized obstruction to the arterial blood flow, e.g. coronary or cerebral thrombosis or embolism. This type of hypoxia is easily recognizable because of the profound effects in the organ involved.

Generalized Hypoxia It is often difficult to be detected especially when it develops slowly. Of all the tissues, the central nervous system is most susceptible to the effects of hypoxia. Moreover in this tissue, the effects of hypoxia are also most serious, and often irreversible. Next in the order of susceptibility and criticality of effects is the myocardium. At the other extreme is the skeletal muscle, which can obtain energy by anaerobic metabolism.

The effect of hypoxia also depends on the rate of its development. Elderly patients with a chronic cardiopulmonary disorder may tolerate the degree of hypoxia which is fatal if due to an acute disorder like pneumonia, when there is no time to adapt to the sudden decrease in oxygen supply.

The symptoms of hypoxia include impairment of judgment, drowsiness, disorientation, headache, excitement and dulled pain sensibility. Anorexia, nausea and vomiting may occur. One of the most important effects of hypoxia is decreased mental proficiency as shown by poor judgment, memory and performance of fine motor activities. Euphoria is often present. Tachycardia and hyperventilation are important signs of hypoxia associated with low arterial pO_2. Cyanosis is another important sign but absent in hypoxia due to severe anaemia or carbon monoxide poisoning. Unconsciousness and death may occur when severe hypoxia develops suddenly, e.g. loss of cabin pressure in an aircraft flying at a height over 30,000 ft. Similarly, poisoning with carbon monoxide and cyanide can kill the person within minutes.

Anaemic Hypoxia is more benign than other types of hypoxia, because at rest, tissue oxygen

Table 19.1: Comparison of different types of hypoxia

	Hypoxic hypoxia	*Anaemic hypoxia*	*Stagnant hypoxia*	*Histotoxic hypoxia*
Arterial pO_2	Sub-normal	Normal	Normal	Normal
Arterial O_2 content	Low	Low	Normal	Normal
Cyanosis	Present	Absent	Present	Absent
Dyspnoea at rest	Present	Absent	Present	Present
Common causes	Hypoventilation Asthma Emphysema Cong. heart disease High altitude	Severe anaemia CO poisoning	Circulatory shock	Cyanide poisoning
Oxygen therapy	Useful except in congenital heart disease	Useless except in CO poisoning	Useless	Useless

requirements are easily met with. At rest, overall tissues extract approximately 5 ml of oxygen from 100 ml of blood. Therefore, even if haemoglobin level is 50% of normal, the arterial blood contains approximately 9.5 ml oxygen per 100 ml of blood—that would be more than sufficient for the body requirements. However, an anaemic patient's capacity for physical work is diminished. At times of increased oxygen demand, the limited oxygen content of blood becomes a problem.

In case of carbon monoxide poisoning, however, even if 50% of haemoglobin is converted to carboxyhaemoglobin, oxygen delivery to the tissues is seriously affected (vide infra).

Carbon Monoxide Poisoning

Minute amounts of carbon monoxide (CO) are normally formed in the body and function as a chemical messenger in the central nervous system synapses. When inhaled in large amounts, CO is highly toxic. It is formed by incomplete combustion of petrol, diesel, coal gas, wood, or charcoal. Exhaust fumes of automobile engines contain 6% or more of CO. That is why a person residing in a city with a large number of automobiles may have up to 10% of haemoglobin as carboxyhaemoglobin in his blood. Cigarette smoke also contains CO.

More serious type of CO poisoning may result from accidental exposure to high concentrations of CO when charcoal or wood is burnt to heat up a closed room in winter or automobile gas fumes are accidentally or deliberately inhaled. Every year, about 500 Americans die of accidental CO poisoning; about 2000 commit suicide by inhaling automobile exhaust fumes.

Carbon monoxide reacts with haemoglobin to form carboxyhaemoglobin (CO-Hb), by combining with the sixth covalent bond where oxygen is normally attached. Since the affinity of haemoglobin for CO is 200 times its affinity for oxygen, CO-Hb becomes useless for oxygen transport. An additional handicap is the fact that presence of CO-Hb shifts the oxygen dissociation curve of the remaining normal Hb to the left (Fig. 19.1). Thus oxygen delivery from even normal haemoglobin is curtailed. That is why an anaemic individual with haemoglobin level 50% of normal can do moderate degree of physical work, but an individual with 50% haemoglobin converted to CO-Hb is seriously incapacitated.

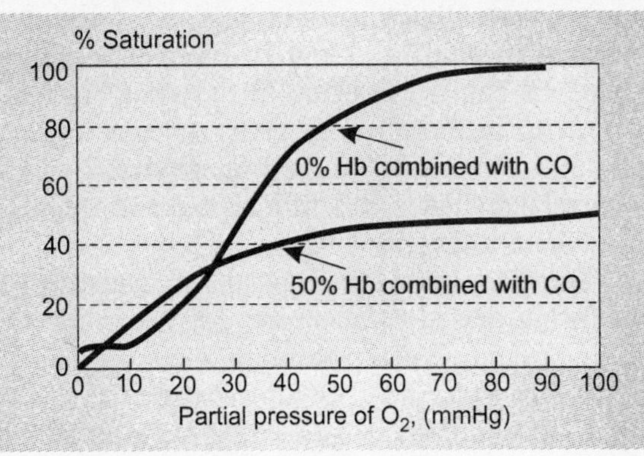

Fig. 19.1: Haemoglobin-oxygen dissociation curve in the presence of 50% as CO-Hb.

Symptoms of CO poisoning are similar to other types of hypoxia, especially headache and nausea, but hyperventilation is not a clinical feature. Absence of hyperventilation is due to the fact that in such type of (anaemic) hypoxia, arterial pO_2 remains normal, and hence the peripheral chemoreceptors are not stimulated. *Cherry red colour* of CO-Hb visible in the skin, nailbeds and mucous membranes is an important clue to the diagnosis of carboxyhaemoglobinaemia. A patient with CO poisoning is treated by:

(i) Immediate termination of exposure to CO.
(ii) Adequate ventilation by artificial respiration, if necessary.
(iii) Ventilation with pure oxygen is preferable to ventilation with fresh air, since it hastens the release of CO from CO-Hb.
(iv) Hyperbaric oxygen therapy, if available, is the most effective treatment.

CYANOSIS (Colour Plate 3, Fig. 4)

Bluish discoloration of the skin and/or mucous membranes is known as cyanosis. It is caused by the presence of *deoxygenated* or an *altered haemoglobin* in sufficient concentration in the blood. Presence of at least 4–5 gm% of deoxygenated Hb in the capillary blood is essential to give the bluish tinge to the skin/mucous membranes. (Normally the capillary blood contains approximately 2–2.5 gm% of deoxygenated Hb.) This is related to the fact that the colour of deoxygenated haemoglobin is bluish purple, in contrast to reddish colour of oxyhaemoglobin. Cyanosis can be detected in the skin, lips, ear lobes, tip of the nose, nailbeds, cheeks and the mucous membrane of the oral cavity. In dark skinned individuals, it is difficult to detect cyanosis till it is very severe.

19

There are two broad groups of causes producing increased concentration of deoxygenated haemoglobin. Correspondingly, cyanosis can be categorized into: (1) central cyanosis caused by hypoxic hypoxia, and (2) peripheral cyanosis caused by stagnant type of hypoxia.

Central Cyanosis is due to a generalized disorder of oxygenation of blood due to a decrease in arterial pO_2. This type of cyanosis is apparent all over the body including mucous membrane of the oral cavity.

Peripheral Cyanosis is due to stagnation of blood leading to greater extraction of oxygen in the peripheral areas like nailbeds, tip of the nose, ear lobes, i.e. peripheral areas of the body where the blood flow even normally is less. In peripheral cyanosis, the extremities are cold in contrast to the normal warm extremities in central cyanosis.

Causes of central cyanosis (all produce hypoxic hypoxia):

(i) Pulmonary disorders like bronchial asthmatic attack, pneumonia, emphysema, pulmonary oedema, etc.
(ii) Congenital heart disease with right to left shunt.
(iii) High altitude (greater than 3000 metres).

Causes of peripheral hypoxia (all produce stagnant hypoxia):

(a) Reduced cardiac output (circulatory shock, congestive heart failure)
(b) Severe cold exposure (severe cutaneous vasoconstriction)
(c) Venous obstruction.

It is absolute rather than relative concentration of deoxygenated haemoglobin that is important for production of cyanosis. In a patient with severe anaemia (haemoglobin concentration 6–7 g%), cyanosis would not occur even if 50% of the haemoglobin is present as deoxygenated form, because there would be only 3–3.5 g% concentration of deoxygenated haemoglobin. On the other hand, in polycythaemia, cyanosis is more easily detected.

Some Uncommon Causes of Cyanosis

As mentioned above, cyanosis is observed when the capillary blood contains 3–3.5 g% of deoxygenated haemoglobin. Presence of much smaller concentrations of altered haemoglobins such as sulphaemoglobin or methaemoglobin produces cyanosis since these blood pigments are very dark in colour. In such cases, the distribution of cyanosis resembles the central type. Such types of cyanosis are rare but may be suspected when cyanosis is observed in the absence of a cardiac or respiratory dysfunction. It may be remembered that CO poisoning does not produce cyanosis because carboxyhaemoglobin is cherry red coloured pigment.

HIGH ALTITUDE PHYSIOLOGY

As we ascend to high altitude, the composition of air does not change. But, because of a decrease in the total barometric pressure, pO_2 of the atmospheric air decreases proportionately. The consequent risk of developing hypoxia concerns permanent residents of high mountains, the mountaineers, armed forces stationed at high altitude and aviators.

The values of total barometric pressure and pO_2 of environmental air and alveolar air at different altitudes are shown in Table 19.2.

Table 19.2: Values of total barometric pressure and pO_2 of environmental air and alveolar air at different altitudes

Altitude (height above sea level)	*Barometric pressure (mmHg)*	*Environmental air pO_2*	*Alveolar air pO_2*
0	760	159	104
10,000 ft	523	110	67
20,000 ft	349	73	40
30,000 ft	226	47	21
40,000 ft	141	29	12

Critical Altitude

At 10,000 ft, some degree of hypoxia is always present but the body can acclimatize to the oxygen lack. An altitude of 18,000 ft is the highest at which permanent inhabitation is possible. Above 20,000 ft, hypoxia can endanger life unless O_2 is added to the inhaled air. Modern aircrafts commonly fly at altitude of about 35,000 ft. The use of pressurized cabins in these aircrafts help to provide an environment similar to that at sea level.

Mountain Sickness

When a person residing at sea level ascends to a high altitude over a short period of 1–2 days, he experiences symptoms of hypoxia, e.g. breathlessness, weakness, headache, dizziness, palpitation, sweating, dimness of vision, partial deafness, sleeplessness and nausea. These symptoms, together known as the *mountain sickness*, disappear gradually over a period of days or a few weeks, due to a number of adjustments in the body (acclimatization) described below.

High altitude pulmonary oedema is one of the more serious and often fatal forms of mountain sickness. Pulmonary oedema occurs particularly in those individuals who ascend rapidly to high altitude and immediately engage themselves in heavy physical activity. The exact mechanism of high altitude pulmonary oedema is not clear. The major contributory factor seems to be pulmonary vascular hypertension. Pulmonary vascular hypertension has been attributed to:

(i) Acute hypoxia related to the high altitude leading to pulmonary vasoconstriction.
(ii) Increased cardiac output because of physical activity at high altitude.
(iii) Cold exposure.
(iv) Excessive secretion of antidiuretic hormone also seems to contribute to water retention and pulmonary oedema.

Acute pulmonary oedema worsens the hypoxia and may lead to death. The patient usually responds to rest, oxygen therapy and return to low altitude.

High altitude cerebral oedema is another serious form of mountain sickness. In the cerebral vessels, in contrast to the pulmonary vessels, acute hypoxia produces vasodilatation and increased cerebral capillary pressure which leads to cerebral oedema. Hypoxic damage to the blood-brain barrier leading to increased capillary permeability seems to be a contributory factor. The transudation of fluid into cerebral interstitial spaces produces cerebral dysfunction characterized by severe headache, mental confusion, hallucinations, ataxia, and bladder dysfunction. These symptoms may progress to coma and death. Hyperbaric oxygen therapy, rest and immediate descent to low altitudes are some of the measures found useful in the treatment of such cases.

Acclimatization to High Altitude

Continued stay at high altitude brings about the following compensatory changes in the body which help to decrease the degree of hypoxia.

Hyperventilation

This is the most fundamental response to hypoxia. Hyperventilation not only brings more O_2 into the lungs but also reduces the gap between the pO_2 of the environmental air and the alveolar air. In other words, pO_2 value of the alveolar air tends to come closer to the pO_2 value of the inhaled air.

The ventilatory response takes 3–4 days to develop fully. Initially, increase in the pulmonary ventilation blows off larger quantities of alveolar CO_2 which reduces the arterial pCO_2. The consequent respiratory alkalosis increases the pH of CSF as well, which opposes the effect of hypoxia on the respiratory centres. Over the next 2–4 days, the compensatory changes in the kidney and CSF (vide infra) restore the pH of the blood and especially CSF to normal. As a result, the respiratory centres respond to the hypoxic stimulus with full force and pulmonary ventilation may increase by as much as 5–7-folds.

Renal Compensatory Changes

The respiratory alkalosis results in greater loss of HCO_3^- in the urine. Plasma HCO_3^- concentration decreases by 1–2 mEq/L. The pH of blood rises initially to 7.5 but later on declines to some extent.

However, the renal compensatory changes are so mild that normal pH of blood is not achieved.

Compensatory Mechanism in CSF

By an active transport mechanism operating at the cerebral capillaries, the concentration of the HCO_3^- in the CSF may be reduced by 5 mEq/L and consequently the pH of the CSF is restored to normal. This compensatory mechanism is far more important in permitting the increase in pulmonary ventilation.

Polycythaemia

Hypoxia stimulates the secretion of erythropoietin leading to an increase in red cell count and haemoglobin concentration. Thus, at high altitude, even though pO_2 of the arterial blood is subnormal, and haemoglobin is not fully saturated, the O_2 content of the arterial blood may not be low.

Increased 2, 3 DPG Concentration

As discussed above, the pulmonary hyperventilation tends to lower arterial pCO_2, leading to respiratory alkalosis. Decreased arterial pCO_2 and the rise in pH of blood (alkalosis) shift the Hb-oxygen dissociation curve to the left (opposite of Bohr effect). This change would interfere with the off-loading of oxygen from haemoglobin in the tissues. This tendency is counteracted by an increase in 2, 3 DPG concentration in the red blood cells induced by respiratory alkalosis. Since 2, 3 DPG decreases the affinity of haemoglobin for O_2 (shifts Hb-oxygen curve to the right), the off-loading of oxygen remains normal respite the existence of respiratory alkalosis.

Tissue Changes

At the tissue level, there is increase in the number of mitochondria and oxidative enzymes such as cytochrome oxidase, which facilitates oxygen utilization by the tissues.

Cardiac Output

The heart rate and cardiac output tend to increase during early days of acclimatization. After a prolonged stay, the cardiac output and heart rate return to normal values.

Work Capacity

At high altitudes, besides the decreased mental efficiency discussed above, the work capacity of the skeletal as well as the cardiac muscle is decreased. At the height of 6000 metres, the work capacity of an unacclimatized individual is 50% of the capacity at sea level. Acclimatization for about 2 months improves the work capacity to approximately 70% of normal.

Permanent residents of very high altitudes in the Himalayas are polycythaemic, short in stature and have barrel-shaped chest. They are so well acclimatized that their physical efficiency is almost similar to the residents at sea level.

Exposure to cold and UV radiations are other hazards of high altitude.

ABNORMAL TYPES OF RESPIRATION

(i) Apnoea Temporary cessation of breathing is known as apnoea. It could be due to: (i) reduced stimulation of respiratory centre, e.g. following voluntary hyperventilation, or (ii) due to active inhibition of respiratory centre, e.g. voluntary breath-holding, or (iii) it could be a part of deglutition reflex or vomiting. *Sleep apnoea* is potentially dangerous.

(ii) Tachypnoea This term denotes increased rate of breathing with no change or even decrease in the depth of breathing. Tachypnoea is seen in pathological conditions like pulmonary congestion, fever, etc.

(iii) Hyperventilation This terms is used to describe increased pulmonary ventilation, e.g. during exercise or hypoxia due to high altitude or other causes. When the hyperventilation involves more than 4–5-fold increase in pulmonary ventilation, an unpleasant sensation or discomfort is felt. This type of breathing is called dyspnoea.

(iv) Dyspnoea Dyspnoea literally means difficult breathing. Normal breathing goes on without reaching our consciousness. When the pulmonary ventilation increases to double the normal value, the subject becomes conscious of the breathing activity. When pulmonary ventilation increases 4–5-folds, the increased respiratory effort is associated with a feeling of discomfort. The level of ventilation at which discomfort is felt is known as dyspnoea point. Dyspnoea is not always pathological. Strenuous exercise is associated with dyspnoea which is physiological. Dyspnoea may develop because of: (a) decreased breathing reserve either because of an increase in pulmonary ventilation or a decrease in maximum ventilatory volume or (b) decreased mechanical efficiency of respiratory system.

(a) Breathing Reserve Normal pulmonary ventilation (PV) at rest is approximately 6 L/minute whereas maximum ventilatory volume (MVV) is 120 L/minute. Therefore, breathing reserve is 120–6 = 114 L/minute.

$$\% \text{ of breathing reserve} = \frac{\text{MVV-PV}}{\text{MVV}} \times 100$$

$$= \frac{120-6}{120} \times 100$$

$$= 95\%$$

When the value of breathing reserve falls below 60%, dyspnoea is generally present.

(b) Mechanical Efficiency Due to disorders of the lungs or the thoracic cage, the patient may have low mechanical efficiency of the act of breathing. Consequently, the patient uses more energy (oxygen) for the work of breathing than a normal individual. Such patients develop dyspnoea even with a small increase in pulmonary ventilation.

Causes of Dyspnoea

1. Disorders of Lungs or Thoracic Cage In lung diseases such as pneumonia, or emphysema dyspnoea results from: (i) decreased maximum ventilatory volume, or (ii) increased pulmonary ventilation because of hypoxia and, (iii) increased work of breathing. During an attack of bronchial asthma, dyspnoea is chiefly because of markedly increased work of breathing.

In disorders of the thoracic cage such as kyphoscoliosis, or poliomyelitis, dyspnoea is mainly due to reduced mechanical efficiency of the respiratory apparatus as well as a decrease in MVV.

2. Disorders of the Heart (Cardiac Dyspnoea) In cardiac failure, dyspnoea is because of pulmonary congestion which causes: (i) increased stiffness of the lungs which decreases mechanical efficiency of the respiratory system, and (ii) stimulation of J-receptors. A characteristic feature of cardiac dyspnoea is orthopnoea ("upright breathing), i.e. dyspnoea becomes worse in supine posture since it causes further increase in pulmonary congestion leading to pulmonary edema and severe hypoxia.

3. Increased Demand of Pulmonary Ventilation Even when cardiorespiratory systems are normal, dyspnoea may develop due to a marked increase in pulmonary ventilation because of: (a) high altitude hypoxia or (b) acidosis (diabetic ketoacidosis, renal failure) or (c) increased body metabolism (fever, thyrotoxicosis).

(v) Cheyne-Stokes Breathing This term is used to describe alternating periods of apnoea and hyperventilation (Fig. 19.2). It may be seen *during sleep* in patients suffering from central type of sleep apnoea syndrome. In an *awake patient*, this type of breathing is seen in severely ill patients with: (a) congestive heart failure, (b) renal failure, or (c) head injury. In such cases, Cheyne-Stokes breathing indicates impending death.

The most common cause of Cheyne-Stokes breathing is reduced sensitivity (elevated threshold) of the respiratory neurons to pCO_2. Apnoea persists till arterial pCO_2 rises to sufficiently high level and arterial pO_2 falls to hypoxemic level. The combination of these stimuli

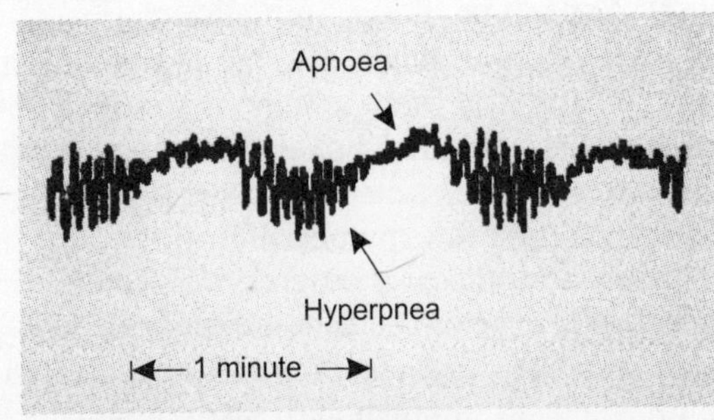

Fig. 19.2: Cheyne-Stokes breathing.

result in a brief period of hyperventilation, which improves the pCO_2 and pO_2 levels to the extent that there is no more adequate stimulus and apnoea occurs once again and the cycle is repeated.

In patients with *congestive heart failure*, another mechanism seems to be responsible for Cheyne-Stokes breathing. Normally, the exchange of gases occurs in the lungs whereas the feedback control of CO_2 is exerted on medullary (central) chemoreceptors, i.e. the depth of breathing corresponds to the pCO_2 in the brain not by pCO_2 of the blood in the pulmonary capillaries where gas exchange occurs. When individuals with slower circulation (chronic CHF) ventilate, they lower the pCO_2 in the lungs, but it takes longer for the brain to appreciate this change. During this time, pCO_2 of the arterial blood is lowered to a subthreshold level and apnoea results. Apnoea lasts till pCO_2 of the arterial blood reaches the threshold level and the cycle is repeated (Fig. 19.3).

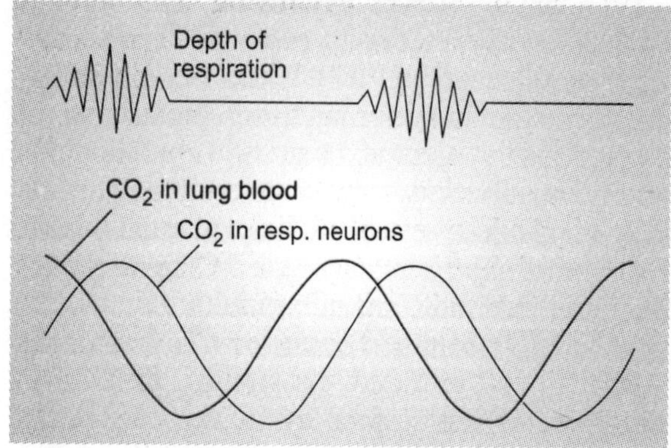

Fig. 19.3: Mechanism of Cheyne-Stokes breathing in congestive heart failure.

(vi) Asphyxia This condition occurs by occlusion of the trachea, i.e. by strangulation, hanging, entry of a foreign body or spasm of the glottis muscles by a fish bone. There is high risk of asphyxia by inhalation of amniotic fluid during delivery and first few minutes after birth.

Asphyxia results in a progressive decrease in arterial pO_2 (hypoxia) and increase in pCO_2 (hypercapnoea). The combination of these two stimuli results in stimulation of respiration which soon progresses to violent respiratory efforts. There is a sharp increase in secretion of ACTH, glucocorticoids and catecholamines, particularly norepinephrine by adrenal medulla. Acidosis becomes pronounced. Blood pressure and heart rate are elevated. When hypoxia and acidosis become very severe, the medullary cardiovascular centre fails; heart rate and blood pressure fall. If breathing is not restored, death occurs within 4–5 minutes.

Drowning is asphyxia caused by immersion in water. In about 10% of the cases of drowning, the contact of water with the glottis produces intense laryngospasm and asphyxia even though water does not enter the lungs. In the remaining 90% of the cases of drowning, water enters the lungs, leaving no scope for gas exchange. Even if rescued in time and resuscitated by artificial respiration, the entry of water into the lungs is likely to produce further complications.

When drowning occurs in *fresh water* or water with low salt content, water is rapidly absorbed by the lung parenchyma leading to plasma hypotonicity, massive intravascular haemolysis with all its complications. Moreover, excess of water in the alveoli interferes with the action of pulmonary surfactant causing collapse of the alveoli. Drowning in *sea water* results in a different type of complications. Ocean water is markedly hypertonic. When present in the alveoli, it draws out water from the pulmonary capillaries causing hypovolemia. Therefore, treatment of a case of drowning should not end with the resuscitation of the patient. The possible late complications should also be attended to.

EMPHYSEMA

This is one of the most serious chronic respiratory disorders. A history of cigarette smoking and recurrent attacks of bronchitis is usually present. Cigarette harms the lungs in a number of ways: (a) Cigarette smoke paralyses the protective ciliary escalator mechanism so that the mucus cannot be easily moved out of the respiratory passages. (b) Cigarette smoke stimulates the mucus secretion which further aggravates the problem. (c) Cigarette smoke inhibits the alveolar macrophage activity.

Respiratory infection attracts leucocytes which release proteolytic enzymes including elastase. A plasma protein α 1-antitrypsin normally inactivates the proteolytic enzymes, but the enzyme is inhibited by cigarette smoke, and by free oxygen radicals released by the leucocytes. The ultimate result is the destruction of the elastic fibres in the lung parenchyma. Alveolar septa are broken down and large air sacs replace the small alveoli (Fig. 19. 4).

Pathophysiological changes in emphysema include:

(a) An increase in physiological dead space.
(b) An uneven alveolar ventilation: perfusion ratio.
(c) Diminished elastic recoil of the lungs. As a result, the chest becomes barrel-shaped and the work of breathing is increased.
(d) Reduced diffusion capacity of the lungs.
(e) Arterial pO_2 is reduced and pCO_2 is increased. In the later stages of the disease, severe hypoxia, polycythaemia and hypercapnoea can be observed.

Arterial pCO_2 as high as 60 mmHg may be observed. Consequently, pulmonary arterial hypertension leading to right heart failure (cor pulmonale) develops.

Pulmonary function tests reveal a decrease in vital capacity, specially FEV-1, an increase in functional residual capacity (FRC), low arterial pO_2 and elevated pCO_2.

BRONCHIAL ASTHMA

Bronchial asthma is characterized by attacks of extreme dyspnoea caused by bronchiolar constriction. The expiration is far more difficult than the inspiration because increase in intrapleural pressure, a normal component of expiratory process, causes further compression of the bronchioles. During an acute attack of asthma, vital capacity is reduced. More important diagnostic feature is reduction in FEV-1. Treatment with bronchodilator drugs relieves the bronchospasm. Repeated attacks of asthma ultimately produce a permanent increase in residual volume and functional residual capacity, i.e. the patient becomes emphysematous. At this stage, bronchodilator drugs fail to produce any relief.

Asthma is due to an allergic response of the bronchi to inhaled allergens like pollen or dust. These individuals produce immunoglobulin E (Ig E) which gets attached to the mast cells lying in the mucosa of the small bronchi and bronchioles. The inhaled antigen reacts with the antibody causing disruption of the mast cells which in release of histamine, bradykinin and some other agents. These substances cause: (a) spasm of the bronchial smooth muscle, (b) local oedema, and (c) increased mucus secretion.

OXYGEN THERAPY

Oxygen therapy is the mainstay of the treatment of respiratory failure or hypoxemia. It often

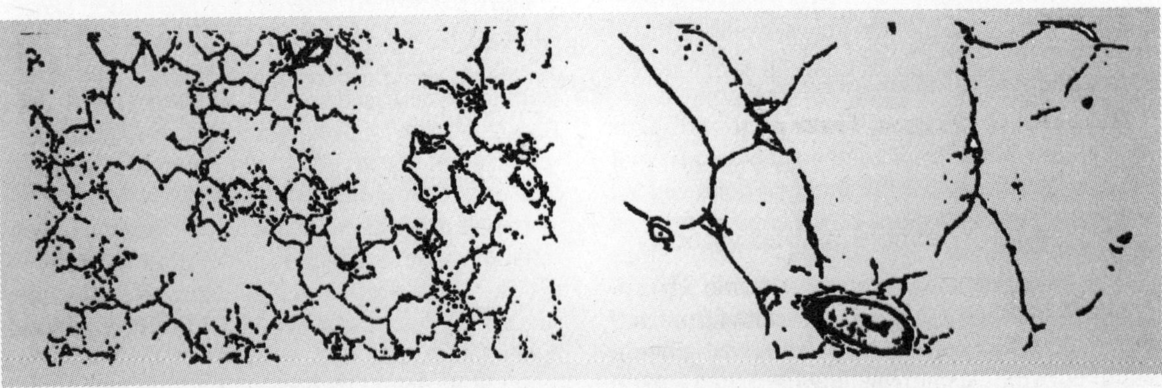

Fig. 19.4: Microscopic appearance of a normal lung (A) and an emphysematous lung (B).

produces dramatic improvement in condition of the patient. However, there are potential hazards associated with its use. Therefore, it is important to understand the physiological principles underlying oxygen therapy.

Effects of Inhalation of Pure Oxygen When fresh air is inhaled, the alveolar air and the arterial blood pO_2 is 100 mmHg. At this partial pressure, each 100 ml of blood contain 0.3 ml of oxygen in dissolved form (0.003 ml / mmHg partial pressure) and approximately 19 ml combined with haemoglobin. Inhalation of pure oxygen increases the alveolar pO_2 to approximately 600 mmHg. At this partial pressure, each 100 ml of blood contains 1.8 ml of oxygen in dissolved form (0.003 × 600), but the amount of oxygen combined with haemoglobin is still 19 ml. In other words, inhalation of pure oxygen improves arterial pO_2. It does not improve the oxygen content of blood to any significant degree.

In view of the facts discussed above, it would be clear that oxygen therapy would be useful in the type of hypoxia in which arterial pO_2 is subnormal, i.e. hypoxic hypoxia. It is useless to administer oxygen to the other types of hypoxia—anaemic (CO poisoning is an exception), stagnant, or histotoxic, because in such cases, arterial pO_2 is already normal.

Emphysematous patients are hypoxic as well as hypercapnic. The arterial pCO_2 may be elevated to the extent that CO_2 causes depression, rather than stimulation, of the respiratory centres. In such patients, hypoxic stimulation of the peripheral chemoreceptors may be the only driving force for respiration. Oxygen therapy in such patients may lead to cessation of respiration and death.

Hyperbaric Oxygen Therapy If 100% is inhaled at a pressure of 3 atmospheres, alveolar pO_2 of approximately 2000 mmHg is achieved. At such pO_2, each 100 ml of blood contain 6 ml of oxygen in dissolved form (0.003 × 2000). Since body requirement of oxygen at rest is only 250 ml/ minute, only 5 ml of oxygen is extracted from 100 ml blood, which can be supplied by the amount dissolved in the plasma. Haemoglobin shall remain saturated even in the venous blood. Indications for hyperbaric oxygen therapy are given below. It may be noted that respiratory failure is not an indication for hyperbaric oxygen therapy.

Indications for Hyperbaric Oxygen Therapy

(i) Carbon monoxide poisoning.
(ii) Gas gangrene: This disease is caused by clostridia bacterium which grows best under anaerobic conditions, e.g. necrotic tissues such as injured muscles. The bacteria produce tissue necrosis and gas locally as well as toxins that cause death by systemic manifestations. Before the use of hyperbaric oxygen therapy, the disease was almost always fatal. These bacteria do not grow if the tissue pO_2 is above 70 mmHg.
(iii) Decompression sickness.
(iv) High altitude cerebral oedema.
(v) Very severe blood loss (before blood transfusion can be arranged).

For hyperbaric oxygen therapy, the patient is placed in a closed chamber in which pure oxygen is pumped under 2–3 atmospheric pressure.

Oxygen Toxicity

Although oxygen therapy is a life-saving measure in patients with severe hypoxic hypoxia, prolonged inhalation of pure oxygen is not without risk. Inhalation of pure oxygen for more than 8 hours produces symptoms of oxygen toxicity:

(a) Respiratory Symptoms. At first the patient complains of irritation in the upper respiratory passages (nasal congestion, sore throat, and cough). Continued pure oxygen inhalation causes damage to the pulmonary alveolar epithelium. There is degradation of pulmonary surfactant leading to increased surface tension in the alveoli. As a result, the lungs have a tendency to atelectasis (collapse of the alveoli), and pulmonary oedema that ends in pulmonary fibrosis.

(b) Neurological Symptoms. They include muscle twitching, dizziness, disturbances of vision, mental irritability, and disorientation. More severe oxygen toxicity may lead to convulsions, coma and death.

(c) Retrolental Hyperplasia. This is one of the extremely serious complications of pure oxygen therapy. It occurs in premature infants suffering from respiratory distress syndrome who had been treated with high concentration oxygen therapy. The basic defect lies in the developmental immaturity of retinal blood vessels which are extremely sensitive to high concentrations of oxygen. In premature infants, the peripheral retina is incompletely vascularized. Exposure to high concentrations of oxygen causes obliteration of these vessels. On stoppage of oxygen therapy, vaso-proliferation begins and extends even into the vitreous. Ultimately, retinal detachment and blindness occurs. The problem can be avoided if the infant is made to breathe air containing less than 30% oxygen.

Administration of oxygen under hyperbaric conditions shortens the duration for which oxygen can be safely administered. If pure oxygen is inhaled under pressure of 4 atmospheres, symptoms of oxygen toxicity may appear within half an hour.

Cellular Mechanism of Oxygen Toxicity

Inhalation of pure oxygen produces toxic effects through production of hydrogen peroxide and free radicals such as super oxide (O_2^-), and hydroxyl radical (OH^-). These agents damage: (i) cellular enzymes, particularly those containing sulphydral (-SH) groups, and (ii) oxidation of polyunsaturated fatty acids, the essential components of the cell membrane and intracellular organelles. It may be mentioned that even normally, some amount H_2O_2 and free radicals are produced in the tissues but are quickly removed by antoxidants like catalases, peroxidases, ascorbic acid, glutathione, etc. During administration of pure oxygen, the concentrations of these toxic agents become so large that natural antoxidants cannot prevent the tissue damage.

EFFECTS OF HIGH BAROMETRIC PRESSURE

Sea divers and caisson workers (who dig tunnels beneath the river-bed or sea-bed) are exposed to high ambient pressure. At sea level, the atmospheric pressure equals 760 mmHg (1 atmosphere). For every 33 ft under the sea, the column of water exerts pressure equal to 1 atmosphere. For example, atmospheric pressure is 2 atmospheres at the depth of 33 ft, 3 atmospheres at 66 ft below the sea level. The inhalation of air under high pressure can lead to the following complication:

Nitrogen Narcosis

Nitrogen constitutes about 80% of the atmospheric air. Its inhalation at sea level pressure does not produce any effect because, due to low solubility coefficient, very small amount is normally dissolved in the plasma. However, when inhaled under high pressure, a large amount of N_2 is dissolved in the blood. When inhaled for sufficiently long period, e.g. working at depth of 100–120 ft for one hour or more, sufficiently large amount of N_2 enters the blood and the nervous tissue producing nitrogen narcosis. Euphoria is the earliest symptom. Later on, drowsiness, light headedness, fixation of ideas, loss of balance, incoordination of movements, and difficulty in concentration occurs. The symptoms of nitrogen narcosis resemble those of alcohol intoxication. Hence, the disorder has been nicknamed: "raptures of the deep." Prolonged work at greater depth may result in hallucinations or even coma. The symptoms of nitrogen narcosis disappear soon after the individual ascends back to the sea surface. However, too rapid ascent may produce a still more serious complication, the decompression sickness, discussed below. The mechanism of production of nitrogen narcosis is not clear. Nitrogen and many other inert gases like helium, argon and neon have anaesthetic property which parallels the lipid solubility of the gases. These gases are believed to act by interfering with ion movement at the water-lipid interface in the mitochondria or the cell membrane of the nervous tissue.

Decompression Sickness (Caisson's Disease)

If a person works under the sea for many hours and then suddenly ascends to the sea surface, he is likely to suffer from decompression sickness. The symptoms include pain in the legs or arms, dizziness, or even paralysis. These symptoms are produced when nitrogen, dissolved in the nervous tissue while under high pressure, is evolved as gas bubbles on sudden ascent to the sea surface. The bubbles may disrupt neuronal pathways in the central nervous system and the peripheral nerves. The bubbling of nitrogen gas in the blood may block the pulmonary capillaries causing dyspnoea and severe pulmonary oedema. Sudden expansion of air in the lungs due to decompression may rupture the pulmonary vessels causing air embolism and death.

The risk of decompression sickness can be eliminated by decreasing the rate of ascent. The safe rate of ascent is determined by the depth at which the person worked and the duration of time he had been there. For example, a person who has worked for 45 minutes at the depth of 300 ft should ascend to the sea surface in 5 hours.

The risks of nitrogen narcosis and decompression sickness are decreased by inhalation of helium-oxygen mixture, instead of normal air (N_2-O_2 mixture).

The molecular weight of helium is 4 as compared to 28 of N_2. Moreover, its lipid solubility is only 40% of N_2. Using He-O_2 mixture, the risk of narcotic effects is totally eliminated and decompression time is shortened.

Oxygen Toxicity

Inhalation of pure O_2 at a depth of 100–120 ft may produce convulsions and unconsciousness within half an hour. Therefore, pure O_2 is seldom used in scuba below the depth of 30 ft.

SCUBA Diving Deep sea diving was earlier restricted to a limited number of individuals such as caisson workers or Navy men, or for harvesting pearls. The individual used a diving helmet connected to a hose pipe through which air was pumped from the sea surface. With the advent of self-contained underwater breathing apparatus (SCUBA), deep sea diving has become a popular recreational activity also. The SCUBA consists of one or two tanks full of compressed air or helium-oxygen mixture. The diver inhales the gas from the tank through a short hose-pipe and a face-mask with breathing valves. The tanks are strapped to the back of the diver. With the more frequent use of SCUBA, nitrogen narcosis and decompression sickness have become more widespread. The preventive measures against such mishaps have been discussed above.

ARTIFICIAL RESPIRATION

In patients with acute asphyxia, artificial respiration may be a life-saving measure. Drowning, electrocution, anaesthetic accidents, carbon monoxide poisoning, etc. cause acute respiratory failure and can be treated effectively by artificial respiration.

Artificial respiration is also useful in patients with self-limiting ventilatory failure, e.g. paralysis of respiratory muscles due to a viral infection (polio).

Mouth to Mouth Breathing

This is the most simple and effective measure of resuscitation. The victim is placed in supine position and his neck is extended by placing one hand under the neck and lifting it and pressing the forehead with the other hand. The victim's mouth is sealed by the operator's mouth while his nostrils are closed by the fingers of the hand on the forehead (Fig. 19.5). About 12–20 times per minute, the operator blows into the victim's mouth about twice of the amount of normal tidal volume. Following each inflation, the operator unseals the victim's mouth allowing expiration to occur passively. Some of the air is likely to enter the stomach through the oesophagus. It can be easily expelled by pressure on the epigastrium.

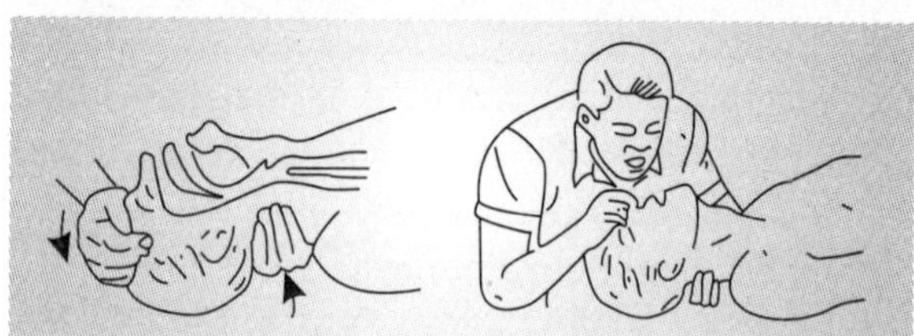

Fig. 19.5: Mouth to mouth artificial respiration.

It may be remembered that expired air of the operator still contains 16% of oxygen which is sufficient to revive the patient.

Mechanical Ventilators

A patient with chronic ventilatory failure, e.g. due to paralysis of respiratory muscles, can be kept alive for months with the help of a mechanical ventilator. Mechanical ventilators are mechanical devices which promote periodic inflow of air (or an air-O_2 mixture) into the lungs. The outflow of air is usually passive due to elastic recoil of the lungs. Two types of mechanical ventilators are available: (a) Negative pressure ventilators in which negative pressure is created around the chest wall which aids inflow of air into the lungs, and (b) positive pressure ventilators which push air into the lungs under positve pressure to produce inspiration.

(a) Tank Respirators (Iron Lung) In this type of respirator, whole body of the patient is inside the tank, only the head protrudes out through a flexible but air-tight collar (Fig. 19.6 A). At the other end of the tank is a motor driven leather diaphragm which moves back and forth to produce periodically negative pressure around the body. Nowadays, this type of ventilators are no more used because of their cumbersome size and weight.

(b) Positive Pressure Mechanical Ventilators These light weight devices are most popular nowadays (Fig. 19.6 B). A cannula is introduced into the trachea in the neck (by tracheotomy) and boluses of air or air-oxygen mixtures from a storage tank are periodically delivered into the lungs under positive pressure. High positive pressure can rupture the lungs (barotrauma). With high quality machines, this risk has been minimized.

PULMONARY FUNCTION TESTS

Pulmonary function tests may be employed in patients with pulmonary disorders for diagnostic or prognostic purposes. They are also used to assess the capacity of the individual to tolerate the risk of surgery. Although a formidable number of pulmonary function tests are feasible, most of them are of interest to a research worker. The information required by a clinician can be provided by a few relatively simple investigations. Pulmonary function may be affected by diseases of the lungs (e.g. asthma, emphysema, diffuse pulmonary fibrosis, pulmonary oedema, etc.) or disorders of the thoracic cage (e.g. kyphoscoliosis) or by neuromuscular disorders (poliomyelitis, myopathy, etc.).

Most of the disorders mentioned above lead to ventilatory defects. Gas transfer factor may be affected in disorders like emphysema, massive surgical resection of the lung or in pulmonary oedema. However, in pulmonary oedema, the clinical picture, and radiological investigations are sufficient to diagnose the disorder. Such patients are not subjected to pulmonary function studies.

Ventilatory Function Tests

Ventilatory performance is tested by spirometry. A typical water-sealed spirometer is shown in Fig. 15.11.

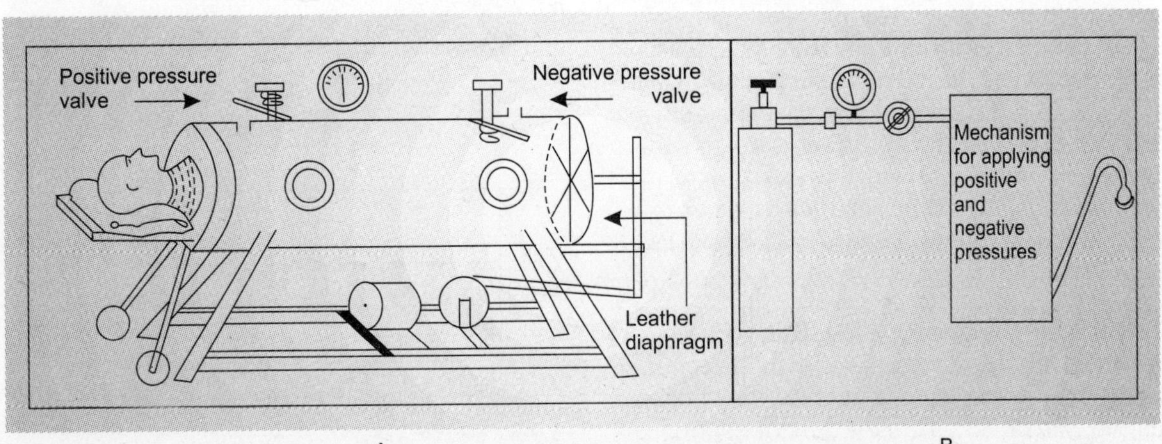

Fig. 19.6: (A) A tank respirator (iron lung); (B) A positive pressure mechanical ventilator.

(i) Vital Capacity and FEV_1 The subject is asked to make a maximum inspiratory effort and then exhale into the mouthpiece attached to the breathing tube. The record may be static (vital capacity) or dynamic [timed/forced expiratory volume (FEV)]. The latter is recorded on a kymograph attached to the spirometer. Normally, 80% of the vital capacity can be expired in the 1st second ($FEV_1\% = 80\%$). Vital capacity varies with age, sex, body size and muscular development. It is greater in males than in females. Normal vital capacity is 2.6 L/m^2 BSA in normal adult male and 2.1 L/m^3 BSA in normal adult female. There is a variation in the ventilatory performance of different age groups. An observed value should be considered abnormal if it is 20% below the predicted normal value for the age and sex group.

Vital capacity is reduced in patients with respiratory obstruction (asthma) emphysema, pulmonary fibrosis, poliomyelitis, etc.

Forced expiratory volume 1st second (FEV_1) and peak expiratory flow rate (PEFR) estimation help to differentiate between obstructive lung disorders like bronchial asthma and emphysema from restrictive lung disorders like pulmonary fibrosis. Vital capacity is reduced in both obstructive as well as restrictive lung disorders. However, in obstructive lung disease, FEV_1 and PEFR are proportionately more affected than the vital capacity.

(ii) Peak Expiratory Flow Rate It is measured by a very simple device known as peak flowmeter (Fig. 19.7). PEFR is defined as the maximum rate of air flow which can be achieved during a sudden forced expiration, from the position of full inspiration. The value obtained is determined mainly by the calibre of the airways. Normal PEFR is 500–600 L/min.

(iii) Mid-Expiratory Flow Rate ($FEF_{25-75\%}$) It is a useful measurement for early detection of small airway obstruction. It measures the flow rate during middle 50% of the expiratory spirogram. It is calculated by measuring the volume of air expired during this period divided by the time

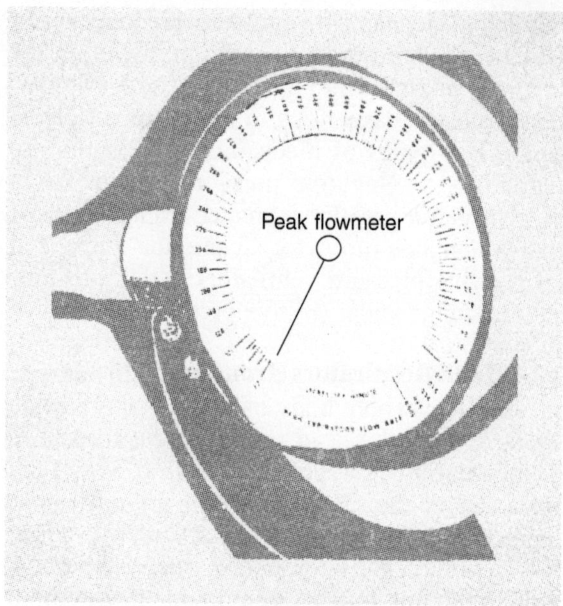

Fig. 19.7: Peak flowmeter.

(Fig. 19.8). Normal range of $FEF_{25-75\%}$ is 1.4–5.5 L/sec in men and 1.4–3.5 L/sec in women.

(iv) Maximum Breathing Capacity (MBC) Maximum breathing capacity of an individual is seldom measured because it is relatively difficult

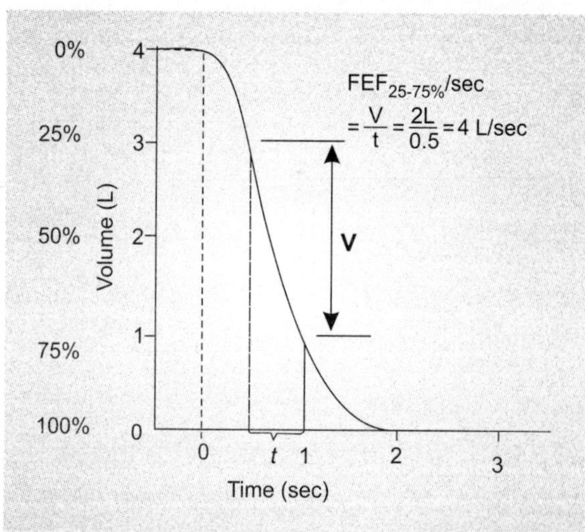

Fig. 19.8: Calculation of $FEF_{25-75\%}$ from a forced expiratory spirogram.

to perform and better information is obtained by measurement of FEV_1 and $FEF_{25-75\%}$ than MBC.

(v) Functional Residual Capacity (FRC) It can be estimated by nitrogen washout method. The subject inhales pure O_2 for 5 minutes and expires into a large gas bag, called Douglas gas bag, washed with pure O_2 (and hence made nitrogen free). The nitrogen content of the gas in the bag would be solely from the subject's lungs. The total amount of gas expired into the bag and its nitrogen concentration is measured. It is assumed that the alveolar air has 80% nitrogen.

$$C_1 \times V_1 = C_2 \times V_2$$

$$80 \times \text{FRC} = \text{Conc. of } N_2 \text{ in bag air} \times \text{Vol. of gas in bag}$$

$$\text{FRC} = \frac{\text{Conc. of } N_2 \text{ in bag air} \times \text{Vol. of gas in bag}}{80}$$

Example: $C_2 = 5\%$
$V_2 = 48{,}000$ ml

$$\text{FRC} = 48{,}000 \text{ ml} \times 5/80 = 3000 \text{ ml}$$

FRC is increased in emphysema.

Blood Gases

The overall function of the respiratory system is to provide adequate amounts of oxygen to the tissues and remove CO_2. Therefore, estimation of arterial pO_2, pCO_2 and pH are most fundamental of all the pulmonary function tests. Use of miniaturised glass electrodes now permits the estimation of all the three parameters within a minute or so, using a single very small sample of blood. The blood sample is usually taken from the radial artery, although a femoral arterial sample can also be taken.

Normal range of arterial pCO_2 in healthy young adults is 33–44 mmHg, normal range of arterial blood pH is 7.35–7.45. Arterial pCO_2 level basically depends on the volume of alveolar ventilation. Hypoventilation causes increased pCO_2 and acidosis (respiratory acidosis). Hyperventilation produces a fall in arterial pCO_2 and a rise in blood pH (respiratoryalkalosis).

The normal range of arterial pO_2 in healthy young adults is 75–105 mmHg. Decreased arterial pO_2 may be due to one of the following reasons:

(i) Alveolar hypoventilation.
(ii) Physiological shunts and increased physiological dead space leading to decreased ventilation/perfusion ratio. These are abnormalities commonly present in emphysema.
(iii) Right to left vascular shunts.
(iv) Diffusion defects.

Transfer Factor

The exchange of gases in the lungs was earlier believed to be dependent merely on the ability of the gases to diffuse across the alveolar respiratory membrane. This concept led to the use of the term *diffusion capacity*. Later, it was realized that many other factors, like ventilation-perfusion balance, pulmonary-capillary blood volume, haemoglobin concentration of the blood and the rate of reaction of gases with haemoglobin, are also involved in the exchange of gases. Therefore, nowadays, the term transfer factor, rather than diffusion capacity is used. Many technical difficulties preclude the estimation of transfer factor for O_2. Instead, transfer factor for CO is usually estimated.

Transfer Factor for CO (TF CO)

Transfer factor for CO can be calculated if the following information is available:

(i) The quantity of CO transferred per minute.
(ii) The pressure gradient of CO across the alveolar membrane. It actually means partial pressure of CO in the alveolar air, since pCO in the blood would be zero.

Single breath method is more commonly used for the estimation of TF CO. The patient takes a measured breath containing known volumes of helium (He) and CO and holds the breath for 10 seconds and then breathes out. From the sample of expired air, the concentrations of He and CO are measured. Computerised calculations yield the informations: (i) and (ii) mentioned above. Thus TF CO can be calculated. Normal TF CO in adults is

20 ml/min/mmHg. From the knowledge of TF CO, transfer factor of any other gas may be calculated. The calculation is based on the fact that the diffusion of a gas through a membrane is directly proportionate to its solubility in water and inversely proportionate to the square root of its molecular weight. On this basis, TF O_2 would be 1.23 times the TF CO. TF CO_2 would be 20.7 times the TF CO.

Exercise Testing

Exercise test provides information about the total cardiopulmonary performance of the individual. Measurement of pulse rate, minute ventilation, O_2 uptake and arterial blood gases tension during graded exercise on a treadmill or a bicycle ergometer is extremely useful, especially when the cause of dyspnoea is obscure.

Section VI

Nerve and Muscle

CHAPTER 20

The Nerve

Our body consists of a number of organ systems. Activity of each organ has to be coordinated with other systems so that they may not act against one another. Moreover, activity of each organ needs to be adjusted to the changes in the internal or external environment. The nervous system serves these functions.

In order to respond to the changes in the environment, a mechanism for detecting the change is essential. The information is communicated to the central nervous system which evaluates the extent of change and sends appropriate signals to one or more organs to compensate for the change. All such adjustments require an efficient and elaborate communication system. The *central nervous system (CNS)*, consisting of the brain and the spinal cord, contains centres for the integration of input signals and for production of output signals. The *peripheral nervous system* consists of *afferent nerves* that carry input signals (nerve impulses) from the tissues to the CNS and *efferent* nerves that carry output signals from the CNS to the peripheral tissues.

The central nervous system is comprised of two major cell types: the *neurons* and the *neuroglial cells*. A neuron is the basic unit of nervous tissue. It is specialized for the function of reception, integration and transmission of information in the body. The neuroglial cells are 10–50 times the number of neurons. They are not directly involved in the transfer of information, but they play a key role in the overall function of the nervous system. The neuroglial cells are discussed in detail at a later stage in this chapter.

NEURON (NERVE CELL)

Morphologically, numerous types of neurons can be seen in the CNS. But the basic structure of a neuron is best studied in a spinal motor neuron. This cell has a cell body (*soma*) with 5–7 small processes called *dendrites*, that branch extensively. In addition, there is a long process called the *axon* that may be a few millimeters to over one metre in length (Fig. 20.1). After fixation and staining with specialized techniques, the neuron cell body is seen to contain a large nucleus with one (or sometimes two) nucleoli but there is no centrosome. The absence of centrosome indicates that the neuron

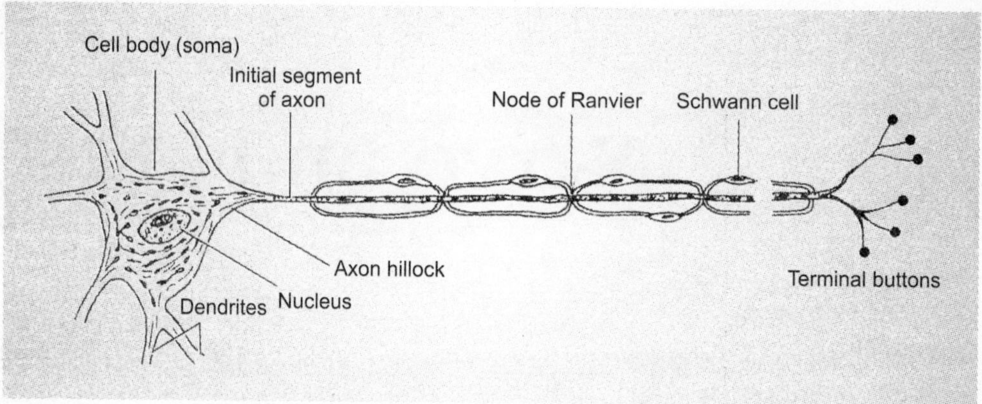

Fig. 20.1: Diagram of a neuron with myelinated axon.

has lost the ability for cell division. Neurons, once destroyed, are replaced by neuroglia only.

The cytoplasm of the soma shows mitochondria, Golgi apparatus, ribosomes, endoplasmic reticulum, Nissl bodies and neurofibrils. The structure and function of these organelles is similar to any other cell. The mitochondria are found not only in the soma but also along the entire length of the axon. The neurofibrils appear as fine filaments which traverse the soma from the dendrites to the axon and extending up to its termination. Nissl granules (bodies) appear as prominent granular masses which take up basic dyes. Chemically, they are composed of ribonucleic acid. They are absent in axon hillock (see below). Nissl granules disintegrate when the soma or its axon is injured.

A neuron may have one or more dendrites but the axon is usually single. The dendrites constitute the receptor zone of a neuron and transmit impulses towards the cell body only. On the other hand, the axon transmits impulses away from the cell body. Within the central nervous system, the dendrites are short and often branched. In the peripheral sensory neurons, the dendrite may be as long as or even longer than the axon.

The neuron cell bodies are mostly located within the grey matter of the CNS. However, some masses of the nerve cell bodies called *ganglia* are also present outside the CNS, e.g. dorsal root ganglia, and autonomic ganglia. The axon may be short and terminate within the grey matter by making contact (synapse) with another neuron. More commonly, the axon is long and either constitutes a part of the long tract of the CNS forming the white matter or leave the brain or spinal cord as peripheral nerve fibre.

The axon originates from the thickened area of the cell body called the axon hillock. The initial segment is the name given to the initial unmyelinated portion of the axon. The axon terminates by dividing into a number of branches, each ending in a number of *synaptic knobs* (*terminal buttons*). Synaptic knobs contain microvesicles in which a chemical transmitter is stored.

Functionally speaking, the neuron can be divided into four zones. (i) The soma and dendrites constitute the receptor zone of the neuron. (ii) The initial segment, where nerve impulse is generated. (iii) The main length of the axon, that transmits the nerve impulse.(iv) The nerve terminals that release the neurotransmitter.

Like any other cell, the cytoplasm of the cell body and the axon is enclosed in a plasma membrane.

NERVE FIBRE

On leaving the grey matter, the axon may acquire a thick layer of myelin sheath to become a *myelinated fibre*. The myelin sheath of peripheral nerves consists of compressed layers of Schwann cells spiralling concentrically and forming a wrapping around the axon (Fig. 20.2). Myelin is a protein-lipid complex which helps to insulate the

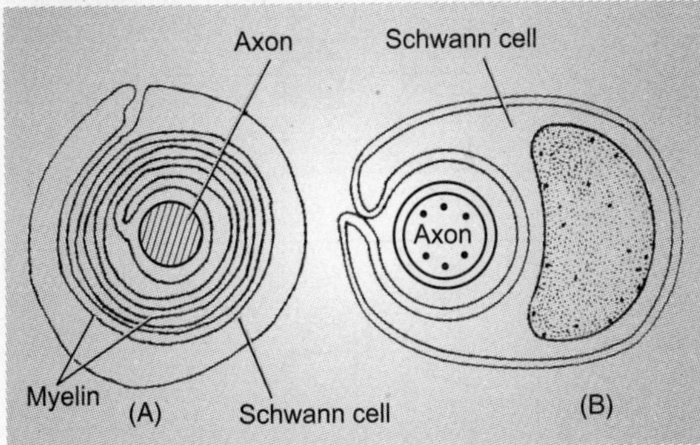

Fig. 20.2: (A) A myelinated nerve fibre with multiple wrappings of myelin produced by a Schwann cell. (B) An unmyelinated nerve fibre.

axon and prevent cross-stimulation of adjacent axons. The nucleus of the Schwann cell is located in the outermost layer of myelin. In the myelinated nerve fibres, constrictions are observed at regular intervals of about 1 mm. These points, called the *nodes of Ranvier*, are due to the absence of myelin (Fig. 20.1). Each internodal segment of the myelin sheath is produced by a single Schwann cell.

Some nerve fibres are of *unmyelinated type*, i.e. the axon is covered by a Schwann cell but there are no multiple wrappings of the membrane which produce myelin.

Within the white matter of CNS, most of the axons are covered with myelin sheath secreted by *oligodendrogliocytes*. Unlike peripheral nerves where each axon has a separate myelin sheath, an oligodendrogliocyte sends processes and forms myelin sheaths around up to 40 axons.

NEURONAL TRANSPORT SYSTEM

Neurons are secretory cells in the sense that they release neurotransmitters at the axon terminals. There are few, if any, ribosomes in the axons or axon terminals. Therefore, all the necessary cytoplasmic proteins (axoplasm), cytoplasmic organelles and neurotransmitters can only be synthesized in the soma, where ribosomes, Golgi apparatus and mitochondria are present. The axoplasm, mitochondria and the neurotransmitter microvesicles have to be transported through the entire length of the axon, that may be more than one metre long. The transport occurs along the microtubules, which appear as neurofibrils under light microscope. Fast and slow axonal transport systems have been described. Fast axonal transport system may show anterograde transport (from the soma to the axon terminals) or retrograde transport (from axon terminals to the soma).

Fast Anterograde Axonal Transport It occurs along the microtubules at a rate of approximately 400 mm per day. The transported materials include the microvesicles containing the neurotransmitters, lipids, proteins, mitochondria and many other cytoplasmic organelles.

Fast Retrograde Axonal Transport It also occurs along the microtubules, but at a rate of approximately 200 mm per day. Materials transported by retrograde transport system include used (empty) microvesicles for recycling or degradation by the lysosomes, and nerve growth factors. Some toxins (tetanus toxin) and viruses (herpes and rabies) may reach the central nervous system by retrograde transport from superficial wounds, etc.

Slow Anterograde Axonal Transport It occurs at a rate of 0.5–10 mm per day. Enzymes for synthesis of small molecule neurotransmitters are transported from soma to the nerve terminals by this system. This system also transports cytoskeleton proteins, neurofilaments and microtubule subunits down the axon.

ELECTRICAL PROPERTIES OF A NEURON

Electrical potentials exist across the plasma membrane of essentially all the cells of the body and seem to have a role in their functions. Only nerve and muscle cells are *excitable tissues, i.e. they are capable of generating* electrochemical impulses (*action potentials*) at their membranes. These two tissues also possess the property of *conductivity,* i.e. the ability to propagate action potentials from the point of generation to the rest of the membrane.

1. EXCITABILITY

Resting Membrane Potential

The study of electrical activity of a tissue has been made possible by the development of microelectrodes (less than 1 μm in diameter), electronic amplifiers and cathode ray oscilloscope (CRO) (Fig. 20.3). The use of an extremely sensitive device like CRO is essential for the recording of an action potential because the potential change is very small (in millivolts) and rapid (in milliseconds). Ordinary galvanometers and pen recorders are not capable of recording an action potential.

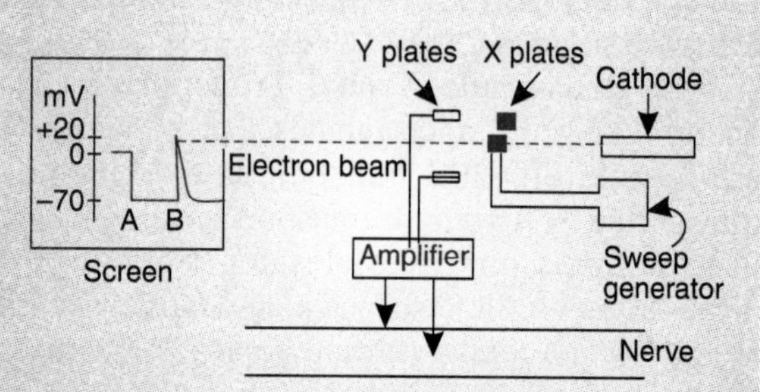

Fig. 20.3: Diagram of cathode-ray oscilloscope.

If two recording electrodes are placed on the *surface* of a nerve fibre and connected to a CRO, no potential difference is observed. However, if one microelectrode is inserted *into* the nerve fibre, while the other remains on the surface, a steady potential difference of 70 mV (inside being negative with respect to the surface) can be observed on the CRO. Since the recording has been made while the nerve is at rest (i.e. not conducting impulses), the potential difference is known as the resting membrane potential (RMP) and expressed as –70 mV (Fig. 20.4).

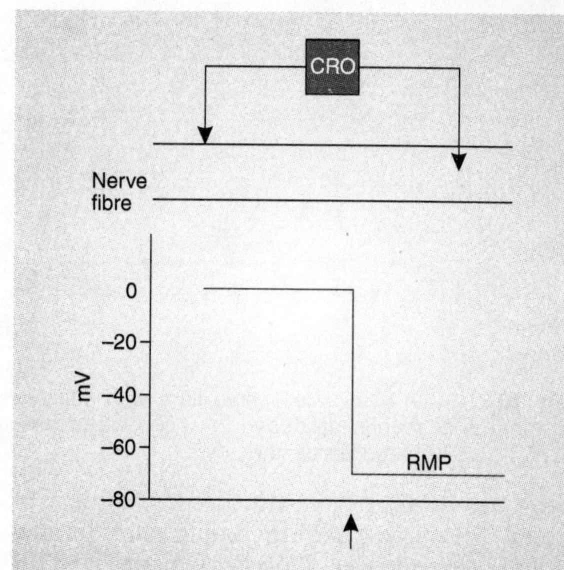

Fig. 20.4: Method to record the resting membrane potential by insertion of a microelectrode inside a nerve fibre (at the time shown by an arrow).

Ionic Basis of Resting Membrane Potential

The selective permeability of the cell membrane produces certain differences in the composition of intracellular and extracellular fluids (Donnan equilibrium). Potassium ion is the dominant intracellular cation whereas Na^+ is the dominant cation in the extracellular fluid. The cell membrane is *impermeable* to chief intracellular anion, the protein. Active transport of Na^+ out of the cell (by Na^+-K^+ ATPase pump) keeps the intracellular Na^+ concentration low (Table 20.1). On the other hand, the cell membrane is very permeable to K^+ and Cl^-.

Table 20.1: Concentrations of important ions inside and outside the neurons

Iron	*Concentration in mEq/L*		*Equilibrium potential (mV)*
	Inside	*Outside*	
Na^+	15.0	150.0	+ 60
K^+	150.0	5.5	– 90
Cl^-	9.0	125.0	– 70

The difference in the concentration of K^+ between inside and outside the cell membrane results in the passive diffusion of K^+ out of the cell along the concentration gradient, through the K^+-leak channels. Since the cell membrane is impermeable to proteins, the chief intracellular anion, the diffusion of positively charged K^+ produces electronegativity inside the cell. An electrical gradient is thus created in which the intracellular negative charge opposes the outward diffusion of K^+. At equilibrium, the inward force on K^+ due to electrical gradient (potential difference) balances the outward force on K^+ due to concentration gradient. The equilibrium potential for a diffusible ion can be calculated by **Nernst equation:**

$$\text{EMF (in millivolts)} = -61.5 \log \frac{\text{conc. of diffusible ion inside}}{\text{conc. of diffusible ion outside}}$$

From the concentrations of K^+ inside and outside the nerve cell membrane (Table 20.1), the equilibrium potential for potassium can be theoretically derived and found to be equal to –90 mV.

$$E_{K^+} = -61.5 \log [K_i^+] / [K_o^+]$$

$$= 61.5 \log \frac{150}{5.5} = -90 \text{ mV}$$

In the calculation given above, the permeability of the membrane to Na^+ and Cl^- has been taken as zero. The actual measurement of resting membrane potential in a nerve fibre gives a value of –70 mV instead of theoretically derived value of –90 mV. Obviously, the K^+ concentration outside the cell is slightly more than that could be explained by passive diffusion only.

It may be noted that only a minute number of K^+ diffuse out of the cell to produce the equilibrium potential. The total concentrations of positively and negatively charged ions are equal in both ECF and ICF, except along the cell membrane. The K^+ which leave the cell because of the concentration gradient remain just close to the cell membrane and produce the positive charge on the outer surface of the cell membrane.

Role of Na^+-K^+ Pump

Na^+-K^+ pump operating continuously at the neuronal cell membrane (and elsewhere) not only prevents the cell from attaining equilibrium potential for Na^+ but also contributes to the resting membrane potential.

Basically, the permeability of the cell membrane to Na^+ is 1/100th of the permeability to K^+. Even then, some Na^+ do enter the cell through Na^+-'leak' channels. However, the intracellular Na^+ concentration is kept low by Na^+-K^+ pump. Na^+K^+ pump is an electrogenic pump which contributes to the resting membrane potential. Na^+-K^+ ATPase catalyses the hydrolysis of ATP to ADP and uses the energy, so liberated, to extrude 3 Na^+ out of the cell in exchange of 2 K^+ into the cell. Thus, the pump maintains net movement of positive charge out of the cell.

Action Potential

At rest, the cell membrane is said to be *polarized,* i.e. the outer surface carries positive charge with respect to the inner surface. When resting membrane potential is being recorded on a CRO, and the nerve fibre is stimulated at a short distance away from the recording electrodes, an action potential can be observed on the oscilloscope (Fig. 20.5). The point of stimulation is shown on the CRO as a mild deflection of the baseline (produced by disturbance of the electron beam) called the *stimulus artefact.* Stimulus artefact is produced by the leakage of electric current from the stimulating electrodes to the

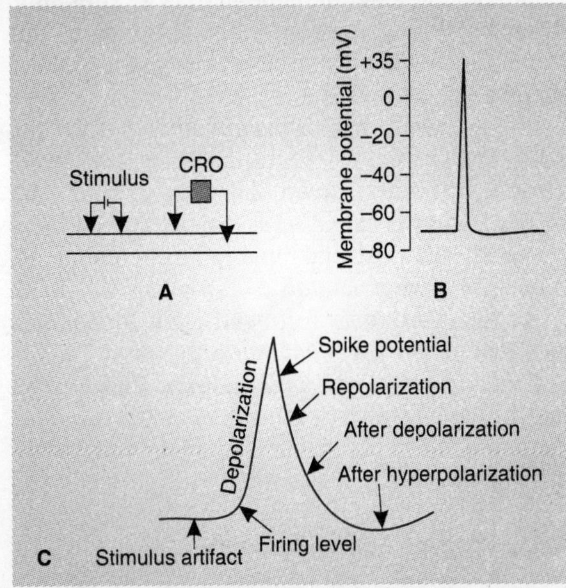

Fig. 20.5: Method to record an action potential of a nerve fibre (A). The action potential recorded is shown in (B). The diagram of action potential has been blown up in (C) to explain its various components.

recording electrodes. A short isoelectric period known as the *latent period* follows the stimulus artefact. Next the electron beam suddenly shoots upwards from — 70 mV (resting potential) to +35 mV potential followed by equally quick reversal of the membrane potential to a value close to the resting membrane potential. Sudden change in the membrane potential of an excitable tissue in response to a stimulus is called an *action potential*. The first phase, i.e. the change in membrane potential from –70 to +35 mV is called *depolarization*, since it represents the loss of original polarity of the cell membrane. The second phase of action potential, i.e. reversal to the nearly original potential is called *repolarization.*

The latent period represents the time taken by the impulse to travel from the site of stimulating electrodes (chiefly cathode) to the site of recording electrodes. Its duration varies directly with the distance between the two sets of electrodes and inversely with the velocity of conduction of impulse in the nerve.

A closer examination of an action potential reveals that the rate of depolarization is initially slow but after membrane potential has reached – 55 mV, the rate of depolarization suddenly increases. *Firing level* is the name given to the potential at which the process of depolarization becomes suddenly fast.

The repolarization also is initially very fast but after about 70% of repolarization has been achieved, it slows down. The slower phase of repolarization is called *after depolarization*. The phases of rapid rise and rapid fall of potential are called the *spike potential*.

Repolarization is followed by a prolonged period of mild *hyperpolarization* (by about 2 mV). It is called *after-hyperpolarization*. Finally, the resting membrane potential is restored. *The duration of spike potential in a neuron is approximately 1 millisecond.*

Ionic Basis of Action Potential

Besides the *Na^+-K^+ leak channels* mentioned above, the neuron cell membrane contains *voltage-gated Na^+ and K^+ channels*. A decrease in the membrane potential between 7–15 mV opens the Na^+ channels partially, whereas 15 mV (firing level) or greater decrease in the membrane potential opens the voltage-gated Na^+ channels fully. In other words, a decrease from –70 to –55 mV potential fully activates the voltage-gated Na^+ channels and positively charged Na^+ rush into the cell following concentration as well as electrical gradients. The cell membrane has a tendency to achieve the equilibrium potential for Na^+ (+ 60 mV). However, within a fraction of a millisecond, the gates close again and the depolarization does not reach a value greater than +35 mV. The closed Na^+ channels now remain in inactivated state and cannot be reopened till the membrane has at least been partially repolarized. In short, the *depolarization is produced by a sudden but brief increase in permeability to Na^+, leading to Na^+ influx* (Fig. 20.6.).

The change in the membrane potential during depolarization results in the *opening of voltage-gated K^+ channels*. The channels open slowly and their closure is rather delayed. The consequent efflux of K^+ (positive charge) out of the cell not only explains repolarization of the membrane, but also mild but prolonged state of hyperpolarization. In short, *repolarization is produced by increase in the permeability of cell membrane to K^+, leading to K^+ efflux* (Fig. 20.6).

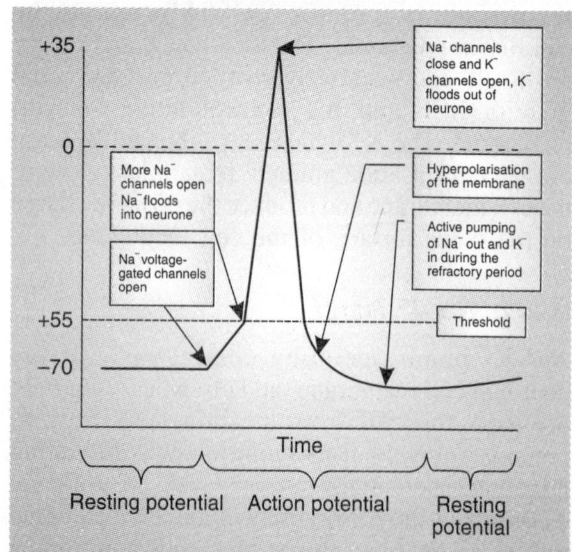

Fig. 20.6: Ionic basis of an action potential.

It would be obvious that, at the end of an action potential, the neuron contains a few extra sodium ions and a little less potassium ions. Ultimately, activation of the Na^+-K^+ pump restores their concentrations to the original state. However, it must be remembered that the number of ions involved in an action potential is infinitely small as compared to the total ions present.

Role of Calcium Ions

Changes in the extracellular calcium ion concentration affect the neuromuscular excitability. A decrease in the extracellular (plasma) Ca^{2+} concentration lowers the threshold of excitation, i.e. even a milder degree of depolarization is sufficient to open the Na^+ channels and produce an action potential. An elevation of plasma Ca^+ concentration has the opposite effect. The exact mechanism by which Ca^{2+} affect the neuromuscular excitability is not known. Probably Ca^{2+} stabilize the gate-proteins of voltage-gated Na^+ channels.

Characteristics of Stimulus

An excitable tissue may be stimulated electrically, mechanically or chemically. For experimental purposes, electrical stimulation is used since it is not only more physiological but also its intensity and duration can be rigidly controlled.

Strength Duration Curve

In the experiment to record an action potential, the stimulus, to be effective, must be of an adequate strength and duration. The minimum voltage necessary to produce a response is called the *threshold intensity*. The stimulus must be applied for a certain minimum duration to be effective. Stimuli of very short duration, no matter how strong, are ineffective.

The relation between the strength and the duration of a stimulus can be studied by varying the duration of a stimulus and finding out the threshold strength for each duration. The record of the results on a semilog graph paper gives the strength-duration curve (Fig. 20.7).

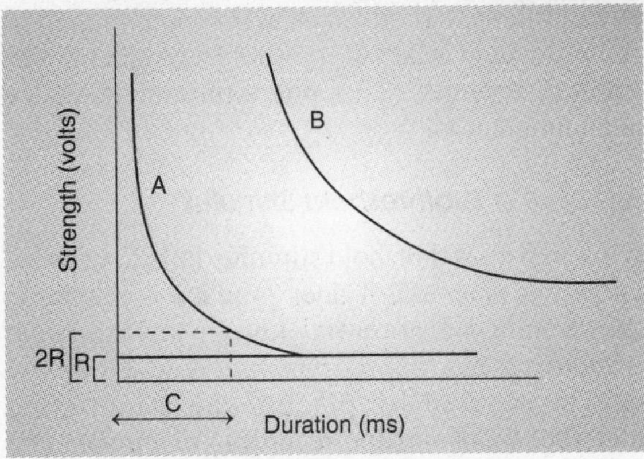

Fig. 20.7: Strength-duration curve of nerve (A) and muscle (B). R = Rheobase; C = Chronaxie.

Rheobase is a *minimum strength* of stimulus which, if applied for adequate time, produces a response. *Chronaxie* is the *minimum duration* for which a stimulus of double the rheobase strength must be applied to produce a response. Chronaxie is an index of excitability of a tissue. A nerve fibre has far shorter chronaxie value than a muscle fibre, indicating greater excitability of the former.

After a nerve injury, the strength duration curve shifts to the right (approaching that of a muscle fibre). As the nerve regenerates, the strength-duration curve gradually shifts to the left (Fig. 20.7). Thus, estimation of chronaxie value is helpful in the assessment of recovery in a patient with nerve injury.

'All or None' Law

If a stimulus of threshold strength is applied, an action potential is produced in a nerve fibre. Further increase in the strength or duration of stimulus does not produce any increase in amplitude or duration of the action potential. In other words, an action potential fails to occur if the stimulus is of subthreshold intensity. When an action potential is produced, it has a constant amplitude and duration, regardless of the strength of the stimulus above the threshold intensity. This property is known as 'all or none' law.

Accommodation

The threshold stimulus must rise to its peak intensity rapidly. A stimulus of slowly rising strength fails to produce an action potential, even if it ultimately achieves threshold strength or even greater strength. This phenomenon is called accommodation.

Effect of a Subthreshold Stimulus

Although a subthreshold stimulus fails to produce an action potential, it does produce a change in the membrane potential known as the *local response* or *electrotonic potential*. Local response can be studied by placing the stimulating electrodes close to the recording electrodes and observing the effect on a CRO. Application of a subthreshold stimulus with cathode produces a depolarizing potential change that rises rapidly and then decays exponentially with time. Anodal current, on the other hand, produces a hyperpolarizing potential (Fig. 20.8). The potential changes at cathode and anode are known as *catelectrotonus* and *anelectrotonus*, respectively.

They are produced by passive subtraction or addition of the charge by a particular electrode. Electrotonic potentials are characterized by the fact that they do not follow 'all or none' law. The degree of depolarization (or hyperpolarization) produced varies with the strength of subthreshold stimulus. When the cathodal current is of sufficient intensity to depolarize the membrane to the firing level, an action potential is fired. From this experiment it would also be clear why stimulation occurs normally at cathode and not at anode.

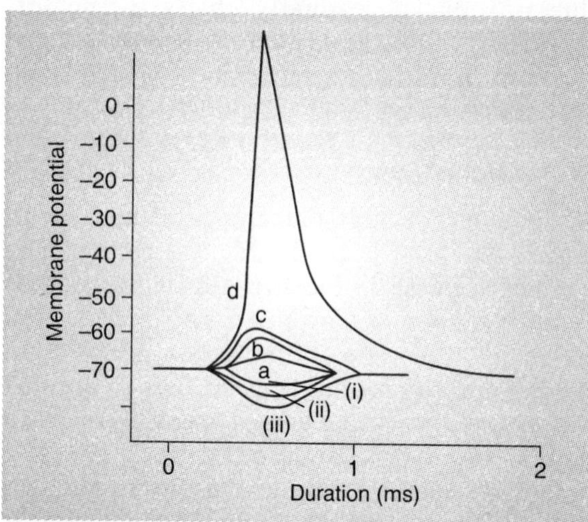

Fig. 20.8: Electrotonic potentials produced by application of subthreshold stimuli. Progressively increasing strengths of stimuli produce responses a, b, c and d at cathode and i, ii and iii at anode. Action potential (d) is fired when catelectrotonus reaches the firing level.

Changes in Excitability of a Nerve Fibre during an Action Potential

During an action potential, the excitability of a neuron is reduced. Application of another stimulus, whatever its strength, during the phase of depolarization or early repolarization fails to produce any response. This period is known as *absolute refractory period*. The later part of the repolarization phase and phase of hyperpolarization is known as the *relative refractory period* (Fig. 20.9), since the threshold of stimulation is elevated and relatively stronger stimulus is required to evoke another action potential. During absolute refractory period, the voltage-gated Na^+ channels are inactivated, which cannot be opened by any stimulus. When the membrane is partly repolarized, there are strong repolarizing forces due to increased potassium conductance (K^+ efflux). Therefore, during this period, only stronger stimuli can increase Na^+ conductance. This period is therefore called relative refractory period.

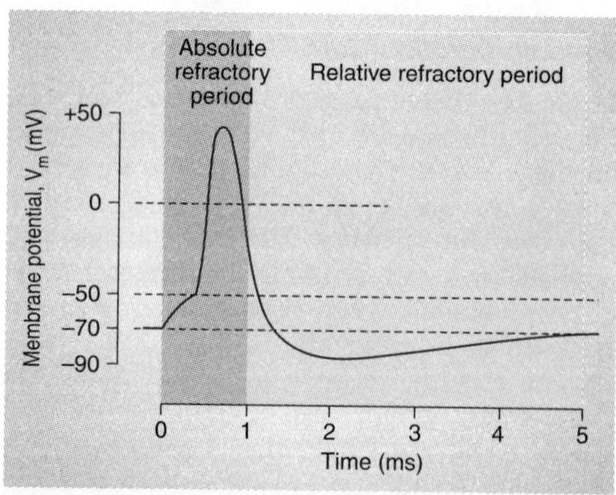

Fig. 20.9: Changes in the excitability of a nerve during an action potential.

2. CONDUCTIVITY

This is another important property of excitable tissues. The action potential (impulse) once generated is propagated (conducted) throughout the length of the neuron. The rate of propagation of the nerve impulse is faster in a myelinated nerve fibre than in unmyelinated nerve fibre.

Propagation of Nerve Impulse

(a) Unmyelinated Nerve Fibre A cell membrane is polarized at rest, i.e. it carries a positive charge outside and negative charge inside the cell membrane. If a threshold stimulus is given at the middle of a nerve fibre (Fig. 20.10), a narrow segment shall undergo an action potential, i.e. transiently, the outer surface becomes negatively charged as compared to the inner surface (segment 'A'). Now the depolarized segment (segment 'A') acts as a current sink for the adjacent segments (segments 'B' and 'C') on either side of segment 'A'. Current is drawn off to such an extent that the membrane potential in segments 'B' and 'C' decreases to the firing level and an action potential is fired in the two segments. By this time, segment 'A' undergoes repolarization. Now, segments 'B' and 'C' act as current sink for segment 'D' and 'E' respectively producing electrotonic depolarization and an action potential. In this fashion, impulse originating at 'A' spreads on either side till it reaches the ends of the nerve fibre. The impulse travels in forward direction only from segment 'A' to 'B', 'B' to 'D'. It cannot come back from segment 'B' to 'A' or from 'C' to 'A' because when segments 'B' and 'C' are undergoing depolarization segment 'A' is in relative refractory period.

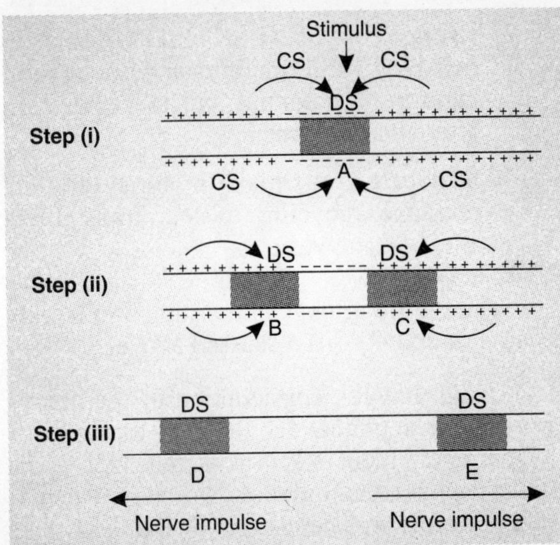

Fig. 20.10: Mode of conduction of a nerve impulse in an unmyelinated nerve fibre. Application of a threshold stimulus at (↓) produces a depolarized segment (DS) (A) which acts as current sink (CS) for the adjacent segments, B and C and electrotonically depolarizes them (Step ii). Segments B and C depolarize segments D and E, respecatively.

In the example given above, the nerve fibre was stimulated artificially in its middle. In the body, an impulse always originates at one end of the neuron and travels to the other end (orthodromic conduction of nerve impulse, see below).

(b) Myelinated Nerve Fibre In the myelinated nerve fibres also, the nerve impulse is propagated basically in the same manner as in unmyelinated nerve fibres, i.e. a depolarized segment produces electrotonic depolarization of the next segment. However, myelin sheath present in these nerve fibres, acts as an effective insulator. Consequently, the action potentials develop at nodes of Ranvier only and one depolarized node of Ranvier causes action potential in the next node of Ranvier and so on (Fig. 20.11). Since the action potential or the impulse jumps from node to node, its propagation is much faster than in unmyelinated nerve fibre. This type of conduction of nerve impulse is known as **saltatory conduction.**

Why the Impulse Jumps from Node to Node? When a given node of Ranvier is depolarized (undergoes action potential), it acts as a current sink for the next node of Ranvier, but has little effect on the internodal segment of the myelinated axon. It may be correlated with the number of voltage-gated Na^+ channels per square μm in various parts of a myelinated axon. The node of

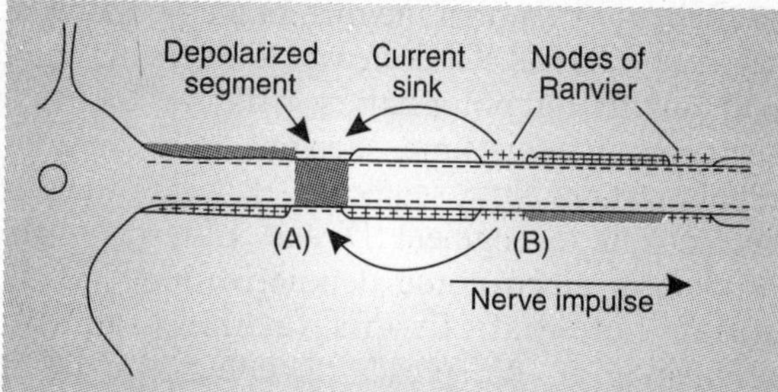

Fig. 20.11: Mode of conduction of a nerve impulse in a myelinated nerve fibre. The depolarized node of Ranvier (A) acting as a current sink depolarizes the next node (B).

20

Ranvier contains 2000 to 12,000 Na^+ channels as compared to less than 25 Na^+ channels over the internodal segments. (At the initial segment of a motor neurons, approximately 350–500 Na^+ channels are present as compared to 50–75 Na^+ channels on the soma; that is why when a motor neuron is excited to threshold level, an impulse is first generated at the initial segment, Chapter 22). The surface of unmyelinated nerve fibres contains approximately 110 Na^+ channels/ square μm area.

Saltatory conduction of nerve impulse is not only up to 50 times faster than in unmyelinated nerve, but also is more energy efficient, since the depolarization and ionic transport occur at each node bypassing the inter-nodal segments of the nerve.

Orthodromic Conduction of Nerve Impulse

Experimentally, a nerve fibre may be stimulated in the middle and the impulse shall travel in both the directions. However, in the intact body, nerve impulse is conducted in one direction only. In the sensory nerve fibre, it is conducted from the sensory receptors towards the cell body (in the dorsal root ganglion). In case of a motor nerve fibre, the impulse travels from the cell body in the CNS towards the skeletal muscle, etc. Such impulse conduction is called *orthodromic conduction* of nerve impulse. Antidromic conduction of nerve impulse (i.e. opposite to the physiological direction) is rare.

In the sensory nerve neuron, the sensory receptor has the lowest threshold of excitation. In the motor neuron, the axon hillock and the initial segment of soma have the lowest threshold of excitation. In the CNS, antidromic conduction of impulse is prevented by one way impulse conduction at the synapses (Chapter 22).

Energy Metabolism of Nervous Tissue

The energy requirements of peripheral nerves and white matter in the central nervous system are rather low. The oxygen consumption of white matter is only 0.2 ml/100 g tissue/min. It may be compared with the oxygen consumption of 3.3 ml/100 g tissue/min in the grey matter. In the soma of a neuron, the high rate of oxygen consumption is related to:

(i) Replacement of intracellular organelles such as mitochondria, Golgi apparatus, ribosomes, etc. (A neuron's lifespan is as long as the individual's lifespan—neurons cannot divide or regenerate).

(ii) Energy cost of Na^+-K^+ ATPase activity involved in the maintenance of resting membrane potential and its restoration after an action potential.

(iii) Synaptic transmission: biosynthesis, reuptake, recycling of neurotransmitters and synaptic vesicles.

In a nerve fiber, oxygen consumption is only because of activity (ii) discussed above.

The high oxygen consumption of the brain's grey matter accounts for the fact that brain's oxygen requirement is approximately 15% of the total oxygen consumption of the body, whereas brain accounts for merely 2% of the total body weight.

Brain cells contain very little glycogen. Therefore their metabolic requirements can be met with only by a continuous supply of glucose from the blood. Nervous tissue accounts for 50–66% of the total glucose utilization in the body.

Action Potentials in a Mixed Nerve

A peripheral nerve contains large number of axons, with varying threshold of stimulation. Myelinated nerve fibres have lower threshold than unmyelinated nerve fibres. A single action potential described above can only be recorded from an individual nerve fibre. If a peripheral nerve is stimulated using a strong stimulus, i.e. stimulus capable of stimulating axons even with highest threshold (= maximal stimulus) and recording electrodes are placed at a distance, an action potential with multiple peaks is recorded (Fig. 20.12). There are three main peaks called 'A', 'B' and 'C'. The peak 'A' consists of four components called α, β, and . The record is called a *compound action potential*. It is produced by summation of individual action potentials of axons with varying conduction velocities. From the site of stimulation, impulses reach the recording electrode sooner in fast conducting fibres and produce the peak 'A'. Peaks 'B' and 'C' are recorded when the impulse reaches the recording electrode through slowly conducting fibres.

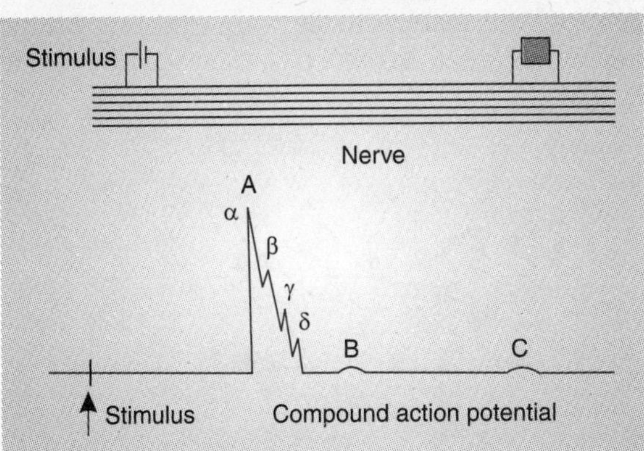

Fig. 20.12: Compound action potential produced by stimulating a mixed nerve containing both myelinated and unmyelinated nerve fibres.

Classification of Nerve Fibres

The number and the amplitude of different peaks in a compound action potential vary in different nerves depending upon the type of nerve fibres present. From the latency value of a particular peak and the distance between the stimulating and recording electrodes, the conduction velocity of the axons responsible for the corresponding peak can be calculated. Based on this principle, mammalian nerve fibres have been classified into groups, A, B and C. Group A nerve fibres are further divided into four subgroups. Aα, Aβ, A and A . The conduction velocity of a nerve fibre is directly proportional to its diameter and degree of its myelination. Type A fibres are thickly myelinated, type B thinly myelinated whereas type C fibres are unmyelinated. The diameters, conduction velocities and functions of different types of nerve fibres are shown in Table 20.2.

Table 20.2: Classification of nerve fibres

Nerve fibre type	*Function*	*Fibre diameter (m)*	*Conduction velocity (m/s)*
A (myelinated)			
α	Proprioception, somatic motor	12–20	70–120
β	Touch, pressure	5–12	30–70
	Motor to muscle spindles	3–6	15–30
	Pain, cold and touch	2–5	12–30
B (myelinated)	Preganglionic autonomic	< 3	3–15
C (unmyelinated)	Post-ganglionic autonomic, pain, temperature	0.3–1.0	< 2.5

Local anaesthesia, hypoxia and pressure can block the conduction of nerve impulses. Relatively, C fibres are more susceptible to the effects of local anaesthetics whereas type A and B fibres are more susceptible to effects of pressure and hypoxia respectively (Table 20.3). Local cooling also decreases conduction velocity

Local Anesthetics These drugs (benzocaine, lignocaine, etc.) produce a reversible blockade of impulses in thin nerve fibres (A and C) carrying pain sensation. Thick nerve fibres (carrying touch or motor impulses) are practically unaffected. Local anesthetics act by blocking fast sodium channels, i.e. inhibiting the process of depolarization. Such drugs can be applied on the skin,

Table 20.3: Susceptibility of nerve fibres to various agents producing conduction block

Agent	*Most susceptible*	*Intermediate*	*Least susceptible*
Hypoxia	B	A	C
Pressure	A	B	C
Local anaesthetic	C	B	A

injected subcutaneously or injected into subarachnoid space via a lumbar puncture.

Sensory nerve fibres are sometimes classified in another manner (Table 20.4).

Table 20.4: Numerical classification of sensory nerve fibres

Type	*Receptor*	*Fibre type*
I a	Muscle spindie (annulospiral endings)	A α
b	Golgi tendon organ	A α
II	Muscle spindle (flower spray ending), pressure, touch	A β
III	Pain, cold, touch	A δ
IV	Pain, temperature	C

NEUROGLIAL CELLS

As mentioned earlier, neuroglial cells are present throughout the central nervous system. Their number is 10–50 times the number of neurons. Though not taking part in conduction of neural signals, the neuroglia play a key role in the normal functioning of the nervous system. Three types of neuroglial cells have been identified: (i) Microglial cells, (ii) Oligodendrogliocytes cells, and (iii) Astrocytes (Fig. 20.13).

Microglial Cells They constitute 20% of the total glial cell population within the brain. These are the scavenger cells of the nervous tissue. Microglia are constantly moving and analyzing the CNS for damaged neurons and infectious agents. These cells are activated by an injury or an inflammatory process. On activation, these cells migrate to the area of tissue damage to become macrophages, and remove the cellular debris.

Microglial cells differentiate from haemopoietic stem cells, which are normally found in the bone marrow. During early development, a group of myeloid progenitor cells travel from the newly formed bone marrow to the brain where they settle and differentiate. In other tissues, macrophages are

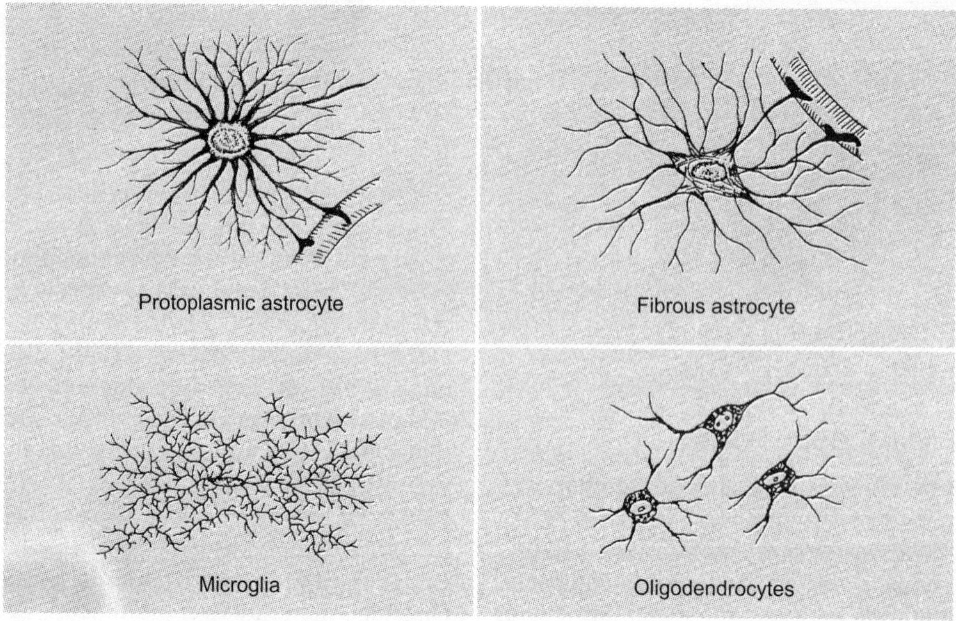

Fig. 20.13: The neuroglial cells.

constantly being used up and replaced by myeloid progenitor cells which differentiate into the needed type. Due to the blood-brain barrier, it is difficult for the body to replace microglia from the bone marrow stem cells. They maintain their status quo while in their quiescent state in the CNS. When activated, they rapidly proliferate in order to keep their numbers up. Activated microglia become large macrophages and remove cellular debris and microbes.

Oligodendrogliocytes They are so called because they possess very few cytoplasmic processes. They are responsible for the formation and maintenance of myelin sheath around the axons in the central nervous system. (In the peripheral nerves, this function is served by Schwann cells). A single oligodendrocyte can extend to up to 50 axons, wrapping around approximately 1 mm of each and forming the myelin sheath; Schwann cells, on the other hand, can only wrap around 1 axon.

Astrocytes They have small cell bodies but have extensively branching processes extending in all directions. Astrocytes are found throughout the CNS and appear to produce substances that are tropic to the neurons. Astrocytes can also take up K^+ and neurotransmitters like glutamate and GABA released into the interstitial fluid by neural activity (Chapter 22).

Thus, astrocytes help to maintain appropriate composition of the interstitial fluid in the CNS. Some processes of the astrocytes are present in close apposition to the cerebral capillaries to form "end feet" and seem to have an important role in the genesis of blood-brain barrier.

Astrocyte Neuron Lactate Shuttle Since long, it has been believed that the astrocytes nourish the neurons, but the mechanism was not clear. Recent researches have revealed the role of astrocytes in the energy metabolism of the neurons (Fig. 20.14). Glucose is the chief substrate for energy production in the nervous system. Glucose entering the neurons directly seems to be sufficient only for its metabolism at rest. At times of increased neuronal activity, the extra energy requirements are met with the help of lactate produced by anaerobic metabolism in the

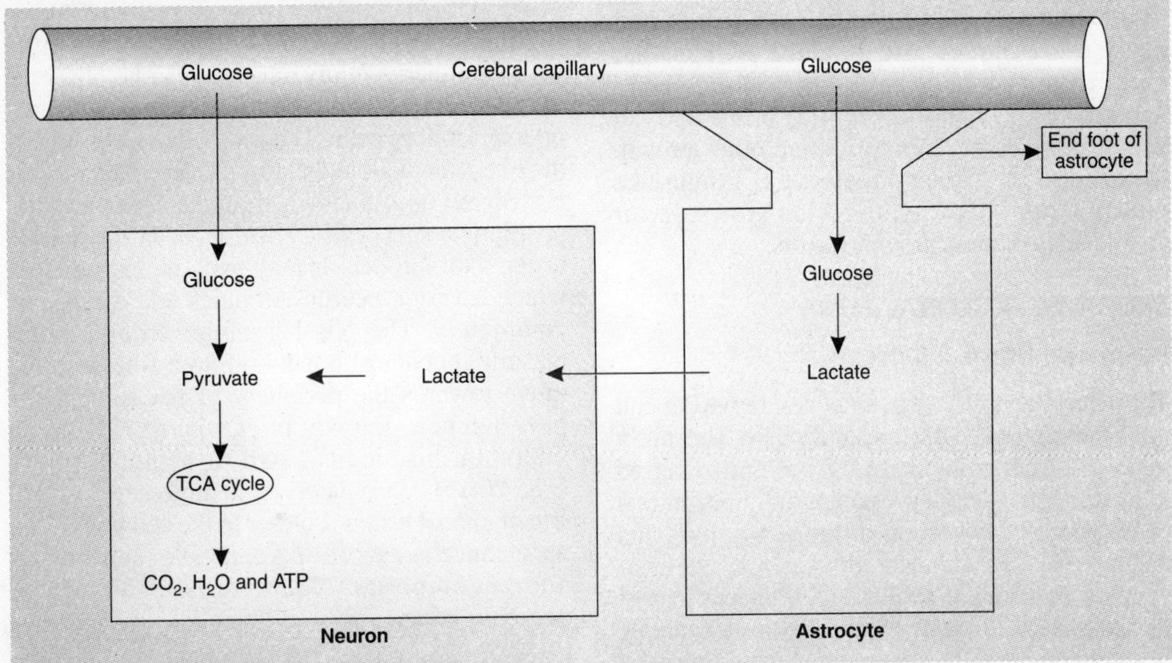

Fig. 20.14: The astrocyte neuron lactate shuttle.

astrocytes. Lactate is transferred from the astrocytes to the nearby neuron, where it is metabolized in the aerobic citric acid cycle to yield a large amount of energy (ATPs). It may be added here that neurons cannot utilize *blood lactate* because lactate does not pass through the blood-brain barrier.

NEUROTROPINS

This name is given to a group of proteins necessary for the survival and growth of neurons. Some of them are synthesized by extraneuronal structures innervated by the neurons, e.g. skeletal muscle innervated by α-motor neurons and tissues innervated by autonomic neurons. Other neurotropins are produced by the astrocytes. From the non-neural tissues, neurotropins are taken up by endocytosis at the nerve terminals and transported to the soma by axonal retrograde transport mechanism.

Nerve growth factor (NGF) was the first neurotropin to be isolated. It is necessary for growth and maintenance of autonomic sympathetic ganglia as well as somatic dorsal root ganglia. A high concentration of NGF has been found in the submandibular salivary glands but, many other tissues also produce NGF. Other neurotropins which have been isolated are neurotropin 3, neurotropin 4/5, brain-derived neurotropic factor (BDNF). Some other growth factors also act as neurotropins, e.g. insulin-like growth factor 1 (IGF-1), fibroblast growth factor and platelet-derived growth factors.

EFFECTS OF NEURONAL INJURY

Peripheral Nerve Injuries

The effects of injury to a peripheral nerve depend upon the degree and the type of damage. The injury may vary from mild pressure for a limited period to crush injury (leaving endoneurial tubes intact) or even complete section of the nerve involving axons as well as endoneurial tubes.

Mild Pressure It results in a transient loss of function only. *Saturday night palsy* is an example of such a problem. This name is given to a transient palsy of radial nerve in a patient who, after a bout of heavy drinking, (common in the West on Saturday nights), sleeps with his/her upper arm resting on the side arm of a chair. The overnight pressure on the radial nerve, where it winds around the humerus, causes anoxic damage to the nerve. The anoxic damage chiefly affects the thick myelinated motor fibres and sensory fibres carrying touch sensation. Pain sensation carried by thin fibres remains relatively intact. The result is a *wrist drop*, along with a feeling of *numbness and tingling and pain in the forearm* in the distribution of radial nerve. The patients recover within a few days without any treatment.

If the nerve has been **crushed or severed**, degenerative changes can be observed not only in the whole length of the axon distal to the site of injury, but also in the cell bodies of the involved axons. These changes are known as Wallerian degeneration.

Wallerian Degeneration

In Wallerian degeneration, changes can be observed both in the soma as well as the axon.

1. *Soma*

Stage of Degeneration Within a few days after peripheral nerve injury, changes can be observed in the soma (cell body) of dorsal root ganglia and/or anterior horn cells. The cell body swells up and may become double the normal size. The nucleus also swells up and moves from the normal central position to an eccentric position, usually opposite to the axon hillock. It may even be extruded, in which case the neuron atrophies and disappears completely. The Nissl granules (rough endoplasmic reticulum) break up into a fine dust and move towards the periphery of the soma. This phenomenon, known as *chromatolysis*, is an important histological sign of neuronal injury (Fig. 20.15). Chromatolysis is more severe if the site of axonal lesion is closer to the cell body. Disappearance of neurofibrils and Golgi apparatus is another important characteristic feature of neuronal injury.

Stage of Regeneration Unless the nucleus has been extruded, the repair begins at about 20 days

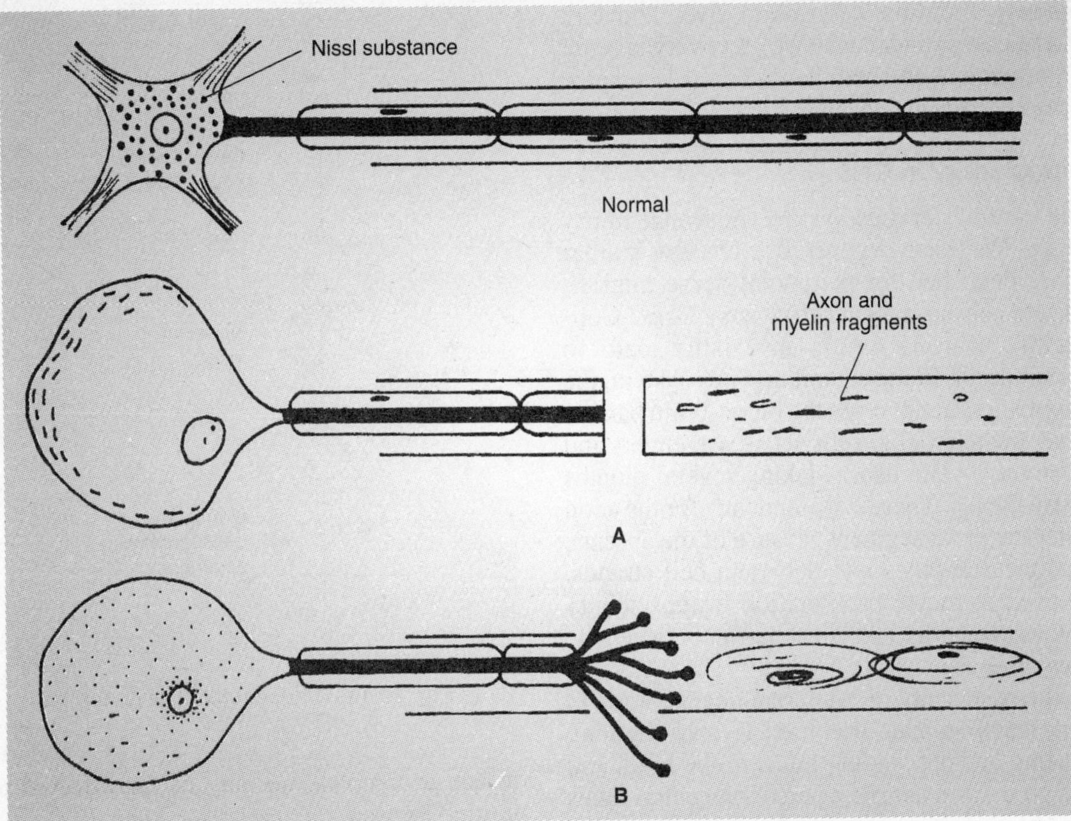

Fig. 20.15: Wallerian degeneration (A) and regeneration (B).

after the injury, and completed in nearly 80 days. The Nissl granules, neurofibrils and Golgi apparatus reappear. The cell regains the normal size. The nucleus returns to its central position.

2. Axon

In the axon, a stage of degeneration lasting about 30 days is followed by stage of regeneration lasting several months to one year.

Stage of Degeneration Distal to the site of injury, the axon and the myelin sheath initially breakup and subsequently degenerate completely (Fig. 20.15). The macrophages of the endoneurium remove the cytoplasmic debris by phagocytosis. The changes become apparent about one week after injury and continue over the next one to two months.

Stage of Regeneration The macrophages and Schwann cells play a crucial role in the regeneration of severed peripheral nerves. The macrophages induce the proliferation of Schwann cells. Moreover, macrophages secrete interleukin-1, which causes synthesis of nerve growth factor and many other neurotropic factors in the actively dividing Schwann cells. The Schwann cells multiply and fill the endoneurial tubes. Further, the central end of the axon begins to elongate and extend into endoneurial tubes at the rate of 2–3 mm per day (Fig. 20.15). If the nerve has been severed, the central axons elongate and extend towards the distal end more slowly. They are guided by the strands of Schwann cells into the distal endoneurial tubes.

Eventually, each endoneurial tube contains an axon extending up to the muscle fibre or sensory receptor, as the case may be. Gradually, the fibre diameter increases to the original size. If the target tissue is not reached, the neuron atrophies completely. From the description given above, it would be easy to understand why recovery is better when a nerve is crushed than when it is severed and the cut ends are separated.

Neuronal Injury in CNS

In the central nervous system, neuronal injury produces Wallerian degenerative changes similar to those described for peripheral nerve injuries, but there are *no regenerative processes*. Consequently neuronal injury invariably leads to neuronal death. In the central nervous system, the macrophages cannot cross the blood-brain barrier. Instead, the microglial cells act as scavengers and remove the myelin debris, taking several months to finish the job. There is no tendency for the axon to enter the distal segment because of the absence of endoneurial tubes and Schwann cell strands. Moreover, astrocyte proliferation in the vicinity of the lesion acts as a physical barrier between the two cut ends.

In the past, study of Wallerian degeneration in experimental animals was used to map the long ascending and descending tracts in the brain and spinal cord. For example, a part of precentral gyrus was destroyed. A few weeks later serial sections of the brain and spinal cord were stained with Weighert's stain. Normal myelinated fibers were stained dark brown leaving pale non-stained areas of degenerating myelin in the tracts affected by the lesion. In this way, the course of pyramidal tracts could be traced. Nowadays, more sophisticated techniques (autoradiography, electrophysiological methods, etc.) are used to trace the tracts.

Transneuronal Degeneration

In the nervous system, the neurons are typically arranged as a series of cells, inter-communicating with each other at synapses. If a neuron is injured, it shows degenerative changes described above. In some cases, similar changes may be observed in another neuron making a synapse with the injured neuron. The degenerative change observed in non-injured neuron is called transneuronal degeneration (Fig. 20.16) or trans-synaptic degeneration. Transneuronal changes are usually mild and reversible but may be serious enough to cause complete atrophy of the affected non-injured neuron.

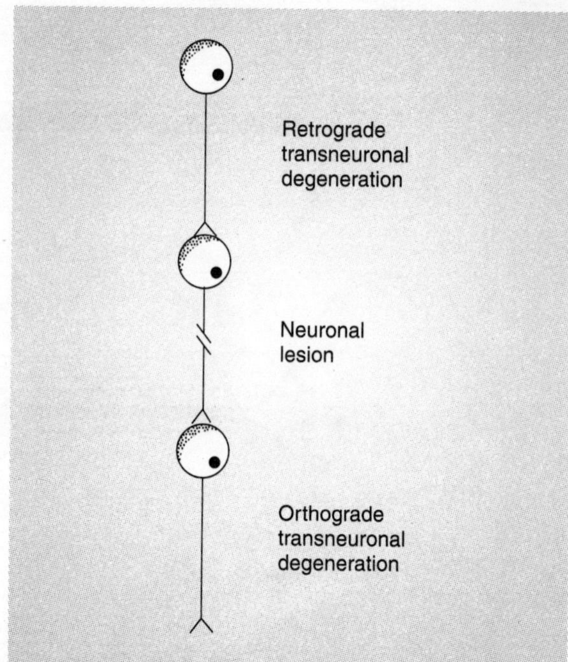

Fig. 20.16: Transneuronal degeneration.

Transneuronal degeneration may *be orthograde* or *retrograde*. The term orthograde transneuronal degeneration is used when degeneration changes occur in non-injured neuron which receives synapse from injured neuron. Degenerative changes in a neuron which makes a synapse with an injured neuron is called retrograde transneuronal degeneration (Fig. 20.16). Transneuronal degeneration is classically observed in visual tracts. A lesion of visual cortex results in degeneration of lateral geniculate body or even retinal ganglion cells (retrograde degeneration). Similarly, optic nerve lesion may produce degeneration in the lateral geniculate body (orthograde degeneration).

The atrophy of skeletal muscle due to a motor neuronal (lower motor neuron) lesion is also an example of transneuronal degeneration.

The reason for transneuronal degeneration is not clear. It may be due to absence of a tropic substance released by the synaptic terminals or by the target tissues.

CHAPTER 21

The Muscle Physiology

Muscle, like neurons, is an excitable tissue but is characterized by the fact that a mechanical contraction follows an action potential. Three types of muscular tissues can be recognized, namely, the skeletal muscle, the cardiac muscle and the smooth muscle. Skeletal muscles are generally under voluntary control. They contract in response to stimulation by a nerve. Cardiac muscle and smooth muscle, on the other hand, are not under voluntary control. They can contract spontaneously.

SKELETAL MUSCLE

Skeletal muscle constitutes nearly 40% of the total body mass. As the name implies, the skeletal muscles are concerned with movement of bones of the skeleton. Most of the skeletal muscles begin and end in fibrous tendons.

A skeletal muscle is made up of numerous skeletal muscle fibres. Each muscle fibre is a long cylindrical multinucleated single cell. Each muscle fibre is surrounded by a membranous sarcolemma which insulates it from the adjacent fibres. Each muscle fibre contains up to several thousand myofibrils, stacked longitudinally throughout the length of the muscle fibre (Fig. 21.1).

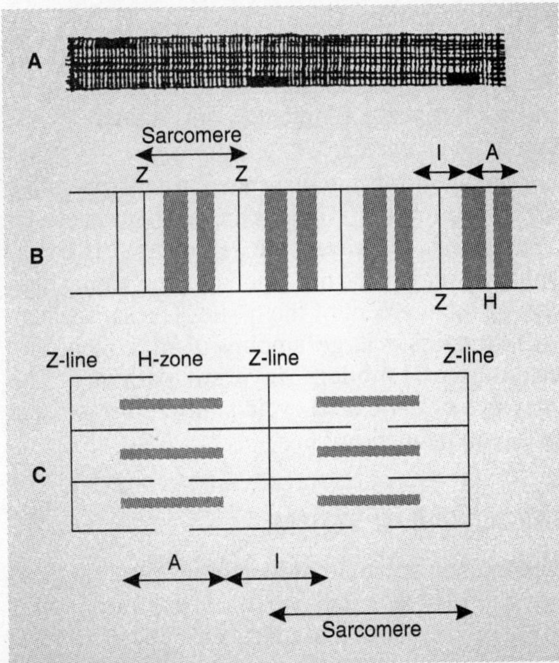

Fig. 21.1: Structure of a skeletal muscle cell (fibre) under ordinary microscope (A), under phase-contrast microscope (B) and under electron microscope (C).

A characteristic feature of skeletal muscle fibre is the well-developed cross-striations. Cross-striations are produced by a difference in the refractive index in the different parts of myofibrils. Some components are *isotropic* while others are *anisotropic* to polarized light. These components, visible as light and dark bands of the myofibrils, are known as *I-bands* and *A-bands* respectively.

Since I-bands and A-bands of adjacent myofibrils are in register with each other, the cross- striations seem to run across the muscle fibre. At a higher magnification, the I-bands are seen to be divided by dark Z-lines and the dark A-bands have lighter H-zones in their centre (Fig. 21.1). The area between two adjacent Z-lines is called a *sarcomere*, which constitutes a unit of skeletal muscle.

Under an electron microscope, each myofibril is seen to contain about *1,500 thick myosin filaments* and *3,000 thin actin filaments*. Actin and myosin filaments partly interdigitate. The light I-bands contain only thin filaments. The dark A-band is seen where myosin filaments are overlapped by actin filaments. When the muscle is relaxed, the actin filaments attached to the opposite Z-lines do not meet each other and a small gap is left where the actin filaments do not overlap the myosin filaments. The gap is seen as H-zone.

Cross-section of a sarcomere shows that the thick myosin filaments are arranged hexagonally and each myosin filament is surrounded by six thin actin filaments.

The myofibrils are suspended in a matrix called *sarcoplasm*, which contains the usual intracellular constituents. However, the sarcoplasm is extraordinarily rich in the mitochondria; indicating high energy requirement of the tissue. The sarcoplasm also contains a large amount of glycogen, and enzymes of Embden-Meyerhof pathway. The enzymes of citric acid cycle pathway are present in the mitochondria.

SARCOTUBULAR SYSTEM

The sarcoplasm contains membranous tubular and vesicular structures surrounding individual myofibrils. These structures constitute the sarcotubular system. It consists of a *T-system* and *sarcoplasmic reticulum* (Fig. 21.2).

The T-system consists of transverse tubules which surround each myofibril at each junction of A- and I-bands, i.e. there are two T-tubules in each sarcomere. The T-tubules are extensions of the sarcolemma and their lumens are in continuity with the extracellular fluid. The T-tubules provide a means of quick transmission of electrical signals (impulses) from the surface of the muscle cell to each sarcomere.

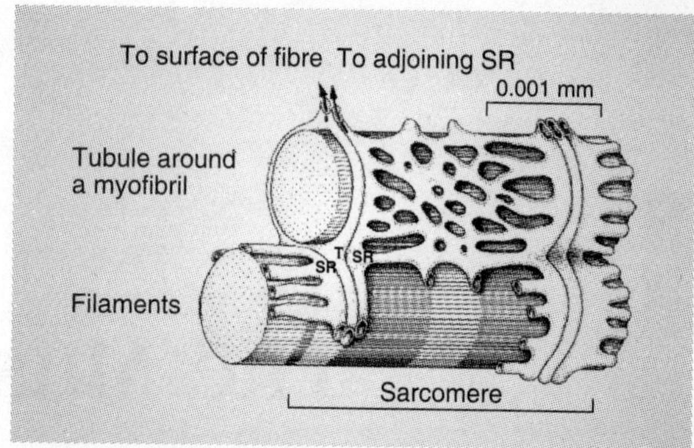

Fig. 21.2: The sarcotubular system. T = Transverse tubules; SR = Sarcoplasmic reticulum.

The sarcoplasmic reticulum (smooth surfaced endoplasmic reticulum) also surrounds the myofibrils. The sarcoplasmic reticulum extends between two T-tubules in a longitudinal fashion. The sarcoplasmin reticulum consists of two portions: central longitudinal portion and enlarged terminal cisterns close to the T-tubes. There is no continuity between the T-tubes and the adjacent terminal cisterns (Fig. 21.3). The sarcoplasmic reticulum is concerned with calcium transport in the sarcomere.

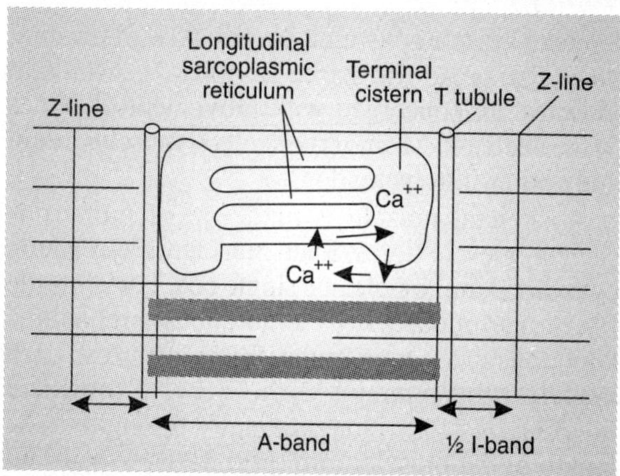

Fig. 21.3: The sarcotubular system. Diagrammatic illustration to show details of sarcoplasmic reticulum and Ca^{++} fluxes during muscular contraction.

Electrical Properties of Skeletal Muscle

Basically, the electrical properties of skeletal muscle are similar to those of a neuron except for some quantitive differences:

1. The resting membrane potential in the skeletal muscle fibre is approximately –90 mV (cf–70 mV in a nerve fibre).
2. The duration of the spike potential is longer, i.e. nearly 5 ms (cf. 1 ms in the nerve fibre).
3. The excitability of the muscle is far less than that of a neuron.
4. The conduction velocity of the action potentials in the skeletal muscle is 3–5 m/s. (In myelinated nerve fibre it can be as high as 120 m/s.)

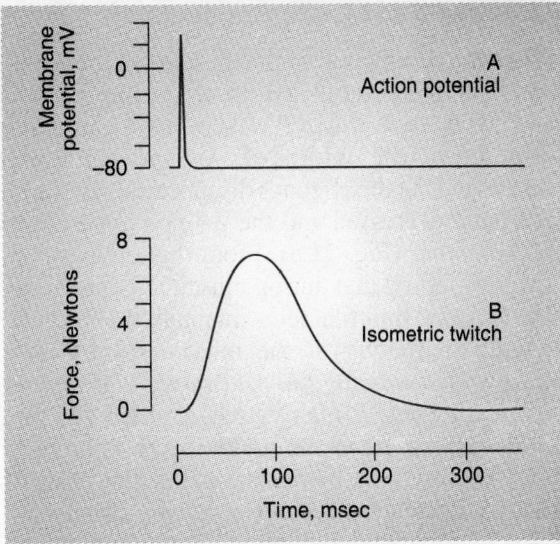

Fig. 21.4: The electrical response (action potential) (A) and the mechanical response (B) of a skeletal muscle following a stimulus.

Mechanical Properties of Skeletal Muscle

The action potential in a skeletal muscle is followed approximately 2 ms later by a brief contraction. This brief contraction following a single stimulus constitutes a *muscle twitch*. Using suitable mechanical levers, the shortening (contraction) of the muscle can be recorded on a kymograph. In Fig. 21.4, the electrical and mechanical events recorded separately have been plotted on the same time scale in order to demonstrate the relation between the two events. The duration of the twitch varies with the type of muscle being tested (see fast and slow muscles).

EXCITATION OF SKELETAL MUSCLE BY A NERVE

Excitation Contraction Coupling

The process by which depolarization of a muscle fibre initiates its contraction is known as excitation contraction coupling. In the body, the skeletal muscles are excited by large myelinated (Aα) motor nerve fibres. In each muscle fibre, a single nerve terminal ends on a specialized part of the sarcolemma called the motor end plate. The junction between the nerve terminal and the motor end plate (neuromuscular junction) is usually situated in the middle of the muscle fibre. Therefore, the action potential from the nerve terminal spreads first to the motor end plate, and then spreads in both directions all over the sarcolemma.

From the sarcolemma, the action potential spreads to each sarcomere through the T-tubules of the sarcotubular system. In this way, all the sarcomeres of the muscle fibre are stimulated almost simultaneously.

The action potential spreads from the T-tubules to the adjacent terminal cisterns of sarcoplasmic reticulum, and cause a rapid release of Ca^{2+} from the cisternal lumen into sarcoplasm. Calcium ions diffuse into the myofibrils, leading to contraction of each sarcomere and hence shortening of the muscle. The muscle would remain contracted as long as the sarcoplasmic Ca^{2+} concentration is high. However, Ca^{2+} pump, operating at the longitudinal sarcoplasmic reticulum, decreases the Ca^{2+} concentration very quickly and the muscle relaxes. From the longitudinal sarcoplasmic reticulum, Ca^{2+} diffuse to the terminal cisterns, to be stored till another stimulus reaches the T-tubules.

21

Mechanism of Muscle Contraction

When the contraction of the muscle was observed under a phase-contrast microscope, it was observed that during contraction, in each sarcomere, the width of A-band remained unchanged but the H-zones disappeared, the width of I-band decreased and the Z-lines came closer to each other (Fig. 21.5). From this observation, it was proposed that during muscular contraction, the thick and thin filaments maintain their normal length. Shortening of the muscle results from *sliding of the actin filaments over the myosin filaments*. Some further details of thick and thin filaments as well as the various muscle proteins must be described before the molecular basis of sliding-filaments mechanism can be discussed.

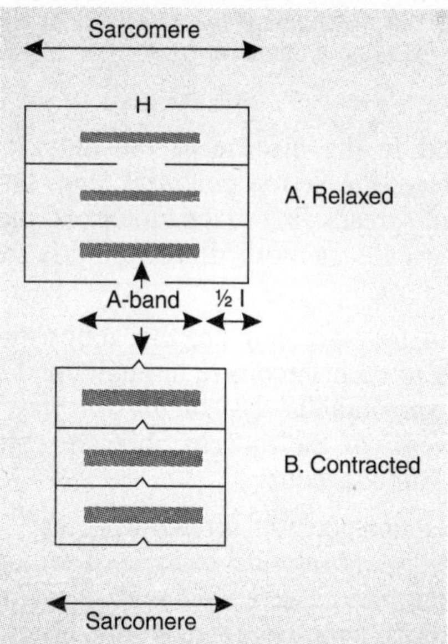

Fig. 21.5: The effect of contraction of skeletal muscle on A- and I-bands. A-band remains constant but the H-zone disappears; the width of I-band decreases.

Muscle Proteins and Filaments

Thick Filaments

Each thick filament is made up of about 200 **myosin molecules**. Each myosin molecule consists of two identical polypeptide chains forming a tail and a globular protein forming the headpiece. The myosin molecules are bundled together into the thick filaments in such a way that middle of the filament contains only the tails whereas the heads protrude out of the outer parts of the filament in a spiral arrangement around the filaments (Fig. 21.6). With this arrangement, the heads of the thick (myosin) filament can make contact with all the six actin filaments surrounding it, by forming crossbridges. The orientation of the heads at the two ends of the myosin filament is also in the opposite direction to each other. Besides the capacity to bind the actin filaments, another important feature of myosin head is that it can act as *ATPase enzyme*.

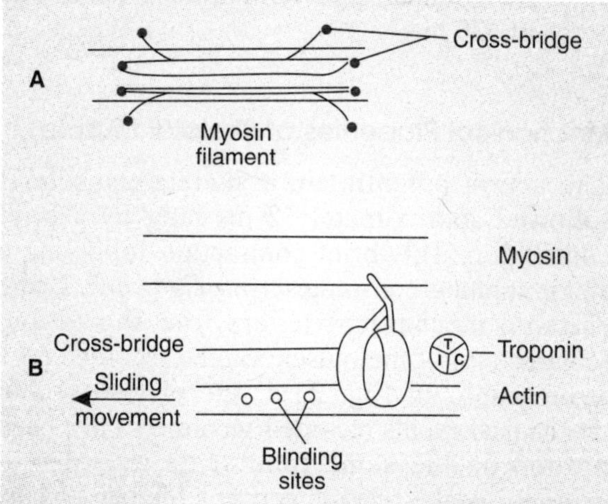

Fig. 21.6: (A) The myosin filament. The heads of the myosin molecules protrude out as cross-bridges. (B) Mechanism of muscle contraction: combination of Ca^{++} with troponin exposes the binding sites on actin filament, myosin cross-bridges attach to the binding sites and bend inwards leading to sliding movement of actin filaments.

Thin Filaments

The thin filament consists of three proteins, the ***actin***, ***tropomyosin*** and ***troponin***. The main body of the thin filament (actin filament) is made up of a double strand of F-actin protein molecule. One end of the actin filament is inserted into Z-disc while the other free end lies in the space between the myosin filaments. At regular intervals, actin filament possesses binding sites for the myosin heads.

In vitro actin molecules exist in two forms: G-actin and F-actin. *G-actin* is a monomeric globular protein with a molecular weight of 46,000. Each monomer contains binding sites for other actin monomers and for myosin, tropomyosin, troponin-I and ATP. *F-actin* is a fibrous polymer, consisting of approximately 300 monomers of G-actin. Thin filament of a sarcomere consists of two strands of F-actin polymers, intertwined in the conformation of a double stranded helix (Fig. 21.7).

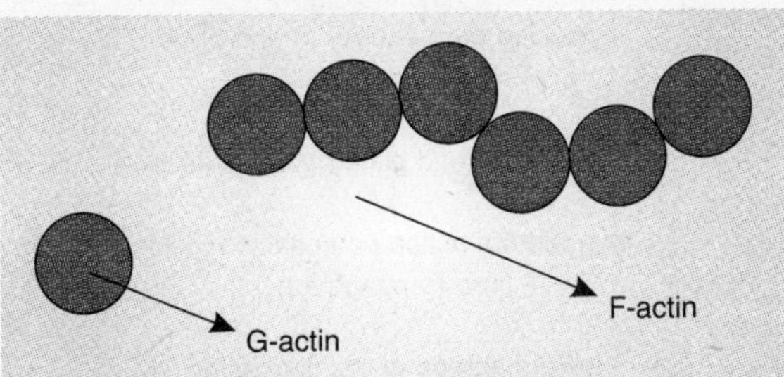

Fig. 21.7: Structure of G-actin and F-actin.

Tropomyosin molecules are polymerized into protein strands that are coiled along the F-actin strands. In resting state, tropomyosin strands cover the binding sites of actin filaments for myosin.

Troponin is a large globular protein consisting of 3 subunits: troponin-I, troponin-T and troponin-C, having strong affinity for actin, tropomyosin and Ca^{2+} respectively. Troponin units are located at intervals along the tropomyosin strands and bound to them by troponin T-subunits. Troponin I is strongly bound to actin and therefore tropomyosin strands are held close to the actin strands.

Sliding Filament Theory of Muscle Contraction

The contraction of the skeletal muscle is initiated by the spread of an action potential from the nerve to the sarcolemma, and then through T-tubules to the terminal cisterns. The Ca^{2+} released from the terminal cisterns bind with troponin-C. The troponin C-Ca^{2+} complex undergo a conformational change leading to lateral displacement of tropomyosin strand (Fig. 21.8).

As a result, the binding sites on the actin filaments are exposed. The myosin heads attach to these exposed binding sites on the actin filaments, forming cross-bridges which bend immediately. The ATP attached to the cross-bridge splits into ADP and energy released is used for mechanical bending of the cross-bridges. *The inward bending of the cross-bridges produces sliding of actin filaments inwards.* Almost

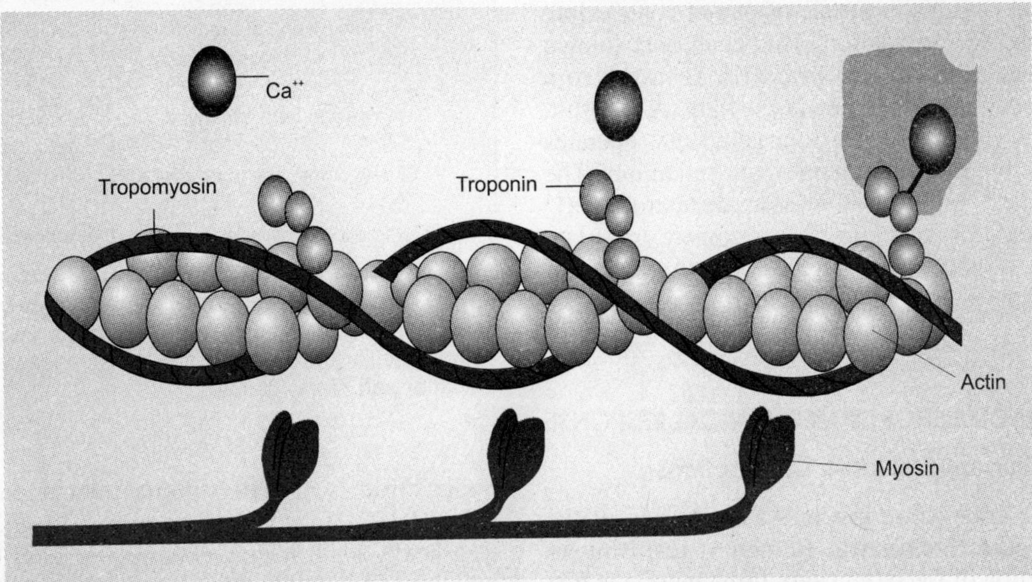

Fig. 21.8: Actin myosin sliding mechanism.

immediately the myosin heads bind another ATP molecule, release actin filament and return to the perpendicular position with respect to the tail of the myosin filament. The cycle of binding, bending, and release is repeated once again. As long as the sarcoplasm contains Ca^{2+}, the process is repeated until the sliding movements of actin filaments bring the Z-lines closer and the muscle shortens. The sequence of events leading to contraction of skeletal muscle is summarized in Fig. 21.9.

Within a few milliseconds after Ca^{2+} release, the Ca-pump operating at the surface of the longitudinal sarcoplasmic reticulum lowers the sarcoplasmic of Ca^{2+} conc. to such an extent that the interaction between actin and myosin filaments stops and the muscle *relaxes* once again.

ATP is consumed not only to produce contraction but also to produce relaxation of the skeletal muscle. Energy is required for mechanical bending of the cross-bridges to produce contraction and for active transport of Ca^{2+} by the longitudinal sarcoplasmic reticulum to produce relaxation.

Experimentally, in vitro, if a muscle is repeatedly stimulated, soon the force of contraction begins to decline. In addition, the muscle fails to relax completely after each contraction. Thus, it remains in a state of partial contraction, without any stimulation. This condition, known as *physiological contracture,* results from deficiency of ATP in the muscle fibre. As a result, there is a failure of calcium pump that operates at the longitudinal sarcoplasmic reticulum. The sustained high level of sarcoplasmic Ca^{++} concentration maintains the sarcomere in a state of sustained contraction. This experiment highlights the role of ATP in relaxation of the muscle.

Stimulation of motor neuron
↓
Impulse reaching motor nerve ending
↓
Inflow of Ca^{2+} into end feet
↓
Release of ACh from microvesicles
↓
Diffusion of ACh into synaptic cleft
↓
Binding of ACh to receptors on the motor end-plate
↓
Increased permeability of end-plate membrane to Na^+
↓
Generation of end plate potential (local)
↓
Generation of action potential in muscle fibre (propagated)
↓
Inward spread of depolarization along T-tubules
↓
Release of Ca^{2+} from terminal cisterns
↓
Diffusion of Ca^{2+} into sarcoplasm
↓
Binding of Ca^{2+} to troponin C
↓
Uncovering of the binding sites for myosin on actin
↓
Crosslinkage between myosin head and actin
↓
Sliding of thin filaments over thick filaments
↓
Contraction of muscle (mechanical response)

Fig. 21.9: Sequence of events leading to contraction of skeletal muscle (The initial 8 steps involving neuromuscular transmission are described in detail in the latter part of this chapter.)

CHARACTERISTICS OF MECHANICAL RESPONSE

Isometric and Isotonic Contractions

Muscle contraction involves a shortening of the sarcomere (contractile elements) resulting in generation of force (tension). If the muscle is free to shorten, e.g. attached to a small load, the contraction is called *isotonic* (same tension) (Fig. 21.10). However, if the muscle is attached to a heavy load, it may contract, develop larger amount of tension but may be unable to shorten. Such a contraction is called *isometric* (same

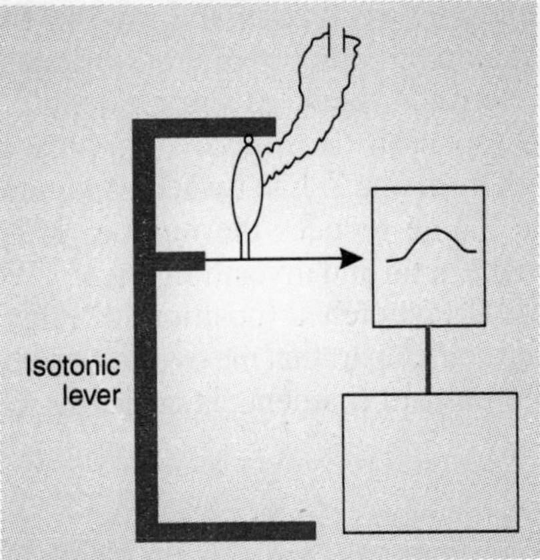

Fig. 21.10: Arrangement for recording an isotonic contraction of a skeletal muscle. The isotonic lever allows free shortening of the muscle.

length) (Fig. 21.11). In this case, the contraction of the contractile elements of the muscle is accompanied by a stretch of its elastic elements (Fig. 21.12). It may be remembered that the skeletal muscle consists of actin and myosin filaments constituting the contractile component, sarcolemma constituting the parallel elastic component; and tendons constituting the series elastic component.

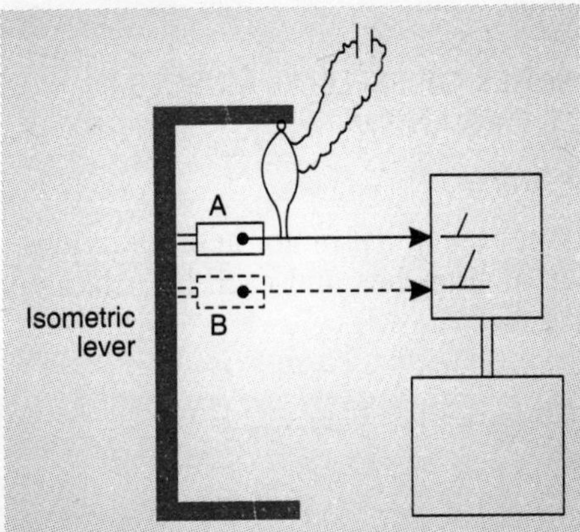

Fig. 21.11: Arrangement for recording isometric contraction of a skeletal muscle. The isometric lever does not allow the muscle to shorten but the tension developed during contraction can be recorded. By shifting the position of isometric lever (e.g. to B), the length of the muscle can be varied and at each length, tension developed can be recorded.

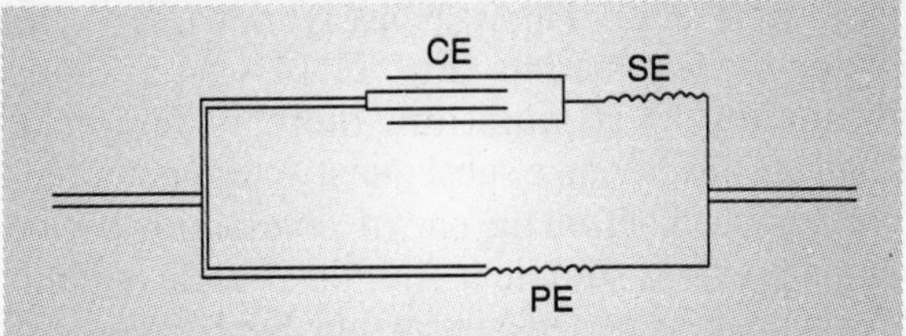

Fig. 21.12: Diagrammatic representation of different components of skeletal muscle. CE = Contractile elements, PE = Parallel elastic elements, SE = Series elastic elements.

In the intact body, lifting a weight off the ground shall involve isotonic contraction of the biceps, and other flexors of the forearm. When the weight is too heavy to be lifted, the effort to lift shall involve isometric contraction of the same group of muscles (Fig. 21.13). Postural muscles also contract isometrically. Since external work is performed during isotonic contraction, greater amount of energy is used than during isometric contraction.

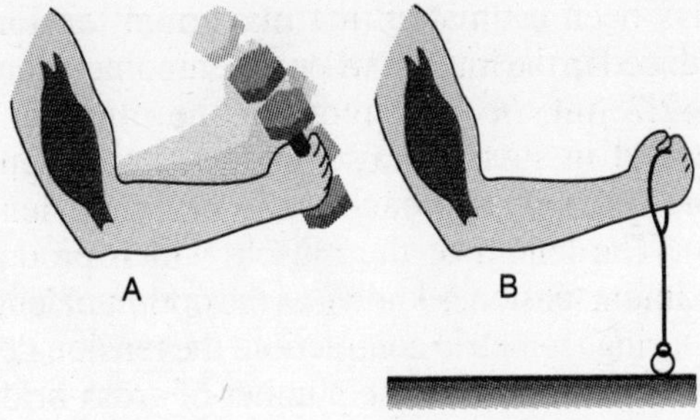

Fig. 21.13: Isotonic (A) and isometric (B) contractions.

Summation of Contractions

The duration of action potential in the skeletal muscle is approximately 5 ms and the refractory period is still shorter. The duration of mechanical response, (simple muscle twitch) is 30–50 ms in mammalian muscle and approximately 100 ms in amphibian muscle. Hence, if the skeletal muscle is stimulated at short intervals, an action potential results with each stimulus, provided each subsequent stimulus falls later than the refractory period of the action potential produced by the previous stimulus. Each action potential results in a mechanical response, i.e. contraction of the muscle. At slower rate of stimulation, the muscle undergoes repetitive contractions separated by partial relaxation. This response is known as *partial* or *incomplete tetanus* (Fig. 21.14). At a higher frequency of stimulation, there is fusion of contractions because subsequent action potentials are produced before the end of contraction period of the previous stimulus. Thus the muscle remains in a state of sustained contraction. Such a response is known as *complete tetanus* (Fig. 21.14). The tension produced during a tetanic response is greater (approximately 4 times) than that produced in simple muscle twitch.

Length Tension Relationship

21

When a muscle is taken out of the body, it shortens considerably. If it is attached to an isometric lever (Fig. 21.11), the isometric tension at different muscle lengths can be recorded by increasing the distance between the two attachments of the muscle. As the muscle is gradually stretched and stimulated, the tension developed gradually increases to a limit and then declines (Fig. 21.15). It has been estimated that maximum tension is produced in the muscle when the sarcomere length 2.0–2.2 μm. *In vivo*, most of the muscles are attached in such a way that the resting length approximately approaches the optimum length (Lo). The length of the muscle which produces maximum tension is known as the optimum length.

During isometric contraction, the tension develops in proportion to the number of cross-bridges formed between actin and myosin filaments.

The effect of muscle length on the tension produced during contraction can be explained by the sliding filaments theory of muscle contraction (Fig. 21.15). At Lo (position 'a'), there is optimum overlapping between actin and myosin filaments so that maximum number of cross-bridges can be formed between them. At muscle length shorter than Lo (position 'b'), the overlapping of actin filaments from one Z-line by actin filament of the opposite Z-line reduces the number of linkages between the actin and myosin filaments. When the muscle is overstretched (position 'c'), the Z-lines are pulled so far apart that the overlapping between actin and myosin filaments is critically reduced.

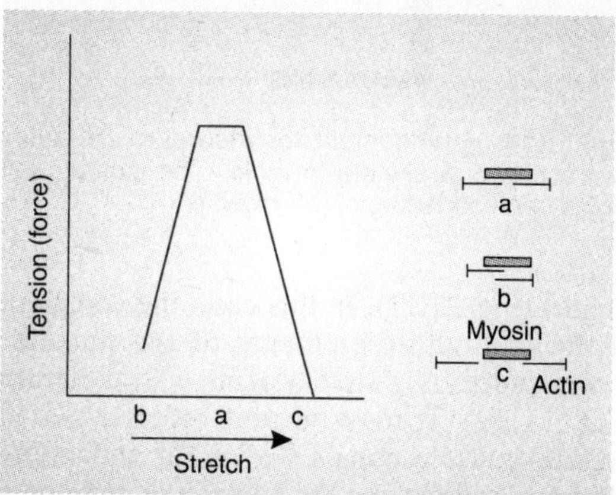

Fig. 21.15: Length: Tension relationship in skeletal muscle. Maximum tension is produced when there is optimum overlapping of actin and myosin filaments (position 'a'). Positions 'b' and 'c' represent under-stretched and overstretched positions of the muscle, respectively.

PROPERTIES OF SKELETAL MUSCLE IN INTACT ORGANISM

Motor Unit

The axon of a spinal motor neuron divides into a number of branches and each branch supplies a

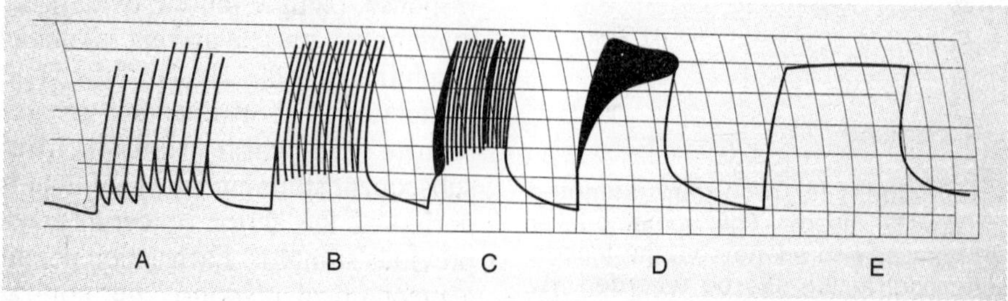

Fig. 21.14: Effect of increase in frequency of stimulation of skeletal muscle. (A) normal contractions and relaxation; (B to D) partial tetanus, (E) complete tetanus.

single muscle fibre. In this way, each motor neuron innervates a number of skeletal muscle fibres. A motor neuron and all the muscle fibres innervated by it constitute a *motor unit*. The number of muscle fibres in a motor unit varies. Muscles involved in fine, graded and precise movements (e.g. those involved in movements of fingers or eyeballs) have only 3–6 muscle fibres in a motor unit (Fig. 21.16). Where only gross movements are required (e.g. muscles of the legs), a motor unit may have as many as 1000 muscle fibres. The muscle fibres of a motor unit are not bunched together. The muscle fibres of different motor units are intermixed so that even when only few motor units are activated, whole of the muscle contracts, though to a mild degree. When more motor units are activated, the muscle gives a stronger pull.

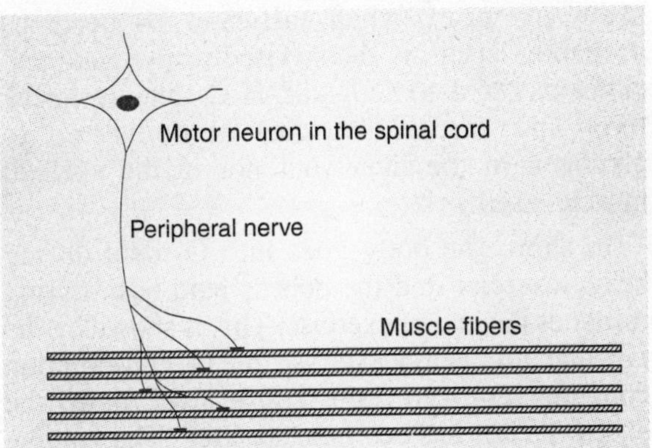

Fig. 21.16: A motor unit.

Fast and Slow Muscles

Different muscles not only vary in the number and the length of the constituent muscle fibres but also in many other features. The diameter of a muscle fibre may vary from 10 to 80 μm. Muscle fibres vary in their ultramicroscopic structure, as well as, in functional properties. Based upon these features, muscle fibres may be classified into 'fast' and 'slow' muscle fibres. Fast muscle fibres have shorter latency and total twitch time than slow muscle fibres (Fig. 21.17).

For example, in mammals, the twitch time is 10 msec, 30 msec, and 100 msec in cases of ocular, gastrocnemius and soleus muscles, respectively. It may be correlated with the fact that these three types of muscles are used for very quick, moderately fast and slow type of movements, respectively.

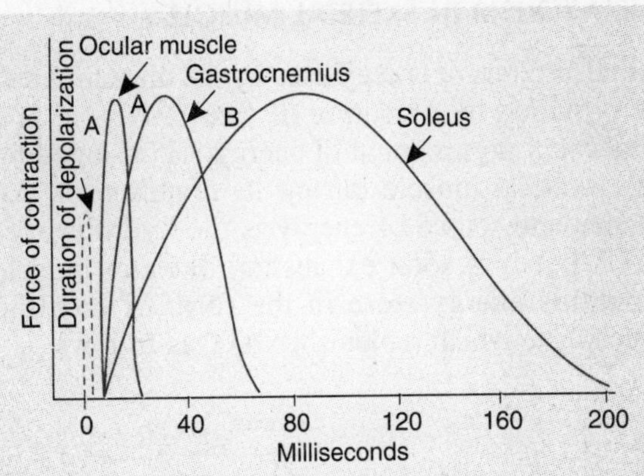

Fig. 21.17: Simple twitch recorded from fast muscles (A) and a slow muscle (B) of a frog.

Fast and slow muscles are also called *white* and *red* muscles respectively, due to greater myoglobin content of the latter. In addition, slow muscles have got larger mitochondrial density than fast muscle fibres. It may be added that no muscle is purely red or white. Muscles like soleus involved in slow postural movements have a larger proportion of slow (red) muscle fibres, whereas those involved in faster movements have a larger proportion of white muscle fibres. (For further details, see Chapter 60).

Gradation of Muscular Power

On different occasions, a skeletal muscle may be required to generate widely different degrees of power. One may lift a pin from a table and the same muscle may be involved in lifting a 10 kg weight. Gradation of muscular power is chiefly achieved by activation (recruitment) of different number of motor units. In addition, an increase in the frequency of discharge in the motor unit also helps to increase the muscular power. However, except during most powerful contractions, muscles are normally stimulated at a subtetanic discharge rate. Asynchronous (out of phase with each other) discharge in different motor units of the muscle helps to convert the jerky response of individual muscle fibres into a smooth pull of the whole muscle.

Human skeletal muscle can produce a maximum tension of 3–4 kg/cm^2 of the muscle, a value common to most of the mammals.

METABOLISM IN SKELETAL MUSCLE

Small amount of energy used by the muscle at rest is provided by oxidation of free fatty acid and glucose. Large amount of energy is consumed by the skeletal muscle during its contraction. An immediate source of energy is the hydrolysis of ATP, but it is soon exhausted. Skeletal muscle contains energy-store in the form of creatine phosphate which replenishes ATP as follows :

$$\text{Creatine phosphate} + \text{ADP} \underset{\text{Rest}}{\overset{\text{Exercise}}{\rightleftharpoons}} \text{(Creatine kinase) creatine} + \text{ATP}$$

Creatine phosphate is limited in amount, and does not allow more than 100 contractions. If the muscle is to contract any further, ATP must be generated by aerobic or anaerobic metabolism of glucose or glycogen.

During contraction, glycogen and glucose (transferred from the blood) are metabolized by glycolytic reactions to pyruvate and finally broken down to CO_2 and H_2O through citric acid cycle. The aerobic citric acid cycle operates when sufficient O_2 is freely available and yields larger amount of energy (38 ATPs for each molecule of glucose). If O_2 is deficient, glucose is metabolised by anaerobic glycolysis to pyruvate, which is reduced to lactic acid, but glycolysis yields only 2 ATPs for each glucose molecule.

Oxygen Debt Mechanism

During heavy exercise, O_2 supply to the muscle may be insufficient for the oxidation of pyruvate in citric acid cycle. Under these conditions, pyruvate is converted to lactate by the following reaction:

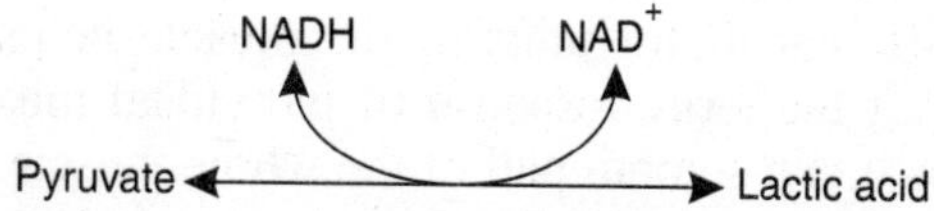

The reaction prevents the accumulation of pyruvate which would inhibit further glycolysis in the series of reversible reactions by the law of mass action. In addition, under anaerobic conditions, a blockade of glycolysis at phosphoglyceraldehyde diphosphoglyceric acid stage is likely to occur since it exhausts available NAD^+ (see Chapter 41). However, as shown above, the reduction of pyruvic acid to lactic acid generates NAD^+ and glycolysis continues. Anaerobic glycolysis generates much smaller amount of energy than the aerobic metabolism of glucose but the chief benefit of the former is that at least for a short period muscular activity can continue even when adequate O_2 is not available.

Lactate produced in the muscle diffuses into the circulation. During recovery (after the end of heavy exercise), when sufficient O_2 becomes available, lactate is reconverted to pyruvate and either oxidised to CO_2 and H_2O (mainly in the liver and cardiac muscle) or converted to glycogen in the liver (but not in the skeletal muscle itself.)

In short, the body goes into O_2 debt during heavy exercise and the debt is paid back during rest after the end of exercise. This is shown by the fact that after heavy exercise, the O_2 consumption does not return to pre-exercise level till all the excess lactate has been metabolised. The volume of O_2 consumed after the end of exercise over and above the pre-exercise consumption level gives the value of O_2 debt (Fig. 21.18).

Heat Production

The efficiency of an engine is calculated as the percentage of energy input that is converted into mechanical work. When the skeletal muscle shortens, only 20–25% of the energy input is converted into muscular work and the rest is wasted as heat. During isometric contraction, no external work is performed and all the energy used by the muscle is converted into heat.

Heat production is increased in the muscle not only during contraction (initial heat), but also for about 30 minutes subsequently (recovery heat).

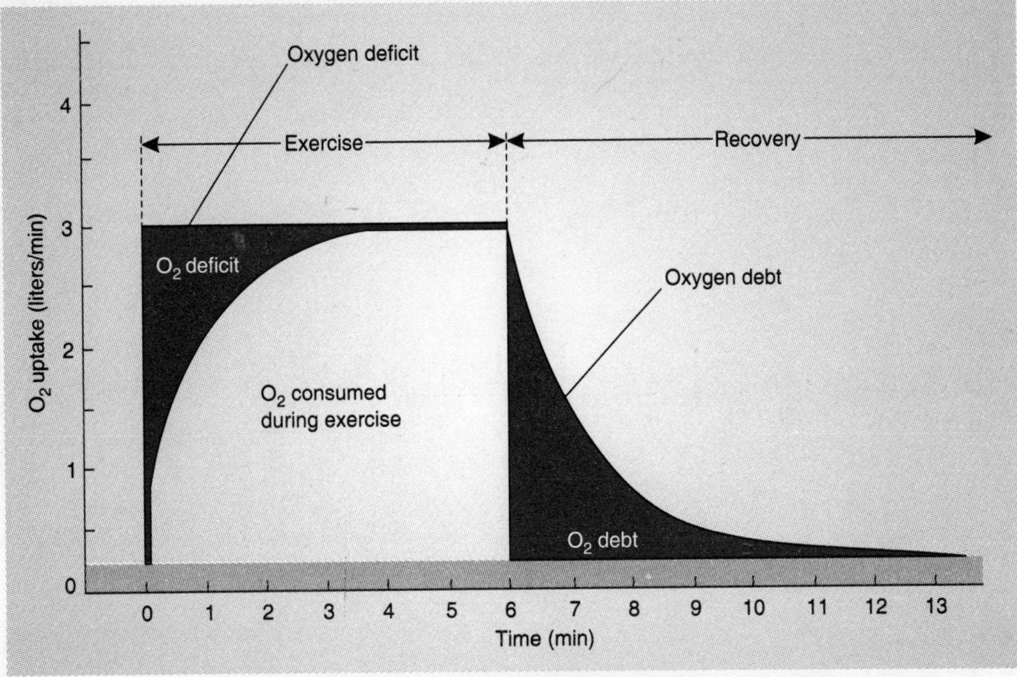

Fig. 21.18: Oxygen debt.

The recovery heat is liberated by the metabolic processes that restore the muscle to the pre-exercise state.

Electromyography

This is a process of recording the electrical activity of a skeletal muscle on a CRO. A surface electrode may be used to pick up the activity of underlying muscle or a needle electrode may be inserted into the muscle to get a more accurate record. The record is called an electromyogram (EMG).

Electromyography is helpful in the diagnosis of many neuromuscular disorders.

Muscle tissue at rest is normally electrically inactive, i.e. a muscle at rest should be electrically silent. When the muscle is voluntarily made to contract, action potentials begin to appear. As the strength of the muscle contraction is increased, more and more muscle fibers produce action potentials. When the muscle is fully contracted, there should appear a disorderly group of action potentials of varying rates and amplitudes (known as the *interference pattern*) (Fig. 21.19A). An EMG of a patient who has myopathic disease shows a decreased amplitude and frequency of action potentials (Fig. 21.19B).

Disuse Atrophy

When a skeletal muscle is not put to use even for a few days, its size and power begin to deteriorate. This change is known as disuse atrophy. The phenomenon of disuse atrophy may be seen when:

(i) A limb is placed in a plaster cast for a few weeks as a treatment for bone fracture.
(ii) Muscle is paralyzed due to damage to its innervation by lower motor neurons (denervation atrophy).

Generalized atrophy of all the limb muscles may occur in:

(a) Chronically bed-ridden patients who do not use their limbs for weight-bearing.
(b) Weightlessness during space flight.

If the muscle function is restored within a few weeks, muscle power and size can be regained by exercise. If the disuse is permanent, e.g. due to

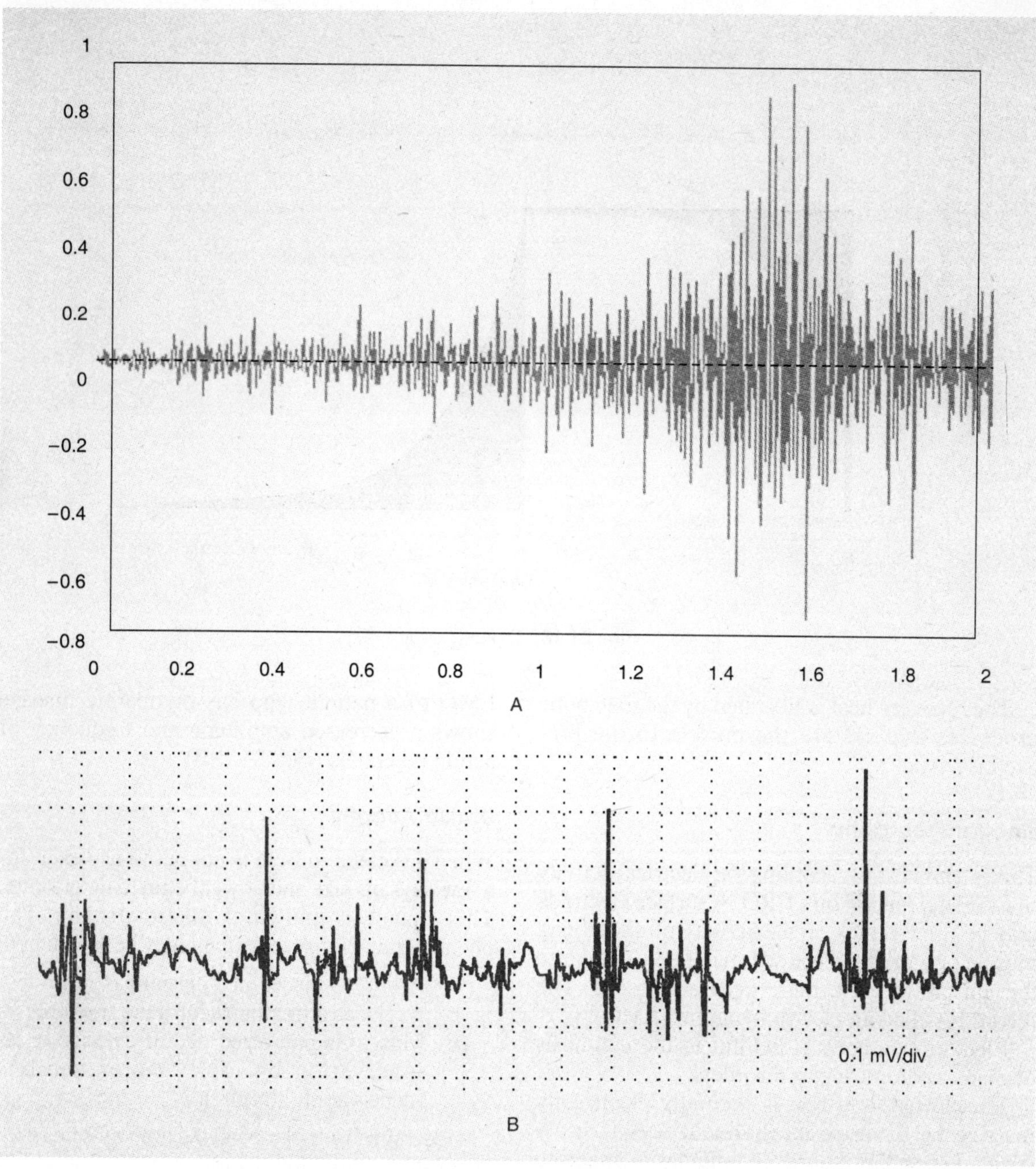

Fig. 21.19: Electromyogram in a normal individual (A) and a patient of myopathy (B).

lower motor neuron paralysis, the muscle fibres are progressively lost and replaced by fibrous tissue. The condition is called *denervation atrophy.* The muscle mass gradually shrinks. This stage is called *muscle wasting.* Further, the fibrous tissue that replaces the muscle fibres has a tendency to shorten progressively (*contracture*) leading to a permanent deformity of the limb.

RIGOR MORTIS

This term is used to describe the permanent shortening and rigidity of skeletal muscles after death. Soon after death, the ATP stores of the skeletal muscle are exhausted. The consequent failure of Ca^{++} pump at the longitudinal sarcoplasmic reticulum increases the cytosolic Ca^{++} concentration that promotes the actin-myosin interaction (sliding). The contraction is irreversible because ATP is not available to undo the actin-myosin interaction, i.e. the myosin heads remain attached to actin filaments in an abnormal and fixed manner. About 24–72 hours later, the rigidity begins to disappear when the muscle fibres decompose and disintegrate due to release of lysosomal enzymes from the muscle fibres.

SMOOTH MUSCLE

Morphologically, smooth muscle cells are characterized by the absence of cross-striations and smaller size. A typical smooth muscle fibre is 50–200 μm long and 2–5 μm in diameter (cf. 1–40 mm length; 50–100 μm diameter of the skeletal muscle fibre). Smooth muscle may be classified into: (a) multiunit smooth muscle, (b) visceral smooth muscle.

Multiunit Smooth Muscle In this case, the smooth muscle is composed of discrete muscle cells (muscle fibres). Each muscle fibre is capable of contracting independently and often each fibre is innervated by an individual neuron. Ciliary muscle and smooth muscle of the trachea, bronchi and iris and piloerector muscles contain multiunit type of smooth muscle fibres. Such muscle fibres can produce discrete and finely graded contractions.

Single Unit (Visceral) Smooth Muscle In this type of smooth muscle, the cells are arranged in sheets and bundles. The cells are in close contact with each other and have many *gap junctions* between the adjoining cells (Fig. 21.20). Due to the gap junctions, large masses of smooth muscle cells are excited simultaneously and therefore whole mass of cells contracts together. Most of the viscera, specially the gut, bile duct, ureter, urinary bladder and uterus contain this type of smooth muscle.

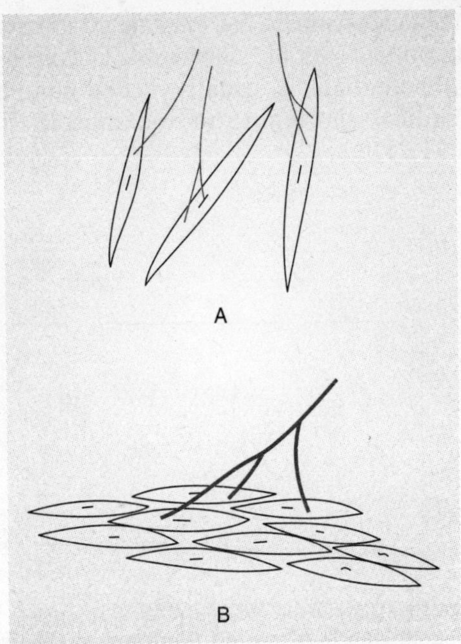

Fig. 21.20: Smooth muscle. A, multiunit type; and B, visceral type.

ELECTROPHYSIOLOGY OF SMOOTH MUSCLE

Resting Membrane Potential (Slow Waves) In the visceral smooth muscle, a constant resting membrane potential is not observed. Instead, mild fluctuations in the membrane potential around a mean value of –50 to –60 mV called *slow waves* are recorded. The slow wave activity (SWA) shifts towards –50 mV when the tissue is active and towards –60 mV when it is inhibited by neural, hormonal or other tissue factors. The lower resting potential in the smooth muscle in due to relatively lower intracellular K^+ concentration. Superimposed on the resting membrane potential are waves of various forms.

Spike Potentials These are characteristically seen in the *visceral smooth muscle* of the gut. Stimuli like neurotransmitters, hormones, or even distension (stretch) of the viscus may increase the magnitude of the sine waves to a threshold level and then many spikes, each lasting 10–50 ms, are superimposed over the sine waves. Occurrence of spike potentials is usually accompanied by mechanical shortening of the muscle fibres (Fig. 21.21).

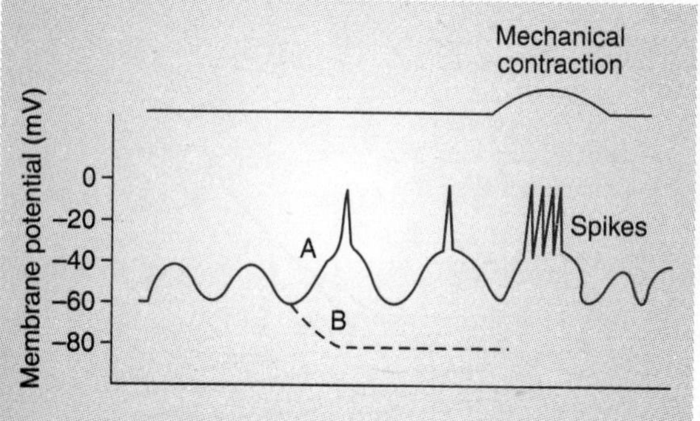

Fig. 21.21: Slow wave activity (SWA) recorded from the smooth muscle of the gut. Stretch or acetylcholine increases the magnitude of SWA as well as cause superimposition of spikes (A). Norepinephrine produces an increase in the transmembrane potential and inhibition of the muscle (B).

Visceral smooth muscle can contract spontaneously, in the absence of any extrinsic innervation, because mere stretch can provoke spike potentials and mechanical shortening.

Multiunit smooth muscle fibres mainly contract in response to neural stimuli. Although true spike potentials or action potentials do not occur in such muscle fibres, autonomic nerve impulses produce local depolarization which is followed by contraction of the muscle.

Ionic Basis of Spike Potentials Smooth muscle cells have far more voltage-gated Ca^{2+} channels and very few Na^+ channels than the skeletal muscle. Therefore influx of Ca^{2+} rather than Na^+ is mainly responsible for the action potential.

Excitation Contraction Coupling

In the smooth muscle, excitation contraction coupling is mediated by Ca^{2+} just as in the skeletal muscle. However, in this tissue, sarcotubular system is poorly developed and ECF is the direct source of Ca^{2+}. The diffusion of Ca^{2+} during action potential and subsequent removal by the calcium pump occurs rather slowly. That explains the long latency as well as prolonged duration of the smooth muscle contraction.

In the skeletal muscle, Ca^{2+} combines with troponin-C to trigger the sliding mechanism. Troponin-C is absent in the smooth muscle. Here Ca^{2+} bind with the protein calmodulin and the Ca^{2+}-calmodulin complex activates ATPase activity of the myosin head.

Molecular Basis of Contraction

Smooth muscle contains both actin and myosin filaments having chemical characteristics similar to but not exactly same as in skeletal muscle. The actin filaments are attached to *dense bodies* (and not to Z discs). The actin filaments radiating from the two adjacent dense bodies overlap a single myosin filament located midway between the dense bodies (Fig. 21.22). The actin myosin filament ratio is 10:1 in smooth muscle as compared to 2:1 in skeletal muscle. The adjacent

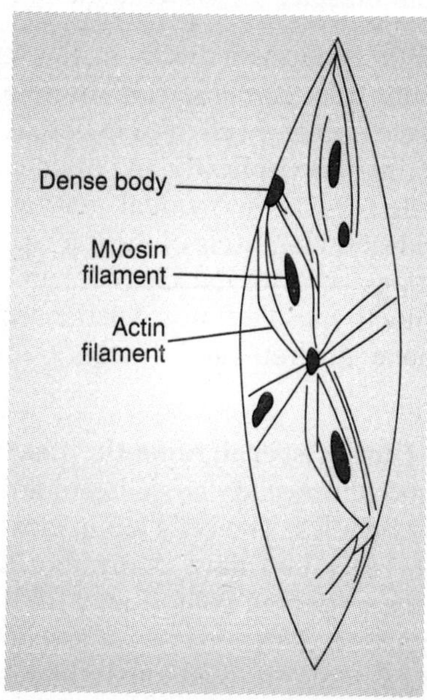

Fig. 21.22: Actin and myosin filaments in a smooth muscle fibre.

actin myosin units are not in register with each other. That is why cross-striations are not seen when smooth muscle is observed under light microscope. The basic mechanism of contraction is same as in skeletal muscle. Formation of cross-bridges between myosin heads and actin filaments is followed by sliding of actin filaments over myosin filament. However, there are some important differences as given below:

Slow Cycling of Cross-Bridges The attachment of myosin heads to actin filaments, their release and reattachment for the next cycle are slower processes in the smooth muscle than in the skeletal muscle. Therefore, full contraction develops more slowly than in skeletal muscle.

Percentage of Shortening Smooth muscle may shorten to one-third (33%) of its stretched length, whereas skeletal muscle can shorten to only 70–75% of the stretched length. Far greater shortening of smooth muscle fibres allows the hollow viscera to change their lumen from very large size to almost zero.

The "Latch" Effect Once smooth muscle contracts, it can maintain its contraction for a prolonged period of time with minimal expenditure of energy, i.e. myosin bridges hold on to the actin filaments like a latch.

The importance of latch effect is that smooth muscle can maintain tonic contraction for hours and hours with very little use of energy and without any further need for excitable neural or hormonal stimuli.

Mechanical Response in Smooth Muscle

In the smooth muscle, the twitch time is rather prolonged. After a latent period of 50–100 ms, the full contraction takes about 1–3 seconds, i.e. about 30 times as long as a single skeletal muscle twitch. Surprisingly, the strength of smooth muscle contraction is approximately equal to that of the skeletal muscle, i.e. 3 kg/cm^2 of the cross-sectional area.

Energy required by a smooth muscle is 1/20th to 1/400th of the energy required by the skeletal muscle to produce similar degree of tension. The economy of energy utilization in smooth muscle is useful because most of the viscera have some degree of resting tone (tonic contraction) all the time.

Factors Affecting Smooth Muscle Contraction

1. Stretch As mentioned above, stretch of the visceral smooth muscle leads to development of spike potentials, contraction and increased tension, even in the absence of extrinsic innervation. However, if the smooth muscle fibres are stretched and held at the stretched length, an initial increase in tension is followed by a decrease to the level that existed before the stretch. This property is referred to as *plasticity* of the smooth muscle. It is best demonstrated in the urinary bladder when it gradually gets filled up with urine.

2. Neural Control Most of the visceral smooth muscle fibres have dual autonomic innervation. The effects of cholinergic parasympathetic and noradrenergic sympathetic nerve fibres are antagonistic in most of the smooth muscle fibres. However, acetylcholine may be excitatory to some smooth muscle fibres (e.g. intestine and urinary bladder) and inhibitory to others (e.g. sphincters in the GIT and urinary bladder). Similarly, norepinephrine causes contraction of smooth muscle in some organs (e.g. sphincters of GIT and urinary bladder) but relaxation of smooth muscle elsewhere (e.g. bronchial smooth muscle). These differences depend upon the type of specific receptor proteins, (excitatory or inhibitory) present on the surface of muscle cells.

3. Local Tissue Factors Many local tissue factors such as lack of O_2, excess of CO_2 and low pH cause relaxation of smooth muscle in the arterioles and precapillary sphincters.

4. Hormones Hormones like norepinephrine, epinephrine, angiotensin-II, vasopressin, oxytocin, serotonin and histamine influence the smooth muscle. The excitation or inhibition depends upon the type of receptor proteins present on the cells. Uterine musculature is particularly sensitive to the effects of oestrogen, progesterone and oxytocin.

NEUROMUSCULAR TRANSMISSION

SKELETAL MUSCLE

Skeletal muscle fibres are innervated by large myelinated (Aα) motor nerve fibres. Each nerve fibre divides, and may make contact with only three to several thousand muscle fibres. The junction of the nerve terminals with the muscle fibre is called the *neuromuscular junction.* As a branch of motor nerve approaches the muscle fibre, it loses its myelin sheath and divides into a number of branches called the *terminal buttons* or the *end-feet*. At the site of contact, the sarcolemma is modified to form a thickened region called *motor end-plate* (Fig. 21.23). Here, the sarcolemma is thrown into folds or palisades. The terminal buttons invaginate into the spaces between the folds of the sarcolemma so that a large surface area of the cell membranes of the neuron and the muscle fibre come in close contact.

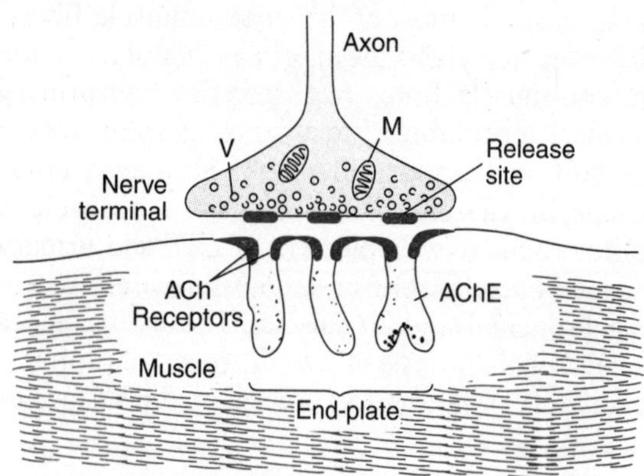

Fig. 21.23: Structure of neuromuscular junction. M: mitochondria, V microvesicles, ACh: acetylcholine, AChE: acetylcholine estrase.

The two cell membranes, however, always remain separated by a *synaptic cleft.* The terminal buttons contain large number of microvesicles full of acetylcholine (ACh). The post-synaptic membrane (motor end plate) not only contains many receptors for acetylcholine, but also is rich in the enzyme, acetylcholinesterase (AChE).

As the nerve impulse approaches the terminal branches of the axon, it increases the permeability of the nerve endings to Ca^{2+}. The Ca^{2+} enter the nerve terminal, bind to microvesicles containing ACh, causing their exocytosis. Acetylcholine released from the microvesicles diffuses across the synaptic cleft to bind with specific receptors on the motor end-plate. As a result, permeability of the motor end-plate to Na^+ (and K^+) increases several thousand times, due to opening of ACh-gated (*ligand-gated*) channels. The influx of Na^+ into the skeletal muscle fibre, at the motor end-plate, produces a depolarizing potential called *end-plate potential.* An end-plate potential of about 30 mV is sufficient to generate action potentials on either side of the end-plate, by current sink mechanism. The action potentials, once generated, are conducted away from the end plate on either side, finally resulting in excitation-contraction coupling and mechanical response.

The end-plate potential is a local response and differs from the action potential in that: (a) it can be experimentally graded (i.e. it does not follow all or none law), (b) it is not propagated, and (c) it can be summated. These properties of end-plate potential have been demonstrated by application of graded amounts of ACh on the surface of motor end-plate (Fig. 21.24). Although an end-plate potential of about 30 mV is sufficient to trigger

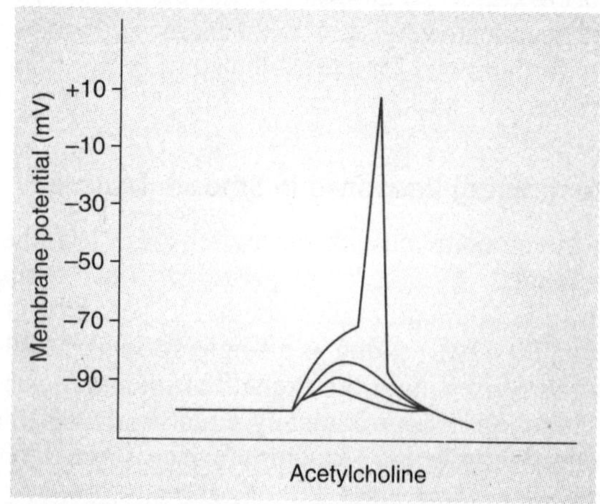

Fig. 21.24: Application of graded concentrations of acetylcholine on the motor end-plate produces graded local responses called end-plate potentials (EPP).

an action potential in the skeletal muscle, but actually, an end-plate potential of 50 to 75 mV is usually produced by the exocytosis of sufficient number of microvesicles. In this way, it is assured that a nerve impulse reaching the muscle is always, without fail, able to produce a contraction.

Physiologically, there is no need for summation of end-plate potentials. There is always 1:1 relation between the impulse rate in the motor nerve and rate of skeletal muscle fibre contraction. The end plate potential is very short lived. Within one millisecond of the release from the axon terminal, ACh is removed, partly by diffusion out of the synaptic cleft, and mostly by destruction by the enzyme acetyl cholinesterase. As a result, the post-synaptic membrane returns to its resting polarity; ready to respond to the next stimulus. The chief benefit of chemical transmission at the neuro-muscular junction is that a small branch of an axon is able to excite a much larger muscle fibre.

During many surgical operations, complete skeletal muscle relaxation is required. This can be achieved by administration of a drug like d-tubocurarine which acts by competing with ACh on the receptor sites on the motor-end-plate. As a result, ACh released from the nerve terminals fails to depolarize the membrane. In other words, the passage of the impulses from the motor nerve to the skeletal muscle is blocked. After the operation, the effect of d-tubocurarine is abolished by administration of anticholinesterase drugs like neostigmine.

Myasthenia Gravis It is a disorder of neuro-muscular transmission. The hallmark of myasthenia gravis is muscle weakness that increases during periods of activity and improves after periods of rest. Muscles that control eye and eyelid movement, facial expression, chewing, talking and swallowing are especially susceptible. The muscles that control breathing and neck and limb movements can also be affected. Asymmetrical ptosis (drooping of one or both eyelids), diplopia (double vision) due to weakness of the muscles that control eye movements are the usual early features of the disease. Death may occur due to the paralysis of the respiratory muscles. Myasthenia gravis is believed to be an auto-immune disease. The patient develops antibodies against his own acetylcholine-gated ion channels (Fig. 21.25). Moreover, the amount of ACh released from the nerve terminals also seems to be inadequate. Consequently, the end-plate potential produced in response to an impulse in the motor nerve is inadequate to generate an action potential in the skeletal muscle. The disorder can be treated by administration of neostigmine, an anticholinesterase agent.

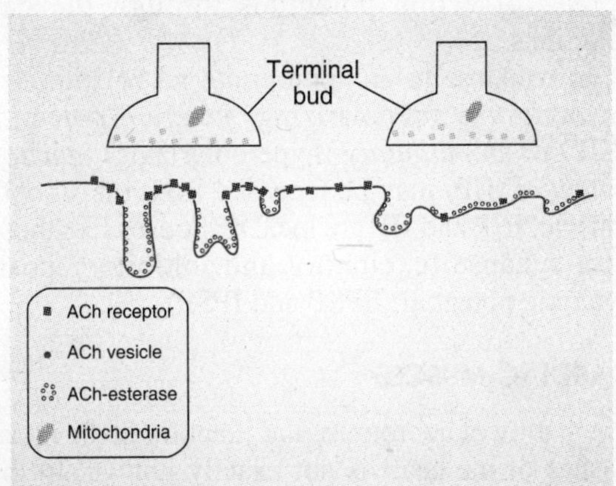

Fig. 21.25: Neuromuscular junction: left: normal, right: in myasthenia gravis.

SMOOTH MUSCLE

As the sympathetic and parasympathetic nerve fibres approach the smooth muscle, they branch extensively and come in close contact with a large number of smooth muscle fibres. The neuronal network has a beaded appearance with large enlargements called varicosities (Fig. 21.26).

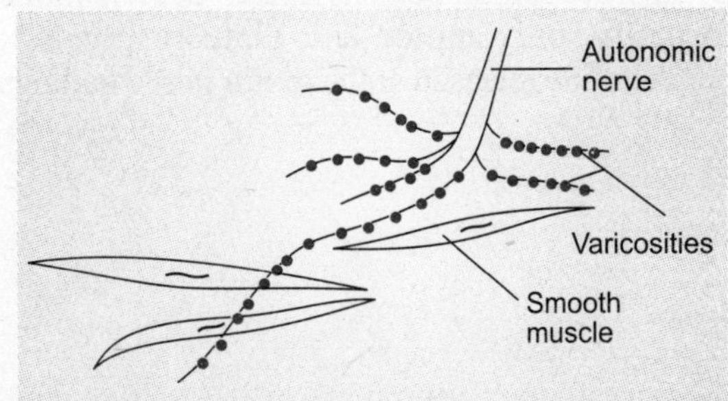

Fig. 21.26: Neuromuscular junction in smooth muscle.

The varicosities contain the neurotransmitter (acetylcholine or norepinephrine). In the smooth muscle, the nerve fibres do not make any special contact (unlike neuromuscular junction formed in the skeletal muscle). Instead, the nerve fibre releases its transmitter from each varicosity into the interstitial fluid close to the muscle fibre. The neurotransmitter then diffuses into a large number of muscle fibres. In a bundle of smooth muscle cells, often only the cells on the surface are innervated. The deeper cells are stimulated by spread of action potentials through the gap junctions.

In response to an appropriate nerve stimulus, an *excitatory* (depolarizing) *junction potential* (EJP) or an *inhibitory* (hyperpolarizing) *junction potential* (IJP) may be recorded from the smooth muscle. EJP and IJP are local responses like those in a synapse (excitatory and inhibitory post-synaptic potential; EPSP and IPSP).

CARDIAC MUSCLE

The nature of neuromuscular junction in the nodal tissues of the heart is not exactly known. In the atrial and ventricular myocardium, the contact between the musculature and the noradrenergic fibres resembles that in the smooth muscle.

DENERVATION HYPERSENSITIVITY

After denervation, tissues generally become more sensitive to the chemical transmitter normally released by the nerve endings. The phenomenon is known as denervation hypersensitivity. For example, after an injury to a motor nerve, the paralysed muscle not only shows disuse atrophy, but also become hypersensitive to acetylcholine. Normally, only motor end plate responds to acetylcholine released at the motor nerve endings. However, denervation results in upregulation of cholinergic receptors throughout the muscle cell membrane. Therefore, the entire muscle cell membrane becomes responsive to even minute amounts of acetylcholine normally circulating in the blood. The result is *fibrillation potentials* which are an important EMG evidence of denervation of skeletal muscle (Fig. 21.27). Only when the muscle atrophies completely, fibrillation potentials disappear.

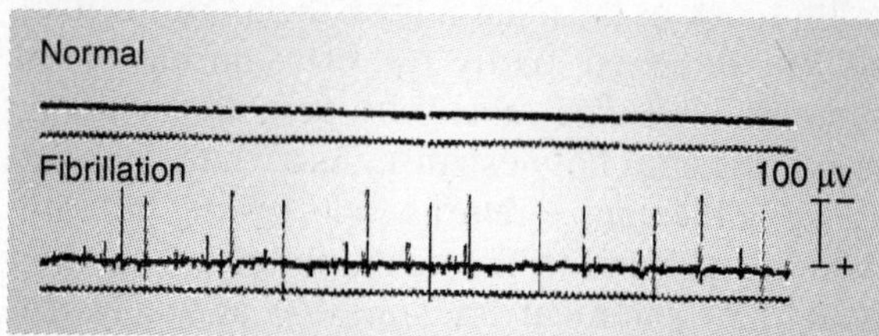

Fig. 21.27: EMG recordings of a muscle at rest showing absence of electric activity in a normal muscle (above) and fibrillation potentials in a denervated muscle (below).

In the visceral smooth muscle, denervation does not produce denervation atrophy, but denervation hypersensitivity is often observed. Experimentally, it can be demonstrated by cutting postganglionic sympathetic fibres to one iris of an animal. After a few weeks, intravenous injection of norepinephrine produces greater pupillary dilatation in the denervated eye than in the normal eye (with intact innervation). Based on this principle, tests for integrity of autonomic innervation of the eye have been devised (Chapter 31).

Besides the upregulation of receptors for the neurotransmitter, an interference with the reuptake of the neurotransmitter by the nerve endings may also contribute to the denervation hypersensitivity.

Section VII

Central Nervous System

22 CHAPTER

Synaptic Transmission

The central nervous system is bombarded with thousands of sensory signals most of the time. But, more than 99% of the signals are ignored. Motor activity occurs only in response to important signals. The processing of information occurs at the synapses. A synapse is the junction between two neurons. At a synapse, a weak signal may be allowed to die out or amplified into a strong signal. Similarly, at a synapse, a signal may be channelized into many directions (divergence) or signals from many sources may be channelized in one direction (convergence).

In mammals, most synaptic transmission is chemical in nature, i.e. a chemical transmitter released from the terminals of one neuron excites the next neuron. The processing of signals at the synapse, e.g. inhibition, amplification, convergence or divergence, is possible because of the chemical nature of the synaptic transmission. (Electrical neural synapses are common in invertebrates only. In this type of synapse, action potentials are coupled from one nerve terminal to another at the gap junctions.)

STRUCTURE OF A SYNAPSE

There is a considerable variation in the manner in which an axon terminates on the cell body of another neuron (Fig. 22.1). Characteristically, an axon terminates into several branches, and each branch end in an enlargement, known as a *terminal button* or a *synaptic knob*. A synaptic knob comes in close contact with the cell body at soma-dendrite junction (e.g. ventral horn cells of the spinal cord). However, a synaptic knob may end on the dendrites only (e.g. pyramidal cells in the motor cortex). Sometimes the terminal branches of the presynaptic axon may encircle the cell body of the postsynaptic neuron in a basket like fashion (basket cells of the cerebellum and in autonomic ganglia) or they intertwine with the dendrites of the postsynaptic cell (climbing fibres of the cerebellum). Around a ventral horn cell of the spinal cord, up to 10,000 synaptic knobs may be present. In a few situations, however, only one axon may terminate on the cell body of another neuron, e.g. fovea centralis of the retina.

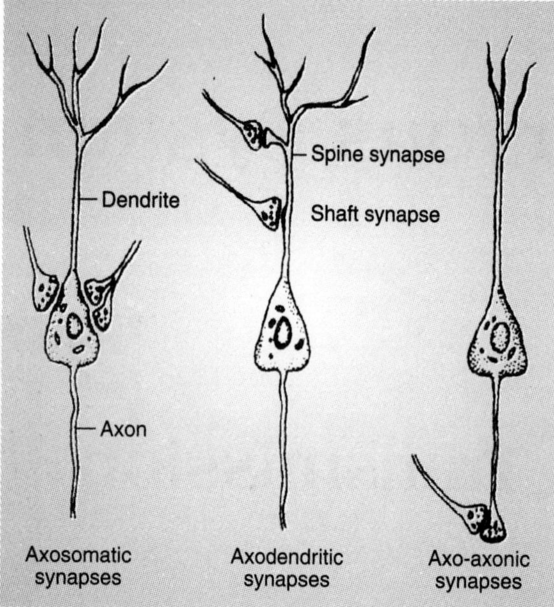

Fig. 22.1: An axon terminal may come in contact with an another neuron in a variety of ways.

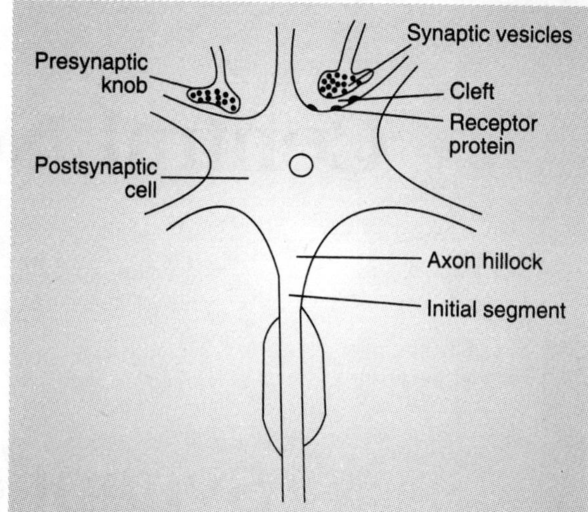

Fig. 22.2: Electron microscopic structure of a synapse (diagrammatic).

22

CHEMICAL TRANSMISSION OF NERVE IMPULSE

Under the electron microscope, synaptic knobs are seen to contain a few mitochondria and a large number of synaptic vesicles containing a chemical transmitter. A synaptic cleft of about 30–50 nm separates the cell membrane of the synaptic knob from the cell membrane of the postsynaptic cell (Fig. 22.2). There are three kinds of synaptic vesicles: *small clear* synaptic vesicles that contain neurotransmitters such as acetylcholine, glycine, GABA , glutamate, etc.; *small vesicles* with *dense core* that contain a catecholamine, and *large vesicles with dense core* that contain a neuropeptide. Different synaptic knobs on a particular postsynaptic cell may contain different neurotransmitters, but generally in a synaptic knob all the vesicles contain only one type of neurotransmitter (see cotransmitters discussed below). In the postsynaptic cell, the part of the cell membrane immediately adjacent to a synaptic knob contains appropriate receptors for the chemical transmitter present in the presynaptic knob.

As the nerve impulse reaches the axon terminal, it opens voltage-gated Ca^{2+} channels. The consequent increase in the intracellular Ca^{2+} concentration causes rupture of the microvesicles by exocytosis. The chemical transmitter released from the vesicles diffuses across the synaptic cleft and binds with the specific receptors on the surface of postsynaptic neuron resulting in the opening of ligand-gated Na^+, K^+ or Cl^- channels. Within 1–2 ms, the action of the chemical transmitter is terminated, either by *diffusion* of the transmitter out of the cleft, or by *an enzymic destruction.* Another important mechanism terminating the action of a chemical transmitter is its active transport back into the presynaptic terminals (transmitter reuptake).

Reuptake of Neurotransmitters In case of many neurotransmitters, most of the amount released into the synaptic cleft is actively transported back into the presynaptic nerve terminals and restored in the microvesicles (Fig. 22.3), e.g. norepinephrine, dopamine, serotonin, GABA, glycine and glutamate. In case of glutamate, the reuptake mechanism involves an active role of astrocytes (Fig. 22.4). Certain drugs can inhibit the reuptake of a specific neurotransmitter and thereby prolong or increase its effect.

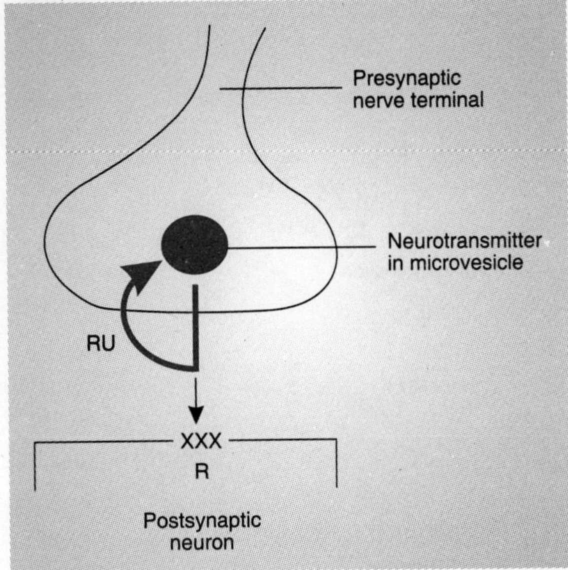

Fig. 22.3: Reuptake of a neurotransmitter. R: receptors; RU: reuptake.

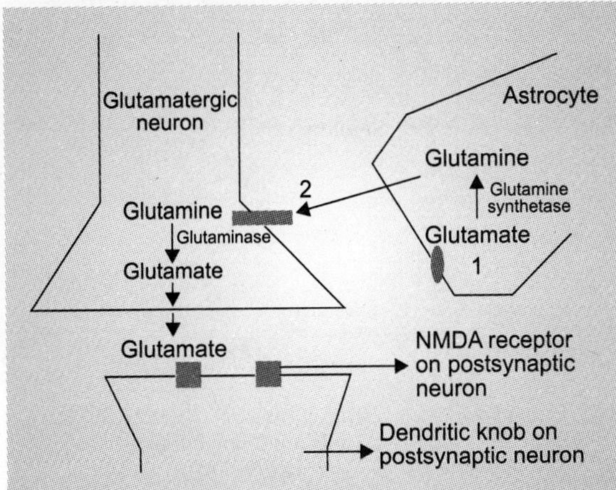

Fig. 22.4: The figure depicts the role of astrocytes in the active reuptake of glutamate from a glutamatergic synapse by glutamate transporters (1). Glutamate is converted to glutamine in astrocytes. Glutamine is actively taken up through glutamine transporters (2) in the terminals of glutamatergic neurons and converted again to glutamate.

Recycling of Microvesicles Small molecule neurotransmitters can be synthesized in the soma as well as terminals of a neuron. However, microvesicles can only be formed in the soma which contains the endoplasmic reticulum. Therefore, the microvesicles which have emptied their contents by exocytosis are reutilized to store the chemical transmitter newly synthesized in the nerve terminals. This is called recycling of microvesicles.

NEUROTRANSMITTERS

Names of some important chemical neurotransmitters are given in Table 22.1. Their chemical structure is shown in Fig. 22.5.

Acetylcholine This neurotransmitter is released by: (i) α-motor neurons at the neuromuscular junction, (ii) all preganglionic autonomic neurons, (iii) postganglionic parasympathetic neurons, (iv) postganglionic cholinergic sympathetic neurons, and (v) cholinergic neurons in many parts of CNS. In the CNS, notable areas rich in such neurons include spinal cord, reticular activating system, corpus striatum and forebrain. In the CNS, cholinergic neurons are mostly *excitatory* in nature even though some cholinergic receptors are muscarinic type while others are nicotinic type. These receptors as well as biosynthesis and catabolism of acetylcholine are described in detail in Chapter 31.

22

Norepinephrine and Epinephrine Norepinephrine is released at most of the postganglionic sympathetic nerve terminals. In the CNS, neurons may secrete epinephrine (adrenalin) or norepinephrine (noradrenalin). These neurons are called adrenergic and noradrenergic neurons, respectively. The CNS contains far more number of noradrenergic neurons than adrenergic neurons. Noradrenergic neurons constitute two major systems in pons and medulla oblongata: (i) locus ceruleus system and (ii) lateral tegmental system. From these neurons, the axons descend to the spinal cord and cerebellum, and ascend to many other parts of the brain. Most of these neurons are *excitatory* in nature. Certain drugs can produce increase or decrease in noradrenergic activity in the CNS leading to elevation and depression of mood respectively. Adrenal medulla releases both norepinephrine and epinephrine. The biosynthesis and catabolism of these two catecholamines is discussed is Chapter 31.

Table 22.1: Names of some important chemical neurotransmitters and their location

Class and neurotransmitter	*Important locations*
I. Acetylcholine	Neuromuscular junction Preganglionic autonomic neurons Postganglionic parasympathetic neurons Postganglionic sympathetic neurons supplying sweat glands, skeletal muscle vessels Many parts of CNS
II. Amines	
Norepinephrine	Most postganglionic sympathetic nerve terminals Many neurons in the brain
Epinephrine	Hypothalamus Thalamus, periaqueductal grey matter of spinal cord
Dopamine	Striatum, hypothalamus, limbic system
Serotonin	Hypothalamus Limbic system Spinal cord GIT
III. Amino acids	
Glycine	All over CNS (neurons mediating direct inhibition)
GABA (Gamma-amino butyric acid)	All over CNS (neurons mediating indirect inhibition)
Glutamate	All over CNS
IV. Polypeptides	
Hypothalamic releasing hormones	Hypothalamus
Substance P	Endings of primary pain afferents Many parts of brain
Encephalins	Substantia gelatinosa in the spinal cord Many other parts of CNS
β-endorphins	Hypothalamus

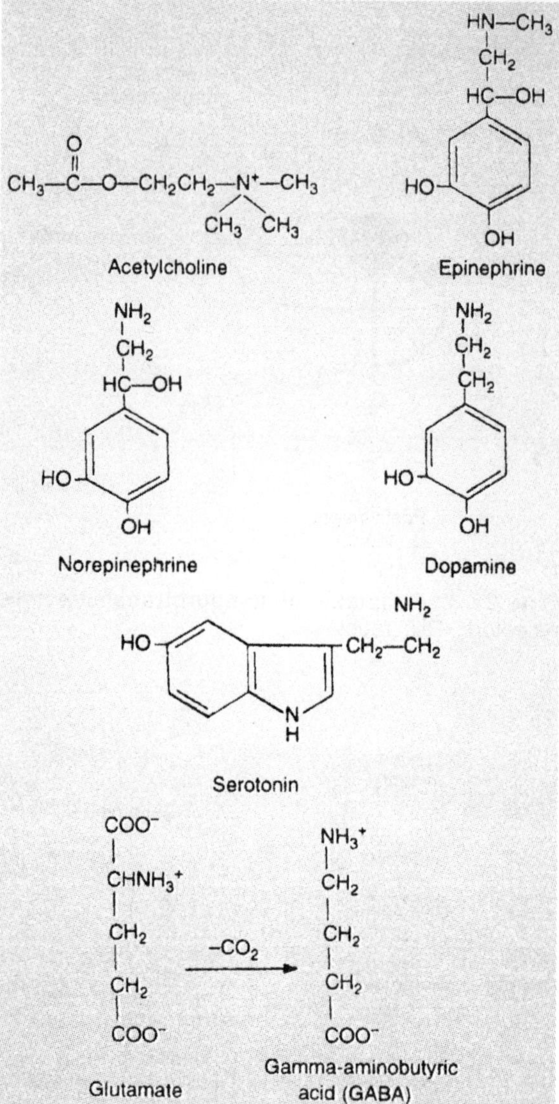

Fig. 22.5: Chemical structure of various neurotransmitters.

Dopamine Dopaminergic neurons are found in the basal ganglia, hypothalamus and limbic system. The biosynthesis and catabolism of this catecholamine is also described in Chapter 31. Degeneration of dopaminergic neurons of the substantia nigra produces Parkinson's disease (Chapter 25). In the treatment of this disorder, dopamine cannot be used since it does not cross the blood-brain barrier. Instead, its immediate precursor L-DOPA is used which can cross the blood-brain barrier. It seems, sufficient amount of the enzyme DOPA-decarboxylase is available within the surviving dopaminergic neurons which convert L-DOPA to dopamine in the basal ganglia.

Serotonin (5-Hydroxytryptamine, 5-HT) It is present in the highest concentration in the blood platelets and GI tract. In the GIT, it is found in the enterochromaffin cells and in myenteric plexus. Lesser amounts are present in the brain. Serotonin is inactivated by monoamine oxidase (MAO) to form 5-hydroxy indolacetic acid (5-HIAA) which is excreted in the urine. In the GI tract, 5-HT receptors facilitate secretions and peristaltic movements. In the brain, serotonergic neurons have their cell bodies in the brainstem and they project to portions of hypothalamus, limbic system, neocortex and spinal cord. Some 5-HT receptors are *excitatory* while others are *inhibitory* in nature. The concentration of 5-HT at CNS synapses can be increased by certain drugs which *inhibit serotonin reuptake* by serotonergic neuron terminals. Such drugs have been found useful in the treatment of *mental depression.*

Histamine Histaminergic neurons have their cell bodies mainly in the posterior hypothalamus and their axons project to all parts of the brain. The exact function of this diffuse histaminergic system is not known as yet.

Glycine Glycine-secreting neurons are the neurons of the brain and the spinal cord which produce *direct inhibition* at the synapses (vide infra). *Renshaw cells* of the spinal cord and *Golgi bottle neurons* of the spinal cord and brain are well known inhibitory neurons which secrete glycine. Strychnine blocks glycine receptors and hence produces uncoordinated muscular hyperactivity known as convulsions.

Gamma-Aminobutyric Acid (GABA) It is the major *inhibitory* transmitter of the CNS. It produces *presynaptic (indirect) inhibition* (vide infra). Two types of GABA receptors are known. GABA-**A** receptor activity produces inhibition by increasing Cl^- conductance, whereas GABA-**B** receptor activity produces inhibition by increasing K^+ conductance. Reuptake of GABA is an important mechanism for its removal from the synaptic cleft. Certain drugs (e.g. diazepam) which inhibit the reuptake of GABA are helpful in the treatment of epilepsy (anticonvulsant action), anxiety neurosis and insomnia (inability to sleep). Tetanus toxin prevents the release of both glycine and GABA and hence produces severe convulsions.

Glutamate and Aspartate Glutamate is the chief *excitatory* transmitter in the brain and spinal cord. It accounts for 25% of excitatory transmission in the brain. Aspartate seems to be the chief excitatory transmitter of cortical pyramidal cells.

Neuropeptides In contrast to the small molecule neurotransmitters described above, neuropeptides have a different mode of synthesis and action. These polypeptides cannot be synthesized in the cytosol of the axon terminals. They can only be synthesized in the ribosome-Golgi body apparatus in the neuronal cell body. They are packaged in large dense core vesicles which release their content by autolysis (i.e. do not undergo recycling). The neuropeptides have a slow but prolonged action since reuptake by axon terminals does not occur. Most of the neuropeptides act as hormones, e.g. hypothalamic releasing hormones, ADH, oxytocin, etc. Two important polypeptide neurotransmitters include *substance P* and *opioid peptides*. Substance P is a polypeptide containing 11 amino acids. It is the transmitter released by primary pain nerve endings in the dorsal horn of the spinal cord. It is also found in the hypothalamus and nigrostriatal system of the basal ganglia. Opioid polypeptides (encephalin, endorphin and dynorphins) have an important role in the central inhibition of pain signals (Chapter 23).

Many other polypeptides have been detected in the CNS, but their function as neurotransmitters has not yet been proved. Such polypeptides include cholecystokinin, gastrin, secretin, motilin, atrial natriuretic peptide, brain natriuretic peptide, etc.

Gases Nitric oxide (NO) and carbon monoxide (CO) have been detected in the CNS synapses. As a neurotransmitter, NO differs from all other neurotransmitters discussed above in a number of ways:

(i) NO is not stored in the synaptic vesicles. It is synthesized and released immediately.
(ii) Its receptors are located inside the soma of postsynaptic cell (not on the surface).
(iii) It acts by forming a second messenger CGMP (not by altering ionic conductance).
(iv) Its action is not unidirectional. It may be released from the presynaptic terminals and act on the postsynaptic cell (as other neurotransmitters) or it may be released by postsynaptic cell body and act on presynaptic neuron terminals.
(v) Its action is not limited to one synapse only. It diffuses out and may act on many synapses as far as 100 μm away.

Nitric oxide is believed to play a modulatory role in the regulation of the action of excitatory neurons as well as in long-term potentiation and depression of synapses and in storage of memory.

Cotransmitters

Soon after the discovery of neurotransmitters, it was proposed that a given neuron is capable of synthesizing only type of neurotransmitter which was released at all of its terminals (Dale principle). Now, it has been shown that although Dale principle is generally true, some neurons can produce more than one neurotransmitter or secrete a neurotransmitter as well as a peptide modulator. The additional transmitter or the modulator is known as cotransmitter. The physiological significance of cotransmitters is not yet clear. The additional transmitter or the modulator may help to potentiate the effect of primary neurotransmitter.

ELECTRICAL EVENTS DURING SYNAPTIC TRANSMISSION

The electrical events occurring during synaptic transmission have been studied by inserting a micro-electrode into a ventral horn cell of the spinal cord and stimulating the sensory nerve fibres in the dorsal root (Fig. 22.6). Application of a single stimulus to the afferent nerve fibres may produce a *mild, transient,* **depolarizing** or **hyperpolarizing** change in the ventral horn cell. These changes in the membrane potential of the postsynaptic cell are called excitatory postsynaptic potential (*EPSP*) and inhibitory postsynaptic potential *(IPSP)*, respectively.

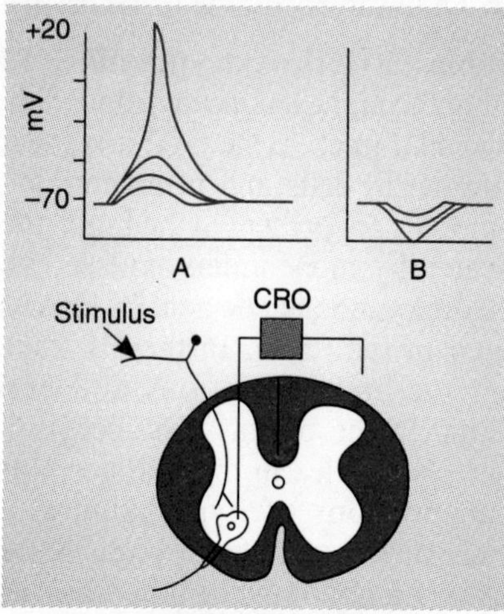

Fig. 22.6: Arrangement for recording excitatory or inhibitory postsynaptic potentials. Application of a stimulus to a dorsal root afferent may produce: (A) a depolarizing local response in the ventral horn cell (EPSP) or (B) hyperpolarizing local response (IPSP) in the ventral horn cell.

Synaptic Excitation (Excitatory Postsynaptic Potentials)

Excitatory postsynaptic potential consists of a depolarizing response in a postsynaptic cell produced by a single stimulus to an appropriate afferent nerve fibre. It begins about 0.5 ms after the nerve impulse enters the spinal cord, reaches its peak in another 1–1.5 ms and then declines exponentially. During this change, the excitability of the neuron to another stimulus is increased, hence the name.

EPSP is a local response. It shows temporal and spatial summations. Application of many stimuli at very short intervals, i.e. before the EPSP due to previous stimulus has decayed, results in a greater degree of depolarization (temporal summation). Simultaneous stimulation of many afferent fibres, each of which individually produces EPSP also results in greater degree of EPSP (spatial summation). If temporal, or more commonly, spatial summation brings the membrane potential of the cell to the firing level, an action potential is fired and propagated in the postsynaptic neuron. There is an interval of 0.5 ms between the arrival of impulse at the presynaptic terminal and development of EPSP in the postsynaptic cell. This interval, called synaptic delay, is due to the time required for the release and action of the chemical transmitter. The number of neurons (synapses) involved in a reflex action can be known from the latency of the response, because at each synapse the latency would increase by 0.5 ms.

Ionic Basis of EPSP

The chemical transmitter which produces EPSP does so by combining with specific receptors on the cell membrane of the postsynaptic neuron in close contact with the synaptic knob. The transmitter-receptor binding results in opening of ligand-gated Na^+ channels leading to increased Na^+ permeability in the post-synaptic cell. However, since a very small area of the postsynaptic membrane develops increased Na^+-permeability, the amount of Na^+ influx so produced is able to produce only a mild degree of depolarization in the entire soma. The depolarization is soon reversed by stronger, natural repolarizing forces.

Firing of Action Potential

As mentioned above, due to temporal or more commonly, spatial summation, the EPSP may reach the firing level of depolarization, resulting in an action potential. The action potential is fired first in the axon hillock and initial segment region of the neuron and not in the area close to the

22

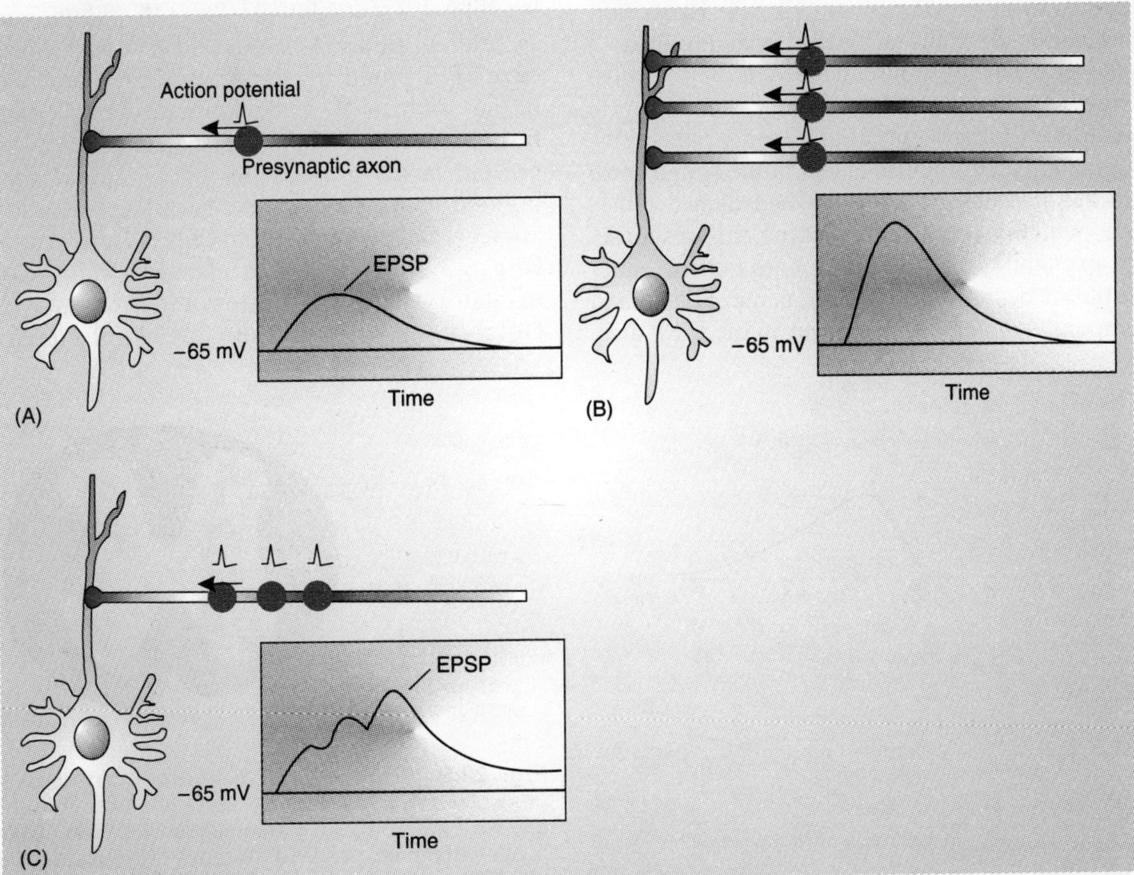

Fig. 22.7: An EPSP in response to a single stimulus (A), Spatial (B), and temporal (C) summations of EPSP.

synaptic knobs. The main reason for the origin of action potential in this area is that it has lowest threshold of excitation, due to presence of a large number of voltage-gated Na^+ channels. The EPSP in the soma depolarizes the axon hillock and initial segment region, by electrotonic (current sink) mechanism, to the firing level and initiates an action potential. Once generated, the action potential travels in both directions, i.e. peripherally in the axon as a nerve impulse and also backwards over the cell membrane of the soma. The passage of action potential over the soma helps to clear the existing EPSP, so that the cell is ready to respond to another set of stimuli.

Synaptic Inhibition

Postsynaptic (Direct) Inhibition

Stimulation of most of the afferent fibres in the dorsal root produces an EPSP. However, stimulation of some afferent fibres produces a hyperpolarizing response in the ventral horn cells. This response, called inhibitory postsynaptic potential (IPSP), begins after a longer latency, 1–1.2 ms after the impulse enters in the spinal cord, reaches its peak in 1.5–2 ms and then declines exponentially (Fig. 22.8). During this response, the excitability of the ventral horn cells to other stimuli is decreased, hence the name. Spatial and temporal summations can occur in the IPSP also.

Ionic Basis of IPSP

The chemical transmitter released from the presynaptic terminals may increase the membrane permeability of the postsynaptic cell to Cl^- *(by opening ligand-gated chloride channels)*. As a result, the influx of negatively charged chloride ions produces mild hyperpolarization which is soon reversed by normal polarizing forces. Mild hyperpolarization can also be produced by *opening of ligand-gated K^+ channels* leading to small efflux of K^+ ions.

Since hyperpolarization of the neuron moves the membrane potential further away from the threshold of excitation (firing level), it is difficult to stimulate such a cell or at least stronger stimulation is required. Hence, the potential change is called inhibitory postsynaptic potential. This type of inhibition of the postsynaptic neuron is called *direct (or postsynaptic) inhibition.*

Afferent fibres in the dorsal nerve root mostly have EPSP producing terminals. IPSP is produced by the terminals of small plump cells called **Golgi-bottle neurons**. The Golgi-bottle neurons are present in the gray matter of the spinal cord, inserted in the pathway between the dorsal-root afferents and the ventral horn cells (an interneuron) (Fig. 22.9). Dorsal-root afferents release an excitatory neurotransmitter and stimulate the Golgi-bottle neuron. The Golgi-bottle neuron

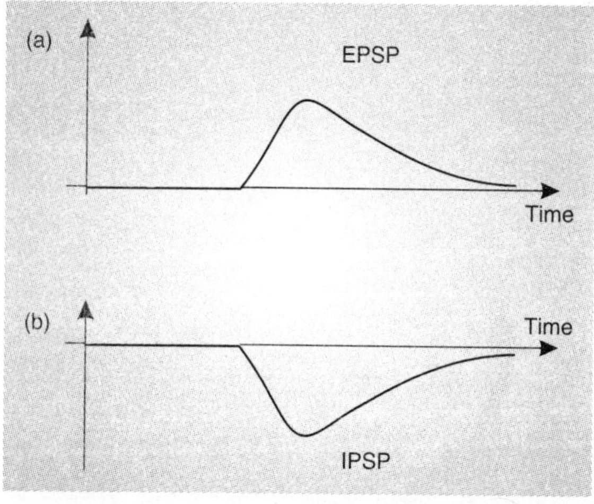

Fig. 22.8: Comparison of EPSP (a) and IPSP (b).

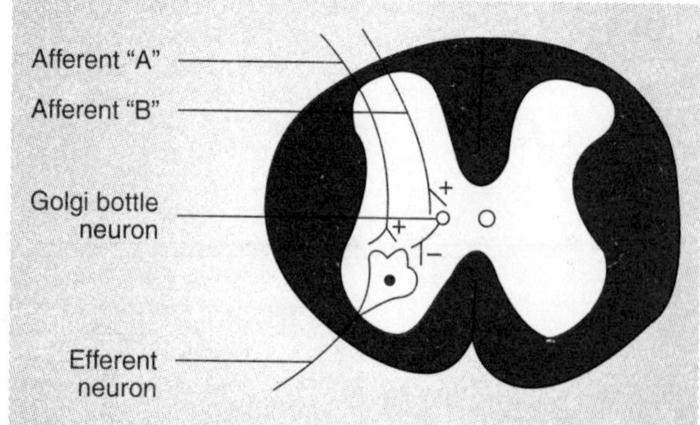

Fig. 22.9: Arrangement of neurons involved in production of EPSP or IPSP. Both afferents A and B release EPSP producing neurotransmitter. Stimulation of afferent B produces IPSP because of the intervention of a Golgi-bottle neuron which releases an inhibitory chemical transmitter near the ventral horn cell.

releases glycine which produces IPSP in the ventral horn cell. Presence of an additional synapse in the pathway explains why latency of IPSP is longer than that of EPSP.

Presynaptic (Indirect) Inhibition

In this type of inhibition, IPSP is not generated in the postsynaptic neuron. Instead, the postsynaptic neuron is indirectly inhibited. In Fig. 22.10, an inhibitory neuron (A) synapses with the terminal of an excitatory neuron (B) by an axo-axonic synapse. Activation of the inhibitory neuron (A) results in a decreased in the amount of excitatory neurotransmitter release by the neuron (B). As a result, the EPSP developing in the post synaptic cell (C) would be smaller than what would have been without the activity of neuron (A).

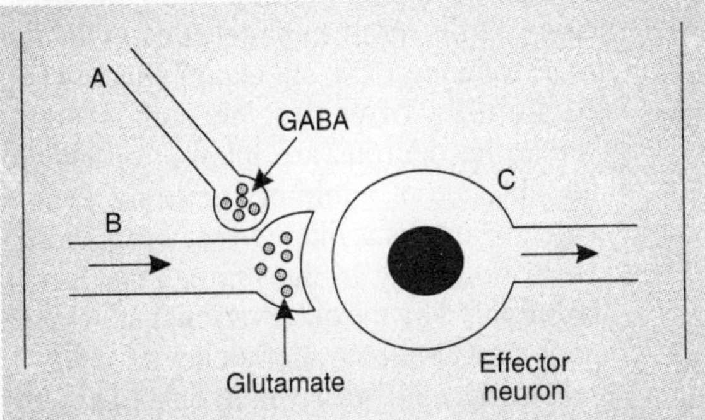

Fig. 22.10: Axo-axonic synapse. Chemical transmitters in the excitatory neuron (B) and a neuron producing presynaptic inhibition (A).

In presynaptic inhibition, the activity of inhibitory transmitter (GABA in this case) results in increased Cl^- or K^+ conductance in the excitatory neuron (B) terminal. As a result, an impulse reaching neuron (B) terminal has smaller amplitude than normal (Fig. 22.11). Therefore, the calcium influx into the neuron terminal (B) would be less than normal. Hence, neuron (B) terminal releases lesser amount of excitatory transmitter (glutamate in this case). Thus, neuron (C) has been indirectly inhibited because it would develop smaller EPSP in response to neuron (B) activity. *GABA* is the most well-known neurotransmitter involved in presynaptic inhibition. In dorsal horn of the spinal cord, the presynaptic inhibition of the first order pain afferents is produced by interneurons secreting *encephalin* (Chapter 23).

Direct inhibition and indirect inhibition, both have inhibitory influence on the effector neuron. So, what is the difference? Postsynaptic (direct) inhibition reduces the excitability of the *effector cell itself* due to the effects of the inhibitory

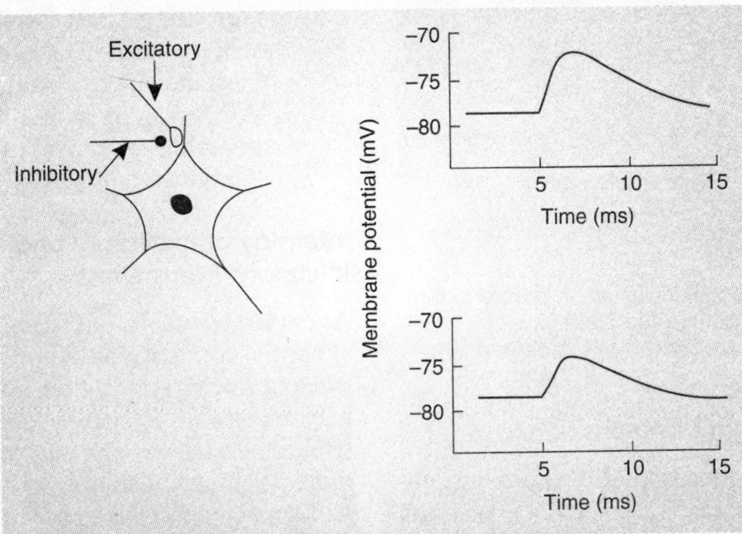

Fig. 22.11: Effect of an impulse discharge on the action potential generated in an excitatory neuron terminal: when stimulated alone (top), and under the effect of presynaptic inhibition (bottom).

transmitter released on its surface. Thus, the effector cell becomes *less responsive to all excitatory inputs*. Presynaptic inhibition is more specific. It *decreases the effect of a particular input* without disturbing the response of the effector cell to other inputs.

Renshaw Cell Inhibition (Feedback Inhibition)

This is basically a postsynaptic type of inhibition. It is classified differently because the inhibitory Renshaw cells (named after its discoverer) are activated by a collateral of the ventral horn neuron rather than an afferent neuron (Fig. 22.12). The axon of a ventral horn cell gives off a collateral branch which secretes acetylcholine and excites the Renshaw cells present in the ventral grey horn of the spinal cord. Renshaw cells secrete glycine and inhibit not only the same ventral horn cell but also other ventral horn cells lying nearby. In this way, firing of an action potential by a motor neuron of the spinal cord is followed by a phase of hyperpolarization (inhibition) of not only the same motor neuron but also many others in the neighbourhood. This type of feedback inhibition is seen in other parts of CNS as well. It serves to limit the excitability of the motor neurons.

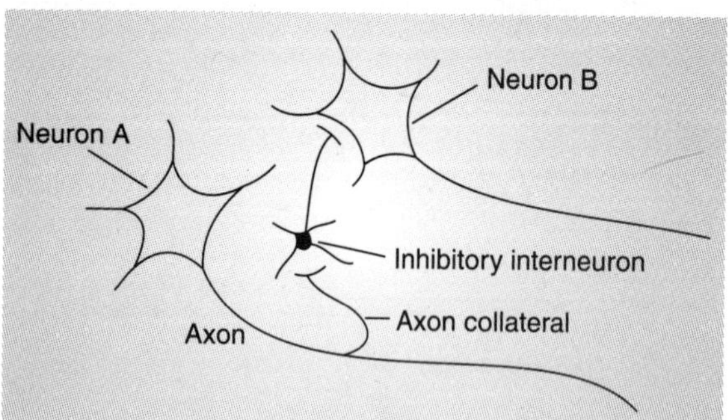

Fig. 22.12: Renshaw cell inhibition. A collateral from an alpha motor (A) excites the Renshaw cell which produces postsynaptic inhibition of the neuron (B).

Function of Inhibitory Neurons

Inhibitory neurons constitute approximately 10–20% of the neuronal pool in the CNS. Whereas the function of the excitatory neurons is easily understood, some difficulty may arise in the appreciation of the importance of inhibitory neurons.

(i) One important function of the inhibitory neurons is to keep the excitability of neurons in check by feedback inhibition (e.g. Renshaw cell inhibition).

(ii) Another, easily understood role is in the reciprocal inhibition of muscles around a joint, i.e. when one group of muscles contract, the antagonistic group of muscles must be inhibited so as to allow the movement.

(iii) A more generalized and far more important role of the inhibitory neurons is in the maintenance of a check on the overall excitability of central nervous system. Since the neurons are interconnected, in the absence of inhibitory neurons, even a single stimulus is likely to set up unending electric activity in the brain. This fact is highlighted by the observation that in some patients of epilepsy, deficiency of GABA-secreting inhibitory neurons has been demonstrated. Moreover, inactivation of inhibitory neurons by a poison, strychnine, leads to over-excitability of the entire nervous system. Even minor stimuli result in convulsions in the whole body.

(iv) Our body is exposed to thousands of sensory stimuli. On entering the CNS, most die out, few produce a response, and still fewer are stored in memory. This is possible because of the activity of inhibitory neurons.

Interplay of Excitatory and Inhibitory Transmitters

As explained before, an efferent neuron may make synaptic connections with a huge number of synaptic knobs. At any time, some synaptic knobs may release an excitatory chemical transmitter while others may release inhibitory chemical transmitter. The final response of the postsynaptic cell will depend upon the sum total of all these influences. That is how chemical transmission at the synapse serves the integrative function in the CNS.

SOME CHARACTERISTIC FEATURES OF SYNAPTIC TRANSMISSION

One-way Conduction At a synapse, an impulse can be conducted in one direction only, i.e. from the presynaptic to the postsynaptic neuron. This happens because only the presynaptic nerve terminals contain the chemical transmitter, whereas the postsynaptic nerve cell body contains the specific receptor sites. If an impulse travels antidromically in an axon, it will die out at the soma due to the absence of the chemical transmitters in the cell body. Thus, the chemical transmission at the synapse is responsible for the orderly conduction of impulse in one direction only.

Convergence and Divergence

The chemical nature of transmission permits one afferent neuron to excite a large number of efferent neurons (Fig. 22.13). This phenomenon is called *divergence of nerve signals*. On the other hand, signals from many sources may converge to a single efferent neuron. For example, ventral horn cells of the spinal cord receive convergent signals from corticospinal tract, reticulospinal tract, rubrospinal tract, and sensory afferent from dorsal root, etc. (Fig. 22.14).

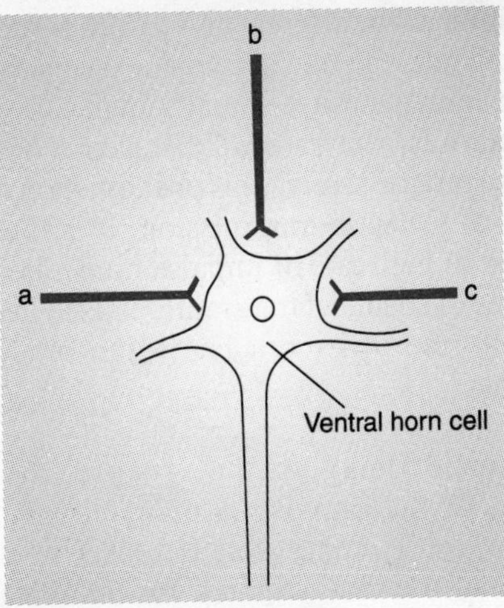

Fig. 22.14: Convergence of signals on a ventral horn cell.

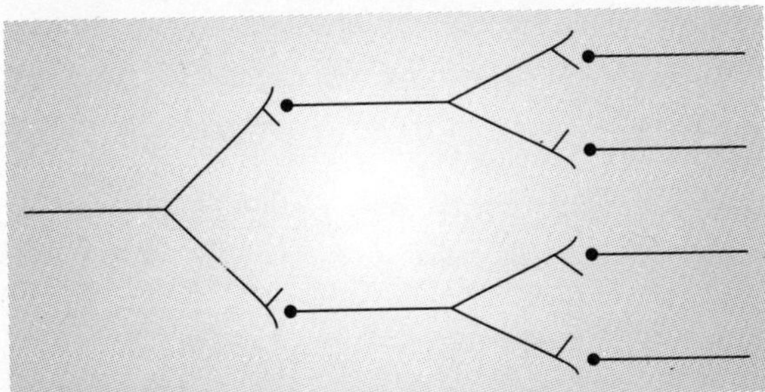

Fig. 22.13: Neuronal arrangement for divergence of nerve signals.

Reciprocal Inhibition An afferent signal may activate excitatory signals to a group of muscles and simultaneously activate inhibitory signals to other, usually antagonistic muscles. For example, when a stimulus causes flexion at a joint, there is excitation of the neurons supplying the flexor muscles of the joint. At the same time, the stimulus causes inhibition of the antagonistic extensor muscles. The neuronal arrangement for this phenomenon, called reciprocal inhibition, is shown in Fig. 22.15. The afferent fibre makes an excitatory synapse with the neurons supplying the flexor muscles. At the same time, a branch of the afferent fibre excites an inhibitory interneuron which synapses with the motor neurons supplying the extensor muscles of the joint.

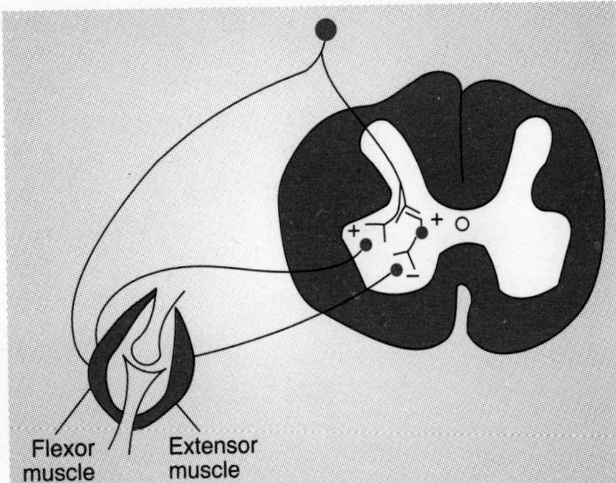

Fig. 22.15: Neuronal arrangement for reciprocal inhibition. A reflex action producing contraction of flexors of a joint causes inhibition of extensors by intervention of an inhibitory neuron.

Fatigue If the afferent nerve fibre is stimulated at a rapid rate, the rate of impulse discharge in the postsynaptic neuron is initially high but within a few seconds, the rate of discharge begins to decrease progressively. This phenomenon is called fatigue of synaptic transmission. It is due to the fact that, at high rate of impulse transmission, the synthesis of chemical transmitter fails to keep pace with the rate of its release at the presynaptic terminals.

Synaptic Delay At the synapse, the transmission of the impulse is delayed for a short duration, i.e. approximately 0.5 ms.This delay is because of the time required for the release and action of the chemical transmitter at the synapse. If an impulse passes through a chain of neurons, it is delayed at every synapse. For this reason, from the duration of reaction time of a reflex action, the number of neurons involved in the reflex can be estimated.

Effect of Acidosis and Hypoxia Both hypoxia and acidosis are highly detrimental to function of the brain, since synaptic transmission is particularly affected by them.

Synaptic Plasticity This term is used to describe the short- and long-term changes in the synaptic function as a result of previous afferent discharge (experience). The change may consist of an amplified or attenuated response of the synapse. Synaptic plasticity forms the basis of learning and memory. Synaptic plasticity may be exhibited as one of the following phenomenon: post-tetanic potentiation, habituation, sensitization, long-term potentiation and long-term depression. This topic is discussed in detail in Chapter 28.

23

CHAPTER

Somesthetic Sensory System

Sensory mechanisms within the human nervous system may be broadly classified into two categories: (1) Special senses and (2) Somesthetic senses. The special senses include vision, hearing, taste, smell and equilibrium and shall be discussed separately. The present chapter is concerned with the discussion on the somesthetic sensations.

Three types of somesthetic sensations can be distinguished by their points of origin.

- *Exteroceptive* sensations arise from the surface of the body and include touch, pain, temperature and pressure.
- *Visceral* sensations arise from the viscera.
- *Proprioceptive* sensations arise from the muscles, tendons and joints which provide an awareness of positions and movements of various parts of the body.

SENSORY RECEPTORS (Fig. 23.1)

Our body reacts to a large variety of stimuli. In each case, the information is carried to the brain in the form of nerve impulses. This is possible because our body contains a variety of sensory receptors, each of which responds to a specific stimulus. Different types of receptors convert different types of energies, e.g. mechanical, thermal, chemical or electromagnetic energy into electrical energy, i.e. the nerve impulse.

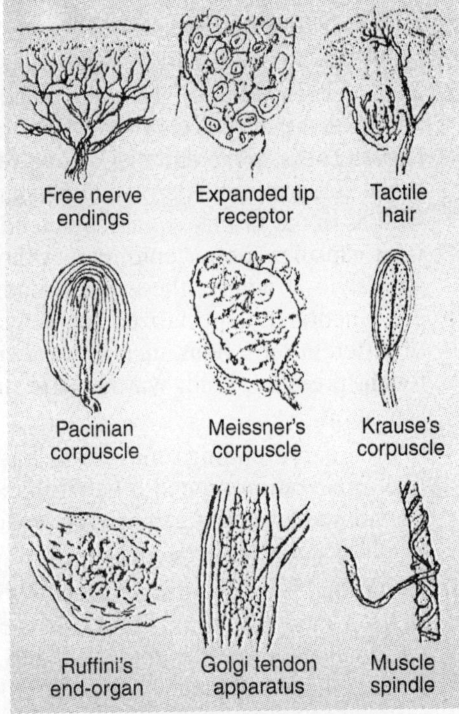

Fig. 23.1: Sensory receptors.

Broadly speaking, sensory receptors may be classified into five categories:

1. **Mechanoreceptors**, which detect mechanical deformation of the tissues.

2. **Thermoreceptors**, which detect changes in the temperature of the tissues.
3. **Nociceptors** (pain receptors), which detect physical or chemical damage in the tissues.
4. **Electromagnetic receptors**, which detect light-waves.
5. **Chemoreceptors,** which detect certain changes in the chemical composition of tissue fluids, e.g. taste, pCO_2, pO_2.

A detailed list of receptors in each of the five categories mentioned above is given in Table 23.1.

Structure of Sensory Receptors

Cutaneous Receptors

Cutaneous sensory receptors are modified terminals of sensory nerve fibres which are specialized for responding to a particular sensation. Cutaneous sensory receptors may be classified into the following three types:

(i) **Free Nerve Endings** These nerve endings belong to either type C or type Aδ afferent fibres. These nerve endings can be found in the epidermis and dermis of the skin, as well as in the fasciae, ligaments, tendons, joint capsules, periosteum, etc. Although similar in structure, these nerve endings are functionally specialized for detection of different sensations such as pain, crude touch, pressure, cold, warmth and tickle sensation.

Free nerve endings may form basket-like arborization around a hair follicle to constitute hair-end organ, a very sensitive touch receptor in the skin.

(ii) **Expanded Nerve Endings: Merkel's disc** in this case the unmyelinated nerve terminals pass into the epidermis and end as disc-shaped structures. Such receptors respond to crude touch.

(iii) **Encapsulated Receptors** An unmyelinated nerve terminal of a myelinated nerve fibre may be covered by a capsule. Meissner's corpuscle (fine touch) and Pacinian corpuscle (pressure) belong to this category.

Table 23.1: Classification of sensory receptors

A. Mechanoreceptors
1. *Cutaneous tactile sensibility (in epidermis and dermis)* (Fig. 23.1).
   Free nerve endings
   Merckel's discs (expanded nerve endings)
   Ruffini's endings (spray endings)
   Meissner's corpuscles (encapsulated endings)
   Krause's corpuscles (encapsulated nerve endings)
   Hair-end organs
2. *Deep tissue sensibility:*
   Free nerve endings
   Merckel's discs
   Ruffini's endings
   Pacinian corpuscles (encapsulated nerve endings)
3. *Muscles and joints:*
   Muscle spindles
   Golgi-tendon receptors.
4. *Hearing:*
   Organ of Corti (cochlea)
5. *Equilibrium:*
   Vestibular receptors
6. *Arterial blood pressure:*
   Baroreceptors

B. Thermoreceptors
1. Cold receptors
2. Warmth receptors

C. Nociceptors
Pain: Free nerve endings

D. Electromagnetic receptors
Vision–Rods and cones

E. Chemoreceptors
Taste receptors
Olfactory receptors
Arterial chemoreceptors (pO_2, pCO_2 and pH)
Central chemoreceptors (pCO_2, pH)

Specialized Sensory Receptors

There are a number of highly specialized sensory receptors such as rods and cones (vision), organ of Corti (hearing), muscle spindles (stretch receptors), taste receptors, olfactory receptors, vestibular receptors, arterial baroreceptors, arterial chemoreceptors, etc. The structure of these receptors has been discussed at appropriate places in the book.

Properties of Sensory Receptors

Transducer Function

Sensory receptors, like transducers, convert different types of energies, e.g. mechanical, chemical, thermal and electromagnetic, etc. into electrical energy.

Pacinian corpuscle is a large-sized receptor which can be easily dissected in experimental animals. Therefore, it has been used to demonstrate how mechanical energy can be converted into an action potential. A pacinian corpuscle consists of concentric lamellae of connective tissue surrounding an unmyelinated terminal portion of a myelinated nerve fibre (Fig. 23.1). The myelin sheath begins inside the corpuscle but the 2nd node of Ranvier is usually outside the corpuscle (Fig. 23.2).

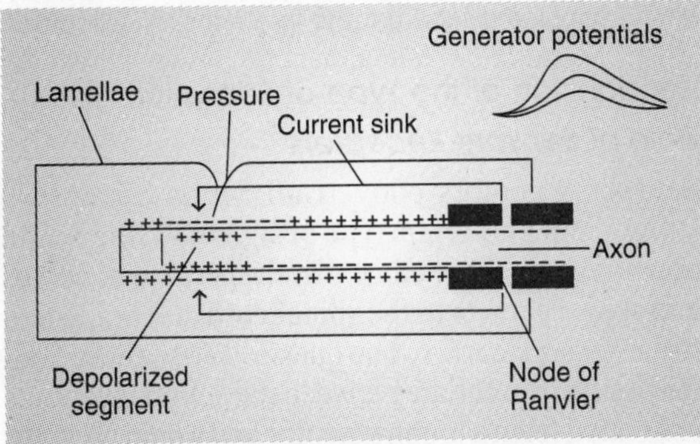

Fig. 23.2: Mechanism of origin of generator potential in a pacinian corpuscle (diagrammatic).

Generator Potentials Recording electrodes (connected to a CRO) are placed on the nerve fibre just as it leaves the Pacinian corpuscle. If a mild pressure is applied on the corpuscle, a mild non-propagated depolarizing potential called the *generator potential* or the *receptor potential* can be recorded. When the pressure is increased in steps, the degree of depolarization increases till the magnitude of depolarization is sufficient (about 10 mV) to generate an action potential, which is propagated in the nerve fibre. The generator potential resembles EPSP and its source is the unmyelinated nerve terminal. The application of pressure causes deformation of a part of the unmyelinated nerve fibre, resulting in the opening of Na^+-channels and depolarization in a segment of the nerve terminal. The increase in Na^+-permeability (and therefore the magnitude of generator potential) is proportionate to the degree of pressure applied. The depolarized segment produces electrotonic depolarization (current sink action) in the 1st node of Ranvier.

When the generator potential reaches a critical level, a propagated action potential is fired in the 1st node of Ranvier. If still greater force is applied on the receptor, the frequency of discharge is proportionately increased.

Generator potentials recorded in a few other receptors like muscle spindles, organ of Corti show a similar mechanism of transduction. However, some sensory receptors may have a different mechanism of transduction. For example, in the rods and cones of the retina, hyperpolarization rather than depolarization causes the generation of an action potential.

Specificity

Each sensory receptor responds only to a particular stimulus. For example, the touch receptor responds to deformation of the skin, thermoreceptors to the change in tissue temperature and rods and cones to the electromagnetic waves.

Adaptation

When a stimulus of constant strength is applied continuously, most of the receptors adapt partially or completely to it, i.e. the discharge rate from the receptor decreases progressively, and in some cases, may cease completely. Some receptors like those for touch (e.g. Meissener's corpuscles) and pressure (Pacinian corpuscles) adapt most rapidly, whereas pain receptors show least adaptation. Muscle and joint receptors also show very little adaptation. Thermoreceptors adapt to a moderate degree (Fig. 23.3). The mechanism of adaptation varies in different receptors.

Sensory receptors like Meissener's corpuscles and pacinian corpuscles are called *phasic receptors*

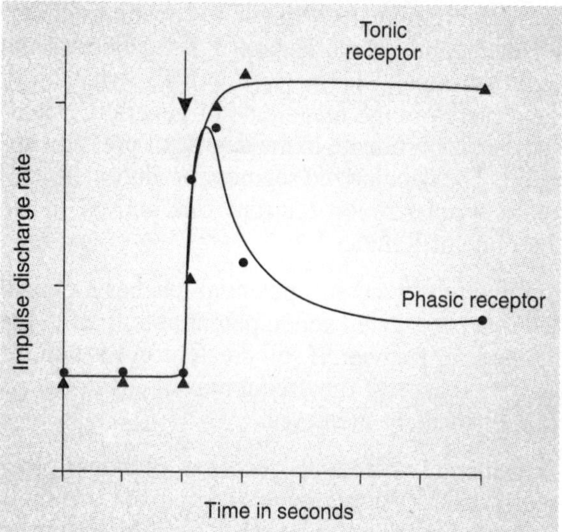

Fig. 23.3: Adaptation in sensory receptors. Frequency of impulse discharge during sustained stimulation in a tonic receptor and a phasic receptor.

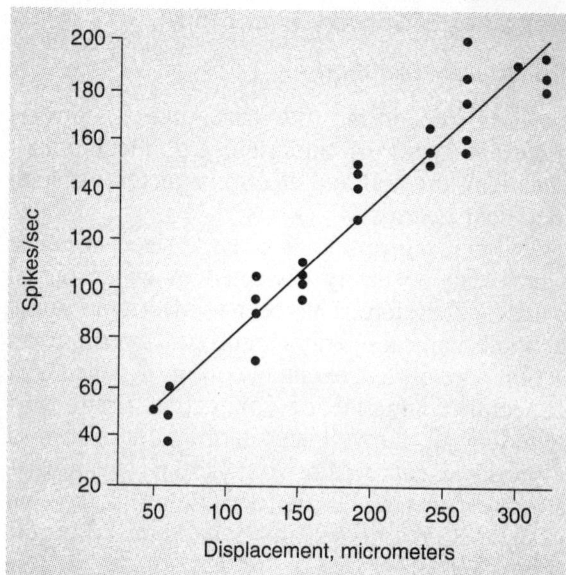

Fig. 23.4: Effect of increasing the strength of stimulus on the impulse discharge rate in a sensory receptor.

whereas those which adapt slowly and incompletely are called *tonic receptors*. Each type has its own functional significance. Phasic receptors discharge while a change is actually taking place. The rate of discharge is directly related to the rate of change. They do not discharge if a stimulus is present continuously, so that the brain is not bombarded with useless sensory information. On the other hand, pain and cold receptors detect potentially noxious stimuli and help to prevent tissue damage. Similarly, information from muscles and joints is continuously required for the maintenance of posture. Therefore, the lack of adaptation in these tonic receptors is highly valuable.

Effect of Strength of Stimulus

Depending upon the strength of stimulus, the frequency of discharge increases in the sensory receptors (Fig. 23.4).

Effect of Extent of Stimulation

When a larger part of the body is stimulated, larger number of sensory receptors are stimulated and therefore impulses are carried in a larger number of nerve fibres.

Recognition of the Type of Sensation

Role of Sensory Receptors

Sensory receptors convert all forms of sensory stimuli into a common type of signal, i.e. the action potentials which are carried by the peripheral nerves and sensory tracts in the spinal cord and brainstem to the sensory cortex. The question arises how does the brain differentiate between the action potentials generated from a touch receptor and a pain receptor and interprets the sensation accordingly. It is believed that the *sensory receptors themselves act as the peripheral analyzers.* The impulses generated are carried by discrete nerve fibres which are specific for each sensation from sensory receptor to the sensory cortex. Integrity of this pathway is essential for an accurate interpretation of the type of sensation. For example, during recovery from a nerve injury, a touch receptor may make connection with a nerve fibre meant for pain sensation. In such a case, a tactile stimulus in the affected region produces intense pain rather than the sensation of touch.

Doctrine of Specific Nerve Energies

If a discrete sensory afferent fibre in the ascending tract of the spinal cord is stimulated electrically, the sensation of touch, pain, cold or warmth may be felt by the subject depending on the type of afferent fibre stimulated. The specificity of sensory pathways from the receptors to the sensory cortex has been called the *Doctrine of Specific Nerve Energies*.

Law of Projection

Due to point to point representation of the body in the somatosensory cortex, the site of origin of each sensation is recognized highly accurately. If the sensory fibres are experimentally stimulated anywhere in their course, the conscious sensation produced is as if it is coming from the area where the receptors are located (*law of projection*). After amputation of a limb, sometimes the patient complains of intense pain in the absent limb (*phantom limb*). The sensation is due to pressure on the nerve terminals at the stump of the amputated limb. The sensation evoked in the brain is projected to the area where receptors used to be.

Recognition of the Intensity of Stimulus

Weber-Fechner law describes the relationship between the physical magnitudes of stimuli and the perceived intensity of the stimuli.

$P = k \cdot \log S$

P: percieved intensity (quantity) of the stimuli
S: actual intensity (quantity) of the stimuli
k: constant factor (to be determined experimentally)

Weber-Fechner law is applicable to few sensations such as hearing and vision. For other sensations, power function more accurately describes this relation.

$P = KS_A$

K and A are constants

TRANSMISSION OF SENSATIONS

SENSORY NERVES

Although each type of sensation has its own importance, some sensory signals must be carried to the brain very fast, while others may be conveyed slowly. Hence, different types of nerve fibres carry sensory signals from the receptors (see Table 20.2). For example, information from the muscle and joint receptors must be carried very fast because their position changes practically every second while running. Hence these sensations are carried by the fastest conducting thick myelinated nerve fibres. Relatively more critical types of sensory signals, e.g. tactile localization or tactile two-point discrimination are also carried in thick myelinated fibres. At the other extreme, the sensation of dull aching pain may be carried rather slowly. Thin unmyelinated (C-type) fibres are involved in this sensation (see Table 20.2).

Bell Magendie Law

Each spinal nerve contains both afferent and efferent nerve fibres. As it approaches the spinal cord, it divides into two roots, the dorsal root and the ventral root. All the afferent fibres enter the dorsal root, whereas the ventral root contains only the efferent fibres arising from the ventral horn cells of the spinal cord (Fig. 23.5). The fact that the dorsal root contains only the afferent (sensory) fibres and the ventral root contains only the motor fibers is known as the Bell Magendie law.

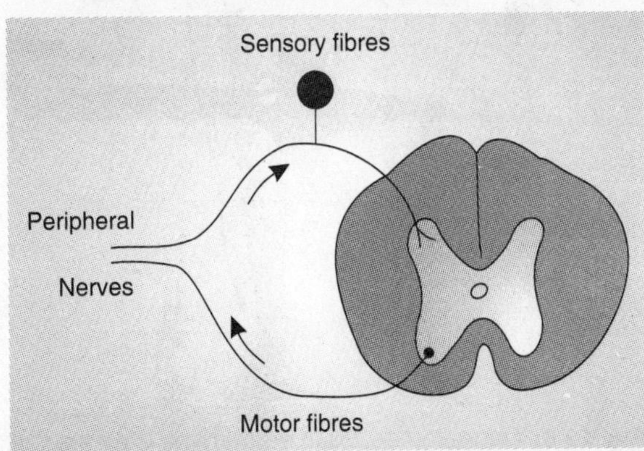

Fig. 23.5: The Bell Magendie law.

DORSAL ROOT

Ultimately, all the sensory fibres enter the CNS through dorsal roots of the spinal cord or their cranial equivalents. On entering the cord, the dorsal root divides into two bundles. A *medial bundle* containing group I, II, III afferents and a *lateral bundle* containing group III and IV afferents.

Dermatomes

The area of the skin supplied by afferent fibres of a single dorsal root (spinal cord segment) is called a dermatome. Dermatomes are quite different from peripheral nerve fields. Often fibres from one dermatome are present in different peripheral nerves (Fig. 23.6).

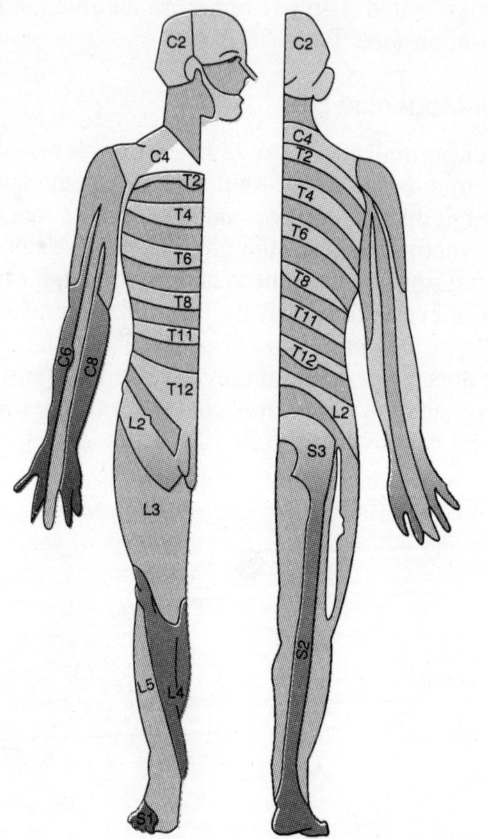

Fig. 23.6: Dermatomes: Each dermatome is an area of skin supplied by afferent fibres from a single dorsal root.

Dermatomes are remnants of orderly metameric arrangement which has survived only in the trunk. Here, the dermatomes consist of a series of 12 narrow overlapping bands running from vertebral column to the midventral line. The bands slope down as they pass around the body. The apparent complexity of the dermatomes in man is simplified if considered in the position of our ancestors, the monkeys (Fig. 23.7). The knowledge of dermatomes is utilized to know the level of spinal cord injury or the level of spinal tumour by mapping the resultant area of altered sensation.

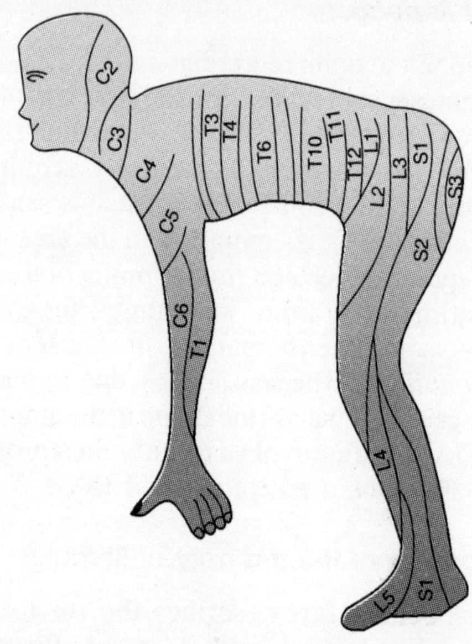

Fig. 23.7: The apparent complexity of human dermatomes is clarified when they are considered in the position of our ancestors, the monkeys.

SPINAL CORD

The dorsal grey horn of the spinal cord has been divided into six laminae on the basis of cyto-architecture. Laminae II and III constitute what was earlier known as substantia gelatinosa.

Some of the large myelinated fibres of the medial division of the dorsal root which carry sensations of fine touch, proprioception, etc. ascend in the dorsal column as such and relay only in the gracile and cuneate nuclei situated in the medulla oblongata. The second order neurons arising from the gracile and cuneate nuclei cross the midline and ascend in the medial lemniscus to terminate in the ventral posterior nucleus of the thalamus.

The remaining fibres of the medial division and those of the lateral division terminate around the cell bodies of the dorsal grey horn.

The dorsal horn cells may be broadly classified into two types of cells.

I. *Interneurons or local neurons* or which synapse with other neurons within the spinal cord. These cells are concerned with spinal cord reflexes.

II. *Relay neurons* that give rise to long fibres which ascend in the sensory tracts of the spinal cord and transmit exteroceptive and proprioceptive information to the brain.

Major ascending tracts in the spinal cord consist of:

1. **Dorsal columns (fasciculus gracilis and F. cuneatus),**
2. **Anterolateral columns [anterior (ventral) and lateral spinothalamic tracts],**
3. **Dorsolateral columns (dorsal and ventral spinocerebellar tracts)** (Fig. 23.8).

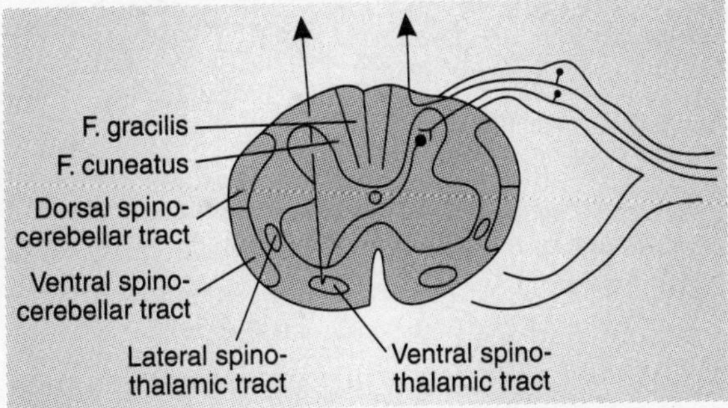

Fig. 23.8: The ascending (sensory) tracts in the spinal cord.

Dorsal Columns (Fasciculus gracilis and F. cuneatus)

Dorsal columns are well developed in man and wholly myelinated. Sensations carried by these tracts include fine touch, tactile localization, sense of two point discrimination, sense of vibration, sense of pressure with intensity discrimination and *conscious proprioception* (sense of position and movement.

Many fibres of the dorsal columns, on their way up, terminate or relay in the dorsal grey horn. In the medulla oblongata, the second order neurons start from the gracile and cuneate nuclei, cross the midline and ascend up as medial lemniscus to terminate in the ventral posterior lateral (VPL) nucleus of the thalamus. From the thalamus, the 3rd order neurons project mainly to the postcentral gyrus of the cerebral cortex (Fig. 23.9).

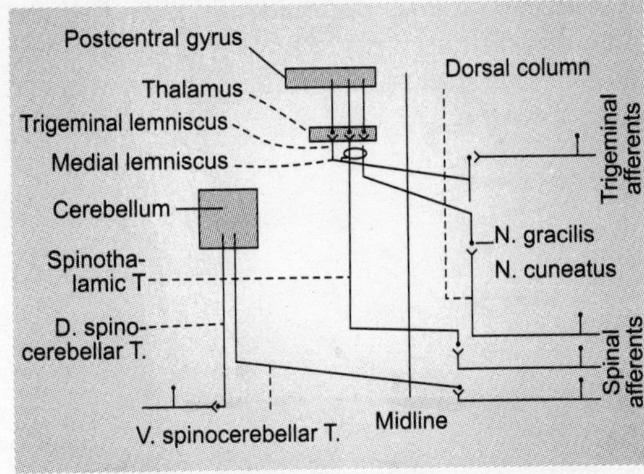

Fig. 23.9: The sensory pathways in the central nervous system.

Spinothalamic Tracts

These tracts carry sensations of pain, warmth, cold, crude touch and pressure without intensity discrimination, tickling, itching and sexual sensation. The first order neurons carrying these sensations terminate in dorsal horn of the spinal cord. Axons of second order neurons cross the midline in front of the central canal and ascend in the anterolateral quadrant as spinothalamic tracts. In general, touch is carried by ventral (anterior) spinothalamic tract, whereas pain and temperature are carried by lateral spinothalamic tract. There seems to be no rigid localization between these two tracts, more so regarding tickling, itching and sexual sensations.

In the medulla oblongata, the spinothalamic tracts join the medial lemniscus to terminate in the ventral posterior lateral (VPL) nucleus of the thalamus.

Lamination in Sensory Tracts

The dorsal columns as well as spinothalamic tracts are formed by addition of fibres from different parts of the body in an orderly fashion. As the dorsal column ascends, the fibres from the sacral region are pushed more and more medially and those from lumbar, thoracic and cervical regions are added in that order from midline to the lateral side. In the lateral spinothalamic tract, because the fibres cross to the opposite side and then enter the tract, sacral fibres are pushed superficially, while those from thoracic and cervical regions are deeper in the tract (Fig. 23.10).

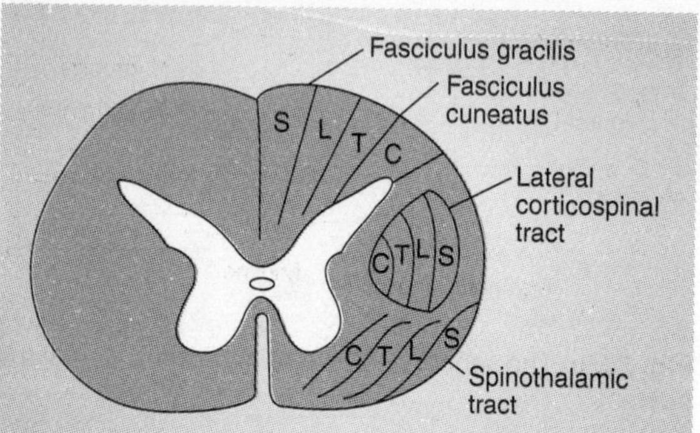

Fig. 23.10: Lamination in sensory tracts in spinal cord.

Spinocerebellar Tracts

These tracts carry *unconscious proprioceptive impulses* arising from the muscle and joint receptors to the cerebellum. The first order axons carrying these sensations ascend in the dorsal white columns for a few segments before entering the dorsal grey horn, where they synapse with large 2nd order sensory neurons located deep in the dorsal grey horn called the Clarke's column. The axons of the 2nd order neurons ascend in the spinal cord as dorsal and ventral spinocerebellar tracts. Dorsal spinocerebellar tract contains ipsilateral (uncrossed) fibres, whereas the ventral spino-cerebellar tract contains contralateral (crossed) fibres.

Face and Oral Cavity

The trigeminal nerve carries sensations of touch, pain and temperature from the face and oral cavity including teeth, and proprioceptive information from the jaw muscles. The cell bodies of the trigeminal sensory fibres are clustered in the trigeminal ganglion on either side. The trigeminal ganglion, equivalent to the dorsal root ganglia in the spinal cord, lies within the skull, ventral to the pons. Different areas of the facial skin are innervated by three branches of the trigeminal nerve: ophthalmic, maxillary and mandibular divisions (Fig. 23.11).

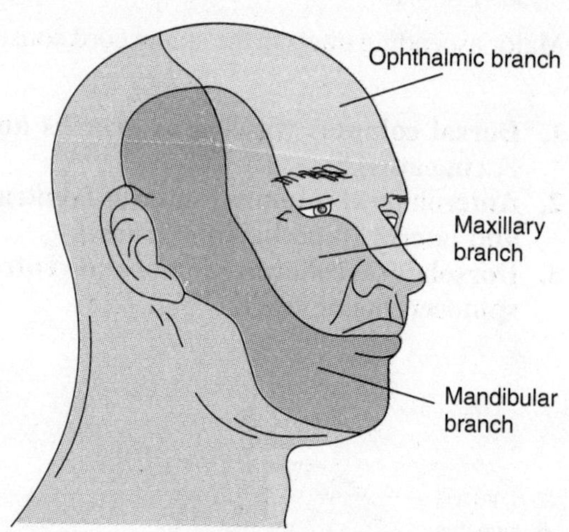

Fig. 23.11: Distribution of areas of the face innervated by ophthalmic, maxillary, and mandibular divisions of trigeminal nerve.

The central fibres of the trigeminal ganglion terminate in the ipsilateral *trigeminal sensory nucleus* which consists of three components: (i) Principal sensory nucleus located in the pons, (ii) an elongated spinal nucleus which extends from pons down to the upper spinal cord and (iii) a mesencephalic mucleus extending into the midbrain (Fig. 23.12).

The tactile sensations from the face are mediated by the principal sensory nucleus whereas pain and temperature sensations are mediated by the spinal nucleus. The proprioceptive information reaches the mesencephalic nucleus. From the trigeminal nucleus, which constitutes the second order sensory neurons, the axons cross to the opposite side and ascend as trigeminal lemniscus to the *ventroposterior medial* nucleus (VPM) of the thalamus.

Afferent impulses from *all other cranial nerves*, e.g. VII (taste), IX and X (thoracic and abdominal

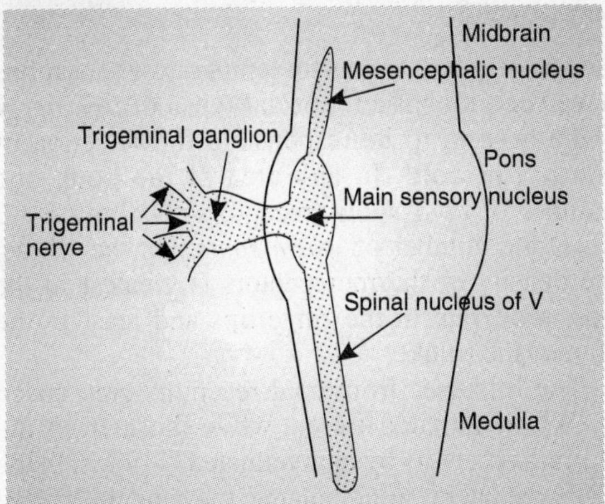

Fig. 23.12: Subdivisions of trigeminal sensory nucleus and their location.

visceral sensations) and vestibular division of 8th nerve are also carried by the *medial lemniscus*.

Thalamus

Medial and trigeminal lemnisci terminate in the ventral posterior nucleus of the thalamus. A topographic representation of the body can be demonstrated in this thalamic nucleus. Fibres concerned with the sensations from the face terminate in the most medial part of the nucleus; those from the arm in the middle and those from the leg in the lateral most part of the nucleus. Pain is perceived in the thalamus itself. All other sensations are transmitted to the cerebral cortex by the 3rd order neurons arising from the thalamus.

SOMATIC SENSORY CORTEX

Sensory signals from the body are projected to two regions of the cerebral cortex: (1) Somatic sensory area-I, located in the postcentral gyrus of the parietal lobe. (2) Somatic sensory area-II, located in the superior wall of the lateral sulcus.

Somatic Sensory Area-I

This area corresponds to Brodmann's areas 3, 1, and 2 (*see* Figs 26.2 to 26.5).

In popular usage, the term somatic sensory cortex is used to mean area-I alone, because the function of the area-II is not yet clear.

A distinct topographic representation of the body can be demonstrated in somatosensory area-I (Fig. 23.13). Each side of the cortex receives sensory information from the opposite side of the body only (contralateral representation). The body is represented upside down in the postcentral gyrus, i.e. the face is represented at the foot of the gyrus whereas the legs and feet are represented at the top extending to the medial surface. Some parts of the body like lips, tongue and fingers have proportionately larger representation than the other areas like the trunk. The cortical representation of the part of the body varies with the number of sensory receptors present in it rather than its size. In turn, the number of sensory receptors varies with the extent to which the part can be used to collect biologically useful sensory information or the skill with which the part is to be used.

The function of somatic sensory area-I can be known from the sensory deficit produced by its destruction (cortical anaesthesia). It is important to appreciate that cortical lesions do not abolish

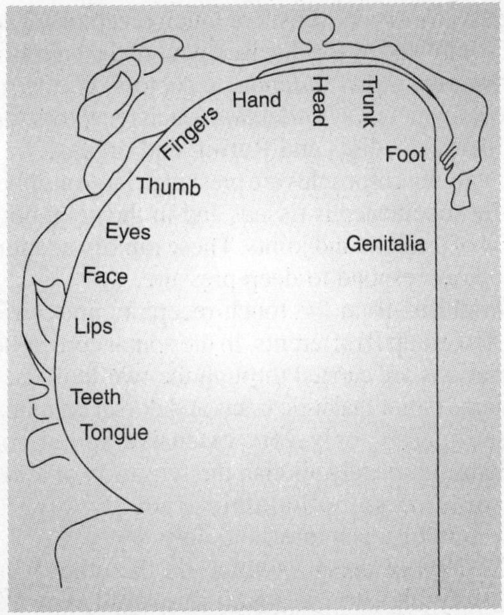

Fig. 23.13: Sensory homunculus on the postcentral gyrus.

all the somatic sensations. Cortical anaesthesia mainly involves loss of proprioception, fine touch, tactile localization, tactile two-point discrimination and stereognosis. Pain and temperature sensations are least affected, but they are poorly localized. Mild differences in the temperature also cannot be appreciated.

From the observations in patients with thalamic syndrome (Chapter 27), it has been inferred that the perception of pain and temperature occurs at (subcortical) thalamic level but their localization probably requires the help of somatic sensory area-I. The function of somatic sensory association area is discussed elsewhere.

SOME SPECIAL ASPECTS OF SENSORY FUNCTION

Touch and Pressure

23

Many types of receptors are involved in the detection of tactile sensation. Meissner's corpuscles are present in large numbers in the cutaneous papillae of the fingertips, lips, nipples and orifices of the body. In the hairy skin, basket-like arborization of unmyelinated nerve endings around the base of the hair follicles (hair end organs) form very sensitive touch receptors. They are stimulated by the displacement of the hair. Both of these are *rapidly adapting* receptors. The dermis also contains *slowly adapting* touch receptors such as Merckel's discs and Ruffini end organs.

Pacinian corpuscles are present in large numbers in the subcutaneous tissues and in the neighbourhood of tendons and joints. These rapidly adapting receptors respond to deep pressure.

Impulses from the touch receptors are carried by Aß (group II) afferents. In the spinal cord, touch sensations are carried through the two leminiscus systems (spinothalamic tracts and dorsal columns). Consequently, only very extensive spinal cord lesions completely abolish the sensation of touch. Lesions of spinothalamic tract produce an elevation of touch threshold only.

Lesions of dorsal column, on the other hand, not only elevate the touch threshold, but also produce loss of tactile localization, two-point discrimination and stereognosis.

Temperature

No specific end-organs for temperature sensations have been identified. Special types of *free nerve endings* seem to be responsible for detection of warmth or cold. In any area of the body, the number of *cold spots* (receptors) is about 3–10 times the number of *warm spots*. On the whole, the density of thermoreceptors is greatest in the lips, moderate in the fingertips and least in the skin of the trunk.

The impulses from cold receptors are carried by Aδ myelinated fibres, while those from the warmth receptors by unmyelinated C-fibres. In the CNS, the lateral spinothalamic tract and the medial lemniscus carry the impulses to the thalamus.

The thermoreceptors respond to the temperature of the subcutaneous tissue surrounding them and not to the environmental temperature as such. That is the reason why cold metallic objects feel colder than wooden objects with the same temperature. The metal being a good conductor, takes away more heat from the skin than a wooden object, and hence, cools the subcutaneous tissues to a greater degree. Similarly, alcohol-induced cutaneous vasodilation gives a feeling of warmth, even when the person is exposed to extreme cold. The inability to appreciate degree of cold exposure can be dangerous.

The cold receptors respond from 10–40°C and warmth receptors from 30–45°C (Fig. 23.14). Between 30 and 40°C, the stimulation of cold and warm receptors to different degrees helps the

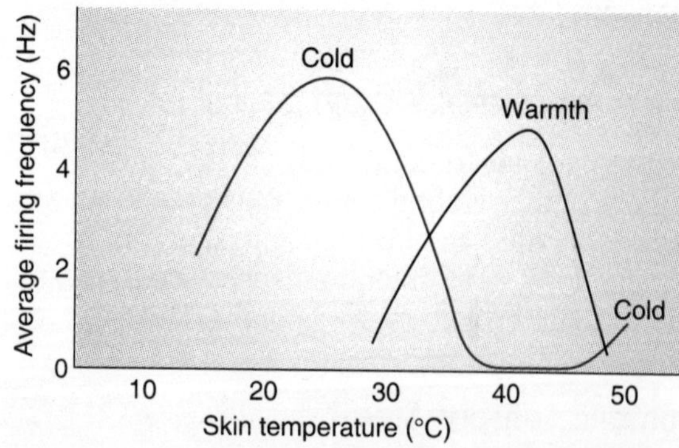

Fig. 23.14: Impulse discharge rate of thermoreceptors at various grades of subcutaneous temperature.

person in the appreciation of fine grades of temperature. Extremes of heat or cold produce tissue damage. Therefore, a sensation of pain rather than temperature is produced.

Thermoreceptors show moderate degree of adaptation. On exposure to cold, the skin temperature begins to fall. Initially, the person feels much colder than at a later stage, even when exposed to same cold environment. Similarly, on sudden exposure to hot environment, the feeling of warmth is more intense in the beginning.

Proprioceptive Sensations

Proprioceptive sensations are those concerned with the physical state of the body, i.e. the sense of position, tendon and muscle sensations, deep pressure and sense of equilibrium. Sense of position includes: (a) sense of static position, and (b) kinesthesia, i.e. conscious recognition of rates of movement of different parts of the body. Receptors for the sense of position are chiefly located in the joint capsules and ligaments around the joint. Ruffini's end organs are the most important receptors for this function. Few Golgi receptors and Pacinian corpuscles are also involved. From these receptors, sensations are carried by thick myelinated nerve fibres (group I and II) in the peripheral nerves and by dorsal columns in the spinal cord. Ultimately, the **conscious proprioceptive sensations** reach the somatic sensory cortex.

Unconscious proprioceptive information arising from muscle spindles, Golgi-tendon organs and joint receptors reaches the cerebellum through group Ia and Ib fibres in the peripheral nerves and through spinocerebellar tracts and dorsal columns in the spinal cord. From the nuclei gracilis and cuneatus, fibres concerned with unconscious proprioception reach the cerebellum as external arcuate fibres. Spinocerebellar tracts enter the cerebellum through inferior peduncles.

PAIN

Pain constitutes one of the most important indications of ill-health. Pain occurs whenever tissues are being damaged. Hence, pain is basically a protective mechanism of the body. It is meant to produce reflex responses which induce the individual to get rid of the injurious stimulus. The danger of lack of pain sensation is best demonstrated in paraplegics due to severe spinal cord injuries. Within weeks, the patient develops ulcers on the pressure points in the lower part of the body (e.g. sacral region and greater trochanters).

Pain receptors are *free nerve endings* of two types of nerve fibres, Aδ and C fibres. High density of pain receptors is present in the superficial layers of the skin and in many deeper tissues like periosteum, joints, arterial wall and falx and tentorium in the cranium. Most other deeper tissues have relatively sparse pain nerve endings, but widespread tissue damage always results in pain, even in these areas.

Pain receptors may be stimulated by excessive mechanical stress, mechanical damage, extreme heat or cold or electrical damage. Visceral pain is often due to excessive tension on nerve endings in the smooth muscle, e.g. pain due to uterine contractions during childbirth or pain due to colics of alimentary, biliary or urinary tracts.

23

Chemical Mediators of Pain

A number of substances, normally present inside the cells, produce pain when released from damaged tissues into extracellular fluid. For example, 5-hydroxytryptamine (5-HT), prostaglandins; K^+, AMP and ADP and acids stimulate pain nerve endings. In addition, plasma and other extracellular fluids normally contain a protein system, from which very potent pain producing plasma kinins can be formed. Bradykinin and kallidin are two well-known kinins produced from a substrate called kininogen (an α-2 globulin) by certain enzymes formed by tissue injury or inflammation.

Transmission of Pain Signals: Fast and Slow Pain

In the peripheral nerves, pain signals are transmitted through two types of fibres: (a) through fast conducting Aδ fibres and (b) through slow conducting C fibres. In the spinal cord, Aδ fibres and type C fibres terminate in the dorsal gray horn. The second order neurons give rise to long axons which cross to the opposite side and ascend as lateral spinothalamic tract. Even in the spinal cord and brainstem, there seems to be a fast-acute pain pathway (composed of myelinated fibres) and a slow-chronic pain pathway (composed of unmyelinated fibres).

Some of the fast conducting fibres terminate in the reticular formation of the brainstem and the rest terminate in the posterolateral ventral nucleus of the thalamus. From thalamus, some fibres relay to the somatic sensory cortex to help in the localization of pain.

Almost all the slow conducting fibres terminate in the reticular formation of the brainstem. However, sensory signals are further relayed to the non-specific intralaminar nuclei of the thalamus, which in turn relay activating signals to all parts of the brain (Fig. 23.15).

23

The transmission of pain signals through two routes explains why a single prick with a sharp needle produces almost immediately sharp localized pain, followed about one second later by slowly increasing painful sensation which lasts many seconds and sometime even minutes.

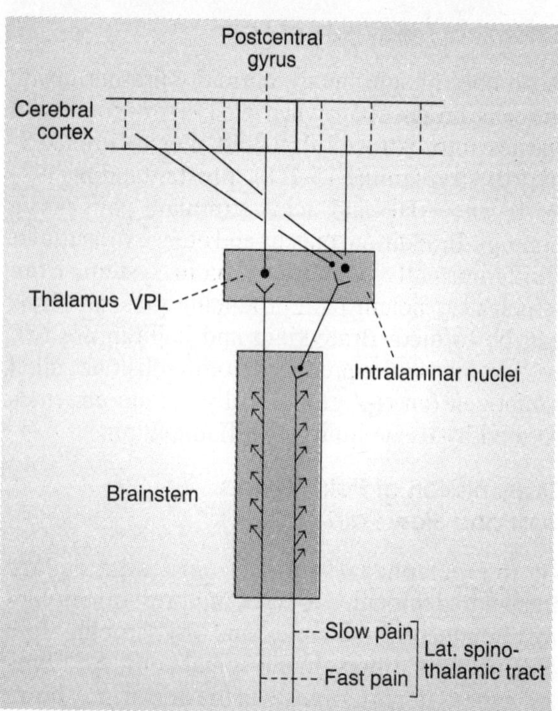

Fig. 23.15: Pathways of slow and fast pain.

Threshold for pain has been estimated by using an instrument producing heat pain. It was observed that the threshold for pain is almost *similar in all the individuals, although different people react differently to pain.*

Perception of Pain

Complete removal of somatic sensory cortex does not abolish the perception of pain. It is believed that pain perception occurs at subcortical levels, i.e. in the thalamus and in the reticular formation of the brainstem. However, *cerebral cortex helps to interpret the quality and localization of pain.*

Pain not only indicates the existence of tissue damage but also may prevent further damage by initiating a withdrawal reflex or forcing the person to give rest to the affected part.

Visceral Pain

Due to high density of pain receptors in the skin, superficial pain is accurately localized. On the other hand, deep somatic pain and visceral pain are poorly localized, due to sparse distribution of pain receptors. It may also be mentioned that the viscera do not have any other sensation except pain and that is partly the reason why visceral pain is poorly localized.

Localized tissue damage in the viscera may not produce any pain at all. If the abdominal wall is infiltrated with a local anaesthetic and opened, localized cuts or burns in the gut do not produce any pain. Diffuse visceral inflammation or distension of the hollow viscera produce intense pain.

Visceral pain sensation is carried by unmyelinated type-C afferents in the sympathetic (from all the thoracic and most of the abdominal viscera) and parasympathetic (from many pelvic viscera) nerves. In the central nervous system, visceral pain fibres accompany somatic pain fibres in the spinothalamic tract and the medial lemniscus.

Neuropathic Pain

Nociceptive pain is the name given to the sensation of pain arising from an area of tissue damage such as physical trauma (sprain, fracture), inflammation, distension of a hollow viscus, etc. In this type of pain, the tissue injury releases algogenic substances (5-HT, prostaglandins, kinins, etc.) which stimulate the pain nerve endings. This type of pain is biologically useful and it responds to common pain killers (analgesics) such as aspirin and other non-steroidal anti-inflammatory agents.

Neuropathic pain results from damage to the peripheral nerves or a part of CNS. Pain occurs without any apparent tissue injury, because the pain nerve fibres are pathologically stimulated. Peripheral neuropathy (diabetes mellitus, chronic alcohol abuse), prolapsed intervertebral disc (PIVD) or nerve entrapment in a cancerous growth are common causes of neuropathic pain. Neuropathic pain is often described as shooting or stabbing type. It does not respond to ordinary analgesics. Even morphine, the most potent analgesic ingredient of opium may be ineffective. This type of pain is biologically useless, but it produces profound psychological effects. Some important differences between the nociceptive pain and neuropathic pain are shown in Table 23.2.

Table 23.2: Differences between nociceptive pain and neuropathic pain

Nociceptive pain	*Neuropathic pain*
Nociceptive stimulus evident.	No obvious tissue damage
Well localized	Poorly localized
Visceral pain may be referred	Not referred
It is "typical" or "has been experienced before"	It is different from the usual somatic or visceral pain
It responds to common analgesics	Only partially relieved by narcotic analgesics

Referred Pain

Pain due to disorder of a deep somatic tissue or a viscus is usually felt in the structure concerned. However, in many tissues, pain may be felt in some other deeper or superficial structure supplied by the same neural (spinal) segments. Such a pain is said to be referred to the second structure. For example, in myocardial ischaemia, pain is referred to the left shoulder and arm. Pain due to a stone in the lower part of the ureter is usually referred to the corresponding testis and inner thigh. Similarly, inflammation of the diaphragm due to pleurisy or severe cholecystitis produces pain at the tip of the shoulder. The site where pain can be referred is determined by the dermatomal rule. Pain is usually referred to a structure with common embryonic origin and hence both are innervated by a common neural (spinal) segment. Embryologically, the heart originates from structures in the neck and upper thorax and hence the visceral pain fibres enter the spinal segments from C_3 to C_5. Important sites where visceral pain is referred are shown in Fig. 23.16.

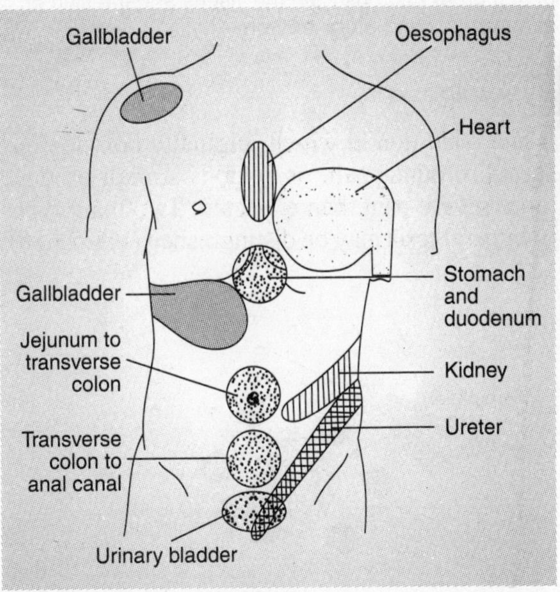

Fig. 23.16: Important sites where visceral pain is referred.

Mechanism of Referred Pain

All the nerve fibres of a given dermatome enter the same spinal segment. Moreover, pain afferents in the peripheral nerves are far more in number than in the lateral spinothalamic tracts. Therefore, many primary pain afferents must be converging on each of the second order neurons of the spinothalamic tract. So when somatic and visceral pain afferents converge on the same second order neuron, pain due to a disorder in the viscus is interpreted as coming from the somatic structure (Fig. 23.17). Pain is more often referred to the anterior than the posterior half of the body. This is probably because we are more conscious of the front than the back of the body.

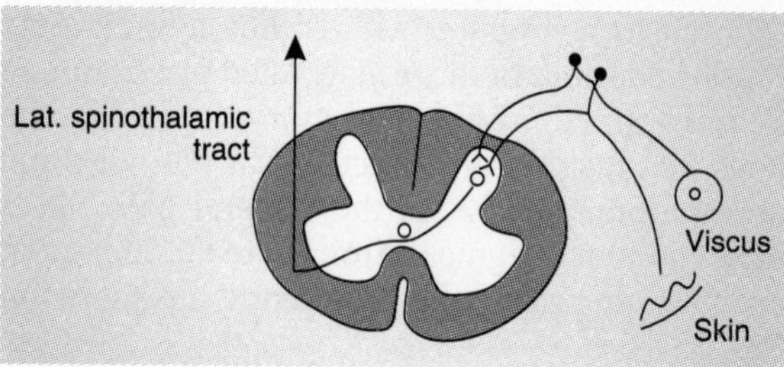

Fig. 23.17: Mechanism of referred pain. Convergence of first order neurons from the viscus and the skin on a common second order neuron.

23

Hyperalgesia

It is a condition in which originally non-noxious stimuli produce pain or noxious stimuli produce more severe pain than expected. Two main types of hyperalgesia may be distinguished (Fig. 23.18).

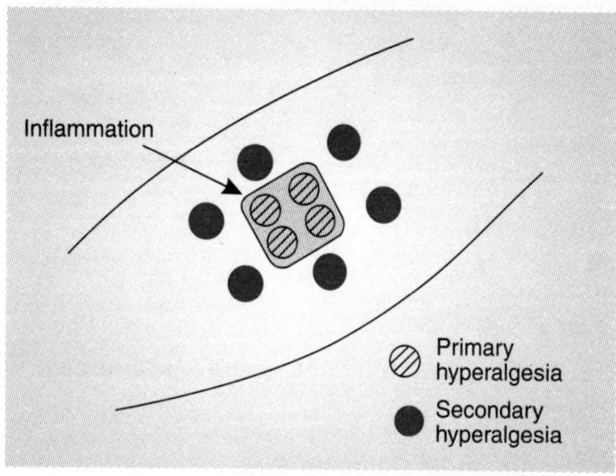

Fig. 23.18: Primary and secondary hyperalgesia.

Primary Hyperalgesia This occurs over an area of tissue damage. The pain threshold is lowered so that, even non-noxious mechanical (touch) or thermal stimuli produce pain. Primary hyperalgesia is due to release of algogenic (pain producing) substances like histamine, 5-HT, plasma kinins and prostaglandins from the damaged tissues.

Secondary Hyperalgesia This may occur in a normal healthy tissue surrounding the diseased tissue. In this condition, there is no lowering of pain threshold. However, noxious stimuli produce far more severe pain than expected in a normal skin. Secondary hyperalgesia may be due to the phenomenon of subliminal fringe. Primary pain afferents from an area of tissue damage not only stimulate the appropriate 2nd order neurons to threshold level, producing pain and primary hyperalgesia, but also excite the 2nd order neurons belonging to nearby area to subthreshold degree (Chapter 24). Hence application of a noxious stimulus produces more intense pain in this area.

CENTRAL PAIN INHIBITORY SYSTEM

Certain experimental observations have demonstrated the existence of a pain inhibitory system in the central nervous system:

(i) Electrical stimulation of nucleus Raphe magnus (NR) situated in the reticular formation of the medulla oblongata causes inhibition of the spinal withdrawal (flexor) reflex evoked by application of a noxious stimulus to a limb.

(ii) Electrical stimulation of the periaqueductal gray matter (PAG) in the midbrain also produced inhibition of withdrawal reflex in response to a noxious stimulus.

(iii) Morphin, the active ingredient of opium is an extremely potent pain killer. A search was made for the morphine-sensitive receptors in the CNS, acting on which morphine (opium) relieves pain. Such receptors, known as *opioid receptors* were found in various parts of CNS, particularly in brainstem and dorsal horn of the spinal cord.

(iv) A number of peptides were found in the brainstem and dorsal horn of the spinal cord which have analgesic (pain-relief) action like morphine. These opioid polypeptides include β-endorphin, met-endorphin, leu-encephalin and dynorphin. Obviously certain neurons in the CNS secrete these analgesic polypeptides. These opioid polypeptides cause presynaptic inhibition of pain sensation either in the dorsal horn of the spinal cord or in the brainstem (Fig. 23.19).

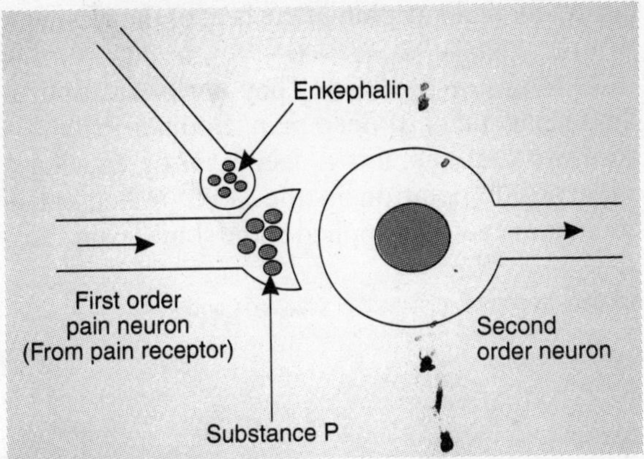

Fig. 23.19: Presynaptic inhibition of pain in the dorsal horn of the spinal cord.

From the observations discussed above, it may be inferred that the *transmission of pain signals in the CNS can be inhibited either at spinal cord level or at brainstem level.*

The PAG and Raphe nuclei constitute the *central analgesia system.* Neurons of the PAG project on and activate the Raphe nuclei. Axons of the Raphe nuclei project on and activate the presynaptic inhibition-producing interneurons in the dorsal horn of the spinal cord (Fig. 23.20). Axons of the Raphe nucleus are serotonergic in nature.

GATE CONTROL HYPOTHESIS

Dorsal horn of the spinal cord may be considered as a gate for the transmission of pain signals into the CNS. The gate may be partially or completely closed, i.e. the transmission of pain signals may be partially or completely blocked by:

(a) Activity of the descending inhibitory pathways from PAG and Raphe nuclei, or
(b) Impulse discharge in the large afferent fibres carrying sensation of touch.

It is a common observation that touching the area of inflammation usually gives partial relief

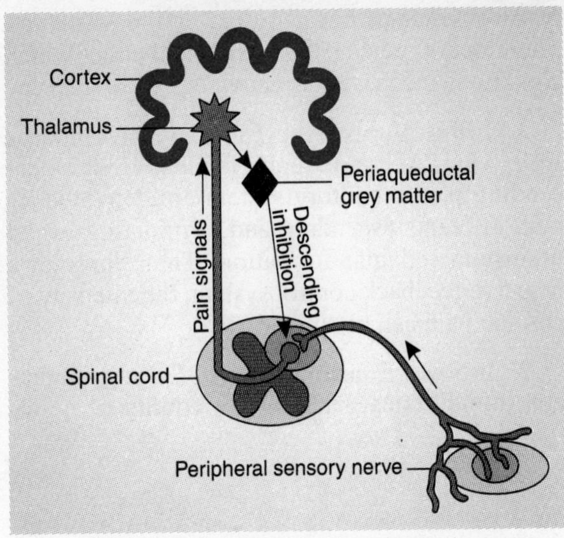

Fig. 23.20: The role of central analgesia system.

from pain. It is believed that touch afferents, as they enter the dorsal columns, give off collaterals that synapse with short interneurons that produce opioid peptides and produce presynaptic inhibition of the second order neurons carrying pain signals (Fig. 23.21).

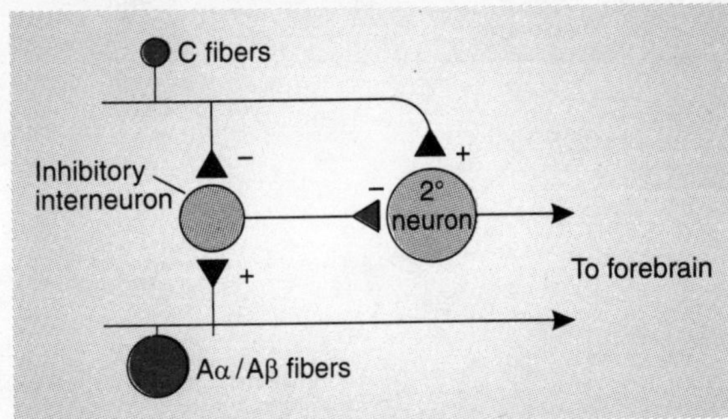

Fig. 23.21: Mechanism of gate control of pain in the dorsal horn of the spinal cord.

When is the Pain Inhibitory System activated?

It is obvious that nature has provided a system by which pain signals can be blocked at the entry point in the spinal cord or/and during their transmission in the brainstem on way to the thalamus. However, pain sensation is basically protective in nature. Therefore, it remains to be explained under which conditions the system is activated.

1. Limitation of the Intensity of Chronic Pain The PAG and Raphe nucleus of the descending pain inhibitory system are activated by pain afferents ascending and terminating in the brainstem reticular formation. Thus, through a negative feedback control system, the intensity of chronic pain can be limited.

2. Intense Emotional State During intense emotional states, sufficient amounts of endogenous endorphins seem to be released, which temporarily inhibit the pain sensation. It has been commonly observed that some athletes sustain serious injury during the sporting event, but it comes to their notice only when the game is over. Similarly, in war, many soldiers are gravely injured but do not feel any pain in the heat of the moment.

3. Counter-irritants They are often used in the management of deep pain. Counter irritant is an *agent* that counters a deep *pain* by causing a superficial irritation in the skin. When these counter irritants are applied to the skin at pain sites,

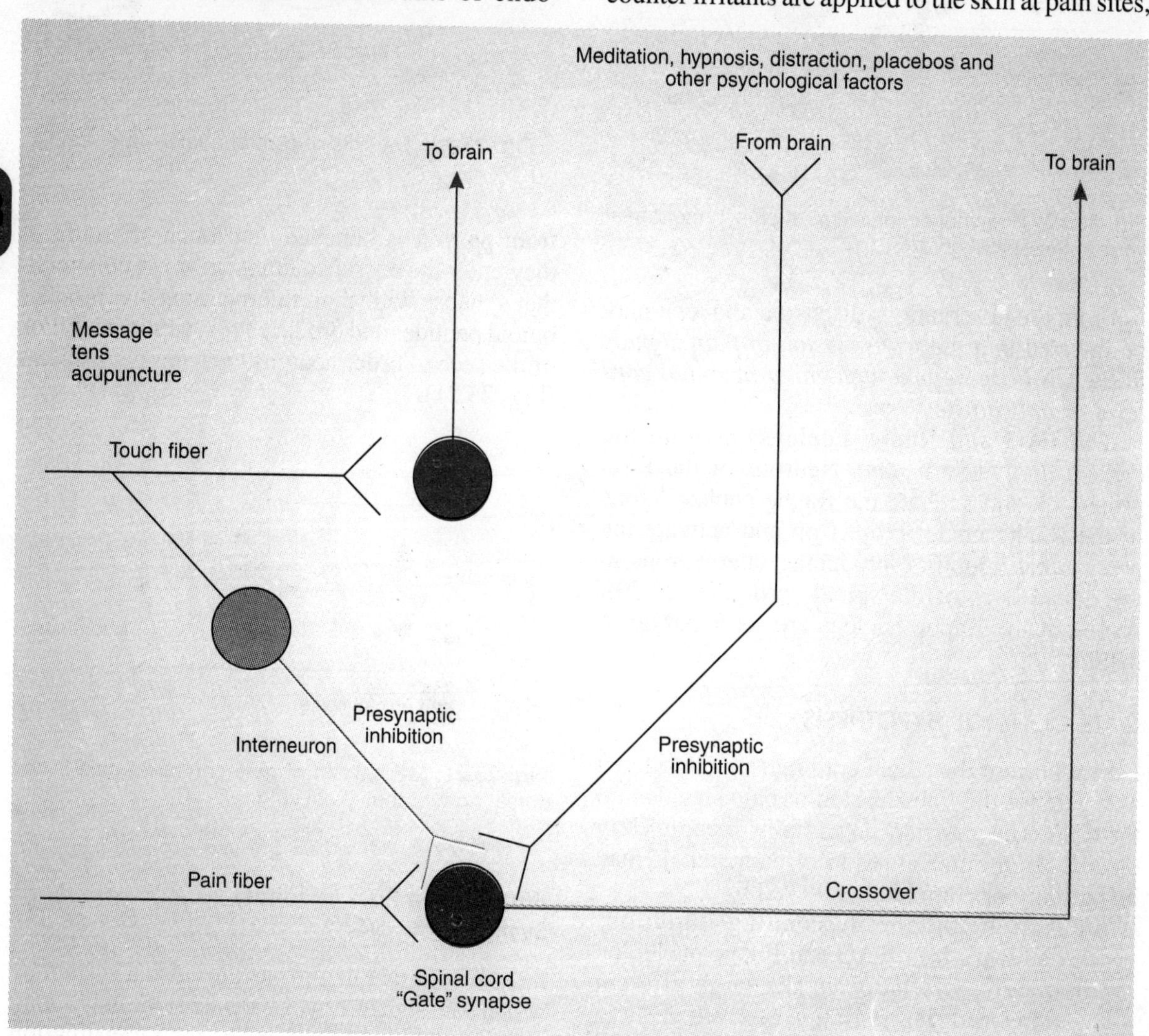

Fig. 23.22: Some tools for the management of pain.

they produce a mild, local and inflammatory reaction, which provides relief at another site that is usually adjacent to, or underlying, the skin surface being treated. Counter irritants are believed to stimulate the large myelinated touch receptors in the affected area leading to closure *of the gate for pain in the dorsal horn* .

4. Mild Transcutaneous Electrical Nerve Stimulation (tens) It is now often found to relieve deep pain. It seems to act like a counter-irritant.

5. Acupuncture It is often used in relief of pain seems to act by releasing endogenous endorphins.

The mechanism of action of some modes of management of pain is shown in Fig. 23.22.

Neurotransmitters Involved in Transmission and Inhibition of Pain

Substance P released by C pain fibres.
Glutamate released by Aδ pain fibres.
Serotonin released by descending pain inhibitory fibres.
Opioid peptides by pain inhibitory neurons in the brainstem and spinal cord.

SYNTHETIC SENSATIONS

The skin contains separate receptors for sensations of touch, pain, cold, warmth and pressure. Combination of two or more of these sensations produces additional information which is sometimes described as "synthetic sensations", e.g. sensations of vibration, two-point discrimination, and stereognosis. The importance of these synthetic sensations lies in the fact that their loss is an important and early sign of posterior column disease or damage to cerebral parietal cortex.

Sensation of Vibration

It is produced by rhythmic stimulation of touch and pressure receptors. It is usually tested by placing a vibrating tuning fork over a bone, e.g. lower end of tibia.

Two-Point Discrimination

The minimum distance by which two touch stimuli must be separated to be perceived as separate stimuli is called 'two-point discrimination'. Two-point discrimination can be determined with a compass that is used to draw circles in geometry. The distance between the points of the compass is decreased until the patient can no longer distinguish two separate punctate stimuli. This distance varies from a few mm on the lips and fingertips to over 60 mm on the back of the trunk. The difference in the distance of two point discrimination seems to be related to the density of touch receptors in different part of the body.

Stereognosis.

The ability to identify objects by handling them and without looking at them is called stereognosis. Normal persons easily identify a pencil, a key or a coin by holding them in a hand. Touch and pressure receptors are involved in this sensation. Somatic sensory association area is also involved in the perception of this sensation, since the subject can identify only the objects he has seen earlier.

23

CHAPTER 24

Somatic Motor Activity: Regulation of Posture

SOMATIC MOTOR ACTIVITY

GENERAL CONSIDERATIONS

The motor component of nervous system is capable of three types of movements as given below.

1. Voluntary Movements such as writing, throwing a ball or playing a musical instrument represent the most complex motor activity. Such movements are characterized by being (i) purposeful and (ii) initiated at will. Such movements can be improved with training. Once learned, they can be executed with minimum voluntary attention.

2. Reflex Responses are rapid, stereotyped and involuntary activities. They are produced in response to specific stimuli, e.g. withdrawal reflex in response to a painful stimulus.

3. Rhythmic Motor Activities such as walking, running or chewing combine the features of the first two types of motor activities. These movements are initiated and terminated at will. However, once initiated, these relatively stereotyped movements may continue in almost reflex-response like pattern.

Since muscles can only pull, not push, each movement depends on balanced contraction of two opposing sets of muscles. The contraction of primary movers (agonists) is counterbalanced by the contraction of the opposite group of muscles (antagonists). A large number of muscles have to contract in a sequence with varying force to execute even a simple act of picking a book from a table. Moreover, all voluntary contractions are performed in the constantly changing background of postural reflex activity.

ROLE OF SENSORY INFORMATION IN MOTOR ACTIVITY

A large amount of exteroceptive information flows back from visual, auditory and cutaneous receptors. These receptors provide information about the position of other objects in space and relationship of our body with respect to them. At the same time, proprioceptive impulses from the muscles, joints and the vestibular apparatus provide information about different parts of the body with respect to each other. Both types of information are essential for proper execution of motor activity. Sensory information is used both as *feedback* and *feed forward* control systems. In the feedback system, the performance is being constantly monitored by sensory system which modifies the output signals to bring the rate, direction or force of movement to the desired end. Feedback system is useful in slow motor activities like touching the nose-tip with finger of an outstretched arm or lifting a book from a table. For fast motor activities, feed forward system is also required. For example, in a cricket match, to catch a ball, the fielder's visual system anticipates the trajectory of the ball and the position of the hands where the ball can be intercepted. The sensory information is fed into the feed forward system which brings about the required motor activity. Complex tasks like writing, singing or playing a musical instrument depend upon feedback and feed forward systems of regulation, both of which require extensive sensory input.

MOTOR NEURONS AND INTERNEURONS

Each spinal segment contains several million neurons. The cell bodies of the 2nd order neurons of the sensory tracts are located in the dorsal horn of the grey matter. The ventral grey horn contains several thousand large neurons whose axons leave the spinal cord through the ventral root and supply the skeletal muscle. They are called alpha (α) motor neurons. Cell bodies of α-motor neurons are largest of all the neurons in the spinal cord.

The diameter of the largest neuron cell body may be as large as 135 μm.

In addition to the α-motor neurons, the ventral grey horn contains much smaller γ-motor neurons. Gamma neurons innervate the intrafusal fibres of the muscle spindles.

Interneurons are present in the grey matter of the brain as well as the spinal cord. In the spinal cord, they are present in the dorsal horn as well as the ventral horn and in the intermediate areas between the two. In the ventral horn, their number is 30 times the number of motor neurons. Interneurons are small and highly excitable cells having numerous interconnections with primary sensory neurons, as well as with the motor neurons. These cells form complex neuronal circuits responsible for the phenomenon of convergence, divergence, repetitive discharge, etc. discussed later in this chapter.

REFLEXES

A reflex is an involuntary response to a stimulus. A reflex action is mediated through a chain of neurons which passes through the central nervous system. The components of a typical reflex arc consist of (i) a receptor organ, (ii) an afferent neuron, (iii) one or more interneurons, (iv) an efferent neuron, and (v) an effector organ (Fig. 24.1).

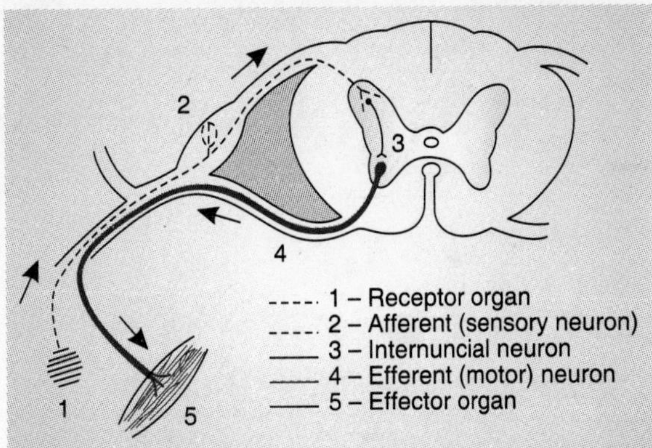

Fig. 24.1: Components of a typical reflex arc. 1: sensory receptor organ, 2: afferent neuron, 3: interneuron, 4: efferent neuron, and 5: effector organ.

In the simplest form, a reflex arc consisting of two neurons : an afferent neuron carries sensory input from the receptor to the CNS and synapses with a motor neuron whose axon supplies an effector organ (Fig. 24.2). Such a reflex arc contains only one synapse and hence called a monosynaptic reflex (e.g. stretch reflex, tendon jerks). Only a few reflexes are monosynaptic.

Most of the reflexes are polysynaptic and involve intervention of a few to hundreds of interneurons between the afferent and efferent

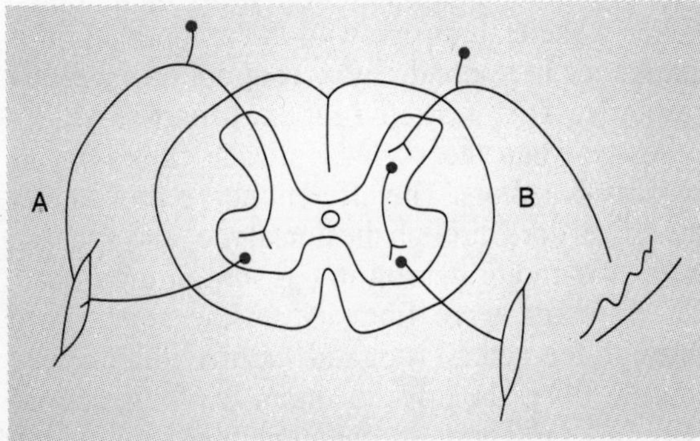

Fig. 24.2: (A) Monosynaptic reflex arc. (B) Disynaptic reflex arc.

neurons (Fig. 24.3). Polysynaptic reflexes may be organized at different levels from the spinal cord to the subcortical centres of the brain.

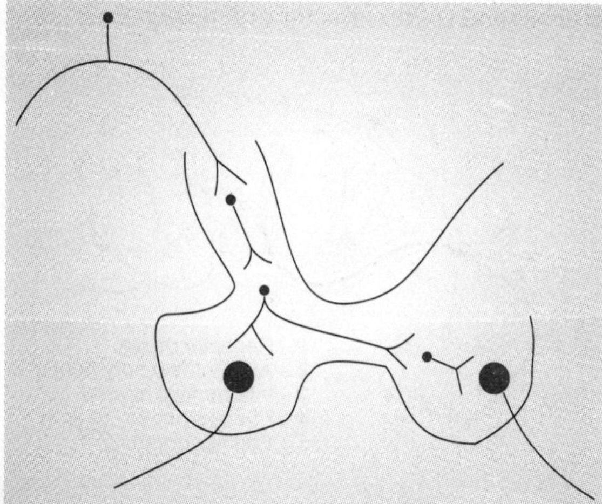

Fig. 24.3: Polysynaptic reflex arc.

24

After entering the spinal cord, sensory signals may follow one or both of the following routes. They may ascend to a higher level of the CNS through the various sensory tracts and reach the thalamus and the somatosensory cortex. On the other hand, they may terminate locally in the grey matter of the spinal cord and elicit local segmental responses. Some signals may ascend a few or more segments and then terminate in the grey matter to produce intersegmental responses.

STRETCH REFLEX

Stretch reflex is the simplest form of a reflex. When a skeletal muscle with intact innervation is stretched, it responds by a contraction, a reflex response. This is stretch reflex. *Muscle spindles* lying between the skeletal muscle fibres act as sensory receptors. The afferent nerve fibres enter the spinal cord through the dorsal root and synapse with A α-motor neuron in the ventral grey horn. The efferent nerve fibre leaves the spinal cord through the ventral root and supplies the skeletal muscle fibre, the effector organ for the response (Fig. 24.4). There is only one synapse in the reflex arc. Hence stretch reflex is known as a *monosynaptic reflex*.

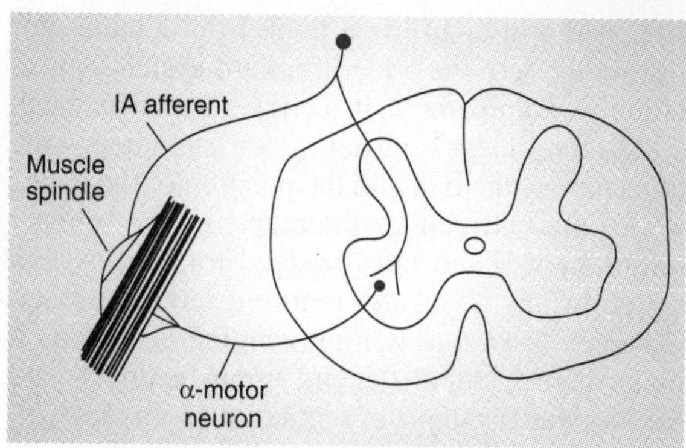

Fig. 24.4: Pathway for a stretch reflex.

Muscle Spindles

Structure

Muscle spindles are *sensory receptors* which detect the degree and rate of stretch of the skeletal muscle. These receptors are spindle-shaped structures, 1–5 mm long present in between and parallel to the ordinary skeletal muscle fibres (average length 30 mm). Either end of the muscle spindle is attached to the endomysium of the skeletal muscle fibre. The number of muscle spindles in a muscle belly varies depending upon the accuracy of movements which the muscle is required to perform (Fig. 24.5).

Each muscle spindle contains 2–10 modified muscle fibres called *intrafusal fibres* (cf. *extrafusal fibres*, the name given to the ordinary skeletal

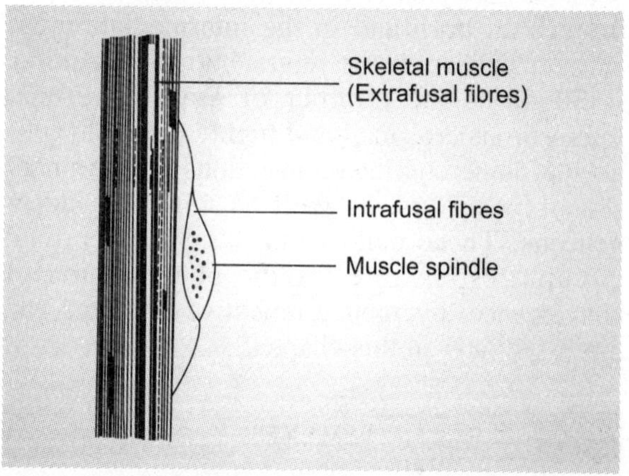

Fig. 24.5: Location of a muscle spindle in relation to a skeletal muscle fibre.

muscle fibres). In the central or equatorial region of the spindle, the intrafusal fibres are surrounded by a fluid contained in a capsule which gives the characteristic shape to the muscle spindle. In the equatorial region of the intrafusal fibres, the nuclei are aggregated whereas striations are relatively well marked on either end (polar region) of the muscle spindle. Stretching or contraction of the polar regions of the intrafusal fibres causes the stretching of the middle part which is noncontractile.

Two types of intrafusal fibres can be identified in a muscle spindle. They are called *nuclear bag fibres* and *nuclear chain fibres*. In the former, the nuclei are collected in the central dilated part as if present in a bag. In the latter, the nuclei are arranged in a single file (Fig. 24.6).

Afferent Nerve Supply

Two types of sensory endings have been observed in the muscle spindle. Group Ia fibre terminals wrap around the centre of the nuclear bag or nuclear chain fibres and are called *annulospiral endings* or *primary endings*. Group II afferent fibre terminals located in the polar region of the nuclear chain fibres are called *flower spray endings* or secondary endings.

Efferent Nerve Supply

The muscle spindles are supplied by a separate type of motor neurons. They are called γ-motor neurons. Their axons are 3–6 μ in diameter as compared to 12–20 μ diameter of the axons of α-motor neurons. The importance of γ-motor neurons may be judged from the fact that their axons constitute 30 of the motor fibres in the ventral root of the spinal cord. Gamma-motor fibres terminate on the polar (contractile) regions of the intrafusal fibres. There are two types of γ-motor fibres: (i) Some of the γ fibres terminate as motor end-plates on the intrafusal fibres, (ii) other, form extensive network (Fig. 24.6).

Muscle Spindle Activation

The discharge rate in the afferent fibres from the muscle spindles increases under two conditions: (1) By stretch of the whole muscle (extrafusal fibres) or (2) by contraction of intrafusal fibres.

When the whole muscle is stretched, the muscle spindles attached to some of the extrafusal fibres are also stretched resulting in increased discharge rate in the spindle afferent fibres.

Increased discharge in the γ-motor neuron produces *contraction of the polar end of the intrafusal fibres leading to a stretch of the non-contractile equatorial region*. Therefore increased γ-discharge also increases discharge in the muscle spindle afferents.

There is a difference in the response of type Ia and type II afferents. In type II afferents, the discharge rate is increased in proportion to the degree of stretch and the higher discharge rate is maintained as long as the muscle remains stretched. This type of response has been called *static response* to differentiate it from the *dynamic response* seen in type Ia afferents (Fig. 24.7). In this type of afferents, the receptors not only respond to the *degree of stretch* but also to the *rate of stretch*. They react strongly when the muscle length is

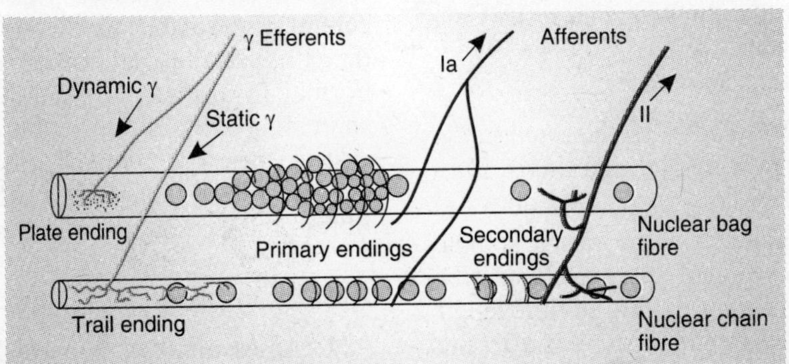

Fig. 24.6: Structure and innervation of intrafusal fibres.

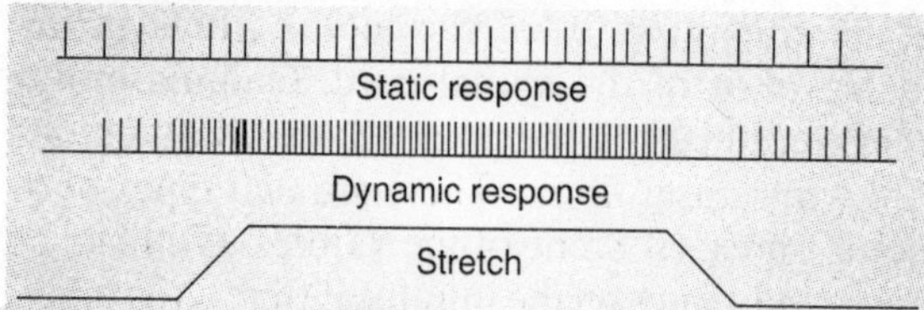

Fig. 24.7: Static and dynamic responses in the muscle spindle during stretch.

changing. When the stretch is being produced there is very high discharge rate which decreases during the stage of maintained stretch and ceases altogether when the stretch is being released.

Central Connections

(a) From the muscle spindles, *unconscious proprioceptive* sensations are carried to the spinal cord where the 2nd order neurons constitute the dorsal and ventral spinocerebellar tracts. Muscle spindles are also involved in the production of *conscious kinesthetic sensations* as produced by joint receptors. For this function, the impulses are carried in the dorsal columns to ultimately reach the somatic sensory cortex.

(b) Type Ia afferent fibres arising from the muscle spindles make direct synaptic connections with A α-motor neuron in the ventral grey horn of the spinal cord. The axons of the α-motor neurons innervate the extrafusal fibres lying close to the muscle spindle (Fig. 24.4). Increased discharge in the Ia fibres by passive stretch of the extrafusal fibres causes increased α-motor discharge and contraction of the extrafusal skeletal muscle fibres (stretch reflex).

Functions of Muscle Spindles

The role of muscle spindles in the *unconscious proprioceptive sensations* and *conscious kinesthetic sensations* has been mentioned above.

Most important function of the muscle spindles is to act as comparator of the extrafusal fibre length. At a normal resting extrafusal fibre length, there is a slight discharge in the type Ia afferents. If the muscle length is passively increased (the muscle is stretched) type Ia discharge is increased. The reflex increase in α-motor discharge causes contraction of the extrafusal fibres and restores their original length. Thus, the muscle spindles, through the stretch reflex, *acts as a feedback device to maintain the skeletal muscle at a certain physiologically useful length*. This action of muscle spindles (particularly in the anti-gravity muscles) is of *fundamental importance in the maintenance of standing posture*.

Role of γ-Efferent Discharge in Muscle Spindles

1. Increased Spindle Sensitivity Gamma-motor activity is regulated by descending tracts from many parts of the brain, particularly by *descending facilitatory* and *inhibitory reticulospinal tracts*. Variations in the γ-motor discharge alter the sensitivity of the stretch reflex. As we know increased γ-motor activity, per se, increases type Ia fibre discharge. In this situation, a given degree of muscle stretch would result in much greater type Ia discharge than would have occurred with normal γ-motor activity. Thus increased γ-discharge increases spindle sensitivity.

2. Role during Voluntary Movements During voluntary movements, active shortening of the extrafusal fibres would relieve tension on the muscle spindles and hence tend to decrease Ia discharge. Thus, proprioceptive information would tend to disappear when it is most needed. However, during voluntary contractions, there is always **alpha-gamma coactivation**. Increased γ-motor discharge always accompanies increased α-motor discharge, because both are fired by the same corticospinal signals. Thus increased γ-discharge maintains central region of the muscle spindle taut even when the extrafusal fibres are contracting. In other words, normal Ia discharge is maintained in spite of shortening of the extrafusal fibres. Muscle spindle system, therefore, remains effective regardless of the momentary changes in length of the extrafusal fibres produced by active contractions.

Clinical Application of Stretch Reflex

1. Assessment of Muscle Tone Assessment of muscle tone is one of the important components of clinical examination of a patient with a neurological disorder. Muscle tone is tested by flexing a limb at various joints, e.g. elbow or knee joint. If the afferent or the efferent nerve to the muscle is damaged (i.e. stretch reflex arc is interrupted), the muscle offers very little resistance to passive stretch, and is said to be *flaccid* or *hypotonic*. A *hypertonic* (also called *spastic*) muscle offers high resistance to the passive stretch. A muscle shows hypertonia when -motor discharge is high. Thus, muscle tone depends on:

(i) Integrity of the stretch reflex arc.

(ii) Discharge in -motor neurons. In turn, -motor discharge is affected by reticulospinal tracts. Through these tracts cerebral cortex, basal ganglia, cerebellum and vestibular nuclei influence the muscle tone.

2. Tendon Jerks The stretch reflex can be demonstrated by striking the patellar tendon with a "reflex hammer". It produces a transient stretch on the quadriceps muscle resulting in a reflex contraction of the quadriceps and extension of the leg at the knee joint (knee jerk). Similarly tapping the Achilles tendon causes contraction of the gastrocnemius muscle (ankle jerk). The tendon jerks are discussed in detail later in this chapter.

Inverse Stretch Reflex

Golgi tendon organs (Fig. 23.1) are high threshold stretch receptors located in the tendons and musculo-aponeurotic junctions. These receptors are located in *series* with the muscle fibres (in contrast to the muscle spindles which are located in parallel). Golgi tendon organs are activated by relatively higher degree of stretch than the muscle spindles. They are also activated by strong active contraction of muscle fibres. The impulses are carried to the spinal cord by type Ib fibres. Increased discharge in the Golgi tendon organs produces inhibition of α-motor discharge to the corresponding skeletal muscle, through intervention of an inhibitory neuron in the reflex arc (Fig. 24.8).

Golgi tendon organs seem to regulate the muscle force in a feedback fashion. If the force of contraction of a muscle becomes too powerful, there is risk of tearing of the muscle or avulsion of the tendon from its attachment to the bone. In such a situation, discharge in the Golgi tendon organs decreases the α-motor discharge to safe limits. The lengthening reaction observed in patients with upper motor neuron type of lesion is also due to activation of Golgi tendon organs (pages 298, 320).

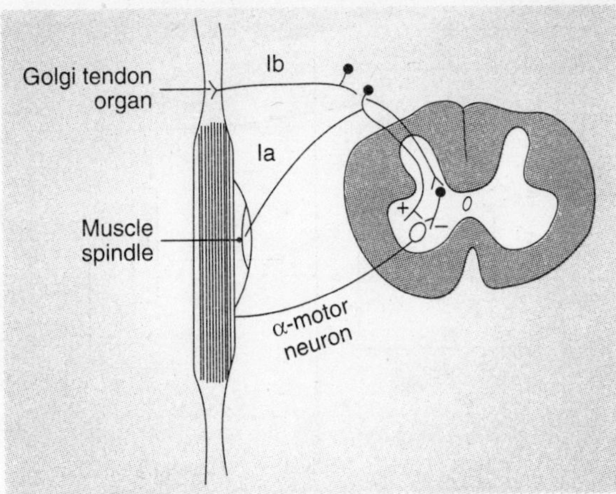

Fig. 24.8: Pathways for stretch reflex and inverse stretch reflex. On stimulation of a muscle spindle, impulses pass through Ia afferents and cause increased α-motor discharge (stretch reflex). On stimulation of Golgi tendon organs, impulses pass through Ib afferents and cause decreased discharge in the α-motor neuron (inverse stretch reflex).

FLEXOR (WITHDRAWAL) REFLEX

As mentioned earlier, most of the reflex activities are mediated through highly complex polysynaptic pathways. Flexor reflex shall be described as an example of polysynaptic reflexes. Application of a noxious (painful) stimulus to a limb produces contraction of the flexor muscles of that limb. As a result, the limb is withdrawn away from the noxious stimulus. This phenomenon is known as flexor reflex or withdrawal reflex.

Flexor reflex is usually demonstrated in spinal animals (produced by a transverse section in the lower cervical region of the spinal cord). In such an animal, application of relatively strong and painful stimulus produces not only flexion of the concerned limb but also extension of the opposite limb (crossed extensor reflex) (Fig. 24.9). Still stronger stimuli may produce a response in all the four limbs, i.e.

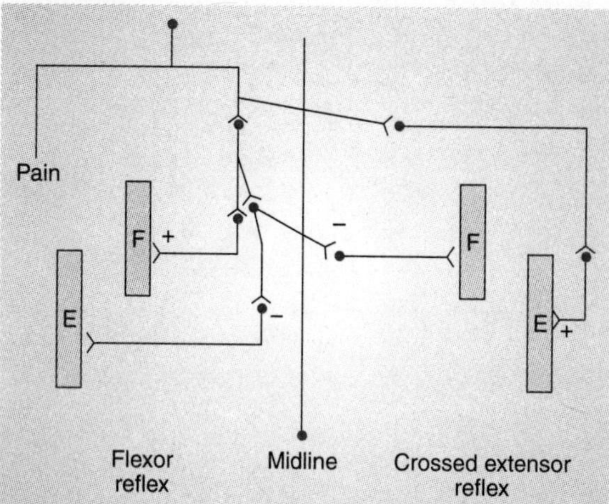

Fig. 24.9: Neural pathways for flexor reflex. Application of a painful stimulus produces contraction of flexor muscles of the limb (flexor reflex). A stronger stimulus produces extension of the contralateral limb (crossed extensor reflex).

24

application of electric shock to one hindlimb produces flexion of that limb, extension of the contralateral hindlimb, extension of the ipsilateral forelimb and flexion of the contralateral forelimb.

The interval between the application of a stimulus and the onset of response is known as the *reaction time*. It is determined, in part, by the time taken by the impulse transmission in the afferent and efferent limbs of the reflex arc (*peripheral delay*). The remaining time spent by the impulse in traversing the spinal cord is called the central delay. The *central delay*, and consequently the reaction time, increases in proportion to the number of synapses involved in the reflex arc. In case of a stretch reflex, the central delay is less than 1 ms, indicating that it is a monosynaptic reflex. In case of flexor reflex, the central delay is much longer. In crossed extensor reflex, the central delay may be longer than 200 ms reflecting the huge number of interneurons involved in the reflex.

Function of Withdrawal (Flexor) Reflex

The flexor reflex is usually initiated by a potentially harmful (nociceptive) stimulus. The flexor response takes the limb away from the source of irritation. The crossed extensor reflex helps to support the body. Flexor reflex is prepotent, i.e. it preempts all other reflex activities taking place at that time in the involved spinal cord segment.

SOME PROPERTIES OF POLYSYNAPTIC REFLEXES

Synaptic Delay

As discussed above, the reaction time of a polysynaptic reflex increases in proportion to the number of interneurons involved in the reflex arc.

Subliminal Fringe

The tension produced in a muscle by simultaneous stimulation of two afferents (say a and b in Fig. 24.10) may be more than the sum of the responses produced separately. This is due to subliminal fringe effect. In the example illustrated in Fig. 24.10, stimulation of afferent fibre 'a' produces two units of tension, due to excitation of motor neurons number 1 and 2. Stimulation of afferent 'b' also produces two units of tension due to excitation of motor neurons number 3 and 4. Interneurons from both these afferents may impinge upon a common motor neuron number 5 and individually may produce only subliminal stimulation. In that case, stimulation of afferents a and b simultaneously produces 5 units of tension rather than the expected 4 units, because the motor neuron number 5 is also excited to the threshold level.

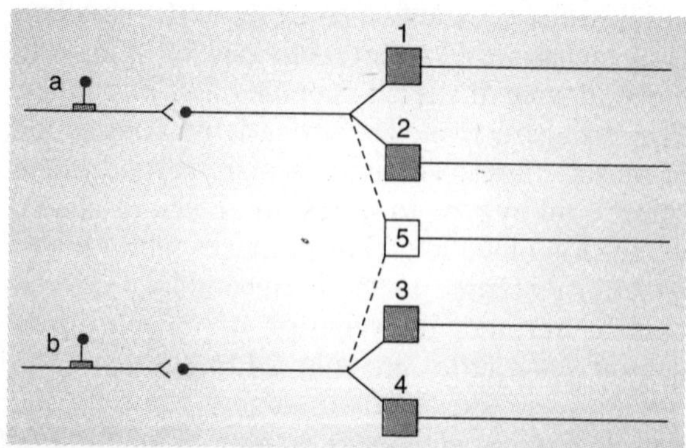

Fig. 24.10: Subliminal fringe. a = 2 unit tension; b = 2 unit tension; a + b = 5 unit tension.

Occlusion

In another situation, stimulation of two afferents (say 'a' and 'b') simultaneously may produce less tension than the sum of tension produced by stimulation of these afferents separately. This phenomenon, called occlusion, is due to the fact that some motor neurons are excited to threshold level by afferent 'a' as well as by afferent 'b' in Fig. 24.11. Stimulation of afferent 'a' excites motor neurons i, j and k giving three units of tension. Stimulation of afferent 'b' excites motor neurons k, y, z, again giving 3 units of tension. But stimulation of afferents 'a' and 'b' together would produce only five units of tension instead of the expected six units.

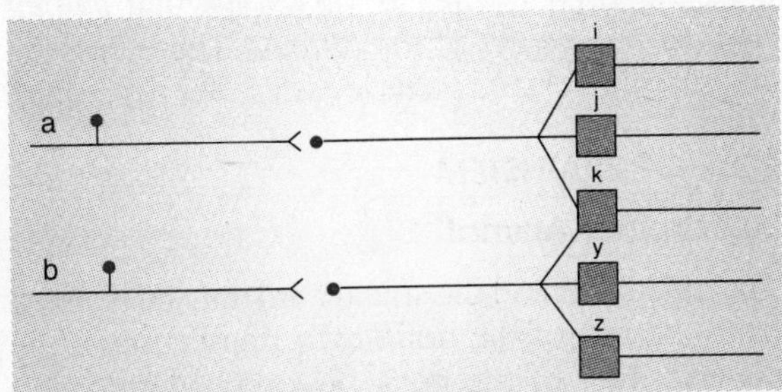

Fig. 24.11: Mechanism of occlusion effect.

Recruitment and After-Discharge

If the motor nerve to a muscle is directly stimulated and the tension produced is recorded, it would be seen that the tension rises immediately and at the end of stimulation, it falls abruptly (Fig. 24.12A). On the other hand, if the same muscle is made to contract by contralateral afferent stimulation (crossed extensor reflex), it would be observed that the muscle tension rises to a peak very gradually. On discontinuation of the afferent stimulation, the contraction continues for several seconds and then gradually declines (Fig. 24.12B). The initial gradual increase in the muscle tension is due to recruitment of more and more motor neurons by gradual increase in the interneuronal activity. The persistence of contraction even after the cessation of afferent stimulation is because of

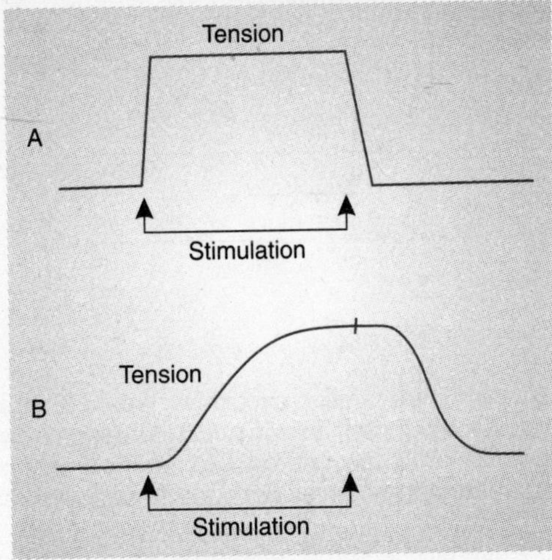

Fig. 24.12: Experimental stimulation of a motor nerve causes abrupt contraction and relaxation of the concerned muscle (A). Crossed extensor reflex causes gradual recruitment of the motor units during stimulation; and gradual decline after the end of stimulation (B).

24

the after-discharge in the motor units. The after-discharge is due to persistent stimulation of the motor neurons by reverberating circuits in the interneurons (Fig. 24.13). The phenomena of recruitment and after-discharge help to make reflex movements smooth at the onset and termination.

Reciprocal Inhibition

Reflex contraction of a muscle is usually accompanied by a reflex relaxation of its antagonist muscle. This phenomenon is due to reciprocal innervation of the antagonist muscles. For example, passive stretch of a muscle illustrated in Fig. 22.15 would increase discharge in Ia nerve fibre leading to the reflex increase in α-motor discharge and contraction of the muscle. At the same time, α-motor discharge to the antagonist muscle would be inhibited. A collateral from the afferent fibre stimulates an inhibitory interneuron which synapses with the α-motor neurons of the antagonist muscle. The reciprocal innervation helps in smooth execution of reflex activity at various joints.

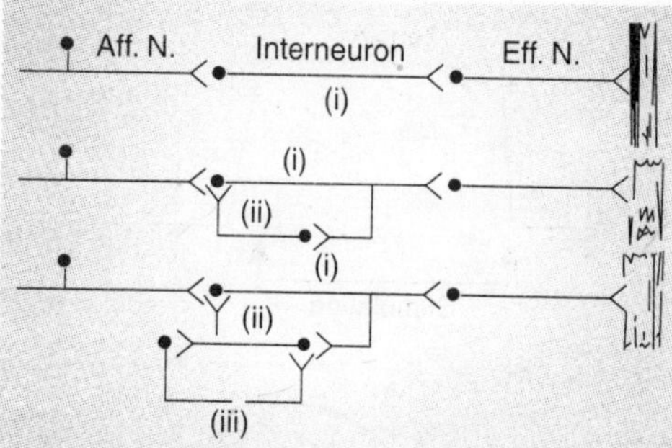

Fig. 24.13: Reverberating circuits. An afferent impulse may pass on to efferent neuron passing through a single interneuron (i). If the neurons constitute a complex network, interneurons may continue to stimulate each other causing continued impulse discharge in the efferent neuron. Neuron (i) stimulates (ii); (ii) stimulates (i) once again. Neuron (iii) stimulates (ii) and neuron (ii) stimulates (i) as well as (iii) once again.

REGULATION OF POSTURE

Erect posture is a prerequisite to most of the somatic motor activities of man and other higher animals. In quadrupeds, extensor muscles are basically the antigravity muscles. In man, the maintenance of erect posture is more difficult because a narrow base of the two feet has to support over 150 cm tall body. A standing man can fall in any direction. The muscles which oppose the fall act as antigravity muscles depending upon the direction of the fall. Therefore, any of the muscles of the trunk and limbs can act as an antigravity muscle. The erect posture becomes further unstable when a man begins to move, and more so during performance of physical work. Afferent input from *muscle and joint receptors*, *vestibular* and *visual* receptors produce a very complex and coordinated reflex activity which provides a stable postural background for the voluntary movements.

The role of different regions of the CNS in the maintenance of posture can be experimentally investigated (usually in a cat) by producing transection in the neuraxis at various levels.

ROLE OF SPINAL CORD: SPINAL ANIMAL

A spinal animal is produced by a transection in the spinal cord below the origin of phrenic nerve, preferably in the midthoracic region. The result is an immediate and permanent inability to perform voluntary movements (paralysis) and loss of sensations below the level of the lesion. In addition, for a period lasting a few minutes in cat to about three weeks in man (with spinal cord injury) all the reflex activities cease. Muscle tone is lost. Urinary bladder and rectum are paralyzed. Blood pressure falls and the degree of change varies with the level of transection. This phase of areflexia is called the *spinal shock*. Spinal shock is due to transient reduction in the excitability of the spinal motor neurons isolated from the supraspinal centres. When the isolated spinal segments regain their reflex activity, the muscle tone recovers to some extent. The flexor reflex, crossed extensor reflex and visceral reflexes can be demonstrated in the spinal animals. However, the *stretch reflex is very weak* and *cannot support the weight of the animal*. Therefore, the animal cannot stand on its legs even for a moment.

ROLE OF BRAINSTEM

Bulbospinal Animal

The hind brain and the spinal cord may be isolated from the rest of the brain by a transection at the upper border of the pons. The procedure called *decerebration* results in an immediate *spasticity* (rigidity) of all the antigravity muscle (decerebrate rigidity). Spinal shock does not develop with lesion at this level or any other higher level.

Decerebrate rigidity is characterized by hypertonia of the antigravity muscles. The tail and the head are hyperextended and the back is concave due to hyperextension of the spine. The limbs are also hyperextended and rigid (Fig. 24.14). The animal can be made to "stand" on its four limbs.

However, it is easily toppled even by a slight push and cannot stand on its own (it has no righting reflexes). The mechanism of decerebrate rigidity would be discussed separately a little later. The following reflexes can be observed in a decerebrate or bulbospinal animal:

1. A strong stretch reflex.
2. Positive supporting reaction.
3. Negative supporting reaction.
4. Crossed extensor reflex.
5. Tonic neck reflexes.

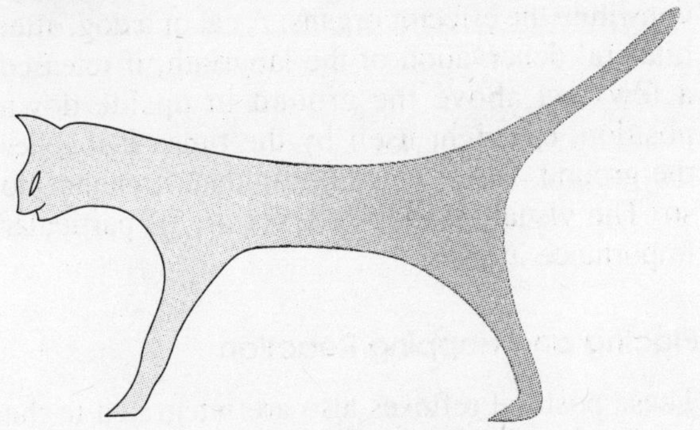

Fig. 24.14: Decerebrate rigidity in a cat.

Positive supporting reaction can be elicited by passive dorsiflexion of the toes of the feet. Reflex contraction of all the flexors and the extensors of the limb converts it into a solid pillar. Passive plantar flexion releases the limb from the positive supporting reaction. This response is called the *negative supporting reaction*. For the positive supporting reaction, the afferents arise from the stretch receptors of the interossei muscles.

Crossed extensor reflex can also be demonstrated in such an animal. It is not difficult to understand how these three reflexes would be helpful in the intact animal. During normal walking, the limbs are alternately extended to support the body and flexed for the forward movement. Moreover, when one forelimb is flexed, the other forelimb is extended.

In decerebrate animal, not only the posture of one limb is adjusted in relation to the other (crossed extensor reflex), but also the position of the limbs is adjusted in relation to the position of the head by tonic neck reflexes.

Tonic neck reflexes are better demonstrated after bilateral extirpation of the labyrinth (to eliminate the role of the latter).

(i) Dorsiflexion of the head produces extension of the forelimbs and flexion of the hindlimbs.
(ii) Ventroflexion of the head produces flexion of the forelimbs and extension of the hind limbs.
(iii) Pressure on the vertebral column in the lower cervical region leads to flexion of all the four limbs.
(iv) If the head is rotated to one side, the "jaw limbs" (the limbs towards which jaw is turned) are extended while the "skull limbs" are flexed. The tonic neck reflexes are integrated in the upper cervical spinal segments.

The proprioceptive receptors located in the muscles and joints of the neck initiate the tonic neck reflexes.

ROLE OF MIDBRAIN: HIGH DECEREBRATE ANIMAL

If the brainstem is transected at the rostral border of the midbrain, the animal not only can stand normally but also typical quadruped walking movements can be reflexly performed. The decerebrate rigidity is present but it disappears when the limb is performing a reflex activity. The chief advance in the postural regulation in mesencephalic animal over bulbospinal animal lies in the presence of *righting reflexes*.

The ability to stay upright is a universal property in the animal kingdom. In higher animals and man, it is dependent upon the presence of specific righting reflexes. If a mesencephalic animal is laid on its side, almost immediately the head rights itself, and then body follows suit, and finally the animal stands erect.

Labyrinthine Righting Reflex

When the animal is lying on one side, asymmetrical discharge from the two labyrinths causes responses in the neck muscles leading to righting of the head.

Body on Head Righting Reflex

The righting of the head is also produced by another reflex called the body on head righting reflex. One side of the body is in contact with the bench while the other is in contact with the air. The asymmetrical discharge from the body surfaces causes righting of the head (body on head righting reflex).

Neck Righting Reflex

Righting of the head because of labyrinthine and/or body righting reflex causes twisting of the neck.

This sets up afferent impulses which reflexly bring the thorax and lumbar region in the upright position.

Body on Body Righting Reflex

The asymmetrical discharge of the body surfaces discussed above not only causes righting of the head but also contributes to the righting of the body, i.e. this reflex can lead to righting of the body even if the head of the animal is held in the lateral position.

The integrating centre for the righting reflexes described above is located in the region of the Red nucleus in the midbrain.

ROLE OF CEREBELLUM

Cerebellum, through its connection with the red nucleus influences the activity of brainstem reticular formation and thereby gamma motor neuron activity. Through its connections with the vestibular nucleus and vestibulospinal tract, cerebellum influences the activity of alpha motor neurons. Thus, normal cerebellar function is essential for the maintenance of normal muscle tone and posture. In humans, unilateral cerebellar disease causes atonia in the skeletal muscles of the same side. It also produces rotation of the face to the opposite side; the trunk is bent with concavity towards the affected side. The deep reflexes show the pendular response.

ROLE OF BASAL GANGLIA

The basal ganglia constitute a relay station for descending extrapyramidal pathways. Parkinsonism is characterised by rigidity of both protagonists and antagonists of the limbs (lead pipe type of rigidity). There is flexion at the knee, hips, and strenomastoids. Arms are adducted and flexed. Due to rigidity, it becomes difficult to elicit the deep reflexes.

ROLE OF CEREBRAL CORTEX

Optical Righting Reflexes

Righting of the head is brought about by visual righting reflexes also. These reflexes are integrated in the calcarine cortex, while the neck muscles constitute the effector organs. A cat or a dog, after bilateral denervation of the labyrinth, if released a few feet above the ground in upside down position, can right itself by the times it touches the ground. But if it is blindfolded, it cannot do so. The visual righting reflexes are of particular importance in man.

Placing and Hopping Reaction

These postural reflexes also are integrated in the cerebral cortex. If a blindfolded animal is suspended in the air, near a table and the snout touches the table, the animal immediately places both the fore-paws on the table (*placing reaction*). When a standing animal is pushed laterally, it makes a hopping movement and brings the legs under the body to support it in upright position (*hopping reaction*).

MECHANISM OF STANDING IN MAN

As mentioned before, a man standing on the narrow base of the feet has very unstable posture and may fall in any direction. It may be presumed that a continued contraction of most of the trunk and leg muscles keeps the posture upright. However, electromyographic studies have revealed very little muscle activity in a person standing quietly upright. The configuration of the hip and the knee joints is such that the force of gravity itself tends to keep these joints extended. However, the balance is very precarious. All the time, one or the other muscle reflexly contracts to oppose the effect of gravity.

When the body sways forward, the extensors of the trunk and flexors of the legs contract and restore the balance. Next moment, the body may sway backwards when recti abdominis and extensors of the legs contract. Tendency to fall sideways is opposed by contraction of contralateral external oblique abdominal muscles. All these changes are reflexly induced by stretch receptors in the legs and the trunk as well as by visual and vestibular afferents. It is obvious that, at any moment, only a few muscles need to contract. Hence, energy required for standing quietly is not very high.

MECHANISMS OF DECEREBRATE RIGIDITY (SPASTICITY)

Decerebrate rigidity is usually produced by a transection in the brainstem at the midcollicular level. However, it may be produced by a transection in the brainstem anywhere above the level of the vestibular nuclei. A section below the level of the vestibular nuclei produces spinal shock and reflex pattern characteristic of spinal animal (hypotonia and weak stretch reflexes) instead of decerebrate rigidity.

The rigidity, produced by midcollicular transection, can be abolished in any limb by cutting the dorsal roots (deafferentation) carrying afferent impulses from the particular limb. Further, in animals with decerebrate rigidity γ-motor discharge has been found to be increased, which can be abolished by deafferentation, or by administration of chlorpromazine (a drug which decreases the activity of ascending reticular formation of the brainstem). From these experiments, it has been concluded that:

1. Decerebrate rigidity is due to over-activity of γ-motor discharge leading to over-sensitivity of stretch reflex.
2. Increased γ-motor discharge is due to over-activity of some centres in the brainstem involved in the regulation of stretch reflex.
3. Vestibular nuclei also contribute to the rigidity.

Brainstem reticular formation regulates γ-motor discharge through *reticulospinal tracts*. A longer *facilitatory area* of the reticular formation discharges "spontaneously" (possibly due to a constant sensory input from the collaterals of the ascending reticular activating system). It receives facilitatory corticobulbar extrapyramidal projection also. A smaller *inhibitory area* of the brainstem reticular formation discharges when driven by impulses arising from suppressor areas of the cerebral cortex or from the cerebellum.

Midcollicular transection cuts off all facilitatory and inhibitory corticobulbar extrapyramidal pathways. Hence bulbar inhibitory area becomes less active since now it is driven by cerebellum only. On the other hand, bulbar facilitatory area remains active, since it is driven by stronger ascending reticular activating system. The resulting imbalance in the discharge between descending facilitatory and descending inhibitory reticulospinal tracts causes increased γ-motor discharge (Fig. 24.15). The interruption of extrapyramidal corticobulbar projection also removes inhibitory influence on the vestibular nuclei. Therefore, greater activity of vestibular nuclei causes increased α-motor activity through the vestibulospinal tract and contributes to the rigidity in the decerebrate animal.

In human patients, the term *spasticity* is used to describe a state of muscular hypertonia, hyperactive tendon reflexes and clonus (repetitive contractions in response to suddenly applied and sustained stretch of a muscle). It is typically observed in patients with hemiplegia due to a vascular lesion in the internal capsule leading to destruction of pyramidal and extrapyramidal

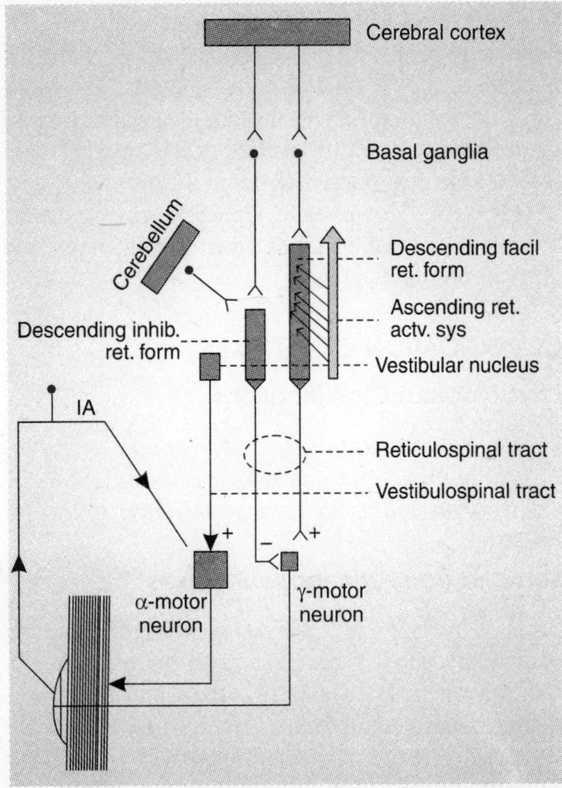

Fig. 24.15: Supraspinal control of stretch reflex.

tracts. The hypertonia is encountered chiefly in the extensors of the lower limb and flexors of the upper limb (antigravity muscles). Like decerebrate rigidity, spasticity is also due to an imbalance in facilitatory and inhibitory reticulospinal projection on the γ-motor neurons leading to hypersensitive stretch reflex activity.

While testing the muscle tone in such patients of hemiplegia, if a limb is passively flexed, initially great resistance is offered by the muscles. If still more force is used, the resistance suddenly disappears. This phenomenon, known as *Clasp-knife effect*, or the *lengthening reaction*, is a characteristic feature of spasticity in a hemiplegic patient. The initial resistance is due to activation of over-sensitive stretch reflex, whereas the sudden decrease in resistance is due to stimulation of Golgi tendon organs and activation of inverse stretch reflex.

Further Discussion on Reflexes

So far, the discussion on reflexes has mainly centered on somatic reflexes and their role in posture regulation. However, the reflex activity occurs in almost all the body systems. We have cardiovascular reflexes, gastrointestinal reflexes, visual reflexes, auditory reflexes and so on. These reflexes are discussed in detail in different chapters in this book. However, it would be profitable to have a review of reflexes from physiologic and clinical points of view.

CLASSIFICATION OF REFLEXES

Physiological Classifications

(i) *Monosynaptic and polysynaptic reflexes.*
(ii) *Somatic and autonomic reflexes.*
(iii) *Conditioned and unconditioned reflexes.*

Somatic and Autonomic Reflexes

Somatic reflexes are the reflexes which involve somatic nervous system, e.g. postural reflexes and withdrawal reflex. Tests of superficial and deep reflexes discussed below are concerned with somatic reflexes. Autonomic reflexes are concerned with autonomic nervous system. These are too numerous to be counted here, e.g. reflex salivary and gastric secretion, baroreceptor and chemoreceptor reflexes involving CVS and respiration, pupillary reflexes, etc. Only some of them can be clinically tested.

In some reflexes, the afferent limb of the reflex arc involves autonomic nervous system whereas the efferent limb involves somatic structures, e.g. cough reflex.

Conditioned and Unconditioned Reflexes

By definition, a reflex action is an involuntary response to a stimulus. The response is inborn and present in all members of the species. All the reflexes mentioned above fall in this category and may be called *unconditioned reflexes*. *Conditioned reflexes* are not true reflexes. These responses occur because of conditioning or experience. Hence, they should better be called *conditioned responses*. However, because of historical usage, the term conditioned reflex is still widely used. For example, sight of tasty food does not produce salivation in a child unless the child has repeatedly tasted the food and liked it. The salivation in response to taste of a food is an unconditioned reflex action, whereas salivation on the sight of food is a conditioned response.

Clinical Classification of Reflexes

Certain reflexes are tested from clinical point of view, i.e. a change from the normal response helps in the diagnosis of a neurological disorder.

These reflexes are further classified as: (i) superficial, (ii) deep and (iii) visceral depending upon the location of sensory receptors involved in the reflex.

Superficial Reflexes

The superfical reflexes are explained in Table 24.1.

Deep Reflexes (Tendon Jerks)

A tendon jerk (deep reflex) is tested by giving a single sharp blow on the tendon of a slightly stretched muscle by a soft rubber hammer (usually called a patellar hammer). The sudden deformation of the tendon results in a transient stretching of the muscle belly leading to the stimulation of

Table 24.1: Superficial reflexes

Superficial reflex	*How tested*	*Result*	*Spinal level where mediated*
Abdominal	Stroking abdominal wall below costal margin, at the level of umbilicus and in iliac fossa	Contraction of abdominal muscles	T7–12
Plantar	Stroking sole of foot	Flexion of toes of foot	L5, S1
Cremasteric	Stroking skin of upper inner thigh	Upward movement of testicle	L1, 2
Anal	Stroking skin near the anus	Contraction of anal sphincter	S3, 4
Bulbocavernosus	Pinching dorsum of glans penis	Contraction of bulbo-cavernosus muscle	S3, 4

muscle spindles in the muscle (not Golgi tendon organs). The consequent synchronous volley of Ia afferent discharge results in monosynaptic reflex activation of alpha motor neurons leading to a brief contraction of the muscle. Thus, when a tendon jerk is being tested, the integrity of stretch reflex at a particular spinal level is under investigation.

Tendon reflexes are diminished or absent with a lesion of any segment of the reflex arc: (a) afferent pathway (e.g. tabes dorsalis), (b) the anterior horn cell (e.g. lower motor neuron disease, poliomyelitis) or (c) both afferent and efferent pathways (e.g. peripheral neuropathy).

Tendon jerks are exaggerated (hyper-reflexia) due to an increase in gamma motor discharge, which may be due to:

(a) Physiological causes like anxiety, nervousness.
(b) Thyrotoxicosis.
(c) Upper motor neuron disease (discussed later).

The deep reflexes usually tested are described in Table 24.2.

Clonus

This clinical sign is usually seen when the stretch reflex is highly sensitized, e.g. in a patient with upper motor neuron lesion. In such a patient, the knee is slightly bent and supported on the left hand, and the other hand is used to suddenly dorsiflex the foot. The sudden stretch of calf muscles results in reflex contraction of calf muscles. If the dorsiflexion of the foot is maintained, the calf muscles go into oscillations of repeated contraction and relaxation. This phenomenon is called clonus.

Table 24.2: Deep reflexes

Deep reflex	*Tendon tapped*	*Response*	*Spinal segment where mediated*
Knee jerk	Patellar tendon	Contraction of quadriceps	L 2, 3, 4
Ankle jerk	Achille's tendon	Contraction of calf muscles	S1, 2
Biceps jerk	Biceps tendon	Contraction of biceps muscle	C5, 6
Triceps jerk	Triceps tendon	Contraction of triceps muscle	C6, 7
Supinator jerk	Blow on styloid process	Supination of elbow	C5, 6

Visceral Reflexes

The reflexes concerned with deglutition, micturition and defecation are enquired into. History of the patient is sufficient indication of the integrity or otherwise of these reflexes. For example, history of regurgitation of food, especially liquids into the nasopharynx during swallowing or history of urinary incontinence are sufficient evidence of lesion in the respective reflex arc.

VESTIBULAR APPARATUS

The vestibular apparatus or the labyrinth consists of three semicircular canals and two sacs, the utricle and the saccule. It helps in the recognition of position and movements of the head. Afferent impulses arising from the vestibular apparatus give rise to *labyrinthine righting reflexes* which play an important role in the regulation of posture.

24

The vestibular labyrinths consist of a system of thin walled ducts and sacs to constitute the *membranous labyrinth* that lies in *a bony labyrinth*—a series of channels in the petrous part of temporal bone. *Perilymph* with the chemical composition resembling ECF (Na^+ 150 mEq/L, K^+ 5 mEq/L) is present in the bony labyrinth surrounding the membranous labyrinth. The membranous labyrinth is filled with a fluid called *endolymph*. It contains very little Na^+ (1.0 mEq/L) but high concentration of K^+ (150 mEq/L). There is no communication point between perilymph and endolymph.

Semicircular Canals

The semicircular canals are known as *lateral (horizontal)*, *superior* and *posterior* canals and are oriented in the three planes of the space at right angles to each other (Fig. 24.16). The lateral canals attain the horizontal plane only when the head is bent 30° forward. Both ends of each semicircular canal open into the utricle. At the end, near its origin from the utricle, each canal has a dilated part called the *ampulla* which contains the receptor organs of the semicircular canals known as the *crista ampullaris*.

Non-dilated ends of the superior and the posterior canals have a common opening in the utricle. Thus, the three semicircular canals open into the utricle by five apertures instead of six.

The *crista ampullaris* is a mound or a ridge of tissue whose upper surface contains tall ciliated columnar sensory hair cells. The cilia or the hair extend upward into a firm gelatinous structure called the *cupula* (Fig. 24.17). The cupula extends across the entire lumen of the ampulla and forms a movable partition in the ampulla. Movements

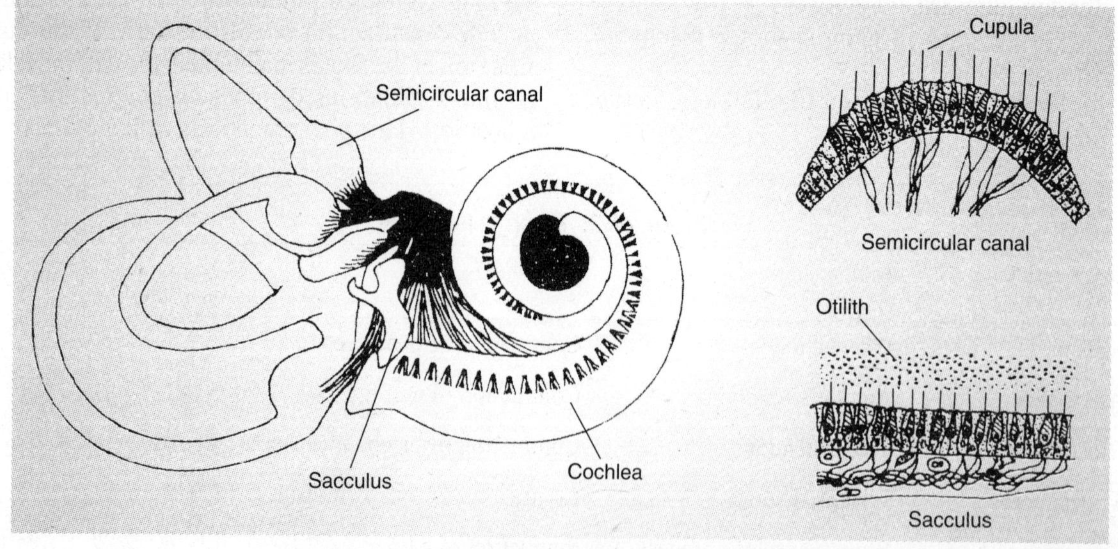

Fig. 24.16: The vestibular apparatus and the cochlea.

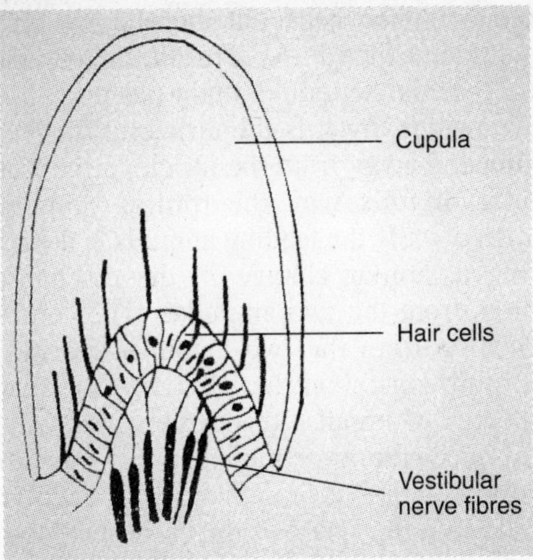

Fig. 24.17: Structure of the crista.

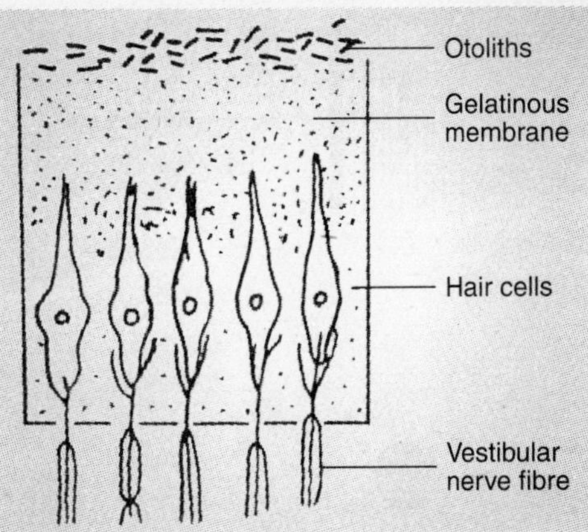

Fig. 24.18: Structure of the macula.

of the endolymph produced by the movements of the head deflect the cupula sideways thereby bending the hair cells. The bases and the sides of the hair cells synapse with the sensory axons of the vestibular nerve.

Otolith Organs

The utricle and the saccule each contain a receptor organ called the *macula.* Each macula is covered by columnar epithelium like the crista. The hair cells are embedded in a thin gelatinous layer covering the epithelium (Fig. 24.18). Many chalky particles or the *otoliths* are embedded in the gelatinous layer. That is why the saccule and the utricle are also known as the otolith organs. When the head is in normal vertical position the macula of each utricle is in horizontal plane while the macula of each saccule lies in vertical plane.

Hair Cells

The columnar epithelium of the crista ampullaris or the macula consists of some supporting cells called *sustentacular cells* and the *true receptor cells called the hair cells*. The basal ends of the hair cells are in close contact with the afferent neuron terminals. About 60–100 rod-shaped processes or hairs project from the apical surface of each hair cell. These are called *stereocilia*. The cores of stereocilia are composed of parallel filaments of actin. Located at one edge of the apical surface is a large process called kinocilium. *Kinocilium* is a true cilium (i.e. it contains 9 pairs of microtubules in its circumference) but it is non-motile. The length of the stereocilia is maximum near the kinocilium and minimum at the opposite end (Fig. 24.19).

The membrane potential of a hair cell is about – 60 mV. Bending of the stereocilia in the direction of the kinocilium depolarizes the cell membrane and increases the discharge rate in the vestibular afferents. The hyperpolarization of the hair cells, produced by the bending of the stereocilia in the opposite direction, decreases the discharge rate in the vestibular afferents. The degree of depolarization or hyperpolarization is proportionate to the degree of displacement of the stereocilia.

Connections of Vestibular Apparatus

The cell bodies of the vestibular afferent nerve are situated in the vestibular ganglion. The central axons of the vestibular nerve enter the medulla oblongata and terminate around four nuclear masses consisting of the large principal nucleus situated in the pons and medulla, the descending nucleus, the superior nucleus and the lateral nucleus. All the four vestibular nuclei seem to have common connections and function. From the vestibular nuclei, the fibres pass to the paleocerebellum, the red nucleus, the brainstem reticular formation, the oculomotor nuclei and to

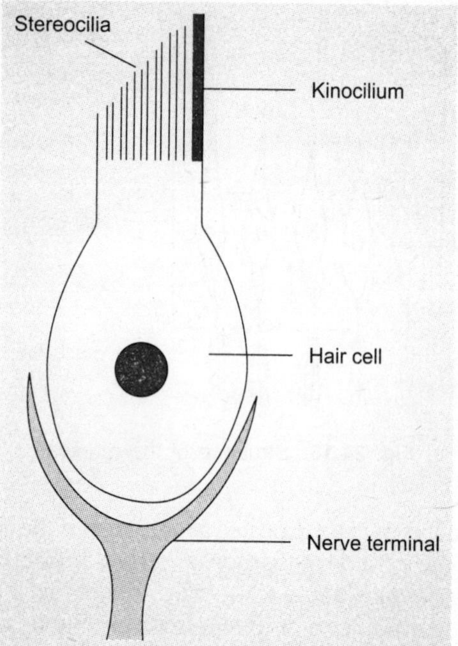

Fig. 24.19: The hair cell of the vestibular apparatus.

24

the opposite thalamus and the temporal lobe. Some fibres of the vestibular nerve pass directly to the cerebellum. The vestibular nuclei receive fibres from the cerebellum as well. The close association between the cerebellum and the vestibular nuclei is important in the regulation of posture. The descending fibres from the vestibular nuclei constitute the vestibulospinal tract which terminates around the α-motor neurons of the spinal cord.

Mode of Action of Semicircular Canals

The semicircular canals are stimulated by rotational acceleration in the plane of the canal. For example, a person is made to sit in a special mechanically rotated chair, and his lateral (horizontal) canals are brought into horizontal plane by bending the head 30° forward. If the chair is rotated in the direction shown in Fig. 24.20, the left ampulla would lead its canal while the right ampulla would be trailing behind the canal. Before the beginning of the rotation, the cupulae of both ampullae would be in the mid-position "a". When the rotation begins the bony and the membranous canals start rotating with the head but the endolymph lags behind due to inertia. As a result, the cupulae in both the ampullae would attain position "b", i.e. cupula swings towards the utricle in the trailing ampulla and away from the utricle in the leading ampulla. In this way the trailing ampulla is stimulated while the leading ampulla is depressed causing a similar change in the discharge of impulses from the two ampullae. The combined information from the two ampullae reaches the brain informing it about the direction of the rotation. The degree of impulse discharge varies with the rate of acceleration of the rotational movement.

If the rotation is continued, the endolymph also takes up the speed of the canal. Due to their own elasticity, the two cupulae swing back to the resting position, and the impulse discharge from both the ampullae comes back to the resting level. On deceleration or sudden stoppage of the rotational movement, the endolymph would continue to move in the direction of the movement and the two cupulae would attain position "c" in Fig. 24.20, i.e. leading ampulla is now stimulated whereas the trailing ampulla is depressed. As a result, for a few seconds, the subject has sensation of rotation in the direction opposite to the actual movement just terminated. Finally, the cupulae regain the resting position once again, and the false sense of rotation also disappears (Fig. 24.21).

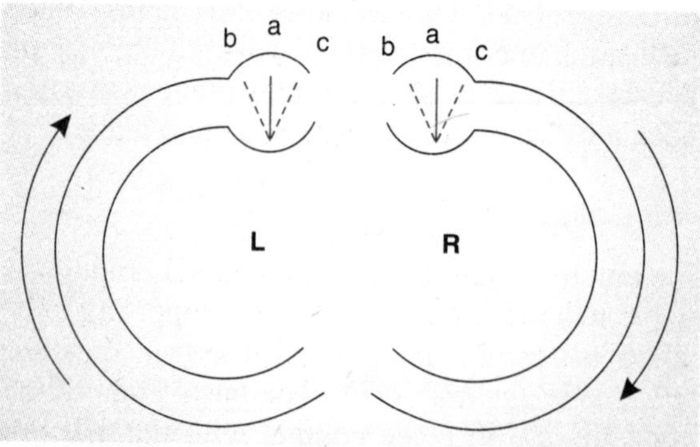

Fig. 24.20: Mode of action of the semicircular canal. The arrows indicate the direction of rotation of the head. The cupula attains position "a" at rest, "b" at the beginning and "c" at the end of rotation.

From the description given above, it appears that acceleration and deceleration, in prolonged angular rotation, can be a source of misinformation leading to inappropriate postural reflexes.

Fortunately, in day-to-day life, such a situation does not arise. However, many aircraft accidents have occurred due to such a problem, when the pilot used his subjective judgment after an instrumental failure.

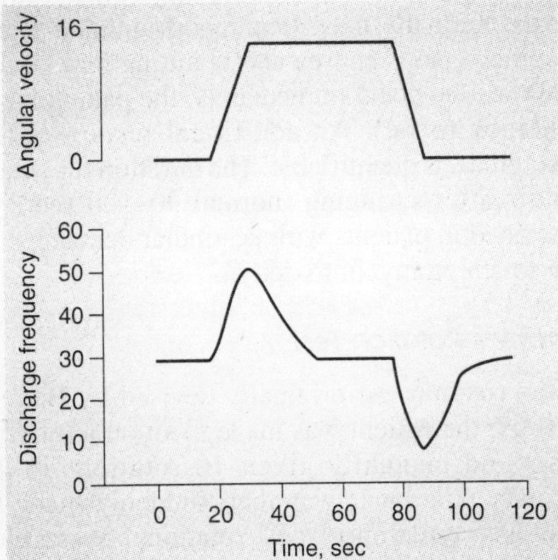

Fig. 24.21: Response of semicircular canals to angular rotation. The semicircular canals are stimulated at the beginning and the end of an angular motion at a constant velocity.

Mode of Action of Otolith Organs

Due to the presence of calcium carbonate crystals, the specific gravity of the cupulae of the maculae is three times that of the supporting tissue.

Consequently, the pull of the gravity deforms the hair cells even under resting conditions. This is in contrast to the semicircular canals, where stimulation of the hair cells is dependent upon the movement of the endolymph. The otolith organs discharge continuously for a given position of the head, providing information about the *head's orientation in space*. The discharge rate from the otolith organs increases by tilt of the head in any direction. The *saccules are affected by lateral tilt of the head*, whereas the *utricles are affected by ventroflexion or dorsiflexion of the head.*

Detection of linear acceleration (not linear motion) is another function of the otolith organs. When the body is suddenly thrust forward, say by sudden forward movement of the car, otolith organs have greater inertia than the surrounding fluid because of their weight and hence fall backwards on the hair cells. The reflex postural response consists of leaning forward to prevent the person from falling backwards. However, otolith organs give very little information regarding the linear motion. Passengers in the aircraft do not have any sensation of movement, even though they are flying at the speed of several hundred kilometers per hour.

Role of Vestibular Apparatus

Postural Regulation

The vestibular apparatus plays a key role in the maintenance of muscle tone and posture. The role of the vestibular apparatus in the righting reflexes has already been discussed. In decerebrate animal, after denervation of $C_{1,2,3}$ nerve roots (to eliminate tonic neck reflexes), changes in the position of the head lead to changes in the muscle tone. If the animal is placed in supine position, maximum tone is present in the antigravity muscles. Minimum tone is present in these muscles when the animal is in prone position and the snout is 45° below the horizontal plane. The purpose of these *tonic labyrinthine reflexes* in the regulation of posture is not clear, but the labyrinth seem to be essential for the regulation of tone and posture. After unilateral extirpation of the labyrinth, skew deviation (one eye rolled upward and outward while the other is rolled downward and outward) and nystagmus can be observed in the eyes. The head shows rotation and lateral flexion. Unilateral labyrinthectomy in the rat causes rolling movement, i.e. continuous effort to "right" itself by rolling along the longitudinal axis of the body.

Vestibulo-Ocular Reflex

Through its connections with the third, fourth and sixth cranial nuclei (via median longitudinal

24

bundle), the labyrinth helps to maintain visual fixation on moving objects by vestibulo-ocular reflex (VOR). If the head is moved to the left, the eyes are moved conjugately to the right, in order to maintain the gaze fixed on an object as the head moves. As the head is rotated to the left, the discharge of the vestibular fibers supplying the left horizontal canal is increased; concurrently, the discharge on the right is decreased. This results in an excitation of the right abducens nerve fibers innervating the right lateral rectus muscle and the left oculomotor nerve fibers innervating the left medial rectus muscle. The ensuing muscle contractions turn the eye to the right. The reflex, of course, also occurs when the head is rotated in the other direction, but the eye movement is in the reverse direction as well.

The vestibulo-ocular reflex (VOR) ensures best vision during head motion by moving the eyes contrary to the head to stabilize the line of sight in space. The vestibulo-ocular reflex operates in both horizontal and vertical planes owing to the arrangement of the three semicircular canals, and it maintains such stability that the observed object does not oscillate until quite high velocities are attained. But for VOR, one would not be able to read a book during a bus ride or read the road signs while traveling in a car moving at a high speed.

Motion Sickness

Severe over-stimulation of vestibular apparatus may be produced by pitching and rolling movements of a ship. It occurs to a variable degree during journey by road especially in the hills. The subject has an unpleasant sensation of rotation accompanied by nausea, vomiting, pallor and cold perspiration. Most of the symptoms and signs are the effects of vestibular stimulation on the medullary autonomic centres.The basic problem producing motion sickness is said to be a disagreement that exists between visually perceived movement and the vestibular system's sense of movement

Clinical Tests of Labyrinthine Function

Caloric Stimulation Test

Vestibular function can be tested by caloric stimulation. Syringing the external ear with hot or cold water sets up convectional currents in the endolymph which stimulate the semicircular canals. Normally, the patient reports giddiness, and in some persons nausea and vomiting may occur. If allowed to stand immediately, the patient has a tendency to fall. An additional response, the nystagmus, is quantifiable. The duration for which it lasts after syringing (normal 90–130 sec.), is shortened in patients with vestibular damage, e.g. due to streptomycin toxicity.

Barany's Rotation Test

In the rotation test originally devised by Barany in 1907, the patient was made to sit on a rotation chair and manually given 10 rotations in 20 seconds. The chair was then suddenly made to stop. The duration of post-rotational nystagmus was noted visually. Nowadays, the test has become very sophisticated. The rotational chair is electrically driven. Nystagmus is recorded by electromyography of the eyeball.

Nystagmus

This term is used to describe the repetitive short jerky movements of the eyeball, slow in one direction and quick or jerky in the opposite direction. Nystagmus may be observed in normal persons after caloric stimulation of the labyrinth. Its absence or shorter duration indicates vestibular damage. Nystagmus may occur spontaneously in patients with vestibular or cerebellar disorder.

25

CHAPTER

The Cerebellum and the Basal Ganglia

CEREBELLUM

The cerebellum lies in the occipital fossa of the skull, dorsal to the medulla and pons. It is connected to the brainstem by three peduncles; the superior, middle and the inferior peduncles. Anatomically, cerebellum is divided into small central vermis and two large cerebellar hemispheres. Many anatomical fissures divide the cerebellum into a number of subdivisions (Fig. 25.1). However, functionally it is preferable to consider cerebellum to consist of three portions called: (a) archicerebellum, (b) spinocerebellum, (c) neocerebellum (Fig. 25.1).

Archicerebellum is phylogenetically the most primitive portion. It consists of flocculonodular lobe. Its chief connections are with the vestibular apparatus and hence it is concerned with the maintenance of equilibrium of the body.

The rest of the vermis along with the adjacent medial portions of the hemispheres constitute the *spinocerebellum*. This region receives the proprioceptive afferents from the body and is therefore concerned with the coordination of movements. The lateral portions of the cerebellar hemispheres, constituting the *neocerebellum,* are phylogenetically the newest portions and are best developed in humans. Neocerebellum interacts with the cerebral motor cortex and helps in planning and programming of the movements. It is also concerned with coordination of movements.

By stimulation of tactile receptors in the skin and recording electrical potentials in the cerebellum, point to point (topographic) representation of the body can be demonstrated in two areas of the spinocerebellum (Fig. 25.2).

AFFERENT CONNECTIONS

Tract	*Input*
1. Dorsal spinocerebellar tract	Ipsilateral proprioceptive impulses from the trunk and leg
2. Ventral spinocerebellar tract	Contralateral exteroceptive and proprioceptive impulses from the trunk and leg
3. Olivocerebellar tract	Proprioceptive impulses from all over the body relayed through inferior olive
4. Cuneocerebellar tract	Ipsilateral proprioceptive impulses from the arms and neck
5. Vestibulocerebellar tract	Ipsilateral vestibular impulses direct and via vestibular nuclei
6. Tectocerebellar tract	Visual and auditory impulses via superior and inferior colliculi
7. Pontocerebellar tract	Impulses from the opposite motor cortex via pontine nuclei
8. Rubrocerebellar tract	Impulses from the opposite red nucleus
9. Reticulocerebellar tract	Impulses from the brainstem reticular formation

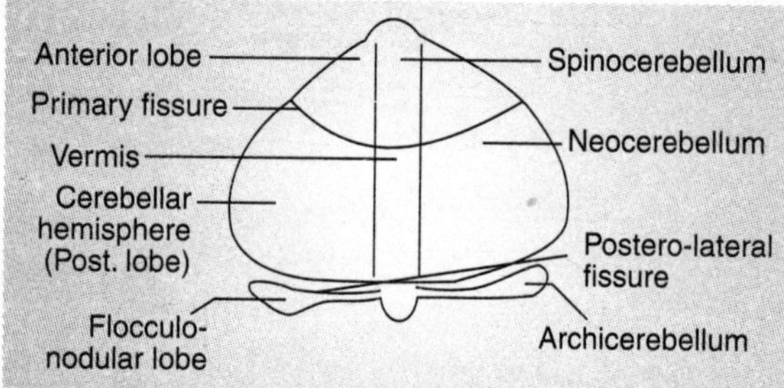

Fig. 25.1: Anatomic (on the left) and physiologic (on the right) division of the cerebellum.

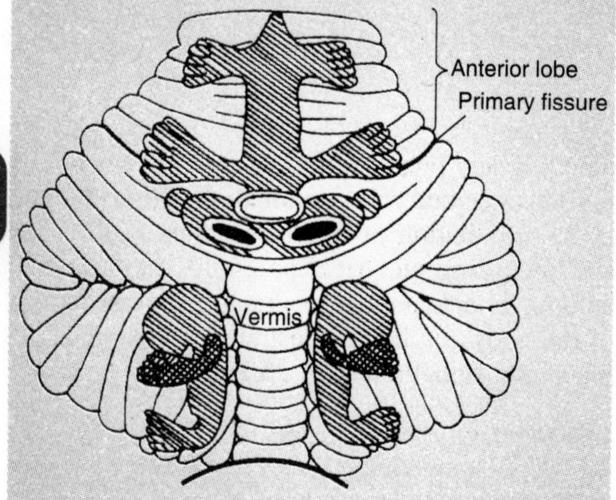

Fig. 25.2: Representation of the body in the cerebellum (cerebellar homunculi).

EFFERENT CONNECTIONS

The cerebellar afferents project on the four deep nuclei in an organized manner as follows: The fastigial nucleus, the globose and the emboliform nuclei receive fibres from the spinocerebellum. The dentate nucleus receives fibres from the neocerebellum.

The *fastigial, globose and emboliform nuclei* give efferents to:

(a) Vestibular nuclei.
(b) Medullary reticular formation.
(c) Third, fourth and sixth cranial nuclei (through medial longitudinal bundle)
(d) Ascending reticular formation.

Through these connections, the spinocerebellum plays an important role in the regulation of posture.

The *dentate nucleus* gives rise to the most important efferent output of the neocerebellum. The efferent fibres go to the opposite (a) red nucleus, and (b) thalamus (ventrolateral nucleus). The thalamo-cortical fibres link the neocerebellum with areas 4 and 6 of the motor cortex (Fig. 25.3). The dentato-thalamo-cortical, cortico-ponto-cerebellar pathways and other connections of the dentate nucleus through rubroreticular and rubrospinal fibres help in the control of motor activity.

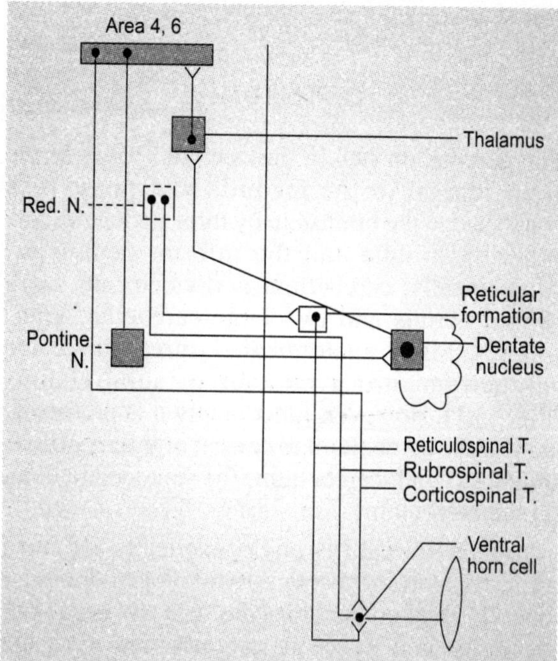

Fig. 25.3: The dentato-thalamo-cortical and cortico-ponto-cerebellar pathways.

The sensory input to the cerebellum is mostly ipsilateral. Since the dentato-thalamo-cortical pathway crosses to the opposite side and the corticospinal tract also undergoes decussation, the *cerebellum regulates the activity of the same side of the body.*

INTRACEREBELLAR NEURONAL CIRCUITS

Histologically, the cerebellar cortex consists of the outer molecular layer, and inner granular cell layer. In between the two layers is a single row of large *Purkinje cells* (Fig. 25.4A). The four pairs of nuclear masses of the cerebellum are embedded deep in the white matter (cerebellar medulla). The neurons of the deep cerebellar nuclei constitute the efferent output of the cerebellum. These neurons are subjected to both excitatory and inhibitory inputs.

Two types of afferent fibres can be identified in the cerebellum: The *climbing fibres* (from the inferior olive) and the *mossy fibres* (all other afferents).

Each *climbing fibre* projects directly on the primary dendrites of *one Purkinje cell*, around which the terminals entwine like a climbing plant.

Each *Mossy fibre* ends on the dendrites of hundreds *of granule cells*. The axons of granule cells reach the molecular layer and bifurcate to form a 'T'. The two branches are straight and run long distances. These branches, called the *parallel fibres*, synapse with the dendrites of a *large number of Purkinje cells* (Fig. 25.4B).

Both types of afferents, either directly (climbing fibres) or indirectly (mossy fibres through granule cells) excite the Purkinje cells. The Purkinje cells release the inhibitory transmitter (GABA) at their terminals on the deep nuclei.

The cerebellar cortex contains three other types of cells, namely, the *basket cells, stellate cells* and the *Golgi cells*. All the three are inhibitory in nature.

The dendrites of basket cells and stellate cells synapse with the parallel fibres and their axons terminate on and inhibit the Purkinje cells. The Golgi cells receive input from the collaterals of the climbing fibres, as well as, from the parallel fibres. Their axons terminate on and inhibit the granule cells.

It is interesting to note that, in spite of the fact that the activity of Purkinje cells is inhibitory in nature, the *output of the deep nuclei of the cerebellum to the brainstem and the thalamus is entirely excitatory.* It is believed that the entire cerebellar circuitry is concerned with modulating excitatory output of the deep cerebellar nuclei.

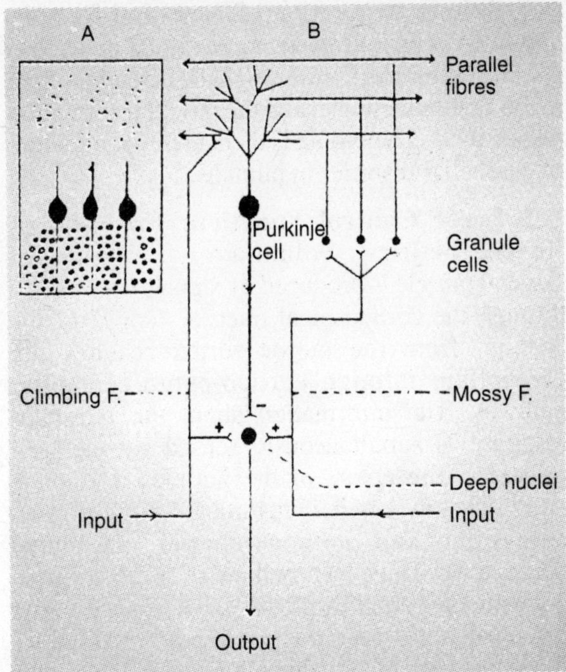

Fig. 25.4: Intracerebellar connections.

FUNCTIONS

In spite of extensive research, it is still difficult to describe the exact functions of the cerebellum. Ablation studies have demonstrated disturbances of equilibrium, muscle tone and posture. There is *no paralysis or sensory deficit but incoordination is prominent in all voluntary movements.*

1. Role in Maintenance of Equilibrium Afferents from the vestibular apparatus reach the *archicerebellum* directly and after relay through the vestibular nuclei. Efferents from the archicerebellum reach the vestibular nuclei. Thus, the vestibular apparatus and the flocculonodular lobe of the cerebellum are intimately connected.

Destruction of the flocculonodular lobe, experimentally in animals, or by a tumour in children produces *trunk ataxia*, i.e. an inability to stand erect and walk.

2. Role in Regulation of Tone and Posture *Spinocerebellum* projects on the alpha as well as gamma motor neurons through the efferent output to the vestibular nuclei and the reticular formation respectively. Hypotonia is a characteristic feature of cerebellar disorder in humans.

3. Error Control Function: Function of Neocerebellum Voluntary contraction of skeletal muscle is produced by signals transmitted through the corticospinal tract. A "copy" of the "order" from the motor cortex reaches the cerebellum through cortico-ponto-cerebellar pathway. The information about the muscular response is simultaneously sensed by the proprioceptive receptors of the muscles and joints and reaches the cerebellum through spino-olivary-cerebellar and spinocerebellar pathways (Fig. 25.5). Thus, cerebellum is a position to compare the "order" with the "performance". Any discrepancy between the two can be rectified by feedback control of cerebellum over the motor cortex through dentato-thalamo-cortical pathway.

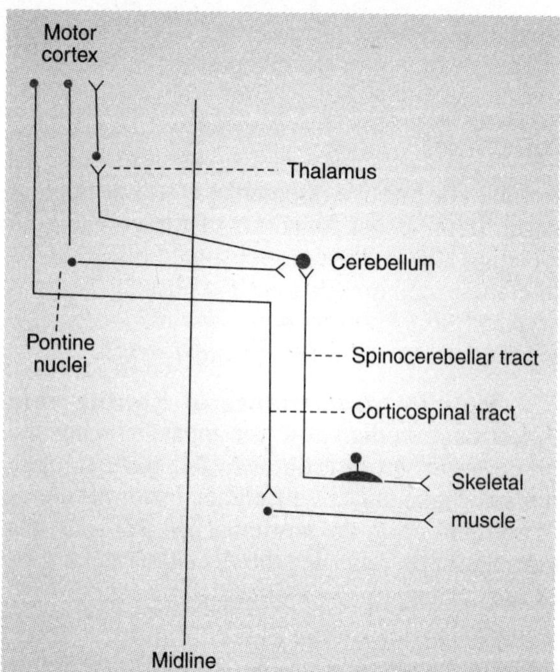

Fig. 25.5: The proprioceptive feedback servomechanism.

4. Planning Function: Function of Neocerebellum The error control function of the cerebellum discussed above plays the role in proper execution of movements initiated by the motor cortex. Some recent researches have shown that impulse discharge in some neurons of the dentate nucleus increases about 80 milliseconds before the onset of muscle activity. This could not be a feedback effect. This observation led to the hypothesis that dentate nucleus may play a role in initiating activity in the motor cortex.

5. Improvement in Performance of Motor Skills Recent researches have revealed that cerebellum is involved in the improvement in motor skills by training. Most of the motor skills involve a sequence of muscular contractions. Repetition makes the performance easier, better and almost automatic. This results from plasticity in the cerebellar neuronal circuitry.

6. Role in Mental Dexterity A number of facts about cerebellum point towards some more important role of cerebellum in human motor as well as non-motor activities: First of all, it contains more neurons than all the rest of the brain combined. Second, it has a more rapidly acting mechanism than any other part of the brain, and therefore it can process quickly whatever information it receives from other parts of the brain. Third, it receives an enormous amount of information from the cerebral cortex, which is connected to the human cerebellum by approximately 40 million nerve fibers. Cerebellum has been compared to a powerful computer, capable of making contributions both to the motor dexterity and to the mental dexterity of humans.

Cerebellar Syndrome

Observations of abnormalities in motor function in a patient with cerebellar disorder (cerebellar syndrome) provide the best insight into the function of the organ. If the lesion in the cerebellum is unilateral, the *motor abnormalities are seen ipsilaterally* (same side of the body).

1. Ataxia (Incoordination of movements). It is the hallmark of cerebellar disorder. There is:

(a) *Decomposition of movements*, i.e. the movements seem to occur in stages at different joints.
(b) *Asynergia*, i.e. lack of coordination between the protagonist, synergist and antagonist muscles.
(c) *Dysmetria*, i.e. the movements are incorrect in range, direction and force.

2. Intention Tremor Coarse tremor can be observed during the execution of movements. The tremor is absent when the limb is at rest (cf. Parkinsonian tremor).

3. Atonia The muscles have little or no tone.

4. Slurred Speech

5. Nystagmus

6. Muscle Power and Voluntary Control Normal.

7. Deep Reflexes: Normal The *knee jerk* is characteristically *pendular*: After the initial reflex response, the leg continues to swing forwards and backwards several times like a pendulum.

The cerebellar dysfunction described above can be demonstrated by the following **clinical tests**:

1. **Finger-nose test**. The patient has great difficulty in promptly bringing the finger of an outstretched arm to touch the tip of his nose. Intention tremor becomes more severe as the hand approaches the face.
2. The patient is unable to rapidly perform alternating movements, e.g. supination and pronation of the forearm. The abnormality is called **adiadochokinesia**.
3. The patient is **unable to walk on a straight line (even with eyes open)**; he follows a zigzag path (drunken gait).
4. **Speech** is slow and slurred (due to incoordination of the muscles of the tongue and larynx).
5. **Nystagmus**.

THE BASAL GANGLIA

The term basal ganglia is used to include three large nuclear masses, namely, caudate nucleus, putamen and globus pallidus, lying in the forebrain, and another two functionally related structures, the subthalamic nucleus of Luys and substantia nigra lying in the mesencephalon. Phylogenetically, the caudate nucleus and putamen are of more recent origin and hence called *neostriatum* as compared to the more primitive globus pallidus (Fig. 25.6).

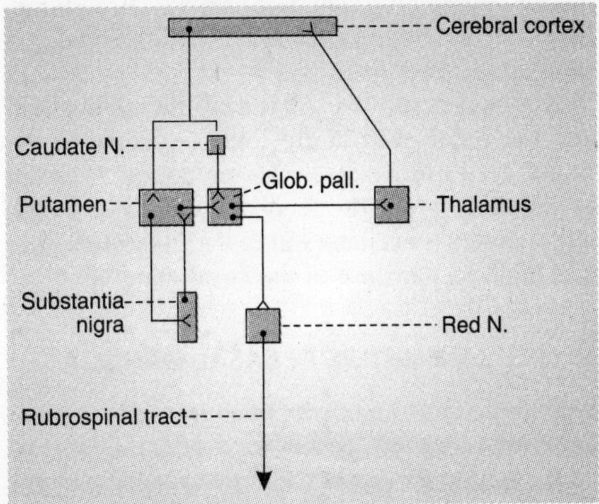

Fig. 25.6: The basal ganglia.

CONNECTIONS

The connections of the basal ganglia may be considered under three headings:

1. Motor Cortex—Basal Ganglia—Motor Cortex Circuit The chief afferents to the basal ganglia include cortico-striate projections which originate from all parts of the cerebral cortex and terminate in the caudate nucleus and the putamen. Fibres proceed from the neostriatum to the globus pallidus and from there to thalamus and thence to all parts of motor cortex (Fig. 25.6). The neostriatum to globus pallidus projection is inhibitory in nature because the nerve endings release GABA. As a result, this circular pathway provides a *negative feedback loop* to control the activity of motor cortex.

2. Neostriatum—Substantia Nigra Interconnections A *GABA* secreting inhibitory pathway projects from the neostriatum to the substantia

25

nigra. In turn substantia nigra has *dopamine* secreting inhibitory projection on the neostriatum.

3. Efferent Projection on the Brainstem Reticular Formation The main efferent outflow from the globus pallidus is to the thalamic nuclei. There is a small indirect efferent projection on the spinal cord, in the form of globus pallidus → substantia nigra → brain stem reticular formation → reticulospinal tract pathway. In addition, there is globus pallidus → red nucleus → rubrospinal tract pathway.

It would be obvious that both the cerebellum and the basal ganglia are interconnected to the motor cortex and help in the regulation of motor activity. However, the feedback control over the motor cortex is excitatory in case of the cerebellum and inhibitory in case of the basal ganglia.

25

NEUROTRANSMITTERS IN BASAL GANGLIA

Although a large number of neurotransmitters have been identified in various parts of the CNS, the basal ganglia are one of the important areas where the pharmacological approach based on the knowledge of neurotransmitters has been helpful. In the basal ganglia, well-defined dopaminergic, GABA-ergic and cholinergic pathways have been identified. Whereas dopamine and GABA are inhibitory neurotransmitters, acetylcholine is excitatory neurotransmitter in the basal ganglia.

The main dopaminergic pathway arises from the substantia nigra and terminates in the neostriatum where the neurotransmitter is secreted by the nerve terminals. Degeneration of the nigral-striatum pathway leading to deficiency of dopamine in the neostriatum has been identified as the chief cause of Parkinson disease.

GABA secreting pathways project from the neostriatum to the substantia nigra. *Cholinergic* pathways have been identified between substantia nigra, globus pallidus and neostriatum.

FUNCTIONS

Experimental researches have shed very little light on the function of the basal ganglia. Lesions of the basal ganglia in experimental animals produce very little effect. Our knowledge of the function of basal ganglia is chiefly based on the clinical observations in patients with pathology of these nuclear masses. Alterations in the muscle tone, akinesia (poverty of movements) and involuntary movements are characteristic features of basal ganglia disorders. A sensory deficit is not present.

1. Planning and Programming Like cerebellum, neuronal discharge in the basal ganglia begins well before the beginning of the movement. Therefore, it is believed that the cerebellum as well as the basal ganglia are involved in the planning and programming of the movements (Fig. 25.7). Bradykinesia (or akinesia), i.e. difficulty in initiation of motor activity is a hallmark of Parkinson disease.

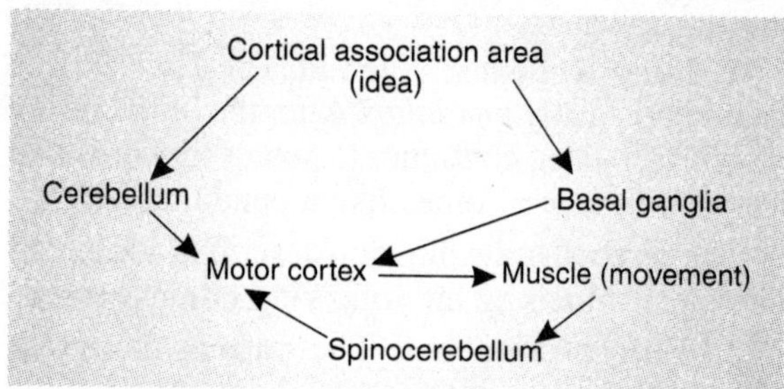

Fig. 25.7: Planning and programming of movements.

2. Regulation of Tone and Posture The cortical inhibitory areas project on the caudate nucleus which, in turn, projects on the bulbar inhibitory reticular formation. Inhibition of spinal reflexes has been observed on stimulation of the caudate nucleus. Moreover, rigidity (lead-pipe type) is a characteristic feature of Parkinson disease. All these observations illustrate the role of basal ganglia in the regulation of muscle tone and posture.

3. Cognitive Function Recent researches have suggested the involvement of basal ganglia not only in motor function but also in neuropsychological processes. Some of the behavioral consequences of basal ganglia dysfunction are disturbances of cognitive processing, in both animal models and human clinical populations. In humans with idiopathic Parkinson disease, deficits in attention, working memory, planning and problem solving are usually evident.

PARKINSON DISEASE

This disorder, observed in middle-aged patients, is due to degeneration of dopaminergic nigral-striatum pathway. The concentration of dopamine in the substantia nigra and the neostriatum is about 50% of the normal. Some of the characteristic features of this disorder are listed below.

Bradykinesia

This term is used to describe the inability to initiate movement due to difficulty selecting and/or activating motor programs in the central nervous system. Poverty of movement is the most characteristic feature of Parkinson disease. The patient has *mask-like facial expression* and an *unblinking reptilian stare*. There is *absence* of normal associated movements, e.g. *swinging of the arms* during walking or change of *facial expression* related to the emotional content of the speech. Even ordinary motor tasks are performed very slowly, taking much longer time than average normal.

Bradykinesia/akinesia are not due to any paralysis. Sensory system is also normal. Still there is great difficulty in initiating voluntary movements. Muscle power is not affected.

Lead Pipe Rigidity

Rigidity mostly involves the proximal muscles of the limbs. It affects both the protagonists and antagonists. During passive movement of a limb, the resistance is observed throughout the effort as if a lead pipe is being bent (i.e. there is no clasp-knife effect). In advanced cases, the rigidity may increase to such an extent that the patient with arms adducted and flexed, knees flexed and the back bent has a *statue-like appearance* (Fig. 25.8). Parkinsonian rigidity (like spasticity of hemiplegia) is due to exaggerated gamma motor discharge. Rigidity may make it difficult to elicit deep reflexes.

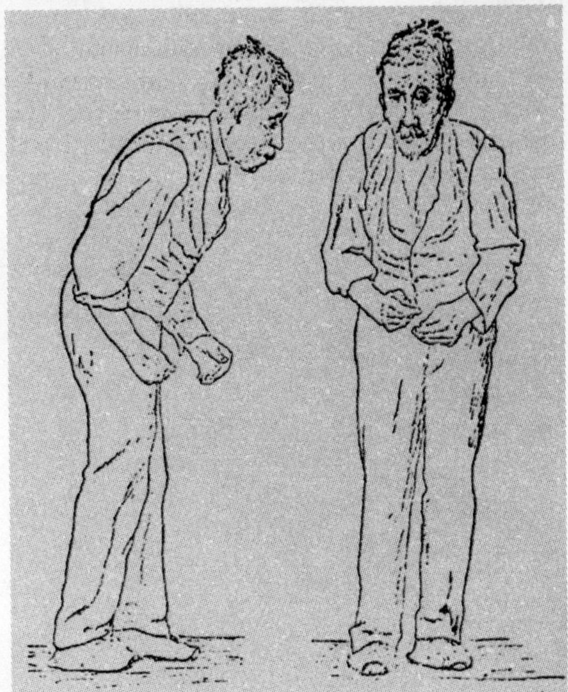

Fig. 25.8: Parkinson disease.

Tremor

Involuntary rhythmic oscillatory movements of the distal parts of the limb or the head are called tremor. Tremor are produced by alternating contraction of the protagonist and antagonist muscles. Parkinsonian tremor occur at a frequency of 4–6/s. Parkinsonian tremor are *present at rest* but disappear during sleep or voluntary activity, hence often called *resting tremor* (cf. intention tremor of cerebellar disease).

As mentioned above, Parkinson disease is due to degeneration of dopamine producing neurons of the substantia nigra. As a result, there is a disturbance of neural balance between the excitatory cholinergic and inhibitory dopaminergic activity of the neostriatum. Administration of drugs like reserpine, which further deplete the dopamine stores in the neurons in patient with Parkinsonism, exacerbate the symptoms and signs of the disease. Physostigmine, which enhances the effect of acetylcholine, also increases the rigidity and tremor. The disorder can be treated by administration of a dopamine precursor like L-dopa which (unlike dopamine), can cross the blood-brain barrier. The residual dopaminergic neurons in the basal ganglia convert L-dopa to dopamine and thus produce relief to the patient.

Chorea and **athetosis** are two other diseases produced by pathological changes in the neostriatum. In chorea, there are spontaneous jerky, irregular "dancing" movements that seem to move randomly from one part of the body to another. Athetosis is characterized by slow, confluent writhing movements.

26

CHAPTER

The Motor Cortex

The cerebral cortex is a highly convoluted and laminated sheet of grey matter containing several billion neurons. In man, it is 2.5–4 mm thick and its surface area is about 2500 cm^2. Histologically, six layers can be identified in 90–95% of the cortical surface (Fig. 26.1). This part is called the neocortex. In the remaining part named allocortex, the six layers are not properly defined. The allocortex includes the cortex of the hippocampus and rhinencephalon. Morphologically, three types of cells may be identified in the cerebral cortex.

1. Pyramidal Cells These cells have triangular or trapezoidal cell bodies with the base downward. Such cells are present in layers II, III and V of the neocortex. Giant pyramidal cells, also called **Betz cells**, are found in V layer of primary motor cortex (Brodmann's area 4).

2. Stellate or Granule Cells These cells have small cell bodies from where the dendrites arise in all directions. Layer IV is packed with such cells and is best developed in the primary sensory cortex.

3. Fusiform Cells Such cells have spindle-shaped cell bodies, and are present in layer VI along with cells of other varying shapes.

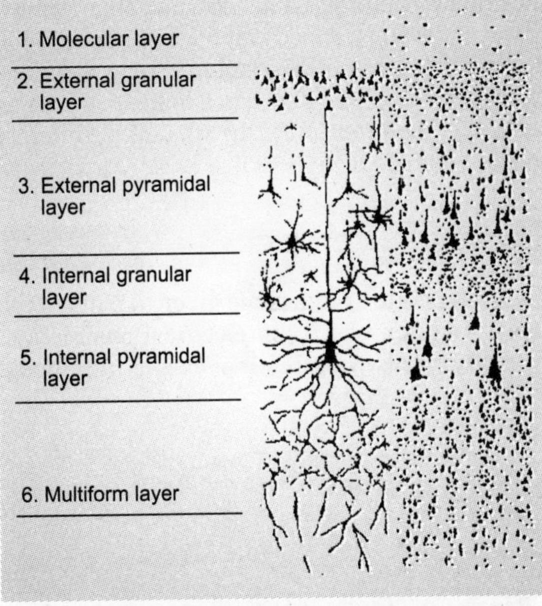

Fig. 26.1: Histologic structure (cytoarchitecture) of neocortex. Left column shows cells stained with Golgi stain. Right column shows cells stained with Nissl stain.

Afferent Connections

The specific thalamocortical afferents ascend through layers VI and V, to form extensive plexus in layer IV. Non-specific thalamocortical projection ends mainly in layer I, but as the fibres ascend, they give collaterals to all other layers of the cerebral cortex. Association and commissural fibres in layer IV terminate mainly in layer II and III.

EFFERENT CONNECTIONS

1. Efferent cortical projection to the **basal ganglia**, **brainstem** and **spinal cord** arises from the pyramidal cells of layer V.
2. The corticothalamic efferent projection arises from the pyramidal and fusiform cells of layer VI.
3. The commissural and ipsilateral corticocortical efferent fibres arise from pyramidal cells of layer II and III.

Brodmann's Areas

On the basis of cytoarchitecture, the cerebral cortex has been divided into a number of areas each having a distinct morphological feature. Based on this, the map of human cerebral cortex prepared by Brodmann is most widely used in experimental and clinical neurology (Figs 26.2 and 26.3). It may, however, be emphasized that the difference in the function of different Brodmann's areas is not as much because of the difference in the cell type as because of the difference in the afferent and efferent connections of the cells in that area.

MOTOR CORTEX

The motor cortex is the name given to parts of the cerebral cortex which, on electrical stimulation, promptly results in discrete movements in the body.

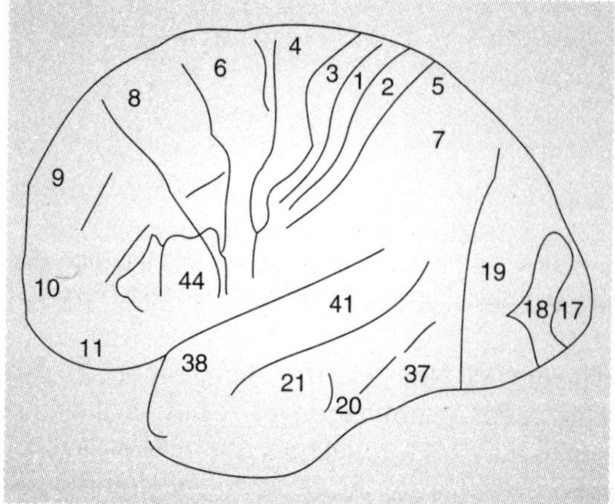

Fig. 26.2: Brodmann's areas of the cerebral hemisphere (lateral aspect).

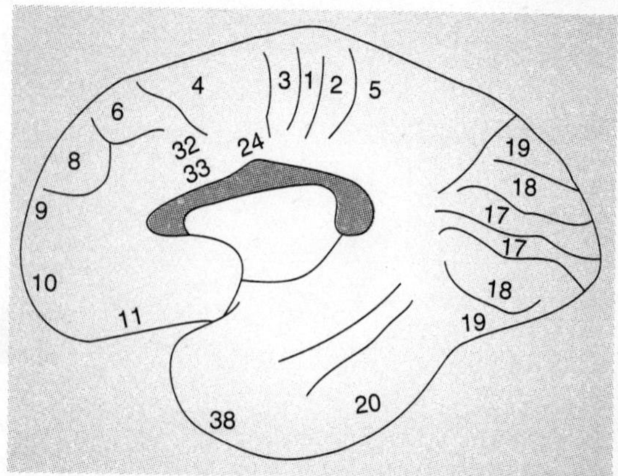

Fig. 26.3: Brodmann's areas of the cerebral hemisphere (medial aspect).

A large part of the cerebral cortex in front of the central sulcus shows such an activity. However, the *precentral gyrus* is called the *primary motor area,* since it has the lowest threshold of stimulation (Figs 26.4 and 26.5).

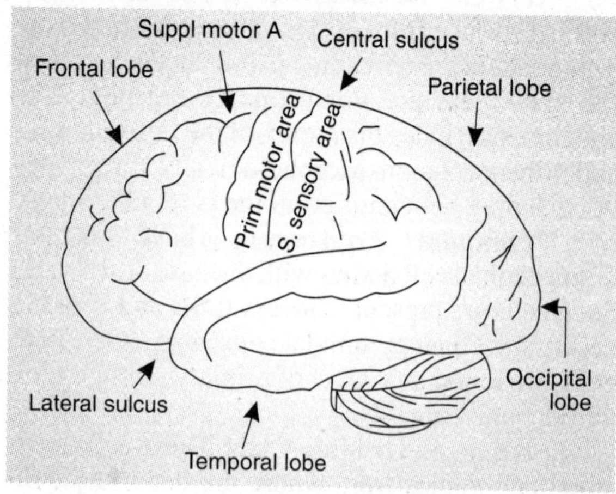

Fig. 26.4: Lateral aspect of the cerebral cortex showing the motor and sensory cortex.

Primary Motor Area (Brodmann's Area 4)

It occupies the whole length of the precentral gyrus and extends on to the medial surface of the cerebral hemisphere. Each primary motor area controls the opposite side of the body. Electrical stimulation of the discrete portions of the primary motor cortex in animals and humans has revealed that:

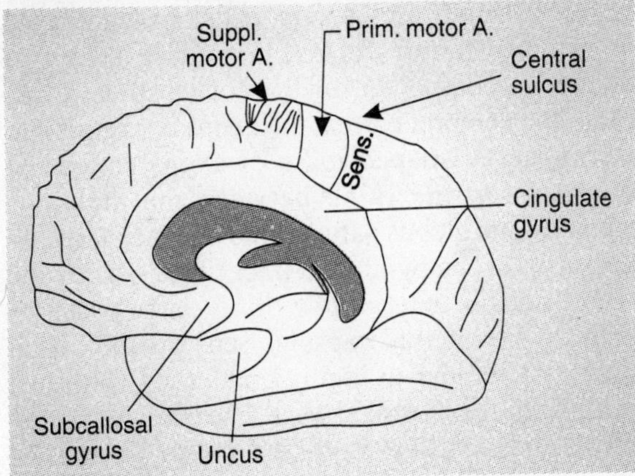

Fig. 26.5: Medial aspect of the cerebral cortex showing the motor and sensory cortex.

(a) The whole body is represented upside down. The face is represented at the bottom of the precentral gyrus, the hip and knee at the top while the leg and foot are represented on the medial surface.

(b) Parts of the body concerned with highly skilled movements have proportionately larger cortical representation. For example, the hands or the tongue and lips have much larger representation than that of the trunk.

A figure of a man may be constructed in such a way that the size of each part corresponds to the amount of cortex represented by it. The result, called a *motor homunculus*, is a highly distorted figure of a man with a very large thumb, relatively large face, enormous tongue, and very small trunk and legs (Fig. 26.6).

(c) Motor cortex is organized in terms of movements rather than individual muscles.

(d) Stimulation of the points representing upper parts of the face, the pharynx and the vocal cords produces bilateral responses.

Primary motor cortex corresponds to Brodmann's area 4. Histologically, the fifth layer of the cerebral cortex, in this part, contains *giant cells of Betz* (mean diameter 16 μ) (Fig. 26.1), which give rise to thick myelinated corticospinal fibres.

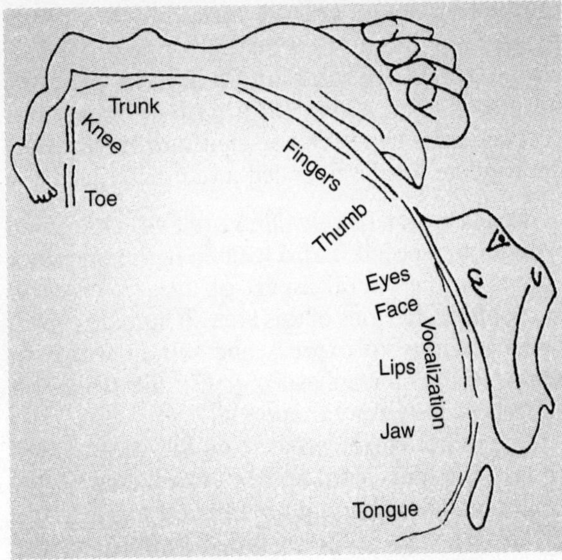

Fig. 26.6: Motor homunculus on the precentral gyrus of the cerebral cortex.

Supplementary Motor Area

This is located on the medial aspect of the cerebral hemisphere, on and above the superior bank of the cingulate sulcus, and extending up to upper region of the lateral surface in front of area 4 (Figs 26.4 and 26.5). For the most part, the supplementary motor area projects to the motor cortex. Supplementary motor area seems to be involved in programming motor sequences. Lesions of this area in monkey result in a difficulty in performance of complicated motor activities, or actions involving coordination between the two limbs.

Premotor Cortex (Brodmann's Area 6, 8, 44)

Electrical stimulation of the cerebral cortex, 1–3 cm in front of the primary motor cortex produces a variety of responses like coordinated movements of the eyes, swallowing, contraction of the parts of the body producing different postural positions and vocalization, etc. This area has been called premotor cortex. It has subcortical connections with primary motor cortex, sensory association area of the parietal lobe and the basal ganglia.

Premotor cortex influences motor behaviour both through extensive connections with primary motor cortex as well as directly via axonal projections through corticobulbar and corticospinal tracts (pyramidal tracts). In general, premotor cortex uses information from other cortical areas to select a sequence of movements appropriate for the intended motor activity.

Broca's area *(Brodmann's area 44)* concerned with motor speech is also located in the premotor cortex on the lateral aspect of the *left cerebral hemisphere.* Lesions of this area, in humans, result in an inability to express one self in words or sentences (motor aphasia), or use the hands for skillful activity (motor aprexia).

The motor cortex projects on the ventral horn cells of the spinal cord or their cranial equivalents in the brainstem through *pyramidal tracts* and a group of tracts collectively known as the *extrapyramidal tracts.*

PLASTICITY IN MOTOR CORTEX

Recent researches have revealed plasticity in the motor cortex, i.e. the cortical representation of a given part of the body is not permanently fixed. It may enlarge if that part of the body is put to greater use. For example, if a person begins training of playing a string instrument (e.g. violin), the finger area of the contralateral motor cortex gradually enlarges. The change is detectable at 1 week and becomes maximum at 4 weeks of training. On the other hand, disuse of a body part reduces its cortical representation. The phenomenon of plasticity can be demonstrated in the somatosensory cortex also.

PYRAMIDAL TRACTS (CORTICOSPINAL TRACTS)

Corticospinal tract is the most important tract through which the motor cortex controls the activity of the ventral horn cells in the spinal cord.

It is also called the pyramidal tract, since it forms a prominent pyramid on the ventral surface of the medulla oblongata.

Corticospinal tract originates from the primary motor cortex, supplementary motor cortex and the premotor cortex. About 40% of the fibres present in this tract arise from the parietal lobe, especially the somatic sensory cortex. Thick myelinated fibres, arising from the giant cells of Betz located in primary motor cortex, constitute the most important component of the corticospinal tract. From the cerebral cortex, the axons converge into a compact V-shaped mass of axons called the *internal capsule* lying between the thalamus medially and globus pallidus and putamen laterally (Fig. 26.7). The pyramidal tract fibres occupy the 'genu' and the anterior two-thirds of the posterior limb of the internal capsule. Sensory and visual tracts are present in highly condensed form just behind the corticospinal tract. The extrapyramidal fibres, descending from the motor cortex lie intermingled with the corticospinal fibres in the internal capsule. In elderly persons, the internal capsule is a common site of vascular lesions

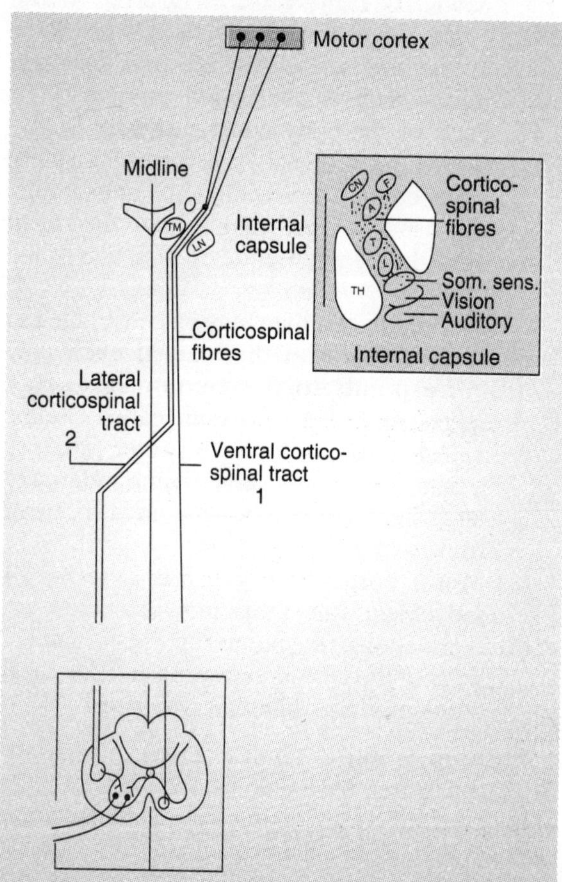

Fig. 26.7: The corticospinal (pyramidal) tracts.

(thrombosis) which produce widespread motor disturbances on the contralateral side of the body (hemiplegia).

As the pyramidal tracts descend in the brainstem, the corticobulbar fibres cross to reach the cranial nerve nuclei of the opposite side. In the medulla oblongata, the remaining corticospinal fibres on either side form a ventrally projecting mass called the *pyramids*. In the lower part of the medulla, about 80% of the corticospinal fibres cross to the opposite side *(pyramidal decussation)* to form the lateral corticospinal tract which descends in the lateral white column of the spinal cord (Fig. 26.8). The remaining 20% fibres descend ipsilaterally as anterior corticospinal tract in the ventral white column of the spinal cord.

In the spinal cord, fibres of the lateral corticospinal tract end directly on the nearby ventral horn cells. Fibres of the anterior corticospinal tract ultimately cross the midline but only near the level they synapse with the ventral horn cells. An interneuron is usually interposed between the anterior corticospinal fibre terminal and the ventral horn cell.

Fibres of the *lateral corticospinal tract* mainly control the activity of the ventral horn cells supplying the *distal muscles of the limbs*. Fibres of *anterior corticospinal tract* mainly control the muscles of the trunk and the *proximal parts of the limbs*.

EXTRAPYRAMIDAL TRACTS

A large number of fibres arise from all parts of the motor cortex, but do not enter the corticospinal tracts. Instead, they relay in the various basal ganglia, red nucleus, tectum and the brainstem reticular formation. Ultimately, they constitute the reticulospinal tract, the rubrospinal tract, the tectospinal tract and the vestibulospinal tract. In contrast to the pyramidal tracts, the extrapyramidal tracts constitute *multisynaptic pathways* regulating activity of the ventral horn cells (Fig. 26.9). Extrapyramidal pathways are chiefly concerned with the regulation of muscle tone and posture. They help to provide appropriate and stable postural background for the muscle activity produced by the pyramidal tracts.

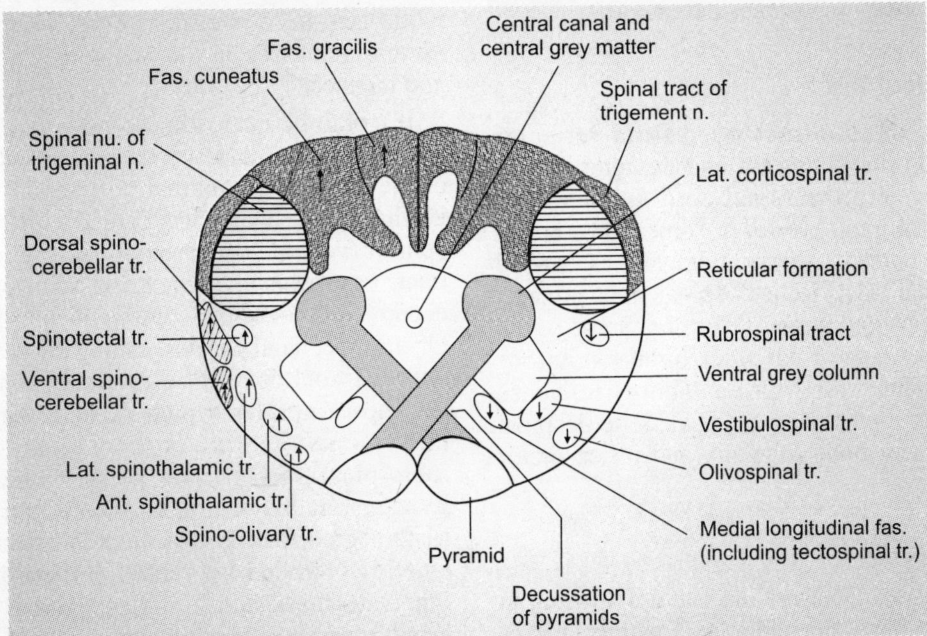

Fig. 26.8: Transverse section through lower region of the medulla showing pyramidal decussation.

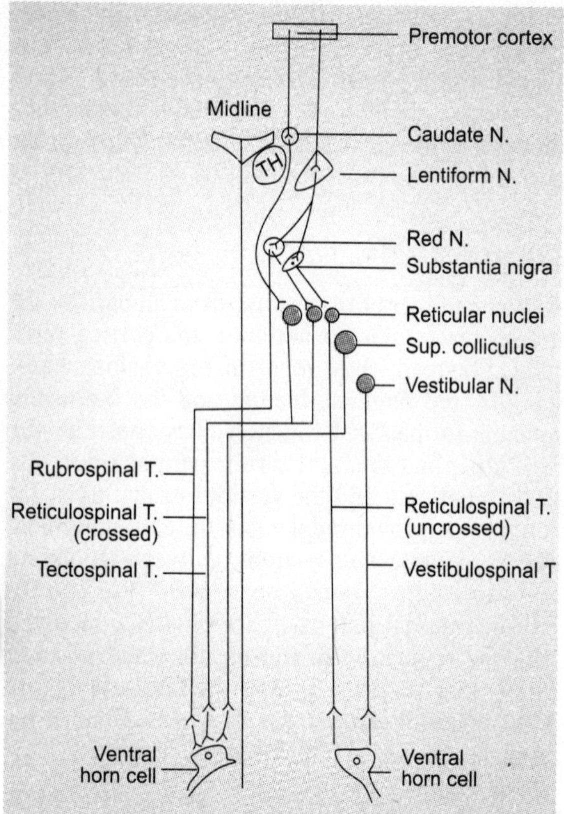

Fig. 26.9: The extrapyramidal tracts.

Reticulospinal Tract

The fibres of this tract arise from reticular formation in the brainstem and descend mostly ipsilaterally into the spinal cord as uncrossed reticulospinal tract. However, some fibres cross-over to the opposite side and descend as crossed reticulospinal tract. Reticulospinal tract projects on the both α- and γ-motor neurons. Some of the fibres of reticulospinal tract have excitatory influence, while others have inhibitory influence on the lower motor neurons. Thus, reticulospinal tract influences both voluntary and reflex motor activity.

Rubrospinal Tract

This tract arises from the red nucleus situated in the upper region of the midbrain. The tract crosses the midline and descends through pons and medulla. In the spinal cord, the tract is present in the lateral white columns and its fibres terminate around the ventral horn cells. The red nucleus has inputs from both the cerebral cortex and cerebellum. Therefore, the rubrospinal tract constitutes an indirect pathway by which cerebral cortex and cerebellum can influence voluntary and reflex motor activity.

Tectospinal Tract

Fibres of this tract arise from the superior colliculi of the midbrain. Tectospinal fibres cross the midline and descend contralaterally. Most of the fibres terminate around the ventral horn cells of the spinal cord, particularly in the cervical region. Tectospinal tract is concerned with the reflex postural activity in response to visual stimuli.

Vestibulospinal Tract

The vestibular nuclei are situated in the pons and medulla. They receive afferents from the vestibular apparatus and cerebellum. The vestibular nuclei give rise to vestibulospinal tract, which descends ipsilaterally (uncrossed), and projects on the alpha-motor neurons of the spinal cord. This tract plays an important role in the maintenance of posture and balance.

It would be interesting to note that pyramidal and extrapyramidal tracts concerned with muscles of the trunk and proximal portions of the limbs, i.e. the muscles mainly concerned with the postural control (ventral corticospinal tract, reticulospinal tract, vestibulospinal tract and tectospinal tract) occupy anterior white column of the spinal cord. On the other hand, the descending tracts concerned with the control of distal muscles of the limbs, i.e. those muscles which mediate fine skilled movements (lateral corticospinal tract and rubrospinal tract) occupy lateral white columns. Even among the ventral horn cells, a medial and a lateral group can be identified. The medial group, chiefly controlled by ventral corticospinal tract, innervates the postural muscles, whereas the lateral group innervates the distal muscles of the limbs (Fig. 26.10).

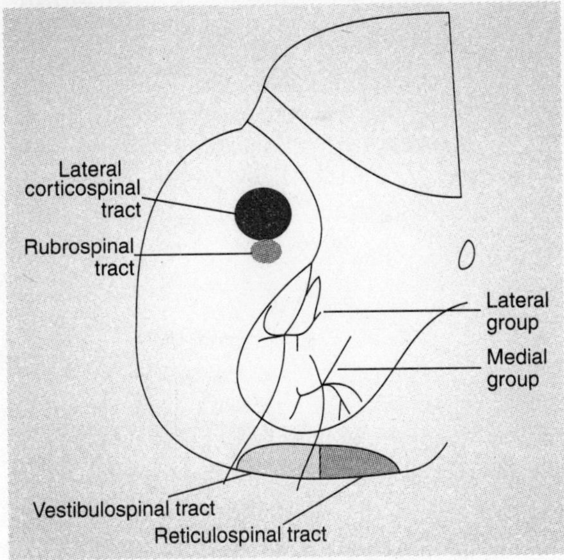

Fig. 26.10: Position of descending tracts and the medial and lateral groups of ventral horn cells.

EFFECTS OF LESIONS

Removal of a small part of primary motor cortex in a monkey results in loss of voluntary control (paralysis) of the movements represented in the area. This disability is especially prominent in the distal muscles of the limb, i.e. hands and fingers.

Experimentally produced unilateral lesions of *pure pyramidal tracts*, e.g. in the medulla oblongata produce *paralysis* of the opposite arm and leg along with *decreased muscle tone and hyporeflexia*.

A lesion in the internal capsule damages both the *pyramidal and extrapyramidal fibres* and the muscle *paralysis is* accompanied by *increased muscle tone (spasticity) and exaggerated tendon jerks*. The difference is due to the fact that the extrapyramidal projection over the ventral horn cells is predominantly inhibitory in nature and its removal produces exaggerated γ-motor neuron activity leading to spasticity and exaggerated tendon jerks.

FUNCTION OF MOTOR CORTEX

From the effects of lesions described above, it may be concluded that the corticospinal and corticobulbar tracts are essential for the execution of voluntary movements. However, it is not yet clear how the motor activity is primarily initiated. The tentative hypothesis has been summarized in Fig. 25.7. The *idea* of performing a voluntary movement arises in the *association areas* of the cerebral cortex. But, the *planning and the programming* seem to occur in the *cerebellum* and the *basal ganglia* and relayed to the primary motor cortex. Finally, the increased impulse discharge in the corticospinal tract and hence in the ventral horn cells produces contraction of the appropriate muscles. Proprioceptive information from the muscles and joints, relayed via the sensory cortex or the cerebellum, helps in the feedback control of the neurons of motor cortex. The degree of control of the motor cortex on the voluntary movement is more prominent in humans and apes than in other animals. Cats and dogs are able to stand, walk or eat after complete destruction of the cerebral cortex, although discrete movements cannot be performed. In these animals, the motor cortex is present but after its lesion, the basal ganglia are able to produce gross motor functions.

Regulation of Spinal Motor Neuron Activity

The corticospinal tract terminates on the ventral horn cells (α-motor neurons), either directly, or indirectly through a small interneuron situated in the spinal segment. The four extrapyramidal tracts named earlier also project on the ventral horn cells. In addition, the ventral horn cells receive afferents from the same, as well as, a few nearby spinal segments. The α-motor discharge to the skeletal muscle depends on the sum total of all the facilitatory and inhibitory inputs received from all of the above mentioned sources.

Signals from the brain are not required for all the α-motor neuron activities. Reflex activity can occur in the spinal cord with minimal higher control, e.g. stretch reflex or flexor reflex. However, complex reflex activities involve coordination by centres located at different levels of the CNS. *Voluntary control of movement is absolutely dependent upon the activity of the corticospinal fibres.*

Upper Motor Neurons and Lower Motor Neurons

Voluntary contraction of a muscle can occur only if signals originating from the primary motor cortex are first transmitted in the corticospinal (or corticobulbar) fibres to the ventral horn cells in the spinal cord (or cranial nerve nuclei in the brainstem), and from where the signals are carried by the efferent fibres to the skeletal muscle. In other words, voluntary control over the skeletal muscle requires activity of the corticospinal as well as ventral horn neurons (α-motor neurons). Lesion of either of these two types of neurons results in paralysis of the muscle. The ventral horn cells, or their cranial equivalents, are often called the lower motor neurons. The corticospinal neurons or corticonuclear neurons are called the upper motor neurons (Fig. 26.11). The terms lower motor neuron or upper motor neuron types of paralysis are used to describe the paralysis due to lesions of ventral horn neurons or cranial nerve nuclei and corticospinal neurons, respectively.

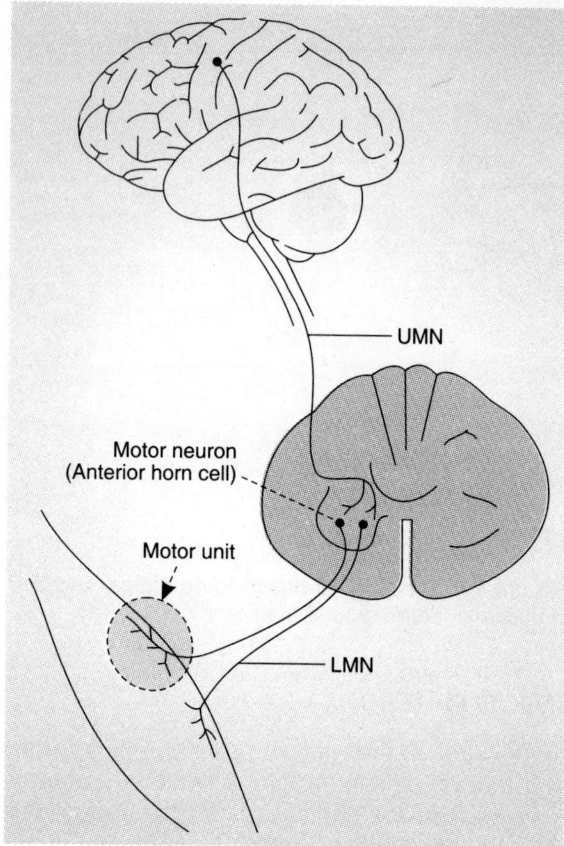

Fig. 26.11: Upper motor neurons (UMN) and lower motor neuron (LMN).

PARALYSIS

Paralysis is the loss of voluntary control on a muscle. In this context, some definitions are given below.

Clinical Classification

Hemiplegia Paralysis of muscles of one side of the body including face, upper limb and lower limb.

Monoplegia Paralysis of the muscles of one limb only.

Paraplegia Paralysis of muscles of both lower limbs.

Quadriplegia Paralysis of muscles of all the four limbs.

Physiological Classification

(a) Upper motor neuron type of paralysis.
(b) Lower motor neuron paralysis.

Upper Motor Neuron Paralysis (UMN Paralysis)

This type of paralysis is due to a lesion of corticospinal tract. The descending extrapyramidal tracts are usually also involved. Some of the clinical signs of UMN paralysis can be attributed to damage to corticospinal tract while others are attributed to damage to extrapyramidal tracts.

Clinical Signs

1. **Loss of voluntary control** of skeletal muscles. Skilled movements performed by the muscles at the distal ends of the limbs are particularly affected.
2. **Spasticity (or hypertonia)** of the muscles.
3. **Clasp-knife reaction** When a sudden passive movement of a limb is attempted, there is a marked resistance. When still more force is used, the resistance suddenly disappears. The initial resistance is because of strong stretch reflex while sudden loss of resistance is because of activation of inverse stretch reflex.

4. **Superficial reflexes** like abdominal, plantar, cremasteric are absent.

5. **Deep reflexes** like biceps jerk, knee jerk, ankle jerk, etc. are exaggerated.

6. **Babinski sign** (see below) is positive.

Pyramidal tract lesion produces signs (1), (4) and (6). Signs (2), (3), (5) are because of damage to extrapyramidal fibres.

Lower Motor Neuron Paralysis (LMN Paralysis)

This type of paralysis is due to a lesion of the ventral horn cells of the spinal cord, anterior root or spinal nerves (or cranial nerves or their nuclei). Following are the clinical signs of a lower motor neuron paralysis.

1. **Loss of voluntary control** over the muscle (s) supplied by the lower motor neuron.

2. **Flaccidity of the muscles** The muscles show extreme hypotonia.

3. **Atrophy (wasting)** of the muscles.

4. **Loss of superficial and deep reflexes** in which the affected muscle is involved.

5. **Muscle fasciculations** This term is used to describe the twitching of the paralysed muscle. This sign is seen only when there is slow destruction of the ventral horn cells, e.g. motor neuron disease.

6. **Muscle contractures** This term means permanent shortening of the paralysed muscle. Contracture often involves the non-paralysed antagonistic muscles whose action is no longer opposed by paralysed muscle.

A lesion in the internal capsule typically produces upper motor neuron type of paralysis (e.g. hemiplegia: see below). However, a lesion in the spinal cord produces a combination of lower motor neuron type of paralysis in some muscles as well as upper motor neuron type of paralysis in others (e.g. complete transaction of spinal cord, see below). A lesion in the brainstem would produce lower motor neuron type of paralysis in the muscles supplied by the cranial nerves as well as upper motor neuron type of paralysis of the upper and lower limb muscles.

Comparison of UMN and LMN types of paralysis is given in Table 26.1.

Table 26.1: Comparison of UMN and LMN types of paralysis

	UMN Paralysis	*LMN Paralysis*
1. Loss of voluntary control (paralysis)	+	+
2. Muscle tone	Increased (spasticity)	Decreased (flaccidity)
3. Tendon jerks	Exaggerated	Absent
4. Superficial reflexes	Absent	Absent in concerned muscle
5. Babinski sign	+	–
6. Muscle fasciculations	–	+
7. Muscle wasting	–	+
8. Muscle contractures	–	+

+ = Present
– = Absent

HEMIPLEGIA

A vascular lesion in the internal capsule is fairly common in elderly individuals. It results in paralysis of the **opposite side of the body**. The clinical picture to be described below is the result of damage to both pyramidal and extrapyramidal fibres passing through the internal capsule. Initially, besides the loss of all voluntary movements, there is severe hypotonia and absence of all the reflexes on the involved side of the body. This condition, resembling the spinal shock, lasts for about 2–3 weeks. Later the paralysis persists but hypertonia and hyperactive deep reflexes form a prominent feature.

1. **Paralysis** The paralysis affects movements of the face, arm and leg. The muscles of the upper face, thorax and abdomen are not paralysed because they have bilateral cortical representation. Movements of the eyeball may be affected if the corticonuclear fibres are also damaged.

2. **Muscle Tone** Hypertonia, (spasticity) is most prominent in the antigravity muscles (flexors of the upper limb and extensors of the lower limb).

3. **Deep Reflexes** Knee jerk, ankle jerk, biceps jerk, triceps and supinator jerks are exaggerated. Ankle clonus is often present.

4. Superficial Reflexes Abdominal, cremasteric and plantar reflexes are absent since these need facilitation by the pyramidal tracts.

5. Babinski's Sign Like all the features described above, this sign can be elicited on the affected side only. It consists of dorsiflexion of the big toe and fanning out (abduction) of the small toes in response to firm scratching of the outer border of sole of the foot (Fig. 26.12). Although physiological significance of Babinski's response is not clear, its clinical importance cannot be overestimated. Except in infancy, Babinski's sign can be elicited only when pyramidal tracts are destroyed. Occasionally, it may be only unequivocal sign of a pyramidal tract lesion.

6. Sensory Deficit In patients with more extensive lesions of the internal capsule, the sensory and visual fibres are also affected. In such patients, besides hemiplegia, contralateral homonymous hemianopia and cortical type of hemianesthesia (of the affected side of the body) may also be observed.

7. Recovery In many patients, considerable degree of recovery occurs. Muscles of the lower limb and proximal muscles of the upper limb show better recovery of voluntary control than fine muscles of the hands and fingers. The recovery may be due to restoration of function in the partially damaged fibres of corticospinal tract, or due to more effective use of extrapyramidal pathways which may escape damage.

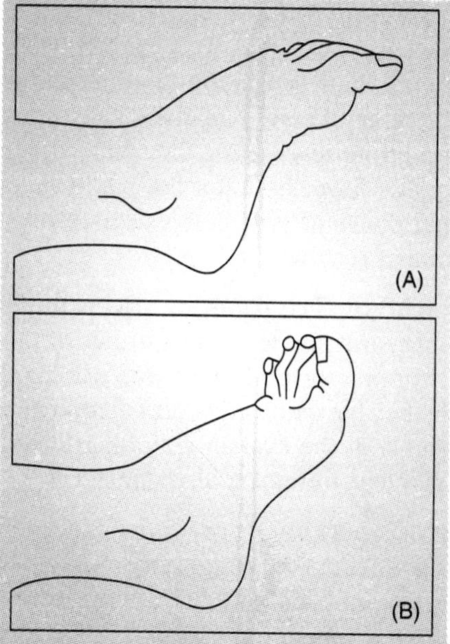

Fig. 26.12: Normal plantar reflex (A), and Babinski's sign (B).

SPINAL CORD LESIONS

Automobile accidents, war injuries or spinal tumours may produce spinal cord lesions of varying severity.

Complete Transection of Spinal Cord

Complete transection of the spinal cord produces an immediate, complete and permanent loss of all sensations and voluntary movement below the level of the lesion (Fig. 26.13). During the stage of spinal shock (lasting 2–3 weeks), all the reflexes are abolished, muscles are flaccid, bladder and rectum are paralysed. Blood pressure may fall if the level of the lesion is upper thoracic segments.

When the spinal shock has passed off, autonomic reflex activity is first to return. Among the somatic reflexes, Babinski's sign is first to appear. Following features constitute the permanent disability.

At the Level of the Lesion

The injury usually involves a few segments of the spinal cord. The muscles innervated by the α-motor neurons arising from these segments show the characteristic picture of lower motor neuron type of paralysis, i.e. loss of voluntary control, flaccidity, absence of tendon jerks, and progressive wasting of the paralysed muscles. All these signs are due to damaged ventral horn cells/ventral root of the spinal cord.

Below the Level of the Lesion

(i) **Bilateral Spastic Paralysis of Muscles** The loss of voluntary control (paralysis) is caused by interruption of corticospinal tract, whereas spasticity is due to damage to extrapyramidal tracts. Spasticity is

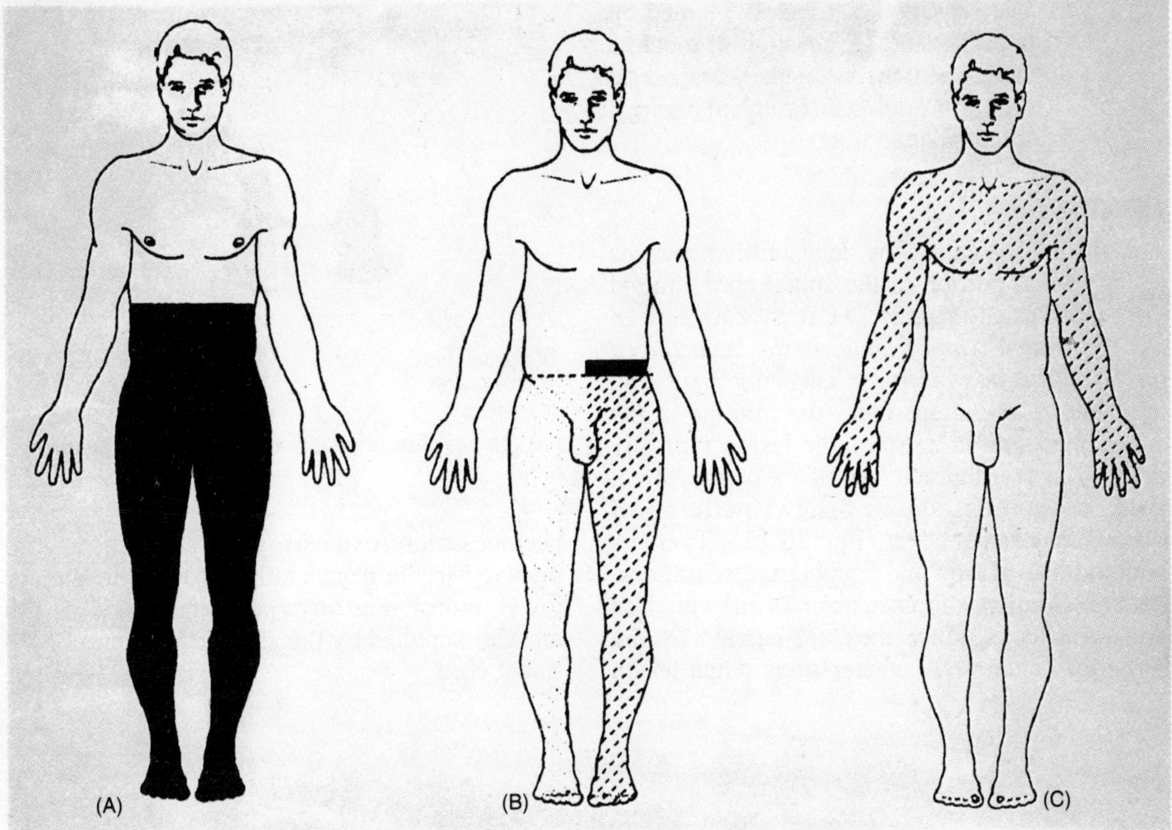

Fig. 26.13: Effect of various lesions on the sensory system. (A) Complete transaction of spinal cord; (B) Hemisection of spinal cord; (C) Syringomyelia.

associated with bilateral absence of superficial reflexes and presence of Babinski's sign on both the sides.

(ii) Bilateral loss of all sensations.

(iii) Loss of voluntary control over bladder and rectum.

Hemisection of Spinal Cord (Brown-Sequard Syndrome)

A tumour of the spinal cord or a traumatic injury may produce lesion of one-half of the spinal cord. Such cases are characterized by (Fig. 26.13):

At the Level of the Lesion

(a) *Ipsilateral* lower motor neuron type of paralysis. This is due to damage to ventral horn cells/anterior root.

(b) Ipsilateral band of total loss of all sensations due to destruction of dorsal roots and dorsal grey horn.

Below the Level of the Lesion

(i) *Ipsilateral* spastic paralysis (UMN type) of muscles.

(ii) *Ipsilateral* positive Babinski's sign.

(iii) *Ipsilateral* loss of superficial reflexes

(iv) *Ipsilateral* loss of tactile discrimination, proprioception and vibration sensation (dorsal column sensations).

(v) *Contralateral* loss of pain and temperature sensation. (The spinothalamic tracts on the affected side carry pain and temperature sensations from the opposite side of the body).

(vi) The sensation of touch is blunted on both the sides. (Sensation of touch is carried by two routes: ipsilateral dorsal columns and contralateral ventral spinothalamic tract).

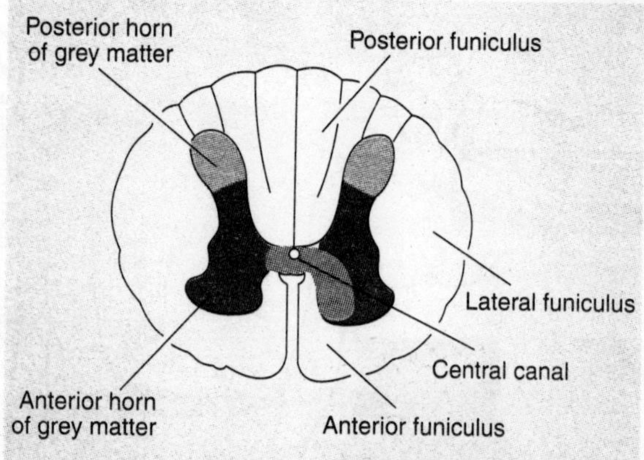

Fig. 26.14: Site of lesion in syringomyelia (darkened area).

Syringomyelia

This disorder is caused by degenerative changes in the central portion of the spinal cord, around the central canal (Fig. 26.14). It is characterized by *dissociated type of anaesthesia in localized parts of the body*. Fibres carrying pain and temperature sensations cross the midline in the anterior commissure. Since the lesion typically involves a few thoracic segments of the spinal cord, the patient shows "shawl pattern" of dissociated anaesthesia (Fig. 26.13). There is bilateral loss of pain and temperature sensations, but the sensations of touch, position and vibration are not affected since they are carried by the posterior columns. At a later stage when lesion becomes more extensive, ventral horn may be involved in the degenerative process, leading to lower motor neuron type of paralysis of the muscles supplied by the affected segments of the spinal cord.

The Thalamus, Reticular Activating System, EEG and Sleep

CHAPTER 27

THALAMUS

The two thalami are ovoid masses of grey matter lying close together rostrally, and joined in the midline by the mass intermedia, and separated only by the third ventricle. Caudally, they diverge to enclose the corpora quardigemina. The external medullary lamina, consisting of thalamocortical and corticothalamic fibres covers the lateral surface of the thalamus and separates it from the internal capsule. An attenuated layer of neurons, called the reticular nucleus, is present between the external medullary lamina and the internal capsule (Fig. 27.1).

The thalamus is divided into the lateral and the medial masses of nuclei by the internal medullary lamina which consists of internuclear thalamic fibres. Rostrally, the internal medullary lamina bifurcates to enclose the anterior thalamic nuclei.

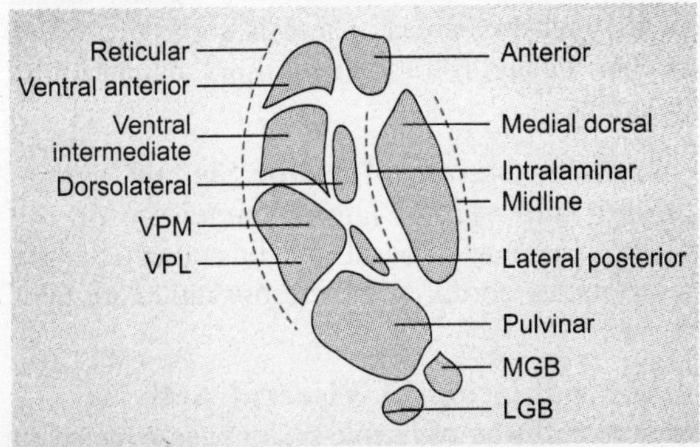

Fig. 27.1: Nuclei of the thalamus.

The medial nuclear mass consists of: (i) intralaminar nuclei; (ii) centromedian nucleus present close to the internal medullary lamina; (iii) extensive dorsomedial nucleus; and (iv) midline nuclei present in the mass intermedia.

The lateral nuclear mass can be divided into the dorsal and the ventral group. The dorsal group consists of the lateral dorsal and lateral posterior group in the middle zone and pulvinar in the posterior zone. The ventral group consists of: (i) ventral anterior; (ii) ventral lateral nuclei in the anterior zone; and (iii) ventral posterior nucleus in the middle zone. The ventral posterior nucleus has two divisions namely, *ventroposterior lateral (VPL)* and *ventroposterior medial (VPM)*. (iv) The lateral and the medial geniculate bodies are present in the posterior zone. The functional classification and connections of the thalamus are as follows:

Thalamic Nuclei associated with Sensory Pathways

1. VPL and VPM Nuclei These are the sites of termination of ascending somatic afferent tracts. The medial lemniscus carrying afferent fibres from the gracile nucleus, cuneate nucleus and the spinothalamic afferents terminate in the VPL, whereas the trigeminal lemniscus terminates in the VPM. Thus, VPL receives sensations of touch, pressure, position, temperature and pain from all parts of the body except the face. VPM receives all these sensations from the face along with the sensation of taste. In the ventroposterior nucleus, a topographic representation of the body can be demonstrated.

Third order neurons arise from the VPL and VPM and project on the postcentral gyrus relaying all sensations except the sensation of pain.

2. Medial Geniculate Body It receives fibres from the auditory nuclei and the inferior colliculi and project on to the auditory area of the cerebral cortex. Medial geniculate body is topographically organized and reflects spatial distribution of the organ of Corti. Destruction of a small part of medial geniculate body produces deafness of a particular band of sound frequency.

3. Lateral Geniculate Body It shows an orderly organized representation of the retina. It receives projection from the superior colliculi also. It projects topographically on the visual cortex. In the lateral geniculate body, the macula is represented in the caudal two-thirds, whereas the remaining retina is represented in the rostral one-third.

Nuclei concerned with Motor Function

1. Ventral Lateral Nucleus It is the chief motor nucleus of the thalamus. It receives the dentato-thalamic fibres from the cerebellum and projects on the primary motor cortex and premotor cortex (area 4 and 6). It receives fibres from the globus pallidus also.

2. Ventral Anterior Nucleus It receives fibres from the cerebellum, globus pallidus and substantia nigra. Efferent fibres go to other thalamic nuclei and premotor cortex.

3. Intralaminar Nuclei They receive afferent from the spinothalamic and dentato-thalamic tracts and project on to the neostriatum and frontal lobe.

Nuclei Concerned with Visceral Function

1. Anterior Thalamic Nuclei They receive afferents from the hippocampus directly via fornix and relayed through mamillary body (mamillothalamic tract) and project on the cingulate gyrus.

2. Lateral Dorsal Nucleus It also has connections similar to that of anterior thalamic nuclei.

3. Dorsomedial nucleus It receives afferents from the hypothalamus and amygdala and projects to the entire frontal cortex rostral to area 6 and 32.

Thalamic Nuclei serving Integrative Function

1. Pulvinar and Lateral Posterior Nucleus They receive fibres from superior colliculus and pretectal nucleus and project extensively to parieto-occipitotemporal cortex intercalated between the somatic, visual and auditory cortex.

2. Reticular Nucleus It receives afferents from the collaterals of corticothalamic and thalamo-cortical fibres traversing between them. Reticular cell axons project on the thalamic nuclei and regulate their activity by a feedback system.

Functions of Thalamus

1. Relay Station of Sensory Signals The specific relay nuclei such as VPL, VPM, lateral and medial geniculate bodies act as relay station of sensory information on way to the cerebral cortex. All sensations (e.g. somatosensory, visual, auditory), except olfactory, have to pass through the thalamus. It is believed that the thalamic nuclei do not merely relay the sensory signals to the cortical sensory areas. There is some degree of modulation and filtration of sensory signals in the thalamus.

2. Relay Station of Motor Signals Ventral anterior and ventral lateral nuclei are on the efferent pathway of basal ganglia and cerebellum to the motor cortex and therefore modulate their activity.

3. Modulation of Visceral Activity The efferent pathway of limbic system passes through thalamus.

4. Perception of Pain Pain sensation is perceived in the thalamus and brainstem reticular formation. However, somatosensory cortex is essential for localization of pain.

5. Perception of Thermal Sensation Crude thermal sensations (cold or hot) can be perceived in the thalamus. Appreciation of fine grades of temperature difference requires somatosensory cortex.

6. Generalised Cerebral Alertness The so-called non-specific thalamic nuclei (intralaminar and midline nuclei) are concerned with generalized arousal of cerebral cortex. (See reticular activating system, vide infra).

7. Thalamo-cortical Unit There are so many interconnections between thalamus and cerebral cortex that the two seem to function as one unit. A cortical area may be rendered non-functional by severing its connection with specific thalamic nucleus.

Thalamic Syndrome

The thalamus constitutes one wall of the internal capsule. Therefore, some of its nuclei are likely to be involved in the vascular lesions of the internal capsule. The term thalamic syndrome is used to describe relatively rare group of symptoms and signs because of a *vascular lesion of thalamus alone*. The characteristic features of thalamic syndrome are given below.

1. Contralateral Hemianaesthesia Due to lesion of VPL and VPM, all somatosensory including pain and thermal sensations are affected. (In a patient with internal capsule lesion, pain and temperature sensations remain intact).

2. Contralateral Hyperalgesia or Causalgesia These clinical features usually become prominent a few weeks after the thrombotic thalamic lesion. The patient has exaggerated and unpleasant or painful sensation resulting from mild cutaneous stimulation by touch, warmth or cold. Such a condition is known as *hyperalgesia*. Attacks of pain may occur in the absence of any stimulus. The clinical feature is known as *causalgia*. (Such features are not seen in a patient with internal capsular lesion).

3. Contralateral Homonymous Hemianopia may be observed if the vascular lesion involves LGB.

4. Complex Motor Disorders resembling cereballar damage (ataxia, intention tremor, muscular atonia) and/or basal ganglia damage (choreoathetosis) may occur on the contralateral side (due to damage to ventral anterior or ventral lateral nuclei).

ELECTROENCEPHALOGRAM (EEG)

The electroencephalogram is the record of spontaneous electrical activity of the brain by using electrodes on the *surface of the scalp*. The electrical activity of the brain can also be recorded from the surface of the brain after opening the skull (e.g. during brain surgery). Such a record is called electrocorticogram.

EEG record may be bipolar or unipolar. A bipolar record shows potential variations between a pair of scalp electrodes. Unipolar recording is the potential difference between a sensitive scalp electrode and an indifferent electrode placed on the ear (Fig. 27.2). A 16-channel polygraph is

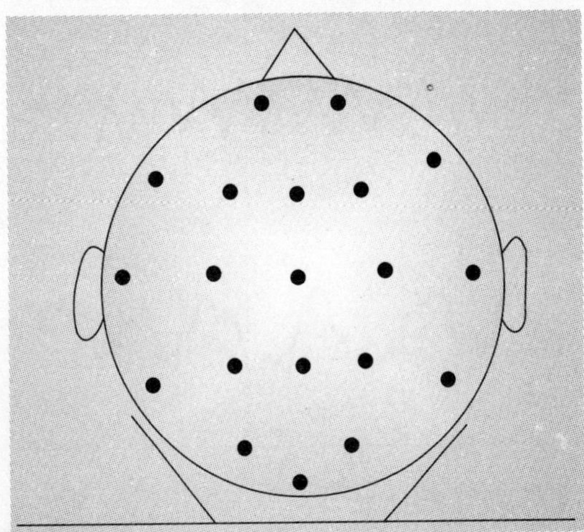

Fig. 27.2: The placement of electrodes on the scalp for EEG recording.

usually used to record the electrical activity from the various regions of the scalp.

The EEG record consists of recurring oscillations in the electrical potential. The oscillations differ in the frequency and amplitude at different points on the scalp and during different stages of mental alertness. The frequency of these oscillations may vary from 1/s to over 50/s. Their amplitude may vary from 50 to 200 μV. Depending on their frequency, the oscillations or the "brainwaves" may be classified as follows (Fig. 27.3).

Frequency (in Hertz)	*Name of EEG wave*
1–3.5	Delta (δ)
4–7	Theta (θ)
8–13	Alpha (α)
14–30	Beta (β)

27

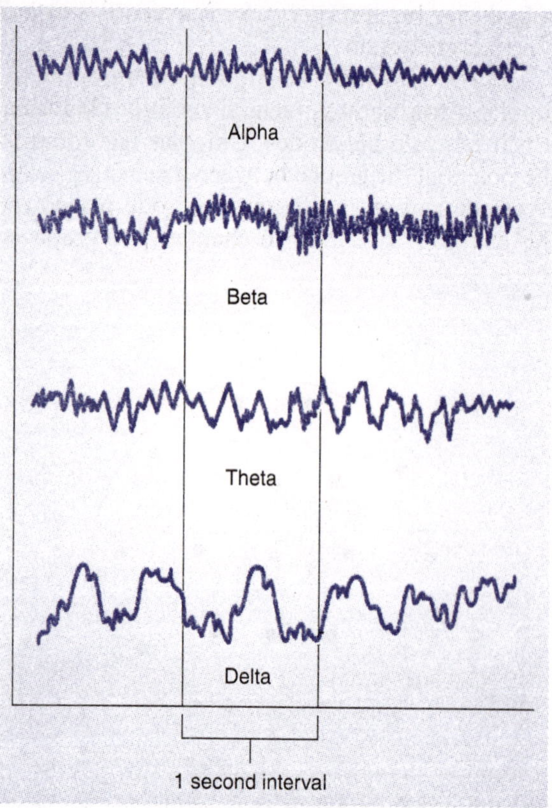

Fig. 27.3: EEG waves.

Alpha Rhythm (8–13 Hz)

In a normal person, at rest and eyes closed, the α-rhythm (8–13 cycles/s) is the dominant frequency in the EEG. It is seen at greatest amplitude in the parietal and occipital region in the adults. The amplitude of these waves slowly waxes and wanes, but the average amplitude is about 50 μV (Fig. 27.4).

The α-rhythm is believed to originate from awake but inattentive brain. The frequency of α-rhythm is *decreased* by: (i) low blood sugar level, (ii) low body temperature, (iii) Addison's disease, and (iv) high arterial pCO_2.

The frequency of α-rhythm *is increased* by (i) high blood sugar level, (ii) high body temperature, (iii) Cushing's syndrome, and (iv) low arterial pO_2. In some patients, latent EEG abnormalities become apparent when the subject is asked to hyperventilate (so as to lower arterial pCO_2).

Alpha Block Any form of sensory stimulation, e.g. opening of the eyes, listening to a clicking sound, cutaneous touch or even mental arithmetical calculations can abolish the α-rhythm. The phenomenon is called alpha block. Instead, a high frequency low voltage, ß-rhythm, (also called desynchronized pattern), is recorded (Fig. 27.5).

Beta Rhythm (14–30 Hz)

Beta rhythm is also seen in adults, more often over the frontal lobe. Beta rhythm is seen all over the brain in an alert mind, busy in mental calculations. In a patient with agitated mind, the beta wave frequency is on the higher side of the beta rhythm range. Beta rhythm is normally seen during REM sleep.

Theta Rhythm (4–7 Hz)

Such waves are normal in children up to the age of 13 years. In adults, theta rhythm is seen during stages I and II of NREM sleep.

Delta Rhythm (1–3.5 Hz)

Delta rhythm is the dominant rhythm in infants up to the age of one year. In adults, such waves

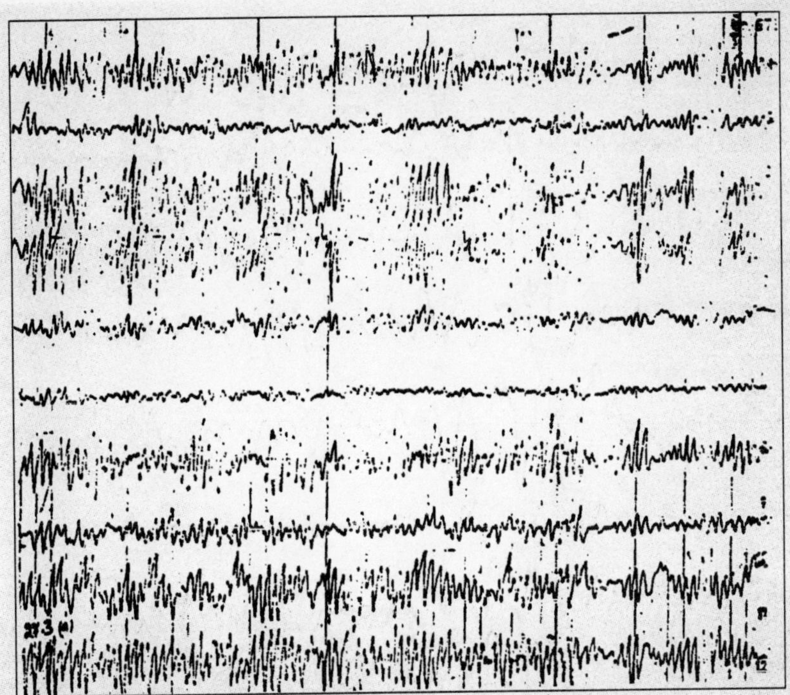

Fig. 27.4: Normal EEG record on a 16-channel recorder.

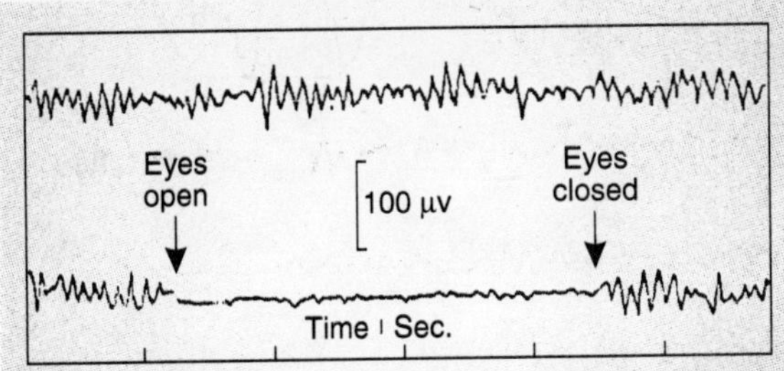

Fig. 27.5: A part of EEG record showing alpha rhythm as well as alpha block (desynchronization).

with average voltage over 100 μV are normally seen in stages III and IV of NREM sleep.

Theta and delta waves are grouped together as *slow waves. Appearance of slow waves in the EEG of an awake adult are always considered pathological.*

Indications for Electroencephalography

1. **Epilepsy** EEG recording remains the *mainstay of diagnosis of epilepsy* (Fig. 27.6).
2. **Brain Tumour** Nowadays, MRI (magnetic resonance imaging) is usually used for the detection of a brain tumour. However, in a few cases, presence of irregular slow waves (θ or δ waves) in a localized area of the scalp may be the only early sign of a cerebral tumour.
3. **Brain Death** Flat EEG in a patient with ischemic or traumatic damage to the brain is one of the important criteria for the diagnosis of brain death. (Drug intoxication, hypothermia and recent hypotension are other causes of flat EEG).

RETICULAR ACTIVATING SYSTEM

Wakefulness and Sleep

The midventral core of the brainstem contains a complex network of cells and fibres which extends into diencephalon above and spinal cord below. Some of the cells constitute large and anatomically well-defined masses, e.g. cranial nerve nuclei, red nucleus and superior olive. These are not included

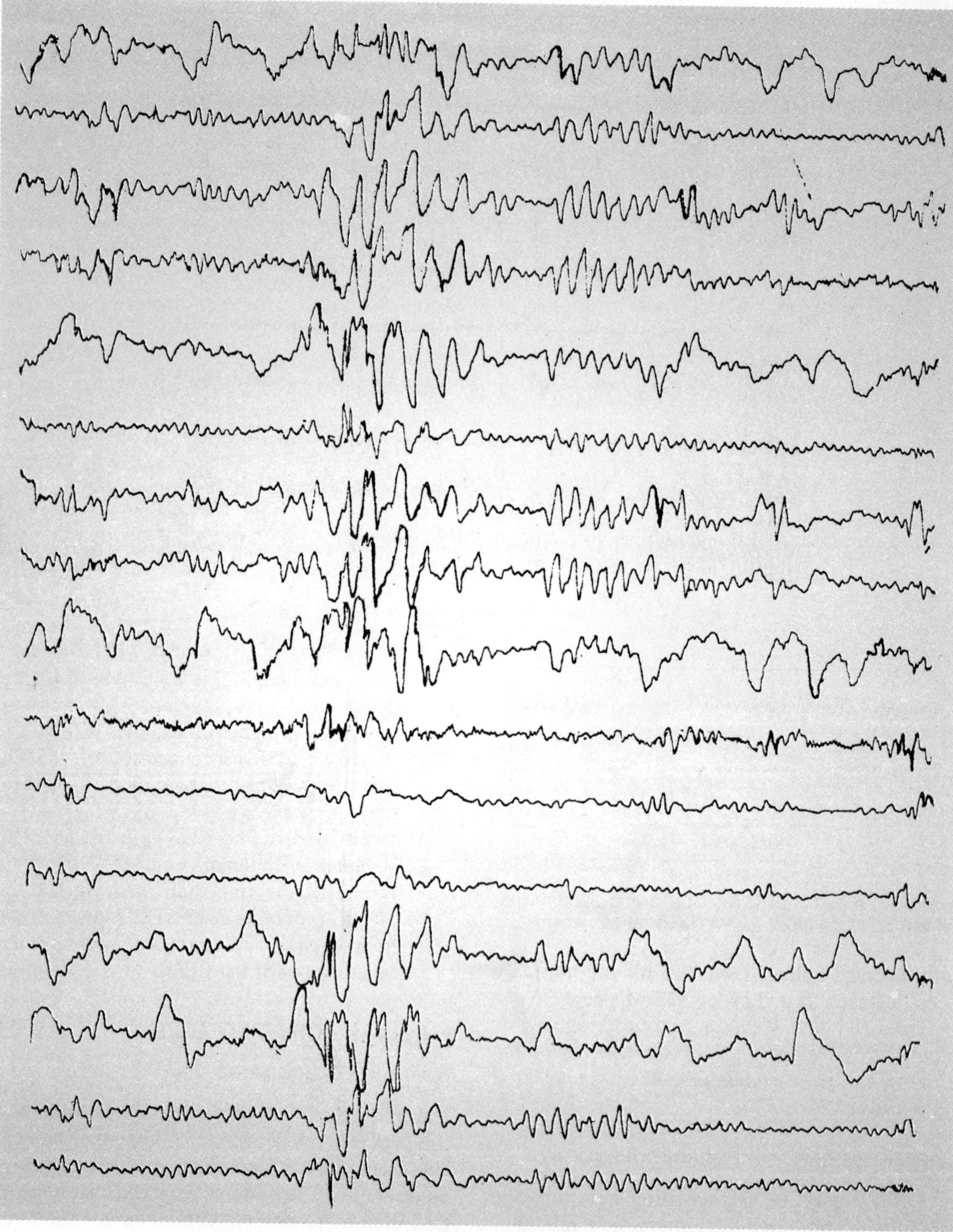

Fig. 27.6: EEG record of a patient of epilepsy showing delta waves.

in the term reticular formation. The term *brainstem reticular formation* refers to:

(i) Many aggregations of cells, though not anatomical entities, have fairly well-defined physiological actions, e.g. centres that regulate respiration, heart rate, blood pressure, etc.

(ii) A highly complex network of interconnected neurons. Some of these neuronal networks give rise to reticulospinal tracts, the important constituents of (descending) extrapyramidal system. Others constitute an ascending system which has an important role in arousal and consciousness. The last group of neurons constitutes the reticular activating system.

Reticular activating system (RAS) is the name given to the ascending polysynaptic pathway that extends from the brainstem reticular formation to non-specific thalamic nuclei (intralaminar and midline nuclei) and projects diffusely to the cerebral cortex. Some of the cortical projection of RAS bypasses the thalamus. The long sensory tracts, as they ascend in the brainstem, give collaterals to the RAS (Fig. 27.7). Thus, the RAS receives inputs from the medial and the trigeminal lemnisci as well as from the visual, auditory and olfactory systems. Therefore, the RAS is a non-specific system which can be excited by any sensation. Stimulation of the RAS causes immediate and marked activation of the cerebral cortex resulting in arousal of the animal (or man) if asleep.

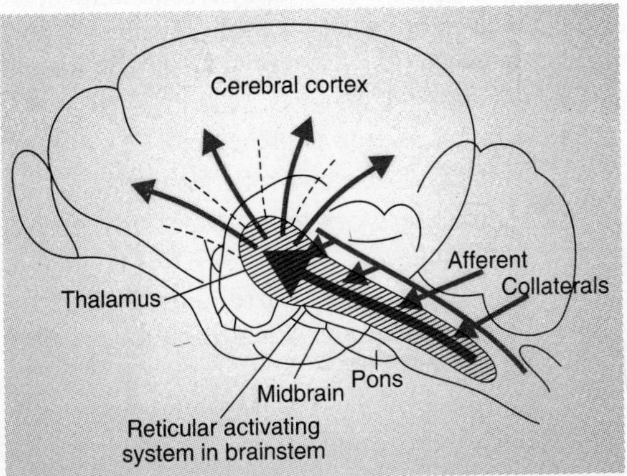

Fig. 27.7: Reticular activating system.

Stimulation of a sensory nerve produces two types of electrical activity in the cerebral cortex. Initially, there is a brief (lasting few milliseconds) and localized response over the specific sensory cortex, e.g. in the "foot area" of the postcentral gyrus, if electric shock is given over the foot or over occipital lobe after photopic stimulation. This initial response is called the *primary evoked potential* which has the latency of about 10 ms. About 50 ms later, there is a *diffuse secondary response* in which the electrical activity can be recorded from most the cerebral cortex. The diffuse secondary response may last as long as 30 seconds. The primary evoked potential is produced by conduction of sensory signals through the specific sensory pathways. The secondary diffuse response is due to spread of impulses through the RAS to the cerebral cortex.

27

Arousal Reaction

In a sleeping animal or man, the characteristic electroencephalogram (EEG) pattern consists of high voltage slow waves (δ waves). The animal or man can be easily awakened by application of any sensory stimulus. This is called the arousal reaction. Although any sensory stimulus can produce arousal reaction, pain and proprioceptive stimuli are more effective than others. On arousal from the sleep, the EEG pattern changes to high frequency low voltage activity (ß-wave activity).

Factors Affecting Arousal Reaction

1. Cortical Stimulation Electrical stimulation of certain portions of cerebral cortex (e.g. superior temporal gyrus) increase the RAS activity leading to arousal and desynchronization of the EEG pattern.

2. Hormones Hormones like epinephrine and norepinephrine increase the alertness of the brain and produce arousal reaction, if asleep. The catecholamines produce these effects by lowering threshold of the neurons of RAS.

3. General Anaesthetics General anaesthetic agents produce unconsciousness by depressing the conduction in the RAS. Various general anaesthetics, although differ in their chemical structure, but have a common property of high lipid solubility. In addition, many of them produce hyperpolarization in the neurons. In contrast to 2–4 synapses in the specific long sensory tracts, the polysynaptic RAS pathway contains hundreds of synapses. Hence, the depressant action of the general anaesthetics is more effective in blocking the conduction in the RAS than in the specific sensory pathways.

Function of RAS

Activity of the RAS is of fundamental importance for the functioning of brain. Although non-specific in nature, it brings the cerebral cortex to such a background level of alertness that other brain functions like motor activity, sensory perception, memory and abstract thinking are possible. RAS is periodically depressed, which results in a state of loss of reactivity to environmental events, known as sleep.

27

SLEEP

Sleep is defined as a state of unconsciousness from which a person can be readily aroused by appropriate sensory stimuli. The loss of reactivity to environmental events, characteristic of unconsciousness, also occurs under anaesthesia, or in coma, but these states are not readily reversible. In adults, the sleep-wakefulness cycle follows a 24 hour (circadian) rhythm. A newborn infant has many cycles of sleep and wakefulness in 24 hours, but by the end of second year of life, a single sleep-wakefulness cycle is established. The sleep cycle consists of about 7–8 hours of sleep and 16–18 hours of wakefulness. During the 1st month of life, an infant sleeps for about 16 hours everyday. The total duration of daily sleep decreases to about 8 hours in adolescents, and 7 hours in adults.

Types of Sleep

Slow Wave Sleep (SWS)/Non-Rapid Eye Movement (NREM) Sleep

It is so-called because of the presence of slow waves (delta waves) in the EEG recorded during this type of sleep. The physiological changes associated with SWS are as follows:

1. Elevation of threshold of many reflexes.
2. Babinski's sign may be present even in a healthy individual.
3. Muscle tone is reduced.
4. Heart rate is reduced and steady.
5. Blood pressure is reduced and steady.
6. Respiratory rate is reduced and steady.
7. BMR is reduced.
8. Increased secretion of growth hormone.
9. Decreased secretion of adrenal medullary catecholamines.
10. Pupillary constriction.
11. Eyeballs rolled up but stationary.
12. Dreams occur but on awakening the individual cannot recall them.

Rapid Eye Movement (REM) Sleep/ Paradoxical Sleep/Desynchronized Sleep

This type of sleep is characterized by bursts of rapid side to side movement of the eyeballs. The characteristic EEG recording is a high frequency, low voltage rhythm (ß-rhythm or desynchronized rhythm). The physiological changes associated with REM sleep are as follows:

1. Threshold for arousal is markedly elevated.
2. Muscle tone throughout the body is markedly lowered.

   Signs (1) and (2) indicate greater depth of sleep than SWS but EEG pattern is that seen in an awake person. Because of this paradox, this phase of sleep is also named *paradoxical sleep*.
3. Babinski's sign is present.
4. Threshold of many reflexes elevated.
5. Heart rate is irregular, especially during dreaming.
6. Blood pressure is irregular, especially during dreaming, when high values may be recorded.
7. Respiratory rate is irregular, especially during dreaming.
8. Dreams occur which can be vividly recalled on awakening.

9. Sexual arousal occurs leading to penile erection or clitoral engorgement.
10. Despite extreme low tone in the skeletal muscle, a few irregular movements occur in the body.
11. Extreme relaxation of pharyngeal muscles predisposes the individual to sleep apnoea syndrome.
12. Pupillary constriction.
13. Decreased secretion of growth hormone.
14. BMR is similar to that of awake state.
15. Body temperature regulating mechanisms totally fail. Greater protection needed against cold or warmth.

Distribution of REM and NREM Sleep

Every 80–100 minutes of SWS is followed by 5–30 minutes of REM sleep. There are about 4–6 bouts of REM sleep every night. Thus, REM sleep constitutes 20–25% of the total sleep time in adults. In infants, REM sleep constitutes 25–50% of the total sleep.

If EEG is continuously recorded in a sleeping individual, the following stages may be identified: Initially, when a person goes to sleep, he goes into SWS. From EEG record, four stages of SWS may be identified (Fig. 27.8).

Stage I It is a stage of very light sleep. Slightly slow α-rhythm is recorded.

Stage II It is characterized by the appearance of *sleep spindles* consisting of α-wave like (10–14 cycles/second, 50 μV) waves superimposed on a low voltage background.

Stage III As the depth of sleep increases further, a few sleep spindles (bursts of α-wave-like activity) are seen to be superimposed on the background of low frequency, 1–2 cycles/second, high voltage (100 μV) waves (δ-waves).

Stage IV Only δ-waves can be seen. The threshold for arousal is markedly elevated. The muscle tone is also decreased.

The stages I, II and III are of very short duration. After 60–90 minutes of stage IV of SWS, the person reverts to the stages III and II and then enters into REM sleep, when the EEG pattern changes to high frequency low amplitude (ß-waves) pattern (Fig. 27.9). After 5–30 minutes of REM sleep, the cycles of SWS are repeated.

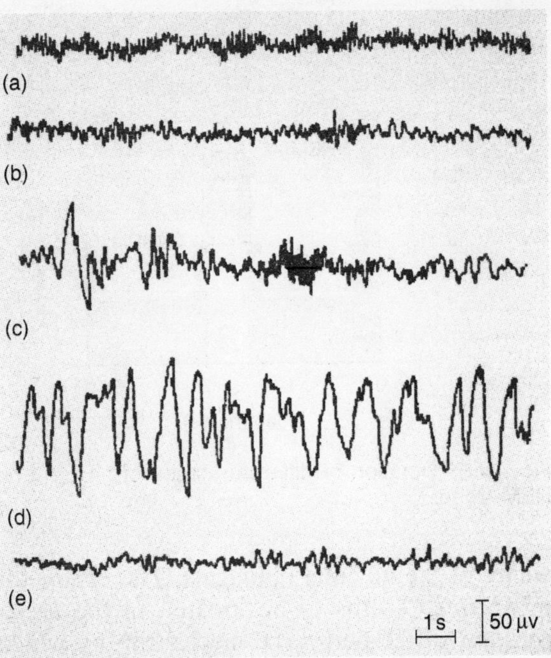

Fig. 27.8: The pattern of EEG in different stages of NREM and REM sleep. (a) to (d) : stages I to IV of NREM sleep; (e) REM sleep.

Neural Mechanism of Sleep

1. Passive Theory of Sleep Up to the middle of the last century, sleep was considered a passive process. The wakefulness/sleep cycles were explained on the basis of the activity/fatigue respectively of reticular activating system (RAS) of the brainstem. This theory was discarded when it was discovered that stimulation of certain areas of brainstem or diencephalon produced sleep in awake animals. Therefore, the active theory of sleep was proposed.

2. Sleep is an Active Inhibitory Process There seems to be certain centres in the brainstem and diencephalon, activation of which produces inhibition of RAS and consequently inhibition of cerebral cortex, leading to induction of sleep. The centre for *SWS* seems to be located in the *Raphe*

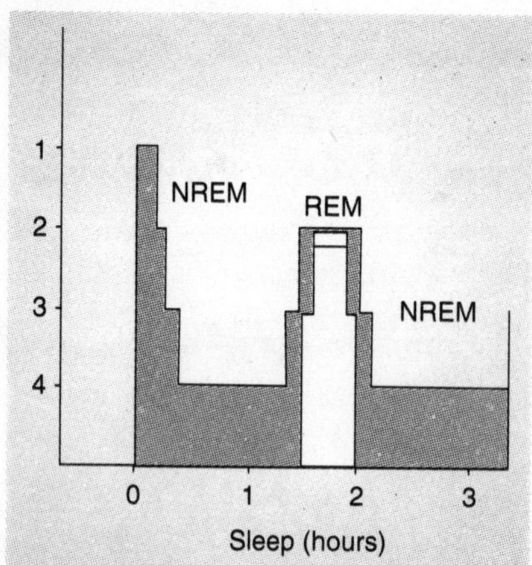

Fig. 27.9: Duration of different stages of NREM and REM sleep.

nuclei of the medulla oblongata. The centre for *REM sleep* seems to be located in the *locus ceruleus* of the pons. The mechanism by which these sleep centres are periodically activated is not yet clear.

Chemical mediators of sleep or neurotransmitters involved in production of sleep are not exactly known. Many chemicals have been implicated, but there are evidences against each.

Significance of Sleep

Although the exact biological role of sleep is not known, there is no doubt that it is essential for the normal physical and mental health. Both REM and NREM types of sleep seem to be required. Experimentally, a person may be selectively deprived of SWS or REM sleep. Subsequently if allowed undisturbed, the person undergoes greater proportion of the sleeping time to the type of sleep deprived earlier.

Sleep deprivation initially affects the higher functions of the brain. More prolonged sleep deprivation may affect subcortical and even visceral function.

Sleep Disorders

Insomnia is defined as an inability to have sufficient or restful sleep despite adequate opportunity for the same.

In **sleepwalking (somnambulism)**, the individual wanders about in the house during sleep without being aware of it. It generally occurs during stage 3 or 4 of *slow wave sleep* - deep sleep. One study showed that the highest prevalence of sleepwalking was 16% for children of 11 to 12 years of age. Sleepwalkers engage in their activities with their eyes open so they can navigate their surroundings.

In **narcolepsy**, there is an irresistible urge to sleep. The person goes to sleep while performing daytime tasks. Narcolepsy is related to the *REM sleep*. Normally when people fall asleep, they experience 90 minutes of non-REM sleep, which is then followed by REM sleep. People with narcolepsy, however, enter REM sleep immediately. In addition, REM sleep occurs inappropriately throughout the day. People with narcolepsy fall asleep suddenly—any-where, at any time, even in the middle of a conversation. These sleep attacks can last from a few seconds to more than an hour.

The physiological basis of all these sleep disorders is yet not clear.

Disorders of Consciousness

1. Syncope (Fainting) It is a sudden and transient loss of consciousness. Most commonly, it is due to cardiovascular abnormalities leading to transient decrease in cerebral blood flow. *Postural hypotension* is one of the important causes of syncope. Another type, called *vasovagal* syncope is reflexive in nature, and associated with pain, fear or other type of emotional stress. In this case, stimulation of autonomic nerves to the circulatory system causes sudden bradycardia, vasodilatation and drop in blood pressure. More serious causes of syncope include sudden decrease in cardiac output due to *myocardial infarction* or *cardiac arrhythmias*.

2. Coma It is characterized by loss of consciousness from which arousal cannot be elicited. Coma is not simply deep sleep. The causes of coma may be:

(a) **Cerebral disorders** (head injury, cerebral thrombosis or haemorrhage or brain tumour).

(b) **Metabolic disorders** (diabetic coma, hypoglycemic coma, hepatic coma, uraemic coma, respiratory failure, heat stroke).
(c) **Narcotic poisoning**.

Brain Death

A patient with ischemic or traumatic damage of the brain may ultimately go into irreversible coma. Such a stage is reached when brain death has occurred, i.e. patient's brain is dead though his life may be maintained by artificial cardio-pulmonary supportive measures. The diagnosis of brain death calls for termination of these supportive measures because the patient would never recover. Moreover, only when brain death has been declared, the removal of viable organs (e.g. kidney) for transplantation can be considered. Loss of consciousness accompanied by flat EEG, fixed dilated pupils, absence of pupillary, corneal and swallowing reflexes are some of the important criteria for diagnosis of brain death.

28 Higher Functions of the Cerebral Cortex

Functions of somatic sensory area and motor area of cerebral cortex have already been discussed. Functions of visual and auditory cortex are discussed elsewhere. "Higher functions" of the cerebral cortex include:

(i) Speech
(ii) Learning and memory;
(iii) Intellectual functions such as insight, imagination; and other functions of mind.

ASSOCIATION AREAS

Human brain is characterized by huge size of the parts of cerebral cortex known as the association areas. Association areas comprise 85% of the human brain as compared to 20% of the canine brain. Most of higher functions of the brain are related to the large parts of cerebral cortex known as the association areas. Various association areas of the brain are shown in Fig. 28.1.

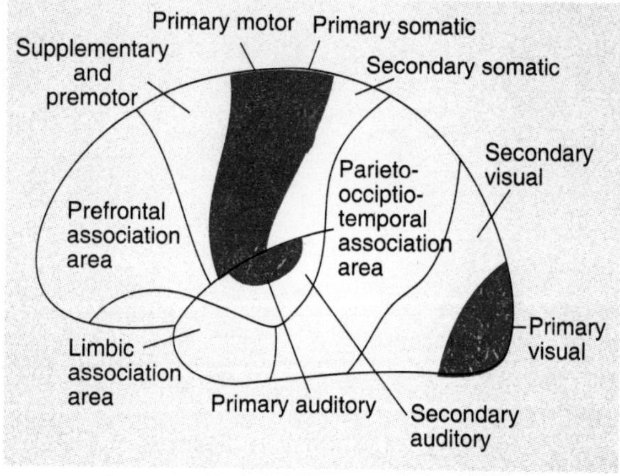

Fig. 28.1: Association areas of the brain.

The primary sensory areas directly receive somatic, auditory, visual, olfactory and gustatory sensations from the peripheral receptors. Sensory stimuli are further processed in association areas that relate to one or more sensations. The sensory association areas provide meaning of the sensation perceived. If one holds an object in one's hand, the sensation of touch would be perceived in the hand area of the somatosensory cortex (Brodmann's areas 3, 1, 2). However, the nature of the object would be interpreted by the somatosensory association area (Brodmann's area 5) from the shape, size and texture, etc. of the object. If one looks at a book, the black or coloured objects against white background shall be perceived by the primary visual cortex (Brodmann's area 17 and 18). Only in the visual association area (Brodmann's area 19), the objects would be identified as various words or pictures, etc. Similarly, the auditory association area (Brodmann's area 42) interprets the meaning of sounds heard.

The premotor and supplementary areas of the motor cortex serve as motor association areas. The functions of the largest association area of the brain, i.e. prefrontal cortex are most complex.

INTELLECTUAL FUNCTIONS

The portion of frontal lobes in front of the motor cortex is known as the **prefrontal area**. This area, like other association areas, is developed better in man than in any other species. However, the function of such a large mass of grey matter seems to be most complex of all the association areas. The highest functions of the human brain such as intellect, imagination, insight, creativity, are believed to be located in the prefrontal area.

Prefrontal lobotomy has been performed in patients with tumours of this region. The consequent *deficits* observed in such subjects gives some indication of the function of the prefrontal area:

(i) Such patients show a difficulty in remembering the temporal sequence of events, i.e. he cannot remember how long ago he saw an event or a picture card.

(ii) The subject is easily distracted in the sequence of thoughts. Hence, any activity involving a number of steps in sequence cannot be performed properly.

(iii) The patient has great difficulty in abstract thinking, e.g. planning for future or considering the consequences of a particular motor activity beforehand.

(iv) The patient may not act within the norms of social or moral behaviour. Months after prefrontal leucotomy, one officer was found peeing into the waste paper basket of his office.

(v) The patient shows total loss of ambition.

LANGUAGE AND SPEECH

Speech is defined as an ability to understand or express oneself by spoken or written words. Visual association area, auditory association area, Wernicke's area and Broca's area of the brain are concerned with the reception, formulation and expression components of speech.

Wernicke's Area The posterior end of the superior temporal gyrus in the *left hemisphere* is called the Wernicke's area. It is the site of integration of secondary somatic, auditory and visual areas and thus acts as the tertiary association area. In response to the words heard or read and interpreted by the secondary auditory or visual sensory areas, the Wernicke's area formulates ideas for the expressive part of the speech and sends signals to the Broca's area via arcuate fasciculus (Fig. 28.2).

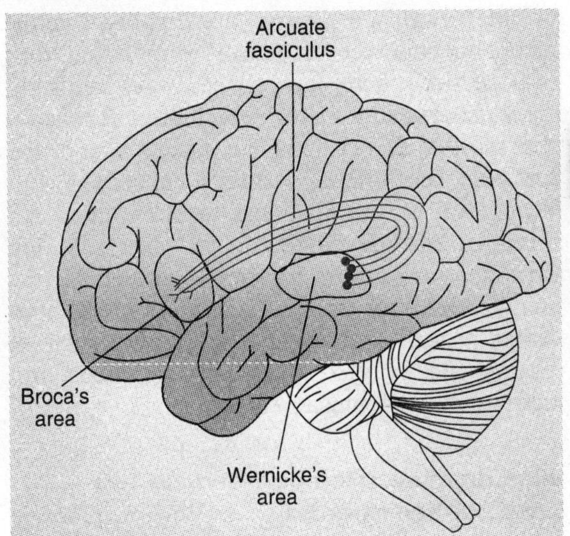

Fig. 28.2: Connection between Wernicke's area and Broca's area.

Broca's Area (area 44) of the *left hemisphere* constitutes the centre for motor part of speech. It is connected to the ipsilateral Wernicke's area. The Broca's area is concerned with the function of spoken speech. The centre for written speech seems to be located close to the Broca's area, and together the two areas constitute the motor speech areas. Motor speech areas project to the primary motor cortex concerned with the control of larynx, lips and tongue for spoken speech and fingers for written speech. Lesions of the Broca's area produce an inability to express oneself by spoken speech (motor aphasia).

Cerebral Dominance for Language

In the human cerebral cortex, the functions concerned with language are predominantly controlled by one of the hemispheres. In a great majority of the individuals, the association areas concerned with the function of speech are located in the left hemisphere, and hence it is often called the "dominant hemisphere". The motor area concerned with the hand movements is closely associated with the centre for speech. That explains the right-handedness in over 90% of the individuals. Among left-handers, only 15% have right-sided cerebral dominance. In 70% of left-handers, left hemisphere is the "dominant" hemisphere.

The Wernicke's area of the dominant hemisphere not only receives sensory stimulation from both the hemispheres through the corpus callosum, it also controls the motor speech area. It may be stressed that although the Wernicke's area of the dominant hemisphere is chiefly concerned with the control of the language function, it is not absent or underdeveloped on the other side. On the non-dominant side, it serves equally important functions of understanding and interpreting non-verbal, visual or auditory experiences such as recognition of visual patterns or faces and interpretation of music, etc.

Intercommunication between the Two Cerebral Hemispheres

Most of the cortical areas of the two cerebral hemispheres are connected to each other by fibres passing through the corpus callosum. In addition, the anterior commissure contains fibres which connect the anterior portions of the two temporal lobes, especially the amygdala. By these connections, information stored in one hemisphere in made available to the other hemisphere.

In some patients of epilepsy, the corpus callosum and the anterior commissure have been sectioned to prevent the spread of epileptic activity from one side of the brain to the other. Such *"split brain" procedures* have shown that each hemisphere has a specific role to play.

The "higher functions" of each cerebral hemisphere are summarized in Table 28.1.

Table 28.1: "Higher functions" of each cerebral hemisphere in a right-handed individual

Left brain	*Right brain*
(i) Right hand control	(i) Left hand control
(ii) Spoken language	(ii) Music awareness
(iii) Written language	(iii) Three-dimensional awareness
(iv) Mathematical skills	(iv) Art awareness
(v) Scientific skills	(v) Insight
(vi) Reasoning	(vi) Imagination

The two-halves of the brain have independent capabilities for consciousness, memory storage and control of motor activities. The corpus callosum is required for the coordination of activities of the two cerebral hemispheres. Similarly, the anterior commissure helps to unify the emotional responses of the two-halves of the brain. In other words, left brain is not really dominant over the right brain. Some specialized higher functions are allotted to each half of the brain and the two-halves have very intimate intercommunication and coordination. Therefore, the terms "dominant" and "non-dominant" have been replaced by categorical and representational hemispheres, respectively.

Speech Defects

Speech defects may be classified into two main categories.

Dysarthria

This term is used to describe a defect in the *articulation (slurring of speech)* which is due *to paresis, or incoordination of the muscles* involved in the production of speech. Dysarthria may be due to lesions of pyramidal tract, cranial nerves, cerebellum or basal ganglia. The comprehension of spoken or written speech is not affected.

Aphasia

This term is used to describe the inability to understand written or spoken speech or express oneself in speech or in writing, in the absence of mental confusion or motor deficit. As discussed earlier, the aphasias are produced by lesions of association areas of cerebral cortex. Word blindness (dyslexia) is produced by a lesion of the secondary visual area (visual association area). Word deafness is produced by a lesion of the secondary auditory area (auditory association area). Motor aphasia, i.e. inability to express oneself in speech or writing is produced by a lesion of area 44 (Broca's area). A lesion of the Wernicke's area of the dominant hemisphere produces *global aphasia* consisting of sensory as well as motor aphasia.

Some workers classify aphasias into fluent and non-fluent types. Lesions of Broca's area produce *non-fluent aphasia*. In this case, the comprehension of written or spoken speech is normal but the person cannot speak. He can utter only a few words with great difficulty. In *fluent type of aphasia*, comprehension of spoken or written speech is disturbed but the motor speech is intact. The patient talks very fluently (or rather excessively) but the speech only sounds normal; it does not make much sense. The patient cannot respond to even simple spoken or written commands.

Aphasias are mostly produced by thrombosis or embolism of a blood vessel in the left cerebral hemisphere. Aphasias are commonly associated with right sided motor and sensory deficit but may occur independently, if the lesion is restricted to cortical association areas.

LEARNING AND MEMORY

Learning and memory are closely related. Learning is defined as the ability to alter behaviour on the basis of past experiences. Memory is the ability to recall the past experiences at conscious or unconscious levels. In the present state of knowledge, it is difficult to fully explain the mechanisms of learning and memory. Certain physiological and psychological experiments form the basis of the following outline of the subject.

Learning (Reflexive Memory)

When a stimulus is repeated many a time, it may produce either habituation or sensitization. When applied for the first time, a stimulus produces a given response. If the stimulus is repeated, the response becomes weaker and weaker and may eventually disappear. This phenomenon, called *habituation,* occurs in neutral types of stimuli. However, if the stimuli are distinctly pleasant or unpleasant, they lead to *sensitization*, i.e. the response increases with repetition of the stimuli. Habituation and sensitization have been called *non-associative types of learning*.

Associative type of learning (also called *conditioned reflexes)* is exemplified by the Pavlov's famous experiment. In this experiment, the ringing of a bell is associated with the presentation of food to the animal. The salivation is produced due to the effect of an unconditioned stimulus (US), i.e. food, on the salivary glands by an innate reflex action. However, if the ringing of the bell is repeatedly associated with the presentation of the food, the ringing of the bell alone (conditioned stimulus, CS) produces salivation. This is called a conditioned reflex. In the animal's brain, the food and the sound of the bell have become associated. A conditioned reflex needs to be reinforced frequently otherwise it dies out. If CS is given repeatedly without US, the conditioned reflex disappears.

Non-associative and associative types of learning as well as learned skills and habits are some times grouped under the heading of *reflexive memory*.

This type of memory is involved in learning to drive a bicycle or a car. Conscious recall is not involved in this process. Encoding of learning (reflexive memory) is believed to occur in the *basal ganglia* and/or the *cerebellum.*

Declarative Memory

Declarative memory involves conscious recall of facts or events that occurred earlier. "I met this man five year ago" or "I met with an accident last year", are declarative types of memory. By repetition, a declarative memory may be converted into reflexive memory, e.g. arithmetical tables.

Memory of an event may last only for a few seconds while of another event may last for months or even years. Declarative memory may be classified into: (1) *Primary or recent memory*, and

(2) *Secondary or long-term memory.* Every moment of our wakeful life, we are exposed to different sensory experiences, but only a few may be recalled after a few minutes (primary memory) or after few days (secondary memory). Events stored in the secondary memory may be recalled even after many years. When we look for a telephone number in the directory, close the directory and dial the number, we are using the primary memory. When we recall an old telephone number, we are using the secondary memory.

Physiological Basis of Memory

1. Primary Memory Primary memory may be due to the entrance of a sensory signal into *reverberating circuits in the sensory cortex*, or between the sensory cortex and the thalamus. Unless the stimulation is strong enough, the reverberating signals are wiped out by newer signals.

28

2. Secondary Memory Secondary memory seems to result from an almost permanent anatomical or biochemical change in the cerebral synapses. Prolonged and intense sensory stimulation has been shown to produce excessive thickening of the concerned primary sensory cortex. Under electron microscope, anatomical changes in the presynaptic terminals have also been observed. Nowadays, *synaptic plasticity* is given fundamental importance in the process of memory storage.

A brain concussion or application of electroconvulsive therapy (ECT) commonly produce retrograde amnesia (i.e. loss of memory of the events immediately prior to the concussion or ECT), without affecting the remote memory. From these observations, it has been concluded that there is a period of encoding or consolidation of memory trace. Any severe cerebral disturbance may erase the trace at this stage. Later on, a more permanent structural change in the brain produces "permanent" memory. Consolidation of memory trace seems to be helped by certain drugs like caffeine, nicotine and amphetamine.

The hippocampus seems to be an important site for the *encoding process involved in consolidation of short-term memory*. Patients with bilateral lesions of hippocampus are unable to establish new long-term memories. Long-term memories are *stored* in various parts of the *neocortex*.

In old age, progressive loss of memory is a normal phenomenon. In certain individuals, the loss of memory starts even at the age of 40–50 years. This serious disorder, called *Alzheimer's disease*, is due to progressive loss of cholinergic neurons in the cerebral cortex and hippocampus.

Synaptic Plasticity

This term is used to describe short- and long-term changes in synaptic function as a result of experience. As a result of afferent stimulation, the synaptic conduction is may be amplified of attenuated. Synaptic plasticity forms the basis of learning and memory. Synaptic plasticity can be exhibited by one of the following phenomena.

Post-tetanic Potentiation

A brief tetanising train of stimuli in a presynaptic neuron results in enhanced postsynaptic potential. The enhancement lasts up to 60 seconds. The tetanising rate of stimuli are believed to cause so much Ca^{++} to accumulate in the presynaptic neuron terminals that their level cannot be lowered to normal by intracellular calcium binding mechanism up to 60 seconds. Increased Ca^{++} concentration in the presynaptic neuron terminals enhances amount of the neurotransmitter released leading to enhanced postsynaptic potential.

Habituation

When a stimulus is benign (neutral, not harmful) and repeated over and over again, the response to the stimulus gradually dies out. On shifting to a house near a railway track, one would be awakened from sleep every time a train passes by. After a few nights, however, one becomes habituated to the noise of the trains, and sleeps soundly despite the noise created by the trains passing by.

Long-term Potentiation (LTP)

It was initially discovered in the hippocampus, but has subsequently been demonstrated in many regions of the cortex. It is defined as a long-lasting increase in synaptic efficacy which follows high-frequency stimulation of afferent fibers. LTP is presumed to have a role in the establishment of long-term memories. In contrast to post-tetanic potentiation which enhances the capabilities of the presynaptic neuron, LTP improves the *postsynaptic cell's sensitivity* to neurotransmitter mainly by *increasing the activity of existing receptors and by increasing the number of receptors on the postsynaptic cell surface.* Moreover, the effect of LTP lasts several months and depends on the synthesis of new proteins.

CHAPTER 29

The Limbic System and the Hypothalamus

LIMBIC SYSTEM

The limbic system is concerned with neural control of emotions and instinctual behaviour. Instinctual behaviour may be defined as actions performed by an animal or man due to an inner urge, and not based on training or learning. Sexual behaviour, protection of young one by the mother, or looking for food when hungry occur in all animals without any training. Migration of certain birds over long distances is also an example of instinctual behaviour. Instinctual behaviour does occur in man, but unlike animals, it is controlled by the neocortex to a large extent.

Emotions have both mental and physical components. For example, when a loud noise is heard it results in awareness of a sensation "I hear a loud noise; is it a bomb blast?" This is called *cognition*. As a result, the person feels frightened. The feeling is called an *affect*. Next, it results in *conation* or an urge to take action. Finally, there is a *physical change*, like running away from the site of noise. Somatic and autonomic changes occur at this stage.

FUNCTIONAL ANATOMY OF LIMBIC SYSTEM

The limbic system consists of a rim of cortical tissue around the corpus callosum, called the cingulate gyrus and the associated structures like amygdala, hippocampus, septal nuclei and mammillary bodies (Fig. 29.1). Phylogenetically, limbic system is an older part of cerebral cortex (allocortex) showing primitive histological pattern.

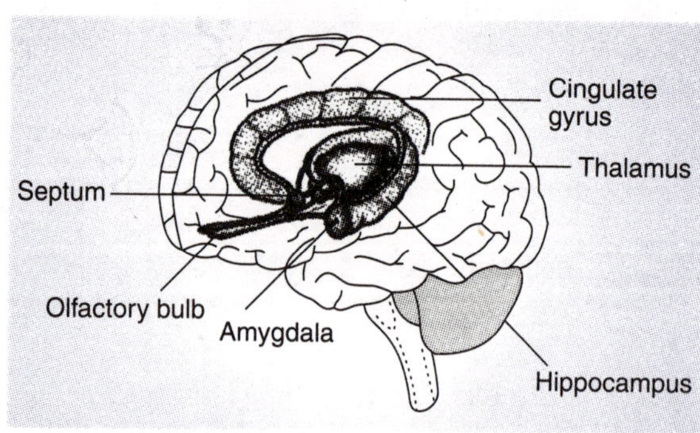

Fig. 29.1: The limbic system.

Connections

Various nuclei of the limbic system are interconnected as follows:

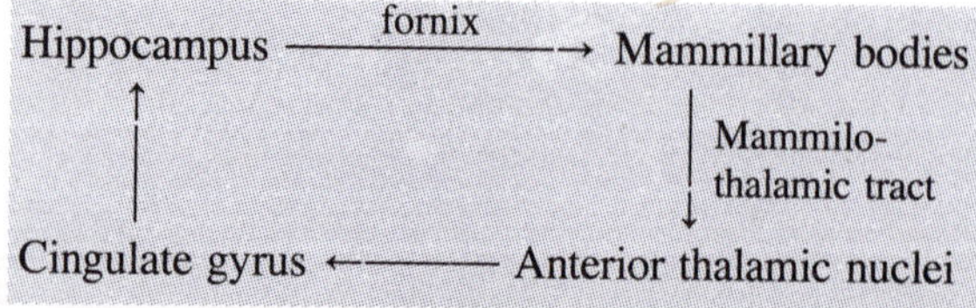

These interconnections constitute a closed circuit known as *Papez circuit*.

Efferent Projection of limbic system is given in Flowchart 29.1.

Flowchart 29.1: Efferent projection of limbic system.

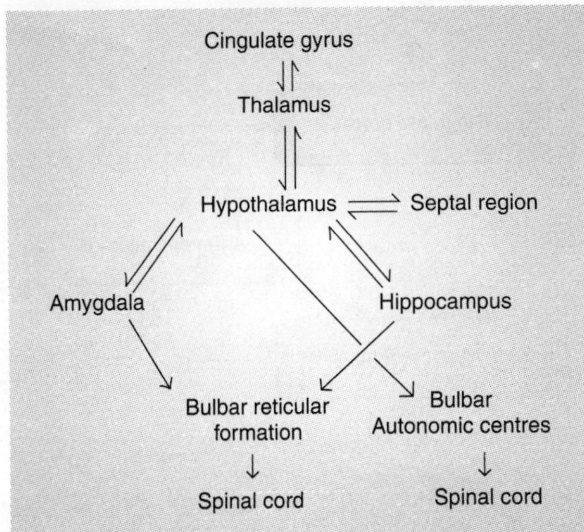

There are two characteristic features of the connections of the limbic system:

(a) There is very little connection with the neocortex. That is why; emotional and instinctual behaviour is not under voluntary control, especially in lower animals.
(b) The anatomic closed circuit (Papez circuit) of the limbic system tends to produce prolonged effect, long after the end of sensory experience (Fig. 29.2).

FUNCTIONS OF LIMBIC SYSTEM

Most of the functions of limbic system are intimately related to the functions of hypothalamus.

Autonomic Responses and Feeding Behaviour

Stimulation of many parts of limbic system produces autonomic responses such as changes in blood pressure and respiration. Such changes are also observed during emotional states.

Stimulation of *amygdala* produces movement of chewing and licking, whereas lesions of amygdala produce moderate hyperphagia (overeating). There may be indiscriminate ingestion of edible or even non-edible materials.

Sexual Behaviour

In adults, sexual interest in the members of opposite sex is as basic an instinctual behaviour as food intake. While the latter is essential for survival, the former is essential for procreation. The final act of copulation is controlled by a series of reflexes integrated in the spinal cord and lower brainstem centres. However, basic urge for sexual activity depends upon certain areas of limbic system and hypothalamus, which in turn, are influenced by gonadal hormones as well as cerebral cortex. The basic responses are innate and therefore present in all the mammals. Successful mating occurs in all adult animals without any previous experience. In humans, the sexual function has been extensively encephalized and hence it is influenced by social and psychic factors to a large extent.

29

Males

Neural Control Stimulation of certain parts of *amygdala* in male animals produces penile erection, copulatory movements of the body and ejaculation. Removal of neocortex, particularly in the frontal region produces inhibition of sexual behaviour. On the other hand, bilateral limbic lesions localized to *piriform cortex* overlying amygdala produce marked intensification of sexual activity. In human males also, such bilateral lesions produce marked hypersexuality (Kluver-Bucy syndrome). The hypothalamus is also involved in the control of sexual activity. In the male rats, anterior hypothalamic lesions abolish sexual interest.

Role of Hormones Gonadal hormones are equally important for the sexual behaviour. In human male, the sexual drive can be correlated with the plasma *testosterone* levels. In adult animals and humans, castration completely abolishes sexual drive, which can be restored by injections of testosterone. Surprisingly, administration of large doses of oestrogens in the

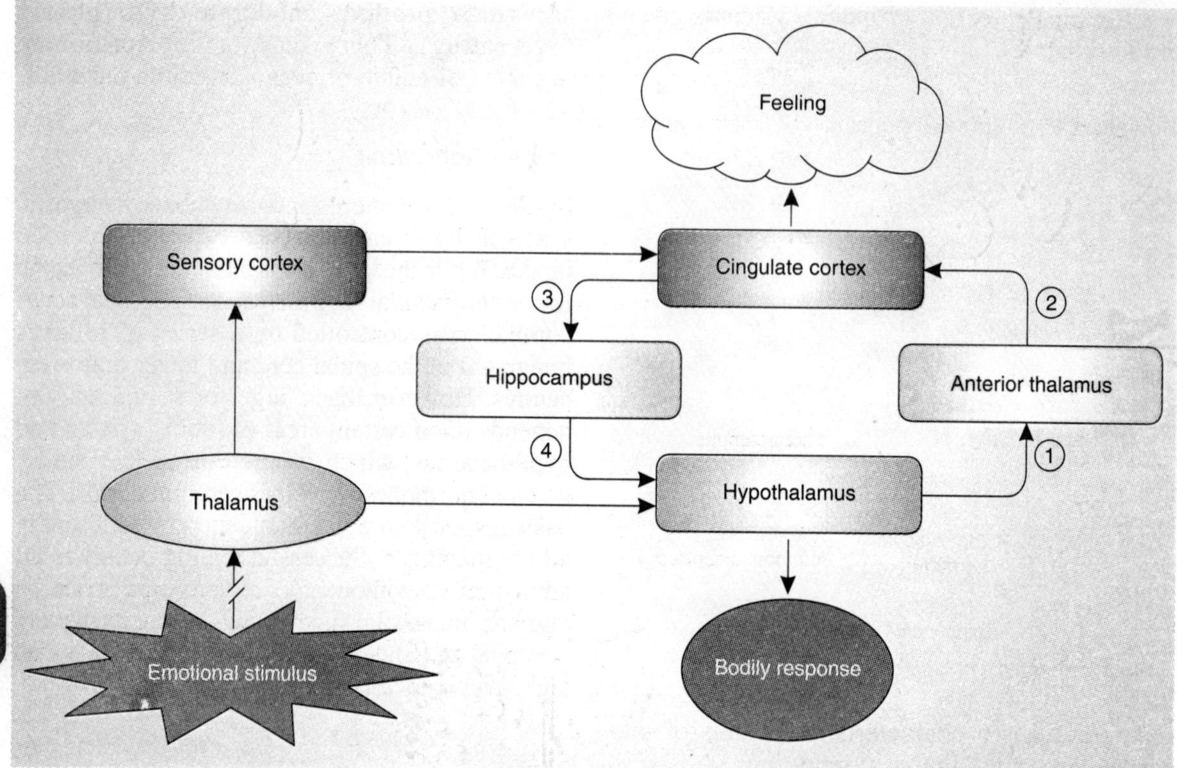

Fig. 29.2: Consequences of entry of an emotional stimulus in the Papez circuit (1–4).

treatment of carcinoma prostate also increases the libido.

Females

Neural Control In male mammals, the sexual interest is continuous process. In female mammals, however, the sexual interest is cyclic in nature. Most of the time, female animal avoids the male and repulses his sexual advances. Periodically, however, there is a change in her behaviour. The female seeks out the male (enticement reaction) and attempts to mate. This short period of sexual interest in the female animals is called *heat* or *oestrus behaviour*. In female animals, removal of neocortex and limbic cortex abolishes the enticement reaction during oestrus without affecting other aspects of "heat". Stimulation of certain areas of amygdala produces ovulation and uterine activity. However, amygdaloidal or periamygdaloidal lesions do not produce hypersexuality in the females. The anterior hypothalamus is involved in the control of sexual activity in females also. Anterior hypothalamic lesions abolish oestrus behaviour.

Role of Hormones In animals, the time of oestrus can be correlated with an increase in plasma oestrogen levels. Implantation of minute amounts of oestrogen in the anterior hypothalamus produces "heat" in ovariectomized rats. Implantation in other parts of the brain is ineffective Thus, like males, anterior hypothalamus regulates sexual behaviour but only when under the influence of gonadal hormones. In human female, sexual activity persists throughout the ovarian (menstrual) cycle, but some studies have shown increased sexual interest at the time of ovulation.

Pheromones These are chemicals substances produced by an animal which act at a distance, through the olfactory mucosa, to produce behavioural or other physiological changes in another animal of the same species.

Pheromones mostly act as sex attractants. In monkeys, sexual drive is greater in the male when exposed to a female at the time of ovulation than when exposed to a female at other times of ovarian cycle. It seems, certain fatty acids present in the vaginal secretions of the monkey send olfactory signals to the male. These fatty acids are present in the human vaginal secretions at about the midcycle. However, the role of pheromones in human sexuality is uncertain. According to the latest reviews on the subject, no pheromonal substance has ever been demonstrated to directly influence *human* behaviour.

Maternal Behaviour

Maternal behaviour is basically concerned with the nursing (breastfeeding) and protection of the offspring by the mother. In the rat, it is manifested by nest building, suckling and licking the pups and retrieving the pups when separated. In animals, maternal behaviour begins just before parturition and continues till the end of lactation. Maternal behaviour is primarily neurogenic, i.e. it depends on olfactory, auditory, visual and thermotactile stimuli arising from the young ones. In the rat, lesions of the cingulate gyrus and retrosplenial portion of the limbic cortex depress maternal behaviour. *Prolactin* and *oxytocin* seem to facilitate maternal behaviour, although these hormones are not absolutely essential for its manifestation.

Fear, Rage and Placidity

Fear and rage are the emotions provoked by exposure to hostile environment. When an animal is threatened, the emotion of *fear* is shown by sweating, pupillary dilatation, cowering and turning the head from side to side or it may produce *rage* or fighting reaction as shown by growling, piloerection, pupillary dilatation, biting and clawing.

Fear reaction can be produced by stimulation of *amygdala* in conscious animals. *Rage* response can be produced by stimulation of *lateral hypothalamus*, or some parts of *amygdala*. Bilateral destruction of amygdaloidal nuclei produces a state of abnormal *placidity*, i.e. the animal remains calm in spite of grave provocation.

Punishment and Reward

By stereotaxic techniques, electrodes can be implanted in specific parts of the brain of an animal, and connected to an electrical system and a pedal (or bar) in the cage. When the animal presses the bar, an electrical stimulus is delivered to the implanted electrodes. If the electrodes are implanted in the *medial forebrain bundle* or in the *lateral* or *ventromedial nuclei* of the hypothalamus, the animal presses the bar again and again. The frequency of bar pressing may be as high as 10,000 times per hour. The animal prefers to keep on pressing the bar rather than eat or drink. What the animal feels cannot be known, but obviously, it must be a very pleasant experience.

Stimulation of some other parts of the brain, especially *lateral portion of posterior hypothalamus,* and *dorsal regions of the mid-brain* produce signs of fear in the animal. After pressing the bar a few times, the animal does not go near it.

The parts of the brain where stimulation produces repeated bar pressing have been called the *reward* (or *pleasure*) *centres*. Those areas, stimulation of which discourages bar pressing are called the *punishment centres*. These experiments have been repeated in some human subjects. According to them, stimulation of the reward centres produces a sensation of pleasure or relief of tension. They also liked to press the bar again and again. Stimulation of punishment centres was reported to produce fear or terror.

Reward and punishment are two most important factors controlling our behaviour. We are motivated to repeat an activity which gives a feeling of pleasure, and avoid the one giving a feeling of punishment.

Memory

Hippocampus has an important role in consolidation of recent memory.

HYPOTHALAMUS

The hypothalamus is a small bilateral structure forming the antero-inferior wall and the floor of the third ventricle of the brain. It extends forwards from the mesencephalic tegmentum to the preoptic area, and is separated from the thalamus by the hypothalamic sulcus. It is an integrative centre for regulation of cardiovascular system, body temperature, food and water intake, endocrine secretion, etc. Usually, bilateral hypothalamic lesions are required to produce complete disruption of any of these functions. Anatomical studies show a large number of well-defined masses of grey matter (nuclei) in the hypothalamus. However, specific physiological role can be assigned to only a few of these nuclei, and mostly the centres for various integrative functions are described as present in anterior, medial, lateral or posterior hypothalamic areas. The anatomical nuclei located in each of these areas are given in Fig. 29.3.

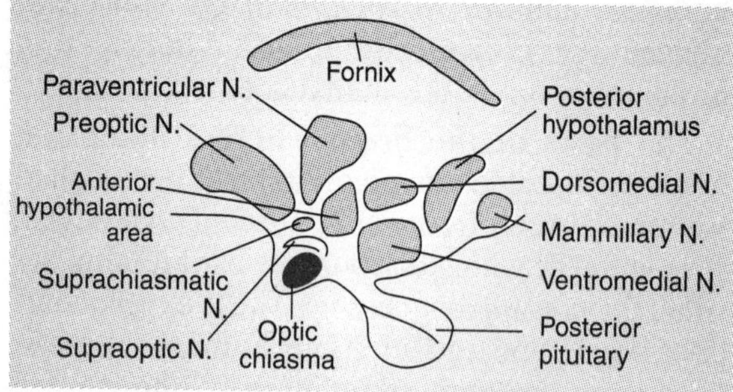

Fig. 29.3: Nuclei of the hypothalamus.

1. Anterior hypothalamus

- Preoptic nucleus
- Supraoptic nucleus
- Paraventricular nucleus
- Suprachiasmatic nucleus
- Anteriorhypothalamic nucleus

2. Medial hypothalamus

- Suprachiasmatic nucleus
- Dorsomedial nucleus
- Ventromedial nucleus
- Arcuate nuclei

3. Lateral hypothalamus

- Lateral hypothalamus nuclei

4. Posterior hypothalamus

- Posterior hypothalamic area
- Mammillary nuclei (medial, lateral, pre- and supra-mammillary nuclei).

Afferent Connections

1. Limbic System From different parts of limbic system, afferents reach the hypothalamus through the medial-forebrain bundle, stria terminalis and fornix and corticohypothalamic tract.

2. Midbrain Tegmentum From the midbrain tegmentum, large number of catecholamine- and serotonin-secreting fibres project to the mammillary nuclei. It is through this indirect route that the ascending sensory pathways project on the hypothalamus.

3. Neocortex There is a minor neocortical projection of the hypothalamus, indirectly through the limbic system.

Efferent Connections

1. Limbic System Via stria terminalis and medial forebrain bundle.

2. Thalamus Via mammillothalamic tract.

3. Tegmental Reticular Formation Descending fibres mostly from the lateral hypothalamic area project on the reticular formation of the tegmentum, and thereby to the motor nuclei of the brainstem and spinal cord. Through this route, the hypothalamus also influences the autonomic nervous system.

4. Posterior Pituitary Gland Via hypothalamic hypophysial tract.

FUNCTIONS OF HYPOTHALAMUS

Regulation of Posterior Pituitary Function

The hypothalamic-hypophysial tract originates from the cell bodies of supraoptic and paraventricular nuclei. Extending through the pituitary stalk, it ends in the posterior pituitary gland. The neurosecretory material synthesized by the neurons of hypothalamic hypophysial tract accumulates in the axon terminals in the posterior pituitary. An increase in the plasma osmolality or a decrease in blood volume increases the discharge rate of neurons in the supraoptic nuclei resulting in the release of antidiuretic hormone (ADH) from the posterior pituitary.

Afferents from the nipple of the breast, stimulated by suckling by the baby, increase the discharge rate of neurons in the paraventricular nuclei leading to release of oxytocin from the posterior pituitary.

Regulation of Anterior Pituitary Function

Unlike posterior pituitary, there is no neuronal link between the hypothalamus and the anterior pituitary gland. Even then, the hypothalamus exerts a strong control over the secretory function of the anterior pituitary. The hypothalamic hypophysial portal vessels provide a vascular link between the two structures. The various neurons of the hypothalamus synthesize certain releasing or release-inhibiting hormones which enter the hypothalamic hypophysial portal vessels in the median eminence. These hormones are carried by the portal vessels to the anterior pituitary where they regulate the secretion of anterior pituitary hormones.

The neural control of anterior pituitary function provides a mechanism for adjusting the hormone secretion in response to the changes in the internal or external environment.

Reproduction

Proper reproductive function depends on both the *gametogenesis*, as well as, the *sexual behaviour*. The secretion of gonadotropin releasing hormone (GnRH) by the hypothalamus causes the release of gonadotropins from the anterior pituitary which regulate the gonadal function.

The sexual behaviour consists of the basic urge to copulate which is accompanied by various physiological and psychological changes. In ovarectomized rats, oestrus behaviour can be induced by implantation of minute amounts of oestrogen in the anterior hypothalamus but not elsewhere. Discrete lesion of this area abolishes sexual behaviour in female, as well as, male rats without affecting the gonadal function.

The male sexual behaviour also depends upon the action of testosterone on the anterior hypothalamus.

Control of Food Intake (Control of Body Weight)

The term *hunger* means a craving for food. Hunger is often associated with a tight or gnawing feeling in the stomach called *hunger contractions*. However, a person feels hungry even after total gastrectomy. Therefore, hunger contractions are not the main cause for the craving for food. *Satiety* is the opposite of hunger. It is a feeling of fulfillment after food intake.

Bilateral lesions of *lateral hypothalamus* (in animals) cause severe decrease in the food intake leading to loss of body weight or even death. On the other hand, animals with bilateral lesions localized *to ventromedial nucleus (VMN)* of the hypothalamus develop hyperphagia (excessive food intake) leading to gross obesity. Based on these observations, the lateral hypothalamus and the VMN have been called the *feeding centre* and the *satiety centre*, respectively. It is believed that the feeding centre is continuously active but its activity is periodically inhibited by the satiety centre activated by the food intake.

Glucostatic Hypothesis

It seems that the VMN acts as a satiety centre by monitoring the blood glucose level. These cells act as glucostats. Their activity is decreased by low blood glucose level, thus allowing the activity of the feeding centre producing hunger, which promotes food intake. The consequent rise in blood glucose level causes increased activity of the satiety centre leading to inhibition of the feeding centre. Even though the brain tissue is not insulin sensitive, it has been shown that glucose transport in the cells of VMN is insulin-dependent. That also explains the increased appetite in patients of diabetes mellitus, in spite of hyperglycaemia.

The mechanism of hunger and satiety given above is rather oversimplification. After lesions of VMN, the animal overeats for a few weeks and becomes over-weight. Then, the amount of food intake levels off to maintain the new higher weight. Therefore, it has been proposed that the hypothalamus acts as a centre for the regulation of body weight.

Lipostatic Hypothesis

In contrast to glucostatic hypothesis mentioned above, some research workers have proposed lipostatic hypothesis for the control of food intake.

29

According to this hypothesis, adipose tissue produces a humoral substance in proportion to the amount of fat stores. The humoral substance acts on the hypothalamus to decrease the food intake and increase energy output. The chemical substance, named **leptin**, is a circulating protein with 167 amino acids. Plasma leptin levels are higher in obese than normal individuals. Many cases of obesity seem to be due to a genetic defect leading to deficiency of receptors for leptin in the hypothalamus.

Role of GIT in Hunger and Satiety

The possible contribution of the stomach in the craving for food (hunger) has been mentioned above. Recent researches have revealed a direct role of stomach in the regulation of food intake and body weight.

Ghrelin It is a polypeptide with 28 amino acids. This hormone is secreted by the epithelial cells of the fundus of the stomach. Injection of this polypeptide in humans produces intense hunger. Plasma ghrelin levels are low in the postprandial period, but gradually increase in between the meals. Grehlin is, nowadays, considered one of the important mediators of hunger and regulation of body weight.

Even satiety cannot be entirely explained by increase in blood sugar level alone. Presence of food in the GIT may also contribute to the feeling of satiety, inhibiting further food intake. Gastrointestinal hormones like CCK, glucagon and somatostatin have been shown to decrease the appetite.

Regulation of Thirst

The hypothalamus contains a "drinking centre" or a centre for the regulation of thirst. It is believed to be situated in a small area slightly anterior to the supraoptic nucleus (Fig. 29.3). Discrete lesions of the drinking centre abolish fluid intake and the animal dies of dehydration. Electrical stimulation of this area in conscious animals (through chronically implanted electrodes), causes the animal to drink water as long as the stimulation continues. Injection of minute amount of NaCl in this area also induces the animal to drink large amount of water. These experiments suggest that the drinking centre monitors plasma osmolality (cf. the osmoreceptors also regulate the secretion of ADH from the posterior pituitary gland).

A decrease in volume of ECF also induces thirst by a separate mechanism. After haemorrhage, the patient feels extreme thirst even though plasma osmolality is normal. It is believed that angiotensin-II produced by hypovolemia (renin-angiotensin mechanism) acts on a separate region of the hypothalamus, known as subfornical organ, and induces drinking behaviour (Fig. 29.4).

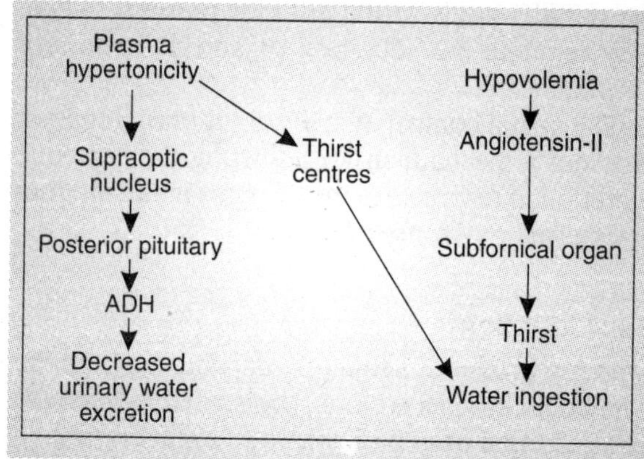

Fig. 29.4: Regulation of water balance.

A thirsty man or animal stops drinking water after an "appropriate amount" of water has been ingested, i.e. the drinking of water stops when it is still in the stomach and plasma still hypertonic. Distension of the stomach by a balloon can also relieve thirst transiently. Dryness of the pharyngeal mucosa, e.g. after injection of atropine sulphate, also induces thirst. These observations suggest that, although the basic craving for water is regulated by the *hypothalamus*, the *stomach* and *pharynx* may also help to regulate the amount of water intake, at least on short-term basis.

Role in Emotions and Instinctual Behaviour

The hypothalamus lies in the efferent pathway of the limbic system, with which it is intimately connected. Hypothalamus seems to be important for the expression of rage. It also contains reward and punishment centres.

Regulation of Body Temperature

The hypothalamus acts as a centre for integration of autonomic, somatic and behavioural mechanisms in the regulation of body temperature. In response to the stimulation of cold receptors, in the skin or elsewhere in the body, the posterior hypothalamus produces cutaneous vasoconstriction, piloerection and abolition of sweating (autonomic effects), shivering (somatic effect) and measures to get away from the cold environment, and wearing woolens (behavioural effects). In response to the stimulation of the warmth receptors in the skin or elsewhere, anterior hypothalamic activity results in cutaneous vasodilatation and sweating.

In experimental animals, lesions of anterior hypothalamus abolish the physiological responses to heat exposure. Electrical stimulation or local warming of this area produces cutaneous vasodilatation, sweating and panting. On the other hand, electrical stimulation of posterior hypothalamus results in cutaneous vasoconstriction and shivering.

A lesion of the posterior hypothalamus abolishes not only body responses to cold but to heat as well, because this area is a final integration centre for all thermoregulatory signals. Final efferent signals for heat production or heat loss emerge from the posterior hypothalamus.

The details of body temperature regulation are discussed in a separate section of this chapter.

Relation to Sympathetic Function

Stimulation of the various regions of the hypothalamus, specially the lateral hypothalamus, produces, changes characteristic of sympathetic stimulation, e.g. increase in heart rate and blood pressure, cutaneous vasoconstriction, piloerection, pupillary dilatation, etc. The hypothalamus seems to be involved in mediating sympathetic responses as components of emotional exteriorization.

Circadian Rhythms

Nervous tissue in general and the hypothalamus in particular is concerned with initiation of appropriate physiological and behavioural responses to minimize or eliminate tissue deficits. Homeostatic regulation is often anticipatory in nature, i.e. regulatory mechanisms are turned on or off before any tissue deficit actually occurs. The rhythmic variations in homeostatic regulatory mechanisms often show 24 hour cycles and hence called circadian (= around a day) rhythms. Many of the rhythms are coordinated with each other. *Suprachiasmatic nucleus* of the hypothalamus is believed to contain the *"biological clock"*, which regulates the circadian rhythms according to the light dark cycles.

Even when the external indicators of time (day-night or light-darkness) are absent, the body's internal clock maintains the rhythm. This may be proved by keeping rats in a permanently darkened laboratory for a few days. Normally, the rats show locomotor activity in the dark (at night) and inactivity in day time. These cycles of locomotor activity and inactivity continue even when the rats are in darkened laboratory with no exposure to sunlight. These cycles can be disrupted by bilateral lesions of suprachiasmatic nuclei. In man, there seem to be two independent oscillator controls. One oscillator regulates slow wave sleep, growth hormone secretion, skin temperature and urinary calcium excretion. The other oscillator controls REM sleep, ACTH and corticosteroid secretion, body core temperature and urinary potassium excretion.

The disturbance of circadian rhythms can occur during high speed jet travel. One may travel several thousand kilometers within a few hours. As a result, the traveler's external clock (day or night) does not coincide with the internal biological clock. That is, the body may be in rest (night) phase while it is day time in the country of destination. It results in irritability, mental depression or even physical illness. The symptoms subside in a few days. The condition is called *jet lag*.

The effects of stimulation and bilateral lesions of some of the hypothalamic areas are given in Table 29.1

REGULATION OF BODY TEMPERATURE

Heat is continuously produced in the body by metabolic processes. Under basal conditions, heat production is about 1 kcal/kg BW/hr or about 1700 kcal/day. Moderate physical activity increases the heat production to about 3000 kcal/day. Therefore, if there was no heat loss, the body temperature would increase by 1°C every hour under basal conditions and by 2°C/hr during moderate activity. Heat may also be gained from the environment by radiation, conduction and convection especially when the environmental temperature is greater than the body temperature. In spite of such a large amount of heat production, the body temperature remains relatively constant because of an efficient mechanism of heat loss. On exposure to extreme cold, heat conservation mechanisms come into action. In fact, even if the body is exposed for several hours to a temperature as low as 10°C or as high as 50°C, the body temperature does not change.

Like humans, other mammals and birds are able to maintain their body temperature within a normal narrow range in spite of wide variations in the environmental temperature. Such animals are called *homoeothermic* or *warm-blooded animals*. In contrast, reptiles, amphibians and fish are called *poikilothermic* or *cold-blooded animals*. Since they do not have an efficient body temperature regulating system, their body temperature fluctuates with the changes in the environmental temperature.

MECHANISMS OF HEAT GAIN

(a) Heat production by metabolic processes of the body. Large amount of heat is produced during muscular contraction (*exercise* or *shivering*).

(b) Heat gain from the environment by *radiation* and *conduction*, especially when the environmental temperature exceeds the body temperature.

Table 29.1: Effects of stimulation and lesion of hypothalamic areas/nuclei

Hypothalamic nuc./area	*Effect of stimulation*	*Effect of lesion*
Supraoptic N	Release of ADH	Diabetes insipidus
Paraventricular N	Relaese of oxytocin	
Preoptic N	Cutaneous vasodilatation, sweating, heat loss	Hyperthermia in hot environment
Suprachiasmatic N	—	Loss of circadian rhythms
Medial hypothalamic area	Secretion of hypophysiotropic homones	Various endocrine deficiencies
Ventromedial N	Cessation of eating, placidity	Voracious eating, obesity, aggressive behaviour
Lateral hypothalamic area	Voracious eating	Weight loss due to lack of food intake.
Posterior hypothalamic area	Cutaneous vasoconstriction, shivering, piloerection, heat production, rage.	Loss of thermoregulation (poikilothermia)
Area anterior to supraoptic N	Water drinking	Hypodipsia, dehydration

(c) *Brown fat metabolism*: In infants, brown fat, because of its very high metabolic rate, is an important source of heat production. It is located between and around the scapulae and neck, behind the sternum and around the kidneys.

MECHANISM OF HEAT LOSS

Heat is lost from the body by *radiation, conduction and evaporation*. When an individual is in cold environment, heat is lost from the body by conduction to objects in contact with him including air and by radiation to distant cold objects. Heat is also lost by evaporation of water from the skin (even in the absence of sweating) and mucous membrane of the respiratory tract. This *insensible loss of water* amounts to about 50 ml/hr in humans and occurs even in cold environment.

(i) The gradient between the temperature of the skin and the environmental temperature determines the cutaneous heat loss by conduction and radiation. The amount of blood flow to the skin determines the amount of heat reaching the surface from the deeper tissues. When the cutaneous blood vessels are dilated, warm blood fills the subcutaneous venous plexus, and the skin temperature approaches the deep tissue temperature. It promotes heat loss. When the cutaneous blood vessels are constricted, e.g. on exposure to cold, the skin temperature, especially of the hands and feet, becomes much lower than the deep tissue temperature (Fig. 29.5). Thus, heat loss is minimized by the decrease in the temperature gradient between the skin and the environment.

(ii) Piloerection Heat loss is further minimized by cold-induced contraction of piloerector muscles leading to erection of the hair. The layer of air entrapped between the hair acts as an insulator.

(iii) Fur/feathers In animals, fur and feathers serve this function more effectively. (Woolens offer better protection against cold than cotton clothes, because of larger amount of air entrapped in the former).

(iv) Subcutaneous layer of fat also acts as an insulator against heat loss. Women have a thicker layer of subcutaneous fat than men. That is partly the reason why, in winters, males are more heavily clothed than females, even though the former produce more heat, because of greater basal metabolic rate (BMR).

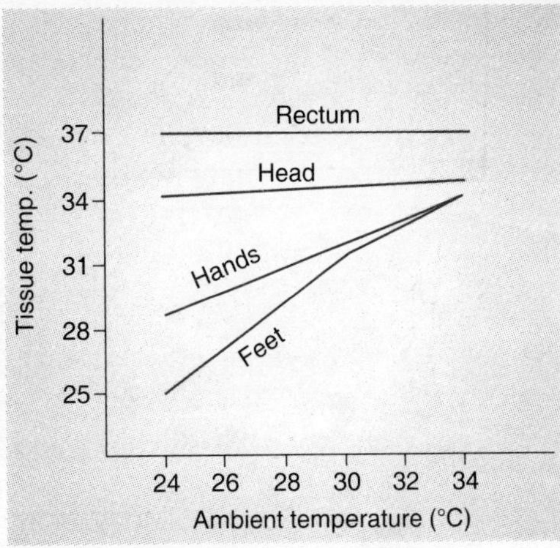

Fig. 29.5: Effect of exposure of a naked individual to low ambient temperature on different parts of the body.

(v) Sweating When the temperature of the environment is greater than that of the skin, the body gains heat from the surroundings, rather than losing it. Under these conditions, evaporation of sweat is the only means of heat loss from the body.

Sweat Glands

A sweat gland consists of a heavily coiled glandular portion lying deep in the dermis that secretes sweat and a duct that passes superficially to the surface of the skin. Sweat glands are of two types: (1) Eccrine, and (2) Apocrine. Most of the sweat glands are eccrine type.

1. Eccrine Sweat Glands These are distributed all over the skin. The coiled secretory portion has diameter of about 0.1 mm, and has a rich blood supply. The duct opens on the surface of the skin independent of hair follicles (Fig. 29.6). These glands have very important role in thermoregulation of the body. The eccrine sweat glands are innervated by cholinergic sympathetic postganglionic nerve terminals. The phenomenon of sweating described in detail below refers to secretory activity of the eccrine glands.

2. Apocrine Sweat Glands These glands are found in the skin of the axillary, pubic, circum-

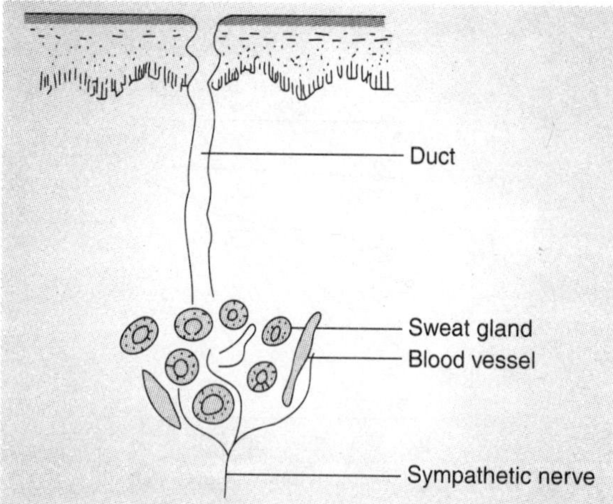

Fig. 29.6: Histological structure of a sweat gland.

areolar and circumanal areas. The coiled secretory portion has about 1 mm diameter. The duct opens into a hair follicle above the opening of the sebaceous gland. These glands do not become active until puberty and involute after menopause or in old age. The axillary apocrine glands produce a hypotonic viscid milky fluid with a pH of about 6, which is odourless when fresh. The characteristic axillary odour of human adult is said to due to bacterial decomposition of apocrine secretions. It is believed to have vestigial sexual attractant role. These glands do not have any thermoregulatory function.

Thermal Sweating

Rate of Sweating

The rate of sweating is practically zero in cold weather. In hot weather, the maximum rate of sweat production is about 0.7 L/hr but it may increase to 1.5 L/hr after acclimatization. In similar conditions of environmental heat stress, men sweat more profusely than women. Body temperature regulation becomes seriously affected on exposure to hot and humid environment because of difficulty in the evaporation of the sweat.

Regulation of Sweating

If the room temperature is gradually raised say from 27°C to 40°C, the body temperature would tend to increase. At a particular room temperature (around 31°C), the sweating starts suddenly, and the rate of sweating progressively increases with increase in environmental temperature. Sweating is induced by the activation of anterior hypothalamic temperature regulating centre by: 1) warm blood reaching it (central action) and 2) by afferent impulses arising from the warmth receptors in the skin (peripheral or reflex action). Activation of the anterior hypothalamic temperature regulating centre increases the impulse discharge in the sympathetic cholinergic fibres to the sweat glands. Bradykinin released from the secretory activity of the sweat glands causes cutaneous vasodilatation providing adequate blood flow for the sweat formation.

Composition of Sweat

The composition of sweat varies with the rate of sweating. The coiled portion of the sweat gland produces the primary secretion by an active secretory process. Its chemical composition is similar to plasma ultrafiltrate. Its sodium concentration is approximately 140 mEq/L and it contains other plasma constituents such as K^+, Cl^-, Ca^{++}, urea, uric acid lactic acid, etc. The chemical composition of the primary secretion is modified as it passes through the straight ductal portion of the gland, but the degree of change varies with the rate of sweating. The modification chiefly involves reabsorption of NaCl from the sweat fluid.

Slow Sweating Rate In such conditions, there is ample time for the NaCl reabsorption, and NaCl concentration may fall to as low as 5 mEq/L. Water is also reabsorbed.

High Sweating Rate When the sweat gland secretory rate is high, (due to stronger thermal stimulation), less time is available for ductal reabsorption of NaCl. Under such conditions, NaCl concentration of the sweat is approximately 60 mEq/L. Thus, heavy sweating in unacclimatized individuals may lead to NaCl deficit in the body.

Acclimatization to Heat

Prolonged exposure to high environmental temperature produces useful adaptations. There is a gradual decrease in the concentration of NaCl in the sweat so that even at high rate of sweating, its Na^+ concentration remains low. Moreover, after acclimatization, sweating starts even with a milder increase in body temperature.

In very hot climate, sweat secretion may be over 10 L/day. Such heavy sweating causes not only loss of body water but also loss of NaCl. Body temperature regulation has priority over regulation of salt and water balance. Therefore, in acute heat stress, a person may die of severe dehydration and salt loss leading to circulatory failure. In unacclimatized individuals exposed to high environmental temperature, 15–20 g of NaCl may be lost in sweat per day. After acclimatization, only 3–5 g of NaCl may be lost per day. The decrease in NaCl concentration in the sweat is brought about by increase in the secretion of *aldosterone,* which decreases Na^+ loss in the sweat.

Emotional Sweating

The eccrine sweat glands are chiefly involved in thermoregulation. As mentioned above, their secretion is regulated by hypothalamic thermoregulatory mechanisms. In response to increased heat production in the body (e.g. during exercise) or exposure to environmental heat, sweating occurs all over the body, even during sleep.

Emotional sweating occurs in the *palms* of the hands, *soles* of the feet, *axillae* and *forehead* only. Emotional sweating is activated by stimuli arising from the cerebral cortex and/or limbic system. Emotional sweating does not occur during sleep. Moreover, whereas thermal sweating is accompanied by cutaneous vasodilatation, emotional sweating is accompanied by cutaneous vasoconstriction. In some emotionally high stung individuals, emotional sweating is so profuse that they avoid shaking hands or a sheet of paper on which they are writing becomes wet. This condition is known as *emotional hyperhidrosis*.

NORMAL BODY TEMPERATURE

In humans, the body temperature is usually measured from the mouth (sublingual) in conscious adults, but in seriously ill adults or in infants it may be recorded from the axilla or the rectum. Average normal human oral temperature is 37°C (normal range 36°C to 37.5°C). The rectal temperature represents the temperature of the body core (pelvic and abdominal viscera). It is usually 0.5°C higher than the oral temperature.

Variations in Body Temperature

(i) There is a *circadian variation* in the body temperature. Body temperature is lowest at about 2.00 AM (during sleep) and highest in the evening. The difference between the two values may be 1°C.

(ii) Due to thermogenic effect of progesterone, the body temperature is higher in the post-ovulatory phase of menstrual cycle than in the preovulatory phase.

(iii) After a bout of heavy exercise, oral temperature up to 38.5°C (rectal temperature up to 40°C) may be recorded.

(iv) Oral temperature changes with the temperature of hot or cold drink . Therefore, soon after a hot or a cold drink, the oral temperature, obviously, should not be measured.

(v) In infants, the body temperature regulation is not very effective. Marked changes in the body temperature may be observed after a cold bath or a bout of screaming.

(vi) In old age, due to decreased activity, the body temperature tends to remain subnormal. In addition, due to compromised circulatory system, older individuals cannot tolerate extremes of environmental temperature.

Concept of "Core" and "Shell" Body Temperature

Although human beings are homoeothermic, the temperature of the whole body is not kept constant around 37°C. Only the temperature of the body "core", i.e., brain and thoracic and abdominal viscera (vital organs) is kept constant. On the other hand, temperature of the body "shell", i.e., the skin and its underlying structures is allowed to vary with the change in the external temperature (Fig. 29.7). In cold weather, the temperature of the shell may be several degrees lower than the core

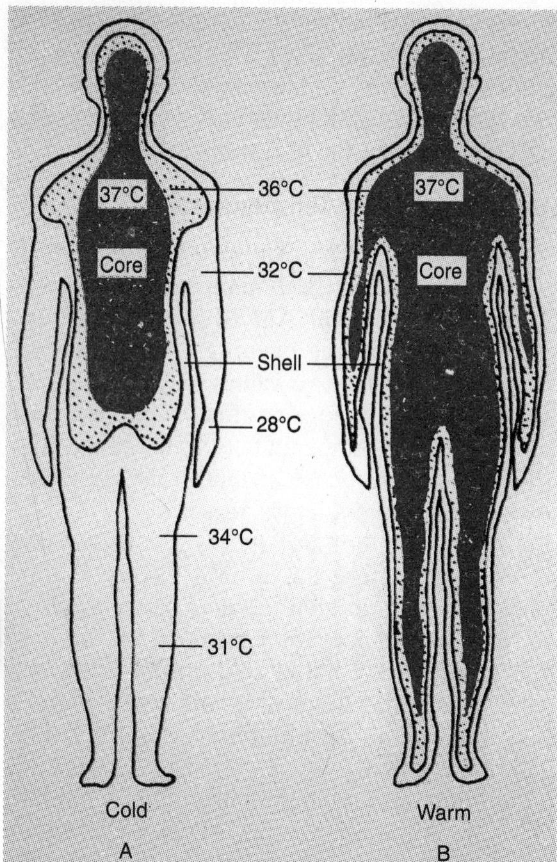

Fig. 29.7: Body core and shell concept. Dark areas—body core; superficial light areas—body shell.

temperature. The lower temperature of the body shell decreases the loss of body heat to the environment by conduction and radiation. In hot environment, the shell temperature approaches the core temperature and this helps in heat loss by conduction and radiation.

BODY TEMPERATURE REGULATORY MECHANISMS

Hypothalamic Thermostat

From the ablation and stimulation experiments in animals on the hypothalamus described elsewhere in this chapter, it was concluded that the anterior hypothalamus responds to heat, i.e. increase in body temperature or exposure to hot environment, whereas the posterior hypothalamus integrates body responses to cold. These responses consist of autonomic, somatic, hormonal, and behavioural mechanisms. The efficiency of hypothalamic thermostatic mechanism can be judged from the fact that the body temperature remains constant over a wide range of environmental temperature, as well as, over a wide range of internal heat production. For example, during heavy exercise, the heat production in the body may increase as much as 20-folds.

Afferents

The skin contains cold, as well as, warmth receptors, but cold receptors are 3–10 times more in number than the warmth receptors. In addition, cold receptors seem to be present in the spinal cord, abdominal viscera and possibly in other internal organs. Thus, *peripheral signals* chiefly activate the hypothalamic response to *cold*. In contrast, receptors for *warmth* seem to be located *centrally*, especially in the preoptic area of the hypothalamus. This centre senses an increase in the temperature of the blood above normal. The cutaneous warmth receptors play somewhat secondary role in temperature regulation.

It may be reiterated that the *cutaneous thermoreceptors respond to the temperature of the skin; not to the temperature of the environment.*

Efferent Mechanisms Activated by Heat

Activation of anterior hypothalamic heat loss centre results in the following.

1. Cutaneous Vasodilatation Inhibition of sympathetic discharge to the cutaneous vessels causes vasodilatation and accumulation of blood in subpapillary venous plexus (Chapter 13). The effect is particularly prominent in the hands, feet and ear lobules. The *AV anastomoses*, present in the skin of these sites, are normally kept closed by strong sympathetic discharge. But, on exposure to heat stress, the decrease in the sympathetic discharge may increase the cutaneous blood flow from 10–15 ml/100 g skin weight/minute to as high as 150 ml/100 g of skin weight/minute. By this mechanism, the warm blood from the deeper tissues is brought to the surface, and heat loss by conduction, radiation and evaporation is facilitated.

2. Sweating This is the most important mechanism for heat loss. It is the only mechanism of heat loss when a person is exposed to the environmental temperature greater than the body temperature. The rate of sweating may vary from practically zero in a cold environment to over 10 L/day in heat stress. In acclimatized individuals, sweat secretion as high as 1.5 L/hr has been recorded during short period of heat stress.

3. Panting In some animals like dogs, which do not have sweat glands, panting is an effective means of heat loss. Panting consists of rapid shallow breathing. Increased vaporization in the mouth and upper respiratory passages facilitates the loss of body heat. There is no disturbance in the arterial pCO_2 or pH since alveolar ventilation is not affected.

4. Anorexia Some degree of anorexia occurs in heat stress. The resulting decrease in food intake may decrease heat production, because of a decrease in specific dynamic action of food.

5. Behavioural Responses include moving into the shade or a cooler place. Moreover certain degree of apathy ("It is too hot to move") decreases muscular activity, causing less heat production in the body.

Efferent Mechanisms Activated by Cold

Heat is being continuously produced in the body. Moreover, hyperthermia is far more dangerous to the body than moderate hypothermia. Probably, that is why physiologically heat loss mechanisms are better developed than the mechanisms against cold. For man, the best mechanism against cold is behavioural, e.g. use of woolens and warm houses. Exposure to cold tends to decrease the body temperature and this activates: (a) measures to conserve body heat; and (b) measures to increase heat production in the body.

Measures for Heat Conservation

1. Cutaneous Vasoconstriction Activation of posterior hypothalamus increases the sympathetic discharge to the cutaneous vessels causing extreme vasoconstriction. The cutaneous blood flow may become as low as 1 ml/100 g skin weight/min. As a result, the practically bloodless skin prevents heat loss by becoming an insulating barrier between the warm core of the body and the cold environment.

2. Piloerection The cold induced piloerection traps air and forms an additional insulating layer to conserve body heat. This mechanism is far more important for protection against cold in animals with fur or feathers.

Measures for Increased Heat Production

1. Shivering When the cutaneous vasoconstriction is insufficient to prevent heat loss, heat production is increased by shivering. Shivering thermogenesis is an increase in the rate of heat production during cold exposure due to *increased contractile activity of skeletal muscles not involving voluntary movements and external work.* Shivering is initiated by the same α-motor neurons that act in voluntary muscle contraction. The difference exists in the motor control, which in voluntary muscle contractions comes from the motor nuclei of the CNS, while in shivering the motor commands originate in the hypothalamus. Incipient shivering progresses from an increase in muscle tone to microvibrations and eventually to clonic contractions or tremor of both flexor and extensor muscles. Shivering closely resembles the normal isometric muscle contractions. Shivering may increase the heat production 4–5–folds.

2. Increased Secretion of Catecholamines The catecholamines increase the rate of cellular metabolism and thereby cause chemical thermogenesis. Increased secretion of epinephrine and norepinephrine occurs as a part of response to cold stress. In adults, heat production is increased by 10–15% by this mechanism. However, in infants increased secretion of catecholamines may increase heat production by 100%.

3. Increased Secretion of Thyroxin After *several weeks of exposure to severe cold*, increased secretion of thyroid stimulating hormone (TSH) and hyperplasia of thyroid gland can be demonstrated. Consequently, thyroxine secretion in winter is somewhat greater than in summer. In infants, even short exposure to cold increases thyroxine secretion.

4. Non-Shivering Thermogenesis In infants, shivering does occur, but non-shivering thermogenesis in the brown fat is far more important means of heat production. Increased metabolism of brown fat, causing heat production, occurs in response to increased sympathetic discharge.

5. Hunger

6. Increased Voluntary Muscle Activity

ABNORMALITIES OF BODY TEMPERATURE REGULATION

Fever

An increase in the body temperature above the normal range is known as fever. It is the most well-known sign of ill-health.

Most commonly, fever is due to an *infection* which may be bacterial (e.g. tonsillitis, abscess), viral (e.g. influenza) or protozoal (e.g. malaria).

However, *tissue destruction* due to any cause (e.g. myocardial infarction, rheumatic fever, neoplasm, etc.) may also produce fever.

As fever develops, heat production is increased by shivering and heat loss is simultaneously decreased by cutaneous vasoconstriction till a new higher body temperature is reached. Now thermoregulatory mechanisms operate to maintain the new temperature level. Thus, the *pathological processes seem to reset the hypothalamic thermostat at a higher level.*

Toxins released from the bacteria act on monocyte macrophages to produce a polypeptide called interleukin-I which disturbs the hypothalamic thermostat. From the area of inflammation, the cytokine factors are released into general circulation. They enter the brain tissue through the circumventricular organ, where the blood-brain barrier is poor. Prostaglandins are the final mediators of interleukin action on the preoptic nucleus. They cause an elevation of the thermostatic set point. Aspirin, a prostaglandin-inhibitor, has pronounced antipyretic action.

Fever may have some protective role, because the growth of some bacteria and viruses is retarded at higher body temperature. However, higher body temperature produces many bad effects such as dehydration, negative nitrogen balance, loss of NaCl in sweat and alkalosis (because of hyperventilation). Very high body temperature, e.g. over 41°C (*hyperpyrexia*, or *malignant hyperthermia*), may produce permanent damage to the brain, liver and kidneys.

Heat Stroke (Sun Stroke)

Heat stroke is a form of *hyperthermia* accompanied by physical and *neurological symptoms:* High body temperature in the absence of sweating, flushed dry skin, mental confusion, disorientation, convulsions may progress to coma and death.

Heat stroke commonly occurs when heavy physical work is performed in hot and humid environment. Prolonged exposure to hot environment may lead to dehydration, salt deficiency and even circulatory shock. As a result, the cutaneous heat loss mechanisms are compromised and body temperature begins to rise sharply. Heat stroke, however, may occur in hyperpyrexia due to any other reason like infections. In the treatment of a person suffering from heat stroke, the reduction in the body temperature is given first priority. Cold water sponging (hydrotherapy) is a simple and very effective measure.

Hypothermia

Hypothermia is the condition when the core (rectal) temperature falls below 35°C. The causes include:

1. Environmental Cold Exposure e.g. after ship-wrecks, or accidents on high altitude. In infants and elderly individuals, it may occur in winters even in homes, if the homes are not adequately warmed.

2. Metabolic Disorders such as hypothyroidism and hypopituitarism.

3. Iatrogenic Hypothermia (21–24°C) may be deliberately induced for a *short duration* during surgery on heart and brain. By decreasing the tissue oxygen requirement, hypothermia helps to prevent hypoxic tissue damage.

Physiological Effects of Hypothermia

The body temperature may decrease to 33°C without any ill-effect. Below 30°C, the glucose metabolism is extremely retarded, heart rate and respiration become very slow.Hypothermia decreases whole body metabolism by about 8% for every 1°C decrease in core temperature. Therefore, at 21–24°C, the tissue demand of oxygen would be considerably reduced and circulatory arrest for 10–30 minutes may be produced without any risk of cerebral damage. Besides decreasing the cerebral oxygen demand, hypothermia protects against hypoxic damage by decreasing the release of neurotransmitters such as glutamate and aspartate. These amino acids are believed to be the mediators of ischemic tissue injury in the brain.

Disorders of Sweating

Hyperhidrosis (excessive eccrine gland sweating) all over the body occurs in patients with hyperthyroidism, pheochromocytoma or some lesions of the hypothalamus.

Palmar, plantar and axillary hyperhidrosis occurs in some individuals with excessive emotional response. Emotional hyperhidrosis is a harmless but socially annoying disorder.

Anhidrosis (absence of sweating) leading to intolerance to heat occurs in some lesions of the hypothalamus. Transverse section of the spinal cord results in anhidrosis below the level of the lesion. Anhidrosis on one side of the face is a component of Horner's syndrome. Patients with diabetic autonomic neuropathy have anhidrosis of the lower limbs and the trunk. Some diabetic patients have profuse sweating in the face and neck at meal time (gustatory sweating). The mechanism of gustatory sweating is not clear.

Hypohidrosis is commonly observed in old age. It is due to a gradual reduction in the number of sweat glands, as well as a reduction in the secretory capacity of each sweat gland. Hypohidrosis causes heat intolerance.

CHAPTER 30

The Cerebrospinal Fluid

The cerebrospinal fluid (CSF) is present in the ventricles of the brain, central canal of the spinal cord and subarachnoid space around the brain and spinal cord. Total volume of the CSF is about 150 ml only. Approximately 22 ml of CSF is present in the ventricles, 45 ml in the cranial subarachnoid space, and the rest in the spinal subarachnoid space and spinal canal.

FUNCTIONS

(i) The brain practically floats in the CSF present in the subarachnoid space. Hence, the fluid acts as a cushion and protects the delicate brain tissue against jolts from blows on the skull.

(ii) Since the brain lies in a rigid cranium, the cerebral blood flow can increase only if volume of some other cranial content decreases. Thus, changes in CSF volume help in reciprocal changes in cerebral blood volume.

(iii) Cerebrospinal fluid provides nutrition to the nervous tissue and drains away the waste products.

(iv) In spite of the existence of blood-brain barrier, some plasma proteins leak out of the cerebral capillaries. From the perivascular spaces, such proteins enter the CSF and are thus drained out of nervous tissue interstitium. (This function is served by lymphatics elsewhere in the body).

FORMATION OF CSF

The choroid plexuses are highly vascular structures chiefly responsible for the production of CSF. Choroid plexus consists of villi-like tufts of choroidal capillaries covered by highly folded layer of ependyma (the epithelial layers covering the entire ventricular system). Tufts of choroids plexus project into each ventricular cavity. The surface area of choroids plexus is further increased by the presence of microvilli on the surface of ependymal epithelial cells. The ependymal cells are connected to each other by *tight junctions*, constituting the blood-CSF barrier.

Cerebrospinal fluid is being continuously produced by the choroid plexus in the two lateral ventricles, and the unpaired third and fourth ventricles. It is produced by an active secretory process in the epithelial cells covering the blood vessels of choroid plexus.

About 30–50% of CSF is formed in the choroid plexuses and the *remainder is formed around blood vessels of the brain, and around ventricular walls*.

There is a free communication between brain interstitial fluid and CSF.

CIRCULATION OF CSF

Cerebrospinal fluid passes from the two lateral ventricles to the third ventricle through foramina of Monro. The third ventricle communicates with the fourth ventricle via the aqueduct of Sylvius. The fourth ventricle is continuous with the long and narrow central canal of the spinal cord. The ventricles and the central canal constitute the *internal system of CSF circulation* (Fig. 30.1).

The cerebrospinal fluid circulates in the *external system* consisting of subarachnoid space around the brain and the spinal cord. Through three openings (the two lateral foramina of Luschka and a central foramen of Magendie), CSF leaves the fourth ventricle, and enters the external system to be reabsorbed by arachnoid villi into dural venous sinuses. The reabsorption is probably a passive process and occurs by diffusion and due to difference in the hydrostatic pressure (Fig. 30.2).

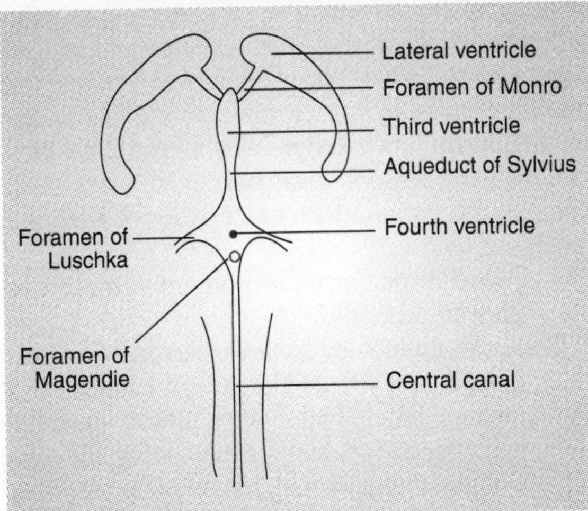

Fig. 30.1: The ventricular system of the brain.

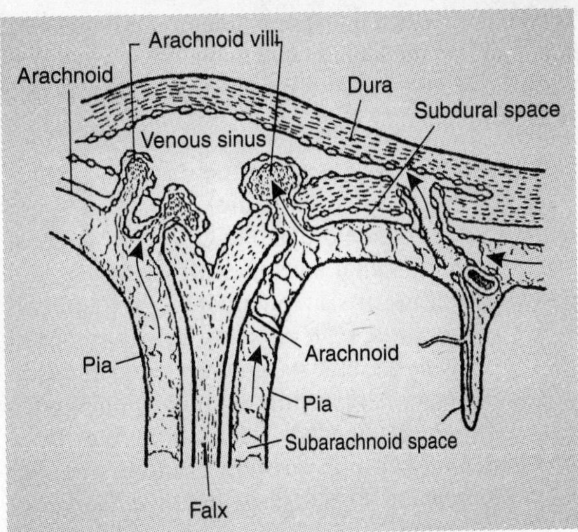

Fig. 30.2: The arachnoid villi, the sites of absorption of CSF into the dural venous sinuses.

COMPOSITION OF CSF

The concentrations of some of the constituents of CSF as compared with plasma are given in Table 30.1. CSF *glucose* level is lower than in plasma. Its *pH* is also lower than plasma pH. CSF *chloride* concentration and pCO_2 are higher than in plasma. *Presence of red blood cells or white blood cells in the CSF is abnormal.*

Table 30.1: Composition of CSF in comparison with plasma

	CSF	*Plasma*
Na (mEq/L)	140	140
K (mEq/L)	2.9	4.6
Ca (mEq/L)	2.3	4.7
HCO_3 (mEq/L)	25	25
Cl^- (mEq/L)	118	99
pH	7.33	7.4
Protein (mg/dL)	20.0	7500
Glucose (mg/dL)	64	100
pCO_2 (mmHg)	50	40

Lumbar Puncture

A sample of CSF can be conveniently obtained by inserting a needle in the subarachnoid space below the termination of the spinal cord, usually between third and fourth lumbar vertebrae. If the needle is connected to a manometer, CSF pressure can also be measured. Normal CSF pressure is about 130 mm H_2O (normal range 60–150 mm H_2O).

Lumbar puncture is performed:

(i) To record CSF pressure.

(ii) To introduce drugs into CSF (e.g. streptomycin, spinal anesthetics).

(iii) For diagnostic purposes. In bacterial meningitis, CSF contains large number of leucocytes and its glucose concentration is markedly reduced. In patients with blockade of CSF circulation, e.g. by a spinal tumour, protein content of CSF, below the level of obstruction, is markedly elevated.

Quekenstedt's Test

While recording CSF pressure, if one internal jugular vein is compressed, there is a sudden rise in CSF pressure (because of decrease in absorption of CSF into the venous system). A block in the circulation of CSF, say by a spinal tumour, is shown by the absence of rise in the CSF pressure.

Variations in CSF Pressure

Around 500 ml of CSF is formed everyday and a similar volume is reabsorbed through the arachnoid villi. Since the rate of formation of CSF is almost constant, the rise of CSF pressure occurs whenever there is blockade in the circulation or reabsorption of the fluid. The arachnoid villi may be blocked by inflammation of the meninges (meningitis) or by a pressure of a large brain tumour. As a result, the reabsorption of CSF is blocked leading to collection of large amount of fluid under high pressure, both inside the ventricles and outside the brain as well. This condition is called *communicating type of hydrocephalus* (excess of water in the cranial cavity). A blockade in the aqueduct of Sylvius causes enlargement of ventricles. This condition is called *non-communicating hydrocephalus* (Fig. 30.3). In infancy, the most obvious indication of hydrocephalus is often a rapid increase in head circumference or an unusually large head size.

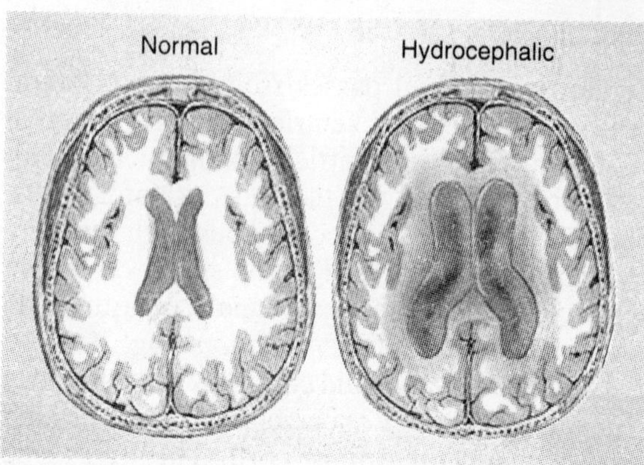

Fig. 30.3: Lateral ventricular size in a normal individual and a patient with hydrocephalus.

Either type of hydrocephalus produces severe brain damage and therefore must be detected and treated at the earliest.

BLOOD-BRAIN BARRIER (BBB)

In most of the tissues, the capillary endothelial cells are so permeable that, except proteins, all other constituents of plasma pass freely across the capillary walls. However, the cerebral capillaries are different. They have such a restricted permeability that a blood-brain barrier is said to exist. Some of the important characteristics of BBB are discussed below.

1. Blood-brain barrier is more impermeable to plasma proteins.
2. Large molecules such as bacteria, viruses, antigens, most of the drugs cannot pass through BBB. That is why, infections of the brain are uncommon. If they occur, they are difficult to control because antibodies present in the blood cannot pass across the BBB.
3. Only substances with high lipid solubility such as CO_2, O_2, alcohol, caffeine and nicotine pass freely across BBB. Substances with low lipid solubility have poor penetration across BBB.
4. Water soluble charged molecules cannot diffuse. They are transported across the cerebral endothelial cells by special transport systems (carrier-mediated transport).

As a result, Na^+, K^+, Cl^-, HCO_3^-, etc. take longer time to pass across BBB. Even urea, the highly diffusible molecule does not pass easily.

5. Glucose, so essential for CNS function, does not diffuse freely across cerebral capillaries. A special transport system GLUT1 is required.
6. Amino acids transfer across BBB also requires specific transport systems.
7. Lactate does not cross BBB.

Anatomical Basis of BBB

Tight Junctions

In most of the tissues, capillaries are characterized by the presence of clefts of approximately 1 μm size between the adjacent endothelial cells. In the cerebral capillaries, electron microscopic picture reveals tight junctions between the adjacent capillaries. The tight junctions constitute the most important element of BBB.

Astrocyte Foot Processes

The foot processes of astrocytes cover over 90% of the surface of cerebral capillaries. These coverings also contribute to the BBB.

BLOOD-CSF BARRIER

The chemical composition of CSF is different from that of plasma in many aspects (Table 30.1). Moreover, changes in the composition of blood are not immediately reflected by changes in the CSF. Hence, a blood-CSF barrier is said to be present in the choroids plexuses, where CSF is formed. Blood-CSF barrier has same characteristics as blood-brain barrier, though the former controls the formation of CSF whereas the latter controls the formation of cerebral interstitial fluid. The similarity in the characteristics of the two barriers may be expected from the fact that in the cerebral tissue, there is a free exchange between CSF and interstitial fluid.

The anatomical basis of blood-CSF barrier, however, is different from BBB. The capillaries of the choroid plexus are actually fenestrated type (highly permeable). The presence of **tight junctions between the adjacent choroidal epithelial cells** forms the basis of blood-CSF barrier.

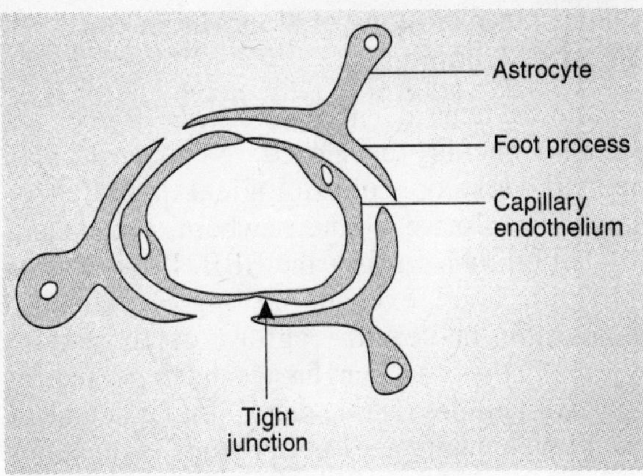

Fig. 30.4: A cerebral capillary with foot processes of astrocytes.

Functions of Blood-Brain and Blood-CSF Barriers

1. Protection against Variations in Electrolyte Composition of Plasma In view of the fact that neuronal function is very sensitive to electrolyte composition of extracellular fluid, cerebral tissue needs better protection than any other tissue. Otherwise, even minor and transient changes in the electrolyte composition of blood would have disastrous consequences.

2. Protection against Circulating Hormones and Neurotransmitters of Non-cerebral Origin Epinephrine, norepinephrine, dopamine, histamine, serotonin, glucagons and somatostatin are present in the blood as hormones. In the CNS, these agents also function as neurotransmitters. Therefore, if these agents could cross the BBB, they would play havoc with the neuronal function.

3. Protection against Circulating Toxins of Exogenous and Endogenous Origin The blood-brain barrier acts very effectively to protect the brain from many common infections. Thus, infections of the brain are very rare. However, since antibodies are too large to cross the blood-brain barrier, infections of the brain which do occur are often very serious and difficult to treat.

Clinical Implications of Blood-Brain and Blood-CSF Barriers

1. In the fetus and neonatal life, BBB does not seem to be fully developed. As a result, if a neonate develops physiological jaundice or hemolytic disease of the newborn, the unconjugated bilirubin crosses the BBB. If the plasma bilirubin level exceeds 18 mg%, bilirubin deposition in certain regions of the brain, especially the basal ganglia, results in permanent motor disabilities (kernicterus). Similar degree of jaundice in adults does not produce kernicterus.

2. Most of the **antibiotics** cannot cross the BBB. Therefore, in a patient with a cerebral infection only an antibiotic which crosses the BBB would be beneficial.

3. Blood-brain barrier may be **disrupted** by hypertension, plasma hyperosmolality, exposure to radiations, trauma, ischemia or inflammations. In all such conditions, brain becomes far more vulnerable to exogenous or endogenous toxins.

4. In the treatment of certain brain tumours, BBB is *deliberately disrupted* by injection of hypertonic mannitol into the carotid and vertebral arteries. Thus, anti-cancer drugs are able to cross the BBB and attack the tumour tissue

Parts of Brain Outside the Blood-Brain Barrier

When an acidic dye is injected into a living animal, all the tissues of the body are stained except most of the brain. This was the observation which led to the concept of blood-brain barrier. However, four small parts of the brain named below are stained like rest of the body. These structures have fenestrated capillaries and are said to be outside the blood-brain barrier. They are also called circumventricular organs (Fig. 30.5).

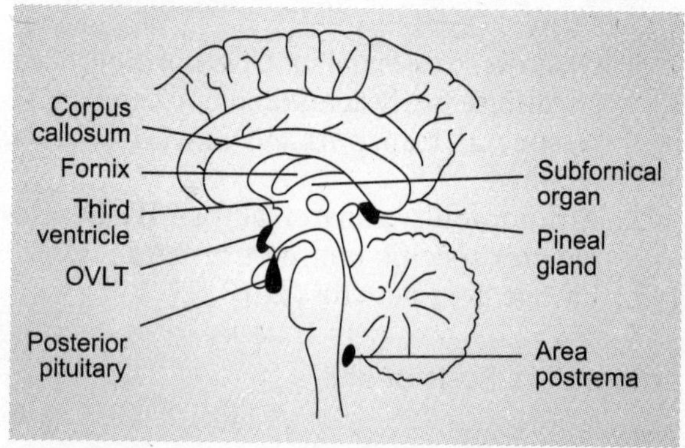

Fig. 30.5: Circumventricular organs (and pineal gland).

1. Neurohypophysis including ventral parts of median eminence.
2. Area prostrema.
3. Subfornical organ.
4. Organum-vasculosum of lamina terminalis (OVLT).

Circumventricular organs contain receptor sites for certain constituents of blood. They mediate various neuroendocrine responses which help in the maintenance of homeostasis. Neurons of neurohypophysis respond to various neurohumoral stimuli and release ADH, oxytocin and hypothalamic hypophysiotropic hormones. Area postrema is a chemoreceptor zone that initiates vomiting in response to certain chemical changes in the plasma. Angiotensin II acts on subfornical organ and possibly on OVLT to induce thirst (water intake). OVLT is the site of osmoreceptors, which control ADH secretion. It seems circulating interleukin-I induces fever by acting on OVLT.

31 CHAPTER

The Autonomic Nervous System

Autonomic nervous system is the portion of nervous system that controls visceral functions of the body, e.g. gastrointestinal motility and secretions, heart rate, blood pressure, sweating, etc. Autonomic nervous system innervates the smooth muscles of the blood vessels, respiratory, excretory and reproductive tracts and pilomotor system. In addition, it innervates the cardiac muscle and the exocrine glands. Autonomic nervous system may be subdivided into sympathetic and parasympathetic systems.

From the word autonomic, one may assume that this part of nervous system is independent of the somatic nervous system. In fact, the somatic and the autonomic nervous systems interact with each other to support the body, by producing various types of somatic and visceral adaptations.

Anatomically, the structures included in autonomic nervous system consist of only efferent neurons. However, it must be stressed that the sensory receptors and afferent neurons are as much important in autonomic nervous system as in the somatic division. Visceral afferents have cell bodies in the dorsal root ganglia or equivalent structures in the cranial nerves. The visceral afferent fibres run chiefly in the vagus, splanchnic and plevic nerves. Their central processes enter the spinal cord or the brainstem to synapse with somatic as well as autonomic efferent neurons. Therefore, the signals originating from the viscera produce responses in visceral as well as somatic structures. Similarly, visceral activity is affected by signals that originate not only from the viscera, but also from the somatic structures.

GENERAL ARRANGEMENT

As traditionally described, the autonomic nervous system is basically a two neuron efferent pathway consisting of a preganglionic neuron and a postganglionic neuron. To understand the general arrangement of autonomic nervous system, one may compare a typical spinal somatic reflex arc with a visceral reflex arc (Fig. 31.1). A somatic

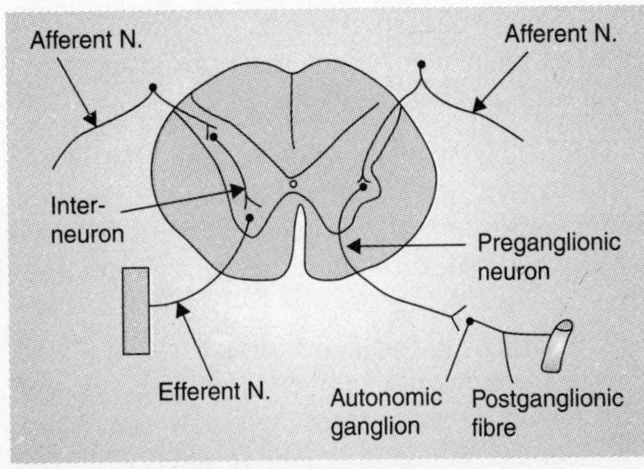

Fig. 31.1: Comparison of a somatic reflex arc (on the left) with an autonomic reflex arc (on the right).

reflex arc consists of an afferent neuron, with cell body in the dorsal nerve root ganglion, an interneuron situated in the gray matter of the spinal cord, and an efferent (effector) neuron, whose cell body is situated in the ventral grey horn of the spinal cord, and the axon (efferent fibre) leaves via the ventral root, to innervate the skeletal muscle. In case of the visceral reflex arc, the afferent neuron has similar location. It synapses with the cell body of the preganglionic neuron lying in the lateral horn of the spinal cord or with certain cranial nerve nuclei in the brainstem. The preganglionic fibre leaves the central nervous system as a thin myelinated fibre that synapses with the neurons present in the peripheral autonomic ganglion. Unmyelinated postganglionic nerve fibres leave the autonomic ganglion to innervate the effector organs, like smooth muscle, cardiac muscle or glands.

31

The peripheral autonomic ganglia are masses of grey matter that have migrated out of the central nervous system during embryonic life. Each ganglion contains cell bodies of a large number of effector cells from which the postganglionic nerve fibres originate.

The sympathetic preganglionic outflow is restricted to all the thoracic and first two lumbar (T_1 to T_{12}, L_1, L_2) spinal cord segments. This is also called the *thoracolumbar autonomic outflow*. The parasympathetic preganglionic outflow consists of two components:

(a) A cranial component consisting of III, VII, IX and X cranial nerves.
(b) A sacral component arising from sacral (S_2 to S_4) spinal segments.

The parasympathetic preganglionic outflow is also known as *cranio-sacral autonomic outflow*. Some important differences between the two subdivisions of autonomic nervous system are given below.

1. In case of sympathetic nervous system (with a few exceptions like pelvic viscera), the ganglia are situated far away from the organ innervated. On the other hand, in parasympathetic nervous system, the ganglia are situated close to the organ innervated. Therefore, the length of the postganglionic nerve fibre is short in case of parasympathetic nervous system and far greater in case of sympathetic nervous system (Fig. 31.2).

2. Another important difference between the two subdivisions of ANS is that in case of sympathetic system, a single preganglionic fibre synapses with as many as 32 postganglionic neurons (Fig. 31.2). There is very little divergence in parasympathetic nervous system, in which preganglionic fibre synapses with usually one or at the most two postganglionic neurons. Consequently, the sympathetic activity tends to be generalized whereas parasympathetic activity is more discrete.

3. The sympathetic system is more widely distributed but the parasympathetic supply is rather restricted in distribution.

4. *Preganglionic neurons* of both the sympathetic and parasympathetic nervous system are *cholinergic*, i.e. acetylcholine is the neurotransmitter released at their terminals. Most of the *postganglionic neurons* of sympathetic nervous system are *noradrenergic*, i.e. norepinephrine is released at their terminals. The exception is the cholinergic sympathetic innervation to the sweat glands and some fibres to the skeletal muscle blood vessels. In contrast, all the postganglionic neurons of parasympathetic nervous system are *cholinergic* in nature.

5. Sweat glands, adrenal medulla and piloerector muscle fibres and majority of the blood vessels receive sympathetic innervation only. On the other hand, the heart, eye, salivary glands, digestive system and pelvic viscera receive both sympathetic as well as parasympathetic innervation.

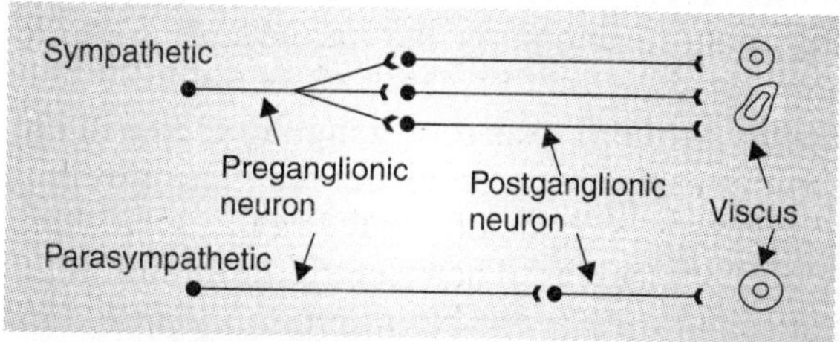

Fig. 31.2: Comparison of sympathetic and parasympathetic nerve fibres.

SYMPATHETIC NERVOUS SYSTEM: FUNCTIONAL ANATOMY

The sympathetic preganglionic neuron cell bodies are present in the lateral grey horn of all the thoracic (T_1 to T_{12}) and the first two lumbar segments (L_1 and L_2). Cell bodies of the ganglionic neurons are present in :

1. Two *paravertebral chains* of sympathetic ganglia.
2. *Prevertebral* sympathetic ganglionic masses called coeliac, superior mesenteric and hypogastric (called inferior mesenteric in animals) sympathetic ganglia.

Each sympathetic chain consists of a series of ganglia interconnected by bundles of nerve fibres. The cervical part of the sympathetic trunk consists of three large masses called superior, middle and inferior cervical ganglia. In the thoracic, lumbar or sacral regions, the number of sympathetic ganglia roughly corresponds to the number of the spinal cord segments (11, 4, 4 respectively).

The thinly myelinated preganglionic sympathetic fibres from each spinal segment pass out in the corresponding ventral root (mixed with the somatic efferent fibres) and enter the mixed spinal nerve. Almost immediately, they leave the spinal nerve as a white ramus communicantes (Fig. 31.3) to enter the lateral sympathetic chain. The preganglionic fibre may end in the adjacent *paravertebral sympathetic ganglion* or may ascend up and end in the cervical sympathetic ganglia. Many preganglionic fibres pass through the lateral sympathetic trunk without relay and terminate in one of the *prevertebral ganglionic* masses.

The unmyelinated postganglionic fibre arising from the paravertebral ganglia may form grey ramus communicantes and re-enter the spinal nerve to supply the blood vessels, sweat glands and erector pili muscle fibres. The postganglionic fibres may pass along the arteries or the cranial nerves. They may also pass out as direct branches and join the autonomic plexus, e.g. the cardiac plexus, coeliac plexus, etc.

The distribution of preganglionic neurons and postganglionic sympathetic fibres is given in Table 31.1 and in Fig. 31.3.

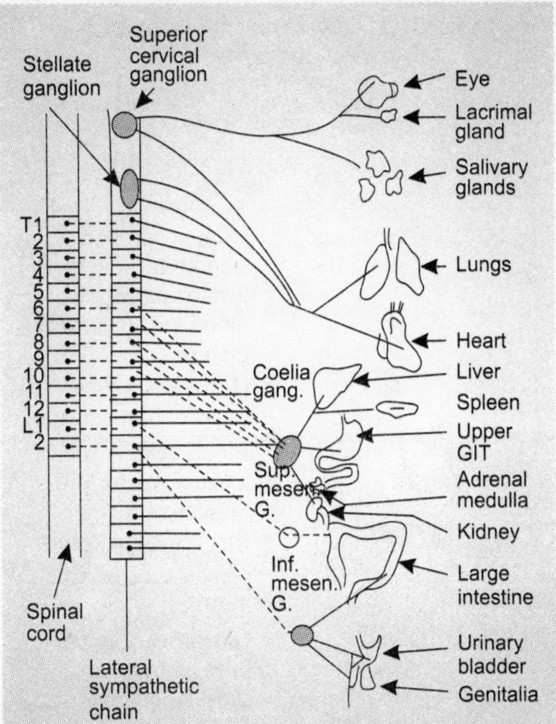

Fig. 31.3: Anatomical distribution of sympathetic nervous system.

PARASYMPATHETIC NERVOUS SYSTEM: FUNCTIONAL ANATOMY

As mentioned above, parasympathetic preganglionic outflow consists of craniosacral outflow. Vagus nerve alone contains about 75% of all the parasympathetic preganglionic fibres and supplies all the thoracic and most of the abdominal viscera. The sacral parasympathetic outflow supplies the pelvic viscera. The distribution of preganglionic cell bodies and final distribution of postganglionic parasympathetic fibres is given in Table 31.2 and in Fig. 31.4.

AUTONOMIC RECEPTORS

The neurotransmitter released by the autonomic, postganglionic nerve fibres is either acetylcholine or norepinephrine. These chemical transmitters produce their effect on the organs by binding with specific protein molecules known as receptors. Such receptors are mostly present in the cell

Table 31.1: Distribution of sympathetic nervous system

Segmental level of preganglionic neurons	*Final distribution of postganglionic fibres*	
T_1 T_2	Head and neck	Dilator pupillae, smooth muscle of levator palpebrae, blood vessels, sweat glands
T_3 T_4	Thoracic viscera	Heart, oesophagus, trachea, bronchi, lungs
$T_{5\text{-}9}$	Forelimb	Blood vessels, sweat glands, erector pili muscles
T_{10}-L_2	Hindlimb	Blood vessels, sweat glands, erector pili muscles
T_6-T_{12}	Upper abdominal viscera	GIT, urinary tract, liver and spleen capsule, adrenal medulla
L_1-L_2	Lower abdominal viscera	Bladder, uterus, fallopian tubes (or testis, vas deferens, seminal vesicles and prostate)
T_1-T_{12}	Thoracic and abdominal parietes	

31

membrane. The binding of neurotransmitters with the receptor may result in:

(a) A change in the membrane permeability due to opening or closing of specific ion-channels. The consequent alteration in the intracellular ionic concentration may alter the organ function.

(b) It may increase the activity of adenyl-cyclase causing the formation of cAMP which initiates various intracellular activities.

A particular neurotransmitter may produce excitation in one tissue and inhibition in another, e.g. norepinephrine produces inhibition of intestinal smooth muscle but causes contraction of the intestinal sphincters. The difference is determined by the nature of receptors present in each tissue.

Table 31.2: Distribution of parasympathetic nervous system

Site of preganglionic cell body	*Final distribution*
Cranial nerve III	Sphincter pupillae, ciliary muscle of the eye
Cranial nerve VII	Lacrimal glands, submaxillary and sublingual salivary glands
Cranial nerve IX	Parotid gland
Cranial nerve X	Heart, bronchi (glands and smooth muscles), alimentary canal (glands and smooth muscles), pancreas
Sacral spinal segments (S_2, S_3, S_4)	Distal part of large intestine, urinary bladder, blood vessels of external genitalia, prostate and uterus

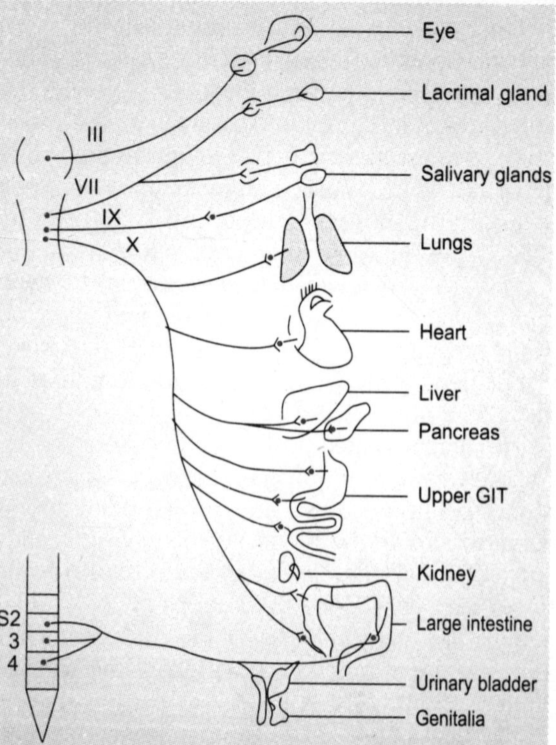

Fig. 31.4: Anatomical distribution of parasympathetic nervous system.

Adrenergic Receptors

The adrenergic receptors can be classified into two main types, namely, the alpha (α) and the beta (ß) adrenergic receptors. These receptors are further divided into α_1, α_2, β_1 and β_2. These adrenergic receptors respond not only to norepinephrine released by adrenergic postganglionic sympathetic nerve endings, but also to the circulating epinephrine and norepinephrine secreted by the adrenal medulla. Both epinephrine and norepinephrine can act on both α as well as ß adrenergic receptors. However, relatively speaking, norepinephrine has greater effect on α-receptors, whereas epinephrine has greater effect on ß-receptors.

The type of adrenergic receptors present in various organs and the effect produced by their stimulation is shown in Table 31.3.

The knowledge of different types of adrenergic receptors has been utilized to develop drugs with specific sympathomimetic or sympatholytic action.

For example, sympathomimetic drugs with action on β_2 receptors can be used as bronchodilators. Alpha-1 blocker drugs are used in the treatment of hypertension. ß-blockers are used in the treatment of cardiac arrhythmias.

Cholinergic Receptors

Cholinergic receptors are those which respond to acetylcholine released at nerve terminals. In the autonomic nervous system, it is released either at *preganglionic sympathetic as well as parasympathetic nerve terminals* or by *postganglionic nerve terminals (mostly parasympathetic)*.

On the basis of their pharmacologic properties, acetylcholine receptors can be classified as *muscarinic* and *nicotinic* types. Muscarine is an alkaloid toxin present in poisonous mushrooms called 'toads-stools'. This toxin acts on the receptors where acetylcholine (ACh) released from the postganglionic parasympathetic fibres normally act, e.g. smooth muscle and glands (Table 31.3). It also acts on the postganglionic sympathetic cholinergic receptors, e.g. sweat glands. All these actions of acetylcholine (ACh) are called **muscarinic actions** and **can be blocked by the administration of atropine.**

Small amounts of *nicotine* stimulate all the *autonomic ganglia* (sympathetic as well as parasympathetic) by acting on receptors in the autonomic ganglionic neurons. These receptors are normally stimulated by ACh released from the preganglionic nerve terminals. Therefore, these cholinergic receptors are called nicotinic type. Nicotinic cholinergic receptors can be blocked by drugs like hexamethonium (**a ganglion blocking agent**) and not by atropine.

In the *motor end plate*, ACh receptors are also *nicotinic type*, i.e. they are stimulated by small amounts of nicotine. However, these receptors can be blocked by drugs like *d-tubocurarin* and not by atropine or hexamethonium.

INTERACTION OF SYMPATHETIC AND PARASYMPATHETIC NERVOUS SYSTEM

The activity of sweat glands, visceral and cutaneous blood vessels and piloerector muscle fibres is regulated by a change in the discharge rate of sympathetic nerves only. However, most of the viscera have dual innervation and have a complex interaction between sympathetic and parasympathetic nerves. The interaction may take many forms.

In the eye, the parasympathetic nerve stimulation produces pupillary constriction whereas sympathetic nerve stimulation produces pupillary dilatation. However, the site of action of the two nerves is different. Parasympathetic nerve causes contraction of the circular constrictor muscle whereas sympathetic nerve causes contraction of the radial fibres of the iris (dilator pupillae). Normally, the discharge rate in both the types of nerves is tonically active and controlled reciprocally.

In the heart, both sympathetic and parasympathetic nerve endings act on the same tissue, e.g. pacemaker of the heart. Stimulation of sympathetic nerve increases the frequency of discharge in the pacemaker whereas the stimulation of parasympathetic nerve decreases the rate of discharge.

The interaction between the two divisions of ANS may occur even at the level of the ganglia. For example, ganglionic cells of the myenteric plexus of the gut make synaptic connections not

Table 31.3: Effects of autonomic stimulation (the type of adrenergic receptors shown in brackets)

Organ	*Effect of sympathetic stimulation (receptor type)*	*Effect of parasympathetic stimulation*
Liver	Glycogenolysis (β_2)	—
BMR	Increased (β_2)	—
Skeletal muscle	Increased glycogenolysis (β_2) and strength (?)	—
Adipose tissue	Lipolysis (β_1) α_1	—
Adrenal medulla	Increased secretion (–)	—
Mental activity	Increased	—
Eye		
Pupil	Dilated (α)	Constricted
Ciliary muscle	Relaxed (β_2)	Contraction
Heart muscle	Increased rate (β_1)	Decreased rate
	Increased force (β_2)	—
Blood vessels		
Coronary	Dilated (β_2)	—
Skin	Constricted (α)	—
Mucous membrane	Constricted (α)	—
Abdominal viscera	Constricted (α)	—
Skeletal muscle	Dilated (β_2)	—
External genitalia	—	Dilated
Pulmonary	Constricted (α)	Dilated
	Dilated (β_2)	Dilated
Lungs		
Bronchial muscle	Relaxation (β_2)	Constricted
Glands	Increased secretion (β_2)	Increased secretion
	Decreased secretion (α)	—
Stomach		
Secretion	Decreased (–)	Increased
Motility	Decreased (α, β_2)	Increased
Sphincter	Contraction (α)	Relaxation
Intestine		
Secretion	Inhibition (α)	Increased
Motility	Decreased (α, β_2)	Increased
Sphincter	Contracted (α)	Relaxation
Gallbladder	Relaxed (β_2)	Contraction
Urinary bladder		
Detrusor	Relaxed (β_2)	Contraction
Internal sphincter	Contraction (α)	Relaxation
Male sex organs	Ejaculation (α)	Erection
Skin		
Sweat glands	Increased secretion	—
Erector pili	Contraction (α)	—
Salivary glands	—	Increased secretion
Lacrimal glands	—	Increased secretion

only with preganglionic parasympathetic fibres but also with the postganglionic sympathetic fibres.

Function of Sympathetic Nervous System

In many instances, the entire sympathetic nervous system discharges as a single unit. Simultaneous discharge of catecholamines from the adrenal medulla not only intensifies but also prolongs the effect of sympathetic stimulation because the circulating catecholamines are removed slowly from the blood. This phenomenon of mass sympathetic discharge usually occurs in response to a life-threatening situation.

Isolated portions of sympathetic system are more commonly activated, e.g. increased sympathetic discharge to the sweat glands on exposure to heat or greater sympathetic discharge to the heart during physical activity.

Function of Parasympathetic Nervous System

Unlike sympathetic nervous system, the effects of parasympathetic stimulation are so varied (e.g. pupillary constriction, bradycardia, increased GIT secretions, micturition, etc.) that they need to be carried out discretely. That is why each function is separately regulated. Parasympathetic nervous system is never activated as a single unit. Acetylcholine, unlike norepinephrine, released from the cholinergic nerve endings is hydrolyzed so quickly after release that it is never found in the circulation. Only in some instances, when the functions are somewhat related, some degree of overlapping does occur. Thus, though salivary secretion can occur without gastric secretion, usually the two occur together.

HIGHER CONTROL OF AUTONOMIC NERVOUS SYSTEM

Earlier it was believed that there are special regions within the central nervous system (autonomic centres) which control all the autonomic functions. As a matter of fact, at every level of central nervous system from the spinal cord to the cerebral cortex, somatic and autonomic nervous systems interact to provide adaptations necessary for the body function.

Medulla Oblongata It is the chief site for modulation of the two divisions of the autonomic nervous system. The reciprocal discharge pattern between the two divisions is also regulated in the medulla oblongata. Moreover, mass sympathetic discharge is also initiated here.

Hypothalamus It is the site of integration of somatic, autonomic and endocrine function. Such integration is essential for the maintenance of homeostasis during exposure to stresses like extreme heat, extreme cold, surgical operation, etc.

The control of **cerebral cortex** over autonomic function is so *little* that the latter is often referred to as involuntary nervous system. Certain experimental evidences suggest that the cerebral cortex adds to the refinement of the control of the autonomic activity.

BIOSYNTHESIS AND FATE OF AUTONOMIC NEUROTRANSMITTERS

Acetylcholine (ACh)

In the cholinergic neurons, ACh is synthesized in the nerve terminals as well as in the cell body. The enzyme *cholineacetyl-transferase* catalyzes the combination of choline with acetyl-coenzyme-A (CoA). Choline is synthesized in the neuron, as well as, actively transported from the blood (Fig. 31.5). ACh is stored in the nerve terminals as synaptic vesicles. During synaptic transmission, it is released into the synaptic cleft to act on the cholinergic receptors present on the surface of

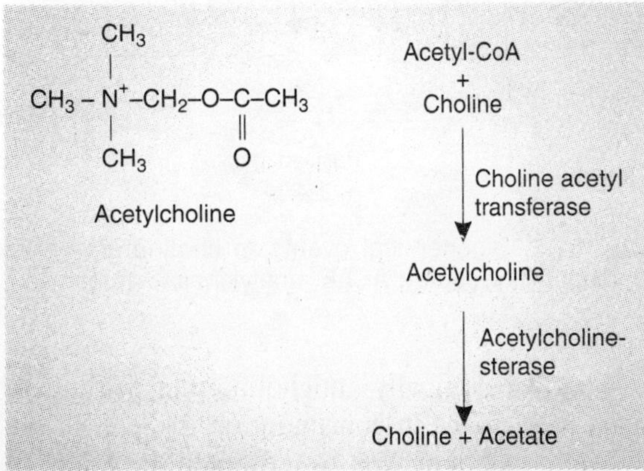

Fig. 31.5: Biosynthesis and catabolism of acetylcholine.

post-synaptic neurons. Within 1–2 milliseconds of its release, ACh is removed from the site of its action. The removal is mainly by hydrolysis by the enzyme *acetylcholinesterase* (AChE). This enzyme is present in high concentration in the synaptic region. The hydrolysis of ACh by AChE is so rapid that ACh cannot diffuse out of the synapse. After hydrolysis, some of the choline is taken back by nerve terminals and used once again in the synthesis of ACh (Fig. 31.6). Reuptake of ACh, as such, does not occur (cf. norepinephrine).

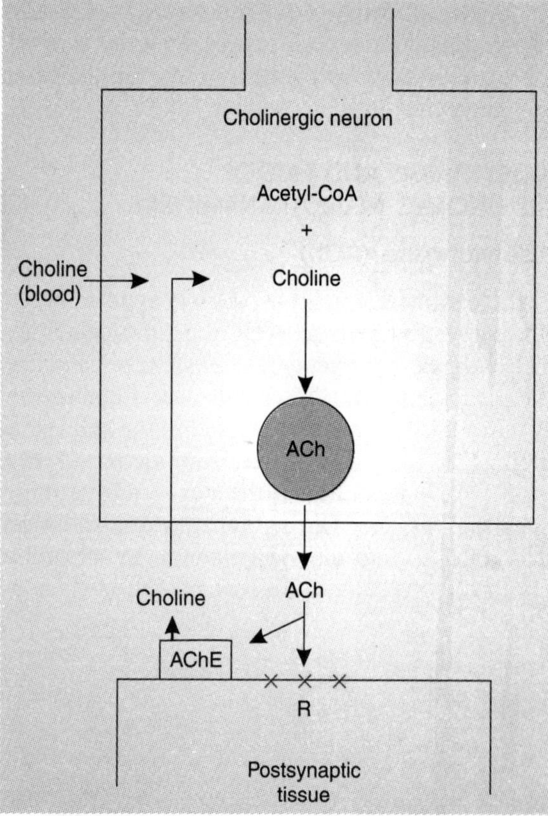

Fig. 31.6: Biochemical events at cholinergic nerve endings. R, receptor; AChE, acetylcholinesterase.

Pharmacologically, anticholinesterase drugs are used to increase in concentration of ACh in the synaptic junctions, e.g. to terminate the effect of d-tubocurarin or in the treatment of myasthenia gravis.

Catecholamines

The postganglionic sympathetic nerve endings release norepinephrine (NE). In the CNS, norepinephrine, epinephrine and dopamine are produced by noradrenergic, adrenergic and dopaminergic neurons, respectively. Adrenal medulla also produces the 3 catecholamines. The biochemical pathways involved in the synthesis of catecholamines from tyrosine are shown in Fig. 31.7. The conversion of phenylalanine to tyrosine occur mainly in the liver. Tyrosine is actively transported into catecholamine-producing neurons or adrenal medullary cells. It is converted to dopamine in the cytosol. Dopamine enters the granulated (dense core) vesicles to be stored as such in dopaminergic neurons or further converted to norepinephrine and finally to epinephrine and stored. The enzyme phenyl *ethanolamine—N—methyl transferase* (PEMT) is essential for conversion of norepinephrine to epinephrine. The enzyme is present in adrenal medullary cells and

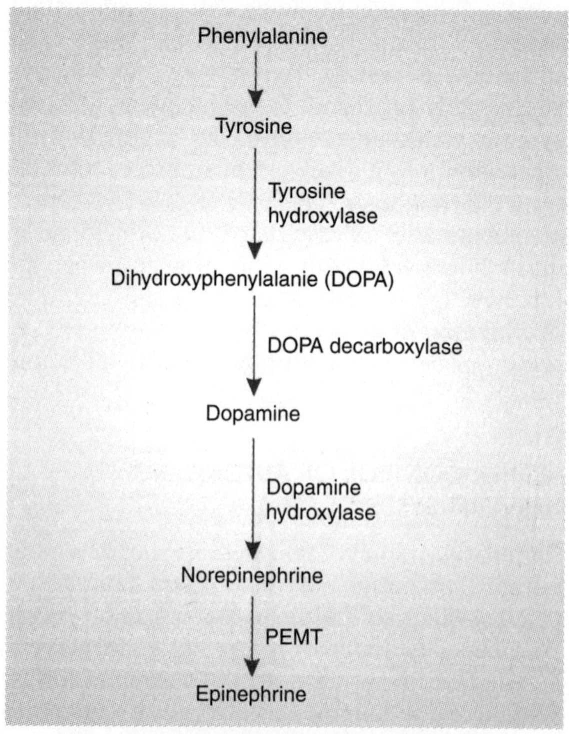

Fig. 31.7: Biosynthesis of catecholamines.

adrenergic neurons of the CNS. It is absent in postganglionic sympathetic neurons and noradrenergic neurons of the CNS.

Release, Reuptake and Catabolism

Norepinephrine (NE) released from the neuronal terminals by exocytosis acts on the noradrenergic receptors in the postsynaptic tissue. Unlike acetylcholine, the major cause of rapid termination of action of NE is its reuptake by the presynaptic neuron itself by an active transport mechanism (Fig. 31.8). A small amount diffuses out of the synaptic cleft into bloodstream. Another small amount is degraded to normetanephrine by the enzyme catecholamine–O–methyl transferase (COMT) present in the postsynaptic tissue. After reuptake, NE is again stored in the presynaptic vesicles. However, before it can be restored, some of it is inactivated (oxidized) by the enzyme monoamine oxidase (MAO) present in the cytosol of the nerve endings to form 3,4-dihydroxymandelic acid (DOMA). Because much of the transmitter is returned unchanged into presynaptic vesicles, *de novo* synthesis of NE is required only to replenish the amount catabolized.

In adrenergic synapses of CNS, epinephrine is similarly removed by mainly reuptake and partly through catabolism by MAO.

The circulating (adrenal medullary) catecholamines are relatively slowly inactivated by COMT present in many tissues, especially the liver. The products normetanephrine and metanephrine are oxidized by MAO to form vanillyl-mandelic acid (VMA) (Fig. 31.9). DOMA released from sympathetic nerve terminals is also converted to VMA by the enzyme COMT in the liver and else where.

Thus VMA is the most plentiful catecholamine metabolite in the urine. The urine also contains small amounts of metanephrine, normetanephrine and unaltered catecholamines. From the discussion given above, it would be obvious why the effects

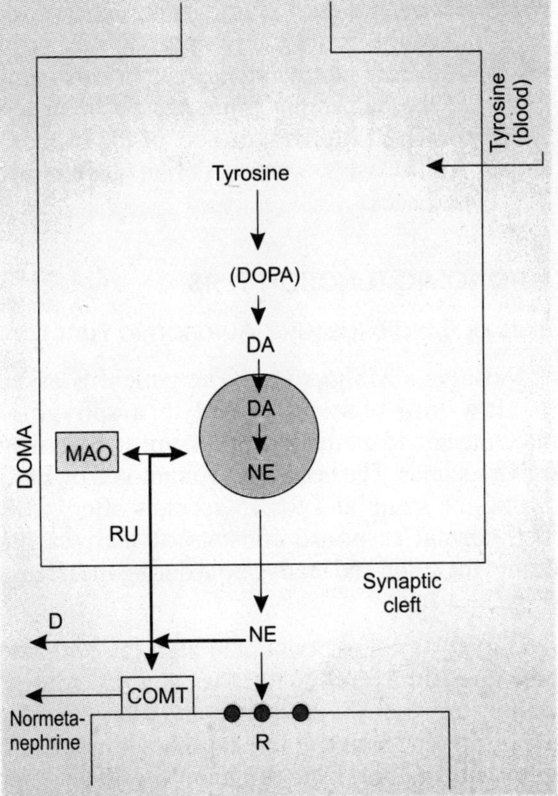

Fig. 31.8: Biochemical events at noradrenergic nerve endings. R, receptor; RU, reuptake; DA, dopamine; MAO, monoamine oxidase; DOMA, dihydroxymandelic acid; COMT, catechol Lamine-O-methyl transferase; D, diffusion into bloodstream.

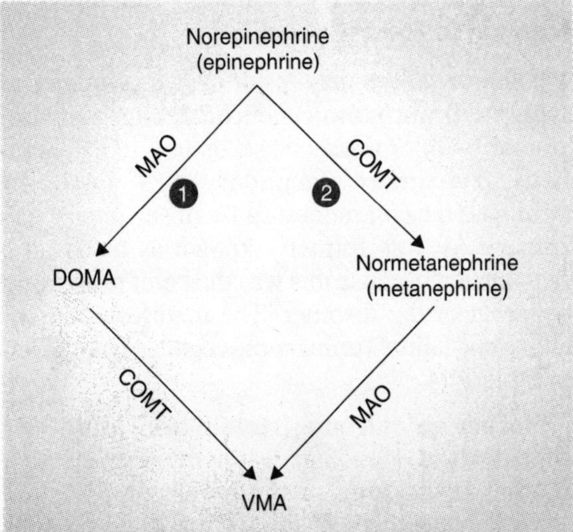

Fig. 31.9: Catabolic pathways for catecholamines. Pathway 1 active in postganglionic sympathetic nerve endings; pathway 2 active in plasma and other tissues (for circulatory catecholamines).

of a brief increase in sympathetic nerve discharge are terminated within a few seconds, whereas the effects of an injection of catecholamines or a brief increase in adrenal medullary secretion persists for 10–30 seconds or even more.

Sympathomimetic Agents

Sympathomimetic agents are the drugs which closely mimic the effects of sympathetic nerve stimulation. Some of these drugs (e.g. epinephrine, norepinephrine, isoprenaline) when injected, act directly on the α and β adrenergic receptors. Many other drugs produce sympathomimetic effect indirectly :

(a) Some of the drugs (e.g. amphetamine) displace NE from the storage sites in the sympathetic nerve ending and hence increase the activity of adrenergic receptors.
(b) Others (e.g. imipramine) inhibit the reuptake of NE by the noradrenergic nerve endings, and hence increase NE concentration in synaptic sites.
(c) Some drugs act as monoamine oxidase (MAO) inhibitor agents and hence decrease the catabolism of NE in sympathetic nerve terminals.

Autonomic Failure (AF)

Autonomic failure may result from a primary (un explained) autonomic neuronal degeneration (primary AF) or it may be secondary to a general medical disorder (secondary AF). Diabetes mellitus is the commonest cause of secondary AF. Primary AF was formerly known as orthostatic hypotension because this was the chief presenting symptom of the disorder. The manifestations of autonomic failure (primary or secondary) are given in Table 31.4.

Table 31.4: Manifestations of autonomic failure

System affected	*Manifestations*
Cardiovascular	Tachycardia, orthostatic hypotension
Sudomotor	Anhidrosis, heat intolerance
Gastrointestinal	Constipation, occasionally diarrhoea, dysphagia
Urinary	Nocturia, frequency, urgency incontinence, retention of urine
Reproductive	Erectile and ejaculatory failure
Ocular	Miosis, anophthalmos

Horner's Syndrome It results from a localized sympathetic dysfunction. It is commonly due to a tumour of the lung or the breast pressing on cervical sympathetic chain. Horner's syndrome is characterized by *unilateral changes* give below.

(i) Small pupil *(miosis)* even in the dark but with normal response to light and accommodation.
(ii) *Ptosis.* It is due to sympathetic denervation of Muller's muscle of upper eyelid.
(iii) Apparent *anophthalmos* due to narrowing of the palpebral fissure caused be denervation of Muller's muscle of the eyelids.
(iv) **Anhidrosis** (sweating deficit) on the face and neck.

AUTONOMIC FUNCTION TESTS

Tests of Cardiovascular Autonomic Function

Valsalva's Manoeuvre The patient is asked to blow into tube connected to a sphygmomanometer and maintain air pressure at 40 mmHg for 15 seconds. The heart rate is monitored by ECG during the strain and for 15 seconds afterwards. The normal response consists of tachycardia during the strain and bradycardia during the release (Fig. 31.10).

During straining period, the high intrathoracic pressure interferes with the venous return, decreasing the CO and arterial BP. The baroreceptor-mediated increase in sympathetic discharge *increases the HR* (and the PR). After the release, the intrathoracic pressure returns to normal causing sudden but transient increase in the venous return leading to increased CO and rise in BP, resulting in baroreceptor mediated *bradycardia.*

The ratio between the longest R-R interval (after the strain) and shortest R-R interval (during the strain) is known as the *Valsalva ratio*. Normal Valsalva ratio is > 1.21. In autonomic neuropathy, Valsalva ratio is < 1.20.

Heart Rate Variation during Deep Breathing (E/I Ratio) The patient is asked to inhale deeply for 5 sec. and exhale during the next 5 sec. This cycle is repeated six times, while the HR is being recorded on the ECG machine. The ratio between longest R-R interval during expiration and the shortest R-R interval during inspiration (E/I ratio) in each respiratory cycle is calculated and averaged for the total record. Normal ratio > 1.20 (Fig. 31.11).

Heart Rate Response to Standing A change of posture from supine to standing results in mild increase in the HR. Normally, the ratio between the HR on standing and in lying posture is >1.04. In autonomic neuropathy, the ratio is 1.00, i.e. there is no change in HR with change of posture.

Blood Pressure Response to Standing Normally, a change of posture from supine to standing causes a decrease in *systolic BP* by not more than 10 mmHg. In autonomic neuropathy, the decrease in blood pressure on change of posture is 30 mmHg or more.

Blood Pressure Response to Sustained Handgrip Handgrip is maintained on a handgrip dynameter at 30% of the maximum voluntary contraction for 5 minutes. Blood pressure is recorded just before the beginning and at the end of the handgrip. Normally, the *diastolic BP* increases by more than 15 mmHg. Blood pressure rise less than 10 mm Hg indicates autonomic neuropathy.

Test of Sudomotor Function

Sudomotor function can be tested by evaluation of sweating response to heat exposure. The subject's body temperature is raised by 1°C by exposure to an electric heater. Areas of sweating are demarcated by using iodine-starch, alazarine red, or quinizarin powders which change colour when moist.

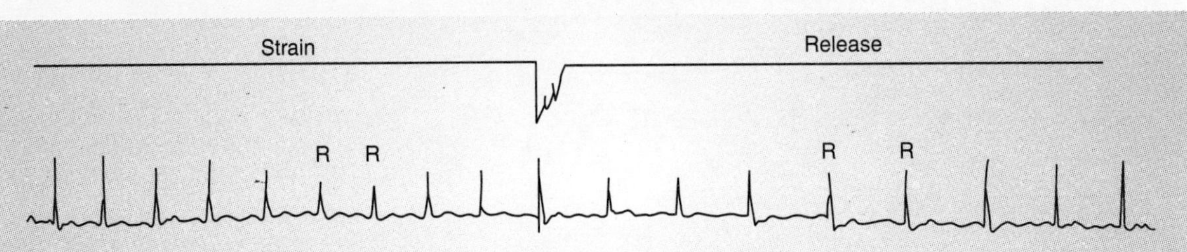

Fig. 31.10: Effect of Valsalva's manoeuvre on the heart rate.

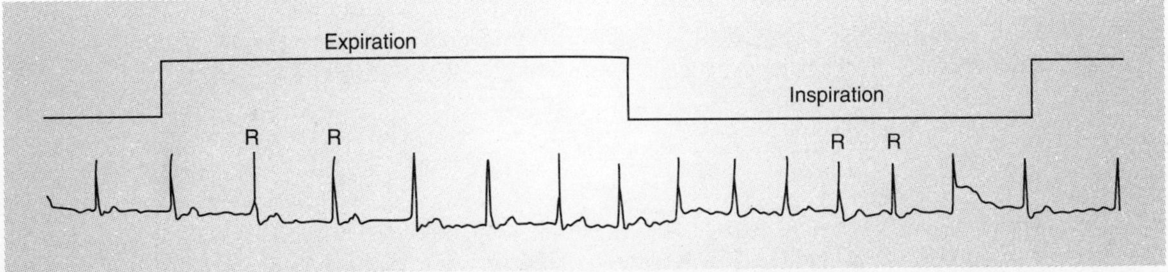

Fig. 31.11: Heart rate variation during deep breathing.

Tests of Pupillary Function

The tests of pupillary function are based on the phenomenon of denervation hypersensitivity. Instillation of *1% norepinephrine* in the eye causes no change in the normal eye but dilatation of sympathetic denervated eye (Fig. 31.12). Similarly, instillation of *2.5% methacholine* produces no change in the normal eye but pupillary constriction in parasympathetic denervated eye.

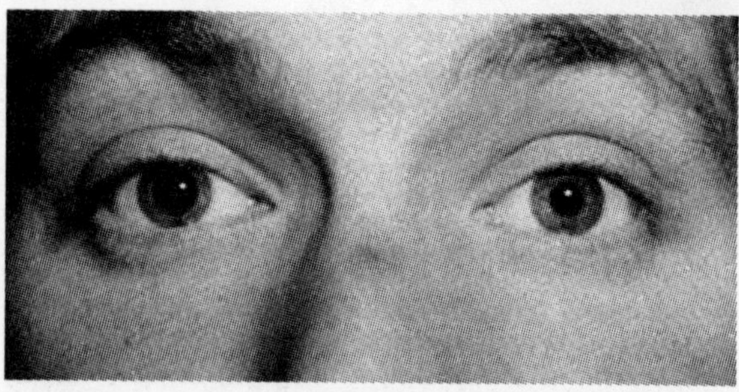

Fig. 31.12: Effect of 1% norepinephrine instillation in the eye. Note dilated pupil (denervation hypersensitivity) on the left.

Test of Bladder Function

A cystometrogram reveals, (i) absence of accommodation of urinary bladder in response to bladder filling and (ii) absent or poor voluntary bladder contraction when asked to micturate. In advanced cases, the bladder capacity may be increased up to one litre.

Section VIII

The Special Senses

32 CHAPTER

Vision

FUNCTIONAL ANATOMY (Colour Plate 3, Fig. 5)

The human eye has the shape of an irregular spheroid. In the three main axes (anteroposterior, transverse and vertical), it has an average diameter of 24 mm each. The eyeball consists of three coats (layers). Sclera, the outermost coat, is fibrous in nature and protective in function. Anteriorly, it is modified into a transparent cornea which permits the light rays to enter the eyeball. Choroid, the middle coat, is a pigmented and highly vascular layer, nutritive in function. Retina, the innermost layer, consists of photosensitive nervous tissue. The three coats enclose a lens, watery aqueous humour between the cornea and the lens, and jelly-like vitreous humour between the lens and the retina (Fig. 32.1).

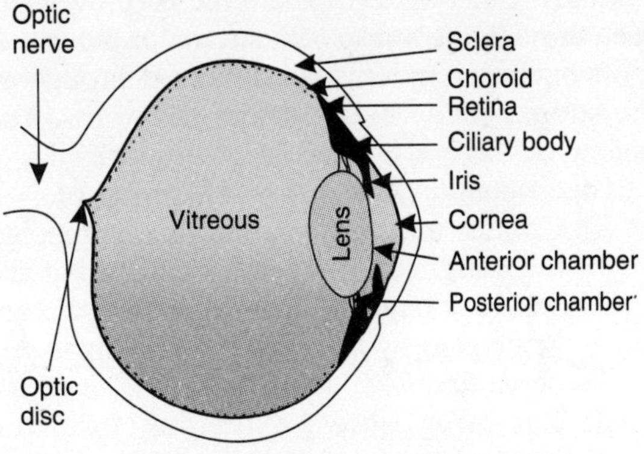

Fig. 32.1: Structure of the eye.

The pigmentation of the choroid prevents internal reflection of rays of light, as well as, prevents entry of extraneous light into the eyeball. Anteriorly, at the sclerocorneal junction, choroid is modified into the ciliary body and the iris.

The ciliary body (Fig. 32.2) contains ciliary muscle consisting of inner circular and outer longitudinal layers of smooth muscle fibres. The ciliary processes are the most vascular part of the eyeball. They are the site of formation of aqueous humour by diffusion as well as by active transport mechanism. The ciliary muscle fibres play an important role in accommodation of the eye.

Iris

The iris forms the circular contractile diaphragm of the eyeball. It is perforated by acentral circular aperture, the pupil. The iris contains loose

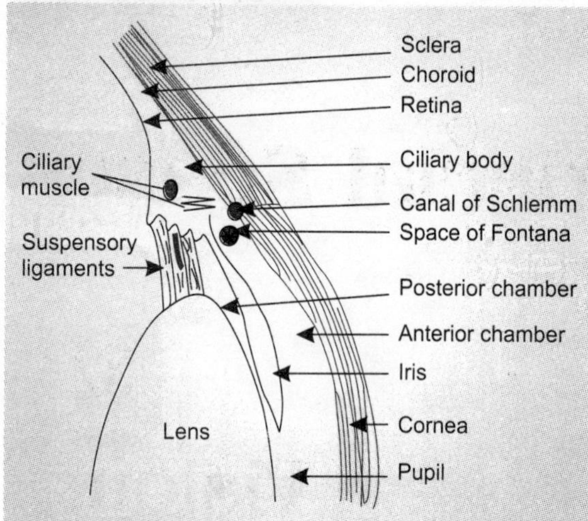

Fig. 32.2: Detailed structure of the eye near the corneo-scleral junction.

connective tissue, melanin pigment and smooth muscle fibres. The amount of melanin determines the colour of the iris. When the pigment is very little, it is present at the posterior aspect of the iris only. Such an iris looks blue or grey when seen through the transparent stroma of the iris. If more pigment is present, it is dispersed throughout the stroma giving brown colour to the iris. The colour of the iris is genetically determined.

The smooth muscle of the iris consists of:

(i) Circular muscle fibres chiefly surrounding the margin of the pupil, constituting the sphincter pupillae. These muscle fibres are innervated by autonomic parasympathetic nerve fibres.

(ii) Radiating fibres, extending from the circumference to the papillary margin, constituting the dilator pupillae. These muscle fibres are innervated by autonomic sympathetic nerve fibres.

The papillary size may vary from 1.5 to 8 mm in diameter. This change can vary the amount of light entering the eye 30-folds. In dim light, the pupils are dilated, but this is not the major mechanism of dark adaptation.

Cornea

The cornea is a highly transparent tissue devoid of blood vessels. Its thickness is less than 1 mm. Its histological structure is shown in Fig. 32.3. The stratified squamous epithelium is not keratinized. The epithelial cells form layers of uniform thickness and great regularity. Substantia propria (stroma) comprises 90% of the whole thickness of cornea. It consist of lamellae of collagen fibres which run the full length of cornea and muco-polysaccharides in the interstitial space. The collagen bundles are parallel to each other. This arrangement accounts for the optic uniformity and transparency of cornea (The sclera is opaque since it contains criss-crossed collagen fibres). Although devoid of blood supply, the cornea consumes oxygen at fairly high rate. Oxygen is consumed by the activity of Na^+–K^+ ATPase present in the endothelium and epithelium. Oxygen is supplied by diffusion from the air and the surrounding tissues. Carbon dioxide leaves by the same routes. Because contact lenses diminish the respiration of cornea, they should be removed for several hours each day. The supply of glucose and elimination of lactic acid involves diffusion through aqueous humour and adjacent tissues.

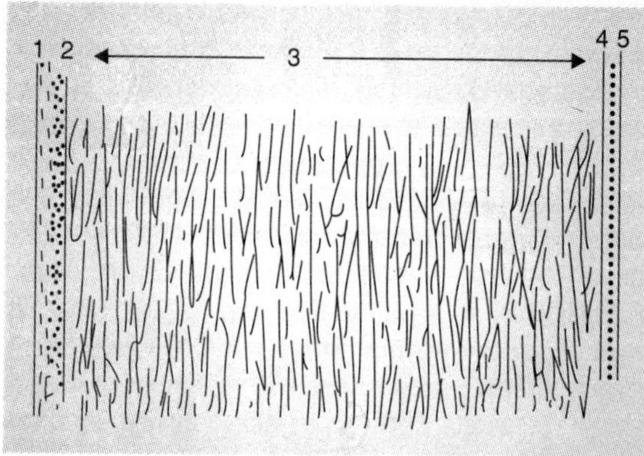

Fig. 32.3: Histological structure of human cornea. 1. epithelium; 2. Bowman's membrane; 3. Substantia propria; 4. Descemet's membrane; 5. endothelium.

Being avascular, corneal grafting has proved relatively easy and very successful, since there is no immunological graft rejection.

Cornea is the most powerful refractive surface of the optical system of the eye. It contributes nearly 44 diopters to the total refractive power, whereas the lens contributes another 15 diopters (Total = 44 + 15 = 59 D).

The refractive power of the cornea depends on its curvature and the fact that it has higher refractive index as compared to air.

Lens

The crystalline lens is an avascular structure composed of transparent collagen fibres enclosed in an elastic capsule. Under the anterior capsule is a layer of epithelial cells which proliferate throughout life. At the periphery of the lens, the cells elongate and become lens fibres, which stretch in an arcuate fashion from anterior to the posterior pole of the lens. Lens fibres are formed throughout life and the new fibres cover the old. New lens stroma is laid down more slowly after 13–14 years of age and water is correspondingly slowly withdrawn, so that size of the lens remains relatively constant. But dehydration process produces a gradually increasing rigidity in the lens leading to a gradual decline in the power of accommodation. This topic shall be discussed in greater detail a little later in this chapter.

Glucose and oxygen reach the lens by diffusion from the aqueous. Glucose is metabolized chiefly through glycolysis and lactic acid is the chief product which diffuses into aqueous. Glucose metabolism generates ATP which is required for the activity of sodium-potassium pump. This pump is essential for maintenance of low sodium and water content of the lens. Relative dehydration of the lens is essential for its transparency.

In old age, the lens often loses its transparency and gradually becomes opaque. The condition is called *senile cataract*. The exact cause of senile cataract is not known. Cataract is associated with swelling and loss of elasticity of the lens and coagulation of lens proteins. Cataract is more common in countries like India and Egypt which have high ultraviolet radiations in the sunlight. But, cataract is seen even in countries with cloudiness throughout the year. Therefore, cataract may be due to cumulative effect of gradually increasing dehydration and damage to lens proteins.

When the cataract is severe enough to impair vision, the condition can be corrected by surgical removal of the opaque lens. The refractive power of the eye can be restored by putting an artificial plastic lens in its place, or by using glasses with powerful convex lenses (+15 D). As expected, the plastic lens cannot have the power of accommodation.

Chromatic and Spherical Aberrations

Like any other optical system, the human eye suffers from slight imperfections. White light is comprised of different wave lengths (or colours like red, green, blue). All lenses, including human lens, have different refractive indices for different wavelengths. Red light with greater wavelength is refracted least, but blue light with shorter wave length is refracted the most (Fig. 32.4). Hence when the eye looks at a white object, the blue rays meet in front of the retina whereas the red rays meet a little behind the retina. However, this type, called *chromatic aberration* has no physiological significance.

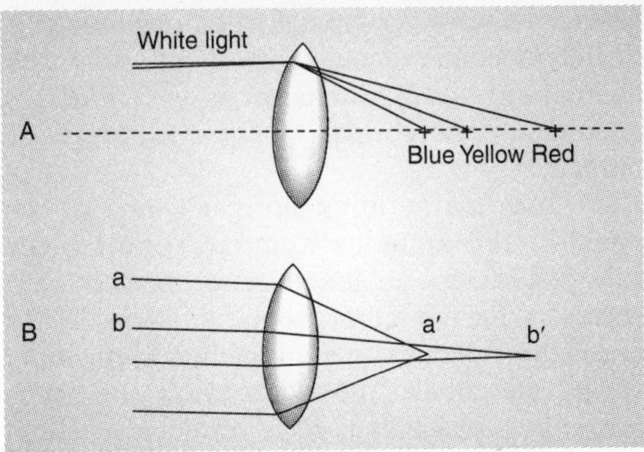

Fig. 32.4: Chromatic aberration (A), and spherical aberration (B).

Spherical aberration in a glass lens results from the fact that peripheral part of the lens possesses greater refractive power than the central part.

Thus, the rays of light which enter the lens at periphery are brought to focus at slightly different depth than those entering near the center of the lens (Fig. 32.4). In the human lens, however, central part has greater power than the remaining part. The spherical aberration is reduced by the iris which covers the outer part of the lens.

Intraocular Pressure

Aqueous humour is a thin watery fluid with a crystalloid composition similar to that of plasma. The viscosity of aqueous humour is low because of its high hyaluronic acid content. It is present in the anterior chamber (between the cornea and the iris), as well as, in the posterior chamber (the narrow circular space between the iris and the lens). After *formation by the ciliary processes*, the aqueous humour passes first into the posterior chamber and then into the anterior chamber through the pupil. It is drained into spaces of Fontana (a network of trabaculae) present at the angle between the iris and the cornea (the angle of filtration). From the *spaces of Fontana,* it is drained into a venous channel called the *canal of Schlemm.*

The normal intraocular tension, about 20 mmHg (normal range 16–22 mmHg), is maintained by the balance between the formation and reabsorption of the aqueous humour (about 2 ml/min). The normal intraocular tension is essential for maintaining the normal spherical shape of the eyeball.

Besides maintaining normal shape of the eyeball, the aqueous humour supplies the substrates (glucose, amino acids, oxygen, etc.) necessary for normal metabolic functions of the avascular structures which it bathes, particularly the lens and cornea. The constant flow of aqueous replenishes nutrients used by these tissues and carries away the metabolic waste products. The enzyme, carbonic anhydrase is involved in the formation of aqueous humour. Local application of carbonic anhydrase inhibitor drugs decreases the formation of the aqueous and hence they are used in the treatment of glaucoma.

Glaucoma is a very serious disorder of the eye. It is caused by an increase in the intraocular pressure, which may result from decreased permeability of the spaces of Fontana (open angle glaucoma) or due to obliteration of the angle (closed angle glaucoma). The angle of filtration may be closed by excessive pupillary dilatation as may occur by the use of atropine in elderly people. The optic nerve is the most susceptible part of the eye to high pressure because the delicate fibers in this nerve are easily damaged. Glaucoma is the leading cause of irreversible blindness.

REFRACTIVE MECHANISMS OF EYE

Dioptric Power

In the human eye, an image of the outside world is formed on the retina. Like a camera, the eye has: (i) a photosensitive surface, the retina; (ii) an aperture, the pupil to regulate the amount of light entering the eye; and (iii) the refractive apparatus consisting of cornea and lens.

The rays of light, as they traverse the eyeball, pass successively through the cornea, aqueous humour, the lens, the vitreous, and finally reaching the retina. As compared to the refractive index of air (1.000), the refractive index of cornea, aqueous humour and vitreous is 1.33. The refractive index of the lens is 1.42. Hence, the rays of light suffer maximum refraction at the cornea (air corneal interface) and to a lesser extent at the lens (aqueous-lens interface); because of lesser difference in the refractive indices of the aqueous humour and the lens than between the air and the cornea.

The refractive power of a lens is expressed in terms of Diopters.

$$\text{Dioptric power (D)} = \frac{1}{\text{Focal length of the lens in metres}}$$

A normal human eye has dioptric power of 59 D. Of this, 15D is contributed by the lens and the rest by the cornea. The importance of lens lies in the fact that its curvature, and therefore, its refractive power can vary. That is how; objects at varying distances from the eye can be brought to a sharp focus at the retina. This phenomenon is called accommodation.

The "Reduced Eye" (Schematic Eye)

It is an optical model of a typical human eye with a single refracting surface substituting the lens and the cornea. The reduced eye has an axial length of 24 mm. The refractive surface (the principal point) is situated 1.5 mm behind the "cornea" (Fig. 32.5). The nodal point, or the optical centre, of the schematic eye is 7 mm behind the cornea. The distance between the nodal point and the retina is (24 – 7 =) 17 mm which is the focal length. The refractive power of such a lens would be 1/focal length (metre) = 1000/17 = 59 D. This simple model, called the "reduced eye", is useful to illustrate the major optical effects in the human eye, as well as, to explain the treatment of the errors of refraction.

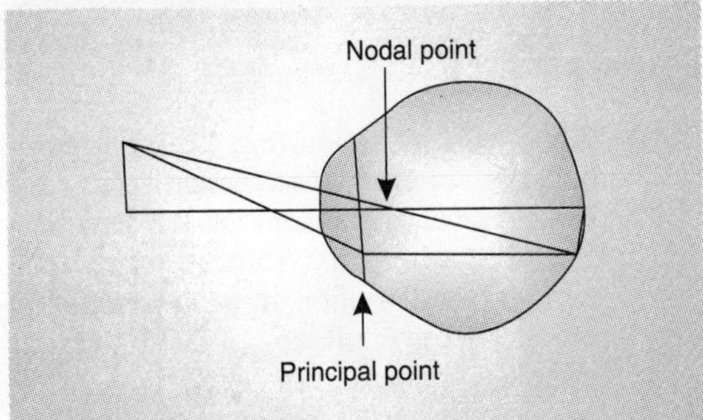

Fig. 32.5: The "reduced eye".

As expected in a lens system, an inverted image of the object is formed on the retina. During the transmission of the nerve impulses in the visual tracts, the image is changed in such a way that the visual cortex perceives it upright.

Accommodation

Mechanism of Accommodation

The ability of the eye to focus an object at varying distances is known as accommodation. This ability depends on the accommodation reflex which results in a change in the curvature of the anterior surface of the lens. During accommodation, the refractive power of the lens may increase from 15 D to approximately 29 D in young children and to lesser extent in adults. The increase in the curvature of the lens is brought about by contraction of the ciliary muscle as explained below (Fig. 32.6).

The lens is composed of a strong elastic capsule filled with transparent proteinaceous fibres. It is held in position by approximately 70 suspensory

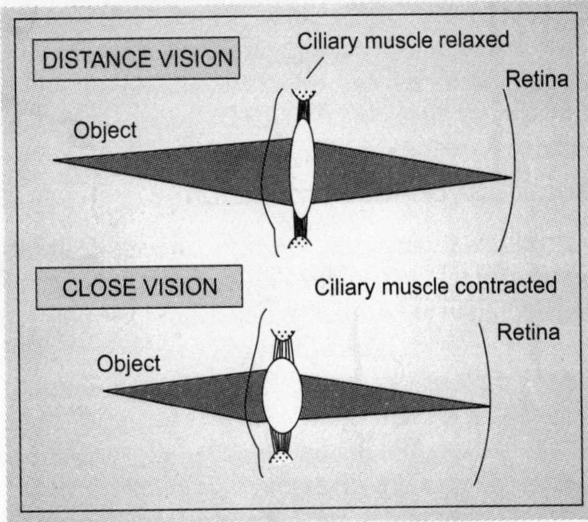

Fig. 32.6: Mechanism of accommodation. A. Non-accommodated eye. Parallel rays of light from a distant object are brought to focus at the retina. B. Accommodated eye. An increase in the convexity of the lens brings the divergent rays of light from a near object to focus at the retina.

ligaments that are attached peripherally to the ciliary body. The tension in the suspensory ligament keeps the lens in a relatively flat shape.

The **ciliary muscle** consists of two types of smooth muscle fibres. The *meridional fibres*, extending from corneoscleral junction to the insertion of suspensory ligaments in the ciliary body, lie 2–3 mm behind the corneoscleral junction. *Contraction of this muscle pulls the ciliary body forwards, loosening the suspensory ligaments*. The other type is the *circular muscle fibres* arranged circularly in the ciliary body. When they contract, a sphincter-like action occurs *decreasing the diameter of the circle of ligament attachments,* which also decreases the tension in the suspensory ligaments. As a result of the combined action of the two types of muscle fibres, the ligaments exert lesser pull on the lens capsule. The elasticity of the lens capsule allows the lens to assume a more spherical shape, particularly on its anterior surface.

Thus, when the ciliary muscle is completely relaxed, the suspensory ligaments are tense, giving relatively flat shape to the lens. With this shape, the lens has refractive power of about 15 D.

Contraction of the ciliary muscle relaxes the tension in the suspensory ligaments so that the lens assumes a more spherical shape, and its refractive power may increase up to 29 D.

Amplitude of Accommodation

For practical purposes, the rays of light from an object more than 6 metres away from the eye are considered to be parallel. When the ciliary muscles are completely relaxed, the refractive power of the combined lens system of the eye (lens + cornea) is such (59 D) that the object is brought to focus on the retina. When the object is closer than 6 metre, the rays are divergent and can be brought to focus only by increasing the refractive power of the lens. The closer the object is to the eye, the more divergent are the rays of light; the greater is the refractive power required. The nearest distance from the eye at which an object can be clearly seen is called the *near point*. It depends on the degree to which the eye can be accommodated. In young children, the near point may be as close as 9 cm. It increases in young adults to about 12 cm. After the age of 40 years there is a rapid decline in the power of accommodation, and the near point may be as far as 50 cm by the age of 50 years, and 100 cm by the age of 70 years. The age-related decline in the power of accommodation is due to a decrease in the elasticity of lens, because of which the lens fails to become more spherical while focusing on near objects. It is not due to any change in the ciliary muscle. This condition, called **presbyopia**, can be easily treated by using convex lenses for near vision.

Accommodation Reflex

The process of accommodation described above is a reflex response to blurring of retinal images. A sudden shift of gaze from a distance to a near object, initially causes blurring, because the lens fails to focus the divergent rays of light on the retina. Within one second, however reflex increase in the discharge of parasympathetic fibres causes contraction of the ciliary muscle leading to relaxation of the suspensory ligaments. The curvature of the lens, consequently, increases. The discharge rate in the parasympathetic fibres is directly proportionate to the degree of initial blurring of the retinal images.

When an individual looks at a near object, besides *accommodation*, there is *pupillary constriction*, as well as, *convergence of the visual axes* of the two eyes. The three components of the accommodation reflex response, accommodation, pupillary constriction and convergence of the eyeballs are together known as the *near response*.

The 3rd cranial nerve contains efferent fibres for all the three components of the near response.

Role of Iris

(i) Pupillary constriction (e.g. during accommodation for near vision) helps to eliminate the spherical aberrations of the lens.

(ii) Probably, the most important role of pupillary constriction in accommodation reflex is in the regulation of depth of focus of the lens system of the eye.

Depth of Focus

Figure 32.7 illustrates two separate eyes A and B that are exactly alike except that the diameter of the pupillary aperture is larger in eye A than in eye B.

In front of each eye, there is a dot-like object. It would be brought to perfect focus on the retina of each eye. If the retina could move slight forward or backward to an out-of-focus position, the size of the image would not change significantly in the eye B and would remain visible as a dot. However in eye A, with large pupil, it would become a blurred circle. In other words, eye B, with narrow pupil has greater depth of focus than eye A. It would be obvious from the laws of refraction, that if the position of retina is fixed and the object is displaced a little away or closer to the eye, it would remain visible in eye B but would go completely out of focus in eye A.

The physiological significance of the above mentioned phenomenon is that, when the pupil is narrow, the power of accommodation of the eye is not required to be altered for minor changes in the position of the object from the eye. It also

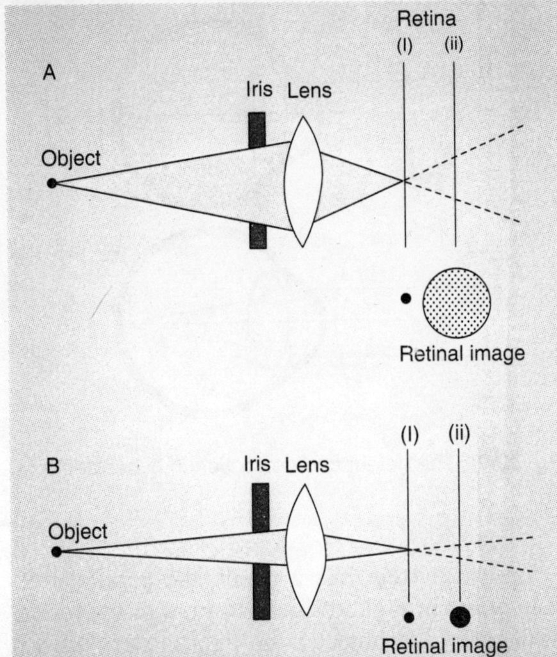

Fig. 32.7: Effect of the diameter of the pupillary aperture on the depth of focus. In position (ii) of retina there is far greater blurring of image when the pupillary aperture is wide (A) than at (B).

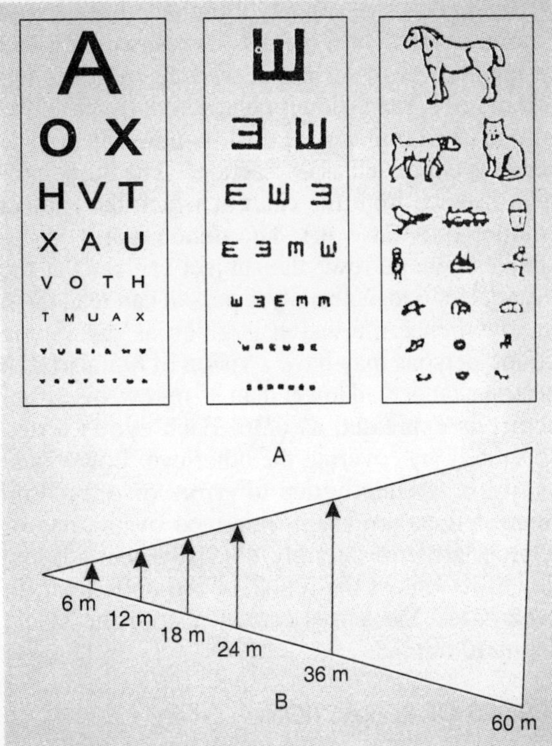

Fig. 32.8: A: Various types of Snellen's charts. B: Principle behind the Snellen's chart. Letters of each line cast an angle of 5 minutes on the eye when seen from the distance mentioned below each line.

explains why persons with errors of refraction can read better in bright light (when the pupil is constricted) than in dim light. Pupillary constriction is one of the components of the near response (accommodation reflex). It helps not only by elimination of the spherical aberrations but also by increasing the depth of focus.

ACUITY OF VISION

The acuity of vision may be measured in many ways. However, a simple way is to estimate the shortest distance by which two lines can be separated and still be perceived as two lines. The Snellen's charts (Fig. 32.8), commonly used for clinical assessment of visual acuity are based on this principle. It consists of eight rows of letters which are black in colour on a white background. From the top to the bottom, the rows of letters are designated as 60, 36, 24, 18, 12, 9, 6 and 5 metres. The size of a letter in each row is such that, when seen from the distance mentioned under it, it subtends a visual angle of 5 minutes at the nodal point in the eye. Each line of the letter subtends the visual angle of 1 minute at the nodal point. These dimensions are based on the fact that the minimum separable distance in a normal eye corresponds to a visual angle of 1 minute (1 minute angle = 1/60th of 1 degree angle of an arc). For example, in the row of letters marked 24 m, each line of the letter shall subtend visual angle of one minute from a distance of 24 metres. Hence, this letter can be read by an emmetropic eye from the distance of 24 metres. Similarly, the other letters of each row can be read from the specified distances.

Snellen's chart, suitably illuminated, is viewed from a distance of 6 metres. The person is asked to read letters in each row, starting from the top (60 m line). The vision is considered normal if the row marked 6 m can be read by the subject. The result is expressed as a "fraction". The numerator is a distance from the chart at which the subject stands (fixed at 6 m). The denominator is the smallest "metre row" the subject can read at the distance of 6 m. Normally, a person can read the 6 m row, hence the vision is given as 6/6. Some young persons may have a vision of 6/5 also. If a person cannot read lower than 36 m row, his visual acuity is expressed as 6/36. Each eye is tested separately by covering the other eye. Low visual acuity is frequently due to errors of refraction. Such defects are easily removed by the use of appropriate lenses. Rarely, the visual acuity is low due to lesions of the retina, or the optic tract. In such cases, the lenses cannot restore the visual acuity to normal.

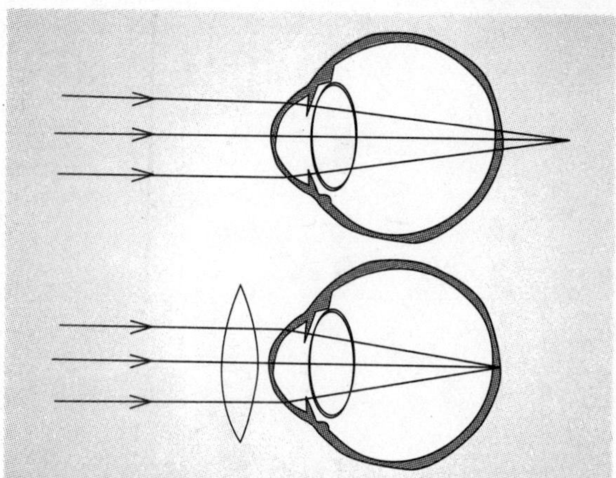

Fig. 32.9: The defect and correction in hypermetropia.

ERRORS OF REFRACTION

The eye is considered normal or *emmetropic* if, when the ciliary muscle is completely relaxed, the parallel rays of light are brought to focus on the retina. If there is a mismatching between the axial length of the eyeball and the focal length of its optical system (cornea and lens), the image may be formed in front or behind the retina.

Hypermetropia (Far-Sightedness)

If the length of the eyeball is too short, the parallel rays of light are brought to focus behind retina. The condition is called hypermetropia. Even distant objects are focussed on the retina by using some degree of accommodation. Therefore, the *near point is farther than normal*. Hence the name *farsightedness*. The problem can be corrected by using spectacles with convex lenses (Fig. 32.9) which converge the parallel rays of light on the retina.

Myopia (Near-Sightedness)

This condition occurs when the axial length of the eyeball is more than the refractive power of its optical system. As a result, the parallel rays of light are brought to focus in front of the retina. Only when the object is brought closer (< 6 m) to the eye, the divergent rays of light can be focused on the retina. Therefore, in such patients the *far-point is closer* and not at infinity as in emmetropes. In severe disorder, the far point may be only a few centimetres from the eye. The condition can be corrected by using glasses with concave (divergent) lenses (Fig. 32.10). These lenses diverge the parallel rays of light so that they are focused on the retina.

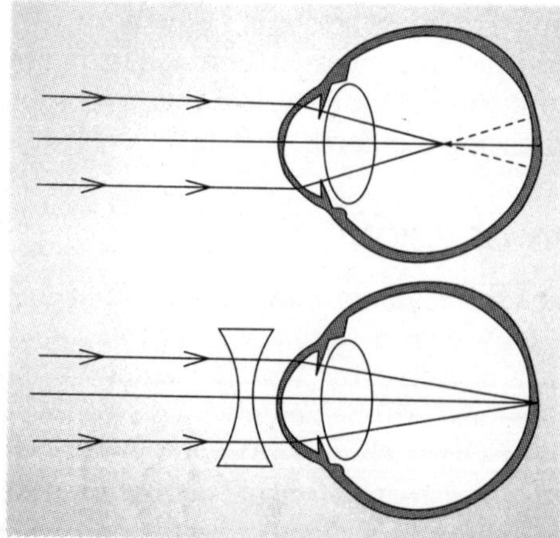

Fig. 32.10: The defect and correction in myopia.

In myopia, the *near point is very close to the eye*. Therefore, such patients require presbyopic treatment very late in life, if at all. In contrast, in hypermetropes, the near point is farther than normal and hence they require presbyopic glasses for near vision at an earlier age than emmetropes.

Astigmatism

As stated above, myopia and hypermetropia result from abnormalities in the axial length of the eyeball. Astigmatism is due to a difference in the horizontal and vertical curvatures of the cornea. A patient with this defect, while looking at a Green's astigmatic chart, finds some lines looking darker than others (Fig. 32.11). This abnormality is treated by using *cylindrical lenses,* whereas the refractive errors described earlier are treated by using *spherical lenses*.

RETINA

The retina is comprised of several layers of which the pigmented layer is the outermost, lying next to the choroid (Fig. 32.12). Next, there are three layers of neurons from out-inwards called the layer of rods and cones, the layer of bipolar cells and the layer of ganglion cells. The axons of the ganglion cells form the innermost layer, called the layer of the optic nerve fibres, lying next to the vitreous. The rods and cones are photosensitive receptors. Thus, the rays of light have to pass through the layer of optic nerve fibres, the layer of ganglion cells, and the layer of bipolar cells to reach the photosensitive zone. The pigmented layer of the retina and the adjacent choroid absorb light rays and prevent reflection of rays back into the eye globe.

In the absence of the pigment, there would be diffuse stimulation of the retina rather than the contrast of light and dark spots essential for acuity of vision. That explains the poor acuity of vision in persons with congenital absence of melanin pigment in the body including iris, choroid and the retina (albinism). The pigment layer also stores large quantities of vitamin A, the important precursor of photosenstive pigments of the rods and cones.

The innermost layer of the retina contains the arteries, the arterioles and the veins supplying nutrition to the ganglion cells and the bipolar cells.

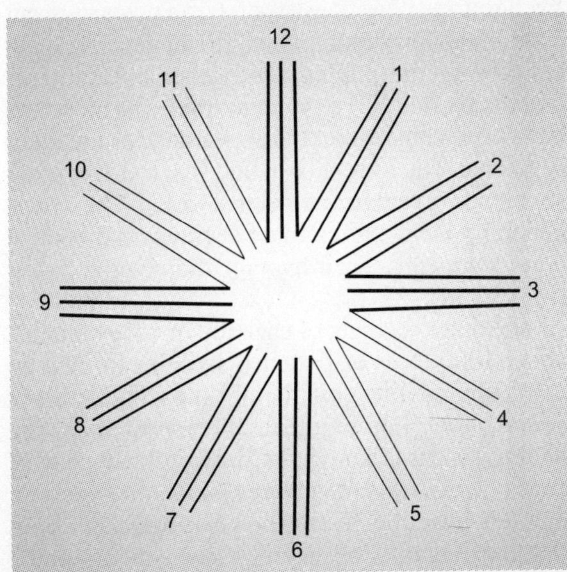

Fig. 32.11: All the lines actually have similar thickness and black colour. The figure shows what a patient with astigmatism would report.

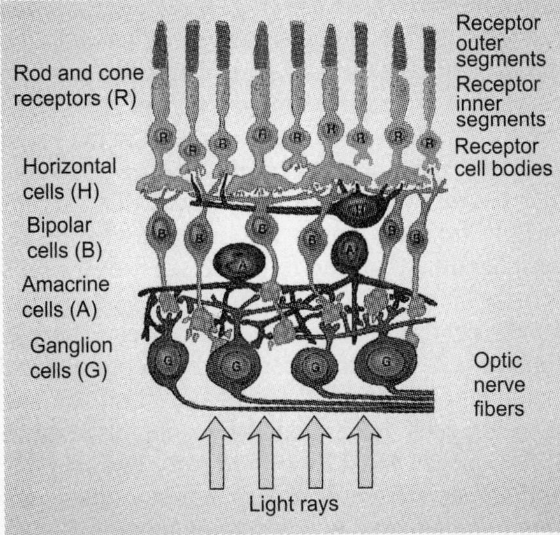

Fig. 32.12: Structure of the retina.

(The rods and cones receive their nutrition from the choroid.)

With the help of an ophthalmoscope, the retinal vessels can be visualized (Fig. 32.13). Retina is the only site in the body where the condition of the blood vessels can be directly observed. That is why ophthalmoscopy forms an important investigation in the diagnosis of certain systemic diseases like hypertension, diabetes mellitus, etc.

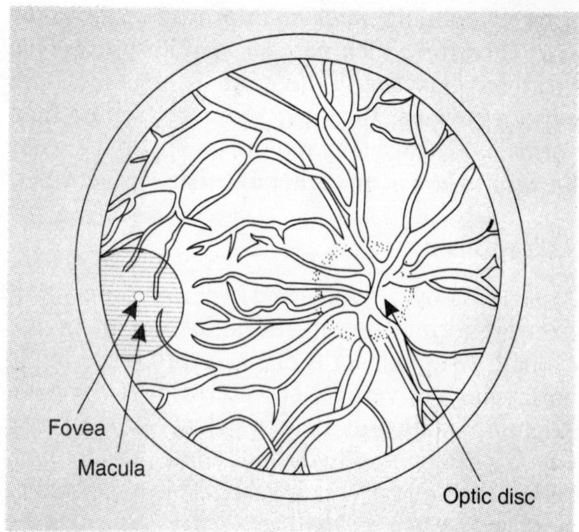

Fig. 32.13: The retina as seen using an ophthalmoscope.

Optic Disc

The optic nerve leaves the eye and the retinal vessels enter through a circular area called optic disc. The optic disc is situated about 3 mm medial to the posterior pole of the eyeball. In this area, the rods and cones are completely absent. That is why a "blind-spot" can normally be recorded in the field of vision.

Fovea Centralis (Colour Plate 3, Fig. 6)

32

All over the retina, the receptor cell layer contains both the rods and the cones. However, one part of the retina called the *macula* contains only the cones. Macula occupies less than 1 mm^2 area. Macular cones are long and thin (average diameter 1.5 μ), whereas elsewhere in the retina, the cones are plumpy (diameter 5–8 μ). The central portion of the macula is about 0.4 mm in diameter and called the *fovea centralis* (Fig. 32.13). In the fovea centralis, the blood vessels, the ganglion cells, the bipolar cells and the axons are displaced away and hence do not interfere with the rays of light. That is why the acuity of vision is sharpest at the fovea centralis. When a small object is being observed, the eyes reflexly move in such a way that the rays of light from the object fall on the fovea. In the peripheral parts of the retina, the density of rods is more than that of the cones. The reverse is true for the central region around the fovea. There is considerable convergence of rods or cones on the bipolar cells, which in turn converge on the ganglion cells. Each human eye contains about 6 million cones and 120 million rods, but only 1.2 million nerve fibres in the optic nerve. Thus, one ganglion cell may be stimulated by as many as 300 rods. The convergence of cones on the ganglion cells is far less (10 : 1). In the fovea, there is no convergence. Each cone synapses with one bipolar cell, which in turn synapses with a single ganglion cell only.

THE PHOTORECEPTORS

Each rod and cone consists of: (i) an outer segment containing the photopigment, (ii) an inner segment containing the nucleus and other cytoplasmic organelles, and (iii) a synaptic zone. The receptors have been named after the appearance of the outer segments. The rods have cylindrical rod-like outer segments (average diameter 2–5 μ). The cones generally have a thick inner segment and conical outer segments. Their average diameter is 5–8 μ (Fig. 32.14).

The outer segment of each rod or cone contains about 1000 discs or flattened saccules formed by infolding of the cell membrane. These discs contain the photopigment. In case of rods, the photopigment is known as *rhodopsin*. In case of cones, *three types of photopigments* are present, but they are collectively known as *iodopsin*. Both rhodopsin and iodopsin are proteins incorporated into the membranes of the discs. The concentration of the photopigment is so high that it constitutes about 40% of the entire mass of the outer segment.

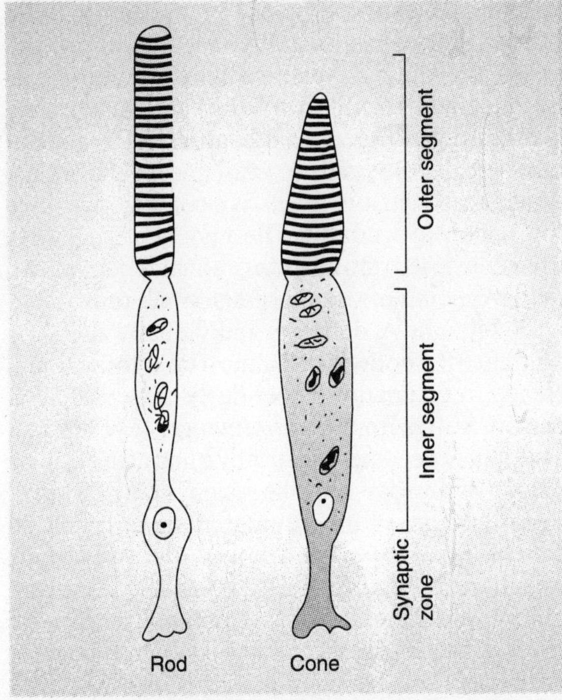

Fig. 32.14: Structure of a rod and a cone.

In both types of photoreceptors, there is a continuous renewal of discs of the outer segment. In the rods, the discs are formed at the base and discarded at the tip of the outer segment. The degenerating discs are phagocytosed by the pigmented epithelium. Abnormality of this phagocytic process produces a serious disorder called *retinitis pigmentosa* causing irreversible loss of vision. In the cones, the renewal process is more diffuse. The inner segment shows the usual cytoplasmic organelles but the mitochondria are in particular abundance.

Photopic and Scotopic Vision

Day light (photopic) vision is a function of the cones, whereas twilight (scotopic) vision is a function of the rods. The cones have much higher threshold of stimulation, but *cone vision is characterized by far greater acuity of vision, as well as, colour vision.* The *rods*, on the other hand, have *very low threshold* but colour or even details of the object cannot be observed. The human photoreceptors respond to light of wavelengths between 400 to 700 nm only.

RHODOPSIN (VISUAL PURPLE)

Rhodopsin is the photosensitive pigment present in the rods. It is composed of a protein called *opsin* (or scotopsin), and *retinene*, an aldehyde of vitamin A. Since vitamin A is an alcohol, the retinene and vitamin A are also known as *retinal* and *retinol,* respectively. Both retinal and retinol can exist as having *11-cis configuration* or *all-trans configuration* (Fig. 32.15). In rhodopsin, the retinene has 11-*cis* configuration. Vitamin A is stored in the pigmented epithelium of the retina as all-*trans* form.

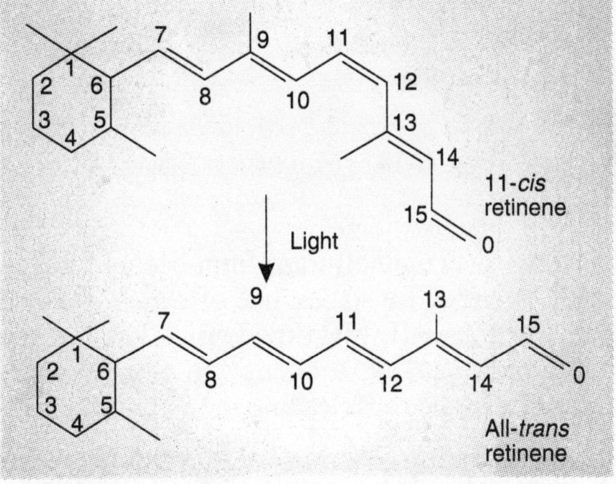

Fig. 32.15: 11-*cis* and all-*trans* isomers of retinene.

Rhodopsin : Decomposition-Regeneration Cycle

Decomposition When light energy falls on rhodopsin, it results in photoactivation of electrons in the retinene so that almost instantaneously the configuration changes from 11-*cis* form to all-*trans* form. The change in physical configuration is such that it cannot hold the protein opsin (Fig. 32.16) and therefore the two are separated. The change from curled up configuration of 11-

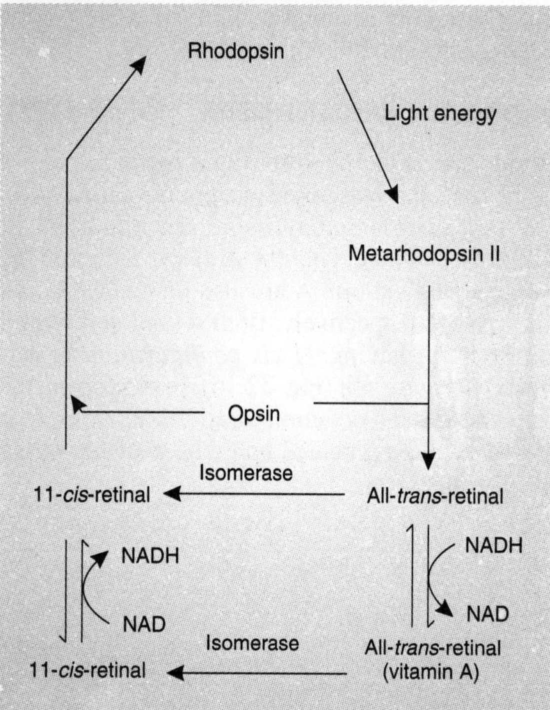

Fig. 32.16: The rhodopsin cycle.

32

cis form to straight all-trans form occurs through many intermediate stages, one of which is called meta-rhodopsin-II. Meta-rhodopsin-II is the key compound causing a change in the Na^+-permeability in the rods, leading to their activation.

Regeneration The first step in the regeneration of rhodopsin is the reconversion of all-*trans* retinal to 11-*cis* retinal. An enzyme *retinal isomerase* catalyses this process. Once reformed, 11-*cis* retinal automatically combines with opsin to form rhodopsin.

The photochemical cycle described above, not only triggers excitation of the rods, but also explains the phenomenon of light and dark adaptation discussed in detail below.

ROLE OF VITAMIN A

Vitamin A is present as all-*trans* retinol in the cytoplasm of the rods, and in the pigment layer of the retina. The all-*trans* retinal produced during decomposition of rhodopsin (on exposure to light) can be reduced to all-*trans* retinol (vitamin A) and stored as vitamin A. When required, vitamin A can be oxidized to all-*trans* retinal. An enzyme alcohol-dehydrogenase essential for this reduction-oxidation cycle is available in the retina. Thus, stored vitamin A acts as a continuous source for rhodopsin synthesis. The amount of vitamin A to be converted into all-*trans*-retinal is determined by the amount of opsin present in the rods.

In vitamin A deficient individuals, adequate amount of rhodopsin cannot be synthesized. Hence, rod function is seriously affected. Such persons suffer from *night-blindness* (nyctalopia). The patient becomes practically blind at dusk, even though during day-time the vision is fairly normal. In early stages of the disorder, normal rod vision can be restored within hours of intravenous injection of vitamin A. Prolonged and severe vitamin A deficiency is associated with more irreversible degeneration of not only rods but also the cones.

Iodopsin

The photochemicals present in the cones are collectively called iodopsin. Iodopsin consists of combination of retinal with different opsins known as photopsins (cf. scotopsin in the rods). The retinal portion is exactly similar in the rods, as well as, the three types of cones. So, the three types of photopigments present in the cones vary in their properties because of the difference in the nature of photopsins. The three photosensitive pigments of the cones consist of blue-sensitive pigment, green-sensitive pigment and red-sensitive pigment. These pigments show peak light absorbance of light wavelengths of 445, 535, and 570 nm respectively. The three types of photopigments are responsible for the colour vision.

DARK AND LIGHT ADAPTATION

The sensitivity of the rods is approximately proportionate to the antilogarithm of the rhodopsin concentration. Prolonged exposure to bright light decreases the concentration of rhodopsin by photogenic decomposition, leading to a marked decrease in the rod sensitivity. Cone sensitivity is also decreased but to a lesser extent. This phenomenon is called **light-adaptation**.

When a person remains in the dark for some time, the resynthesis of rod (and cone) photopigments gradually increase the sensitivity of the eye to light. This phenomenon is called **dark adaptation**. Between the limits of maximum light adaptation and maximum dark adaptation, the sensitivity may change up to 1 million times.

The phenomenon of dark adaptation can be easily observed by suddenly moving from a brightly lit room to a dark room. Initially, nothing is visible but after sometime visibility is markedly increased. The reverse, light-adaptation can be appreciated when one leaves a cinema-hall into the sunlight. Initially, one is dazzled by the bright light but gradually the eyes become less sensitive and the discomfort disappears.

When the changes in visual threshold (minimum amount of light that elicits a sensation of light) are plotted against time (Fig. 32.17), it is apparent that dark adaptation is almost complete in about 20 minutes. The dark adaptation curve shows two distinct limbs. The initial decrease in the visual threshold is rapid but small in magnitude. It is due to adaptation of cones. Subsequently, there is a slow but marked decrease in the visual threshold due to adaptation of the rods.

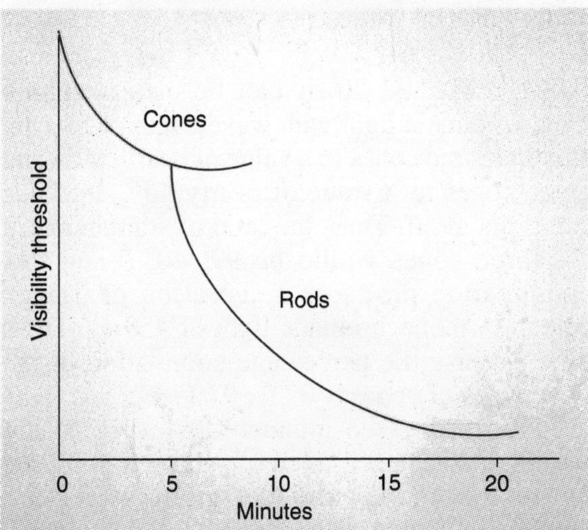

Fig. 32.17: Dark adaptation of the eye markedly decreases visual threshold (increase visual sensitivity).

Red light (wavelength about 600 nm) does not decompose rhodopsin in the rods to a significant amount (Fig. 32.18). Therefore, after wearing red-coloured glasses, one may work in bright light and still remain adapted for dark. By this method, a radiologist can maintain normal visibility even when working in rooms with widely different luminosity.

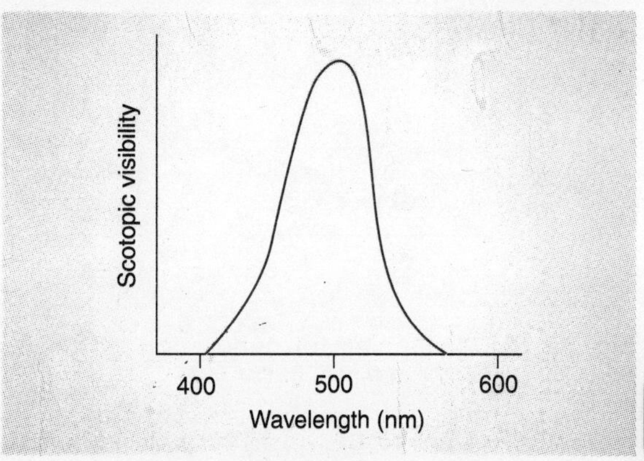

Fig. 32.18: Absorption spectrum of rhodopsin (rods).

Excitation of Rods

Rods and cones are unique among the sensory receptors. Excitation leads to hyperpolarization in the rods and cones, whereas depolarization is the characteristic response in all other sensory receptors.

The sodium pump operates normally at the cell membrane of the *inner segment* of the rods and maintains negative charge in the interior of the cell. However, in the dark, the *outer segment* is permeable to Na^+. Sodium ions enter the rods from the outer segment and neutralize much of the electronegativity produced by the sodium-pump (Fig, 32.19). Consequently, the resting membrane potential in the rods is about –30 mV only.

Exposure to light results in decomposition of rhodopsin. Meta-rhodopsin-II formed during this process decreases the sodium conductance in the outer segment. Consequently, the electronegativity of the rods increases from –30 to –90 mV, i.e.

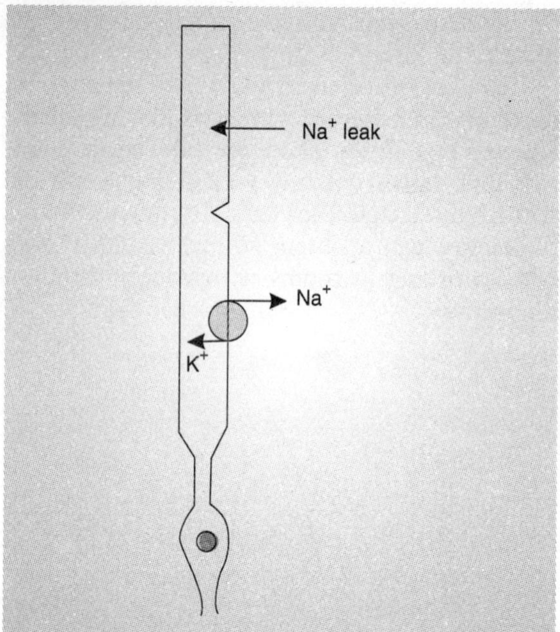

Fig. 32.19: Mechanism of generation of hyperpolarizing receptor potential in the rods.

32

exposure to light results in hyperpolarization in the rods.

In the dark, there is a steady release of neurotransmitter from the synaptic end of the rod. The hyperpolarization induced by light *decreases the release* of the transmitter which somehow excites the bipolar cells.

The electrophysiological response in the cones is similar to that in the rods.

The response of the bipolar cells can be hyperpolarization or depolarization. Propagated action potentials are produced in the ganglion cells only.

The impulses are conducted through the visual pathways to the visual cortex.

COLOUR VISION (Colour Plate 3, Fig. 7)

Human eye can perceive colours with light wavelength varying from 400 to 700 nm (the visible range of spectrum). Long ago, it was observed that all the grades of visible colours can be produced by mixing monochromatic red, green and blue (primary colours) lights in different proportions. This led Young and Helmholtz to advance a theory that the human retina contains three types of cones, each of which responds to one of the three primary colours named above. Subsequent studies proved the validity of this theory. Three types of photopigments have been isolated and their light absorbance have been identified. The red-sensitive pigment (**erythrolabe**), green-sensitive pigment **(chlorolabe)** and blue-sensitive pigment (**cyanolabe**) have peak absorbance at 570, 535 and 445 nm, respectively (Fig. 32.20).

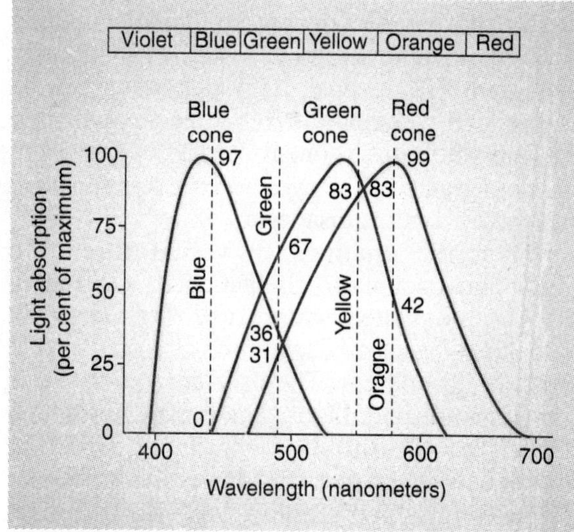

Fig. 32.20: Absorption spectrum of the 3 types of cones (or their photopigments).

From Fig. 32.20, it can be observed that monochromatic light with wavelength of 580 nm stimulates red cones to a value of nearly 99% and green cones to a value of nearly 40% and blue cones not at all. Thus, the ratio of stimulation of the three cones would be 99: 40: 0 and this combination produces a sensation of orange colour. A monochromatic light of 450 nm looks blue because the percentage stimulation of the three types of cones is 0 : 0 : 97%.

If red and green monochromatic lights are equally mixed, a sensation of yellow is produced because both red and the green cones are stimulated to a similar degree. Almost equal stimulation of all the three types of cones produces the sensation of white.

Colour-Blindness

About 8% of male population and 0.4% of female population is colour blind. The sex difference in the incidence of colour-blindness is due to the fact that genes for the red and green sensitive pigments of the cones are located on the X-chromosome and the abnormalities of these genes are inherited as recessive sex-linked characteristics. If only one chromosome is abnormal, the female (X´X) is the heterozygous carrier for the defect but the male (X´Y) is colour-blind. A female can be colour-blind if both the X-chromosomes carry abnormal gene for colour vision. The gene for blue-sensitive cone pigment is located on chromosome 7 (not on X-chromosome). That is why colour-blindness to blue colour is rare.

Colour-blindness may vary from total colour blindness to weakness of one of the primary colours. Colour blind individuals have been classified in various ways but the following classification is commonly employed.

I. Monochromats : Total colour-blindness.	
II. Dichromats :	Protanopia (Red blind) Deuteranopia (Green blind) Tritanopia (Blue blind)
III. Trichomats :	Protanomaly (Red weakness) Deuteranomaly (Green weakness)

The prefixes, 'prot'-, 'deuter'- and 'trit'- refer to the defects of red, green and blue cone systems, respectively. The suffix 'anopia-' refers to colour blindness, whereas the suffix 'anomaly' refers to colour-weakness.

The monochromats do not see any colour; they see the world as black and white and different shades of grey (e.g. black and white TV in contrast to the natural colours seen in the colour TV set). Dichromats have two types of cones. In protanopia, the red cone is absent, in deuteranopia, green cone is absent. Hence persons with these disorders are insensitive to red and green colours respectively. Blue insensitivity (tritanopia) is very rare.

Trichromat colour-blind person has, like a normal individual, all the three types of cones but he has weakness of one of the primary colours. Protanomalous subject is less sensitive to the red colour and hence needs more of red for proper matching, whereas deuteranomalous individual is less sensitive to green.

For obvious reasons, colour-blind persons should not be issued a driving license, or employed as railway-engine drivers, pilots or navigational engineers. Defects of colour vision are usually tested by using Ishihara charts (Colour Plate 3, Fig. 8), Holmgren's skeins of coloured wool or Edridge Green lantern.

VISUAL PATHWAYS

The visual pathways extend from the retina to the visual cortex. The axons of the ganglion cells, the 3rd order neurons of the retina converge on the area called optic disc to constitute the optic nerve. The optic nerve fibres of the two eyes undergo partial decussation in the optic chiasma and continue in the optic tract. A great majority of the fibres of the optic tract terminate in the lateral geniculate body of the thalamus. The fibres of geniculo-calcarine tract (the 4th order neurons) constitute the optic radiations. The optic radiations terminate in the primary visual cortex situated in the occipital lobe.

A smaller number of fibres of the optic tract end in the superior colliculus or in the nearby pretectal area of the midbrain (Fig. 32.21). These fibres are concerned with the visual reflexes (e.g. light reflex) and not with the conscious vision.

Topographically, the retina may be subdivided into a central area called the macular region and the rest known as the peripheral retina. A vertical straight line, the vertical meridian, passes through the centre of the fovea dividing retinal surface into a smaller temporal half and larger nasal half because of the eccentric position of the fovea. A horizontal line or the horizontal meridian divides each half into the dorsal and the ventral quadrants. Fibres from the four quadrants of the retina, macular as well as peripheral region maintain their relative position in the optic nerve. In the optic

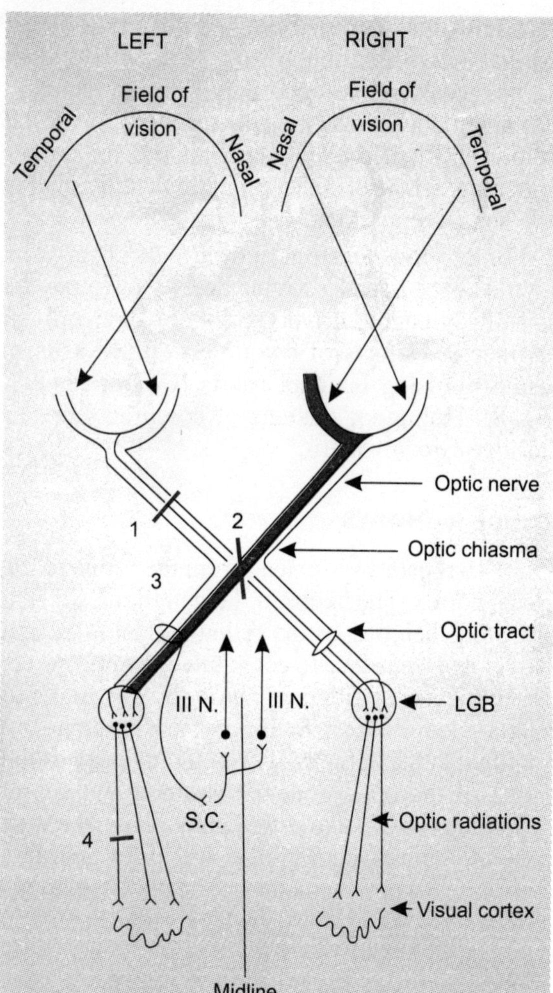

Fig. 32.21: The visual pathways. The effects of lesions at 1 to 4 on the visual fields are shown in Fig. 32.25. SC = Superior colliculus. LGB = Lateral geniculate body.

chiasma, the fibres from the nasal half of retina of each eye cross to the opposite side. Fibres from the temporal half maintain their ipsilateral course into the optic tracts. Each half of the retina receives light rays from the opposite half of the visual fields.

Field of Vision

A visual field is defined as the bounded portions of the external world visible to a stationary eye. Field of vision in each eye is recorded on a chart

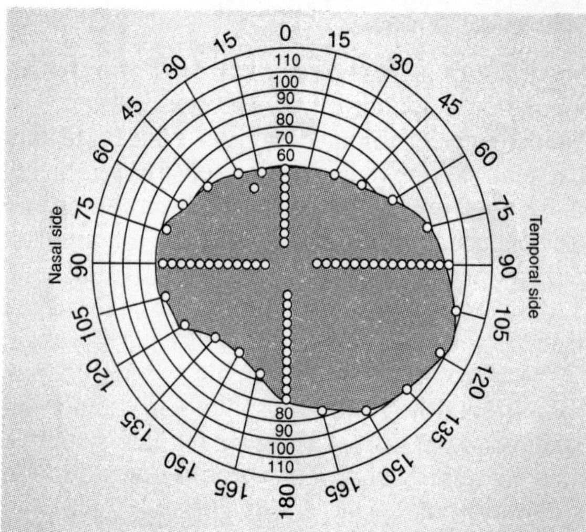

Fig. 32.22: Record of field of vision of right eye using a perimeter.

by a procedure called perimetry (Fig. 32.22). The external boundaries of the normal visual fields are limited by the nose bridge, eyebrows, and the cheek bones. On the superior, nasal, inferior and temporal sides, the normal field of vision extends approximately to 60°, 70°, 80° and 105°, respectively.

Left optic tract contains fibres from the temporal half of the left eye and nasal half of the right eye. Thus, fibres of the left optic tract are responsible for right half of the field of vision of each eye (nasal half of the field of the left eye and temporal half of the field of the right eye). Similarly, fibres of the right optic tract are responsible for left half of the field of vision of each eye. Fibres from the macular region also behave in the ame way as the peripheral retina, i.e. fibres from the nasal half of the macular region decussate but those from the temporal half do not.

Lateral Geniculate Body

In the lateral geniculate body of the thalamus, six layers of grey matter separated by bundles of fibres can be identified. These layers have been numbered 1 to 6 from out inwards. Layers 1, 4 and 6 receive fibres from the contralateral nasal half of the retina. Layers 2, 3 and 5 receive fibres from the ipsilateral temporal half of the retina. About one-third of the fibres in each optic tract are derived from the maculae. A similar proportion of the lateral geniculate body is devoted to the macular representation. Pairing of the layers from the two eyes probably plays a major role in fusion of vision and also may be a part of the mechanism for stereoscopic depth perception.

Primary Visual Cortex

The axons of the cells of the lateral geniculate body constitute the optic radiations. Optic radiations pass through the posterior limb of the internal capsule, sweeping along the lateral wall and posterior horn of the lateral ventricle, terminate wholly in the ipsilateral primary visual cortex.

In the internal capsule, the fibres are situated between the somatic sensory and auditory fibres.

Primary visual area is located bilaterally on the medial aspect of each occipital lobe, both above and below the calcarine fissure (area 17 of Brodmann) (Fig. 32.23). The macular representation is relatively very large and occupies posterior part of the visual cortex. The peripheral parts of the retina are represented in concentric arcs progressing forwards. The upper quadrants of the retina are represented above the calcarine fissure, whereas the lower quadrants are represented below the fissure. Region of the occipital lobe surrounding the primary visual cortex (area 18 of Brodmann) and posterior parietal region are believed to act as secondary visual area or visual association area (*see* Fig. 28.1).

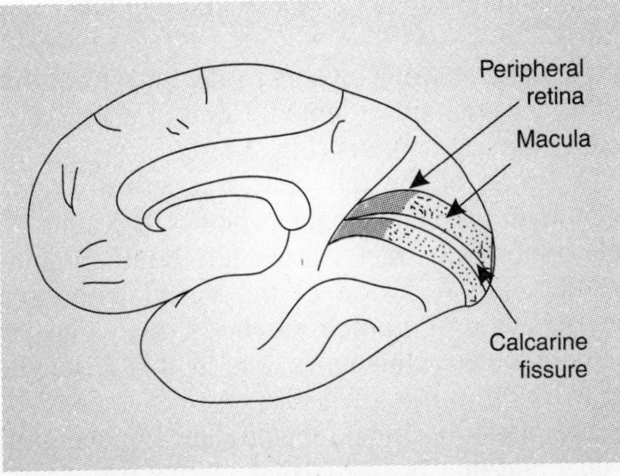

Fig. 32.23: The primary visual cortex.

Pupillary Reflexes

When light is flashed into an eye, the pupil of that eye constricts. This response is called *direct pupillary light reflex*. The pupil of the other eye also constricts and this response is called *consensual light reflex*. The afferent fibres concerned with these reflexes leave the optic tract to end in superior colliculus and pretectal region of the midbrain (Fig. 32.24). Neurons from these areas synapse bilaterally with the neurons in the Edinger-Westphal nuclei, the parasympathetic components of the 3rd cranial nerve nuclei.

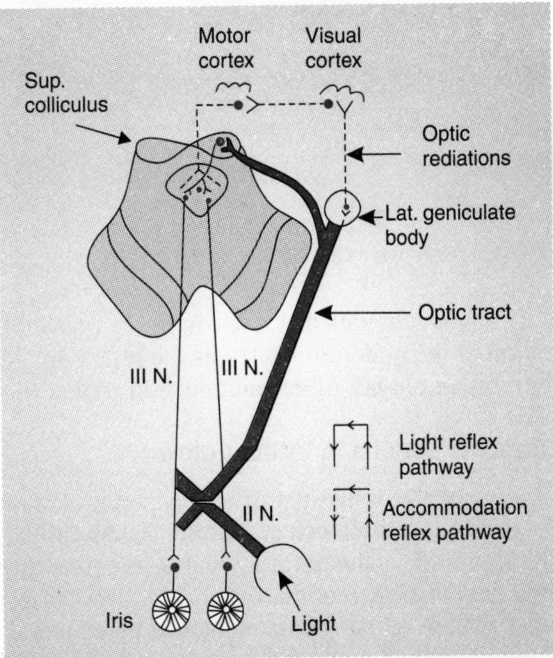

Fig. 32.24: Pathways of pupillary light and pupillary accommodation reflex (near response).

Pupillary constriction also occurs as a component of the near response. In patients with a lesion in the pretectal area, the pupil constricts during accommodation to near object, but not in response to light. Such a pupil is called **Argyll Robertson pupil**.

For the accommodation reflex (near response) the reflex arc is as given in Flowchart 32.1.

Flowchart 32.1: Reflex arc for the accommodation reflex.

Retina ⟶ Optic nerve ⟶ Optic chiasma ⟶ Optic tract
↓
Primary visual cortex ⟵ Lateral geniculate body
↓
Motor cortex → 3rd nerve nuclei (Edinger-Westphal nucleus)
↓
3rd cranial nerve

As mentioned above, the reflex arc for the light reflex is given in Flowchart 32.2.

Flowchart 32.2: Reflex arc for the light reflex.

Retina → Optic nerve → Optic chiasma → Optic tract
↓
Superior colliculus and pretectal region
↓
Edinger-Westphal nucleus → 3rd cranial nerve

It will be obvious that a lesion in the pretectal region of the midbrain interrupts the reflex arc of light reflex but not of accommodation reflex.

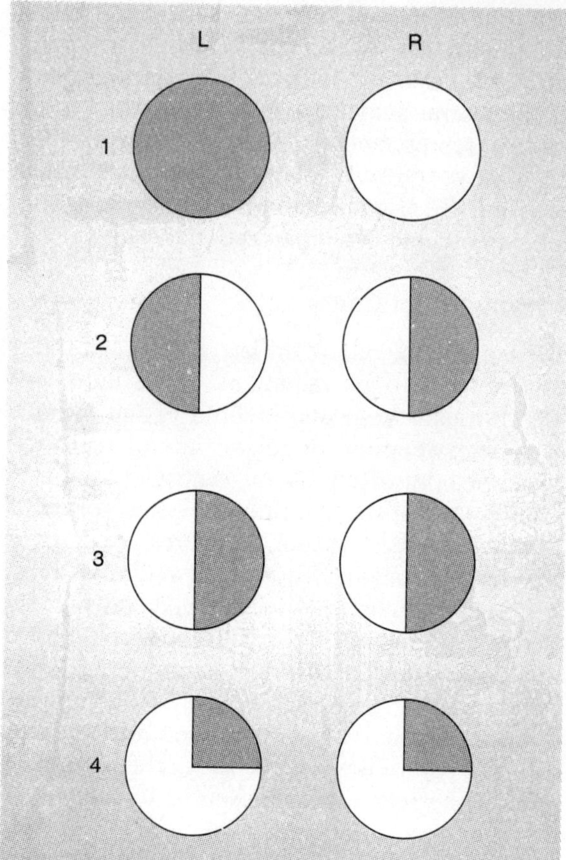

Fig. 32.25: Effect of lesions in the visual pathway on the visual fields. The numbers on the left represent different sites of lesions in the visual pathways shown in Fig. 32.21. Lesion at 1 produces blindness of the left eye. Lesion at 2 produces bitemporal hemianopia. Lesion at 3 produces right homonymous hemianopia. Lesion at 4 produces right homonymous quadrantanopia.

Effects of Lesions in Visual Pathways

Lesions of the visual pathways can be localized by observing their effect on the visual fields. Hemianopia is the term used to describe the blindness of the half of the visual field from causes other than in retina. Hemianopia can be temporal or nasal (Fig. 32.25). *Homonymous* is the term used to describe the blindness of the right halves or left halves of both the fields of vision. When non-corresponding halves of the visual fields are affected, the hemianopia is called *heteronymous* (e.g. bitemporal or binasal hemianopias). A lesion of the central part of the optic chiasma where the nasal fibres of both the retinae decussate results in bitemporal hemianopia. Binasal hemianopia would occur if the lesion involves outer margins of the optic chiasma on either side. Lesions of the optic chiasma are commonly due to a pressure from pituitary tumours (Fig. 32.21).

A lesion of the left optic tract causes right homonymous hemianopia, whereas a lesion of the right optic tract causes left homonymous hemianopia. A lesion of the visual pathways beyond lateral geniculate body also causes homonymous hemianopia, but in this case the light reflex is not affected.

Lesions of occipital lobe produce blindness of a quadrant of a field. Macular sparing (blindness of peripheral field with intact macular vision) also occurs probably because the macular representation is larger and separate from the representation of the peripheral retina.

BINOCULAR VISION

Binocular vision is vision in which both eyes are used together. Having two eyes confers at least four advantages over having one.

(i) It gives us a spare eye in case one is damaged.
(ii) It gives a wide field of view. For example, a human has a horizontal field of view of approximately 200° with two eyes but only 160° with one.
(iii) It gives binocular summation in which the ability to detect faint objects is enhanced. Binocular summation means that the detection threshold for a stimulus is lower with two eyes than with one.
(iv) It can give stereopsis in which parallax provided by the two eyes' different positions on the head give precise depth perception.

Some animals, usually prey animals, have their two eyes positioned on opposite sides of their heads to give the widest possible field of view. Examples include rabbits and buffalos. In such animals, the eyes often move independently to increase the field of view. Even without moving their eyes, some birds have a 360° field of view.

Other animals, usually predatory animals, ape and man have their two eyes positioned on the front of their heads, thereby reducing field of view in favour of streaopsis (depth perception).

If the visual fields of the two eyes are mapped on a single perimeter chart, it will be obvious that the central portions of the fields of vision of two eyes coincide. Objects in this region are observed with both the eyes. The phenomenon is called binocular vision (Fig. 32.26). Because our eyes are separated by about 65 mm, the world seen by each retina is slightly different. The difference is great for objects nearby. The two images formed at the retinal level are fused into a single image at the level of the visual cortex. The points of the two retinae on which the image of an object must fall if it is to be seen binocularly as a single object

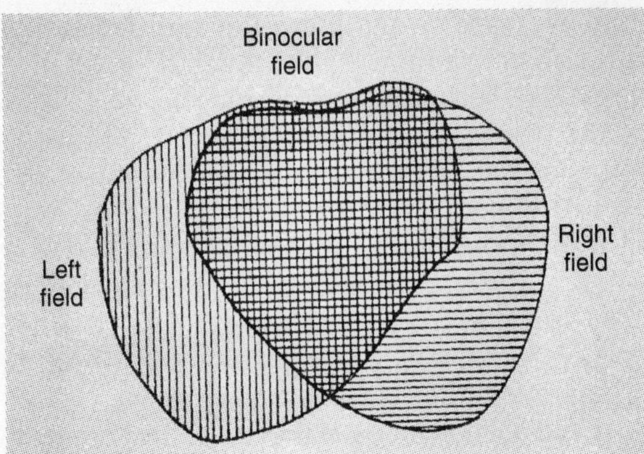

Fig. 32.26: Binocular vision. The visual fields of the two eyes have been plotted together. The central area represents the binocular vision.

are called the corresponding points. If two images of a single object fail to fuse, the condition is known as double vision or *diplopia.*

Depth perception in monocular vision is not very accurate. This can be appreciated by trying to thread a needle with one eye closed. However, even with one eye relative distance between the two objects can be perceived to some extent by moving the eye from side to side and noticing how the objects move in relation to each other. Close objects move, distant objects seem to stay still. Relative size of the images of known objects also helps to some extent to appreciate the relative distance.

EXTRAOCULAR MUSCLES

The innervation and the actions of the extraocular muscles are given in Table 32.1

Adduction and abduction refer to rotation of the eyeball around a vertical axis leading to movement of the pupil towards or away from

Table 32.1: Innernation and the actions of extraocular muscles

Muscle	*Nerve supply*	*Actions*	
		Primary	*Secondary*
Superior rectus	III C. Nerve	Elevation	Adduction, Intorsion
Inferior rectus	III C. Nerve	Depression	Adduction, Extorsion
Medial rectus	III C. Nerve	Adduction	—
Lateral rectus	VI C. Nerve	Abduction	—
Superior oblique	IV C. Nerve	Depression	Intorsion, Abduction
Inferior oblique	III C. Nerve	Elevation	Extorsion, Abduction

midline, respectively. Elevation and depression refer to movement of the eyeball around a transverse horizontal axis leading to movement of the pupil upward or downward respectively. Intorsion and extorsion refer to rotation of the eyeball around an anteroposterior horizontal axis. In these movements, the eyeball rotates like a wheel towards the nose (intorsion) or away from nose (extorsion). Torsion movements are not possible voluntarily but occur as a part of reflex response to tilting of the head.

In full abduction, the superior and inferior recti act as pure elevator and depressor, respectively. In full adduction, the superior and inferior oblique muscles act as pure depressors and elevators, respectively. Therefore, the function of extraocular muscles can be assessed more accurately if they are tested first in midposition of the gaze and subsequently in both full adduction and full abduction of the eyeball.

MOVEMENTS OF EYE

Extraocular muscles are involved in 5 different types of movements of the eyeball.

1. Saccadic movement
2. Smooth pursuit movement
3. Vergence movement
4. Vestibular movement
5. Visual fixation

1. Saccadic Movements These are rapid eye movements occurring voluntarily or involuntarily. For example, when one observes a painting or meets a person for the first time, one's gaze shifts from one point of interest to another and then another. Similarly, when traveling in a car, the eyes gaze on different objects one after another. In other words, these movements refer to the *jumping of gaze from one point to another*. The jumps may occur 2–3 times per second. During saccadic movement, 90% time is spent on gazing the points of interest and only 10% in shifting the gaze. Involuntary saccadic movements may be produced by visual or auditory stimuli.

2. Smooth Pursuit Movements These movements occur when one fixes one's gaze on a moving object; the eyes may follow displacement of an object up to 30° per second. Pursuit movements depend on visual information from areas 17, 18 and 19 and from superior colliculi. The movements of the eyeball follow the velocity of the moving object. In these and all other types of movements named above, the corticonuclear fibres project on the cranial nuclei of III, IV and VI nerves in the brainstem.

3. Vergence Movements Vergence or disjunctive (non-conjugate) eye movements enable the subject to fixate at varying distances in the visual field. There may be convergence or divergence of the eyeball, depending upon the distance between the object and the eyes. Vergence movements are slower than saccadic or pursuit movements. The stimuli for vergence movements are:

(a) Blurring of images at the retina leading to accommodation-convergence reflex.

(b) Displacement of images from the fovea. Cortical area 19 or 22 seems to be involved in the production of vergence movements.

4. Vestibular Movements These ocular movements are initiated by disturbances of visual fixation caused by movement of the head. Impulses arising in semicircular canals or the otolith organs travel via vestibular nuclei and median longitudinal bundle to the nuclei of III, IV and VI cranial nerves (vestibulo-ocular reflex).

5. Visual Fixation This type of muscular contraction helps to maintain an object on the fovea once it has been placed there by voluntary movements of the eyeball. The initial voluntary fixation is controlled by a small area in the premotor cortex of the frontal lobe. The involuntary fixation is controlled by areas 17, 18 and 19 of the occipital cortex.

LACRIMAL FLUID

Normal function of the eye depends on the presence of a thin film of tear fluid (lacrimal fluid) on its corneal surface. The tear fluid serves a number of functions:

(i) It helps in optical function by maintaining optically uniform corneal surface. Minor trauma to the exposed corneal surface is inevitable but the surface cells are quickly regenerated. The living state of these cells depends on the presence of watery fluid on their exposed aspect. The thin even film also compensates for minute irregularities present on the surface of cornea.

(ii) It serves a mechanical function of lubricating the inner layers of the eyelids.

(iii) It is important for the nutritive function for the outer layers of the avascular cornea.

(iv) Lacrimal fluid has an important defence function:

(a) It flushes out cellular debris, dust particles and other foreign materials which enter the conjunctival sac.

(b) It has antibacterial action due to presence of immunoglobulins, lysozymes, and some other antibacterial proteins.

The tear film consists of three layers:

1. Outermost is a thin (0.1 mm) oily layer derived from Meibomian glands and accessory sebaceous glands of Zeis.
2. A relatively thick (7 mm) tear fluid secreted by lacrimal gland and the accessory lacrimal glands of Krause and Wolfring (Fig. 32.27).
3. The innermost layer is extremely thin (0.02 mm) consisting of mucus secreted by the goblet cells of the conjunctiva. This layer is in contact with the cornea.

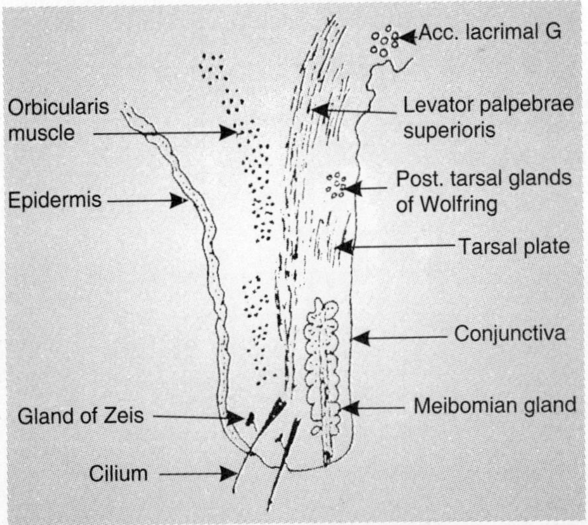

Fig. 32.27: Histological structure of the upper eyelid.

COMPOSITION OF TEAR FLUID

In the Table 32.2, the concentrations of some of the important constituents of the tear fluid have been compared with those of the plasma. It would be obvious that the fluid is produced by an active secretory mechanism and not merely by ultrafiltration.

Table 32.2: Concentrations of important constituents of tear fluid and plasma; a comparison

Constituents	*Tear fluid*	*Plasma*
Na^+ (mEq/L)	140	140
K^+ (mEq/L)	2.5	4.6
Cl^- (mEq/L)	130	99
HCO_3^- (mEq/L)	25	25
Total proteins (gm%)	0.7	7.5
Glucose (mg%)	2.5	100
pH	7.4	7.4

REGULATION OF SECRETION

As mentioned before, the tear fluid is a mixture of the secretions of the lacrimal gland, the accessory lacrimal glands of Krause and Wolfring and mucous glands of the conjunctiva. The main lacrimal gland is situated in the superior temporal angle of the orbit. A number of small ducts release the secretion into the conjunctival sac, mostly in the upper temporal region.

Under ordinary circumstances, the secretion of accessory lacrimal glands along with that of glands of Zeis and conjunctival goblet cells is sufficient to provide the basic requirements of the tear fluid. The chief lacrimal gland is seen to be activated only when the secretion of tears is reflexly increased.

The lacrimal gland is innervated by parasympathetic fibres present in the VII cranial nerve and sympathetic fibres coming from the superior cervical ganglion. The afferent fibres for the reflex secretion of tears arise from the cornea, conjunctiva and nose, and reach the CNS through the fifth cranial nerve. Intense retinal stimulation may also provoke the secretion of tears. The production of tears during emotional disturbances is due to psychogenic stimuli arising from the limbic system. Psychogenic secretion of tears is unique to humans in the animal kingdom.

32

ELIMINATION OF TEAR FLUID

At normal secretory rate, the tear fluid is confined to the conjunctival sac by the oily secretion of the tarsal glands (Meibomian glands) distributed along the lid margin. Tear fluid spills out of the lid margain only when either there is excessive secretion (reflex/psychogenic) or the drainage system is blocked.

About 10–25% of the tear fluid is lost by evaporation; the remainder is drained out of conjunctival sac into the nose through the lacrimal excretory system consisting of the superior and inferior canaliculi, the lacrimal sac and the nasolacrimal duct (Fig. 32.28). The tear fluid enters the canaliculi through the superior and inferior puncta present in the inner margins of the two eyelids. The drainage is helped by blinking.

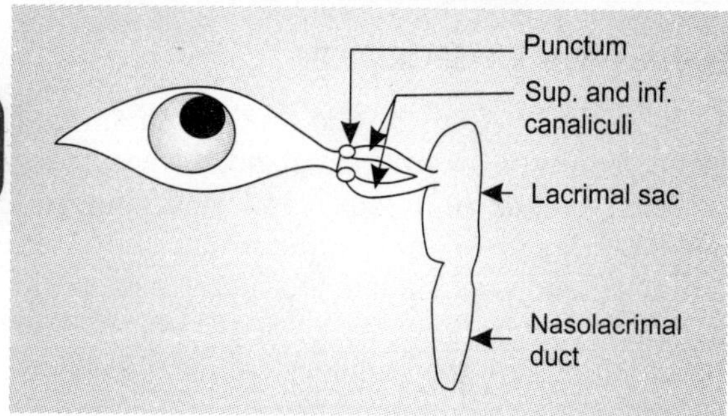

Fig. 32.28: The lacrimal excretory apparatus.

Blinking is produced by involuntary contraction of orbicularis muscle. It occurs approximately 30 times per minute (but at a far lesser rate when reading). Blinking results in:

1. Spreading the tear fluids over the eye and movement of tear fluids towards the puncta. Tear fluid enters the puncta due to capillary action but subsequently the fluid is propelled through the canaliculi into the lacrimal sac by the action of blinking.
2. Contraction of orbicularis muscle during blinking also draws the lacrimal sac laterally, creating negative pressure. As a result, the tear fluid is sucked from the canaliculi into the sac. When the orbicularis muscle relaxes, the sac collapses and the accumulated fluid in the sac is pushed down the nasolacrimal duct.

ELECTRORETINOGRAPHY

Electroretinogram (ERG) is an action potential evoked in the retina on exposure to a flash of light. It is recorded by placing an active electrode embedded in a contact lens on the cornea and a reference (indifferent) electrode on the forehead and connecting them through an amplifier to a polygraph. A flash of light produces an initial negative small a-wave followed by a large positive b-wave (Fig. 32.29A). The a-wave originates from the retinal receptors whereas b-wave originates from bipolar cells. ERG may be recorded in a dark adapted eye by a single flash or in a light adapted eye with 10 Hz flicker.

ERG is abnormal in congenital or acquired disorders of retina (Fig. 32.29B). It is of particular importance in the diagnosis of such disorders: (i) when a dense cataract in the lens prevents direct visualization of the retina by ophthalmoscopy or (ii) in very young children.

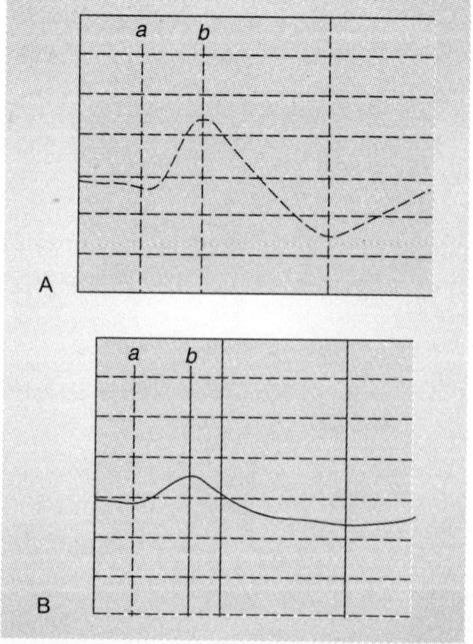

Fig. 32.29: Electroretinogram (ERG) in a normal individual (A), and a patient with retinopathy (B).

33 CHAPTER

Hearing

EXTERNAL AND MIDDLE EAR (Fig. 33.1)

The external ear leads into the tympanic membrane (eardrum). The sound waves strike the tympanic membrane and set it into vibrations. The vibrations of tympanic membrane cease immediately after the end of sound, i.e. the tympanic membrane is critically damped.

The sound waves are communicated to the internal ear by the ossicular system of the (air filled) middle ear (Fig. 33.2). The ossicular system consists of three delicate bones namely, the malleus, the incus and the stapes. One of the important functions of the tympanic membrane and the three ossicles is to provide a mechanical link between the transmission of sound energy in the air, with very low impedance and the fluid medium in the internal ear, with very high impedance. This function of the tympanic membrane and the ossicles is known as *impedance matching*.

The handle of the malleus is attached to the centre of the tympanic membrane. At the other end, the malleus is tightly bound to the incus by a ligament; so both the ossicles move in unison with

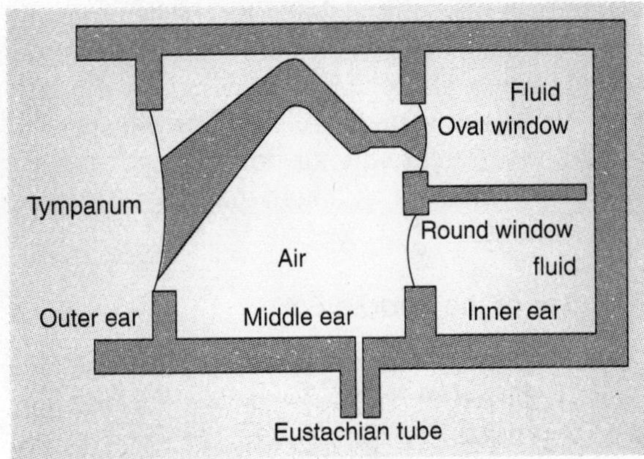

Fig. 33.2: Diagrammatic representation of the ear.

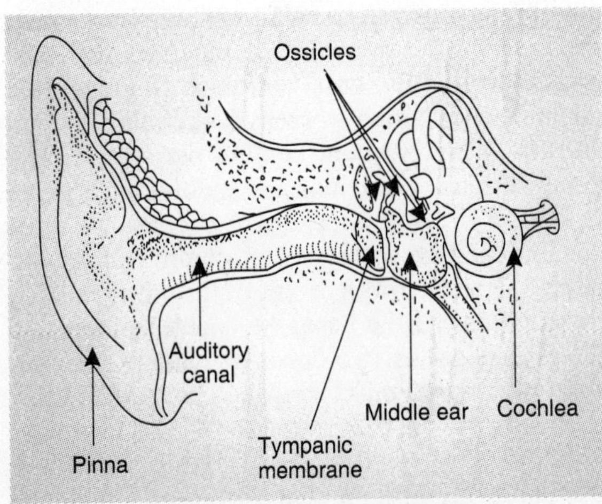

Fig. 33.1: Structure of the ear.

the vibrations of the tympanic membrane. The other end of the incus articulates with the head of the stapes. The oval base of the stapes fits into the oval window at the cochlea where it is attached by the annular ligament.

The mechanical advantage provided by the lever system of the middle ear ossicles increases the force of movement by 1.3 times. Moreover, the surface area of the tympanic membrane is approximately 50 mm^2 whereas the surface area of the oval window is only 3 mm^2. The difference in the two surface areas increases the pressure on the oval window 17-folds. Thus the pressure exerted by the sound waves on the oval window is 22 times (17 × 1.3) the pressure exerted on the tympanic membrane by the sound waves. In this way, the impedance mismatching between the air and the fluid medium for the transmission of sound is mostly compensated for. If the tympanic membrane and the ossicles are removed, and the sound waves strike the oval window directly, even very loud sounds are heard as whispers. It would be apparent why air-borne sounds are not heard by swimmers with both the ears submerged under water.

Muscles of the Middle Ear

The middle ear contains two striated muscles namely, the *tensor tympani* and the *stapedius*. The tensor tympani is attached to the neck at the malleus and keeps the tympanic membrane taut. Contraction of tensor tympani tends to pull the handle of the malleus inwards, whereas contraction of the stapedius pulls the stapes outwards. Both the muscles are reflexly activated by loud sounds (*tympanic reflex*). The threshold of activation of tympanic reflex is a sound of 70 decibel intensity. The force of contraction increases with the increase in the intensity of sound up to 100 decibels. These muscles seem to offer a degree of protection to the cochlea against excessively loud sounds like jet aircraft or loud music. Since, the latent period of the tympanic reflex is about 40–60 ms, the reflex does not protect the cochlea against sudden intense sounds, e.g. by gun shots.

The muscles of the middle ear are also activated just before vocalization or chewing. It seems, the muscles of the middle ear provide a mechanism to produce maximal senstivity to the environmental sounds and minimum senstivity to the self-produced sounds.

EUSTACHIAN TUBE

The Eustachian tube connects the middle ear with the pharynx. It is normally closed but opens up during chewing, swallowing and yawning. When open, the tube serves to equalize the pressures on the two sides of the tympanic membrane. Eustachian tube may be blocked as a result of throat infection. In such a case, the air trapped in the middle ear is partly absorbed causing inward retraction of the drum, accompanied by pain and temporary loss of hearing.

COCHLEA

The human cochlea consists of a spiral canal 35 mm in length. The canal makes two and a half turns around a bony pillar called the modiolus. The cochlear canal is 3 mm in diameter in the first turn but narrows down progressively towards the apex. A thin bony lamina, the osseous spiral lamina projects from the side of the modiolus into the canal. Throughout its length, two membranes, the basilar membrane and the Reissner's membrane, divide the lumen of the cochlea into three chambers called *the scala vestibuli, scala media* and the *scala tympani* (Fig. 33.3). The Reissner's membrane separates scala vestibuli from scala media; the basilar membrane separates the scala media from the scala tympani. Scala media contains endolymph whereas both scala vestibuli and the scala tympani contain perilymph. The composition of perilymph and endolymph is given in Table 33.1. At the apex of the cochlea, the scala vestibuli and the scala tympani communicate with each other through a small opening called helicotrema. At the base, the cochlea opens into the middle ear by two openings namely, the *oval window* and the *round window*. The oval window is covered by the base of the stapes and the round window is covered by the flexible secondary tympanic membrane. The organ of Corti, the structure containing the auditory receptors or the

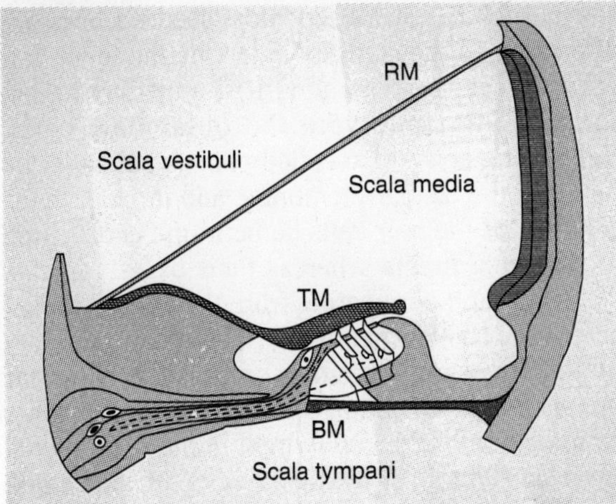

Fig. 33.3: Section of cochlea. RM: Reissner's membrane, TM-tectorial membrane, BM-basilar membrane.

hair cells lies on the basilar membrane. The base of the stapes is rather loosely attached to the oval window by the annular ligament.

The sound waves move the base of the stapes, which alternately moves into and away from the oval window. When the base of the stapes is *pressed into* the oval window, the pressure is transferred to the perilymph in the scala vestibuli and then through the Reissner's membrane to the endolymph in the scala media, pushing the basilar membrane downward. Finally, the pressure is communicated to the perilymph in the scala tympani causing secondary tympanic membrane to *bulge outward* into the middle ear (Fig. 33.2). Outward movement of the base of the stapes produces changes opposite to those mentioned above, ultimately leading to bulging of the secondary tympanic membrane into the internal ear.

Table 33.1: Composition of perilymph and endolymph (mEq/L)

	Perilymph	*Endolymph*
Na^+	150	1
K^+	5	150
Cl^-	125	130

The Reissner's membrane is so thin that, for the purpose of sound transmission, the scala vestibuli and scala media act as one chamber. Therefore, pressure waves in the oval window always set the basilar membrane into vibration. The chief function of the Reissner's membrane is to separate the endolymph of scala media from the perilymph of the scala vestibuli which is essential for the proper functioning of the organ of Corti.

Basilar Membrane Resonance

Although the cochlea narrows from its base to the apex, the width of the basilar membrane is minimum at the base and maximum at the apex (Fig. 33.4). The basilar membrane is composed of about 25,000 transversely arranged stiff elastic reed-like fibres that project from the bony spiral lamina to the spiral ligament on the opposite wall. The length of the basilar membrane fibres increases progressively from 0.1 mm near the oval window to 0.5 mm at the helicotrema. The stiff short fibres near the oval window vibrate at high frequency, whereas the long fibres near the apex tend to vibrate at low frequency.

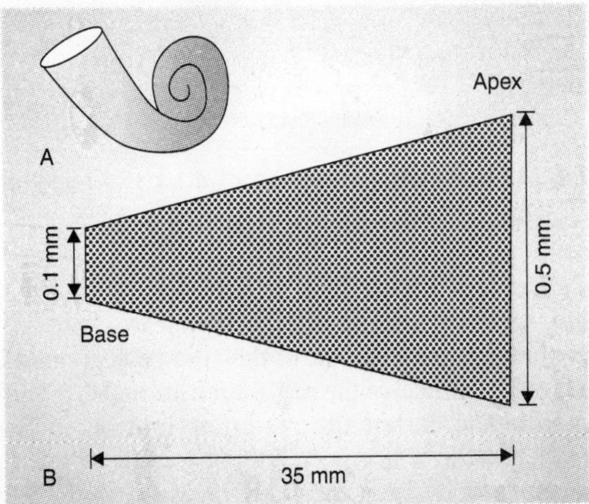

Fig. 33.4: (A) The cochlea (shown partially uncoiled) has a wide base which tapers to the apex. (B) The width of the basilar membrane (shown uncoiled) progressively increases from the base of the cochlea to its apex.

33

Organ of Corti

The organ of Corti is located on the surface of the basilar membrane. It consists of two rods of Corti and the hair cells. The hair cells are the receptors for the sensation of hearing. In relation to the rods of Corti, two types of hair cells can be differentiated. Internal to the inner rod is a single row of *inner hair cells*. External to the outer rods are 3–4 rows of *outer hair cells.* The inner and the outer hair cells are present on the surface of the spiral basilar membrane throughout the cochlea. Thus there are about 3,500 inner hair cells and 20,000 outer hair cells (Fig. 33.5).

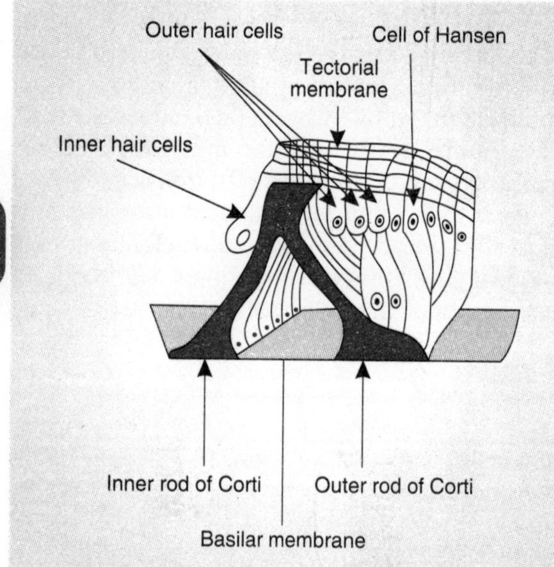

Fig. 33.5: Detailed structure of a part of cochlea showing the organ of Corti (the auditory receptor cells).

The structure of the hair cells is similar to the hair cells of the vestibular apparatus. In the cochlea, the minute hair or the cilia project out of the upper surface of the cell, pierce through a tough membrane called the reticular lamina to be embedded in a thin viscous but elastic *tectorial membrane* lying in the scala media (Fig. 33.5). The cochlear nerve afferents arborise around the bases of the hair cells. The spiral ganglion containing the cell bodies of the cochlear nerve is located within the modiolus.

About 90% of the cochlear nerve fibres are afferents and they chiefly innervate the inner hair cells whereas the remaining 10% are efferents and they mainly innervate the outer hair cells. Supporting cells (also called phalangeal cells) lie between the basilar membrane and the hair cells. The tips of the hair cells bathe in the endolymph of the scala media whereas their bases bathe in the perilymph permeating from the scala tympani across the basilar membrane. The impermeability of the Reissner's membrane and the reticular lamina help to maintain the difference in the ionic composition of the endolymph in the scala media from perilymph in the scala vestibuli and scala tympani.

Mode of Stimulation of Hair Cells

The basilar membrane is not taut. It is easily depressed into the scala tympani by pressure waves in the scala vestibuli. As mentioned above, sound waves set up a series of waves in the perilymph of the scala vestibuli. As the wave rises into the cochlea, its height reaches a maximum and then declines. The part of the cochlea where the height of the pressure wave reaches its maximum varies with the frequency of the sound. *High frequency sound waves produce waves of maximum height near the oval window, whereas low frequency sounds produce waves of maximum height near the helicotrema.* Correspondingly, the basilar membrane near the oval window vibrates in response to high frequency sounds. As the distance of the basilar membrane from the oval window increases, there is a gradual decrease in the frequency of sounds to which the membrane responds. Near the helicotrema, the basilar membrane responds to very low frequency sounds.

Upward movement of the basilar membrane moves the hair cells as well, causing bending of their cilia or hair against the tectorial membrane.

Movement of the hair produces a change in the membrane potential of the hair cells proportionate to the degree of displacement (generator potential).

Changes in the membrane potential of the hair cells seems to excite the cochlear nerve endings by releasing a chemical transmitter at the synaptic junction of the hair cells with the afferent nerve endings. Ultimately, the sensation of sound is transmitted as action potentials in the auditory pathways.

Efferent Control of Cochlea

The cochlear nerve not only contains auditory afferents but also an olivo-cochlear bundle containing inhibitory efferent fibres from the superior olivary nucleus. These cholinergic efferent fibres branch extensively and innervate the hair cells, particularly the outer hair cells. The central inhibitory control over the cochlea seems to provide a mechanism for improving the quality of hearing. The inhibitory mechanism selectively eliminates spontaneous activity among the auditory neurons and also excludes the background noise which interferes with the sound one is keen to hear.

Function of Inner and Outer Hair Cells

As mentioned above, the inner hair cells are one-fifth the number of outer hair cells but receive 90% of the nerve fibres present in the cochlear nerve.

The far more numerous outer hair cells are innervated by fewer nerve fibres which are mostly efferent fibres from the superior olive (olivo-cochlear fibres).

The *inner hair cells* are the *primary auditory receptor cells* which respond to movement of the basilar membrane and generate action potentials in the auditory nerve. The outer hair cells seem to play an important but indirect role in transduction of sound. The length of the outer hair cells varies in response to sounds as well as efferent discharge in the olivo-cochlear fibres. By changing their length, these cells vary the distance between the basilar membrane and the tectorial membrane. Hence, they change the sensitivity of the inner hair cells to a given movement of the basilar membrane. That is why, *outer hair cells* are said to act as *cochlear amplifier*. Their importance in the perception of sound can be judged from the fact that certain antibiotics (e.g. kanamycin) produce deafness even though they damage only the outer hair cells, leaving the inner hair cells intact.

QUALITIES OF SOUND

Loudness and Pitch

Sound consists of waves of alternating condensation and rarefaction of an elastic medium such as air (Fig. 33.6). Hearing is the subjective experience of exposure to sound waves. Normal human ear can hear sound waves of frequencies ranging from 20 to 20,000 cycles/second (Hertz). Some animals like bats and dogs can hear sounds with higher frequency also.

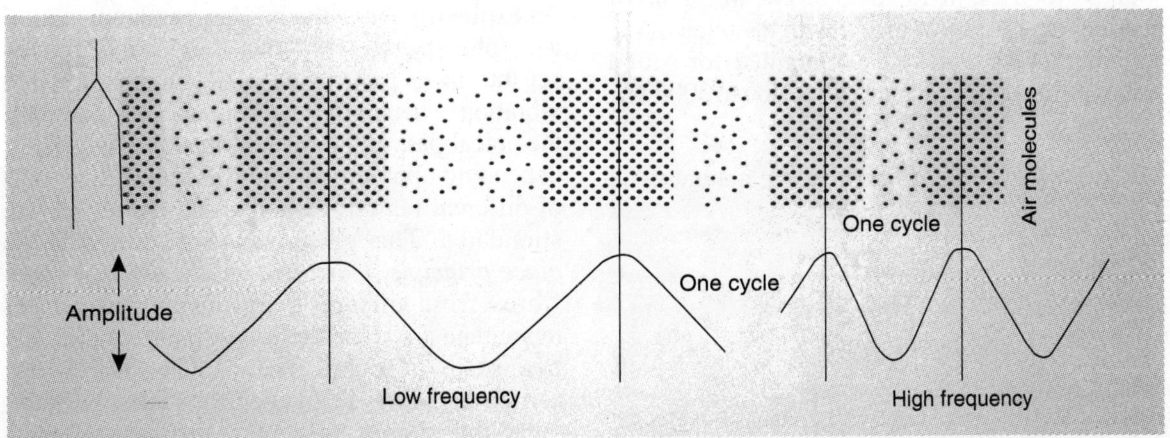

Fig. 33.6: Sound waves : periodic variations in air pressure.

For hearing of normal conversation, sound frequency between 200–4500 Hz is important. Vibrations above 16,000 Hz are called the ultrasonic waves.

Loudness of a sound is a function of amplitude of the sound waves. The *pitch* of a sound depends on the frequency of its waves. The high pitched female voice has an average frequency of 250 Hz as compared to the low pitched male voice with an average frequency of 120 Hz.

Human ear can respond to an extremely large range of sound intensities. The ratio of maximum sound intensity that can be heard without damaging the ear to the minimum sound intensity that can be detected is approximately 10^{12}. To describe such a large range of sound intensities, a log scale has been used. The unit of sound intensity is called bel. The 10-fold increase in the sound intensity is described as one bel increase, whereas 100-fold increase in the sound intensity is described as increase by two bels. Thus, an increase of 12 bels would cover the entire range of intensities of hearing of a normal human ear.

To provide a more refined index of sound intensities, a decibel scale has been used. One decibel (dB) is equal to 0.1 bel. Human ear can appreciate approximately 1 decibel change in the sound intensity. *Sound intensity just perceptible to a normal human ear (threshold of hearing) is called 0 decibel.* Using this as a reference standard, other sound intensities have been compared on a decibel scale. The intensities of some common sounds are given in Table 33.2. The threshold of hearing varies to some extent with the pitch of the sound. Lowest threshold is obtained for sound waves of frequency ranging from 1000 to 3000 Hz.

Table 33.2: Intensities of some common sounds (dB)

Sound	*Intensity (dB)*	
Hearing threshold	0	
Whisper	20	
Normal conversation	40–60	
Heavy traffic	80	Risk of deafness
Loud music	100–120	Risk of deafness
Jet plane	160	Risk of deafness

In this range the threshold of hearing is about 0.0002 dynes/cm^2 sound pressure (Fig. 33.7).

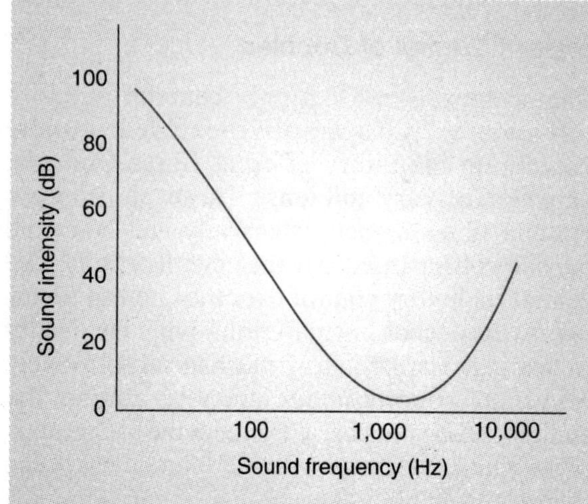

Fig. 33.7: Relation between frequency of sound and threshold of hearing.

NEURAL TRANSMISSION OF SOUND

Acting as a transducer, the cochlear hair cells convert the sound energy into electrical impulses. It remains to be explained how the two qualities of sound, the intensity and the pitch are transmitted along the neural pathways.

Determination of Pitch

As explained above the basilar membrane acts as a peripheral analyzer of pitch. High pitched sound set the lower part of the basilar membrane into vibration, whereas the low frequency sounds make the apical part of the membrane to vibrate. Thus, depending upon the pitch of the sound, hair cells of different regions of the basilar membrane are stimulated. This phenomenon is known as the *place principle*. Correspondingly, afferent nerve fibres from different regions of the basilar membrane are stimulated in response to different frequencies of sounds. The spatial organization is carried all the way in the cochlear nuclei, the brain-stem, the inferior colliculus, medial geniculate body and finally in the cerebral auditory cortex.

Initially, the place principle was proposed by Helmholtz in 19th century. But, he proposed that different parts of the basilar membrane resonate in response to different frequencies of sound (*resonance theory*). However, when the vibrations of the basilar membrane were visualized *in situ*, it was observed that each sound does not lead to resonance of a narrow segment of the basilar membrane. Instead, each sound initiates a wave which tends to travel along the entire length of the basilar membrane, from the oval window to the apex of the cochlea (*traveling waves theory*). There is a difference in the peak amplitude of the movements at different points along the basilar membrane. With low frequencies of sound, the peak amplitude of motion is near the apex of the cochlea. As the frequency of sound increases, the peak amplitude of vibration occurs closer to the base of the cochlea (Fig. 33.8). Thus, although the basic "place principle" was found to be correct, the traveling wave theory has replaced the resonance theory.

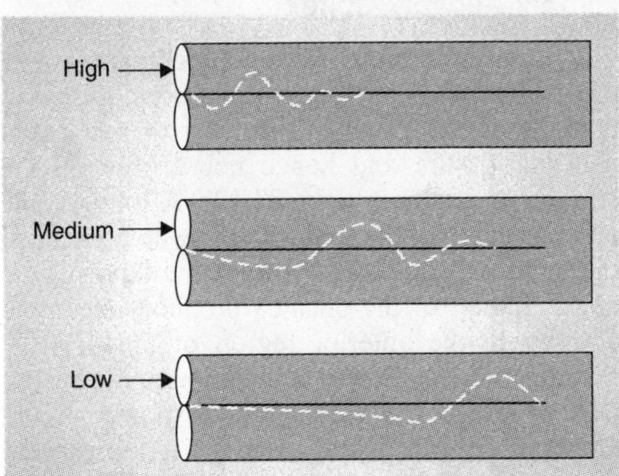

Fig. 33.8: Traveling waves of a basilar membrane in response to sounds of high, medium and low frequency.

The Volley Effect An additional factor seems to be involved in pitch perception of sound frequencies less than 200 Hz. Low frequency sounds are said to produce a proportional change in the frequency of action potentials. When the frequency is very low, the nerve fibres begin to discharge an impulse in response to each cycle of the sound waves (Fig. 33.9). The importance of this "volley effect" is, however, limited. The frequency of action potentials in a given auditory nerve fibre is determined by loudness rather than the pitch of sound (see below).

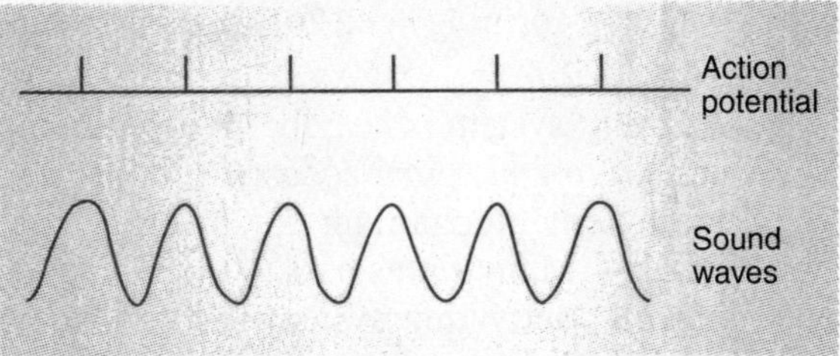

Fig. 33.9: The volley effect. The auditory neuron fires an action potential in response to each sound wave.

Determination of Loudness

The amplitude of vibrations of the basilar membrane increases with the intensity of sound. An increase in the amplitude of vibrations of the basilar membrane not only results in an increase in the frequency of afferent nerve discharge but also causes stimulation of a greater number of afferent nerve fibres (Fig. 33.10). Hearing with two ears is significantly better than hearing with one. At moderate sound intensities, there is summation of the effect. Subminimal stimuli for one ear may reach audible threshold level when heard by both the ears.

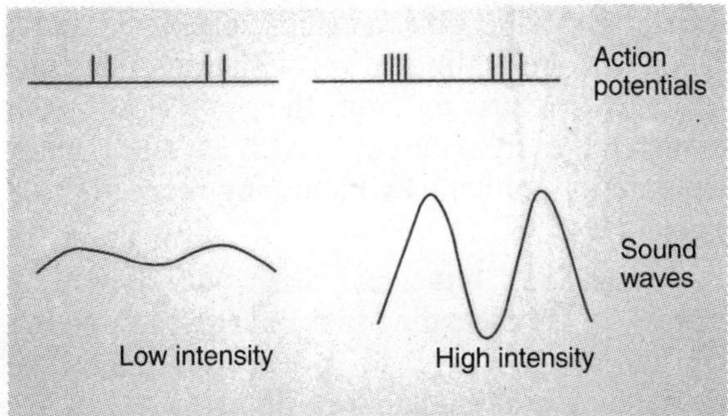

Fig. 33.10: Effect of intensity of sound waves on action potential in cochlear nerve fibres.

AUDITORY PATHWAYS

The auditory pathways are characterized by the following features:

1. Impulses from either ear are transmitted through the auditory pathways bilaterally with only slight preponderance in the contralateral pathways.
2. There is not only an ascending auditory pathway but also a significant descending pathway forming feed-forward and feed-back loops.
3. Auditory system is heavily involved in the brainstem and spinal acoustic reflexes and brainstem mechanism for audio-visual reflexes. Many fibres pass to the brainstem reticular activating system and produce a general arousal.
4. A high degree of spatial organization is maintained at all levels of the auditory pathways. Tonotopic organization can be demonstrated not only in the auditory cortex but also in the medial geniculate body, inferior colliculus, superior olivary nucleus and the cochlear nuclei.

All the fibres arising from the spiral ganglion of the organ of Corti enter the dorsal or ventral cochlear nuclei located in the upper part of medulla oblongata. Second, third and fourth order neurons ascend up and relay successively in the superior olive, inferior colliculus, medial geniculate body of the thalamus and the fifth order neurons finally terminate in the primary auditory area of the cerebral cortex.

The trapezoid bodies and the nuclei of the lateral lemniscus are additional relay stations for some of the fibres arising from the ventral cochlear nuclei. Fibres from the dorsal cochlear nuclei reach the inferior colliculus without any relay in these nuclei (Fig. 33.11).

The superior olive serves not only as a relay station for the ascending fibres but also as a centre for the integration of the ascending afferent and descending efferent auditory fibres.

Inferior colliculus is the most important centre in the brainstem for the integration of the afferent and the efferent auditory signals. The integration of visual and auditory information occurs due to interconnection of the superior and the inferior colliculi. The auditory pathways in the brainstem

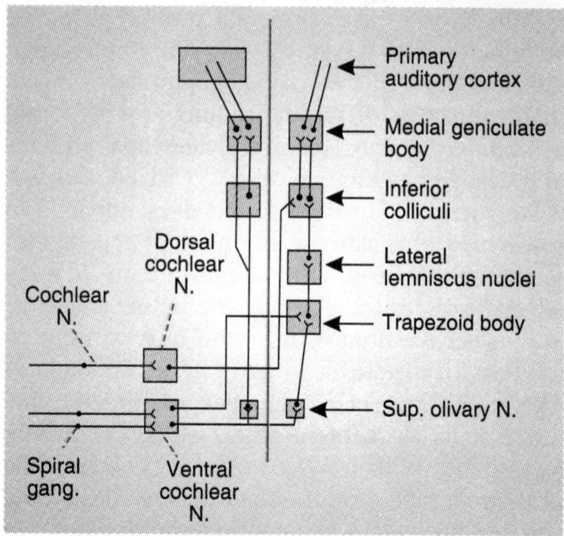

Fig. 33.11: The auditory pathways.

give collaterals to the reticular formation and the cerebellum.

Primary Auditory Cortex

The primary auditory cortex (Brodmann's area 41) is located in the superior temporal gyrus. In humans, it is located in the floor of the lateral cerebral fissure and hence not visible on the surface of the brain (Fig. 33.12). A tonographic representation of the cochlea can be demonstrated in the primary auditory cortex. Stimulation of the apical region of the cochlea produces electrical activity in the anterior region of the primary auditory cortex whereas stimulation of the basilar part of the cochlea produces response in the posterior region. Since, each ear is represented bilaterally in the auditory pathways, from the medulla up wards; the deafness is hardly ever produced by the cortical lesions.

The auditory association area, located around the primary auditory cortex, extends to the lateral surface of superior temporal gyrus.

Localisation of Sound in Space

A person can detect fairly accurately the direction from which a sound is coming. The detection seems to depend upon two cues. First is the time

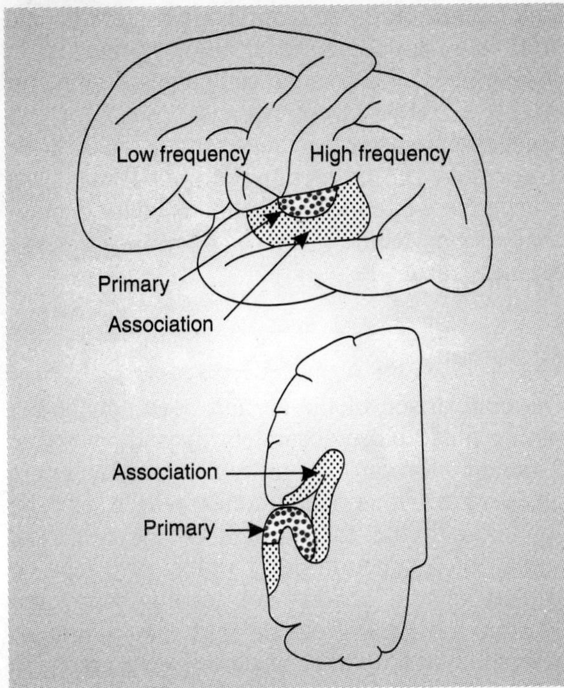

Fig. 33.12: The auditory cortex.

lag between the entry of sound waves in the two ears. For example, if a sound originates from the right side of a person, it reaches the right ear earlier than the left ear. Secondly, there is difference in the intensity of the sound in the two ears. The first cue is rather more important especially for frequencies below 3000 Hz.

Masking

It is a common knowledge that conversation is difficult in noisy surroundings. This is due to the fact that the presence of one type of sound decreases the ability of ear to hear another type of sound. The phenomenon is known as masking. Masking represents the inability of the auditory mechanism to separate the simultaneous stimulation into separate components. Masking is more effective for sounds with similar frequencies than with sounds for widely different frequencies.

EFFECT OF NOISE ON HEARING

The harmful effect of noise pollution has attracted attention recently. Continued exposure to high intensity noise causes hearing loss. The degree of hearing loss and its position on the tonal spectrum is related to the intensity and duration of noise exposure and the frequency range of the noise. Industrial noise and automobile noise is as much dangerous as music system played over 80 dB.

Deafness

Hearing loss may occur due to damage to the tympanic membrane or ossicles or due to a pathological fixation of the stapes in the oval window (otosclerosis). These types of deafness are grouped under the heading of *conduction deafness*. The other type of deafness, called the *nerve deafness*, is due to damage to the cochlea or the auditory nerve.

Two simple tests using a tuning fork with a frequency of 250 Hz are commonly used to differentiate *unilateral* conduction deafness from unilateral nerve deafness. These tests are based on the comparison of the perception of sound when conducted through the bone as compared to that conducted through air.

Air Conduction and Bone Conduction of Sound

Sound waves can stimulate the cochlea through:

1. Tympanic membrane → ossicles → cochlea (air conduction)
2. The conduction of sound waves through the bones of the skull (bone conduction).

Due to gross mismatching of the impedance between the air-bone and the bone-cochlear fluid, very little sound energy can be transmitted to the basilar membrane from the air by *bone conduction*. Therefore, this route may play a role in the perception of extremely loud sounds only. However, considerable "sound conduction" occurs if a *vibrating tuning fork* is applied directly to the skull. Even then, in normal individuals, air conduction is better than the bone conduction. In conductive type of deafness, air conduction of sound is affected but the "bone conduction" remains normal. In such patients, "bone conduction" seems better than air conduction. In nerve type of deafness, since the defect is in the cochlea/auditory nerve, both air conduction and bone conduction are affected. However, because of inherent difference between the air conduction and the bone conduction, the former remains better than the latter even in such patients.

TESTS OF HEARING

Weber's Test

In this test, base of a vibrating tuning fork is placed on the vertex of the skull of the subject. A normal person hears sound equally on both the sides. However, a patient with conductive type of deafness hears sound louder on the diseased side, because on the normal side the sound of tuning fork reaching through bone is masked by louder environmental noise reaching through air conduction. In nerve deafness, the sound of tuning fork is heard louder in the normal ear than the affected ear.

Rinne's Test

In this test, base of a vibrating tuning fork is placed on the mastoid process. When the subject no longer hears the sound, the tuning fork is held in air close to the external auditory meatus. In normal individuals, sound can be heard in the air after the bone conduction is over, i.e. air conduction is better than bone conduction: Rinne's test positive. In conduction deafness, Rinne's test is negative, i.e. bone conduction is better than air conduction. Rinne's test is positive in nerve deafness also.

Audiometry

The comparison of the air and bone conduction can be made more accurately by audiometry in a soundproof room. The instrument produces pure tones of various frequencies which can be delivered to the ear through an earphone for testing air conduction or by a vibrator placed on to the mastoid process for testing bone conduction. At each frequency, the threshold of hearing is determined and plotted on a graph. In this way not only the *degree of deafness* but also the *specific frequency range most affected* can be detected (Figs 33.13A–C). This information is of particular importance for the prescription of a hearing aid.

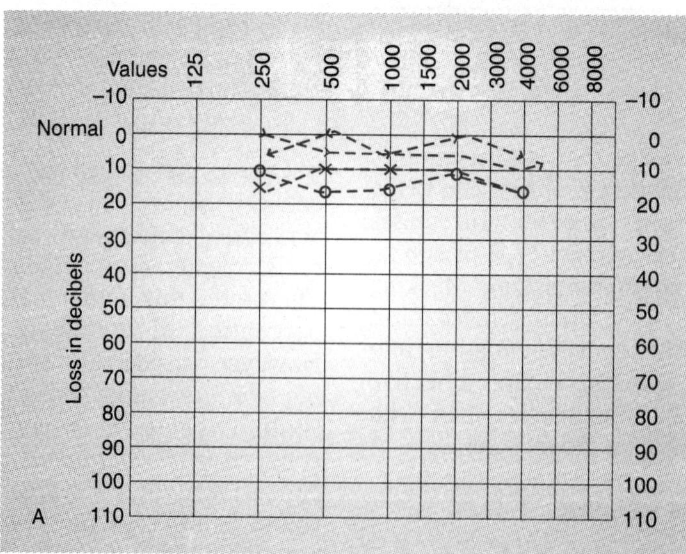

Fig. 33.13A: Normal audiograms.

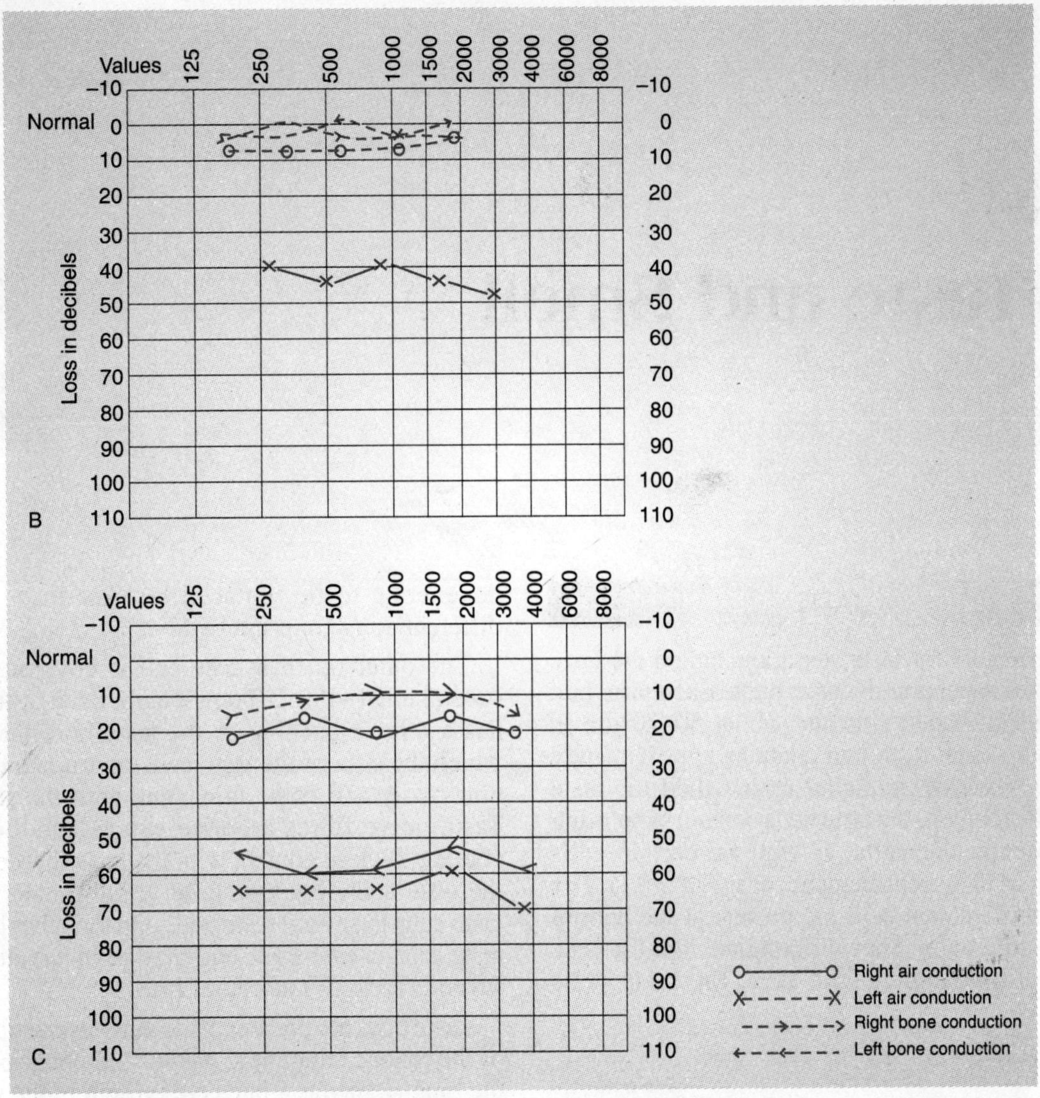

Fig. 33.13B, C: Audiograms. (B) Middle ear deafness, left side. (C) Neural deafness, left side. A 0 dB hearing loss implies normal threshold of hearing for air or bone conduction.

CHAPTER 34

Taste and Smell

TASTE

The receptors for taste sensation, called the taste cells, are located in the taste buds. Each taste bud is a barrel-shaped structure, about 50–70 μm in diameter. Each taste bud contains approximately 40–50 *modified epithelial cells* called the taste cells. In addition, the taste buds contain supporting or sustentacular cells, as well as, certain cells known as basal replacement cells (Fig. 34.1). The basal replacement cells are present at the bottom of the taste buds. They differentiate into the taste cells. After about eight days, the taste cells degenerate to be replaced by new taste cells differentiating from the basal cells.

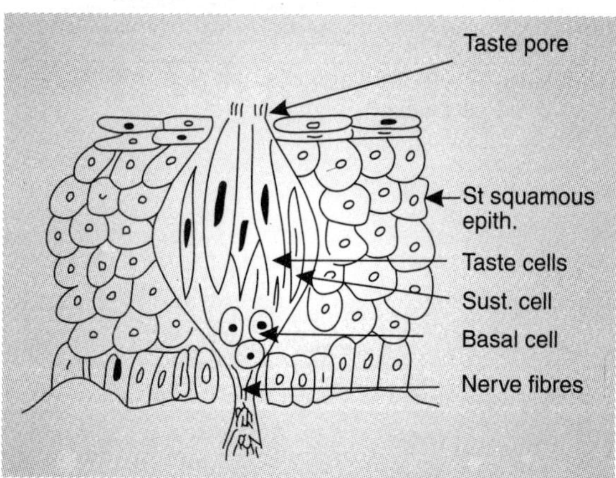

Fig. 34.1: A taste bud.

The outer tip of a taste cell is covered with several microvilli, 2–3 μ in length. Each taste bud has a minute opening or the taste pore through which the cilia of the taste cells protrude into the oral cavity and come in contact with the saliva. Taste nerve fibres arborise extensively before coming in close contact with the basal borders of the taste cells. Each taste nerve fibre innervates taste cells in several taste buds. On the other hand, taste cells in each taste bud may be innervated by several (up to 50) afferent fibres.

Taste buds are present in the mucous membrane of the tongue, epiglottis, palate, and pharynx. On the tongue, the taste buds are present in the walls of circumvallate and fungiform papillae. The circumvallate papillae are largest of all the papillae on the tongue. They are 7–12 in number, situated in a V-formation at the back of the tongue (Fig. 34.2). Each circumvallate papilla contains numerous taste buds. Each papilla is surrounded by a circular groove. Ducts of one or more serous glands open into the groove.

Fungiform papillae are smaller in size but far more numerous than the circumvallate papillae. They are especially numerous near the tip and the margins of the tongue. Each fungiform papilla contains a few taste buds.

In humans, the total number of taste buds is about 10,000. After the age of 45 years, the number of taste buds gradually decreases, resulting in blunting of taste sensation. The earlier belief that there are separate areas on the surface of the tongue where different tastes are best appreciated (Fig. 34.2) is no more held valid. All the taste sensations are sensed equally all over the tongue because all the taste buds practically respond to all the five types of tastes.

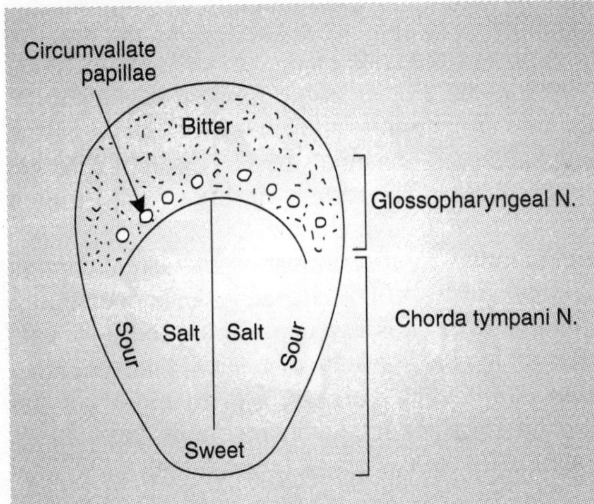

Fig. 34.2: An outdated concept of the areas of the tongue where the four tastes are best appreciated: Bitter substances are tasted on the back of the tongue, sour along the edges, sweet at the tip and salt on the dorsum anteriorly.

TASTE PATHWAYS

The afferent fibres for the taste sensation from the anterior two-thirds of the tongue are carried initially by the *lingual nerve,* a branch of V cranial nerve, which also carries general sensations like touch, pain and temperature from the tongue. Taste fibres leave the lingual nerve and enter the *chorda tympani nerve,* a branch of VII cranial nerve. Taste fibres from the posterior one-third of the tongue are carried by IX cranial nerve and those from the epiglottis, palate and pharynx by the *vagus*. Taste fibres in all these nerves are slowly conducting, thin, myelinated type. Ultimately, all the taste fibres traveling in different cranial nerves join the tractus solitarius to synapse with the neurons in the nucleus of the tractus solitarius. From here, the axons of the second order neurons join the ipsilateral medial lemniscus and relay in the ventroposterior medial nucleus of the thalamus. From here, the axons of third order neurons proceed to terminate in the inferior part of the ipsilateral postcentral gyrus (somatosensory cortex) (Fig. 34.3).

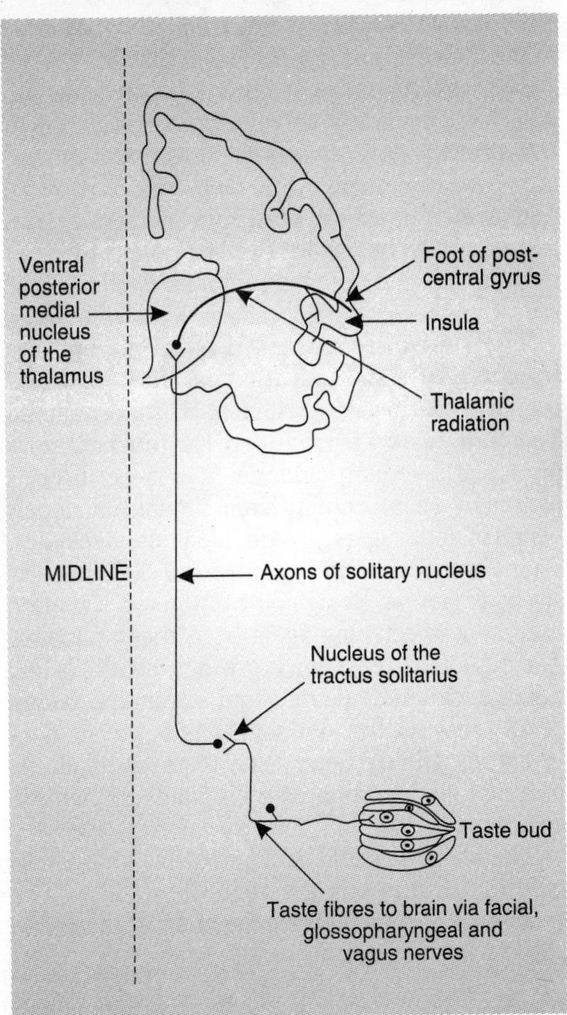

Fig. 34.3: Diagram of taste pathways.

TYPES OF TASTE

In humans, there are four well-known primary taste sensations, namely, **sweet, salt, sour** and **bitter.**

Now for over a decade, fifth primary taste sensation has been recognized. It is called **umami** (pronounced: oomomee) **taste** sensation. This sensation depends on the presence of the amino acid glutamate in the food stuffs. It gives "meaty" taste to the non-vegetarian dishes like chicken, ham or pork. The amino acid is present in some vegetarian food stuffs also, e.g. tomatoes, mushrooms. A salt of glutamate, monosodium glutamate (MSG) is a popular ingredient of most of the Chinese and Japanese cooking.

We can differentiate hundreds of different types of tastes. They result not only from stimulation of five primary taste sensations in different quantitative combinations, but also by addition of sensation of olfaction, heat, cold and texture, etc. *Flavour* is the best word to describe the complex sensation arising from the combination of all these sensations.

The sour taste is caused by acids and the intensity of taste sensation is approximately proportionate to the logarithm of H^+ concentration. The salt taste is produced by ionized salts particularly sodium chloride. The sweet taste is caused by a number of different organic chemicals which include sugars, glycols, alcohols, aldehydes, esters, etc. Saccharin is a chemical 600 times as sweet as sucrose. Being non-calorigenic, it is often used as a sweetening agent by diabetic patients. The bitter taste sensation is given by alkaloids like quinine, caffeine, nicotine and strychnine. Many deadly poisons, found in some plants, are alkaloid in nature. Highly bitter taste of these alkaloids prevents the ingestion of such plants by humans and animals.

The taste threshold of some of the substances mentioned above is given in Table 34.1. The sensitivity of taste buds for the bitter taste may be particularly noticed.

TRANSDUCTION IN TASTE RECEPTORS

Taste sensation can be evoked only after a substance has been dissolved in the saliva. The microvilli of the taste cells bathing in the salivary secretion of the oral cavity respond to various substances by production of a generator potential. Different substances seem to produce depolarization of the taste (receptor) cells by different mechanisms. For example, in case of sour taste, the depolarization of the cells is produced by the blockade of K^+ channels by H^+. Sodium chloride produces depolarization by influx of Na^+ through the *ungated* passive channels.

Table 34.1: Taste threshold of some substances

Substance	*Taste*	*Threshold concentration (μmol/L)*
Hydrochloric acid	Sour	100
Sodium chloride	Salt	2,000
Glucose	Sweet	80,000
Sucrose	Sweet	10,000
Saccharine	Sweet	23
Quinine	Bitter	8

The intensity discrimination by taste receptors is rather crude. A 30% change in the concentration of the substance is essential for appreciation of a change in the intensity of taste. Taste receptors also adapt very quickly, e.g. to maintain the sensation of sweet taste, lozenges have to be continually moved about in the mouth.

Functions of Taste Buds

The sensation of taste provides a source of pleasure—the pleasure of a tasty meal. It is interesting to note that sour or even bitter taste, at very low concentrations may make certain food stuffs tasty. The role of taste sensation in the secretions of saliva and gastric juice, etc. is described elsewhere.

To some extent, taste sensation may play a role in the maintenance of nutritional balance. Animals with salt deficiency show a definite preference for salt. The role of bitter taste in preventing the ingestion of many poisons has already been pointed out.

Phenylthiocarbamide (PTC) It is a chemical substance with extremely bitter taste. In most of the normal individuals, its threshold concentration for bitter taste is 20 μmol/L. But in a small percentage of normal individuals called non-tasters for PTC, the threshold is markedly elevated. *This "abnormality" has no clinical significance since* *no other taste sensation is affected.* However, inability to taste PTC is inherited as autosomal recessive trait and has been used in the studies of human genetics.

Absence of taste sensation is called ageusia whereas diminished taste sensibility is called hypogeusia.

SMELL

Sensory receptors of olfaction are located in the olfactory mucous membrane. In humans, the olfactory neuro-epithelium appears as a yellowish patch about 2.5 cm^2 in area in the roof of each nasal cavity, extending medially over the septum, and laterally over the superior concha (Fig. 34.4). In animals like dogs, with sharper sensation of smell, the olfactory mucous membrane occupies a larger area than in man. Such animals are called macrosmatics whereas humans with relatively poor sense of smell are known as microsmatics.

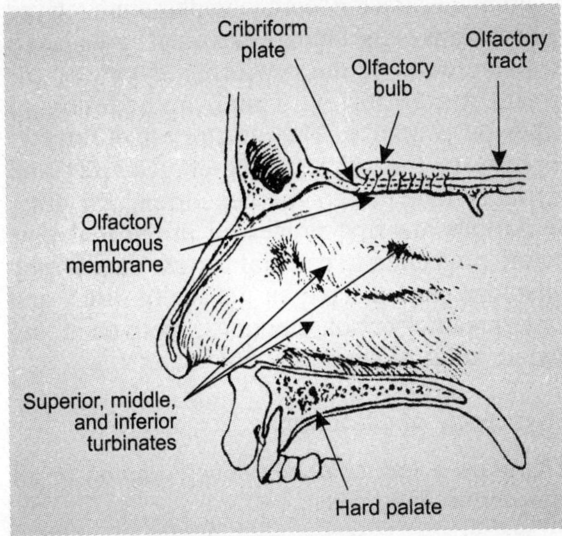

Fig. 34.4: Anatomical location of the olfactory mucosa.

Histologically, olfactory mucous membrane contains 10–20 million olfactory cells lying between the sustentacular cells. The superficial ends of each sustentacular cell contains many microvilli which secrete mucus. The superficial end of each olfactory cell forms a knob from which 6–12 fine cilia project and form a dense mat in the mucus secreted by the sustentacular cells (Fig. 34.5). The Bowman's glands lying just under the basement membrane also secrete mucus.

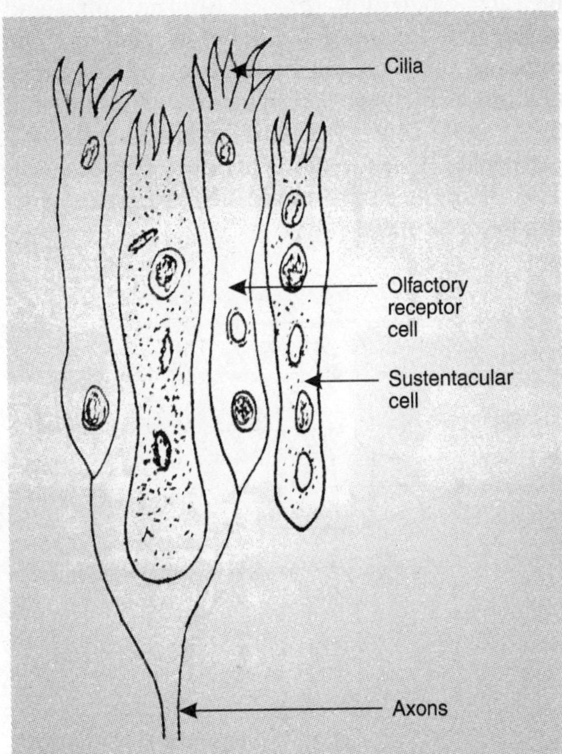

Fig. 34.5: Histological structure of the olfactory mucosa.

The olfactory neuron cell bodies are different from other sensory neurons in many ways: (i) They are the only sensory neurons whose cell bodies are directly exposed to the outside world. In contrast, other sensory neurons are sheltered in the ganglia and send long dendrites to the periphery. (ii) Olfactory neurons undergo a natural turnover every few weeks. They are unique in this aspect.

OLFACTORY PATHWAYS

The deeper axons of the bipolar olfactory neurons pierce the cribriform plate on either side to reach the olfactory bulb.

The olfactory bulb contains mitral cells as well as tufted cells. The axon terminals of the olfactory neurons form synapses with the dendrites of the mitral cells and tufted cells to constitute complex globular masses called olfactory glomeruli. On an average, about 26,000 olfactory axons converge on each glomerulus (Fig. 34.6). The mitral and tufted cells constitute the 2nd order neurons. The olfactory bulb contains two types of inhibitory neurons, namely the periglomerular (PG) cells and the granule cells. The periglomerular cells also participate in the formation of olfactory glomeruli. The dendrites of granule cell synapse with dendrites of mitral cells.

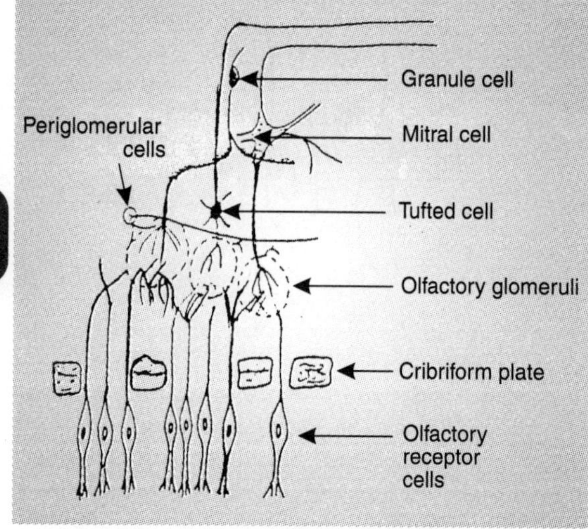

Fig. 34.6: Detailed structure of the olfactory mucosa.

The axons of the mitral and tufted cell run in the *olfactory tract*. Posteriorly, the tract divides into the medial and the lateral olfactory *stria*.

The axons of the lateral olfactory stria terminate in the ipsilateral olfactory cortex including the uncus. The axons of the medial olfactory stria cross the midline in the anterior commissure to synapse with the glomerulus cells of the opposite olfactory bulb (Fig. 34.7).

The olfactory cortex includes the anterior olfactory nucleus, prepyriform cortex, olfactory tubercle and the amygdala. All these are parts of the limbic system.

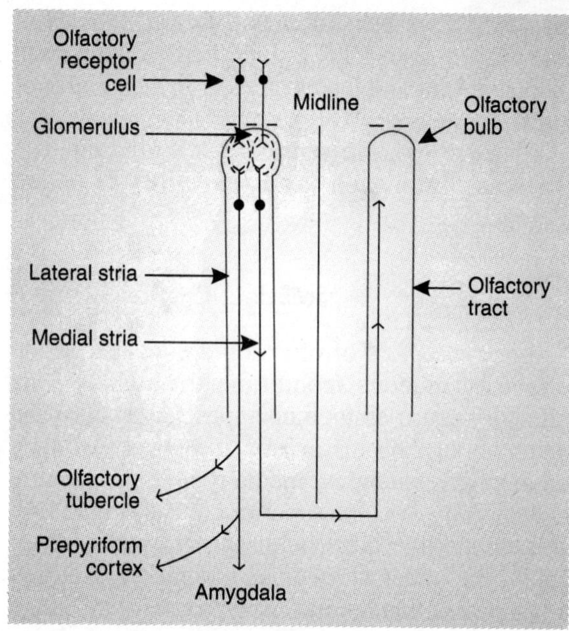

Fig. 34.7: The olfactory pathways.

From the olfactory cortex, impulses are relayed to other parts of the limbic system and via thalamus to many parts of the neocortex especially the orbitofrontal cortex. Thus, the anatomy of olfaction is unique. The olfactory tract projects directly to the primitive cerebral cortex and through thalamus to the neocortex. All other sensations are first processed in the thalamus before projection to cerebral cortex. That is why olfactory stimuli have an unusually direct and widespread effect on emotions, motivation and certain kinds of memory.

Physiology of Olfaction

There are a few characteristics common to all odoriferous substances:

(i) They are all volatile.
(ii) They are water soluble as well as lipid soluble.
(iii) Odoriferous molecules are small and contain only 3–20 carbon atoms.

There seem to be *over 50 primary smell sensations* (in contrast to 3 primary sensations of colour and 5 primary sensations of taste).

Humans can distinguish between 2,000–4,000 different odours. The odoriferous molecules dissolve in the mucus of the nasal mucosa and then bind with the cilia of the olfactory receptors. The consequent opening of Na^+ channels results in an influx of Na^+ and generation of a receptor potential. The receptor potential depolarizes the initial segment of the axon to the firing level. The impulse is then transmitted through the olfactory pathways. The olfactory threshold for some of the substances is given in Table 34.2.

Methyl mercaptan, a substance which gives garlic its characteristic odour has extremely low threshold. Like taste receptors, the intensity discrimination by olfactory receptors is rather crude. A 30% change in the concentration of the odoriferous substance must occur before any change in odour can be appreciated.

Table 34.2: Threshold concentrations of some substances for the sense of olfaction

Substance	*Concentration (mg/l) of air*
Ethyl ether	5.83
Chloroform	3.30
Oil of peppermint	0.02
Iodoform	0.02
Methyl mercaptan	0.0000004

Olfactory neurons adapt very rapidly. The perception of even most disagreeable smell, if constantly present, gradually decreases and may disappear altogether. Unlike adaptation of touch receptors, the adaptation of olfactory receptors may not be always functionally useful.

Sniffing

During quiet breathing, the air passes through lower parts of the nasal cavity. Through eddy currents, however, some air does reach the olfactory epithelium. The amount of air reaching the region of olfactory mucosa can be increased by sniffing. Sniffing is a semireflex response which occurs when a new odour is encountered.

Abnormalities of Olfaction

Absence of sense of smell (called anosmia) is rare. In Kallman's syndrome, congenital hypogonadism is associated with anosmia. Diminished sense of smell (hyposmia) is fairly common in old age.

Section IX

The Gastrointestinal Tract

CHAPTER 35

Functional Organization of GI Tract

The digestive system consists of an alimentary canal extending from the mouth to the anus, the salivary glands, the liver, and the exocrine part of pancreas (Fig. 35.1). The major function of the digestive system or the gastrointestinal tract (GIT) is to transfer nutrients, minerals and water from the external environment to the circulating body fluids for distribution to all the tissues. Most of the foodstuffs are taken in the mouth (ingestion) as large particles of polysaccharides, proteins and fats, which cannot cross the cell membranes. In the GIT, they are broken down into smaller molecules like monosaccharides, amino acids and fatty acids by the process of *digestion.* These small molecules cross the cell membrane of the intestinal epithelium to enter the blood circulation, or the lymph, by the process called *absorption.* Finally, the nutrients are either *assimilated* in the tissues or metabolised for the production of energy.

Different parts of the GIT are specialized for performing different functions aimed at digestion and absorption. For example:

(a) The oesophagus for transport of food from the mouth to the stomach.

(b) The stomach for temporary storage and digestion.

(c) The small intestine for digestion and absorption.

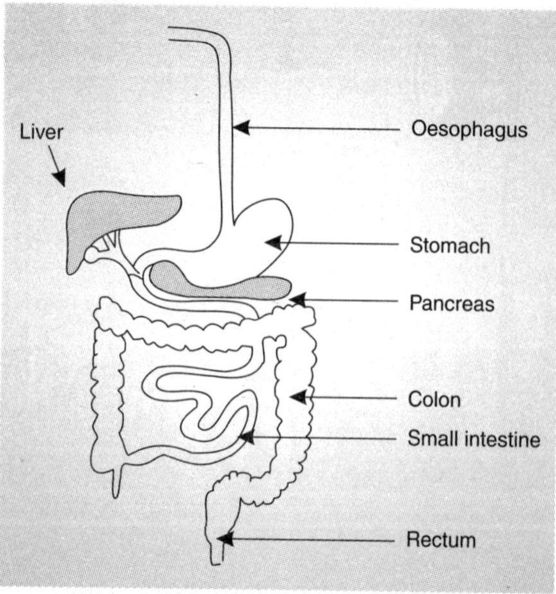

Fig. 35.1: The gastrointestinal tract.

(d) The large intestine for absorption of water and electrolytes.

Some components of the GIT have non-digestive functions. For example, the lymphoid tissue in the tonsils, adenoids and Peyer's patches constitutes an important part of body's immune system. It provides both the humoral and cellular immunity, which is especially effective against the microorganisms trying to enter the body from the alimentary canal.

PHYSIOLOGICAL ANATOMY OF GI TRACT

The gastrointestinal tract is basically a muscular tube, measuring approximately 4.5 m in length in adults. At either end, the lumen is continuous with the external environment. The general structural organization of gut has been illustrated in Fig. 35.2. Histologically, four different coats (layers) can be identified in the wall of the gut from inside outwards.

1. The Mucous Coat The mucosa consists of :

(i) The surface epithelium lining the luminal surface.

(ii) The lamina propria or the connective tissue layer containing tubular exocrine glands, small blood vessels, lymphatics and nerve fibres.

(iii) The muscularis mucosa: A thin layer of smooth muscle which separates the mucosa from the underlying tissue.

The luminal surface is generally highly convoluted due to the presence of many folds (valvulae conniventes) which increase the surface area available for absorption.

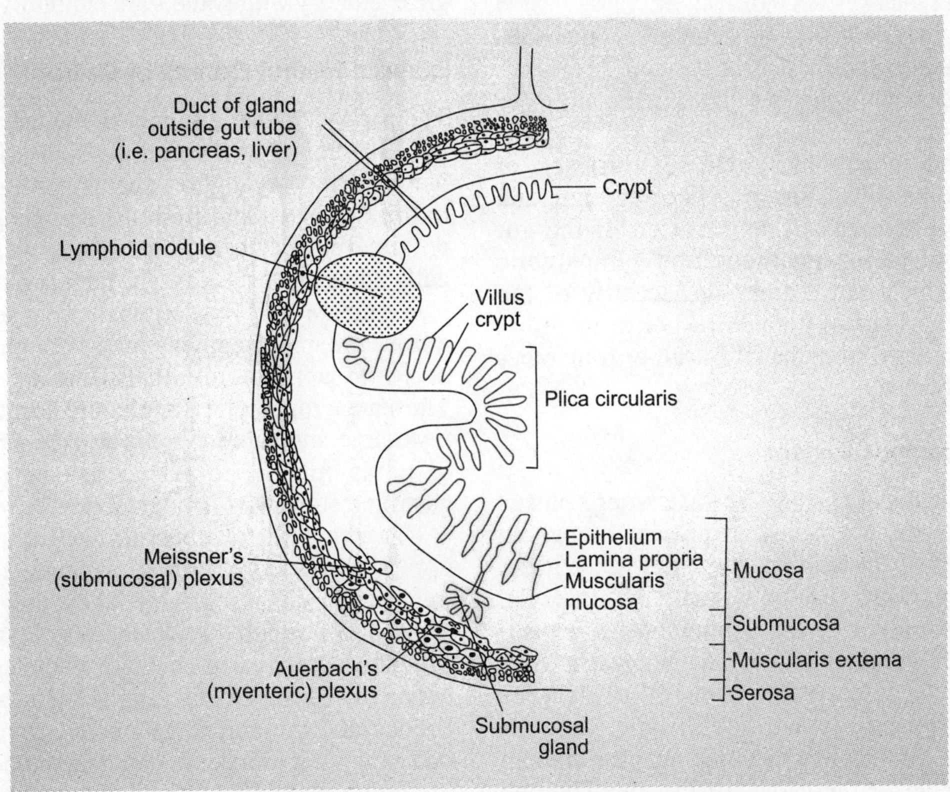

Fig. 35.2: Cross-section of the alimentary canal.

2. Submucous Coat Outside the mucosa is a layer of connective tissue, the submucosa, which contains a network of nerves cell and fibres called the *Meissner's plexus.*

3. Muscle Coat A thick layer of smooth muscle surrounds the submucosa. Actually, the muscle coat consists of two layers of muscle fibres, an outer layer of longitudinally arranged muscle fibres and an inner layer of circularly arranged fibres. An extensive network of nerve cells and fibres named, *Auerbach's plexus (myenteric plexus),* is located between the longitudinal and circular layers of the smooth muscle fibres.

4. Serous Coat This is the outermost layer consisting of a layer of connective tissue.

INNERVATION OF GI TRACT

The gastrointestinal tract is innervated by an *intrinsic nervous system* as well as by *extrinsic nerves*. The intrinsic nervous system, called the enteric nervous system, consists of:

(a) Meissner's plexus situated in the submucosa and
(b) Auerbach's plexus situated in the muscular coat.

The enteric nervous system controls most of the gastrointestinal functions like secretion and motility. The extrinsic innervation of the gut consists of parasympathetic and sympathetic nerves, which can modify the activity of the intrinsic nervous system in response to reflex activity initiated from the GIT itself or from other parts of the body.

Enteric Nervous System

The two neuronal plexuses, the Meissner's plexus and the Auerbach's plexus, are present throughout the length of the alimentary canal (except the oesophagus which has only Auerbach's plexus). They are present in the submucous layer and between the longitudinal and circular muscle layer, respectively. Each plexus consists of neurons forming synaptic junction with other neurons within the plexus or terminating near the smooth muscle fibres or the glands of the gut. The two plexuses are also interconnected with each other. In both the plexuses, the axons branch profusely, so that stimulation of one region produces a widespread response in the GIT.

The **Meissner's plexus** mainly controls the secretory activity and the blood flow of the gut. It also serves the sensory function receiving signals from the mucosal epithelium and from stretch receptors in the wall of the alimentary canal.

The **myenteric plexus** mainly controls the motility of the gut. Stimulation of this plexus results in an increased tone of the gut wall as well as increase in the rate and intensity of its rhythmic contractions.

There is a vast variety of neurons in the enteric nervous system. Besides the usual autonomic transmitters, namely acetylcholine and norepinephrine, the neurons of this system also contain many other neurotransmitters like vasoactive intestinal polypeptide (VIP), substance-P, somatostatin, etc.

Some of the neurons of enteric nervous system are excitatory while others are inhibitory in nature.

Extrinsic Neural Control of GI Tract

The parasympathetic supply to the gut is divided into the cranial and sacral divisions. The vagus nerve carries preganglionic parasympathetic fibres to the gut, extending from the oesophagus to the proximal part of the large intestine, as well as, to the gallbladder and pancreas. The sacral preganglionic parasympathetic fibres originate from second and third sacral spinal segments, pass through the pelvic nerves, to supply the distal half of the large intestine. The parasympathetic ganglia are located in the myenteric and submucosal plexuses. Stimulation of parasympathetic nerves causes *increased* gastrointestinal *motility* and *secretory activity*.

The sympathetic fibres to the gut arise from eighth thoracic (T_8) spinal segment to second lumbar (L_2) spinal segments. These preganglionic fibres pass through (but do not relay in) the lateral sympathetic chain, to continue as the splanchnic nerves. The sympathetic ganglia are located in the coeliac and mesenteric autonomic ganglia. The postganglionic fibres run along the blood vessels, to terminate mainly on the neurons of the enteric nervous system. Stimulation of sympathetic nerve fibres causes *vasoconstriction* and *inhibition of motility in the gut.*

REGULATION OF GASTROINTESTINAL MOTILITY AND SECRETION

In other parts of the body, the control systems chiefly regulate some variables in the extracellular fluids. But in the gut, the control systems regulate the conditions in its lumen. Correspondingly, majority of the receptors for these systems are located in the walls of the intestinal tract especially in its mucosa. These receptors are stimulated by one or more of the following factors:

a. Distension of the gut by luminal contents.
b. Acidity of the chyme.
c. Osmolality of the chyme.
d. Products of protein, fat and carbohydrate digestion, e.g. peptides, fatty acids, etc.

Stimulation of the receptors mentioned above produces reflexes whose effector cells are located in the gut itself, i.e. smooth muscle and the exocrine glands of the gut. The reflex activities maintain optimal conditions for digestion and absorption of the food stuffs. For example, increased acidity of the duodenal contents may be caused by rapid gastric emptying. It produces a reflex inhibition of gastric motility as well as gastric secretion, thereby maintaining optimum pH required for the activity of pancreatic enzymes and bile in the small intestine. These reflexes are mediated through neural and hormonal mechanisms.

Neural Regulation

The intrinsic or the enteric nervous system is involved in the regulation of motility as well as the secretory activity of the gut. The basic propulsive movements of the GIT depend on the integrity of enteric nervous system. The activity of this system may be modified by mechanoreceptors, chemoreceptors or even osmoreceptors located in the mucous coat of the gut. As a result, the peristaltic activity can be modified. These sensory signals arising from one part of the gut may modify the secretory activity of another part of the gut, e.g. low pH of the chyme in the duodenum decreases the acid secretion in the stomach.

The extrinsic innervation is involved in regulation of GIT motility and secretion in response to changes in the environment, e.g. effect of emotions, smell or taste on the gastric secretion and motility. Extrinsic innervation is also involved in the long-loop reflexes in the gut, e.g. gastroileal reflex.

Hormonal Regulation

Gastrointestinal secretions (or even motility to some extent) are regulated by a group of local hormones known as the gastrointestinal hormones.

These hormone-secreting cells are individually scattered in the epithelium of the stomach and small intestines and not in the form of clusters of cells as in the endocrine glands. The luminal surface of the cell responds to various chemical substances present in the chyme and causes release of a local hormone from the opposite surface into a blood capillary. Through blood circulation, the hormone reaches the target tissue situated in the nearby regions of the GIT. For example, the hormone gastrin is released by G cells present in the mucous membrane of pyloric part of stomach in response to the presence of peptides in the chyme. It reaches the body of the stomach via blood circulation to increase the acid secretion as well as the motility of the stomach.

Gastrointestinal hormones are characterised by two facts :

(i) Each hormone even at physiological concentration may affect more that one target tissue. For example, secretin increases the secretion of not only pancreatic juice but also of bile.
(ii) Each target organ is usually responsive to more than one gastrointestinal hormone. For example, acid secreting cells of gastric gland are stimulated by gastrin but inhibited by secretin.

Gastrointestinal Hormones

1. Gastrin

This gastric hormone is secreted by **G cells** (gastrin cells) present in the lateral walls of the mucous glands of the pyloric antrum. Three types of gastrins, namely G-34, G-17 and G-14 have been isolated. They have been named after the number of amino acid residues in each. G-17 is the principal form concerned with the gastric secretion. These gastrins differ not only in the number of amino acids but also in the sequence of the amino acids. Besides the stomach, gastrin has been found in the anterior pituitary, brain and peripheral nerves. The role of gastrin in these extragastric tissues is not clear. Pathologically, large amount of gastrin may be secreted by tumours called gastrinomas which may occur in the stomach and duodenum but are mostly found in the pancreas. The following discussion on gastrin pertains to G-17.

Actions

1. *Acid and pepsin secretion* Gastrin acts on the oxyntic as well as chief cells of the gastric mucosa and causes increased secretion of hydrochloric acid and pepsin respectively.
2. *Gastric motility* It increases gastric motility by increasing gastric peristaltic activity.
3. *Trophic action* It stimulates the growth of mucosa of not only stomach but also small and large intestines.
4. *Insulin secretion* After a protein meal, circulating gastrin increases insulin secretion by the islets of Langerhans. (Carbohydrate meal has no effect.)

Regulation of Secretion The release of gastrin is increased by:

(i) Distension of the pyloric antrum;
(ii) Presence of peptides and amino acids in the gastric contents;
(iii) Vagal stimulation;
(iv) Alcohol and caffeine.

The secretion of gastrin is inhibited when pH of the gastric contents falls below 2.0. The inhibitory effect of acid on gastrin secretion is partly by a direct action on G cells and partly through the release of somatostatin by the D cells of the stomach. Somatostatin is a potent inhibitor of gastrin secretion. This *negative feedback effect* of acid on gastrin secretion helps to maintain pH of gastric contents around 2.0, the optimum pH for digestive function of the stomach. Gastrin secretion is also inhibited by intestinal hormones like secretin, GIP and VIP.

2. Cholecystokinin (CCK)

Initially, it was believed that an intestinal hormone called cholecystokinin produced contraction of the gallbladder whereas a separate intestinal hormone called pancreozymin increased the secretion of pancreatic juice rich in enzymes. Later on, the chemical structure of the two hormones was found to be identical. Therefore, now it is clear that a single hormone released by the upper small intestine has both the properties. Hence, the hormone is now called cholecystokinin-pancreozymin (CCK-PZ) or more commonly as cholecystokinin (CCK).

A number of CCK hormones have been identified in different tissues, e.g. CCK-4, CCK-8, CCK-12, CCK-33, CCK-39, and CCK-58. These hormones differ in the length of their amino acid chains (macrohetrogenicity) as well as in the sequence of amino acids (microheterogenicity). In the duodenum and jejunum, CCK is secreted by **"I" cells**. It is a mostly CCK-8 and CCK-12. Their actions and regulation of secretion are described below. These and other types of CCK hormones have been detected in the brain and nerves but their function is not known.

Actions

(i) Secretion of pancreatic juice rich in enzymes.
(ii) Potentiation of the effects of secretin in the production of bicarbonate-rich pancreatic juice.
(iii) Trophic action on growth of exocrine pancreatic acini.
(iv) Contraction of gallbladder.
(v) Inhibition of gastric motility
(vi) Contraction of pyloric sphincter.
(vii) Increased intestinal motility.
(viii) Increased secretion of glucagon by islets of Langerhans.

Regulation of Secretion The secretion of CCK from the small intestine is increased by the presence of products of digestion particularly

(i) peptides and amino acids and (ii) long chained fatty acids. The release of CCK causes entry of bile and pancreatic juice into the duodenum leading to digestion of protein and fats. Thus, CCK secretion is further increased, providing a sort of *positive feedback action*. Positive feedback action is terminated when products of digestion move into ileum.

3. Secretin

In 1902, Bayliss and Starling demonstrated for the first time that a humoral factor (a chemical messenger) arising from the small intestine reaches the pancreas via blood circulation and increases the secretion of pancreatic juice. Thus secretin was the first hormone to be discovered.

Secretin is a polypeptide with 27 amino acids. Only one form of secretin is known. It is secreted by **S cells** located among epithelial cells of the duodenum and upper jejunum.

Actions

(i) Production of bicarbonate-rich watery pancreatic juice.
(ii) Potentiation of the action of CCK in the production of pancreatic enzymes.
(iii) Secretin increases the bicarbonate content of bile produced in the liver.
(iv) In the stomach, secretin decreases gastric acid secretion and increases the contraction of pyloric sphincter.

Regulation of Secretion Acidity of duodenal contents is the most important stimulus for the secretion of secretin. Products of protein digestion also increase its secretion.

4. Gastric Inhibitory Peptide (GIP)

GIP contains 43 amino acid residues. It is produced by **"K" cells** in the mucosa of the duodenum and jejunum.

Actions GIP was given this name because it was found to inhibit gastric secretion and motility. However, later on, it was realized that this action occurred only with high doses of the peptide. It has no gastric inhibitory activity at blood levels of the hormone normally seen after a meal. With such blood levels, GIP stimulates *insulin secretion* by ß cells of islets of Langerhans.

5. Vasoactive Intestinal Polypeptide (VIP)

VIP contains 28 amino acid residues. It is primarily a gastrointestinal *neurotransmitter* since it is found in the intrinsic nerve fibres of the GIT. It is included among the gastrointestinal hormones since it is also found in the blood. VIP has been found in the brain and autonomic nerve fibres in other parts of the body.

Actions

(i) It causes marked stimulation of intestinal secretion of electrolytes and water.
(ii) It causes relaxation of intestinal smooth muscle.
(iii) It causes inhibition of gastric acid secretion.
(iv) It causes dilatation of peripheral blood vessels.

6. Motilin

Motilin is a polypeptide containing 22 amino acids. It is secreted by **"M" cells** of the duodenal mucosa. It is also secreted by enterochromaffin cells of the intestine. Motilin causes contraction of gastrointestinal smooth muscle. It seems to be a regulator of gastrointestinal motility during the *interdigestive period*.

7. Somatostatin

This polypeptide exists in two forms, somatostatin-14 and somatostatin-28. Both forms are secreted into blood by **'D' cells** present in the islets of Langerhans and gastrointestinal mucosa.

Actions Somatostatin inhibits the secretion of gastrin, VIP, GIP, secretin and motilin. It inhibits pancreatic exocrine secretion, gastric acid secretion and motility and gallbladder contraction.

8. Serotonin

In the gastrointestinal tract, serotonin is secreted by enterochromaffin cells as well as by nerve endings. So it is both a local hormone and a neurotransmitter. It increases gastrointestinal motility.

9. Glucagon

It is secreted by **'A' cells** in the mucosa of the stomach and duodenum. Entero-glucagon seems to be a trophic hormone which stimulates the intestinal epithelial cell proliferation and renewal.

10. Neurotensin

It is a 13-amino acid polypeptide. It is produced by endocrine cells in the mucosa of the ileum. It inhibits gastrointestinal motility. It increases ileal blood flow. The release of neurotensin is increased by the presence of fatty acids in the lumen of the ileum.

36 CHAPTER

The Mouth and Oesophagus

In the mouth, solid food is mixed with saliva, chewed by the teeth and swallowed into the oesophagus. The chewing action of the teeth helps to break up large particles of food, as well as, break-down the indigestible cellulose membrane present in most of the raw vegetables and fruits.

The incisors provide a strong cutting action, whereas the molars have a grinding action. As a result, the bolus of food becomes a homogenized mixture of small food particles, salivary water and mucus, which is easy to swallow. The digestion of food is also facilitated by this process since digestive enzymes act mainly on the surface of food particles and cannot penetrate deep into large chunks of food. Moreover, increased surface area of the food particles is made available for the action of digestive enzymes.

SALIVARY SECRETION

The saliva is secreted by three pairs of major salivary glands, namely, the parotid glands, submandibular glands and sublingual glands, as well as, by many small groups of acini (Fig. 36.1) scattered in the mucous membrane of buccal cavity. The salivary glands secrete approximately 1500 ml of saliva per day. Saliva consists of 99% water and only 1% solids. The organic components of the solids include *mucus* and an enzyme called *salivary amylase.*

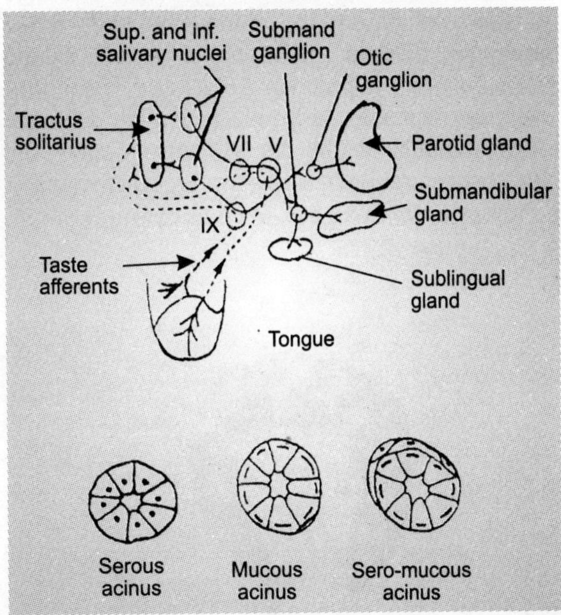

Fig. 36.1: The three salivary glands. (A) The neural pathways involved in the reflex salivary secretion. (B) Different type of acini in the salivary glands.

The important inorganic constituents include Na^+, K^+, Cl^-, HCO_3 and Ca^{2+}. The salivary pH is around 6.4–7.0. Under resting conditions, the concentrations of Na^+ and Cl^- in the saliva are always lower than that in the plasma. Consequently, the saliva is always hypotonic. On the other hand, concentrations of K^+ and HCO_3^- are higher than those in plasma. The saliva secreted by the parotid gland is a *serous fluid* containing the enzyme amylase. The sublingual gland secretes a *mucoid type* of fluid containing mucus. The secretion of submandibular gland is seromucus.

The ionic composition of saliva varies with its rate of flow, as explained below.

Mechanism of Salivary Secretion

Saliva is formed as a result of primary acinar secretion, followed by its modification in the ducts of the salivary glands. The primary secretion contains organic, as well as, the inorganic constituents. This fluid is isotonic with plasma. As the secretion passes through the ducts, the ductal cells actively reabsorb Na^+ and in exchange transfer some K^+ into the lumen (Fig. 36.2). Since the ductal epithelium is impermeable to H_2O, the saliva becomes hypotonic. As the rate of salivary secretion increases, less time is available for the ionic exchange in the ducts. Consequently, the NaCl concentration of salivary secretion increases. Its tonicity increases but, even at the highest rate of flow, saliva remains hypotonic with respect to plasma. At high rates of salivary secretion, the secretory rate of HCO_3^- also increases. Hence, the salivary pH tends to increase from the resting value of about 6.4 to a value of about 7.8 (Fig. 36.3).

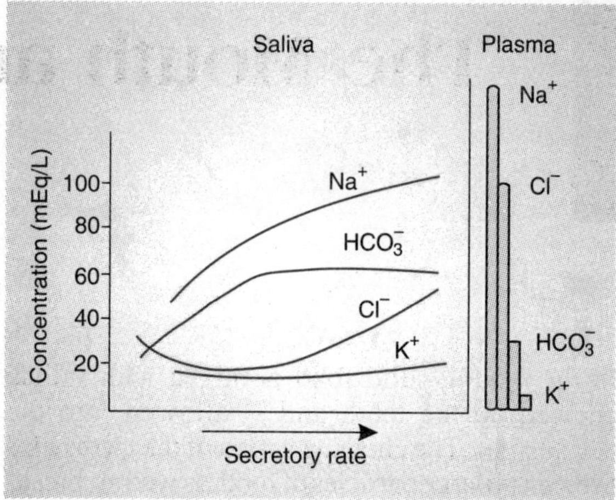

Fig. 36.3: Effect of secretory rate on the ionic composition of the saliva.

Fig. 36.2: Mechanism of secretion of saliva.

Aldosterone, a mineralocorticoid secreted by adrenal cortex, decreases the salivary concentration of Na^+ by an action on the ductal cells. Like renal tubules, Na^+ is exchanged for K^+ ion in the ductal cells. Therefore, the K^+ concentration of the saliva is secondarily increased. Aldosterone is secreted in response to salt deficiency or hypovolemia. It acts on the renal tubules and helps to maintain normal salt and water balance of the body. Since all the saliva secreted by the salivary glands is swallowed along with the food, any change in its Na^+ concentration would not affect the Na^+ balance of the body at all. Therefore, the action of aldosterone on the human salivary secretion is of academic interest only.

Neural Regulation of Salivary Secretion

Under resting conditions, about 0.5 ml of saliva is secreted per minute. Presence of food in the mouth reflexly increases the rate of salivary secretion up to 8 ml/min. Both taste and tactile stimuli from the tongue and other parts of the buccal cavity increase the salivary secretion. The afferent fibres are carried by V, VII, IX and X cranial nerves to the **superior and inferior salivary nuclei** situated in the brainstem. VII cranial nerve carries parasympathetic efferent fibres arising from the superior salivary nucleus to the submandibular and sublingual gland, whereas IX cranial nerve carries parasympathetic efferent fibres arising from the inferior salivary nucleus to the parotid gland (Fig. 36.1).

Sympathetic fibres to the salivary glands arise from thoracic 1 and 2 segments and relay in the superior cervical ganglion.

Experimental stimulation of parasympathetic fibres to the salivary glands causes secretion of a large volume of watery saliva, i.e. saliva poor in organic constituents. It also results in vasodilatation in the salivary glands in an indirect manner. On the other hand, stimulation of sympathetic fibres causes vasoconstriction in the salivary glands and transient secretion of a very small amount of thick viscid saliva rich in organic constituents. *Essentially, the salivary secretion is controlled by parasympathetic innervation.* After parasympathetic nerve resection, the salivary secretion ceases and the glands atrophy. In contrast, resection of sympathetic fibres has no effect on the salivary secretion.

Salivary secretion is increased by:

1. Presence of Food in the Oral Cavity The reflex secretion is mediated by stimulation of taste buds via the reflex arc described above. Stimulation of certain taste receptors (e.g. for sour taste) causes more profuse salivation than other taste receptors. This type of salivation is an *unconditioned response, i.e. it is a true reflex.*

2. Tactile Stimulation of Oral Cavity Presence of even non-edible material in the mouth may cause profuse salivation, e.g. surgical instruments during dental treatment or even smooth surfaced pebbles.

3. Conditioned Salivary Secretion Sight, smell or even thought of tasty food may increase salivary secretion (makes the mouth water). This is a type of conditioned response, i.e. previous experience of the unconditioned stimulus (taste of food) is a pre-requisite for the response. Impulses originating from visual, olfactory or limbic cortex act on the medullary salivary nuclei and increase parasympathetic discharge to the salivary glands.

4. Reflux of Gastric Juice into lower end of oesophagus reflexly increases the salivary secretion.

Unlike other gastrointestinal glands, there is no hormonal regulation of salivary secretion.

Under resting conditions, the small amount of saliva is chiefly secreted by the submandibular gland. On stimulation, there is greater increase in secretion of the parotid gland and the two glands are responsible for 90% of the total salivary secretion (Table 36.1).

Table 36.1: Percentage contribution of different salivary glands under resting and stimulated conditions

Gland	*Resting*	*Stimulated*
Parotid	20%	45%
Submandibular	70%	45%
Sublingual	2%	2%
Accessory glands	8%	8%

FUNCTIONS OF SALIVA

1. The role of salivary amylase in the **digestion of polysaccharides** is limited by the short duration of salivary action. When the bolus of food reaches the stomach and mixes with the gastric juice, the gastric acidity (pH 2) stops the action of salivary amylase (optimum pH 6.5–7).

2. Saliva serves a far more important function, i.e. the **maintenance of oral hygiene.** Saliva helps to *wash away the food particles* that remain in the oral cavity at the end of a meal. (A thorough rinsing of mouth with water or brushing of the teeth are still better). In this way, growth of the harmful bacteria in the oral cavity is prevented. Moreover, saliva contains *several proteolytic enzymes and antibodies* that have bactericidal action.

3. Saliva not only partially **liquefies** the solid food but also its mucus content **lubricates** the bolus of food assisting in its *deglutition.*

4. Saliva serves as **a solvent** for the molecules to reach the **taste** receptors in the taste buds.

5. By keeping the mouth, lips and tongue moist, saliva helps in **speech**.

DEFENCE MECHANISMS OF THE MOUTH

In spite of exposure to environmental microorganisms, especially from the ingested uncooked vegetables and fruit, oral cavity is seldom ulcerated by the bacterial infections. A number of innate and acquired factors are responsible for the defence of the oral mucosa.

1. Epithelial Barrier The oral mucosa is lined with stratified squamous epithelium which is keratinized to a varying degree in different regions of the cavity. Such epithelium is an effective barrier against infections.

2. Epithelial Cell Renewal The superficial cell layers of the oral mucosa are constantly being shed and replaced by cells from the deeper epithelial layers. Thus, if any pathogenic microorganisms tend to colonize on the surface cells, they are soon shed off, swallowed and destroyed by the gastric juice.

3. Mechanical Washing by Saliva Saliva helps in the removal of the desquamated epithelial cells loaded with non-pathogenic bacteria normally present in the mouth or with any pathogenic bacteria trying to colonize. The cells and the bacteria are washed away into the stomach.

4. Microbial Antagonism The presence of a large number of non-pathogenic bacteria creates an environment, which is non-conducive for the growth of pathogenic microorganisms. This phenomenon of microbial antagonism may be due to removal of some nutrients or production of some factors toxic to the bacteria not normally present there.

5. Lysozyme Salivary lysozyme seems to inhibit the growth of pathogenic bacteria without affecting the growth of the normal bacterial flora.

6. Antibodies The oral mucosa is covered with a coat of mucus which contains IgA, the immunoglobulins secreted by the salivary glands.

Oesophagus

The oesophageal secretions are mostly mucoid in nature. The mucus helps in the propulsion of food during deglutition. The mucosa of the lower end of the oesophagus contains many large compound mucous glands. The secretion of these glands protects the oesophagus from digestion by strong gastric acid which often regurgitates into the lower end of the oesophagus.

Deglutition

Deglutition or **swallowing** is a three stage process that transfers the chewed food from the mouth to the stomach. The first or the oral stage is voluntary. The next two stages, namely, the pharyngeal stage and the oesophageal stage are reflex in nature. The reflex activity is coordinated by a *swallowing centre located in the medulla oblongata and lower pons.*

Oral Stage

When the chewed food is ready for swallowing, it is voluntarily rolled back into the pharynx by the backward and upward pressure of the tongue against the palate. This initiates the involuntary or the reflex mechanisms of swallowing.

Pharyngeal Stage

Oral opening of the pharynx, specially the *tonsillar pillars*, *soft palate* and *epiglottis* contain *sensory receptors* for the swallowing reflex. *The afferent fibres* pass via V and IX cranial nerves to the tractus solitarius in the brainstem. The *swallowing centre* consists of a group of neurons located in the reticular formation of the medulla and lower pons. This centre brings about coordinated and sequential contraction of a number of striated and smooth muscles in the pharynx and oesophagus. The *efferent fibres* involved in this reflex are carried by V, IX, X and XII cranial nerves constituting a pharyngeal plexus.

In the pharyngeal stage of swallowing:

(i) The soft palate is elevated, sealing the nasopharynx and preventing the food from entering it.
(ii) The larynx is elevated and thus the epiglottis closes the superior opening of the larynx.
(iii) The vocal cords are approximated and the breathing is temporarily stopped (*deglutition apnoea*).

The multiple responses mentioned above leave no chance for the food to enter the respiratory passages. At the same time, upper 3–4 cm of the oesophagus (normally under tonic contraction constituting the upper esophageal sphincter) relaxes. A rapid peristaltic wave starting in the pharyngeal muscles, passes into the oesophagus, thereby propelling food into the upper part of oesophagus. Once the bolus of food has passed in to the oesophagus, normal breathing is resumed and the upper oesophagus goes into tonic contraction once again. This stage is completed in 1–2 seconds.

Oesophageal Stage (Colour Plate 3, Fig. 9)

The peristaltic wave, which begins in the pharynx, travels down the oesophagus up to its lower end, pushing the bolus of food ahead of it (Fig. 36.4).

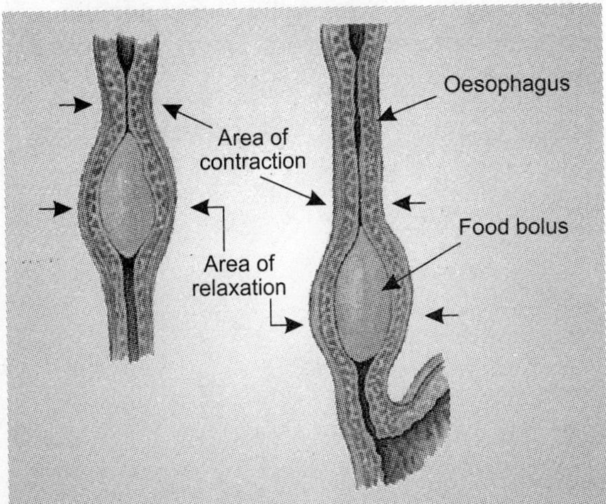

Fig. 36.4: Peristaltic wave in oesophagus.

The lower 2–5 cm of oesophagus normally remains tonically contracted constituting the lower oesophageal sphincter. As the peristaltic wave approaches this segment, the sphincter relaxes and the bolus of food enters the stomach without encountering any resistance. This stage is completed in 5–10 seconds.

In the upright position, the liquids and semisolid foods, under the effect of gravity, reach the lower end of oesophagus ahead of the *primary peristaltic wave* described above. A bolus of solid food may require one or more *secondary peristaltic waves* for its transfer to the stomach.

The primary peristaltic wave always starts from the pharynx as a part of the swallowing reflex. It may not be able to push a bolus of solid food all the way down the oesophagus. In that case, the secondary peristaltic waves are initiated by the distension of oesophagus by the bolus of food. The secondary peristaltic waves can originate in any part of oesophagus depending on the position of the residual bolus of food. One or more secondary peristaltic waves may be required to transfer the bolus into the stomach.

Upper and Lower Oesophageal Sphincters

At the upper and the lower ends of the oesophagus, the tonic contraction of its smooth muscle converts these regions into *physiological sphincters*. These regions are normally closed and open only during deglutition, when the peristaltic waves pass over them. However, histologically, no difference can be detected between the region of sphincteric action and the rest of oesophagus.

The upper oesophageal sphincter serves to prevent the entry of air into the oesophagus during normal respiration. The principal function of *lower oesophageal sphincter* (also called the cardiac sphincter) is to prevent regurgitation of gastric contents (food, gastric juice and air) into the oesophagus. If the intragastric pressure is markedly raised, e.g. after a heavy meal or ingestion of carbonated drinks, the resistance of cardiac sphincter is overcome and air escapes into the mouth (belching).

The local hormone, gastrin, increases the tone of cardiac sphincter which may help to keep the sphincter more tightly closed during digestion.

Achalasia

This oesophageal disorder is characterised by failure of the lower oesophageal sphincter to relax during swallowing. The fundamental defect lies in the degeneration of Auerbach's plexus especially of VIP secreting neurons, in the lower oesophagus. During each meal, food tends to collect in the oesophagus, from where it slowly passes into the stomach. Ultimately, marked dilatation of oesophagus results. Achalasia can occur at any age, but is more common in adults over 25. The chief symptom of the disorder is *dysphagia* (difficulty in swallowing). Patients typically describe food sticking in the chest after it is swallowed. Dysphagia occurs with both solid and liquid food. Moreover, the dysphagia is consistent, meaning that it occurs during virtually every meal. Regurgitation of food that is trapped in the oesophagus can occur, especially when the oesophagus is dilated.

Gastro-oesophageal Reflux Disease (GORD)

The reflux of products of gastric digestion (chyme containing acid, pepsin or even bile) into the oesophagus produces a substernal burning sensation that moves up and down the chest. These symptoms are usually described as *heart burn.* The repeated exposure to the reflux material produces oesophageal erosions, ulceration or even cancer of the lower end of oesophagus.

Even in the empty stomach, normal intragastric pressure is higher than the intra-oesophageal pressure. Straining or coughing cause marked increase in intra-abdominal and intra-gastric pressures, especially after a large meal. In spite of the favourable pressure gradient, gastro-oesophageal reflux does not normally occur because of the tonic contraction of lower oesophageal sphincter. The basic problem in cases GORD is weak basal tone of the lower oesophageal sphincter. Recent studies show that the opening in the diaphragm through which the oesophagus enters the abdomen acts as an additional sphincter around the lower end of the esophagus. In older age group patients, hiatus hernia is often present. A hiatus hernia is an enlarged opening in the diaphragm where the esophagus joins the stomach. The hernia can allow the uppermost part of the stomach to bulge through the diaphragm into the chest area, interfering with the action of lower oesophageal sphincter.

The symptoms of GORD are worse at night because in day time, the acid reaching the oesophagus is quickly removed, by peristalsis and gravity, back to the stomach. Moreover, reflex salivary occurs and the saliva quickly neutralizes the acid. During sleep, the salivary secretion ceases. In the lying posture, the role of gravity also disappears. Therefore, any acid regurgitating to the oesophagus remains for longer duration and severe oesophageal mucosal injury is repeatedly each night.

CHAPTER 37

The Stomach

FUNCTIONAL ANATOMY

The main anatomical divisions of the stomach are illustrated in Fig. 37.1. Surface of the gastric mucosa is covered with columnar epithelial cells those secrete mucus and an alkaline fluid, both of which protect the epithelium from gastric acid and mechanical injury by rough food. The surface is studded with gastric pits. Each pit is the opening of a duct into which one or more gastric glands empty. The gastric pits also are lined with mucus-secreting columnar cells.

The gastric mucosa can be divided into three regions based on the structure of the glands:

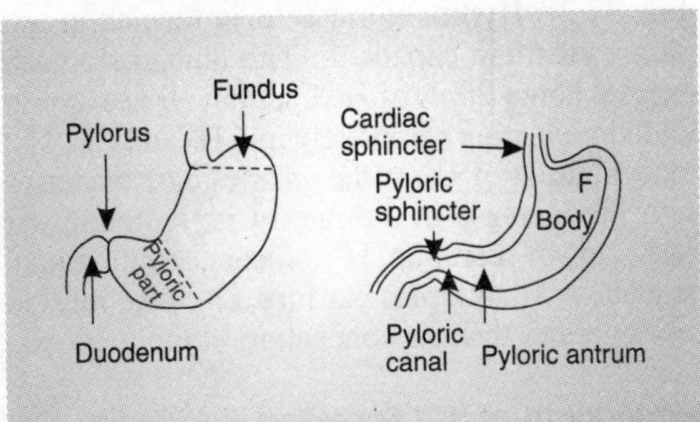

Fig. 37.1: Anatomy of stomach. (A) Surface view. (B) Longitudinal section showing lumen of the stomach.

(i) Cardiac Glandular Region It is a few centimetre wide area just below the lower oesophageal sphincter. It contains tortuous *mucus-secreting* glands (Colour Plate 4, Fig. 10).

(ii) Oxyntic Glandular Region Mucosa of the fundus and body of the stomach containing acid secreting cells is called the oxyntic glandular region. It occupies about 80% of the total gastric mucosa. The tubular exocrine glands of this region contain two types of cells:

(a) Parietal (oxyntic) cells which secrete *hydrochloric acid* and the *intrinsic factor of Castle.*
(b) Chief (peptic) cells which secrete *pepsinogens.*

The neck of the glands is lined with *mucus* secreting columnar cells. Several of the glands open into a common chamber called gastric pit.

(iii) Pyloric Glandular Region The mucosa of the pyloric part of stomach is called pyloric glandular region. It occupies about 20% of the total gastric mucosa. This region is characterized by deep gastric pits. The exocrine glandular portion contains *mucus-secreting* cells. Scattered among them are certain endocrine cells called *G cells* which secrete a local hormone called gastrin into the bloodstream.

Somatostatin-secreting endocrine paracrine type of cells ('D'cells) are also present scattered among other type of cells in the oxyntic and pyloric regions. These cells have long cytoplasmic extensions through which they are believed to exert an inhibitory control over parietal cells, chief cells and G cells. Some other endocrine paracrine cells present in the mucosa of the stomach and small intestine include 'A' cells which secrete glucagon and enterochromaffin cells which secrete serotonin.

Parietal (Oxyntic) Cells

The parietal or the oxyntic cell is pyramidal or triangular in shape and relatively large in size (25 μm diameter). The cell is deeply acidophilic due to the presence of large number of densely packed mitochondria. The mitochondria are involved in the production of large amount of energy required for gastric acid secretion. The most characteristic electron microscopic feature of a parietal cell is the extensive tubulo-vesicular intracellular canalicular systems. The canaliculi course through the cytoplasm but have a common outlet on the luminal surface of the cell (Fig. 37.2). Numerous microvilli line the surface of the canaliculi. An enzyme H^+-K^+ ATPase is located within the cell membrane of the intracellular canaliculi. The parietal cell also contains small amount of endoplasmic reticulum (possibly involved in the synthesis of the intrinsic factor) and a small Golgi apparatus.

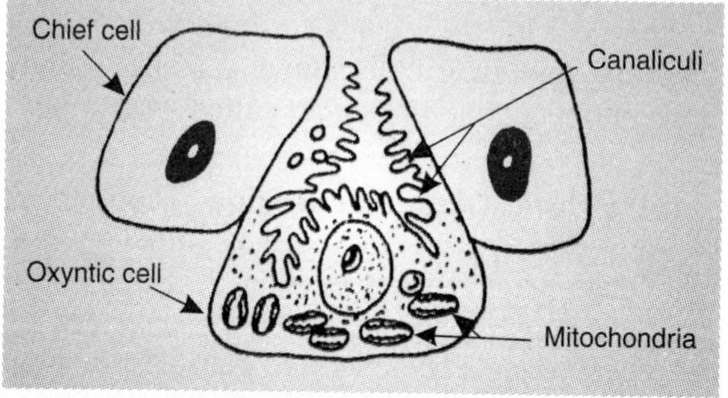

Fig. 37.2: Electron microscopic structure of an oxyntic cell.

Chief (Peptic) Cells

These cells are characterized by basophilic cytoplasm due to the presence of abundant rough endoplasmic reticulum involved in the synthesis of pepsinogens. Another important histological feature is the apically located zymogen granules which contain pepsinogen. Secretory stimuli like vagal stimulation or the local hormone gastrin causes discharge of zymogen granules into the lumen of the gastric glands.

Nerve Supply

Extensive Meissner's and myenteric plexuses are present in the stomach as components of enteric nervous system. In addition, stomach is supplied with extrinsic parasympathetic nerve fibres through vagus and sympathetic fibres through the coeliac plexus.

GASTRIC JUICE

COMPOSITION

In humans, about 2500 ml of gastric juice is secreted daily. Its important constituents include hydrochloric acid (HCl), and organic constituents like pepsinogens, mucus, intrinsic factor of Castle and lipase. It also contains inorganic constituents such as Na^+, Mg^{2+}, SO_4^{2-}, and HPO_4^{2-}.

Secretion of HCl

Under electron microscope, the parietal cells show a complex network of intracellular canaliculi (Fig. 37.2). Hydrochloric acid is formed at the surface of these canaliculi. The human stomach secretes about 2.5 L of HCl per day. It is a strong acid; dissociating completely into H^+ and Cl^-. The concentration of H^+ in the gastric juice increases with the increase in the rate of its secretion. At high rates of secretion, H^+ ion concentration may be as high as 150 mEq per litre, i.e. three million times greater than its concentration in the blood.

Mechanism of HCl Secretion

The parietal cells are known to be particularly rich in the enzyme carbonic anhydrase. This enzyme causes hydration of CO_2 to form H_2CO_3 (Fig. 37.3) which further dissociates into H^+ and HCO_3^-. The H^+ is secreted into the canaliculi of the parietal cells by an active transport mechanism (H^+–K^+ ATPase). Thus H^+ are extruded into the canalicular lumen in exchange for K^+ and the energy released by ATPase is utilized to pump H^+ against the steep concentration gradient. Bicarbonate is released at the basal border of the parietal cell by an HCO_3^-–Cl^- exchange. Therefore, during gastric secretion, the venous blood leaving the stomach is more alkaline than the arterial blood entering it. (This is in contrast to most other tissues where venous blood is more acidic than the arterial blood). Due to the transfer of HCO_3^- into the blood, the urinary pH tends to increase after a meal. This phenomenon is called the alkaline tide. Chloride ions are transferred to the canalicular lumen by a separate mechanism. Finally, water passes into the canaliculi passively.

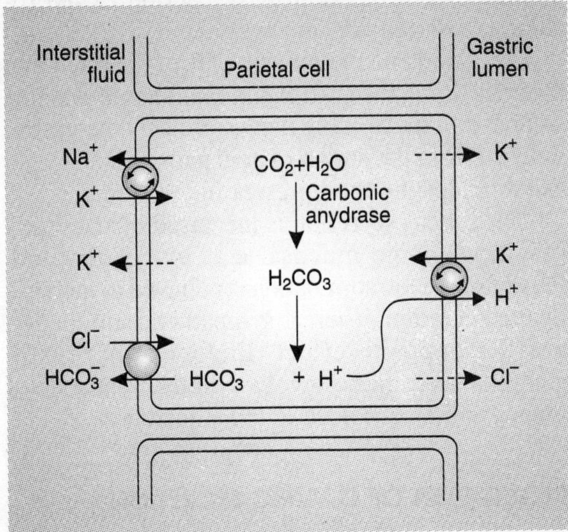

Fig. 37.3: Mechanism of HCl secretion in the oxyntic cells of the stomach.

Acid secretion is increased by histamine, acetylcholine and gastrin (Fig. 37.4). Parietal cells have receptors for each of the three mediators of HCl secretion. Acetylcholine acts on M_1 muscarinic receptors whereas gastrin acts on specific gastrin-receptors located on the surface

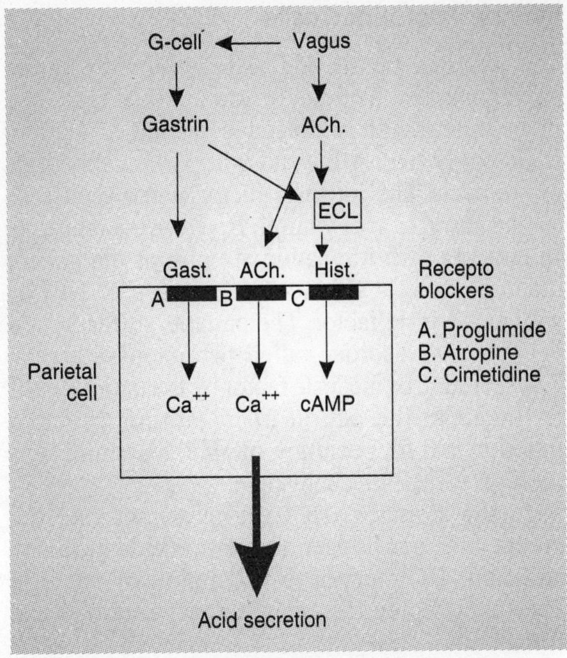

Fig. 37.4: Interaction of neural and humoral factors on the 3 types of receptors of the parietal (oxyntic) cells.

of parietal cells. Both M_1 receptors and gastrin receptors act by increasing intracellular Ca^{2+} which acts as the second messenger. Vagus stimulation leads to release of acetylcholine from the postganglionic parasympathetic nerves supplying the parietal cells of the stomach.

37

The exact role of histamine in the secretion of HCl from the parietal cells is not clear. Histamine is released from enterochromaffin-like (ECL) cells in the gastric mucosa and diffuses to the parietal cells. It has been suggested that gastrin not only acts on the G receptors on the parietal cell, but also on ECL cells causing the release of histamine. Blockade of H_2-receptors does decrease the acid secretion. The drug cimetidine, an H_2-receptor blocker, has been successfully used in the treatment of hyperacidity and peptic ulcer. Theoretically, atropine can also be used to decrease the acid secretion by blocking the M_1 receptors. However, it is not used clinically for this purpose, because of its unpleasant side effects [due to blockade of other muscarinic (M_1) receptors in the body] like tachycardia, dry mouth and constipation.

Intrinsic Factor of Castle

The **intrinsic factor of Castle** is secreted by the parietal cells. The secretion of this factor, a glycoprotein with a molecular weight of 45,000, is probably one of the most important functions of stomach. The intrinsic factor is indispensable for the absorption of vitamin B_{12} from the intestine. In patients with idiopathic atrophy of the gastric mucosa, there is absence of secretion of HCl as well as intrinsic factor. The patients suffer from a very serious disorder called pernicious anaemia. The secretion of intrinsic factor by the parietal cells is linked to the action of histamine. For this function and for secretion of HCl, histamine acts through cAMP mechanism.

In the stomach, HCl serves to activate the proenzyme, pepsinogen to pepsin (vide infra). In addition, HCl serves to kill many of bacteria ingested with food, especially raw vegetables and fruit.

Pepsinogen Secretion

The chief cells of the main gastric glands secrete pepsinogen, an inactive precursor (proenzyme) of pepsin, the major enzyme of the gastric juice. Like many other secretory cells, the proenzyme is synthesized and stored as zymogen granules in the apical region of the chief cells. Secretory stimuli like vagal stimulation, gastrin release or histamine cause the discharge of pepsinogen granules into the lumen of the glands. Pepsinogen with a molecular weight of 42,500 is converted to the active proteolytic enzyme pepsin (mol. wt 35,000) by the cleavage of a peptide from the molecule. The cleavage is produced by HCl or preformed pepsin.

$$\text{Pepsinogen} \xrightarrow{\text{HCl}} \text{Pepsin}$$

$$\downarrow$$

$$\text{Pepsinogen} \longrightarrow \text{Pepsin}$$

The pepsinogen secreted by the chief cells in the main gastric glands is known as pepsinogen-I. Pyloric glands secrete a small amount of another proteolytic proenzyme called pepsinogen-II. Pepsinogen-I and pepsinogen-II can be differentiated by immunochemical methods but the physiological significance of the difference is not known.

Pepsin hydrolyses the peptide bonds adjacent to the aromatic amino acids like tyrosine, and phenylalanine. It splits proteins into proteoses, peptones and polypeptides. Since the optimum pH for the action of pepsin is 2.0, acid secretion by the stomach is as essential as pepsinogen secretion for the digestion of proteins in the stomach.

Secretion of Mucus

The surface of the gastric mucosa is lined with mucus secreting cells. These cells secrete such a viscid *visible mucus* that it forms a gel-like coat over the mucosa. Mucus is chemically a glycoprotein. These cells also secrete bicarbonate, so that the alkaline mucus with pH of 7 forms an extremely important protective layer saving the stomach from the destructive action of hydrochloric acid and pepsin.

The glands of the pyloric part of stomach and the cells lining the gastric pits also secrete alkaline *soluble mucus*. Soluble mucus protects the gastric mucosa from the action of acid and pepsin as well as lubricates the food present in the stomach.

The mucus secretion is increased by the direct irritation of the mucosa, e.g. by rough food. Parasympathetic stimulation is believed to increase mucus secretion, whereas sympathetic stimulation has the opposite effect. Endogenous prostaglandins seem to be involved in the synthesis of mucus and bicarbonate in the stomach.

REGULATION OF GASTRIC SECRETION

Gastric secretion, i.e. secretion of the main gastric glands, is regulated by both neural as well as hormonal mechanisms.

Neural Control

Neural control over the gastric glands is exerted by local enteric plexus and the vagal (extrinsic) innervation. Stimulation of vagus increases the secretion of HCl by the parietal cells and pepsinogen by the chief cells. Acetylcholine released from the postganglionic parasympathetic fibres acts on the parietal as well as the chief cells. Besides this direct action, vagus increases the gastric secretion indirectly also by acting on G cells and promoting the release of the local hormone, gastrin.

Hormonal Control

Gastrin is a local gastrointestinal hormone secreted by G cells (gastrin cells) of the pyloric glands. These flask-shaped cells are located in the lateral walls of the glands in the antral portion of gastric mucosa. The broad base of the G cell contains many granules of gastrin. Many microvilli project from the narrow apical surface of the cell into the lumen of the pyloric glands. The microvilli contain receptors mediating gastrin release in response to gastric contents.

Three types of gastrins, namely, G-34, G-17 and G-14 have been isolated. Besides the difference in their amino acid number, they also differ in the sequence of amino acids. The three types of gastrins have been named after the number of amino acid residues in each of them. G-17 is the principal secretory product of the G cells. It contains 17 amino acids.

The release of gastrin is increased by: (i) distension of the pyloric antrum by food, (ii) presence of peptides and amino acids in the gastric contents and (iii) vagal stimulation. Atropine blocks the action of vagal stimulation on the oxyntic cells but does not affect the release of gastrin from the G cells. It has been postulated that a different neurotransmitter called *gastrin releasing peptide,* rather than acetylcholine is released at the parasympathetic nerve endings on the G cells.

The secretion of gastrin is inhibited when the pH of the gastric contents falls below 2.0. Thus by a feedback control system, the pH of the gastric contents is maintained around 2. In addition, a number of intestinal local hormones like secretin, GIP, VIP also inhibit the release of gastrin.

Gastrin is secreted by the G cells into the blood circulation (and not into the gastric juice). It reaches the stomach through the arterial circulation and stimulates the secretory activity of the parietal cells and chief cells. *Other actions of gastrin* are summarized in Chapter 35.

PHASES OF GASTRIC SECRETION

In the interdigestive period, the secretion of gastric juice is minimal. Its secretion *is markedly increased on ingestion of food,* when secretory rate may be as high as 3 ml/min. After food intake, gastric secretion can be described as three overlapping phases: cephalic phase, gastric phase and intestinal phase.

Cephalic Phase

Stimulation of taste buds by the food not only produces reflex stimulation of salivary glands, but also causes a reflex increase in gastric secretion. The vagus carries efferent fibres of the reflex arc to the stomach. The vagally mediated response increases the secretion of parietal and chief cells by: (i) a direct action, (ii) increasing the secretion of gastrin from the G cells. Even the sight, smell or thought of food may increase the gastric secretion by conditioned reflex mechanism.

Emotions also influence the vagally-mediated gastric secretion. Anger and hostility are associated with increased gastric secretion and motility. Fear and depression decrease the gastric secretion and motility. In high-strung and aggressive individuals, increased vagal discharge produces gastric secretion even during non-digestive period leading to hyperacidity or even peptic ulceration.

Gastric Phase

The presence of food in the stomach further accelerates the rate of gastric secretion. Gastric secretion is increased by two overlapping mechanisms.

Neural Mechanism

Gastric distension is a potent stimulus for the secretion of parietal and chief cells. Stretch receptors located in the wall of stomach act through the Meissner's plexus and increase the postganglionic parasympathetic discharge to the gastric glands. The secretion of *gastrin* is also increased by this neural mechanism.

Hormonal Mechanism

Presence of food in the stomach induces gastric secretion by a hormonal mechanism also. The increase in the gastrin secretion brought about by the contents of the chyme present in the gastric lumen constitutes the hormonal or chemical phase of gastric secretion. Products of partial protein digestion, as well as alcohol and caffeine are potent stimuli for the release of local hormone gastrin by the 'G' cells present in the pyloric glands.

Feedback Control

As a result of cephalic and gastric influences, the increased secretion of HCl in the stomach lowers the pH of gastric contents to as low as 2.0. Any further decrease in the pH of gastric contents is prevented by the inhibition of gastrin secretion from the G cells. On the other hand, if the pH of the gastric contents rises above 3.5 (due to the buffering action of food), the release of gastrin begins once again. In this way, the negative feedback control over gastrin release maintains the pH of gastric contents near 2.0, the optimum pH for the action of pepsin. At the same time, the feedback control protects the gastric mucosa from more severe and potentially harmful acidity.

INTESTINAL INFLUENCES (PHASE)

Earlier, it was called the intestinal phase because in experimental animals with empty stomach, presence of peptides in the upper intestine led to a moderate secretion in the stomach. During normal digestion of food, in contrast to the excitatory cephalic and gastric influences, the intestinal influence on the gastric secretion is chiefly inhibitory in nature. The presence of acid, fats and products of protein digestion in the duodenum cause the release of several *intestinal hormones* like secretin, cholecystokinin (CCK), vasoactive intestinal peptide (VIP) and somatostatin. These local hormones not only promote the secretion of alkaline pancreatic juice and bile but also *inhibit* the *gastric secretion* and *motility*. The stimuli mentioned above inhibit the gastric secretion by triggering an intrinsic reflex called *enterogastric reflex* also (neural mechanism). Thus, the regulation of gastric emptying by upper small intestine *serves to limit the amount of chyme (rich in acid) leaving the stomach* to the extent which is ideal for the digestive and absorptive function of the intestine (see gastric emptying, vide infra).

The inhibitory influences discussed above *help to terminate the gastric secretion* when all the food has left the stomach.

FUNCTIONS OF STOMACH

Functions of the stomach may be discussed under three headings: (A) Secretory functions, (B) Motor functions, (C) Absorptive functions.

Secretory Functions

1. Gastric Acid

(i) Gastric acid serves to destroy the bacteria ingested especially with uncooked (raw) vegetables and fruits.

(ii) Hydrochloric acid activates the proenzyme pepsinogen into an active proteolytic enzyme, pepsin, thus helping in the digestion of dietary proteins.

(iii) By converting dietary iron complexes (with phytate, phosphate, etc.) into more soluble form, gastric acid promotes intestinal absorption of dietary iron. Patients with achlorhydria tend to suffer from iron deficiency as well as more frequent gastrointestinal infections.

2. Pepsinogen Dietary proteins undergo partial digestion in the stomach by the action of pepsin.

3. Intrinsic Factor of Castle Intrinsic factor of Castle is essential for intestinal absorption of vitamin B_{12}. Gastric atrophy or gastric resection is followed by pernicious anaemia within a few months.

4. The Mucus and HCO_3 secreted by the pyloric antral glands help to protect gastric and duodenal mucosa from autodigestion by the gastric juice.

Motor Functions

The motor functions of the stomach include:

(i) Storage of large quantity of food until it can be transferred to the intestine.

(ii) Mixing food with gastric juice until a semifluid mixture known as chyme is formed.

(iii) Slow transfer of food from the stomach to the intestine (gastric emptying) at a rate suitable for proper digestion and absorption in the small intestine.

Storage Function

The empty stomach has a volume of about 50 ml only and the diameter of its lumen is only slightly more than that of the small intestine. But, during a meal, as each bolus of food reaches the stomach, the smooth muscle of the body of stomach relaxes a bit, allowing the volume of stomach to increase without any significant increase in its intraluminal pressure. This phenomenon called **receptive-relaxation of stomach** is due to a vagally mediated reflex. The receptors for this reflex are located in the pharynx and oesophagus. The passage of each bolus of food stimulates these stretch receptors. By the end of the meal, the smooth muscle of the stomach relaxes to such an extent that 1 litre or more of the food can be accommodated.

Mixing of Food

The mixing of food with the digestive juice of the stomach takes place slowly by the peristaltic waves (mixing waves). The gastric peristalsis has a frequency of approximately three per minute. The rhythmicity of gastric peristalsis is determined by the basic electrical rhythm (BER), i.e. cyclic mild depolarization of smooth muscle of the stomach, at the rate of three per minute (slow waves). Certain pacemaker cells among the longitudinal smooth muscle in the fundus of the stomach undergo spontaneous depolarization at the rate of 3/min and the depolarization is conducted to smooth muscle of the remaining part of stomach via the gap junctions. However, in the absence of other inputs, the slow wave depolarization is too weak to induce mechanical contractions of the stomach. Certain neurotransmitters like acetylcholine or hormone gastrin cause generation of depolarizing spikes at the peak of BER cycles resulting in mechanical contractions (peristalsis). The number of spikes fired in a slow wave determines the strength of each peristaltic contraction (Fig. 37.5). In other words, although the frequency of gastric peristalsis does not vary, the force of peristaltic waves is under neural and hormonal control. Distension of the stomach or increased gastrin secretion increase the force of gastric peristalsis.

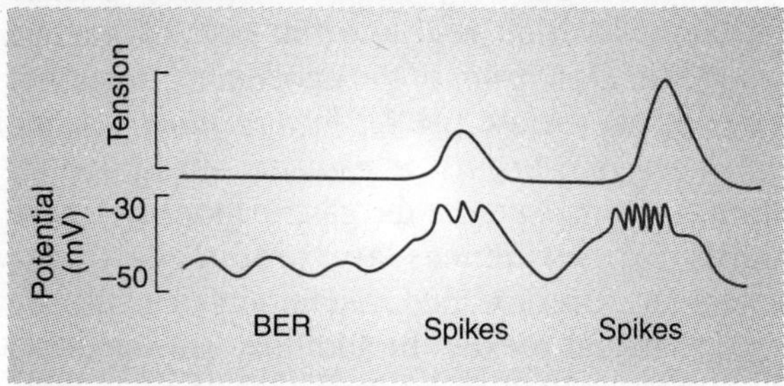

Fig. 37.5: Membrane potentials in the smooth muscle of the alimentary canal and their relation to the mechanical response.

As the gastric peristaltic wave passes down the stomach, the ring of contraction propels the food towards the antrum but simultaneous antral contraction *closes the pyloric sphincter also*. As a result most of the antral contents are forced back into the body of the stomach and only a small amount of chyme passes into the duodenum (Fig. 37.6). The back and forth movement of the gastric contents with each peristaltic wave helps to mix the food with gastric juice converting it into a semiliquid chyme.

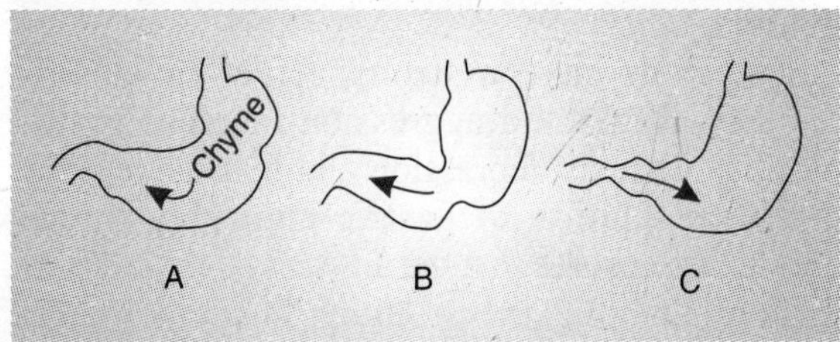

Fig. 37.6: Gastric peristaltic activity and its effect on the gastric contents.

Gastric Emptying

The rate at which the stomach empties into the duodenum depends on the quantity and the type of food ingested. Basically, the rate of gastric emptying is determined by the strength of gastric peristalsis. Distension of the stomach triggers long (vagally mediated) and short (intrinsic neural plexus mediated) reflexes leading to strong peristaltic waves and increased rate of gastric emptying. The local hormone gastrin also increases the rate of gastric emptying.

Certain signals from the duodenum have a more important regulatory control over the gastric peristalsis which regulate the rate of gastric emptying. *Distension* of the duodenum, *acidity* of its contents (below pH 4), *hyperosmolar chyme* or *chyme rich in fats or proteins* are important stimuli which *decrease* the gastric motility. These inhibitory influences are produced by the enterogastric reflex, mediated through the intrinsic enteric neural plexus. In addition, the duodenal factors mentioned above cause secretion of local hormones like secretin, cholecystokinin (CCK), VIP and somatostatin from the duodenal mucosa which decrease the gastric motility by inhibiting the release of gastrin. Fatty meals are particularly known to prolong gastric emptying time.

Therefore, when a mixed meal is taken, fluids begin to leave the stomach almost immediately. Solids begin to leave after a lag period during which they are broken down to smaller particles by gastric movements. Fats, highly acidic or hyperosmolar fluids leave the stomach far more slowly (Fig. 37.7). If one litre of water is drunk alone, most of it leaves the stomach in less than 30 minutes (Fig. 37.8). After a normal meal, the normal *emptying time* of the stomach is about *3 to 4 hours.*

Emotions have a strong effect on gastric motility. Anger and aggression increase gastric motility whereas depression and fear decrease it.

The regulation of gastric emptying by the duodenum ensures that the amount of chyme (rich in acid) leaving the stomach is ideal for the digestive and absorptive function of the intestine, i.e. excessive acidity or osmolality of the duodenal contents is not allowed to occur.

Absorptive Function

Very few substances like alcohol and certain drugs can be absorbed in the stomach.

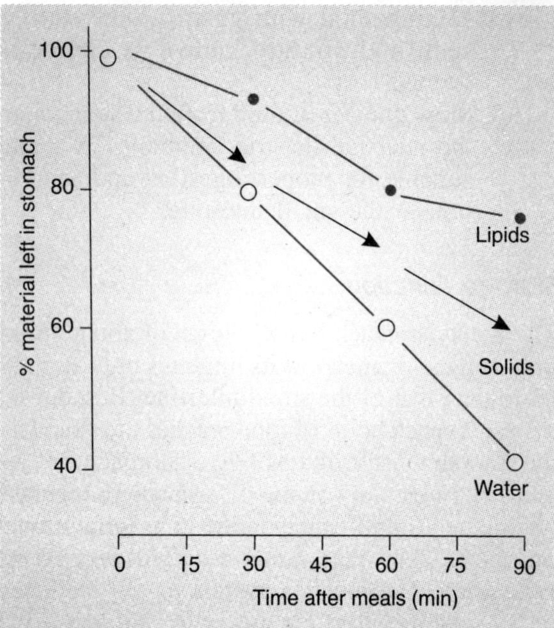

Fig. 37.7: Gastric emptying of 3 different components of a mixed meal.

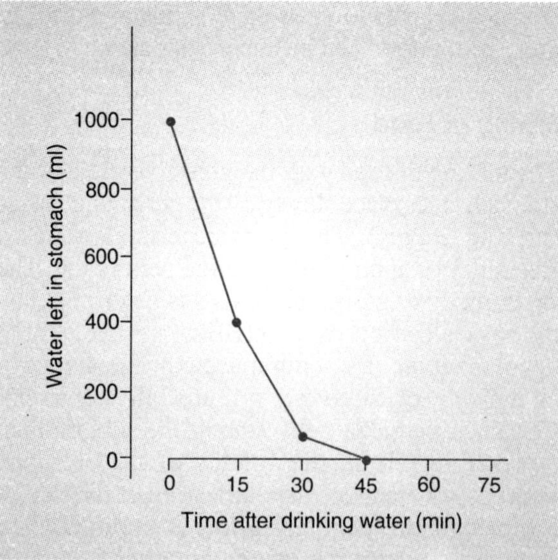

Fig. 37.8: Gastric emptying of one litre of water.

VOMITING

Vomiting usually occurs in response to over-distension or excessive irritation of any part of the gut. Impulses are transmitted via vagus and sympathetic nerves to the vomiting centre situated in the reticular formation of the medulla oblongata, near the vagal nucleus. Efferent impulses are transmitted via V, VII, IX, X and XII cranial nerves to the upper GIT and through spinal nerves to the muscles of respiration.

At the onset of vomiting, glottis is first to be closed and it remains so till the end of the act. Next the pyloric part of stomach contracts firmly and its contents are transferred to flaccid body of the stomach. Now, the simultaneous contraction of the abdominal muscle and the descent of the diaphragm raise the intra-abdominal pressure to such an extent that all the gastric contents are squeezed out of the stomach, into the oesophagus. A reflex relaxation of the lower sphincter of the oesophagus occurs at this moment. Positive intrapulmonary pressure and antiperistaltic waves in the oesophagus help to expel the material from the oesophagus into the mouth.

Just before the actual act of vomiting, the whole sequence of events described above, accompanied by nausea, salivation and sweating may occur repeatedly for a couple of minutes. This condition is called *retching*. Retching is soon followed by actual vomiting.

Besides the upper GIT, afferents from many other parts of the body like the heart and the vestibular apparatus may also stimulate the vomiting centre. Many drugs like morphine and digitalis induce vomiting by acting on certain cells in the medulla oblongata called the chemoreceptor trigger zone, an area which is outside the blood-brain barrier. This type of vomiting is called *central vomiting* to differentiate vomiting induced by stimulation of *peripheral* receptors in GIT, heart, vestibular apparatus, etc.

GASTRIC MUCOSAL BARRIER

It is a physiologic marvel that the gastric juice can easily digest the swallowed piece of meat but it has no corrosive action on the gastric mucosa itself. Several factors seem to be involved in the protection of gastric mucosa from autodigestion. These factors are collectively referred to as the gastric mucosal barrier.

1. Mucus Secretion As mentioned above, the surface epithelial cells and the mucous neck cells of the gastric mucosa secrete a thin layer of mucus.

Mucus consists of a water-insoluble visco-elastic gel, with a diffusion coefficient for H^+ that is one-fourth that of water. This gel is impermeable to pepsin also.

2. Bicarbonate Secretion The surface epithelial cells contain carbonic anhydrase. These cells secrete bicarbonate into the boundary zone of the adherent mucus, creating a relatively alkaline microenvironment immediately adjacent to the cell surface. Bicarbonate secretion is increased by luminal acid, mild irritants, vagal stimulation and prostaglandins.

3. Epithelial Barrier Mucosal epithelial cells are bound to each other by intercellular tight junctions which prevent any back diffusion of hydrogen ions. Surface epithelial cells have profuse regenerative capacity. Mitosis in the neck cells leads to replacement of entire gastric mucosal surface every 2 to 6 days.

4. Mucosal Blood Flow The gastric mucosa is highly vascular. A rich blood supply helps to provide oxygen, bicarbonate and nutrients to the epithelial cells. Mucosal blood flow increases whenever acid secretion is stimulated. Blood flow may be adversely affected during severe medical or surgical stress. These factors are well known causes of acute or chronic peptic ulcers.

5. Neural Component Afferent neurons within the mucosa of the stomach and duodenum can trigger a protective reflex vasodilatation when toxins or acid breach the epithelial barrier.

6. Prostaglandins Endogenous prostaglandins are involved in the synthesis of mucus and bicarbonate in the gastric and duodenal mucosa. They also participate in maintenance of mucosal blood flow and promote epithelial cell renewal in response to mucosal injury.

Alcohol and aspirin (and other non-steroidal anti-inflammatory agents) tend to produce gastritis by eroding the mucous barrier. The mucus coat is soluble in alcohol, while aspirin inhibits the formation and secretion of mucus and bicarbonate.

Therefore, alcohol abuse, or excessive use of aspirin, can permit hydrochloric acid to attack the stomach lining, which leads to bleeding.

Individuals who are highly anxious do not experience proper parasympathetic activation when eating, and consequently do not produce sufficient mucus. Therefore, given the presence of other triggers for ulcer formation (and specifically infection with bacteria of the *Helicobacter pylori*, anxious individuals are often susceptible to peptic ulcers.

Pathophysiology

Peptic Ulcer

Peptic ulcers are chronic lesions that occur in portions of gastrointestinal tract exposed to corrosive action of acid-peptic juice. They are more commonly seen in the first part of duodenum and pyloric antrum of the stomach. The most characteristic feature of peptic ulcer is *epigastric pain* with severity *relating to mealtimes*, i.e. after around 3 hours of taking a meal in case of duodenal ulcers. Pain is relieved by food. In case of gastric ulcers ingestion of food exacerbates pain.

37

Gastric acid and pepsin are requisites for all peptic ulcerations ("no acid, no ulcer"). Excessive secretion of hydrochloric acid (**hyperchlorhydria**) can be demonstrated in many cases of peptic ulcer (Fig. 37.9).

Stimuli which increase gastric acid secretion are well-known predisposing factors for peptic ulceration. Thus, peptic ulcer is more common in persons with aggressive personality, psychogenic stress or who consume very hot and spicy food.

Infection of the gastric mucosa with bacterium *Helicobacter pylori* can be demonstrated in about 90% of the patients with duodenal ulcers and 70% of gastric ulcers. Ulceration seems to results from the action of bacterial urease which generates ammonia and a protease which breaks down the glycoproteins in the gastric mucus. Breakdown of mucus barrier allows the corrosive action of gastric acid and pepsin on the mucosa.

Gastric mucosal barrier is damaged by exposure to any type of **stress**, or by inhibition of prostaglandin synthesis, e.g. by prolonged use of

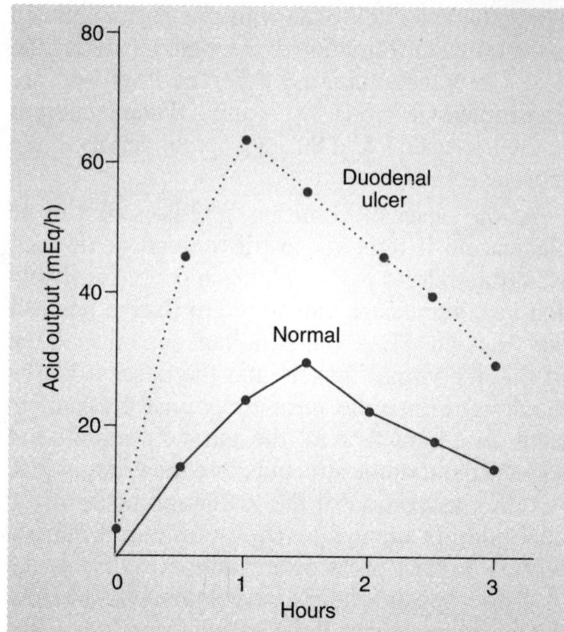

Fig. 37.9: Gastric acid secretion after a protein-rich meal in a normal person and a patient of duodenal ulcer with hyperchlorhydria.

pharmocologic doses of **glucocorticoids** or **nonsteroidal anti-inflammatory drugs** like aspirin. These are well-known causes of peptic ulcer. Thus, peptic ulcer may even occur in patients in whom acid and pepsin secretion is within the normal range.

The medical treatment of peptic ulcer aims at neutralization of gastric acid secretion, promotion of mucus secretion and inhibition of acid secretion.

A variety of antacids which contain aluminium or magnesium hydroxide *neutralize* the gastric acid.

Acid secretion can *be inhibited* by administration of H_2-receptor blockers like cimetidine or ranitidine or by H^+-K^+ ATPase *(proton pump) inhibitor*, omeprazole. Another drug, *sucralfate* increases the resistance of the mucosa by forming adherent protein complexes. Infection by *H. pylori* is treated by *antibiotics.*

Severe duodenal or pyloric ulcers, some times, need surgical treatment. It consists of bilateral vagotomy near the lower end of oesophagus (the cardiac innervation is thus spared) combined with resection of gastrin-producing pyloric part of stomach.

Zollinger-Ellison syndrome is characterized by multiple gastric ulcerations and marked hyperchlorhydria. The disease is caused by gastrin secreting tumours (gastrinoma) in the stomach or duodenum or more commonly in the pancreas.

Gastric Function Tests

Pentagastrin Test

In a fasting individual, overnight gastric juice is aspirated (with the help of a long catheter called Ryle's tube) and discarded. Now, the **basal acid output** is measured by collection of gastric juice every 15 minutes for one hour. H^+ concentration of each sample is separately estimated. Normal basal output is less than 5 mEq H^+/hour. Estimation of basal acid output is particularly useful in the diagnosis of Zollinger-Ellison (ZE) syndrome in which the stomach secretes maximally even at rest (15–50 mEq H^+/hour).

Peak Acid Output It is next estimated after subcutaneous injection of pentagastrin (a synthetic polypeptide with gastrin-like activity) in the dose of 5 μg/kg body weight. The stomach is aspirated every 15 minutes for the next one hour. Each sample is analyzed separately for H^+ concentration.

H^+ secretion reaches the peak value within the first 15 min and is maintained for another 15 minutes approximately. It gradually declines, during the next 30 minutes. Normal peak acid output is less than 45 mEq H^+/hour in males and less than 35 mEq H^+/hour in females. Higher values are seen in patients of Zollinger-Ellison Syndrome and in many (but not all) patients of peptic ulcer. In *pernicious anaemia*, basal acid secretion is nearly absent and there is no increase in acid secretion after injection of pentagastrin *(achlorhydria)*.

Insulin Test

This test is performed only to confirm the success of vagotomy operation. An intravenous injection of a small dose of insulin produces hypoglycemia which leads to hypothalamic stimulation and hence increased vagal discharge. Thus, insulin injection is followed by increased gastric secretion rich in acid and pepsin in normal individuals; but not in those with successful bilateral vagotomy. In other words, secretion of acid in response to insulin injection after vagotomy indicates that the surgical operation has not been successful.

Plasma Gastrin Estimation

This is a diagnostic test for ZE syndrome. Normal plasma gastrin concentration is less than 300 pg/ml. Patients with ZE syndrome have plasma gastrin level above 1000 pg/ml.

Upper Gastrointestinal Contrast Radiography

Barium "meal" Study is performed in patients suspected of having peptic ulcer or gastric carcinoma. The patient is given barium sulphate suspension orally and a radiogram of the upper abdomen is taken (Fig. 37.10). The peptic ulcer is seen as an ulcer crater whereas carcinoma is seen as a filling defect.

(The colon can be visualized by taking a radiogram of the abdomen after administration of barium sulphate through the rectum).

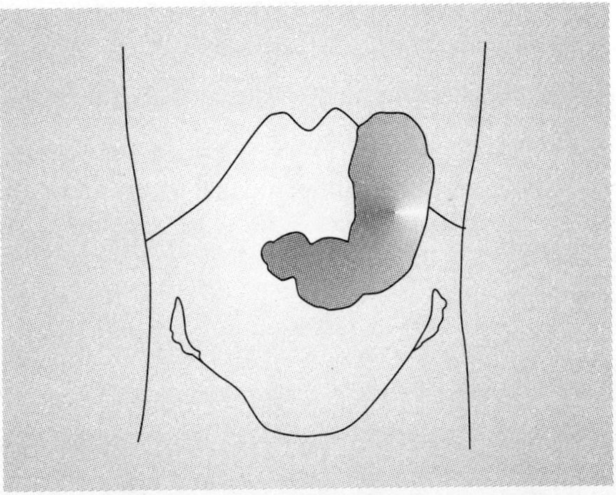

Fig. 37.10: Barium 'meal' study.

Endoscopy

An ulcer or cancerous growth in the stomach can be visualized by endoscopic examination (Fig. 37.11). During the procedure, a biopsy of the suspected site can also be taken. At present, endoscopy is the most important investigation for the diagnosis of peptic ulcer or gastric carcinoma.

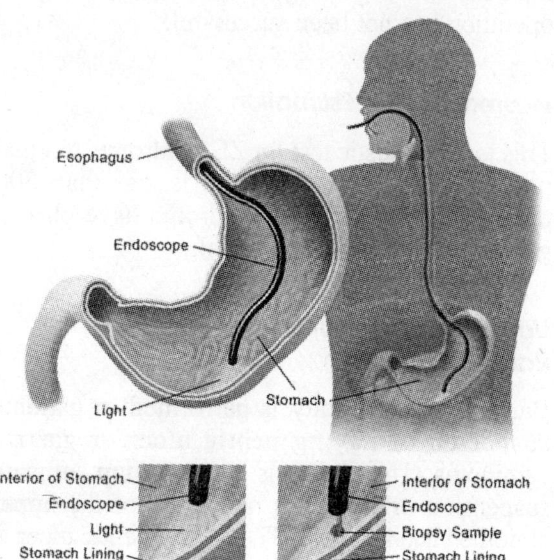

Esophagogastroduodenoscopy (EGD or upper ensoscopy)

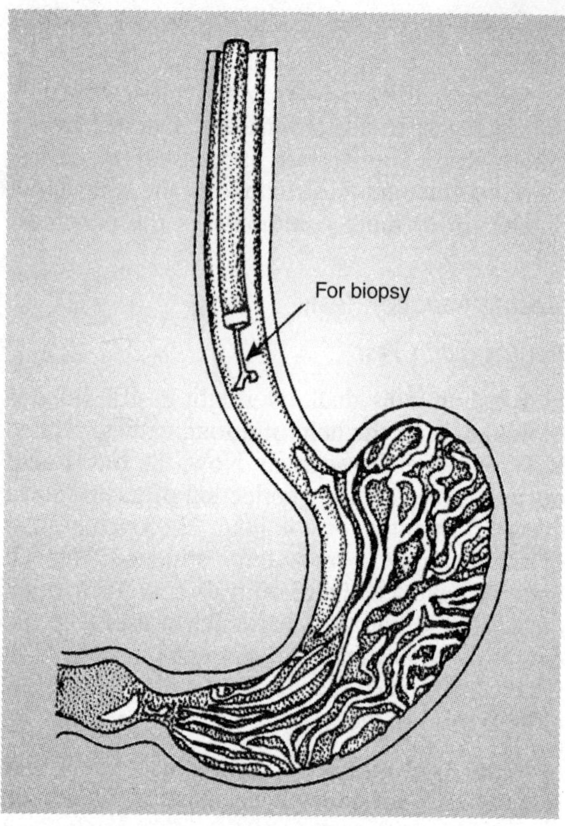

Fig. 37.11: Gastric endoscope with arrangement for a biopsy.

38

CHAPTER

The Pancreas, Liver and Gallbladder

PANCREAS

Functional Anatomy (Colour Plate 5, Fig. 11)

The exocrine pancreas is a highly lobulated gland consisting of clusters of secretory cells forming acini and a complex branched ductal system. The pancreatic acini consist of pyramidal-shaped cells with their apexes projecting towards the lumen of a minute duct. The acinar cells are typical protein secreting cells. Highly basophilic basal region contains the nucleus surrounded by extensive endoplasmic reticulum (Fig. 38.1). The Golgi apparatus is located in supranuclear position. Apexes of the cells are filled with acidophilic zymogen granules. The smallest excretory ducts starting from the acini are lined with centroacinar cells. The secretion is drained into ducts of progressively increasing size and finally into the main pancreatic duct. The main pancreatic duct joins the common bile duct to form ampulla of Vater, which opens into the duodenum. The ductal epithelium consists of cuboidal cells that are devoid of zymogen granules and have very little endoplasmic reticulum. The centro-acinar cells and cell lining the smaller ducts contain carbonic anhydrase, the enzyme required for synthesis of bicarbonate.

COMPOSITION OF PANCREATIC JUICE

About 1500 ml of pancreatic juice is secreted per day. Its inorganic constituents include Na^+, K^+, Cl^-

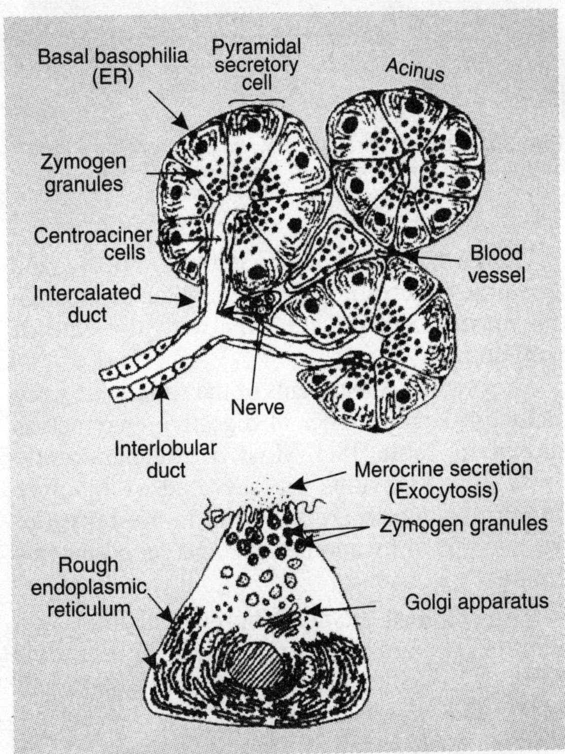

Fig. 38.1: Exocrine pancreas.

and HCO_3^-. It is alkaline in nature with a pH of about 8.0, due to the presence of HCO_3^- in high concentration. The concentration of HCO_3^- in the pancreatic secretion is rather high (80 mEq/L), even at low rates of secretion. At higher secretory rates, the concentration of HCO_3^- may increase up to 120 mEq/L. A reciprocal relationship between the HCO_3^- and Cl^- concentration of the pancreatic juice can be demonstrated (Fig. 38.2).

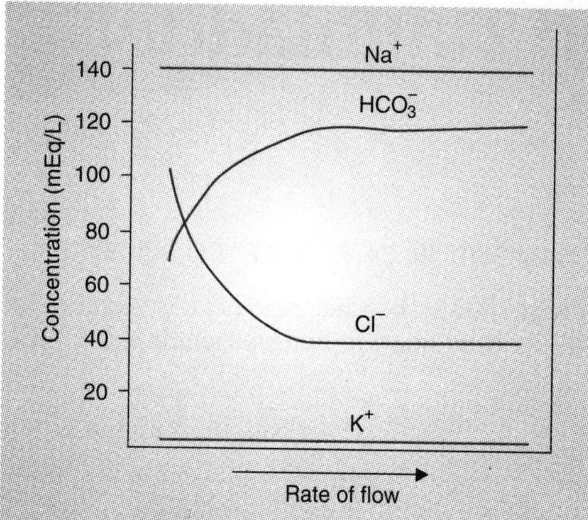

Fig. 38.2: Effect of rate of flow of pancreatic secretion on the ionic composition of the pancreatic juice.

Unlike the saliva, the concentrations of Na^+ and K^+ in the pancreatic juice are similar to those in the plasma and do not vary with the rate of secretion.

The organic constituents of the pancreatic juice include a large number of digestive enzymes as shown in Table 38.1 Most of the pancreatic proteolytic enzymes are secreted as inactive *proenzymes* which are activated in the lumen of the duodenum by another enzyme called enterokinase.

Enterokinase (a brush-border enzyme) is a proteolytic enzyme embedded in the cell membrane of epithelial cells of the proximal small intestines.

It splits off a part of trypsinogen forming the active enzyme trypsin. Trypsin, once formed, activates not only more of trypsinogen but also all other proenzymes present in the lumen.

Table 38.1: Various pancreatic enzymes and their actions

Enzyme	*Substrate*	*Action*
Trypsin	Protein	Breaks peptide bonds adjacent to arginine and lysine.
Chymotrypsin	Protein	Breaks peptide bonds adjacent to aromatic amino acids.
Carboxy-peptidase	Proteins	Splits terminal amino acids of the amino acid chains.
Lipase	Trigly-cerides	Hydrolysis of triglycerides.
Amylase	Polysa-ccharides	Hydrolysis of polysaccharides.
Ribonuclease	RNA	Splits RNA into nucleotides
Deoxyri-bonuclease	DNA	Splits DNA into nucle-otides.
Elastase	Elastin	Splits bonds adjacent to aliphatic amino acids.
Colipase	Fat	Facilitates action of lipase.

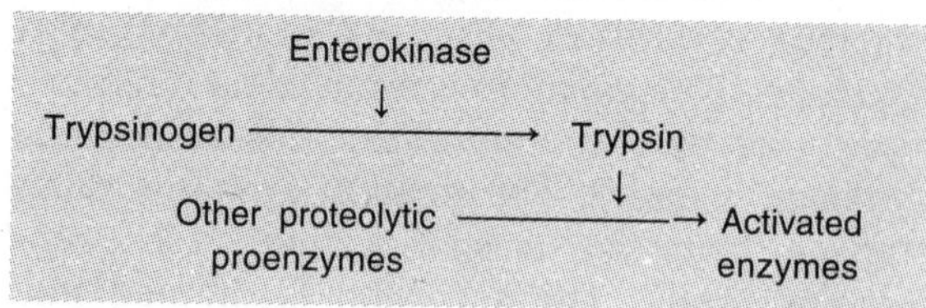

Trypsin and chymotrypsin are *endopeptidases*, i.e. they attack peptide bonds in the interior of proteins forming peptide fragments. Carboxypeptidase is an *exopeptidase* which splits off terminal amino acids from the proteins and peptides.

The pancreatic bicarbonate neutralizes the gastric acid entering the duodenum, thereby providing the optimum pH (6.0–7.0) for the action of pancreatic enzymes in the upper intestine.

Mechanism of Secretion

The pancreatic enzymes are synthesized in the acinar cells. The enzymes are synthesized in the rough endoplasmic reticulum and packaged into the zymogen granules to be released into ductal lumen by exocytosis.

The inorganic components, especially bicarbonate and water are chiefly contributed by the ductal cells. Although the exact mechanism of secretion of inorganic components is not clear; a tentative hypothesis is given below:

The mechanism of bicarbonate secretion is basically similar to that proposed for hydrochloric acid secretion in the oxyntic cells of the stomach. However, the crucial difference is that in the pancreas, H^+ is added to the blood and HCO_3^- to the lumen of the duct. The bicarbonate is derived from hydration of carbon dioxide in the presence of carbonic anhydrase. Bicarbonate is transferred to the ductal lumen by an HCO_3^-/Cl^- antiport operating at luminal border of the cells.

REGULATION OF PANCREATIC SECRETION

The regulation of pancreatic secretion is predominantly under hormonal control; the neural control is relatively less significant.

Neural Control

The reflex increase in vagal discharge due to stimulation of taste buds increases not only gastric secretion but also the pancreatic secretion to some extent. It results in secretion of a small amount of an enzyme-rich pancreatic juice. Enteropancreatic vago-vagal reflexes also increase enzyme secretion.

Hormonal Control

The presence of acid-rich chyme in the duodenum causes secretion of two local hormones, secretin and cholecystokinin (CCK) into the blood circulation. These hormones act on the ducts and the acini of the pancreas respectively, producing a large volume of pancreatic juice rich in HCO_3^- and enzymes.

Secretin

Secretin is a polypeptide with 27 amino acids. It is released by the **S cells** located among the epithelial cells of the duodenum and upper jejunum. The S cells are located in the transition zone of the epithelial lining between the crypts and the villi. Secretin acts on the exocrine pancreas, producing a large volume of pancreatic juice rich in HCO_3^- (Fig. 38.3). Acidity of the duodenal contents is the most important stimulus for the release of secretin. A fall of pH below 4.5 causes a prompt increase in the secretion of secretin. This feedback mechanism helps to neutralize the gastric acid reaching the duodenum. As a result, the pH of the upper intestine remains optimum for the action of the digestive enzymes. Products of protein digestion also increase secretin secretion. Other actions of secretin are summarized in Chapter 35.

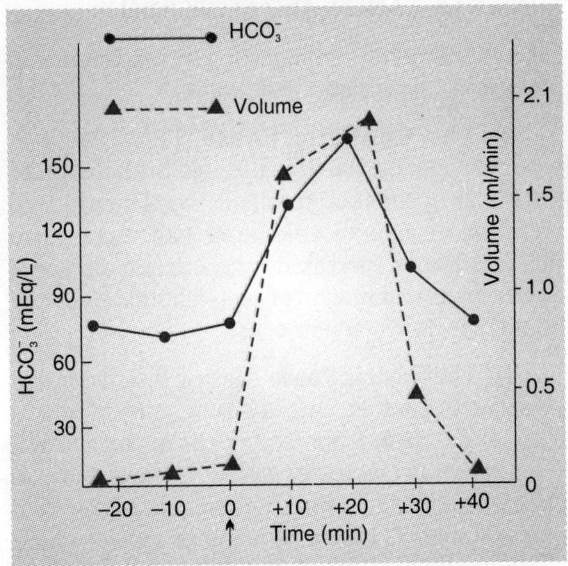

Fig. 38.3: Effect of a single dose of secretin on the HCO_3^- concentration and volume of pancreatic juice. Secretin injected at time 0

Cholecystokinin

The presence of food in the upper small intestine causes release of another hormone called cholecystokinin (CCK), a polypeptide containing 8/12 amino acids. Fats and products of partial protein digestion (proteoses and peptones) are potent stimuli for the release of CCK. This hormone acts on the pancreatic acini leading to the secretion of the enzymes into the pancreatic juice. Other actions of CCK are summarized in Chapter 35.

Gastrin

Gastrin released during the gastric digestion acts not only on the stomach but also on the pancreatic acini. In the pancreas, it stimulates the acinar cells to secrete the enzyme component of the pancreatic juice.

Somatostatin

Somatostatin is secreted by D cells in the gastrointestinal mucosa. It inhibits secretion of gastrin, secretin, VIP and GIP.

PHASES OF PANCREATIC SECRETION

Like gastric secretion, ingestion of food results in 3 phases of pancreatic secretion.

(i) The Cephalic Phase This phase is brought about by chewing of food. Stimulation of taste buds by the food results in vagally-madiated secretion of a small volume of pancreatic juice rich in enzymes. Increased vagal efferent discharge causes direct stimulation of acetylcholine receptors on the pancreatic acinar cells.

(ii) The Gastric Phase Gastric distension and presence of peptones in the gastric antrum causes release of gastrin from the G cells of the antrum. Gastrin not only increases gastric secretion but also causes secretion of a small amount of enzyme-rich pancreatic juice. Like gastric secretion, this phase also is partly neural in nature. Distension of stomach seems to stimulate vagal afferents resulting in a vago-vagal reflex which promotes pancreatic enzyme secretion.

(iii) The Intestinal Phase Quantitatively, this is the most important phase of pancreatic secretion. It is mediated both through hormones (secretin and CCK) as well as through entero-pancreatic vago-vagal reflex. Secretin is the most important mediator of ductal secretion of bicarbonate and water.

However, ductal cells contain acetylcholine- and CCK- receptors also. Hence neural stimuli as well as CCK potentiate the action of secretin on the ductal cells. The acinar secretion of enzymes is mediated through CCK, whose action is further potentiated by enteropancreatic vago-vagal reflexes.

PATHOPHYSIOLOGY

In a normal person, pancreatic enzymes do not digest the pancreas itself because of two reasons: (i) The enzymes are stored and secreted as proenzymes and normally activated only in the small intestine. (ii) Pancreatic acini produce a trypsin inhibitor which surrounds the zymogen granules. It inactivates any trypsin formed auto-catalytically in the acinar cells or the pancreatic ducts. These protective mechanisms fail in acute inflammatory condition of the pancreas.

Acute Pancreatitis It is a very serious and sometimes fatal inflammatory disease of the pancreas. The pancreatic enzymes leak out of the acini causing destruction of the adjacent tissues. The clinical picture is characterized by severe epigastric pain radiating to the back. Marked elevation of plasma amylase and trypsin levels is diagnostic.

Chronic Pancreatitis or the chronic inflammatory disorder of the pancreas results in the deficiency of the pancreatic secretions. The digestive disturbance mainly affects the fats. Increased faecal fat content is indicative of pancreatic insufficiency or intestinal malabsorption. To differentiate between the two causes of fat malabsorption, a double-lumened tube is introduced into the stomach and the duodenum. Gastric juice is aspirated from one lumen so that uncontaminated pancreatic juice can be collected from the other. An intravenous injection of secretin and CCK results in a prompt increase in a bicarbonate and enzyme rich pancreatic juice in normal individuals or those with intestinal malabsorption. The pancreatic secretion does not increase in patients with chronic pancreatitis. This test is known as the *secretin-cholecystokinin test*.

LIVER AND GALLBLADDER

FUNCTIONAL ANATOMY

(Colour Plate 5, Fig. 12)

The histology of the liver is shown in Fig. 38.4A. The hepatic cords radiate centrifugally from the central vein like spokes of a wheel. Branches of portal vein, hepatic artery and bile duct (portal triad) can be seen in the triangular islands of loose connective tissue in the periphery of each lobule. A central vein can be observed in the centre of each lobule.

Large blood sinusoids can be seen separating the cords of hepatocytes. Blood from branches of portal vein and hepatic artery enters the sinusoids to be drained by the central vein into the hepatic vein. Kupffer cells, the tissue macrophages, are present among the endothelial cells lining the hepatic sinusoids. There are large gaps between the endothelial cells of hepatic sinusoids. Therefore, the sinusoids are most permeable blood vessels.

A small bile canaliculus is present between the adjacent hepatic cells of each hepatic cord (Fig. 38.4B). The hepatic cells secrete bile into the canaliculus which is drained into the branches of bile duct located in the portal triad. Two hepatic ducts, one from each lobe of the liver, drain the bile secreted by the hepatocytes. The two hepatic ducts join to form a common hepatic duct (Fig. 38.5). Common bile duct is formed by the union of the common hepatic duct and the cystic duct of the gallbladder. The common bile duct is joined by the pancreatic duct to form the ampulla of Vater. The ampulla opens into the duodenum, where the opening is surrounded by a ring of smooth muscle cells called the sphincter of Oddi.

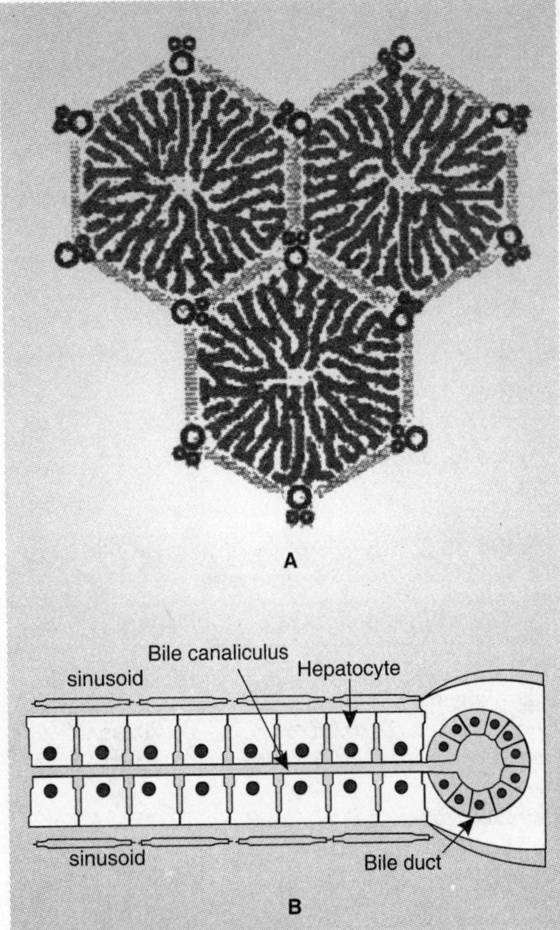

Fig. 38.4: (A) Histological structure of liver. (B) Detailed structure of a hepatic cord.

COMPOSITION OF BILE

Small amount of bile is continuously synthesized in the liver. It is transferred to the gallbladder through the cystic duct, because during the interdigestive period, tone of the sphincter of Oddi is so high that bile cannot enter the duodenum. About 700–1200 ml of bile is secreted by the liver per day. In the gallbladder, bile is stored and concentrated. After a meal, contraction of the gallbladder transfers a large volume of bile into the duodenum.

The composition of bile collected from the hepatic ducts and from common bile duct is shown in Table 38.2. *Inorganic constituents* include Na^+, K^+, Cl^-, HCO_3^-, Ca^{++}. In the gallbladder, water, NaCl, and other inorganic constituents are reabsorbed. Consequently, the organic components of bile become 5–6 times concentrated. The gallbladder contains about 60 ml concentrated bile which can be poured into the duodenum during digestion.

38

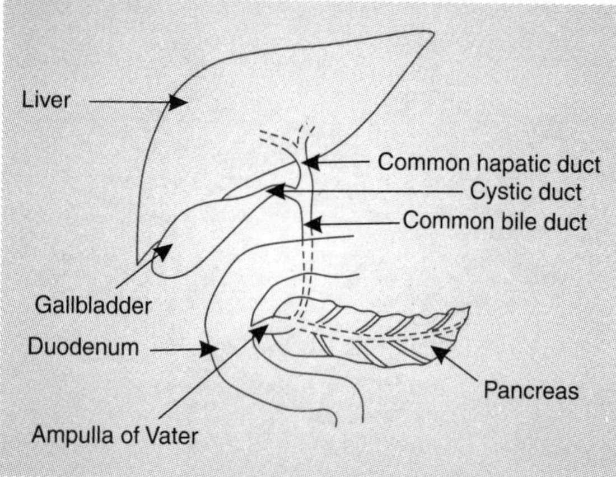

Fig. 38.5: Anatomy of the biliary tract.

Table 38.2: Components of hepatic bile and gallbladder bile

	Hepatic bile (%)	*Gallbladder bile (%)*
Bile salts	1.93	9.14
Bile pigments	0.53	2.98
Cholesterol	0.06	0.26
Lacithin	0.04	0.30
Fatty acids	0.14	0.32
Inorganic salts	0.84	0.65
Total solids	3.54	13.65
Water	97.5	86.40
pH	8.2	7.40

38

Organic Constituents

Bile Salts

Bile salts are the most important constituents of the bile. They are sodium and potassium salts of bile acids, conjugated to amino acids, glycine or taurine. The important bile acids formed in the liver include cholic acid and chenodeoxycholic acid. They are derived from cholesterol; therefore contain cyclopentano-perhydro-phenanthrene nucleus.

Bile salts help in digestion as well as absorption of fat and indirectly help in the absorption of fat soluble vitamins. Since the pancreatic lipase is a water-soluble enzyme, only the surface of a lipid droplet is accessible to its action. In the lumen of the upper small intestine, bile salts break up large lipid droplets into smaller droplets by a process

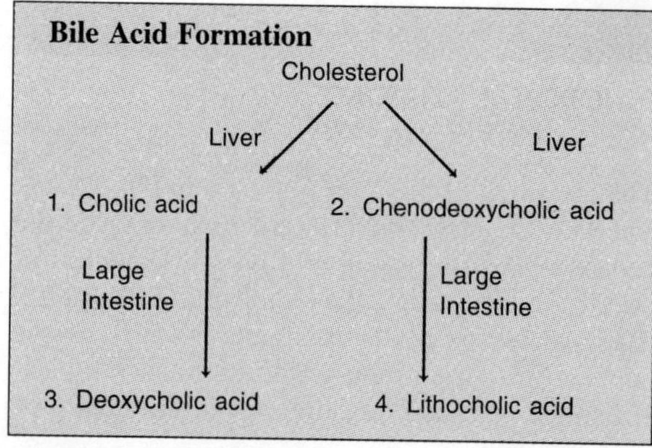

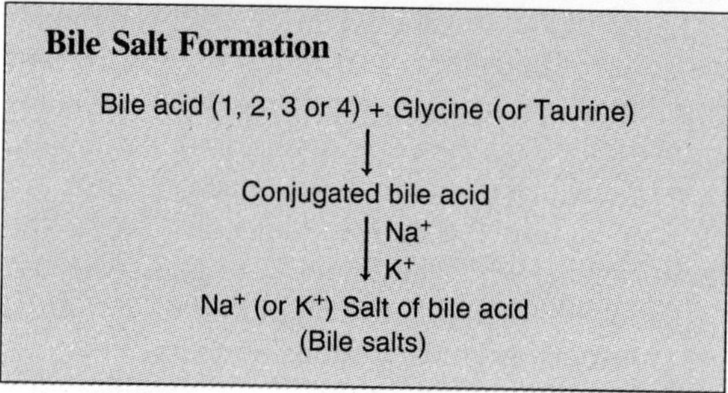

known as *emulsification*, thereby facilitating the digestive action of water soluble lipase. They also combine with the products of hydrolysis of triglycerides to form small water-soluble particles called *micelles* and transport them to the brush border of the epithelial cells for absorption.

From the ileum, 95% of the bile salts are reabsorbed into the portal blood to be resecreted into the bile on reaching the liver. By this **entero-hepatic circulation of bile salts** (Fig. 38.6), about 4–8 g of bile salts reach the duodenum during each meal although the total bile salt content of the body is only 3.5 g. Less than 5% of the bile salts reaching the intestines are degraded and excreted into the stools. That is why the normal rate of bile salt synthesis is approximately 0.2–0.4 g/day only.

Bile Pigments

Bile pigments, the other important constituents of bile have no digestive function. They are the excretory products of haemoglobin breakdown. They give the characteristic golden yellow colour to the bile. The bile pigments are mono- and di-

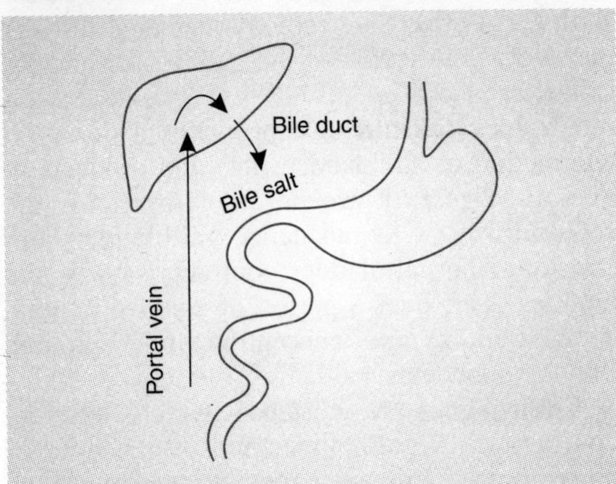

Fig. 38.6: Enterohepatic circulation of the bile salt.

glucuronides of bilirubin and biliverdin. The hepatic cells extract bilirubin (yellow) and biliverdin (green) from the blood, conjugate them with glucuronic acid and transfer them into the bile canaliculi by an active transport mechanism. An enzyme glucuronyl transferase is essential for this function (Fig. 38.7). Hepatocellular dysfunction or obstruction of the biliary passages cause accumulation of bile pigments in the blood producing hepatic or post-hepatic jaundice, respectively.

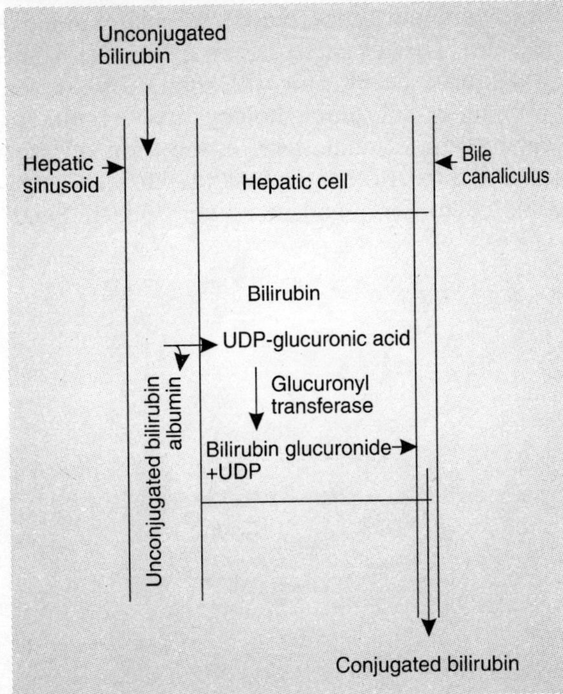

Fig. 38.7: Bile pigment metabolism in the hepatocyte.

Cholesterol

This is another important constituent of bile that does not have any digestive function. Bile serves as the only route of excretion of cholesterol ingested in food or synthesized in the body. Bile salts and lecithin help to solubilize cholesterol present in the bile. A disturbance in cholesterol: bile salts/lecithin is believed to be the cause of precipitation of the former as **gallstones** (large, sand like particles found in the gallbladder of some patients).

Other Excretory Products

Biliary excretion permits the organism to eliminate certain hydrophobic substrates that cannot be eliminated via renal excretion. Certain endogenous waste products, toxins, drugs and heavy metals (e.g. copper) are excreted in the bile.

Functions of Bile

1. Digestive Functions

(a) Bile salts help in digestion of fat in the intestine.
(b) Bile salts help in intestinal absorption of digested fat.
(c) Bile salts help in intestinal absorption of fat-soluble vitamins.
(d) The alkaline pH of bile helps to neutralize the gastric acid.

2. Excretory Functions. Bile is an important route of excretion of:

(i) Bilirubin
(ii) Cholesterol.
(iii) Many other endogenous waste products, drugs etc.

Regulation of Bile Secretion

(i) Neural control The secretion of bile by the liver is increased by *vagal activity* reflexly induced by stimulation of taste receptors in the mouth.

(ii) Secretin secretion also stimulates the formation of bile in the liver.

(iii) Bile salts themselves constitute the most important stimulus for the secretion of bile (Fig. 38.8). Thus, they act as **choleretic agents**—the substances which increase the secretion of bile by the hepatic cells. As the bile salts are recycled in the entero-hepatic circulation, they maintain high level of bile secretion during digestive period. The secretion of bile increases about 1 hour after a meal (when the gastric emptying starts). The maximum rate of bile secretion is achieved 3–5 hours after the intake of food.

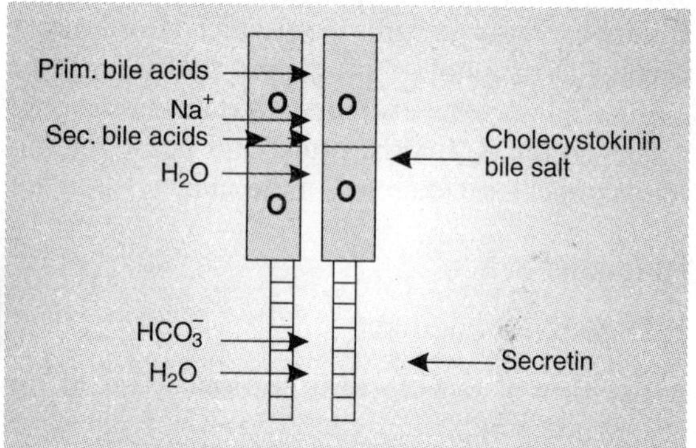

Fig. 38.8: Regulation of secretion of bile.

As the digestive process is completed, the tone of sphincter of Oddi increases once again, the recycling of bile salts stops and the choleretic action comes to an end.

Regulation of GallBladder Function

In between the meals, the rate of secretion of bile by the liver is low. The pressure in the common bile duct is too small to overcome the high resistance of sphincter of Oddi. Consequently, the bile is diverted to the gallbladder through the cystic duct, where it is stored and concentrated.

Shortly after the beginning of a meal, the gall-bladder contracts and the sphincter of Oddi relaxes. Both these effects are reflexly mediated through the *vagal innervation* of the gallbladder and the sphincter of Oddi.

Cholecystokinin also produces a powerful contraction of gallbladder. Fats and products of protein digestion are potent stimuli for the secretion of CCK and hence gallbladder contraction. The gallbladder contracts slowly and empties itself over a period of about one hour. Thus, about 60 ml of concentrated bile is poured into the duodenum.

Cholegogues are substances which cause the contraction of gallbladder and the transfer of concentrated bile into the duodenum. Thus, whereas bile salts act as choleretics, dietary fats and proteins act as cholegogues.

Pathophysiology of Gallstones

Cholesterol is insoluble in water. In the bile, bile salts and lecithin combine with cholesterol to form ultramicroscopic micelles which are water soluble. In the gallbladder, as the bile gets concentrated, the bile salts and lecithin are normally concentrated in the same proportion as cholesterol and hence, the latter remains soluble in bile. However, excessive secretion of cholesterol or chronic inflammation of the gallbladder (chronic cholecystitis) results in precipitation of cholesterol in the form of large sand-like particles. The sand particles may coalesce to form gallstones (Fig. 38.9). Small

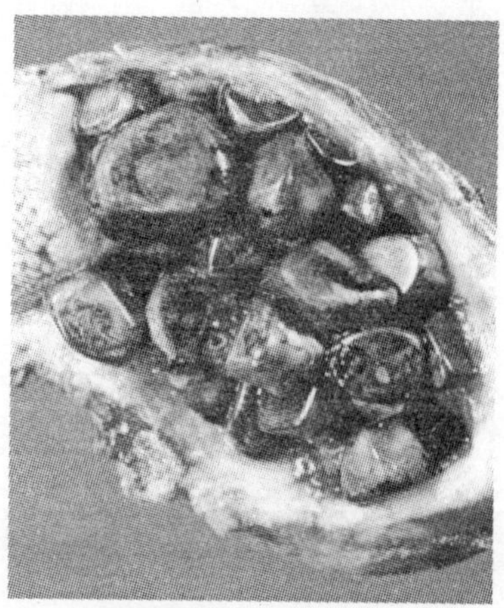

Fig. 38.9: Gallstones.

stones may slip into the common bile duct and cause acute pain (biliary colic) and obstruction of the duct. Obstruction of the common bile duct leads to regurgitation of bile into the liver and thereby in the general circulation causing obstructive jaundice. Absence of bile from the intestine causes impairment of digestion and absorption of fat and fat-soluble vitamins A, D and K. Deficiency of vitamin K may lead to haemorrhagic disorder. Most gallstones, unlike renal stones, do not contain calcium and hence are radio-translucent (cannot be seen in plain X-ray of abdomen). The function of the gallbladder is commonly investigated by oral cholecystography.

Oral Cholecystography

In this test, a radio-opaque dye is given orally to the patient in the evening. The dye is excreted by the liver into the bile and concentrated in the gallbladder. About 14–16 hours later (next morning), the gallbladder shadow can be observed on an X-ray picture of the upper abdomen. *Gallstone*, if present, may be detected as "filling defects" in the gallbladder shadow. The subject is then given a fatty meal (a glassful of cream) and another X-ray picture is taken 30 and 60 minutes later. Normally, the gallbladder shadow shrinks to about one-third of the previous shadow (Fig. 38.10). A failure of the shadow to shrink indicates poor gallbladder contraction in response to fatty meal. This is taken as a sign of *chronic cholecystitis*. In long-standing cases of this disorder, the concentrating power of the gallbladder is decreased to such an extent that even the last X-ray may not show proper gallbladder shadow.

Effects of Cholecystectomy

The gallbladder may have to be removed in patients with gallstones or chronic cholecystitis. In the absence of the storage site (gallbladder) small amount of dilute (hepatic) bile is discharged into the intestine continuously rather than during the digestive period only. After cholecystectomy, the patient has difficulty in the digestion of a heavy fatty meal; otherwise the digestive function is almost normal.

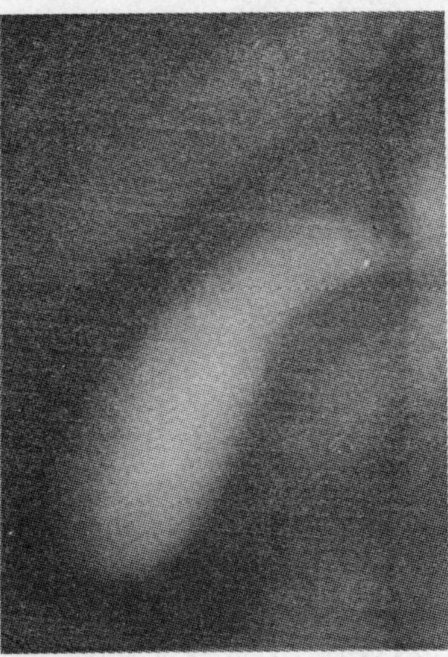

Fig. 38.10: X-ray photographs of the gallbladder after oral administration of a radio-opaque dye in the evening and a cup full of cream next morning.

FUNCTIONS OF LIVER

The functions of the liver are so numerous and varied that they can only be enumerated here.

1. **Synthesis of Bile** This function has been discussed above.
2. **Storage Function** Storage of glycogen, proteins, fats, vitamin A, and vitamin B_{12}, iron.
3. **Metabolic Functions**
   a. Carbohydrate metabolism
      i. Storage of glycogen.
      ii. Regulation of blood glucose.
      iii. Neoglucogenesis.
   b. Fat metabolism Synthesis of fatty acids, cholesterol, ketone bodies, etc.
   c. Protein metabolism
      i. Synthesis of plasma proteins like albumin, carrier proteins, coagulation factors, etc.
      ii. Transamination, deamination and synthesis of urea.

   The liver plays a pivotal role in the metabolism of carbohydrates, fats and proteins. The role of liver mentioned above in these metabolic processes is highly abbreviated. For full details, the chapters on the concerned metabolism should be consulted.

4. **Destruction of old RBCs** (by the Kupffer's cells)
5. **Hydroxylation of vitamin D_3** to 25-OH vitamin D_3.
6. **Inactivation/detoxification** of many hormones, drugs and other toxic products.

PATHOPHYSIOLOGY

Hepatocellular Failure

Hepatocellular failure may occur in acute viral hepatitis or in cirrhosis of the liver. In early stages, indigestion, weakness, muscular wasting and jaundice may be observed. The stage of precoma is characterised by drowsiness, intellectual deterioration, confusion, personality change, tremor, slow and slurred speech. Ultimately, unconsciousness (hepatic coma) sets in, ending in death.

Hepatic coma and precoma have been attributed to the effects of ammonia and other toxic nitrogenous products on the brain. These toxic products are the result of bacterial degradation of nitrogenous substances (proteins) in the gut. These products are normally detoxified in the liver. In hepatocellular failure, the detoxification fails to occur and the toxic nitrogenous products (chiefly ammonia) accumulate in the blood and reach the brain (Fig. 43.3).

Disturbance of plasma glucose, electrolyte levels, and acid-base balance may also contribute to the pathophysiology of hepatocellular failure.

Jaundice (Colour Plate 5, Fig. 13)

Acute viral hepatitis is a common cause of jaundice (hepatic jaundice). In addition, jaundice may be due to non-hepatic causes like excessive haemolysis (haemolytic jaundice or prehepatic jaundice) or obstruction of the common bile duct (obstructive or post-hepatic jaundice). In the latter two types, the hepatocellular function is usually normal and only bile pigment metabolism is disturbed. Thus, the liver function tests may be required for the differential diagnosis of a patient of jaundice or to establish the existence of chronic hepatocellular damage.

Investigations for differential diagnosis of jaundice Observations on various tests for the differential diagnosis of jaundice are summarized in Table 38.3.

Table 38.3: Differential diagnosis of jaundice (liver function tests)

Investigation	*Normal range*	*Jaundice*		
		Pre-hepatic	*Hepatic*	*Post-hepatic*
1. Plasma bilirubin (total)	0.2–1 mg%	↑	↑	↑
2. Plasma bilirubin (conjugated)	0.1–0.4 mg%	→	↑	↑
3. Faecal stercobilinogen	40–280 mg/24 h	↑	↓	↓
4. Urinary bilirubin	Zero	–	++	+++
5. Urobilinogen	0–4 mg/24 h	↑	↑↓	↓
6. Plasma albumin	3.5–5.5 g%	→	↓	→
7. Plasma transaminases	5–14 IU/L	→	↑	→
8. Plasma alkaline phosphatase	3–13 KAU%	→	↑	↑

Plasma Transaminases

Measurement of these enzyme helps to monitor the degree of acute or chronic hepatic cell injury. The test does not reflect any cellular function as such. These enzymes are released into the circulation from the damaged liver cells. Therefore, their levels in the plasma reflect the extent of hepatic cell injury. Serum glutamic-oxaloacetic transaminase (SGOT) and serum glutamic-pyruvic transaminase (SGPT) and isocitrate dehydrogenase enzymes are usually tested.

39 CHAPTER

The Intestines

SMALL INTESTINE

FUNCTIONAL ANATOMY

(Colour Plate 6, Fig. 14)

The small intestine measures about 3 m in length during life. (At autopsy, it seems to be much longer due to loss of smooth muscle tone). The ligament of Treitz demarcates the jejunum from duodenum. Below the duodenum, the upper 40% of the small intestine is known as the jejunum and the lower 60% as the ileum. There is no anatomical boundary between the jejunum and the ileum.

The mucous membrane of the small intestine is characterized by the presence of finger-like projections known as the villi. There are about 20–40 villi per square millimetre. Each villus is covered by a single layer of epithelial cells. The core of each villus contains a network of blood capillaries, a single blind-ended lymph vessel called a lacteal and a few smooth muscle fibres extending from the muscularis mucosa (Fig. 39.1).

The luminal surface of each epithelial cell shows small multiple projections of the cell membrane called the microvilli or the brush border (Fig. 39.2). The villi, the microvilli and the valvulae conniventes increase the surface area of the small intestine by about 600 folds.

Throughout the length of the small intestine, deep invaginations of the surface epithelium form simple tubular intestinal glands, known as crypts of Lieberkuhn. In the duodenum, compound mucous glands called the Brunner's glands are also present mainly between the pylorus and papilla of Vater. These mucous glands are mostly present in the submucosa of the duodenum.

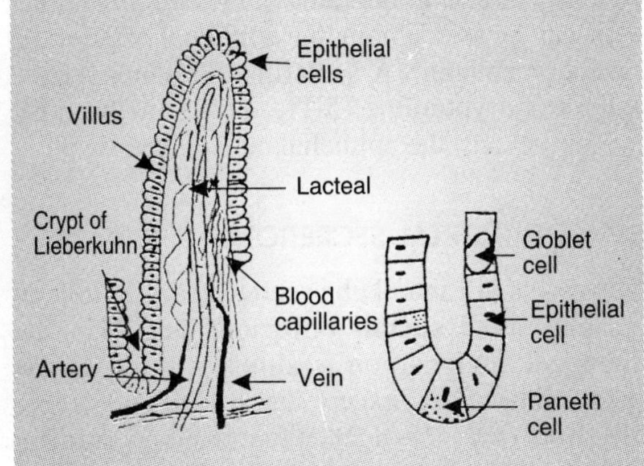

Fig. 39.1: (A) Histological structure of the small intestinal mucosa. (B) Detailed structure of the crypt.

The cells of the lower parts of the crypts undergo active mitotic division. The newly formed cells migrate up to the tips of the villi to be sloughed off into the lumen of the intestine. The total cycle of cell migration from the base of the crypts to the tip of the villus takes about five days.

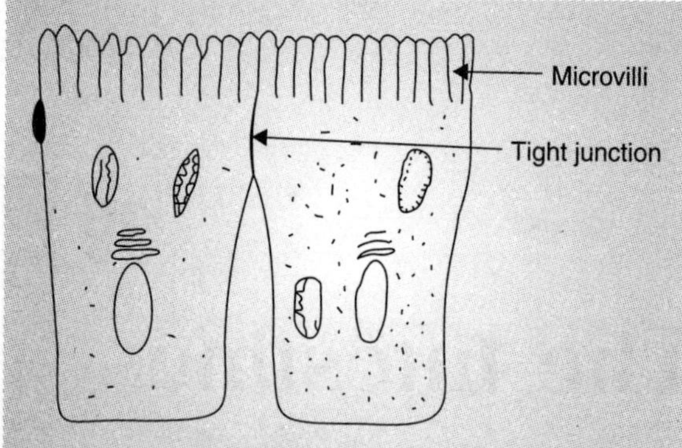

Fig. 39.2: Electron microscopic structure of epithelial cell of the intestinal mucosa.

Thus, about 17 billion cells containing nearly 3 g of proteins are shed into the intestine per day.

Fairly large number of mucous secreting goblet cells can be seen among the epithelial cells of the mucous membrane. Argentaffin cells which secrete 5-hydroxytryptamine (5HT, serotonin) are also present among the epithelial cells of the crypt.

39

SMALL INTESTINAL SECRETIONS

The crypts of Lieberkuhn secrete about 2 litres of a fluid called **succus entericus** per 24 h. Its chemical composition is almost similar to the extracellular fluid, except that it is slightly more alkaline (pH 7.5–8.0). This fluid is rapidly reabsorbed by the intestinal villi. The circulation of this fluid from the crypts to the villi supplies a watery vehicle for absorption of food stuffs from the small intestine.

Digestive Enzymes

If the secretions of the small intestinal glands are collected without the addition of cellular debris, no enzyme can be detected in it. However, the epithelial cells of the small intestine do contain a large number of digestive enzymes. These enzymes are present in the brush border of the epithelial cells. It is believed that these **brush border enzymes** produce final hydrolysis of the food stuffs on the surface of the epithelial cells prior to the absorption of the end products like amino acids, monosaccharides and fatty acids into the cell. The following digestive enzymes have been identified on the brush border:

(i) Three types of **disaccharidases**, i.e. sucrase, maltase and lactase which split the respective disaccharides into the monosaccharides.
(ii) Several **peptidases** that split polypeptides into amino acids.
(iii) Small amount of **intestinal lipase** that splits triglycerides.
(iv) **Enterokinase** that activates trypsinogen.

The *Brunner's glands* secrete thick alkaline mucoid secretion into the duodenum that helps to protect the duodenal mucosa against the acidic chyme coming from the stomach. The *goblet cells* of the surface epithelium secrete mucus throughout the small intestine which helps to lubricate the chyme.

Regulation of Small Intestinal Secretion

Secretion of the crypts of Lieberkuhn is regulated mainly by the *local neural reflexes* initiated by distension of the intestine or irritation of the mucosa by the chyme. The local hormone called *vasoactive intestinal polypeptide (VIP)* also increases the secretion of the crypts of Lieberkuhn.

The secretion of the *Brunner's glands* is increased by: (i) vagus stimulation, (ii) direct tactile stimulation or irritation of the duodenal mucosa, and (iii) secretin. The protective role of the Brunner's glands would be obvious from the fact that the alkaline pancreatic juice can neutralize the acid-rich chyme only in the second part of duodenum. In other words, the first part of the duodenum would remain unprotected against the gastric acid but for the secretions of the Brunner's glands. This may also explain the relation between psychogenic stress and the common occurrence of peptic ulcer in the first part of duodenum.

MOTILITY OF SMALL INTESTINE

Two types of movements can be observed in the small intestine: Segmentation movements and paristaltic movements.

Segmentation Movements

These are non-propulsive type of intestinal movements. Segmentation movements consist of alternate contraction and relaxation of the rings of smooth muscle of the intestine. Each contracting segment is 1–4 cm long. The contraction lasts for about 5 seconds after which the contracting segment relaxes whereas the previously relaxing segment undergoes a contraction (Fig. 39.3). As a result, the chyme moves back and forth but there is no net movement of the chyme towards the large intestine. Segmentation movements help in: (i) digestion by mixing the chyme with the intestinal juices; and (ii) absorption by bringing the products of digestion in contact with the ever-changing absorptive surface of intestinal mucosa. The frequency of segmentation movement is determined by the frequency of the BER (the slow wave activity). In the small intestine, unlike the stomach, the BER is generated spontaneously from multiple foci. The frequency of BER decreases from about 12/min in the duodenum and upper jejunum to about 9/min in the lower ileum.

Peristaltic Movements

Peristaltic movements are superimposed over the segmentation movements. Peristalsis is a propulsive movement which moves the chyme towards the large intestine. A peristaltic wave consists of deep circular ring of contraction which passes down the intestine at the rate of 0.5–2.0 cm/second (Fig. 36.4). Each peristaltic wave travels for a variable but short distance and then dies out. A new wave of contraction is now initiated from a site little distal to the site of origin of the previous wave. In this fashion, the chyme moves along the intestine at a rate of about 1 cm/min. It takes about 3–5 h for the chyme to move from the pylorus to the ileo-caecal valve.

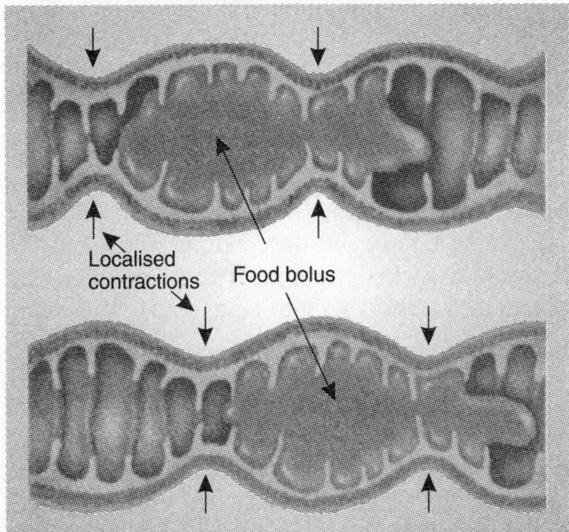

Fig. 39.3: Segmentation movements of the small intestine.

Mechanism

The coordinated peristaltic activity is dependent on the integrity of the **enteric nerve plexus.** Circumferential stretch of the intestine stimulates the stretch receptors which produce a local myenteric reflex leading to contraction of the longitudinal muscle. The reflex activity causes a circular contraction behind the stimulus (stretch) and an area of relaxation in front of it.

Functions

Peristaltic movements *propel the chyme* and also *help in the digestion and absorption* of the food stuffs because different types of nutrients are digested and absorbed in different segments of the small intestine.

The peristaltic waves always travel from the oral end towards the aboral end of the intestine. This phenomenon is known as the *law of the intestines*.

The law of the intestines has been attributed to the descending rate of rhythmicity of BER.

Regulation

The magnitude of segmentation movements and the peristalsis is affected by a number of neural and hormonal influences. Parasympathetic stimulation increases the intestinal motility whereas the sympathetic stimulation decreases it (Fig. 39.4). Intestinal motility is also increased by 5-hydroxytryptamine (5-HT, serotonin) and thyroxine.

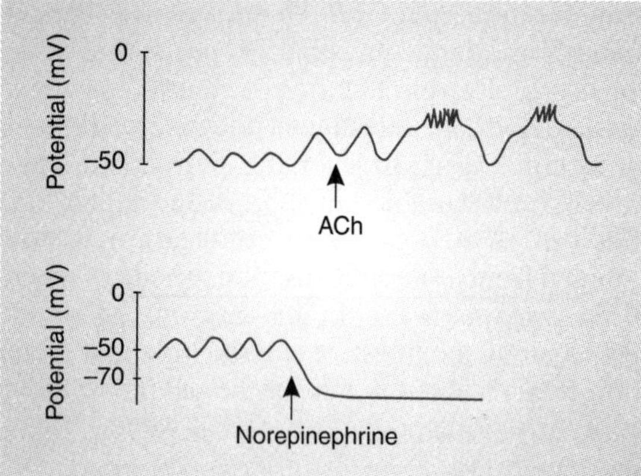

Fig. 39.4: Effect of autonomic neurotransmitters on the membrane potential of the gut.

Emotional states of an individual influence the intestinal motility. Fear decreases the motility, whereas hostility and anger increase it.

ILEO-CAECAL VALVE

39 At the ileo-caecal junction, the ileum is invaginated into the caecum. The ileal opening is very small (2–3 mm in diameter) and offers resistance to the passage of ileal contents into the caecum. The principal function of the ileo-caecal valve is to prevent back flow of faecal matter from the caecum to the ileum. Increased caecal pressure tends to close the ileal opening.

In the terminal part of the ileum, extending over several centimetres, immediately preceding the ileo-caecal valve, the circular muscle coat is thickened to constitute the *ileo-caecal sphincter*. The sphincter normally remains closed and slows down the emptying of the ileal contents into the caecum. In this way, the ileo-caecal sphincter helps in complete absorption of nutrients in the ileum.

GASTRO-ILEAL REFLEX

The gastro-ileal reflex increases the motility of terminal ileum after each meal. The gastro-ileal reflex is initiated by the gastric emptying and helps in increasing the peristaltic activity in the terminal ileum. The gastric hormone, gastrin, also seems to produce a direct relaxation of the ileo-caecal sphincter. Gastro-ileal reflex is mediated through the vagus nerve.

Gastrointestinal Motility in Interdigestive Period

The movements of small intestine described above are seen after ingestion of a meal. In a fasting state, or about six hours after a meal, the pattern of gastrointestinal motility is different. During this period, the gastrointestinal motility is characterized by bursts of intense electrical and contractile activity lasting 1–5 minutes separated by long quiescent periods lasting about 90 minutes. During the active phase, the contractions are more vigorous and more propulsive than contractions that occur after ingestion of food. These interdigestive movements *sweep the stomach and small intestine clear* and empty their contents into the caecum. The cyclic electrical phenomenon starts in the stomach and migrates to the terminal ileum. Hence it has been called **migrating myoelectrical complex (MMC).** The exact genesis of MMC is not clear. It may be mediated through the vagus nerve. The gastrointestinal hormone **motilin**, secreted by endocrine cells of the small intestine, may also be involved in its genesis.

COLON (LARGE INTESTINE)

The colon is a tube about 6 cm in diameter and 100 cm in length. It consists of a blind-ended pouch, the caecum, the ascending colon, the transverse colon, the descending colon and the terminal S-shaped sigmoid (pelvic) colon which opens into a short rectum (Fig. 39.5). The ileum opens into the caecum.

The longitudinal muscle layer is not uniformly distributed in the circumference of the colon. Instead, these muscle fibres are collected into three thick longitudinal bands called the teniae coli. The length of the teniae coli is shorter than the length of the large intestine. Consequently, the thin walls of the colon form numerous out-pouches **(haustra)** (Fig. 39.6). The mucosa of the large intestine is

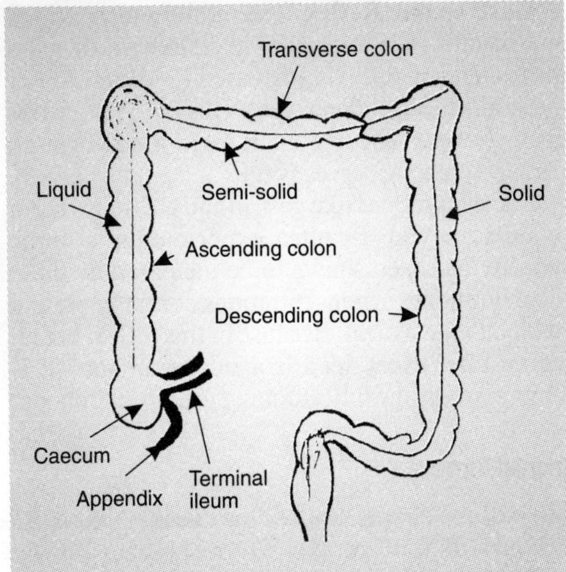

Fig. 39.5: Consistency of faecal contents in different segments of the large gut.

characterized by the presence of simple tubular glands (crypts of Lieberkuhn), the absence of villi and the presence of huge number of goblet cells among the surface epithelial cells.

LARGE INTESTINAL SECRETIONS

Mucus is the chief secretion of the glands of large intestine. It helps to lubricate the faecal matter. Its alkaline nature (pH 8.0) is due to the presence of HCO_3^- which serves to neutralize the acids formed by bacterial action on the faecal matter. Colonic bacteria cause production of gases like CO_2, H_2S and methane (CH_4) but most of the flatus passed from the rectum consists of nitrogen from the air swallowed during deglutition.

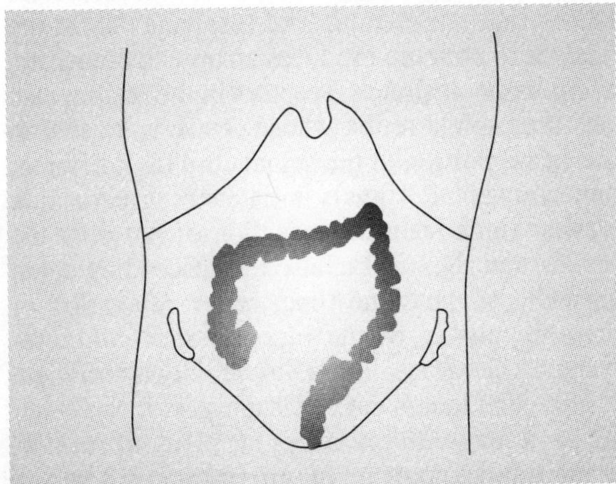

Fig. 39.6: Barium enema: showing haustra.

The secretory activity of the large intestine is increased by the tactile stimulation of the mucosa. The effect is produced by a direct action on the surface epithelium and through local neural mechanism which increase the secretion of the crypts of Lieberkuhn. The physiological role of extrinsic innervation in colonic secretions is not significant. However, pathologic stimulation of pelvic parasympathetic nerves causes marked increase in mucus secretion as well as motility of the colon. That may explain diarrhoea and passage of large amount of mucus in some patients with intense emotional disturbance.

Functions

1. **Absorption of Water and Electrolytes** It is the chief function of the proximal half of the colon. After absorption of the food stuffs in the small intestines, about one litre of isotonic chyme containing residual matter, salts and water reaches the colon. Large intestine can absorb Na^+, Cl^-, and H_2O but *cannot absorb amino acids, fatty acids or* Ca^{2+}. By absorption of the salt and fluid, about 200–300 ml of semi-solid faeces are left.

2. **Certain Vitamins**, e.g. vitamin K and a number of B complex vitamins are **synthesized** by the normal colonic bacteria. They are also absorbed in the large intestine. Broad-spectrum antibiotics, when administered for treatment of infections, kill these harmless (rather useful) bacteria. Hence the body need of vitamin B complex is increased. That is why vitamin B complex is always prescribed along with broad-spectrum antibiotics.

3. **Storage Function** The faeces are stored in the pelvic colon until they can be expelled by the process of defaecation.

Faeces

The stools consist of undigested plant fibre, inorganic material (mostly calcium and phosphate), small amount fat and water. Small amounts of nitrogenous material, mostly of non-dietary origin (desquamated epithelial cells of the mucosa of the intestines) are also present. The faeces contain a large amount of bacteria (most of which are dead), bile pigments and desquamated epithelial cells. If vegetable and coarse cereals are excluded from the diet, the faeces have a fairly uniform composition, i.e. water 65%; solids 35% (inorganic salts 15%, ether soluble substances 15%, nitrogen 5%). When the diet contains a large amount of unabsorbable cellulose due to ingestion of vegetarian food, the bulk of the faeces is markedly increased.

MOTILITY OF LARGE INTESTINE

Segmentation movements occur in the large intestine also. They help in the function of absorbing water and salts. The frequency of movements in the large intestine is only 1–2/min. Segmentation movements result in greater prominence of haustrations. Segmentation movements of the large intestine differ from those in the small intestine:

(i) The regularity of the segments (haustra) is far greater.

(ii) Large length of the large intestine shows haustra at a given time.

Slow wave activity can be observed in the colon but the frequency is only 9/min near the caecum and increases to 16/min in the sigmoid colon. Thus, the frequency of slow wave activity gradually increases down the large intestine, in contrast to gradually decreasing frequency of SWA in the small intestine.

The peristaltic activity can be observed in the large intestine which slowly propels the contents towards the rectum. In the colon, another type of peristaltic activity produces what is called the mass movement **(mass peristalsis)**. During such a contraction, which lasts for about 3 minutes, a marked rise of intraluminal pressure occurs over large segments of the colon. As a result, the colonic contents are propelled towards the sigmoid colon. These contractions occur 3–4 times a day, generally after meals. They seem to be induced by the gastrocolic reflex.

Gastro-colic Reflex The motility of proximal and distal colon as well as the strength of mass movements is reflexly increased by distension of the stomach, e.g. after a meal. This is due to gastro-colic reflex. The reflex is mediated through parasympathetic nerves (vagus and pelvic nerves).

Local hormones like gastrin and CCK also seem to be involved. In vitro experiments, colonic motility has been shown to be increased by these local hormones at concentrations normally present in blood after a meal. Because of this reflex, defaecation after every feed is a rule in infants. It is suppressed by the toilet training in early childhood.

Transit Time

Most of the chyme reaches the caecum within 8–9 hours of food intake. From the caecum the residual (faecal) matter is transported more slowly. It takes another 8–14 hours to reach the sigmoid colon. Vegetarian food (with large amount of cellulose) and spices shorten the transit time. Non-residual food prolongs it.

Defaecation

The mass movements of the large gut generally do not drive the faecal matter into the rectum. The rectum normally remains empty except during defaecation. The junction between the sigmoid colon and the rectum acts as a weak sphincter. Usually, once a day, as a result of strong gastro-colic reflex activity, a mass movement forces the faeces into the rectum. The resultant rise in the intrarectal pressure produces an urge to defaecate. Stimulation of stretch receptors in the rectum also sets up a spinal reflex whose centre is located in the sacral portion of the spinal cord (S_2). Efferent parasympathetic signals initiate strong peristaltic waves which lead to evacuation of not only the rectum and sigmoid but also the descending colon as well. At the same time, reflex relaxation of smooth muscle of the internal anal sphincter occurs. The defaecation reflex activity is sufficient to expel the faeces out of the anus (as it can occur in patients with paraplegia). But normally, defaecation is assisted by respiratory muscles. A deep inspiratory effort is followed by closure of the glottis and contraction of abdominal muscles. The consequent marked rise in intra-abdominal pressure forces down the contents of colon.

Contraction of the muscles of the pelvic floor also helps to evacuate the faeces out of the anus. Except in infants, defaecation is under voluntary control. The external anal sphincter is innervated by pudendal nerve. Normally, it remains closed. Moderate increase in rectal pressure causes further contraction of the external sphincter. If the external sphincter is not voluntarily relaxed, the defaecation reflex dies out after a few minutes and does not recur for several hours.

PATHOPHYSIOLOGY

Diarrhoea It is characterized by *increased water content of the faeces*. It is usually accompanied by increased frequency of defaecation. It can be caused by a number of bacterial, protozoal and viral infections of the intestinal tract. Loss of water, K^+ and HCO_3^- are serious consequences of severe diarrhoea, which may lead to death (specially in infants) due to dehydration. Oral rehydration therapy (ORT) is a life-saving and easily available measure against dehydration.

Constipation It is a fairly common problem. It is frequently caused by irregular bowel habits. If the sensation of fullness of rectum is repeatedly ignored, adaptation occurs. Progressively increasing weakness of the defaecation reflex makes constipation worse.

The symptoms of constipation include headache, loss of appetite, nausea and abdominal distension. These symptoms are not due to absorption of any toxic substance from the colon. These symptoms can be reproduced by inflating a balloon in the rectum. Moreover, in constipated patients, the symptoms disappear immediately after the evacuation of rectum. Constipation is best treated by increasing the ingestion of raw vegetables which contain large amounts of cellulose. Cellulose adds to the bulk of the faeces. The increased bulk of the faecal matter aids in colonic peristalsis by distension.

CHAPTER

40 Digestion and Absorption

Human diet consists of complex macromolecules of carbohydrates, fats and proteins. These large complex molecules cannot be absorbed in the alimentary canal as such. They need to be broken down to simpler and smaller units, by the process of **digestion.** These small units as well as vitamins, minerals and water cross the mucosal epithelium and enter into the blood circulation or lymph **(absorption)**. The small intestine is the major site of the processes of digestion and absorption.

The various digestive enzymes involved in the process of digestion of various foodstuffs are summarized in Table 40.1.

CARBOHYDRATES

Plant starch is the chief source of carbohydrates in human food. It is a high molecular weight **polysaccharide.** Small amounts of sucrose and lactose (the **disaccharides)**, and glucose and fructose (the **monosaccharides)** are also ingested (Fig. 40.1). Glycogen (the animal starch) may be ingested in non-vegetarian diet.

Starch consists of branched chains of glucose monomers. The glucose units are linked by **1,4-α-glycosidic linkage.** Starch consists of about 80% amylopectin and 20% amylose. The two polysaccharides differ only in the fact that amylose consists of unbranched chains whereas amylopectin is composed of branched chains with 24–30 glucose residues. The branching occurs at points where 1,6-α-glycosidic linkages are present. Glycogen basically has similar structure as starch with 1,4-α-linkages all over and 1,6-α-linkages at the branching point. However, the branching pattern of glycogen is far more complex than that of amylopectin (Fig. 40.2).

The vegetables and cereals contain another polysaccharide, cellulose, with β-glycosidic linkages. Since human gastrointestinal secretions contain only α-amylase, cellulose is not digested in the human gut. Cellulose is one of the major components of dietary fibre.

Digestion

The digestion of carbohydrates begins in the mouth. The salivary α-amylase acts on the starch and attacks the internal 1,4-α-glycosidic linkages. The principal products of α-amylase action are maltose and branched oligosaccharides, since, α-amylase cannot attack 1,6-α-linkages or the terminal glycosidic linkages. The optimum pH of the action of salivary amylase is 6.7. Food remains in the mouth for a very short period but the action of salivary amylase continues for 20–30 minutes even in the stomach till the highly acidic gastric juice mixes with the food and terminates its action. Thus considerable digestion of starch occurs with the help of salivary amylase but it is not essential.

Table 40.1: Principal digestive enzymes (Proenzymes are written in brackets)

Source	*Enzymes*	*Substrate*	*Catalytic function or products*
Salivary glands	Salivary α-amylase	Starch	Hydrolyses 1,4- α-linkages
Stomach	Pepsin (pepsinogen)	Proteins and polypeptides	Cleaves peptide bonds adjacent to aromatic amino acids.
Exocrine pancreas	Trypsin (trypsinogen)	Proteins and polypeptides	Cleaves peptide bonds adjacent to arginine or lysine.
	Chymotrypsin (chymotrypsinogen)	Proteins and polypetides	Cleaves peptide bonds adjacent to amino acids that have aromatic side chains.
	Elastase (proelastase)	Elastin	Cleaves carboxy-terminal amino acids with aliphatic chain.
	Carboxypeptidase A (procarboxypeptidase A)	Proteins and polypeptides	Cleaves carboxy-terminal amino acids with aromatic or branched aliphatic side chain.
	Carboxypeptidase B (procarboxypeptidase B)	Proteins and polypeptides	Cleaves carboxy-terminal amino acids with basic side chain.
	Pancreatic lipase	Triglycerides	Monoglycerides and fatty acids
	Pancreatic esterase	Cholesterol esters	Cholesterol
	Pancreatic α-amylase	Starch	Hydrolyses 1,4 α-linkages
	Ribonuclease	RNA	Nucleotides
	Deoxyribonuclease	DNA	Nucleotides
	Phospholipase A	Lecithin	Lysolecithin
Intestinal mucosa	Enterokinase	Trypsinogen	Trypsin
	Aminopeptidase	polypeptides	Cleaves N-terminal amino acid from peptide
	Dipeptidase	Dipeptides	Two animo acids
	Maltase	Maltose, maltotriose	Glucose
	Lactase	Lactose	Galactose and glucose
	Sucrase	Sucrose	Fructose and glucose
	α limit dextrinase	α-limit-dextrins	Glucose
	Nuclease	nucleic acids	Pentoses, purine and pyrimidine bases.
Cytoplasm of mucosal cells	Di-tri- and tetra-peptidases	Di-, tri- and tetra-peptides	Amino acids

Pancreatic amylase can digest all the starch even if the salivary amylase is completely absent.

Pancreatic α-amylase has an action similar to salivary amylase. But its concentration in the pancreatic juice is much greater. Like salivary amylase, it also attacks 1,4-α-glycosidic linkages. Within 10–15 minutes of its arrival in duodenum, most of the starch is hydrolysed to maltose, the disaccharide, maltotriose, the trisaccharide and α-limit dextrins, the branched polymers containing about 8-glucose molecules. Further digestion of carbohydrates occurs by enzymes located in the brush border of the epithelial cells of the small intestine.

The brush border of the small intestine contains the following digestive enzymes:

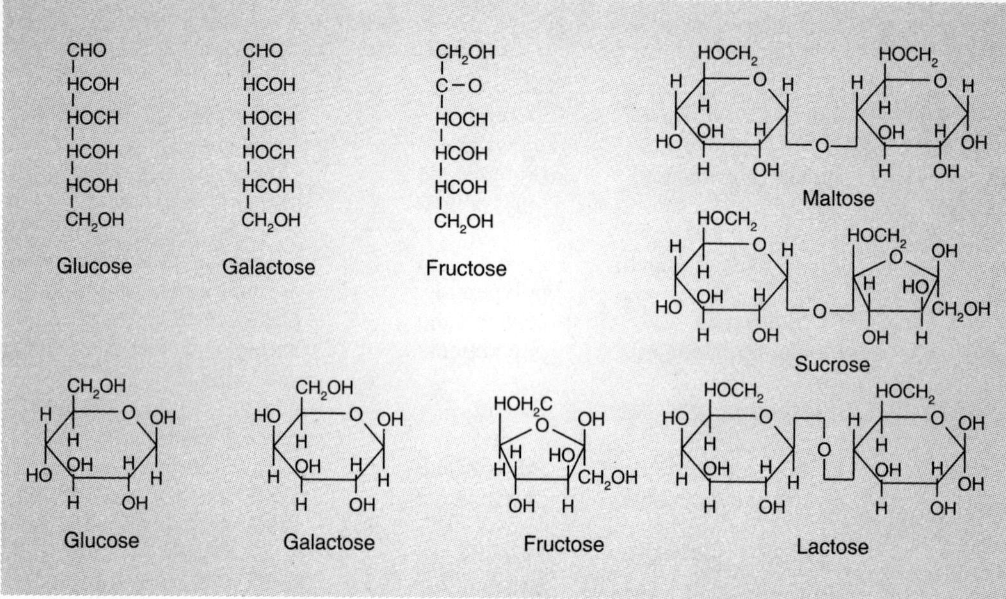

Fig. 40.1: Structures of mono- and disaccharides.

(i) α-limit dextrinase, the only enzyme in the GIT which attacks 1,6-α-glycosidic linkage, at the branching points of α-limit dextrins. This enzyme also attacks 1,4-α-glycosidic linkages resulting in sequential removal of glucose monomers from the dextrins.
(ii) Maltase
(iii) Sucrase
(iv) Lactase

The last three enzymes hydrolyse the corresponding disaccharides as follows:

$$\text{Maltose} \xrightarrow{\text{Maltase}} \text{Glucose + Glucose}$$

$$\text{Sucrose} \xrightarrow{\text{Sucrase}} \text{Glucose + Fructose}$$

$$\text{Lactose} \xrightarrow{\text{Lactase}} \text{Glucose + Galactose}$$

The monosaccharides so formed at the brush border or ingested as such (e.g. glucose, fructose in fruits) are absorbed into the epithelial cell by specific carrier proteins. The activity of these brush border enzymes is high in the upper jejunum and gradually declines in the rest of the small intestine (Fig. 40.3).

Absorption

Glucose is absorbed into the epithelial cell by an active transport mechanism called *secondary active transport* or *Symport.* Glucose and sodium share a common carrier protein (Fig. 40.4). The carrier protein has two binding sites for sodium and one binding site for glucose (or galactose). The intracellular sodium concentration of the epithelial cell is kept very low by the Na^+-K^+ ATPase pump operating at the basolateral border of the epithelial cell. Consequently, Na^+ moves into the cell at the brush border down the electrochemical gradient. The flow of sodium ions down the gradient is so forceful that glucose (or galactose) molecules attached to the carrier molecule enter the cell even against the concentration gradient for the sugar. Ultimately, glucose/galactose leaves the epithelial cell at its basal border by diffusion or facilitated diffusion.

Due to the common carrier protein, the entry of glucose/galactose into the epithelial cell is favoured

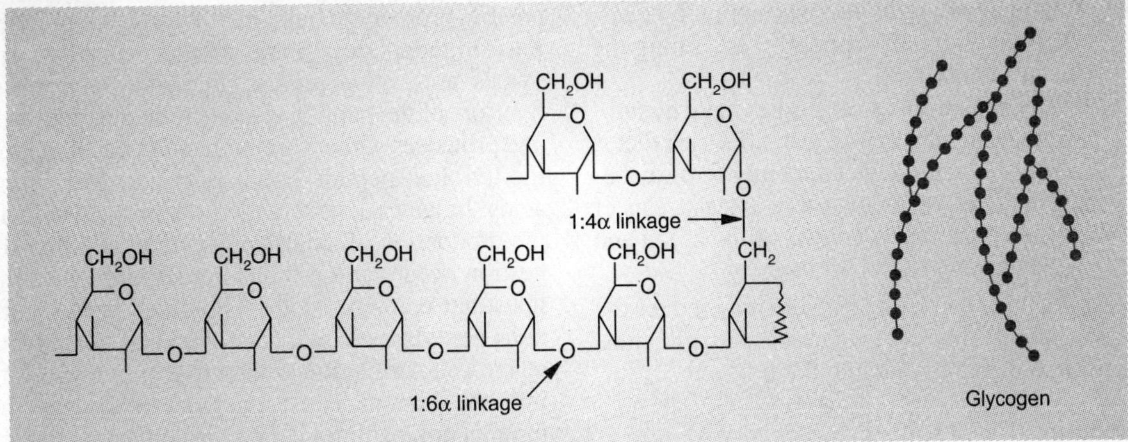

Fig. 40.2: Structure of glycogen.

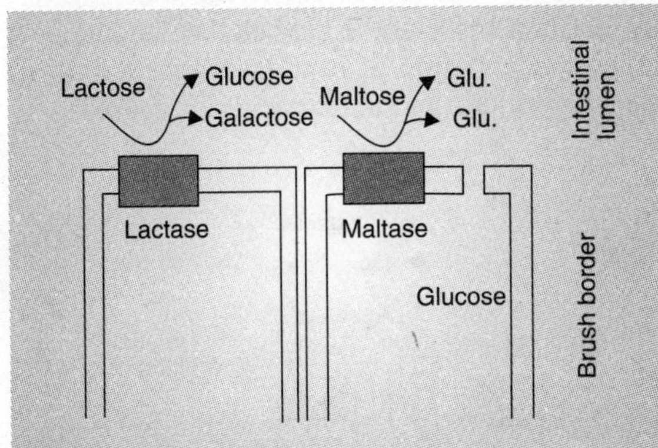

Fig. 40.3: Role of brush border disaccharidases.

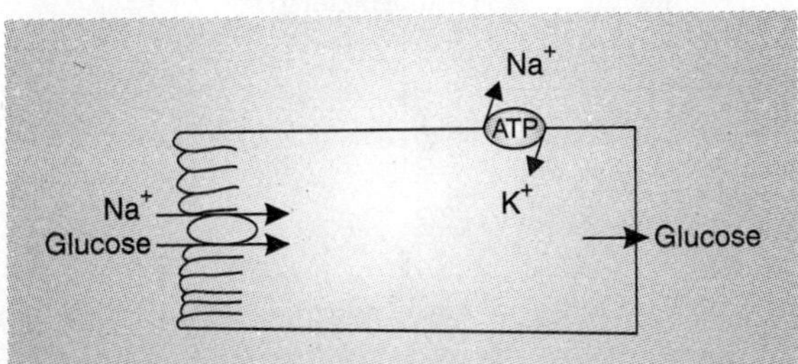

Fig. 40.4: Mechanism of absorption of glucose in the small intestinal mucosa.

by the presence of Na^+ ion in the intestinal lumen. Similarly, presence of glucose and galactose in the lumen favours the absorption of Na^+.

Fructose is rapidly absorbed into the intestinal epithelial cell but not through Na^+-glucose carrier protein. Moreover, the absorption of fructose is not affected by the presence of glucose, galactose or Na^+ in the intestine.

DIETARY FIBRE

This term denotes all the plant cell-wall components mainly non-starch polysaccharides, which cannot be digested in human gastrointestinal tract. It includes cellulose, hemi-cellulose, pectin, gums, etc. In herbivorous animals, intestinal micro-organisms breakdown these polysaccharides into acetate, propionate and butyrate, which are absorbed into the portal blood and utilized for energy production. These polysaccharides contain β-glycosidic linkages. Therefore, they cannot be digested by α-amylase present in human saliva and pancreatic juice.

Even though not a source of energy, the dietary fibre seem to serve many useful functions in the human body.

(i) By adding bulk to the food, it slows down gastric emptying. Therefore, the postprandial rise of blood sugar is attenuated, decreasing the insulin requirement.

(ii) It retains water and therefore makes the faeces larger in amount and softer. Consequently, the large intestinal movements are stronger and constipation does not occur.

(iii) It has a cholesterol lowering action by interfering with its absorption by adsorbing the dietary cholesterol.

(iv) Many epidemiological studies have demonstrated that intake of dietary fibre-rich diet is associated with reduced incidence of diabetes mellitus, coronary artery disease, cancer of the colon, diverticulosis of the colon and gallstones.

On the other hand, dietary fibre may reduce the bio-availability of some vitamins and minerals, e.g. iron and zinc by binding them.

PROTEINS

The protein content of diet varies with the socio-economic status of the individuals. Meat, fish, eggs, cheese and other milk products are the chief sources of dietary proteins with high biological value. Beans, wheat and other pulses are also fairly good sources of proteins in vegetarian diet. In addition, 10–30 g of proteins reach the intestine through gastrointestinal secretions. Another 10–30 g of proteins reach through the desquamated epithelial cells of the gut. Practically, all of these proteins are completely digested and absorbed in the small intestine. The faecal nitrogen content is due to the presence of proteins derived from the colonic bacteria, colonic mucus and desquamated colonic epithelial cells.

Digestion

In the stomach, the pepsin hydrolyses 15% of the dietary protein into peptones. But they cannot be absorbed in the stomach. Stomach can absorb alcohol, and a few drugs only.

Pancreatic juice contains a large number of proteolytic enzymes like trypsin, chymotrypsin, carboxypeptidase, elastase, etc. These enzymes are released into the duodenum as inactive proenzymes. Trypsinogen is converted to trypsin by *enterokinase,* a brush border enzyme. Trypsin can catalyze the conversion of trypsinogen and all other proteolytic proenzymes into active enzymes.

The pancreatic juice contains very high concentrations of proteolytic enzymes. It can digest all the proteins even if gastric pepsin is absent. The pancreatic proteolytic enzymes hydrolyse proteins into oligopeptides. Some of the pancreatic enzymes are *endopeptidases,* i.e. they attack the interiors of the peptide chains producing peptones and proteoses. Others are *exopeptidases,* attacking the terminal peptide bonds releasing free amino acids. In general, pancreatic proteolysis results in the production of small polypeptides. Further digestion occurs at the brush border and inside the intestinal epithelial cells. The brush border contains peptidases which are an integral constituent of the cell membrane with active sites projecting into the lumen. These enzymes hydrolyse the luminal polypeptides coming in contact with them forming di-, tri-, and tetra-peptides and some amino acids. The small peptides and amino acids are absorbed into the cell by active transport mechanism. The cytosol of the epithelial cell contains a larger concentration of peptidases which hydrolyse the peptides into amino acids (Fig. 40.5).

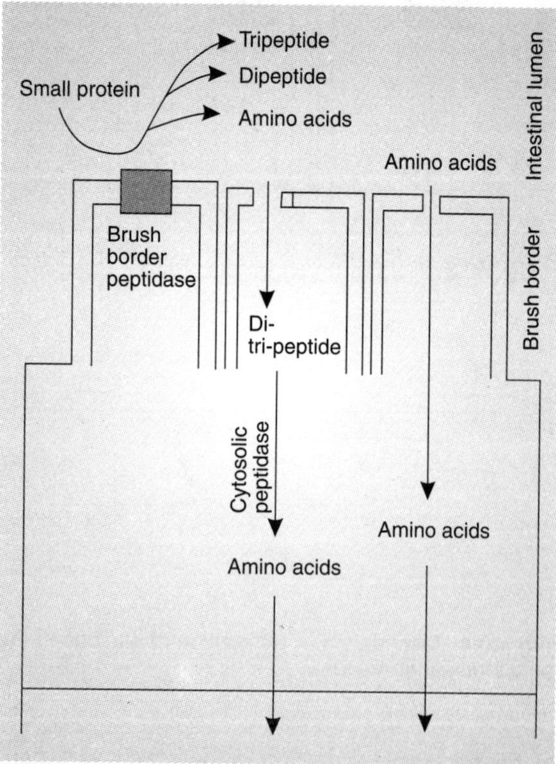

Fig. 40.5: Digestion and absorption of small proteins in the small intestine.

Absorption

From the small intestinal lumen, amino acids are absorbed by specific transport systems. Some of these carriers are sodium-dependent (Na^+-amino acid cotransport) mechanism while others act independently. At the basal border of the epithelial cell, amino acids are transported by facilitated diffusion or by simple diffusion.

As mentioned above, small peptides are also absorbed across the brush border. A single transport carrier system seems to be responsible for absorption of all the small peptides. The transport is secondarily linked to the transfer of Na^+ transport system.

Large proteins cannot be absorbed into the epithelial cells as such. Small amounts may occasionally manage to cross the cell membrane by endocytosis and provoke immunological/allergic reactions. In newborn infants, immunoglobulins present in the colostrum are absorbed in the intestinal mucosa by endocytosis and impart passive immunity to the neonate.

FATS

The diet contains fats of vegetable and animal origin. Mostly, it is in the form of neutral fat (triglycerides). Small amount is present as phospholipids, cholesterol and cholesterol esters. Because of their water-insolubility the digestion and absorption of dietary fats is a far more complicated process than carbohydrates or proteins.

Digestion

The action of gastric lipase is so insignificant that practically digestion of all the dietary fat occurs in the small intestine. The pancreatic juice contains high concentrations of three lipolytic enzymes namely:

(a) *Pancreatic lipase* (glycerol ester-hydroxylase) which hydrolyses triglycerides to produce two fatty acids and a 2-monoglyceride.

(b) *Cholesterol esterase* which hydrolyses cholesterol esters to produce cholesterol and a fatty acid.

(c) *Phospholipase-A$_2$* which hydrolyses the phospholipids. Since most of the dietary fat consists of triglycerides, most of the discussion on digestion and absorption of fats would be centred around it.

Pancreatic lipase is a water soluble enzyme. Therefore, its activity is limited to the oil-water interface of the fat droplet. The surface area available for the action of lipase is increased many thousand times by the emulsification of fat in the intestinal lumen by bile salts.

Emulsification of Fats

The bile salts act as detergents, i.e. they have surface tension lowering action. With the low surface tension of the fats, the segmentation movements of the small intestine break up large fat globules into fine droplets (1 μm in diameter). This process called emulsification of fat exposes much larger surface area of triglyceride molecules to the action of pancreatic lipase. Bile salt molecules have polar and non-polar ends. The hydrophilic polar ends separate the fat droplets from the aqueous phase (Fig. 40.6). The emulsifying action of bile salts is greatly enhanced by the presence of lecithin in the bile. Lecithin has a stabilizing action on the emulsions.

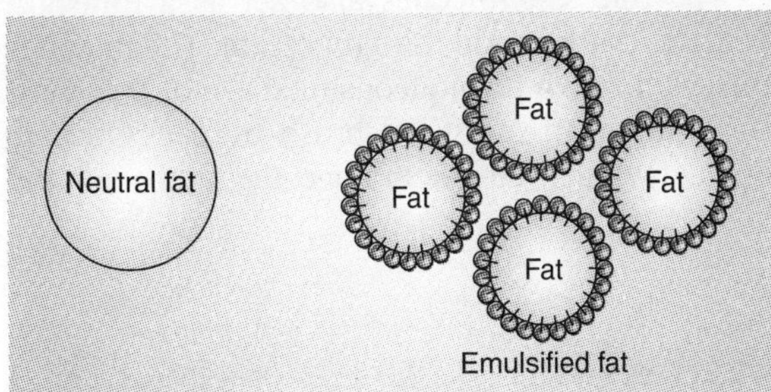

Fig. 40.6: Role of bile salts in the emulsification of fats.

Role of Colipase

Although the emulsification of fat basically helps in its hydrolysis but the bile salt membrane around the fat droplet inhibits the activity of lipase. Colipase, a protein with molecular weight of 10,000 present in the pancreatic juice, displaces the bile salts from the fat droplet and allows the action of lipase.

Absorption of Fat

Transport of Fatty Acids to the Intestinal Epithelial Cell—Formation of Micelles The hydrolysis of fat is a highly reversible process. The accumulation of products of fat hydrolysis (fatty acids and 2-monoglycerides) would tend to stop the reaction by the law of mass action, unless the products of hydrolysed fat are quickly removed from the intestinal lumen. The water insolubility of the products prevents their diffusion to the cell membrane of the intestinal epithelial cell. However, the problem is solved by the presence of bile salts in the intestinal lumen.

Bile salts have the property of forming micelles consisting of small globules of about 2.5 nm diameter. Each micelle is composed of 30 molecules of bile salts. They tend to aggregate in the form of a small globule with their lipid soluble non-polar ends in the centre and water-soluble polar ends fanning out to cover the surface of the micelle. The fatty acids and monoglycerides released from the digestion of fat are quickly incorporated into the central fatty portion of the micelle forming what are known as the **mixed-micelles** (Fig. 40.7). In this fashion, the bile salts allow the lipolytic action to continue.

40

The bile salt micelles also act as a transport vehicle for the products of digestion. The micelles diffuse through the aqueous medium of the intestinal lumen to reach the brush border. Once in contact with the cell membrane, the fatty acids and monoglycerides diffuse freely into the cell. The bile salts are released into the lumen to repeat the process (Fig. 40.8).

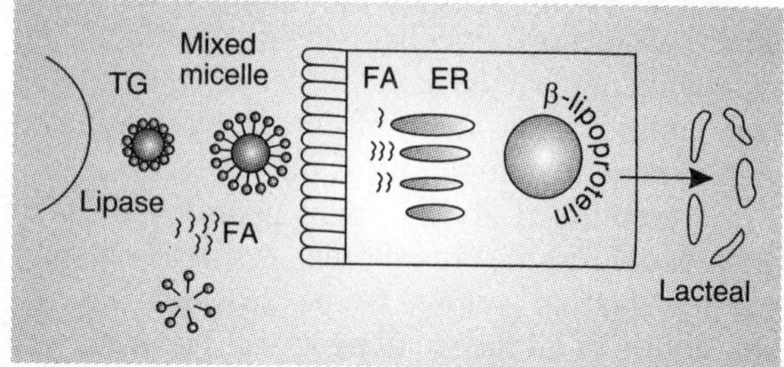

Fig. 40.8: Role of mixed micelles and chylomicrons in the digestion and absorption of triglycerides (TG) FA = fatty acids. ER = Endoplasmic reticulum.

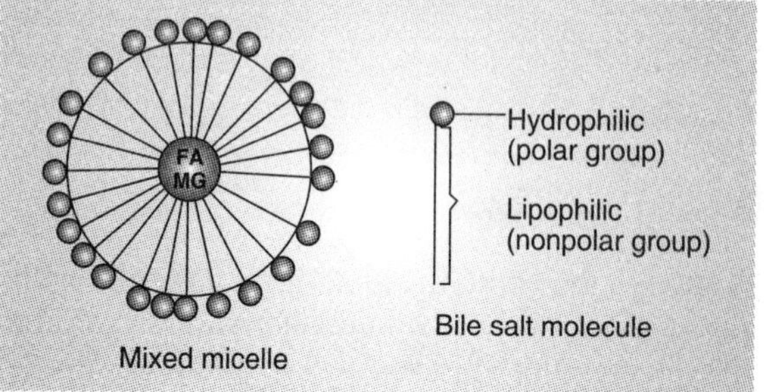

Fig. 40.7: Mixed micelle consists of the products of fat digestion namely fatty acids (FA) and monoglycerides (MG) enclosed in a globule of bile salt aggregate.

The bile salts must be present in certain minimum concentration called *critical micelle concentration* before micelles can be formed. Under physiological conditions, bile salts are always present in the duodenum in more than the critical micelle concentration.

Cholesterol esters and phospholipids are also digested and transported into the cell in the same way as triglycerides.

Formation of Chylomicrons In the mucosal cell, the small chain fatty acids (with less than 10 carbon atoms) are able to diffuse across the basal border and enter the portal blood as free fatty acids. Fatty acids with larger chains are re-esterified into triglycerides in the intestinal epithelium and transported to the lymph capillaries (the lacteals) as chylomicrons (Fig. 40.8). Cholesterol also is re-esterified in the intestinal epithelium. All these steps of re-esterification occur in the smooth endoplasmic reticulum of the epithelial cell. Free fatty acids and 2-monoglycerides involved in the process of re-esterification are mostly those absorbed from the intestine. However, some of the absorbed fatty acids may be attached to the glycero-phosphate produced *de novo* from glucose metabolism by glycolysis.

The absorbed phospholipids form a membrane around small fat globules containing triglycerides and cholesterol esters. The membrane has water-soluble polar ends on the surface and fatty portions inside. This makes the fat globules to diffuse freely in the aqueous medium of the cytosol. A small amount of β-lipoproteins synthesized by the endoplasmic reticulum is also incorporated into the membrane of the fat globule. The globules measuring 60–75 nm in diameter are called chylomicrons. The chylomicrons are too large to diffuse across the basal border of the epithelial cell. Instead, by exocytosis, they are released into the *lacteals*, the large fenestrated lymph capillaries present in the intestinal villi.

The chylomicrons pass into the lymph and ultimately enter the blood circulation through the thoracic duct.

Fate of Bile Salts

The absorption of dietary fat is completed in the jejunum. Bile salts, although helping in digestion and absorption of fat, are not absorbed along with the products of fat digestion. Instead, they are absorbed in the terminal part of the ileum. Conjugated bile acids seem to be absorbed by secondary active transport utilizing sodium-carrier protein. Non-conjugated bile acids seem to be absorbed by simple diffusion.

Absorption of Water

Besides nearly 2 L of water ingested per day with food, another 8 L of water enter the alimentary canal as gastrointestinal secretions (Table 40.2).

Table 40.2: Water balance in the GIT

Input (in litres)		*Absorption (in litres)*	
Water ingested	2.0	Stomach	Nil
Saliva	1.5	Small intestine	9.5
Gastric juice	2.5	Large intestine	0.4
Bile	0.5	Total	9.9
Pancreatic juice	1.5		
Small intestine secretions	2.0	Faecal excretion	0.1
Total	10.0		

In the small intestine, most of the water absorption occurs in the jejunum. Water is absorbed by passive diffusion. It follows the absorption of NaCl, sugars and amino acids. Hence, there is no osmotic gradient between the luminal fluid and the blood.

Absorption of Sodium

About 5–10 g of sodium is ingested with the food per day. In addition, 20–30 g of sodium reaches the alimentary canal in gastrointestinal secretions. All of it is reabsorbed. Sodium can be absorbed in the entire length of the intestine. However, absorption of Na^+ is favoured by the presence of glucose, galactose or amino acids in the intestinal lumen. These substances are absorbed by secondary active transport mechanism mostly in the jejunum. Hence, most of the Na^+ is also absorbed in the jejunum. Whatever left is absorbed in the ileum. Sodium can be absorbed in the large intestine against a larger electro-chemical gradient than in the jejunum. In the small intestine, Na^+ is absorbed by all the processes described for reabsorption of Na^+ in the renal tubules (page 627).

Chloride Absorption

In the jejunum and proximal ileum, chloride is reabsorbed by passive diffusion. It is absorbed by the electrical gradient created by absorption of Na^+.

In the distal ileum and large intestine, however, chloride is absorbed through an active transport system involving a Cl^--HCO_3^- pump. Whereas, Cl^- is absorbed into the intestinal cell, HCO_3^- is secreted into the intestinal lumen (Fig. 40.9). Bicarbonate secretion may help to neutralize the acidity produced by bacterial action in the colon.

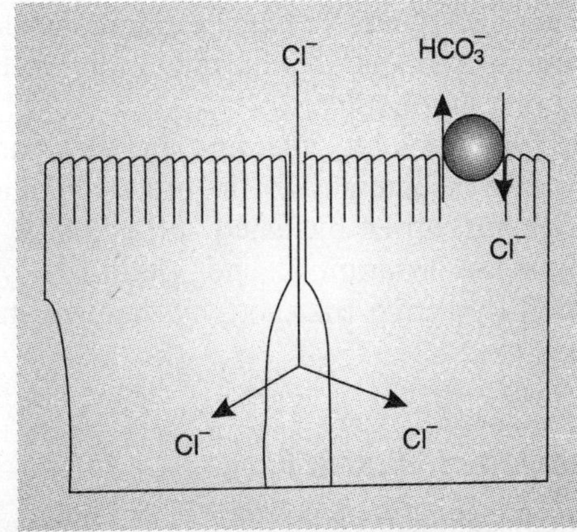

Fig. 40.9: Absorption of chloride in the gut.

Absorption of Calcium

Milk and milk products are important sources of dietary calcium. With the dietary intake of 1000 mg of calcium, only 10% is absorbed. However, when the dietary content of calcium is chronically low (in the range of 400–500 mg per day), even 20–25% of the dietary calcium can be absorbed. The exact mechanism of this adaptation is not clear, but it could be due to increased synthesis of parathormone and 1,25-dihydroxy vitamin D_3.

Calcium is absorbed in the duodenum and jejunum. The exact mechanism of absorption is not clear. A calcium-binding protein present in the cytosol of intestinal epithelium seems to be important for this process. A correlation between the calcium binding protein level in the epithelial cell and the absorptive capacity of the intestine for calcium has been demonstrated. Increased synthesis of intestinal calcium-binding protein is one of the a few well-established functions of 1,25-dihydroxy vitamin D_3.

Dietary phosphates and oxalates, present in cereals and vegetables, grossly interfere with the absorption of calcium by forming insoluble salts. On the other hand, dietary proteins promote intestinal calcium absorption.

Absorption of Vitamins

The absorption of fat soluble vitamins A, D, E and K occurs in the jejunum along with triglycerides and other dietary fats. In the intestinal epithelium, they are incorporated into the chylomicrons to be transported into lymph.

The water soluble vitamins are also mostly absorbed in the jejunum by the process of simple diffusion or carrier mediated diffusion. A few vitamins like vitamin C and vitamin B_{12} are absorbed by active transport mechanism in the ileum.

Absorption of Vitamin B_{12}

Cyanocobalamin or vitamin B_{12} is absorbed in the ileum. A specific cobalamin-binding protein [the *intrinsic factor of Castle* (IF)] is necessary for its absorption. The intrinsic factor is a glycoprotein with a molecular weight of 45,000. It is secreted by the parietal cells of the gastric glands. The secretion of IF parallels the rate of HCl secretion.

In the lumen of the small intestine, IF forms a complex with vitamin B_{12}. Vitamin B_{12}-IF complex binds with a specific receptor protein on the surface of the epithelial cells of the ileum. As a result, free vitamin B_{12} is transported into the cytosol of intestinal epithelium, leaving behind IF at the brush border. At the basal border of the epithelium, vitamin B_{12} enters the portal circulation after binding with a plasma globulin called *transcobalamin-II.* Vitamin B_{12} is stored in the liver after combining with another globulin called *transcobalamin-I.* The storage of a water soluble vitamin is unique to vitamin B_{12}.

Absence of the intrinsic factor may occur due to an autoimmune disease leading to atrophy of the gastric mucosa. In such patients, the gastric juice is completely devoid of HCl (achlorhydria), pepsin and IF. Administration of the most potent stimulus, histamine, fails to produce gastric acid secretion. Deficiency of vitamin B_{12} in the body causes serious haematological and neurological defects called pernicious anaemia. Earlier this disorder was invariably fatal, but nowadays, the condition is easily cured by regular parenteral administration of vitamin B_{12}.

Summary The site of absorption of various food stuffs in the gastrointestinal tract is given in Table 40.3.

PATHOPHYSIOLOGY

Malabsorption syndrome is the name given to multiple nutritional deficiency states produced by a wide variety of digestive and absorptive defects in the gastrointestinal tract. Deficient absorption of amino acids, fats and carbohydrates results in generalized weakness. Malabsorption of water-soluble and fat-soluble vitamins produces anaemia and signs of multiple hypovitaminosis. Water and electrolyte depletion also occurs. The fat and nitrogen content of the stools is increased.

Table 40.3: Site of absorption of various food stuffs in GIT

Stomach	*Duodenum and jejunum*	*Ileum*	*Colon*
Alcohol	Sugars	Vitamin B_{12}	Na^+
Some drugs	Amino acids	Bile salts	Cl^-
	Water soluble vitamins	Na^+	Water
	Fat soluble vitamins	Water	
	Fatty acids		
	Na^+		
	K^+		
	Ca^{2+}		
	Fe^{2+}		
	Cl^-		
	Water		

Consequently, the stools become bulky, pale, greasy and foul smelling (steatorrhoea).

Chronic pancreatitis, obstruction of the common bile duct and gastric surgery are important digestive disorders leading to *secondary* malabsorption syndrome. Malabsorption can be due to a *primary defect* in the mucosa of the small intestine known as the coeliac disease.

Coeliac Disease

This malabsorptive disorder is produced by a congenital absence of an enzyme *gluten hydrolase* in the intestinal mucosa. As a result, gluten, the principal protein of wheat, is not properly hydrolysed. Instead a toxic polypeptide, *gliadin* is formed from gluten. Gliadin causes degenerative changes in the intestinal mucosa resulting in severe malabsorption. Withdrawal of wheat from the diet results in rapid recovery.

Lactose Intolerance

Congenital deficiency of the enzyme *lactase* causes milk intolerance. Lactose, the milk sugar cannot be digested. Undigested lactose reaches the colon where it is metabolized by bacteria producing gas, and toxic products which increase the colonic motility. The diarrhoea may lead to life-threatening dehydration and electrolyte imbalance. The infant can be cured by feeding commercial milk containing sucrose instead of lactose. *Secondary lactase deficiency* occurs far more commonly in *adults*. It produces intestinal distension, diarrhoea and flatulence.

Faecal Fat Test

The patient is given a diet containing approximately 100 g of fat per day for 3–5 days and the stools are collected. In normal individuals, faecal fat excretion is less than 5 g/day. Patients suffering from primary malabsorption syndrome, chronic pancreatitis or obstructive jaundice show excessive excretion of fats in the stools. Secretin-cholecystokinin test helps to differentiate the patients of chronic pancreatitis from those with malabsorption due the small intestinal disorder. Xylose excretion test is also helpful in the differential diagnosis.

Xylose Excretion Test

Xylose is a pentose sugar completely absorbed from the small intestine as such but it is neither metabolised, nor stored in the body. It is freely excreted into the urine. After an oral dose of 25 g of xylose, the urinary excretion of xylose is more than 4.5 g in the next 5 hours in normal individuals. Lesser excretion indicates intestinal malabsorption. The diagnostic value of this test is compromised if the patient's kidney function is subnormal.

Section X

Metabolism and Nutrition

CHAPTER 41

Carbohydrate Metabolism

METABOLISM

Our body utilizes carbohydrates, fats and proteins as sources of energy production. Energy is used in the tissues to performs such diverse functions as contraction of the muscle, conduction of nerve impulse, secretion of glands, beating of cilia and synthesis of compounds required for growth, reproduction and repair. The sum total of all the processes in which energy is made available and utilized is called *metabolism* of the body. The chemical changes by which energy is liberated are grouped under *catabolism*. Catabolic processes are usually oxidative or hydrolytic and they result in the conversion of either food or body tissues into CO_2 and water. The term *anabolism* is used to describe the processes which take up energy and lead to synthesis of proteins, fats or complex carbohydrates for storage in the body.

HIGH ENERGY INTERMEDIARY COMPOUNDS

Adenosine triphosphate (ATP) is a labile chemical substance present in all the cells. It consists of adenine, ribose and three phosphate radicals. The last two phosphate radicals are connected to the remainder of the molecule by what is known as high energy bonds indicated by the symbol "~". Removal of each of these high energy phosphate bonds (~P) releases 12,000 colories (12 kcal). After loss of one ~P from ATP, the compound left over is called adenosine diphosphate (ADP). Loss of another high energy phosphate bond (~P) results in the formation of adenosine monophosphate (AMP).

$$ATP \underset{\nwarrow \text{ 12 kcal}}{\overset{\text{12 kcal } \nearrow}{\rightleftharpoons}} ADP + PO_4 \underset{\nwarrow \text{ 12 kcal}}{\overset{\text{12 kcal } \nearrow}{\rightleftharpoons}} AMP + PO_4$$

All the cells contain ATP in their cytoplasm and nucleoplasm. Energy required for all the physiological processes is derived from ATP as the immediate source. ATP is regenerated by using energy derived from oxidation of food stuffs. Thus, ATP is the ultimate form in which energy is transferred from food stuffs to the energy dependent cellular mechanisms.

Triphosphate derivatives of guanosine (GTP), uridine (UTP) and cytidine (CTP) also have energy-rich phosphate bonds and serve as intermediary compounds for transfer of energy.

Role of Phosphocreatine

Phosphocreatine contains one high energy phosphate bond. On hydrolysis, it releases 13 kcal per molecule. Phosphocreatine, unlike ATP, cannot act as a coupling agent for the transfer of energy between the food stuffs and cellular mechanism. However, it can exchange energy with ATP.

Food stuff — Energy — ATP (↘ ADP) — Phosphocreatine + ADP (stored) (↘ Creatine)

Phosphocreatine + ADP = ATP + Creatine

The importance of phosphocreatine as a high energy compound lies in the fact that most of the cells have only limited stores of ATP. Some tissues like skeletal muscles have, in addition, a large store of creatine phosphate. When extra amount of energy is available in the muscle, after saturation of ATP, the extra energy is stored in the form of creatine phosphate. Whenever muscles consume energy from ATP stores, it is transferred rapidly from creatine phosphate to ADP, thereby maintaining the muscle cells always saturated with ATP.

ATP is the form in which energy is captured during oxidation of food stuffs. Again ATP is the form in which energy is utilized for various metabolic processes. That is why, ATP has been called energy currency of the cells.

Oxidation of food stuffs, whether carbohydrates, proteins or fats, leading to generation of ATP occurs in the mitochondria. That is why, mitochondria have been called the power house of the cells. The cytosol of a cell contains a series of enzymes which can breakdown carbohydrates, fats and proteins to acetyl-CoA. This metabolite is finally oxidized to CO_2 and H_2O in the mitochondria.

The enzymes of citric acid cycle produce H^+ or electrons, oxidation of which yields ATP.

Glucose ↘
Fatty acids ⟶ Acetyl-CoA ⟶ (Citric acid cycle) 2 H ⟶ (O_2) H_2O
Amino acids ↗
ADP ⟶ ATP

The combination of H_2 and O is a rather complicated process. It requires a series of enzymes called the respiratory chain (Fig. 41.1). These

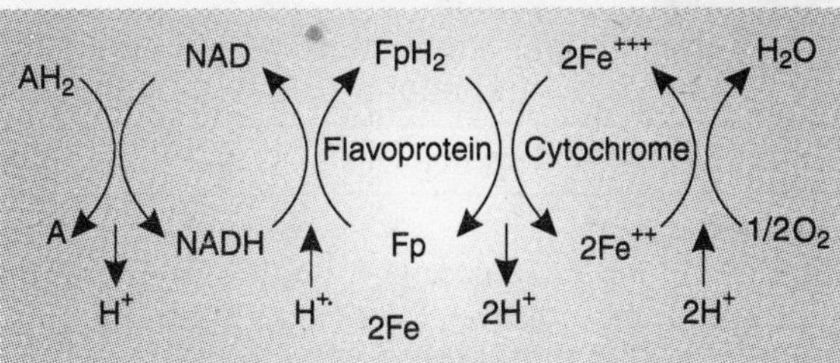

Fig. 41.1: The respiratory chain.

enzymes include nicotinic acid, flavoproteins and cytochromes. The substrate "A" may be oxidized through NAD-flavoprotein-cytochrome chain or through flavoprotein-cytochrome chain only. In the first case, 3 molecules of ATP are generated. In the latter case, 2 molecules of ATP are generated.

GLUCOSE METABOLISM

Glucose is the most abundant final product of carbohydrate digestion in the alimentary canal. Small amounts of fructose and galactose may also be produced. All the three monosaccharides (hexose sugars) are carried by the portal blood to the liver for further metabolism. The metabolism of fructose and galactose is discussed briefly in the later part of the chapter.

Glucose Transport into the Cells

Glucose is transported across the cell membrane by the process of insulin dependent *facilitated diffusion,* i.e. carrier-mediated transport downs the concentration gradient. This is true of tissues like skeletal muscle, adipose tissue and other insulin dependent tissues (GLUT 4).

In the neurons and RBCs, the transport of glucose is not insulin dependent but it occurs by a *carrier-mediated* facilitated diffusion (GLUT 1).

In the epithelial cells of intestinal mucosa and renal tubules, glucose is transported by an *active transport mechanism,* i.e. it is an energy dependent process and glucose can be transported against the concentration gradient (SGLT 1). It would be apparent that different type of transport carrier proteins are involved in the transport of glucose in different tissues (Table 41.1).

The liver cells are permeable to glucose. It is an insulin-sensitive tissue. However, the rate of

Table 41.1: Various types of glucose transporters

Transfer	*Function*	*Site*
Active transport		
SGLT 1 (Sodium glucose cotransporter 1)	Secondary active glucose transport	Small intestine Renal tubules
Facilitated diffusion		
GLUT 1	Basal glucose uptake	Brain, red cells, placenta
GLUT 2	Transport out of intestinal and renal epithelial cell	Liver, small intestine, renal tubules
GLUT 4	Insulin-stimulated glucose uptake	Skeletal muscle, cardiac muscle, adipose tissue, etc.
GLUT 5	Dietary glucose absorption	Jejunum

glucose transport is limited by the rate at which glucose can be converted to glucose-6-PO_4 inside the liver cells. Insulin accelerates the activity of glucokinase involved in this reaction. Thus, insulin indirectly increases the transport of glucose into the hepatic cells. In muscle, adipose tissue and many other insulin-sensitive cells, the rate limiting factor for glucose transport is the permeability of the cell membrane which is directly influenced by insulin.

Metabolism of Glucose

Immediately after glucose enters a cell, it is phosphorylated to glucose-6-phosphate by a non-specific enzyme, *hexokinase* present in all the cells. In the liver, a specific enzyme **glucokinase** is responsible for this reaction. Phosphorylation of glucose is not a reversible reaction except in the liver, intestines and renal tubules where the enzyme *glucose-6-phosphatase* is available to generate glucose from glucose-6-phosphate. In all other tissues, the cell membrane is impermeable to glucose-6-phosphate. Hence, once glucose has entered a cell and phosphorylated, it must be metabolised in one of the four pathways, as follows:

(i) Used for synthesis of glycogen, e.g. in the liver and skeletal muscle.
(ii) Catabolised through glycolytic pathways followed by oxidation in citric acid cycle to yield energy, e.g. in most of the cells specially the skeletal muscle.
(iii) Metabolised through glycolytic pathways but leading to synthesis of fats, e.g. in the liver and adipose tissues.
(iv) Metabolised through hexose-monophosphate shunt (HMP-shunt).

Glycogenesis

Glycogen is a large polymer of glucose. All the cells of the body contain some glycogen. But the liver and skeletal muscle can store large amounts of glycogen. It may constitute 5–8% of dry weight of liver and 1–3% of skeletal muscle. The chemical reactions involved in the synthesis of glycogen are summarized in Fig. 41.2.

Insulin promotes glycogenesis in the liver as well as skeletal muscle.

Glycogenolysis

Degradation of glycogen by the enzyme phosphorylase yields glucose-6-PO_4. Phosphorylase is activated by hormones like glucagon and catecholamines and inhibited by insulin. In the liver, an

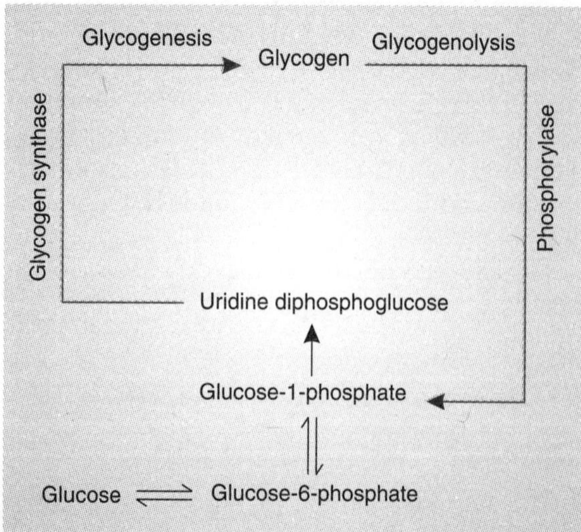

Fig. 41.2: Steps of glycogenesis and glycogenolysis.

enzyme glucose-6-phosphatase is present which splits glucose-6-phosphate to glucose. Hence, in the liver, the end result of glycogenolysis is glucose which enters the blood circulation to maintain blood glucose level. In other tissues, specially the skeletal muscle, the enzyme phosphatase is absent. Therefore, the glycogenolysis results in production of glucose-6-PO_4 which can *only be catabolised* by glycolytic pathways. Thus, in the skeletal muscle, the effect of phosphorylase activity is to produce greater glucose utilization rather than generation of blood sugar.

Glycolytic Pathways

The breakdown of glucose to pyruvic acid or lactic acid is called glycolysis. Glycolysis chiefly occurs via Embden-Meyerhof pathway.

Embden-Meyerhof Pathway

The various steps of glycolysis via Embden-Meyerhof pathway are summarised in Fig. 41.3.

Glycolysis is an anaerobic process. The breakdown of each glucose molecule to pyruvic acid yields only 2 moles of ATP. However, its importance lies in the fact that: (*i*) This process is prerequisite for the subsequent oxidative metabolism which yields much larger amount of energy. (*ii*) Pyruvic acid represents a central branching point in the intermediary metabolism and it can be converted into a number of compounds like fatty acids. (*iii*) Pyruvic acid can be further metabolised (reduced) to lactic acid as follows:

Glyceraldehyde 3-phosphate + Phosphate → 1, 3-diphosphoglyceric acid; NAD^+ → $NADH + H^+$; Pyruvic acid → Lactic acid ($NADH + H^+$ → NAD^+)

Due to this reaction, glucose continues to be metabolised and generate energy (although small in amount) even in lack of oxygen. The conversion of pyruvic acid to lactic acid generates NAD^+ which is essential for the conversion of glyceraldehyde-3-phosphate to 1,3-diphosphoglyceric acid. If there was no conversion to lactic acid, the absence of NAD^+ would have blocked glycolysis at this step.

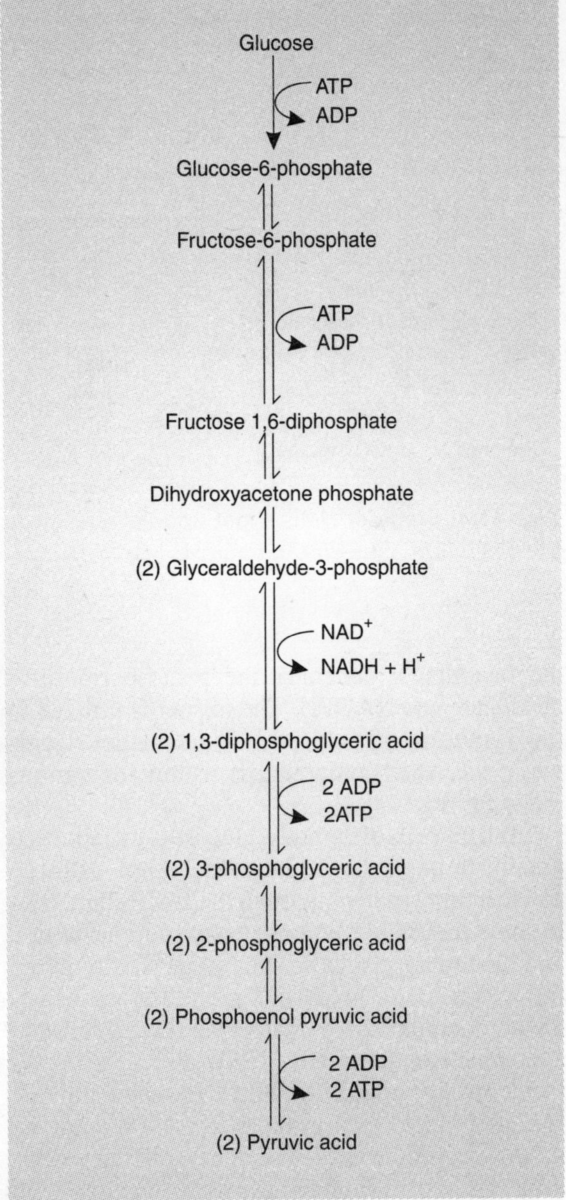

Fig. 41.3: Steps of Embden-Meyerhof pathway.

Hexose-Monophosphate Shunt (HMP Shunt)

The HMP shunt for glycolysis is shown in Fig. 41.4. The HMP shunt or the oxidative pentose pathway includes a group of reactions in which glucose-6-phosphate is oxidised and converted to pentose-phosphate. The importance of this pathway lies in

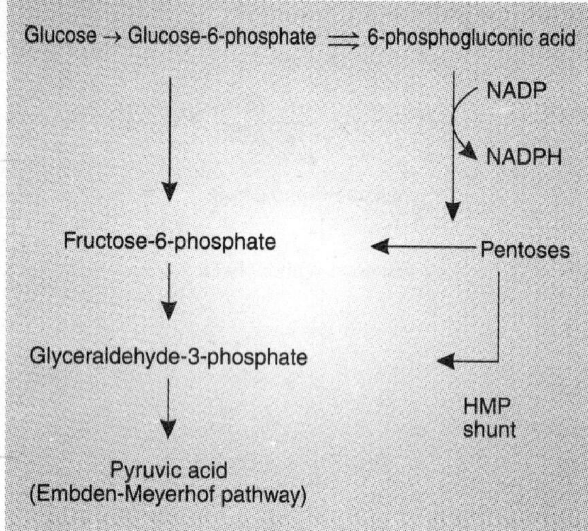

Fig. 41.4: Steps of HMP shunt and its relation to Embden-Meyerhof pathway.

the fact that it generates the pentose ribose-5-phosphate and NADPH. The former is utilized in the synthesis of nucleotides and nucleic acids while the latter compound is useful for various reducing reactions.

41

In all the cells of the body, glucose is metabolised mainly through the Embden-Meyerhof pathway and to a minor extent through the HMP shunt. But in some tissues like adipose tissue, adrenal cortex and mammary glands where NADPH is required for synthesis of lipids and steroids, glucose is metabolised through oxidative pentose pathway to a greater extent. In the RBCs also, glucose is metabolised through the HMP shunt to provide NADPH so as to keep haemoglobin and glutathione in the reduced state. The metabolic reactions involved in both Embden-Meyerhof pathway and HMP shunt occur in the extra-mitochondrial (cytosol) compartment of the cell.

Citric Acid Cycle

Under aerobic conditions pyruvic acid is metabolised to CO_2 and H_2O through citric acid (Krebs) cycle. Before pyruvic acid can enter the citric acid cycle, it has to enter the mitochondria and get converted into acetyl-Co-enzyme A (acetyl- CoA). Acetyl-CoA combines with oxalo-acetic acid to form citric acid. Citric acid now undergoes a series of reactions in which two carbon atoms are split off and oxaloacetic acid is formed once again (Fig. 41.5).

During each cycle, five pairs of hydrogen atoms are generated which undergo oxidative-phosphorylation reaction and yield large amount of ATP. If the H-atoms pass through NAD^+, FAD^+, cytochrome chain, oxidation of each pair of H-atoms yields 3 moles of ATP. If, however, H-atoms pass through FAD, cytochrome only (e.g. succinic acid-fumaric acid reaction) only 2 moles of ATP are generated by oxidation of each pair of H-atoms. In this way, as shown in Fig. 41.5, 15 moles of ATP are generated by oxidation of each mole of pyruvic acid through citric acid cycle.

When oxygen is available, during glycolysis (glyceraldehyde-3-phosphate 1,3 diphosphoglyceric acid), 2 H-atoms are available for oxidation which yield 3 moles of ATP by entering into

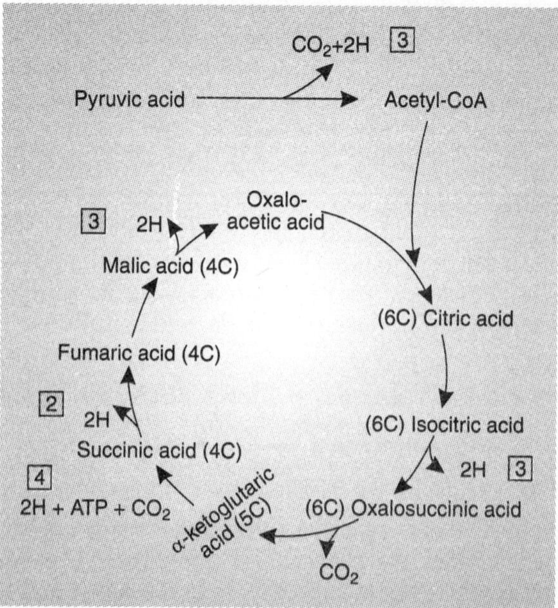

Fig. 41.5: Citric acid cycle. The numbers in the bracket '( )' indicate the number of carbon atoms in each of the acid. The numbers in the square indicate the moles of ATP produced by ADP-ATP reaction or through oxidative phosphorylation of H-atoms. Total moles of ATP generated from each molecule of pyruvic acid is 15.

electron transport chain. Thus, under *anaerobic conditions,* the metabolism of 1 mole of glucose yields only 2 moles of ATP. Under aerobic conditions an additional 36 moles of ATP [(15 + 3) × 2] are produced making a total of 38 moles of ATP for each mole of glucose oxidised.

Besides carbohydrates, other substances like fatty acids and certain amino acids can also be metabolised to acetyl-CoA and degraded in the citric acid cycle. Thus the citric acid cycle occupies a pivotal position for degradation of all metabolites for energy production.

Energy yield during glucose metabolism through HMP shunt is variable. As explained earlier, this pathway generates a large amounts of $NADPH^+$ which are utilized for various synthetic processes. If, however, some NADPH is converted to NADH and oxidised, the amount of ATP generated would depend upon the amount of NADPH oxidised.

Importance of Anaerobic Metabolism of Glucose

Normally, oxygen is available to the tissues for various oxidative reactions. Occasionally, it may transiently become non-available or the cardio-pulmonary system may not be able to supply oxygen appropriate to the metabolic demand of the tissue. Under these circumstances, glucose can be metabolised up to pyruvic acid only. During glycolysis, very little ATP is generated (only 2 ATPs instead of 38 under aerobic conditions for each mole of glucose). However, the release of energy by glycolytic reaction may be a life-saving measure for a few minutes till adequate supply of oxygen is made available.

Formation of Lactic Acid

During glycolysis (anaerobic), pyruvic acid and $NADH^+$ accumulate in the tissues. By the law of mass action, excess of these metabolites would stop the glycolytic process within seconds and no more ATP would be generated. However, the end products react with each other to form lactic acid.

$$\text{Pyruvic acid} \xrightarrow{\text{NADH} \;\to\; \text{NAD}} \text{Lactic acid}$$

Lactic acid diffuses readily out of the cells into blood circulation. Thus, pyruvic acid disappears and NAD is made available to continue the glycolytic reaction. Subsequently, when oxygen is available, lactic acid is converted back to pyruvic acid mainly in the liver and either oxidised or converted to glycogen (Cori's cycle) (Fig. 41.6). Normal blood lactic acid level is 5–20 mg%. Elevated blood lactic acid levels are seen in severe exercise, or in circulatory shock.

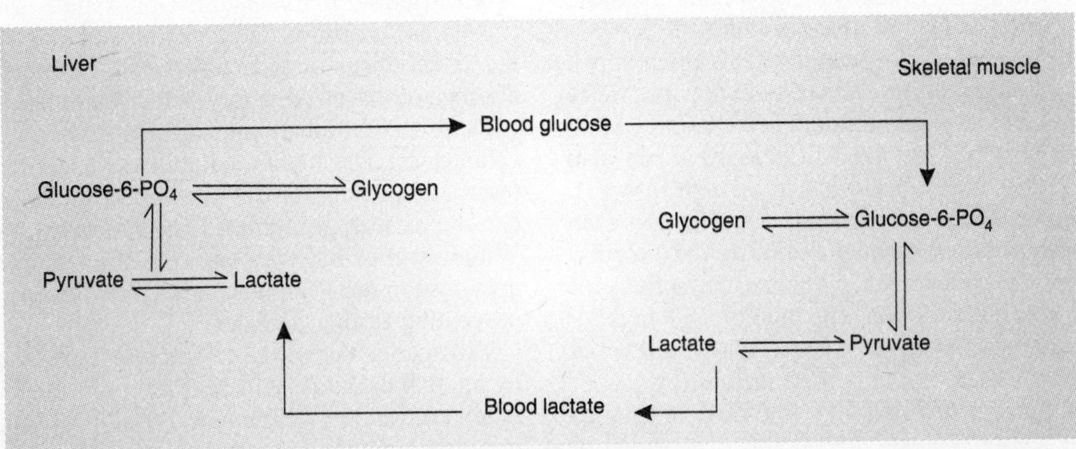

Fig. 41.6: Cori's cycle.

Gluconeogenesis

In addition to being a critical source of energy, particularly for certain tissues like brain, glucose is necessary for the production of many vital intermediates:

(i) Pentose-phosphate derived from glucose metabolism through HMP shunt is used in the synthesis of nucleotides and nucleic acids.
(ii) HMP shunt produces NADPH which is required for many synthetic processes.
(iii) Dihydroxy-acetone-phosphate formed during glycolysis yields glycerol-phosphate which is required for the synthesis of triglycerides.
(iv) The production of mucopolysaccharides and glycoproteins also depends on hexosamines and uronic acid derived from glucose.

The examples given above illustrate the fact that maintenance of continued normal function of the organism requires a continuous supply of glucose even if dietary intake of carbohydrate is insufficient. This is made possible by the process of gluconeogenesis, i.e. conversion of non-carbohydrate nutrients or intermediate metabolites into glucose or glycogen. Gluconeogenesis occurs at moderate rates even normally but the process is accelerated several folds in the presence of certain hormones. The chief precursors of gluconeogenesis are amino acids (like alanine, glutamate, aspartic acid) as well as pyruvate, lactate and glycerol. Amino acids are at first deaminated and then converted to either pyruvate or one of the dicarboxylic acids of the citric acid cycle. In this way, they enter the citric acid cycle and lead to gluconeogenesis.

The process of gluconeogenesis is essentially a reversal of glycolytic pathway and occurs chiefly in the liver and to some extent in the kidney. Most of the enzymes involved in glycolysis can also lead to gluconeogenesis by reversal of the process. However, some enzymes are specific for each pathway and factors which determine the direction of glucose metabolism modulate the activity of these specific enzymes. The ratio of ATP to ADP and AMP, the level of acetyl-CoA and the level of pyruvate/lactate are important factors (by law of mass action) influencing the rate of gluconeogenesis/glycolysis. Elevated concentration of AMP in a cell enhances glycolysis whereas excess of ATP enhances gluconeogenesis. An increased level of acetyl-CoA stimulates gluconeogenesis and inhibits glycolysis. Free fatty acids decrease glycolysis and increase gluconeogenesis.

Glucocorticoids promote gluconeogenesis. They stimulate the release of amino acids from proteins providing the critical substrate for gluconeogenesis. They also induce the synthesis of enzymes specific for gluconeogenesis.

METABOLISM OF HEXOSES OTHER THAN GLUCOSE

Galactose is released as a result of digestion of lactose. Fructose is partly ingested as such and partly liberated by the digestion of sucrose.

Galactose can be converted to glycogen through the following pathway (Fig. 41.7).

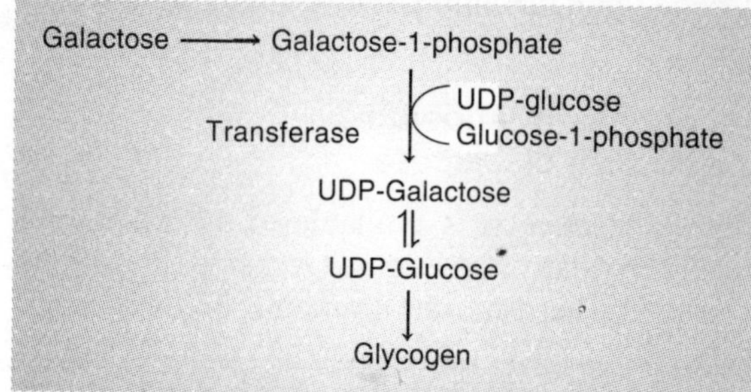

Fig. 41.7: Conversion pathway-Glactose to glycogen.

Galactosaemia is an inborn error of metabolism in which the enzyme galactose-1-phosphate-uridyl-transferase is absent. This enzyme is required for the metabolism of galactose-1-PO_4. Congenital absence of this enzyme results in accumulation of galactose-1-phosphate causing mental retardation, cataract, etc. Due to the availability of a laboratory test for the enzyme, uridyl-transferase, the disorder can be readily diagnosed at an early stage. Withdrawal of milk (lactose, the chief source of galactose in diet) can be an effective measure for preventing further damage.

Fructose is converted to fructose-1-phosphate by an enzyme, fructokinase, present in the liver. After conversion to fructose-1,6-diphosphate, it enters the Embden-Meyerhof's pathway for further metabolism.

42

CHAPTER

Lipid Metabolism

LIPIDS

Compounds are classified as lipids on the basis of their solubility in organic solvents and their relative insolubility in water. The following compounds are included under the term lipids.

1. Free fatty acids.
2. Triglycerides or glycerol esters of fatty acids.
3. Phospholipids.
4. Sphingolipids.
5. Cholesterol, other sterols and steroids.

1. Fatty Acids

The chemical structure of some of the important fatty acids is given in Table 42.1.

Table 42.1: Chemical structure of some important fatty acids

Fatty acid	*Chem. formula*	*Characteristic*
Palmitic acid	$CH_3 (CH_2)_{14} COOH$	(C_{16}) Saturated
Stearic acid	$CH_3 (CH_2)_{16} COOH$	(C_{18}) Saturated
Oleic acid	$CH_3 (CH_2)_7 CH = CH(CH_2)_7 COOH$	(C_{18}) Unsaturated

The fatty acids found in the animal body are monocarboxylic acids with an even number of carbon atoms. They contain long hydrocarbon chains which may be saturated or unsaturated.

2. Triglycerides

Triglycerides are esters of glycerol with different fatty acids.

CH_2OH | $CHOH$ | CH_2OH	+	3–R–COOH	=	CH_2–COO–R | CH–COOR + $3H_2O$ | CH_2–COO–R
Glycerol		Long-chained fatty acid		Triglyceride

R = aliphatic chain of various lengths and degree of saturation.

3. Phospholipids

These are complex lipids containing phosphoric acid.

Lecithin and cephalin are esters of glycerol with two fatty acids and a derivative of phosphatidic acid.

4. Sphingolipids

Like phospholipids, sphingolipids are also complex lipids. Sphingomyelins contain fatty acids, phosphate and a complex base, sphingosine. Cerebrosides contain galactose, fatty acid and sphingosine. Compound lipids (3) and (4) are integral parts of the general cell structure. They are present in large amounts in the central nervous system. Phospholipids are constituents of lipoproteins.

5. Sterols

Sterols include cholesterol and various steroid hormones. These compounds do not contain fatty acids but they have a sterol nucleus cyclopentanoperhydrophenanthrene.

PLASMA LIPIDS

In the post-absorptive state, i.e. about 12 hours after the last meal, the average level of lipids per 100 ml of the plasma is as follows :

Triglycerides	125 mg
Cholesterol	180 mg
Phospholipids	180 mg
Free fatty acids	15 mg
Total	500 mg

Free fatty acids (FFA) are bound to albumin. All other lipids circulate as lipoproteins. Plasma lipids arise from several sources which include the lipids absorbed from the alimentary canal, the lipids released from the liver and those released from the adipose tissue.

Chylomicrons

42

The products of fat digestion in the intestine are absorbed into the epithelial cells of the jejunum where the chylomicrons are formed. Chylomicrons are formed by the combination of proteins with lipids like triglycerides, cholesterol, cholesterol esters with phospholipids, small amount of fatty acids and fat soluble vitamins. Chylomicrons are released into the intestinal lymph and transported through the thoracic duct to the systemic circulation. The turbidity of the plasma after a fatty meal is due to the presence of chylomicrons. But in plasma obtained from the blood sample taken about one hour later, the turbidity cannot be observed since the chylomicrons have been removed from the blood as it passes through the capillaries of the liver and adipose tissue. An enzyme *lipoprotein lipase* (also called the *clearing factor*) is bound to the endothelial cells in the liver and the adipose tissue. It catalyses the hydrolysis of triglycerides of the chylomicrons into fatty acids and glycerol. The fatty acids being highly miscible with the cell membranes diffuse rapidly into the cells where they are re-esterified. Heparin is an important co-factor for the action of lipoprotein lipase. Chylomicrons represent the exogenous triglycerides freshly absorbed from the intestine and being transported to the liver. The endogenous fats like triglycerides and other lipids released from the liver and being transported to the tissues are represented by very low density lipoproteins (VLDL).

Free Fatty Acids

Fats stored in the adipose tissue can be mobilized and transported by the blood to be used in the tissues for the production of energy. An enzyme called *hormone-sensitive lipase* (or tissue lipase) present in the adipose tissue promotes the hydrolysis of triglycerides into glycerol and fatty acids. The fatty acids released from the adipose tissue circulate in the blood bound to plasma albumin and are called free fatty acid (FFA) or non-esterified fatty acids (NEFA). (In contrast, other fatty acids present in the blood are in the form of esters of glycerol or cholesterol, etc.)

The concentration of FFA in the plasma in the resting conditions is very small (about 15 mg %), but their turnover is so fast that even this concentration of FFA is sufficient to provide over 50% of the energy requirement of the body. Their half-life is a few minutes only. Most of the tissues can oxidise FFA to CO_2 and H_2O. Therefore, they are the major source of energy in most of the tissues particularly the myocardium. The mobilization of lipids into FFA is enhanced by epinephrine as well as by glucagon, glucocorticoids, thyroxine and norepinephrine. All these hormones activate the tissue lipase (hormone-sensitive lipase). Tissue lipase is inhibited by insulin.

Lipoproteins

Since lipids are insoluble in water, their transport in the body fluids poses a problem. They are transported in association with polar phospholipids and proteins which are concentrated on the periphery of macro-molecules called lipoproteins.

On the basis of their density, they have been classified as follows.

i. Very Low Density Lipoproteins (VLDL) This fraction of lipoproteins contains nearly 90% of the lipids, consisting of high concentrations of triglycerides and moderate concentration of both phospholipids and cholesterol.

ii. Low Density Lipoproteins (LDL) This fraction of lipoproteins contains 70–80% of lipids consisting of relatively few triglycerides but very high concentration of cholesterol (being transported from the liver to the tissues).

iii. High Density Lipoproteins (HDL) It consists of about equal amounts of proteins and lipids (cholesterol and phospholipids). The cholesterol in HDL is being transported from the tissues to the liver.

Cellular Lipids

Lipids as a part of cell membrane are present in all the cells. Adipose tissue constitutes the fat depots where neutral fats are stored until they are needed for energy production elsewhere in the body. The fat cells of the adipose tissue may contain 80–95% of their volume as triglycerides. The fat stored in the fat cells is not static or an inert lump. Fat is continuously being broken down and resynthesized so that in a particular fat cell, the triglycerides are completely renewed every 2–3 weeks.

FATTY ACID OXIDATION (β-OXIDATION)

The degradation and oxidation of fatty acids occurs in the mitochondria. Free fatty acids can enter the cell membrane freely. But their transport into the mitochondria requires a carrier called **carnitine.** The first step in the oxidation of fatty acids is the combination with CoA. Then over a series of reactions acetyl-CoA is liberated and the fatty acid chain becomes shorter by two carbon atoms. The process is repeated again and again until the entire fatty acid is split into acetyl-CoA.

Oxidation of Acetyl-CoA

The molecule of acetyl-CoA produced by β-oxidation enters the citric acid cycle and is degraded to CO_2 and H-atoms. Hydrogen atoms are oxidised by oxidative phosphorylation to yield energy in the form of ATP. Complete degradation of stearic acid (C_{18} compound) yields nine units of acetyl-CoA by repetition of 5 steps of β-oxidation eight times. Degradation of nine molecules of acetyl-CoA in the citric acid cycle yields 108 ATPs (12 × 9). In addition, 38 ATPs are generated during β-oxidation of the fatty acid (C_{18}) to acetyl-CoA. Thus, the total degradation of stearic acid molecule to CO_2 and H_2O yields 146 ATPs.

Formation and Utilization of Ketone Bodies

Large amounts of fatty acids are degraded in the liver to acetyl-CoA, but only a small fraction of it is used up to produce energy by oxidation in the citric acid cycle in the hepatocytes. The remaining molecules of acetyl-CoA condense to form aceto-acetic acid (a four carbon compound) as shown in Fig. 42.1.

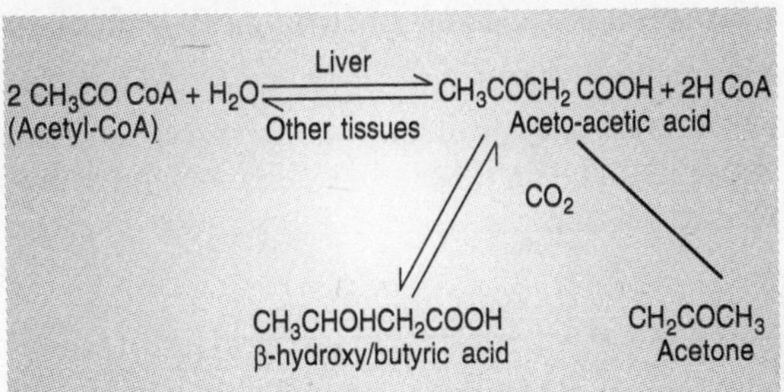

Fig. 42.1: Formation of aceto-acltic acid.

A large percentage of aceto-acetic acid is converted into β-hydroxy-butyric acid and the remaining small percentage is converted into acetone. These three products, namely, aceto-acetic acid, β-hydroxy-butyric acid and acetone are together known as *ketone bodies*. Ketone bodies diffuse out of the hepatocytes and are transported via blood to other tissues where aceto-acetic acid and β-hydroxy-butyric acid are reconverted to acetyl-CoA and oxidized in the citric acid cycle. It is interesting to note that the liver itself cannot oxidize the ketone bodies.

The extra-hepatic utilization of ketone bodies is a normal process in most of the tissues except the brain. Skeletal muscles are particularly adapted to use the ketone bodies as fuel. Normally, the utilization of ketone bodies keeps pace with their rate of hepatic synthesis. Therefore, the plasma level of ketone bodies remains nearly constant at about 1 mg%. Less than 1 mg of ketone bodies are excreted in the urine per 24 hours. However, during prolonged starvation, diabetes mellitus or intake of high fat-low carbohydrate diet, the production of ketone bodies in the liver may exceed their extrahepatic utilization. The consequent accumulation of ketone bodies in the blood is known as **ketosis.** Under such conditions, large amount of these metabolites are excreted in the urine *(ketonuria).* The common features of conditions producing ketosis are deprivation of glucose utilization coupled with utilization of large amounts of fatty acids for energy production. Accumulation of keto acids in the blood results in metabolic acidosis which may be fatal, e.g. diabetes ketoacidosis.

Hormonal Regulation of Fatty Acid Utilization

The release of free fatty acids from the adipose tissue is regulated by the enzyme hormone-sensitive lipase. A number of hormones regulate the action of this enzyme.

42

Neutral fat —Horm. Sens. Lipase→ FFA

Insulin (–)
GH (+)
Glucagon (+)
Catecholamines (+)
Glucocorticoids (+)

After ingestion of a carbohydrate rich meal, the secretion of insulin inhibits HS lipase decreasing the production and utilization of FFA. In fasting state or under stressful conditions, release of hormones like glucagon, catecholamines and glucocorticoids increase the activity of HS lipase. Consequent increase of plasma FFA level increases FFA utilization in peripheral tissues particularly the heart and skeletal muscle.

Synthesis of Fat

Whenever the ingestion of carbohydrates exceeds the amount required for immediate energy production, the rest is stored as glycogen in the liver and skeletal muscle. When the glycogen stores are saturated, the excess of carbohydrates are converted into triglycerides and stored in the adipose tissue. Liver is the chief site of synthesis of triglycerides whereas adipose tissue is the chief site of their storage. (Small amounts of triglycerides are synthesized in the adipose tissue also.) After synthesis in the liver, triglycerides are transported to the adipose tissue as lipoproteins and stored as triglycerides. They can be reconverted to free fatty acids and poured into blood circulation.

The importance of conversion of carbohydrates into fats and storage lies in the fact that the body can store not more than a few hundred grams of glycogen whereas several kilograms of fat can be stored in fat depots. Moreover, oxidation of each gram of fat produces 9 kcal as compared to 4 kcal produced by carbohydrates. Due to these differences, the energy stored as fat may be 200 times the energy stored as glycogen.

Besides carbohydrates, deamination of certain amino acids results in the formation of acetyl-CoA. In this way, even proteins may be converted into fats.

PROSTAGLANDINS

Linolenic acid, linoleic acid and arachidonic acid are poly-unsaturated fatty acids. These have been called *essential fatty acids* since it was shown in the rat that their deficiency in early life caused growth failure, infertility and lesions in the skin and kidney. Such a deficiency disorder has not been observed in humans but still it is believed that dietary intake of these essential fatty acids is indispensible for normal functioning of the human body.

Arachidonic acid is the precursor of prostaglandins. Prostaglandins are a series of closely related 20-C unsaturated fatty acids containing cyclo-pentane ring (Fig. 42.2). They were first isolated from the semen. They were believed to come into the semen from the prostate gland, hence the name. Actually, seminal vesicles are the chief source of prostaglandins in the semen. It is now known that almost all the organs of the body can synthesize prostaglandins.

Besides the prostaglandins, essential fatty acids, particularly arachidonic acid are precursors of a number of local hormones, namely prostacycline, thromboxanes, lipoxines, and leucotrienes. Since all of them are derivatives of 20-C arachidonic acid, they have been grouped under the name of *eicosanoids* (eicosa=20). These substances mainly act on the tissues in which they are produced.

An outline of biosynthesis of various eicosanoids is given in Fig. 42.2.

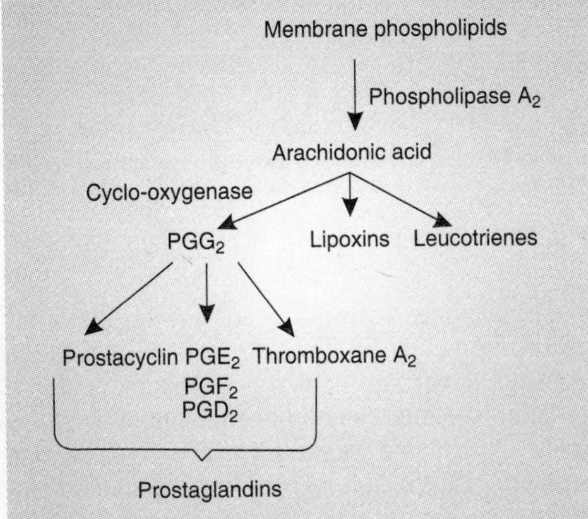

Fig. 42.2: Outline of biosynthesis of various eicosanoids.

Thromboxane-A_2 It is synthesized by the platelets. It is involved in vasoconstriction and platelet aggregation in response to injury to the platelets.

Prostacyclin It inhibits platelet aggregation and also acts as a vasodilator. It is produced by endothelial cells lining the blood vessels. Injury to a blood vessel produces thromboxane from the platelets which causes vasoconstriction and platelet aggregation, and clotting of blood. These steps help to minimise the blood loss and finally stop the bleeding. At the same time, the nearby endothelial cells release prostacyclin which prevents undue extension of the clot.

Leucotrienes These are mediators of allergic and inflammatory responses. Leucotrienes are released when an allergen combines with IgE antibodies on the surface of mast cells. Leucotrienes produce bronchoconstriction, vasoconstriction and increased capillary permeability. They also attract neutrophils and eosinophils to the site of inflammation.

Prostaglandins PGD_2, PGE_2, PGF_2 have been shown to produce such a variety of actions that no unifying role can be assigned to them. For example, prostaglandins produce:

- Decreased gastric acid secretion
- Regression and degeneration of corpus luteum
- Induction of abortion when injected intra-amniotically during mid-pregnancy
- Induction of labour when injected near full term
- Stimulation of renin secretion
- Stimulation of lipolysis
- Vasodilatation and increased blood flow in the kidney
- Release of gonadotropin releasing hormones from the hypothalamus

Of the actions mentioned above, prostaglandins have been therapeutically used to induce abortion during mid-pregnancy.

42

Role of Prostaglandins in Inflammation

Inflammatory exudate contains prostaglandins which produce pain either by direct stimulation of pain nerve endings or by sensitizing the pain nerve endings to the action of other pain producing polypeptides. Prostaglandins also contribute to the production of itching, vasodilatation, increased vascular permeability and cellular infiltration at the site of inflammation.

Prostaglandins produce fever when injected into the cerebral ventricles. It is believed that besides the bacterial pyrogens, prostaglandins released from site of inflammation contribute to the production of fever.

Inflammatory processes primarily help to protect the body against infections, etc. However, in certain diseases, the inflammatory response is so strong and destructive that it may produce permanent damage in the tissues, e.g. in the joints, valves of the heart and cornea. In patients suffering from such disorders, steroids are very effective in suppressing the inflammatory response. But steroids also produce potentially dangerous side effects. Due to this reason, non-steroidal anti-inflammatory drugs (NSAIDs) are more often used to suppress inflammation. Aspirin and indomethacin belong to this category. They inhibit synthesis of prostaglandins by inhibition of cyclo-oxygenase. That is why inhibition of prostaglandin synthesis is not accompanied by inhibition of leucotriene synthesis. Steroids inhibit the synthesis of prostaglandins, as well as leucotrienes because they act by inhibition of phospholipase A_2.

CHOLESTEROL METABOLISM

Cholesterol is a component of all the cell membranes as well as the membranes of the cellular organelles. The physical integrity of the cell depends on the presence of lipids like cholesterol, phospholipids, triglycerides and certain structural proteins. Cholesterol is also a precursor of steroid hormones and bile salts.

Dietary cholesterol (exogenous cholesterol) is absorbed from the intestine and incorporated into the chylomicrons. The adipose tissue removes the triglycerides with the help of lipoprotein lipase and the chylomicron remnants bring cholesterol to the liver. Endogenous cholesterol is synthesized mainly in the liver although most of the other tissues of the body can also synthesize it. Average endogenous synthesis of cholesterol in adult is 1.5–2 g/day as compared to less than 300 mg of cholestrol taken in diet. Eggs and animal fat are chief sources of dietary cholesterol.

Whenever dietary intake of cholesterol is high the synthesis of endogenous cholesterol by liver is decreased and vice versa. However, the feedback control is not tightly regulated and low cholesterol diet does lead to a moderate fall in the plasma cholesterol level. The feedback control is exerted by the inhibitory action of cholesterol on the enzyme HMG CoA reductase (Fig. 42.3).

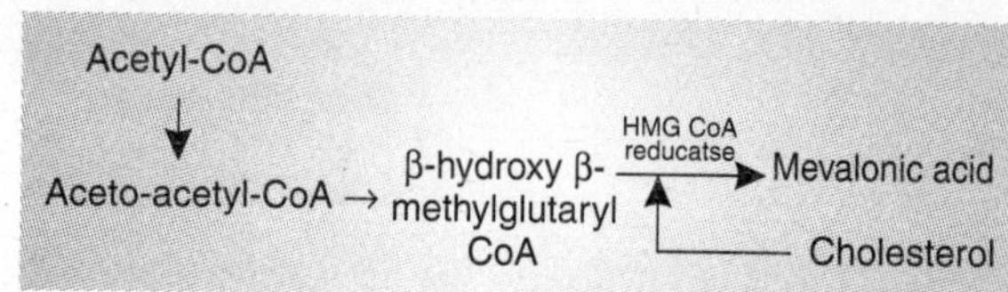

Fig. 42.3: Feed-back control of cholesterol synthesis.

The enzyme can be inhibited by drugs like com-pactin and mevinolin. These drugs have been found useful in lowering the blood cholesterol level.

Of all the dietary components, cholesterol has probably attracted maximum attention of research workers. Infiltration of cholesterol in subend-othelial region of the arteries leads to the rigidity and narrowing of the blood vessel. The condition, called atherosclerosis, predisposes to coronary and cerebral thrombosis. Elevated levels of plasma cholesterol and LDL (low density lipoproteins) are chiefly responsible for the development of atherosclerosis.

43

CHAPTER

Protein Metabolism

PROTEINS

Proteins are components of all the cells of the body. They constitute over 50% of the dry weight of an animal. All the enzymes and many hormones are proteins. Many proteins serve as neuro-transmitters. They also serve as transport proteins. They constitute the contractile component of the muscles. The gene expression is mediated through a specific modification of protein synthesis. In short, proteins are a pivot of animal structure and function.

AMINO ACIDS

Proteins are polymers of amino acids that are linked to each other by peptide bonds. All amino acids contain one or more of carboxyl (—COOH) and amino (—NH_2) groups. The peptide linkage is formed between carboxyl-carbon atom of one amino acid and amino-nitrogen atom of another amino acid.

$$\underset{\text{Amino acid}}{R_1\text{—}\overset{O}{C}\text{—}[OH} \quad \underset{\text{Amino acid}}{H]\text{—}\overset{H}{N}\text{—}R_2}$$

$$R_1\text{—}\underset{\text{(Peptide bond)}}{\overset{O}{C}\text{—}\overset{H}{N}}\text{—}R_2 + H_2O$$

Dipeptide

The carboxyl or the amino groups of the dipeptide can form a peptide bond with another amino acid, at either end constituting a tripeptide. In this way, amino acid chains can be extended. In proteins, the number of amino acids may vary from less than 10 to many thousand, all linked by peptide bonds.

A protein macro-molecule may consist of a single polypeptide chain or it may contain several polypeptide chains held together by covalent bonds. The sequence of amino acids in the chain is called the **primary structure** of the proteins. Depending upon the chemical nature of the amino acids, the polypeptide chain may form a coil (helix) or a zig-zag chain. This physical structure of a polypeptide is called its **secondary structure.** Additionally, the total chain may coil over itself to produce various types of three-dimensional conformation, like globular form or fibrous form, etc. This constitutes the **tertiary structure** of a protein. Further some proteins are made up of distinct subunits, e.g. haemoglobin. This arrangement of the subunits constitutes the **quaternary structure.**

CLASSIFICATION OF AMINO ACIDS

Based on the chemical structure, the 20 known amino acids are classified as given in Table 43.1.

Table 43.1: Classification of amino acid—based on chemical structure

Neutral amino acids

Amino acids with unsubstituted chains
- Glycine (Gly)
- Alanine (Ala)
- Valine (Val)
- Leucine (Leu)
- Isoleucine (Ile)

Hydroxyl substituted amino acids
- Serine (Ser)
- Threonine (Thr)

Sulphur-containing amino acids
- Cysteine (Cys)
- Methionone (Met)

Aromatic amino acids
- Phenylalanine
- Tyrosine (Tyr)
- Tryptophan (Trp)

Acidic amino acids

Mono-amino acids containing 2 or more carboxyl groups
- Aspartic acid (Asp)
- Asparagine (Asn)
- Glutamic acid (Glu)
- Glutamine (Gln)
- α-Carboxy glutamic acid (Gla)

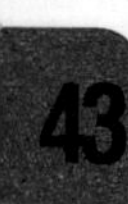

Basic amino acids

Diamino carboxylic acids
- Arginine (Arg)
- Lysine (Lys)
- Hydroxylysine (Hyl)
- Histidine (His)

Imino acids

Contain imino group but no amino group
- Proline (Pro)
- 4-Hydroxy proline
- 3-Hydroxy proline

Of the various amino acids mentioned above, about 10 can be synthesized in the body by transamination of keto acids produced from carbohydrate metabolism. Therefore, they may not be an essential component of diet. On the other hand, the other 10 amino acids cannot be synthesized in the body or the amount synthesized is insufficient for the body requirement. These amino acids have to be essentially supplied regularly in diet. The regular supply of these amino acids is required because they cannot be stored. These two groups of amino acids are known as *non-essential* and *essential* amino acids, respectively. Arginine and histidine are called *semi-essential* amino acids because they are not essentially required from exogenous source in normal adult human being. During growing period and pregnancy, their demand is so much increased that the enhanced demand can only be met with by dietary sources. The essential and non-essential amino acids are listed in Fig. 43.1.

Deamination and Transamination

Amino acids may be converted to α-keto acids by oxidative deamination or transamination reaction. Transamination is a reversible reaction consisting of the transfer of an α-amino group from an amino acid to α-keto acid. All amino acids axcept threonine, lysine and proline can undergo transamination with α-keto glutarate. The following two transaminase reactions of great clinical importance.

$$\text{1. Glutamate + Oxaloacetate} \xrightleftharpoons{\text{Trans-aminase}} \alpha\text{-Ketoglutarate + Aspartate}$$

$$\text{2. Glutamate + Pyruvate} \xrightleftharpoons{\text{Trans-aminase}} \text{Alanine + }\alpha\text{-Ketoglutarate}$$

The enzymes, glutamate-oxaloacetate transaminase (GOT) and glutamate-pyruvate transaminase (GPT) catalyse the reactions (1) and (2) mentioned above respectively. By clinical experience, it has been observed that the serum level of GOT (SGOT) enzyme is elevated in patients with acute damage to myocardium (myocardial

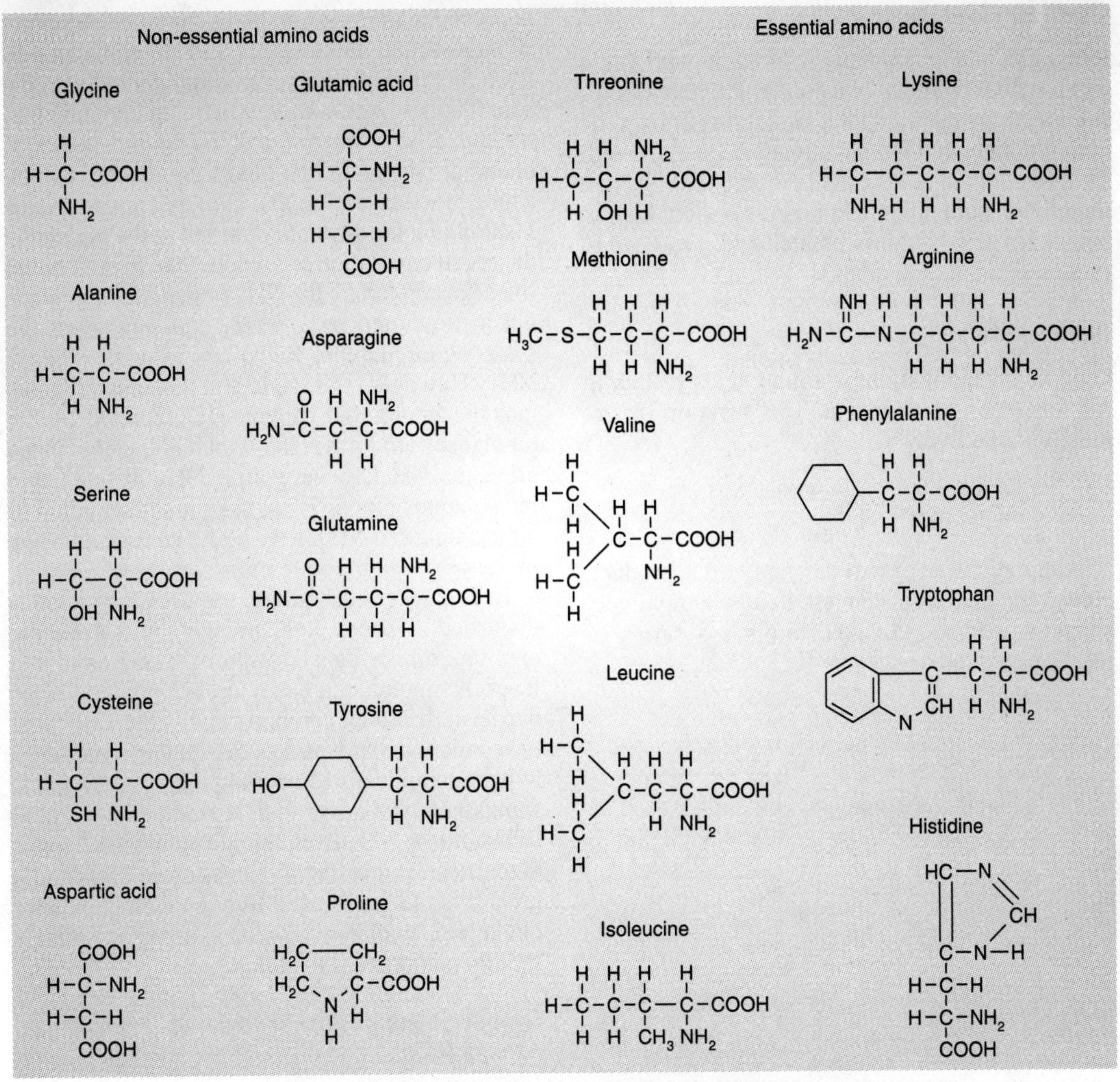

Non-essential amino acids

Glycine

Glutamic acid

Alanine

Asparagine

Serine

Glutamine

Cysteine

Tyrosine

Aspartic acid

Proline

Essential amino acids

Threonine

Lysine

Methionine

Arginine

Valine

Phenylalanine

Tryptophan

Leucine

Histidine

Isoleucine

Fig. 43.1: Structure of essential and non-essential amino acids.

infarction). The serum level of enzyme GPT (SGPT) is elevated in patients with acute liver damage.

Amino Acid Pool

The normal concentration of amino acids in the plasma is 35–65 mg%. The dietary proteins are digested and absorbed into the blood as amino acids. Amino acids are also being formed endogenously by hydrolysis of tissue proteins. Both these sources contribute to the amino acid pool from where amino acids are withdrawn for the various needs of the body. The urinary excretion of amino acids in normal individuals is almost negligible. Even in the stools only a very small amount of unabsorbed proteins of digestive juices and colonic mucus is lost.

Common Metabolic Pool

Pyruvates and intermediates of citric acid cycle form a common metabolic pool for carbohydrates, fats and proteins. The interconversion of carbohydrates and fats has already been discussed. Different amino acids can also enter the common metabolic pool after deamination. Conversely, keto acids may be transaminated and converted to non-essential amino acids.

Urea Synthesis

Oxidative deamination of amino acids results in the formation of ammonia. This reaction occurs mostly in the liver.

$$\text{Amino acid} \xrightarrow[\text{2H}]{} \text{Keto acid} + NH_3$$

Ammonia so released is a highly toxic product. However, liver can convert it into a relatively harmless compound, urea, through a series of reactions, called *urea cycle* (Fig. 43.2).

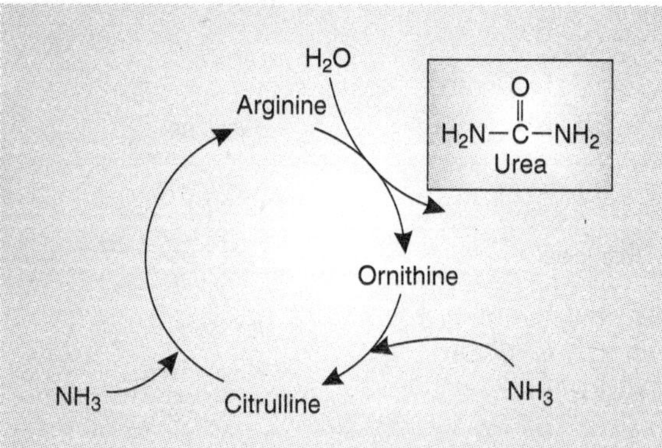

Fig. 43.2: The urea cycle.

In man, urea is the chief product of protein-nitrogen metabolism and the liver is the *only* site for its synthesis. The amount of urea produced per day varies with the amount of daily protein intake in diet. After synthesis, urea is poured into general blood circulation and excreted by the kidneys.

As mentioned above, the deamination of amino acids in the liver is the chief source of ammonia (NH_3). Other sources of ammonia include NH_3 produced in the large gut by bacterial deamination of unabsorbed amino acids and proteins derived from diet and exfoliated mucosal cells. From the blood, small amount of urea diffuses into lumen of the gut. It is converted to NH_3 by the action of bacterial urease. When blood urea level is high, significant amount of NH_3 may be formed in this fashion. All the ammonia formed in the gut enters the portal circulation and reaches the liver. Normal liver can convert all the NH_3 formed there or in the gut to urea, and hence NH_3 does not reach the systemic circulation. Renal tubules also produce NH_3. However, this NH_3 immediately diffuses into the lumen and captures H^+ secreted by the tubular cells to form NH_4^+ which is excreted in the urine (as NH_4Cl); very little NH_3 diffuses into renal venous blood. Thus, in spite of formation of large amount of NH_3 in the body, its concentration in the systemic blood remains very low.

In hepatocellular failure, the urea formation is disturbed. Hence, NH_3 escapes into systemic circulation causing elevation of blood ammonia level. Ammonia can easily cross the blood-brain barrier and produce cerebral toxicity (hepatic coma or hepatic encephalopathy). In liver cirrhosis, portal hypertension leads to opening of portal-systemic shunts near the lower end of oesophagus. These shunts allow NH_3 from the gut to bypass hepatic detoxification leading to elevation of blood NH_3 level (Fig. 43.3). Thus in liver cirrhosis, elevated blood NH_3 level may develop even with relatively little hepatocellular dysfunction.

Gluconeogenic and Ketogenic Amino Acids

After deamination, amino acids enter the common metabolic pool. For example, deaminated glycine and methionine are ultimately converted to pyruvate which may be converted to glucose by the reversible glycolytic reactions. Pyruvate may also be converted to acetyl-CoA which may either be oxidized in the citric acid cycle to yield energy or form fatty acid by condensation reactions. The conversion of amino acids into glucose or glycogen is called gluconeogenesis. Eighteen of the twenty amino acids can be converted to glucose after deamination.

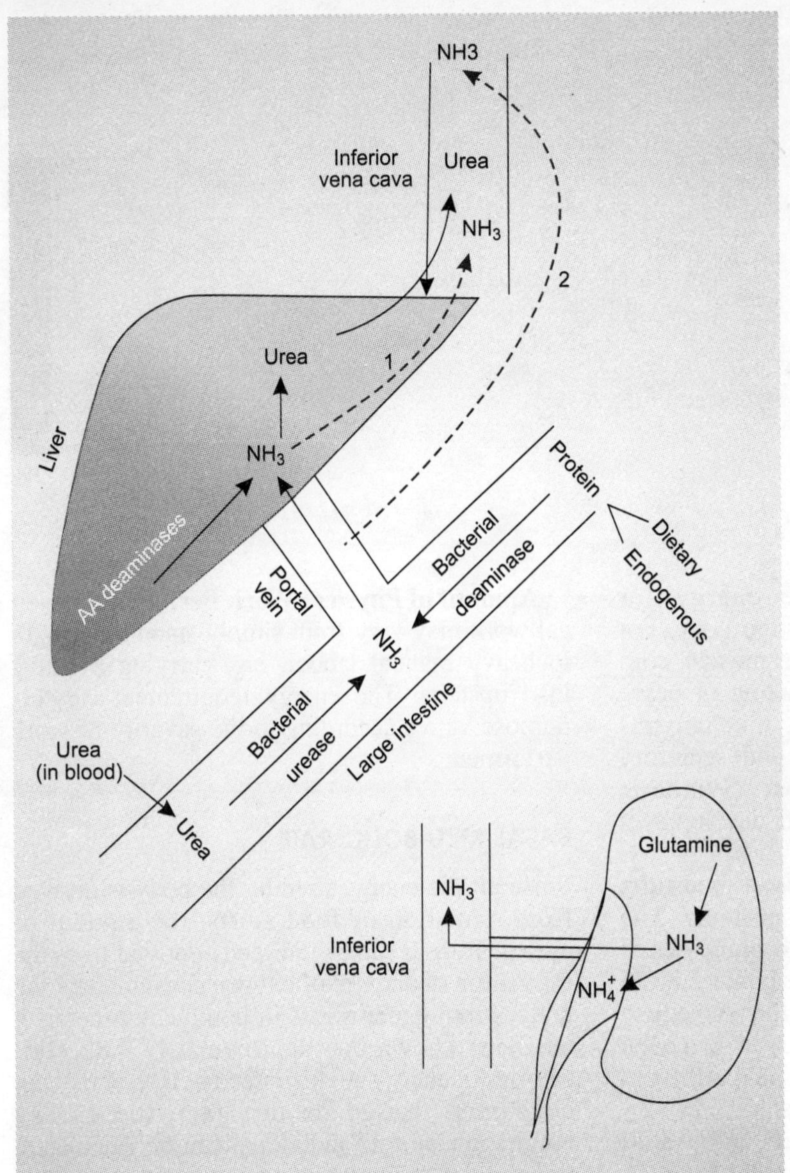

Fig. 43.3: Normal (continuous arrows) and abnormal (dashed arrows) routes taken by NH_3 formed in the body: 1. Hepatocellular failure; 2. Portal systemic shunting. AA, amino acids.

The conversion of amino acids to fatty acids is called ketogenesis. Only few amino acids like leucine, isoleucine, phenylalanine and tyrosine are ketogenic.

When the dietary intake of carbohydrates and fat is normal, only 10% of the total energy requirement is derived from proteins. Excessive intake of carbohydrates decreases the degradation of proteins for the purpose of energy production (*protein sparing action*). However, at least 20–30 g of proteins are always degraded every day, which has been called **obligatory loss** of proteins. That is why even though the external losses of proteins are very little, our diet must contain at least 20–30 g of proteins every day. Larger amounts of proteins may be degraded for energy production when almost all the stores of carbohydrates and fats are exhausted by prolonged starvation. Only under such circumstances, plasma proteins and tissue proteins are sacrificed for energy production.

CHAPTER 44

Nutrition

All living organisms require energy for maintenance of vital functions of the body. For example, energy is required for muscle contraction. It is required for conduction of nerve impulses. All active transport mechanisms involved in various absorptive and secretory processes are energy-dependent. Synthetic reactions involved in growth and development are also energy-dependent.

Energy is generated by oxidation of foodstuffs such as carbohydrates, fats and proteins. The energy liberated by the oxidative processes is trapped as "high energy phosphate bonds." If the energy generated is greater than the immediate requirement, it is stored in the body as glycogen and fat, which, when required, can be oxidized to yield high energy phosphate bonds.

The energy requirement of an individual depends on:

(i) The basal energy requirement and
(ii) The amount of physical work performed.

Basal Energy Requirement Energy is required for various metabolic processes occurring in the body even at rest, such as cardiac contraction, conduction of nerve impulses, hepatic metabolism, active transport mechanisms, etc. Such energy requirement is known as basal metabolic rate (BMR).

Amount of Physical Work Performed Physical work may vary from simply standing upright to heavy manual labour, e.g. carrying a heavy load upstairs. The energy requirement for this purpose varies according to the severity of work performed.

BASAL METABOLIC RATE

Since all the energy used by the body is derived from oxidation of food stuffs, the amount of energy utilized can be indirectly derived from the estimation of amount of oxygen consumed by the body. From experiments in bomb-calorimeter, it has been known that approximately 4.82 kilocalories of energy are liberated per litre of oxygen consumed. Based on this fact, the energy requirements of an individual can be calculated, under conditions of rest, and various grades of physical activity.

For the calculation of basal metabolic rate, oxygen consumption of an individual is estimated if the person fulfils the following criteria:

(a) The subject is in post-absorptive state (12–18 hours after the last meal).

(b) The subject is in complete physical and mental relaxed state.

(c) The investigation is conducted in thermo-neutral surroundings (25–27°C).

Estimation of BMR

Oxygen consumption of the individual is estimated for 6 minutes using a Benedict-Roth apparatus (also called a metabolator). The apparatus is basically an oxygen-filled spirometer having a CO_2 absorbing system containing soda lime, a one way breathing valve and an attached pen writing on a kymograph (Fig. 44.1).

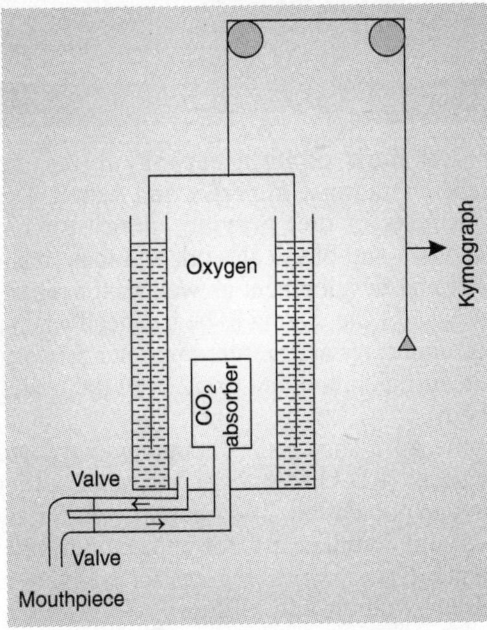

Fig. 44.1: A Benedict-Roth apparatus.

The amount of oxygen consumed per minute is corrected to standard temperature and pressure. From the corrected value of oxygen consumption, energy produced or consumed by the body can be known, since 1 litre of O_2 is equal to 4.82 kilocalories.

Basal metabolic rate is expressed as kilocalories per hour per square metre body surface area, i.e. kcal/h/m^2 BSA. Average normal BMR is 40 kcal/h/m^2 BSA in adult males and 37 kcal/h/m^2 BSA in adult females. Values 10% above or below the normal average are considered to be within the normal range.

Factors Affecting Basal Metabolic Rate

1. Body Surface Area (BSA) Metabolic rate is more closely related to body surface area than to the height or weight alone of an individual. When the height and weight of an individual are considered together, the body surface area can be calculated from the nomograms.

2. Sex Even with similar body surface area, males have higher BMR than the females. This is probably because of a larger percentage of subcutaneous fat (metabolically less active tissue) in females.

3. Age Children have higher BMR than adults. For example, at the age of 2 years BMR is 55 kcal/h/m^2 BSA and it gradually falls to the adult level by the age of 18 years. In old age, the BMR gradually declines. Even at the age of 60 years BMR is 5 kcal/h/m^2 BSA less than in adults.

4. External Temperature Exposure to cold increases the metabolic rate. It may be due to shivering or non-shivering thermogenesis. Exposure to high external environmental temperature also increases the metabolic rate because lot of energy is spent in the cooling mechanisms of the body.

5. Endocrines Thyroxine is the chief endocrine regulating the metabolic rate of an individual. In state of hyperthyroidism, BMR may be increased by 100%. In hypothyroidism, BMR may be decreased by 40%. Catecholamines also increase BMR.

6. Effect of Food Intake Ingestion of food increases BMR. The effect is more marked with protein diet than with carbohydrates or fats. After intake of 100 g of proteins, metabolic rate may be elevated by 20% during the next 4–6 hours. The effect is called *specific-dynamic action of food* (thermogenic effect of food). Why the digestion and assimilation of proteins should increase the metabolic rate is not clear.

7. Sleep During sleep, BMR falls by 10–15% specially during non-REM sleep.

8. Body Temperature For every rise of body temperature by 1°C, the metabolic rate increases by 14%. Thus, during high grade fever, the metabolic rate may be increased by over 50%.

9. Physical Activity Physical activity increases the metabolic rate in proportion to the degree of muscular effort (Table 44.1).

Table 44.1: Metabolic rate in different grades of activity in a male

State of body	*Metabolic rate (kcal/h/m² BSA)*
Awake, relaxed, supine (basal state)	40
Sitting	62
Walking slowly	150
Walking fast	284
Climbing stairs	312

10. Anxiety and Tension Even when lying in the bed, an anxious or tense individual has higher metabolic rate due to involuntary contraction of skeletal muscles as well as release of catecholamines.

11. Pregnancy During pregnancy, specially in the later months, the metabolic rate of the mother is increased because of the burden of fetal metabolism.

44

12. Starvation During prolonged starvation, the metabolic rate gradually decreases, partly because of decreased lean body mass, and partly because of decreased thyroxine secretion.

13. Reading and Other Mental Activities They do not affect the metabolic rate unless accompanied by tension.

TOTAL CALORIC REQUIREMENTS

Total caloric requirements of an individual can be calculated by adding the basal metabolic requirements to the energy required for the nature of his profession and other recreational/household activities. A sedentary worker, like a bureaucrat, requires much less energy than a farm-labourer or a rickshaw-puller. According to ICMR (Indian Council of Medical Research), an average sedentary male requires 2400 kcal per day. A sedentary female requires 80% of this value.

If the caloric requirement of a sedentary male (2400 kcal/day) is taken as a unit, the caloric requirements of other type of male and female workers may be calculated as follows:

Adult male sedentary work	1.0
Adult male moderate work	1.2
Adult male heavy work	1.6
Adult female sedentary work	0.8
Adult female moderate work	0.9
Adult female heavy work	1.2

BALANCED DIET

Our diet must contain carbohydrates, fats, proteins, vitamins, minerals and water. These constituents of diet provide energy for basal metabolism and physical work and materials for growth and development as well as for repair of the tissues. A diet is said to be balanced when the various nutrients are present in proper proportion and in sufficient amount to meet all the needs of the body.

Table 44.2 shows the recommended dietary allowances (RDA) of calories and other nutrients for Indian population. The figures given for adult males and females are for those involved in moderate type of work. Figures for pregnant and lactating women and children of various age groups are also given in the table.

The constituents of some of the important food stuffs are shown in Table 44.3.

CARBOHYDRATES

Carbohydrates constitute the cheapest dietary source of energy. They fulfill over 50% of the total caloric requirement (the rest of the caloric requirement is provided by oxidation of fats and proteins). Although carbohydrates can be synthesized in the body, yet a minimum intake of 50–100 g of carbohydrates per day is essential to prevent the development of ketosis and loss of muscle protein. Moreover, in the absence of

Table 44.2: Recommended dietary allowance (RDA) for Indian population (Indian Council of Medical Research, 1992)

	Energy (kcal)	*Protein (g)*	*Calcium (mg)*	*Iron (mg)*	*Vit.A μg*	*Vit.C mg*	*Folic acid μg*	*Vit. B_{12} μg*
Men (Adult)	2875	60	400	28	600	40	100	1.0
Women (Adult)	2225	50	400	30	600	40	100	1.0
Pregnancy	2525	65	1000	38	600	40	400	1.0
Lactation	2775	75	1000	30	950	80	150	1.5
Infants								
0–6 m	108 kcal/kg	2.05 g/kg	500	–	350	25	25	0.2
6–12 m	98 kcal/kg	1.65 g/kg	500	–	350	25	25	0.2
Children								
1–3 Y	1240	22	400	12	400	40	30	1.0
3–6 Y	1690	30	400	18	400	40	40	1.0
6–9 Y	1950	41	400	26	600	40	60	1.0
Boys								
10–12 Y	2190	54	600	19	600	40	70	1.0
13–15 Y	2450	70	600	28	600	40	100	1.0
16–18 Y	2640	78	500	30	600	40	100	1.0
Girls								
10–12 Y	1970	57	600	34	600	40	70	1.0
13–15 Y	2060	65	600	41	600	40	100	1.0
16–18 Y	2060	63	500	50	600	40	100	1.0

dietary carbohydrates, excessive ingestion of fats is required to provide energy which may expose the individual to the risk of atherosclerosis and coronary heart disease.

In general, in the Indian diet, most of the carbohydrates are ingested in the form of starch. However, in the Western diet, approximately 50% of the carbohydrate calories are derived from sucrose, e.g. candies, ice cream, colas, pastries, chocolate, etc. Such foods are consumed in large amounts by children of the more affluent segment of the Indian population also. The ingestion of sucrose in large quantities is harmful in a variety of ways:

1. Sucrose rich foods are tastier than starch-rich food. *It predisposes to obesity*.

2. The digestion of sucrose is quicker than that of starch. Therefore, ingestion of sucrose causes greater hyperglycemic effect than that of starch, causing a greater load on the beta cells of the islets of Langerhans. *This factor predisposes to diabetes mellitus.*

3. Sucrose is a suitable substrate for the metabolism of a number of bacteria in the oral cavity. Ingestion of sucrose-rich foods, especially that stick to the teeth, e.g. chocolates, promotes the bacterial growth in the oral cavity. The acids produced by bacterial metabolism of sucrose have a corrosive action on the dental enamel, leading to the *development of dental caries*. Thorough rinsing of the oral cavity immediately after consumption of sweets can provide protection against dental caries.

Dietary Fiber This term denotes all the plant cell-wall components consisting mainly of non-starch polysaccharides, which cannot be digested

Table 44.3: Important components of some common foodstuffs in 100 g of each

	Protein g	*Fat g*	*Carbohydrate g*	*Energy kcal*	*Minerals g*	*Calcium mg*	*Phosphorus mg*	*Iron mg*
Cereals								
Rice	7.5	1.0	76.7	346	0.9	10	190	3.2
Wheat flour	12.1	1.7	69.4	341	2.7	48	355	4.9
Pulses								
Bengal gram	17.1`	5.3	60.9	360	3.0	202	312	4.6
Green gram	24.0	1.3	56.7	334	3.5	124	326	4.4
Peas (dry)	19.7	1.1	56.5	315	2.2	75	298	7.0
Rajmah	22.9	1.3	60.6	346	3.2	260	410	5.1
Soyabean	43.2	19.5	20.9	432	4.6	240	690	10.4
Leafy vegetables								
Cabbage	1.8	0.1	4.6	27	0.6	39	44	0.8
Cauliflower	5.9	1.3	7.6	66	3.2	626	107	40.8
Mustard leaves	4.0	0.6	3.2	3.2	1.6	155	26	16.3
Spinach	2.0	0.7	3.8	46	2.1	53	91	10.9
Roots and tubers								
Carrot	0.9	0.2	10.6	48	1.1	80	530	1.03
Onion	1.2	0.1	11.1	50	0.4	46.9	50	0.6
Potato	1.6	0.1	22.6	97	0.6	10	40	0.48
Nuts								
Almonds	20.8	58.9	10.5	655	2.9	230	490	5.09
Coconut dry	6.8	62.3	18.4	662	1.6	400	210	7.8
Groundnut	25.3	40.1	26.1	567	2.4	90	350	2.5
Cashew nut	21.2	46.9	22.3	596	2.6	50	450	5.81
Fruit								
Apple	0.2	0.5	13.4	59	0.3	10	14	0.66
Banana	1.2	0.3	27.2	116	0.8	17	36	0.3
Grapes	0.6	0.4	13.1	58	0.9	20	23	0.5
Mango	0.6	0.4	16.9	74	0.4	14	16	1.3
Tomato	0.9	0.2	3.6	20	0.5	48	20	0.6
Meat and poultry								
Fish	20.9	3.1	13.9	167	1.1	98	152	1.8
Goat meat (lean)	21.4	3.6	–	118	1.1	12	193	–
Chicken meat	25.9	0.6	–	109	1.3	25	245	–
Egg	13.3	13.3	–	173	1.0	60	220	2.1
Milk and milk product								
Cow's milk	3.2	4.1	4.4	67	0.8	120	90	0.2
Buffaloe's milk	4.3	6.5	5.0	117	0.8	210	130	0.2
Cheese	24.1	25.1	6.3	348	4.2	790	520	2.1

in the human gastrointestinal tract. It includes cellulose, hemi-cellulose, pectins, gums, etc. (Chapter 40).

FATS

Fats are the most compact form of food. One gram of fat, on oxidation, yields 9 kcal as compared to 4.5 kcal in case of carbohydrates and proteins. However, fats are far more expensive source of energy than carbohydrates. The value of dietary fat lies not only in the supply of essential fatty acids but also in increasing the palatability of food and producing sense of satiety after intake of food. Moreover, dietary fats act as a vehicle for the supply and absorption of fat soluble vitamins.

Vegetable Fat vs. Animal Fat

In India, the use of animal fat like butter and ghee is considered a valuable and essential component of food in most of the households. Animal fat is the only source of essential fatty acids like linoleic acid, linolenic acid and arachidonic acid. Essential fatty acids are a component of cell architecture as well as precursors of prostaglandins. However, since animal fat chiefly consists of saturated fatty acids, its heavy consumption has been shown to promote increase in plasma cholesterol level leading to increased risk of atherosclerosis and associated disorders like coronary artery disease and cerebral strokes. Even if the animal fat constitutes only 1–2% of total fat intake, it is sufficient to provide the essential fatty acids. In India, till recently only poor people were using vegetable oils in the form of hydrogenated venaspati ghee.

Vegetable oils are not only cholesterol-free but also contain a large percentage of polyunsaturated fatty acids, which have a plasma cholesterol-lowering action. Coconut oil is an exception to this statement, since it contains saturated fatty acids only. The percentage of saturated and unsaturated fatty acids in various types of edible oils is given in the Table 44.4. The cholesterol-lowering action of vegetable fats is lost after hydrogenation. Hydrogenation of vegetable oils raises the melting point to give the consistency of ghee (animal fat) at room temperature. However, hydrogenation converts all the unsaturated fatty acids present in the vegetable oils into saturated fatty acids. Therefore to obtain any benefit, only non-hydrogenated vegetable oils should be consumed.

Table 44.4: Polyunsaturated content of various types of fats

Edible fat	*% polyunsaturated fatty acids*
1. Coconut oil	1
2. Corn oil	57
3. Cotton seed oil	47
4. Ground nut oil	30
5. Mustard oil	29
6. Rapeseed oil	33
7. Palm oil	9
8. Palmolin	11
9. Rice bran oil	33
10. Sunflower oil	79
11. Butter	2

Eggs and organ meat are rich sources of dietary cholesterol. The cholesterol content of eggs (500 mg /100 gm) may be compared with that of liver (440 mg/100 gm), Kidney (800 mg/ 100 gm) and brain (200 mg/100 gm).

Recommended Intake

Fats are basically used as a source of energy and hence can be replaced by carbohydrates. Except for the provision of essential fatty acids, and fat-soluble vitamins, intake of fats is not necessary. Fat intake is also important for the sake of palatability. It has been estimated that fat intake of about 20 gm animal fat / day is sufficient in an adult.

PROTEINS

Proteins are indispensable constituent of diet. Proteins constitute most of the exocrine and endocrine secretions (except steroid hormones). Plasma proteins and haemoglobin synthesis also requires proteins. Proteins are required for growth during childhood and during pregnancy. The normal wear and tear of the tissues is repaired with the help of dietary proteins. The importance of dietary protein intake lies in the fact that almost 50% of the amino acids cannot be synthesized in the body, i.e. leucine, isolucine, lysine, methionine, phenylalanine, threonine, tryptophan, valine, hidtidine and arginine. These amino acids, called essential amino acids, have to be provided in the diet. Proteins are available from both animal and vegetable sources. Some of the vegetables, e.g. soya beans have greater protein content (43%) than meat (21–26%).

Animal proteins like egg, fish, meat and milk have amino acid composition almost similar to that of human tissues. Hence, when ingested, they can be economically used in the body. Such proteins are said to have *high biological value.* Individual proteins of vegetable origin are deficient in one or more of the essential amino acids and hence cannot be used economically in the body. Such proteins are said to have *low biological value (BV)*. The biological value of a protein is expressed as follows:

$$BV = \frac{\text{Nitrogen retained in the body}}{\text{Nitrogen absorbed}} \times 100$$

The biological value of milk protein (casein) or egg albumin is 100%. Biological values of proteins of some of the common foods are compared in Table 44.5

Table 44.5: Biological values of some of the dietary proteins

Food	*Biological value*
Egg	100
Milk	100
Meat	74
Wheat	66
Rice	80
Bengal gram	74
Fish	80
Soybeans	90

However, vegetable proteins, though of lower biological value than animal proteins, are seldom consumed individually. When a mixture of vegetable proteins is ingested, it usually provides all the essential amino acids. A classical example is the consumption of a meal consisting of cereals and pulses. The lysine deficiency of cereals is made up by the pulses, whereas methionine deficiency of pulses is made up by the cereals. Another problem of vegetable proteins is regarding its efficiency of utilization. Since the efficiency of utilization of vegetable proteins is about 65% of the efficiency of animal proteins, the amount of vegetable protein intake has to be proportionately greater than consumption of animal proteins.

Daily protein intake should be spread over all the major 2–3 meals of the day. Amino acids that are not incorporated into tissues are deaminated and excreted as urea. Therefore, occasional intake of high protein diet is not as beneficial as regular intake of moderate amount of protein.

Recommended Intake

According to the Indian Council of Medical Research, the protein intake in an adult, in terms of mixed vegetable proteins should be at least 1 gm /kg body weight /day. If the protein intake is in the form of animal proteins, in view of better bioavailability, protein intake of 0.6 gm /kg body weight/day would be sufficient. Greater intake of proteins is required in infants and children in view of the protein requirement for growth.

MINERALS

Iron

The body of a healthy adult contains 4–5 g of iron in the following forms:

(a) Blood haemoglobin (about 2.5 g).
(b) Iron stored in tissues as ferritin and haemosiderin (1–1.5 g).
(c) Myoglobin in skeletal muscle (0.2 g).
(d) Intracellular enzymes like cytochromes oxidases, catalases and peroxidases (0.1 g).

The functions of iron in the body include:

(i) Oxygen transport by hemoglobin.
(ii) Small oxygen reserve as myoglobin.
(iii) Cellular oxidation as oxidative enzymes.
(iv) Bacterial killing by phagocytes.
(v) Immune function.

Dietary Sources

Our diet contains only about 10 mg of iron per day. Iron may be present in the diet as:

(i) Haem iron or
(ii) Inorganic iron salts

Haem iron is present in meat, fish, liver or chicken. Non-haem iron is present in green leafy vegetables, cauliflower, dried beans, nuts, cereals, and egg.

Absorption

Only about 1–10% of non-haem iron can be absorbed in the gut. On the other hand, about 10–20% of haem iron can be absorbed.

Absorption of non-haem iron is decreased by a number of factors which lead to formation of insoluble and non-absorbable complexes with dietary iron:

(i) High fiber diet (contains phytates)
(ii) Tea or coffee if taken with food (contain polyphenols and tannic acid).
(iii) High calcium content of food.
(iv) Oxalates : Spinach is rich in iron content, but it also contains large amount of oxalates. Therefore, bioavailability of iron from spinach is poor.

Absorption of non-haem iron is favored by simultaneous ingestion of:

(i) Foods containing reducing agents like ascorbic acid (citrus fruit, tomatoes). Non-haem iron is mostly present in Fe^{3+} form, where as only Fe^{2+} form of iron can be absorbed in the gut. Reducing agents convert Fe^{3+} form dietary of iron to Fe^{2+} form.
(ii) Gastric acid. The iron-phytate complexes are more soluble at lower pH. Therefore, gastric acid helps in iron absorption. Iron deficiency anemia is a common feature in patients with partial gastrectomy.
(iii) Ingestion of some haem form of iron with vegetable sources of iron.

Mechanism of Intestinal Absorption

Intestinal absorption of iron occurs mainly in the duodenum and upper jejunum. The mechanism by which the large iron molecule crosses into the epithelial cell is not exactly clear. The following hypothesis is widely accepted at present.

Haem Iron A *haem transporter protein* helps the transfer of haem iron across the intestinal brush border. In the cytoplasm of the epithelial cell, an enzyme, haem oxygenase removes iron from the porphyrin ring and adds it to the Fe^{2+} pool of the epithelial cell.

Non-haem Iron As mentioned earlier, non-haem iron is mostly present as Fe^{3+}. It is first reduced to Fe^{2+} by a brush border enzyme, ferric reductase. Next free Fe^{2+} is transported across the brush border with the help of a transport protein called *divalent metal transporter-1* (DMT1). Reductase activity is a component of DMT1 activity.

In the cytosol of the intestinal epithelial cell, Fe^{2+} can take one of the two possible routes:

(i) It may cross the basolateral border of the epithelial cell into the bloodstream. This step requires a transport protein *ferroportin* (Fig. 44.2), or another transport protein called hephaestin (HP). In the plasma, Fe^{2+} is converted to Fe^{3+} and gets attached to a plasma protein *transferrin* for transport in blood.
(ii) Some cytosolic Fe^{2+} are converted to Fe^{3+} and combine with a storage protein called *apoferritin* to constitute *ferritin*. This form (ferritin) of iron cannot cross the basolateral border of the epithelial cell. Within a few days, it is lost from the body along with the desquamated intestinal epithelial cells.

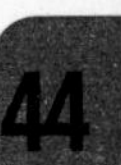

The fraction of absorbed iron that *forms ferritin* and that *crosses the basolateral border* into the blood circulation varies with the status of the iron stores of the body. When the body iron stores are saturated, most of the absorbed iron becomes ferritin in the intestinal epithelial cells and therefore does not enter the body. In iron deficiency states, a larger percentage of absorbed iron enters the circulation and only a small amount becomes ferritin in the epithelial cells. This regulatory control over intestinal absorption of iron is known as the **mucosal block theory** of intestinal iron absorption. It is of critical

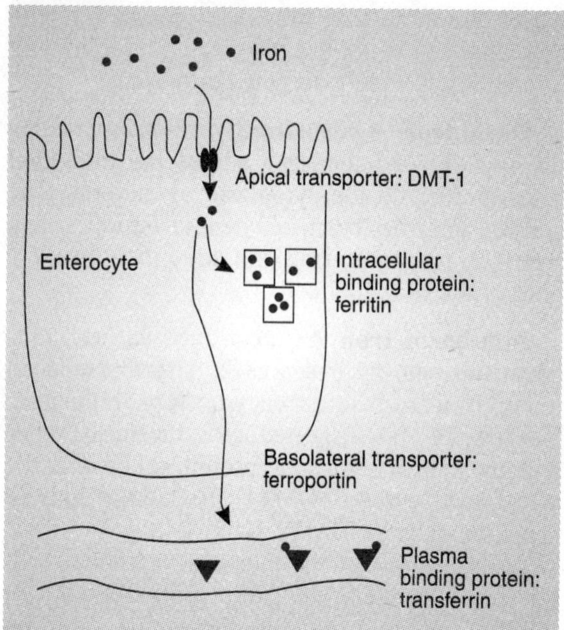

Fig. 44.2: Absorption of iron in the intestinal epithelial cell.

importance in maintaining normal iron balance of the body, since once it enters the circulation; there is no way for the excretion of iron. That is why intravenous iron administration for the treatment of severe anemia, or multiple blood transfusions for the treatment of thalassemias carry a risk of iron overload.

Transport

In the blood, iron is transported as Fe^{3+}, bound to a β-globulin, transferrin. Transferrin-bound iron is readily available for various roles in the body, e.g. formation of haemoglobin, oxidative enzymes, etc. The average plasma concentration of iron is 130 μg/100 ml in males and 110 μg/100 ml in females. *Plasma concentration of transferrin* is also known as *total iron binding capacity (TIBC)* of plasma. Normal value of TIBC is 250–450 μg/dl. Normally, it is about 33% saturated with iron.

Storage

Iron is stored in the body in hepatic parenchymal cells as well as mononuclear macrophages of the bone marrow, liver, and spleen. In these cells, iron is stored as ferritin, i.e. as apoferritin—Fe^{3+} complex. Iron released from the senescent red blood cells is also stored in these cells as ferritin. In these iron stores, larger aggregates of ferritin constitute *hemosiderin*. Under light microscope, presence of hemosiderin can be detected as yellow to brown granules. Ferritin can be identified only under electron microscope. Iron stored either as ferritin or as hemosiderin can be readily mobilized for use in erythropoiesis, etc.

Excretion

In males, 0.5–1 mg of iron is lost per day in urine, sweat, hair and nails. The loss is 1–2 mg per day in women of reproductive age because of additional losses in menstruation, or pregnancy and lactation. Iron excreted in the faeces consists of unabsorbed dietary iron and that present in desquamated mucosal cells. There is no regulatory control over the excretion of iron.

Pathophysiology

Due to poor iron content of most of the food stuffs as well as poor bioavailability of dietary iron (about 10%), iron deficiency anemia is common world wide. It is more common in females of the reproductive age group because of their increased iron losses in menstruation, pregnancy and lactation.

Parameters of Iron Status of the Body

1. **Serum iron level:** Normal 80–180 μg/dl.
2. **Total iron binding capacity, (TIBC):** Normal 250–450 μg/dl.
3. **TIBC saturation:**

$$\frac{\text{Serum iron concentration X 100}}{\text{TIBC}}$$

(Normal 33% saturation)

4. **Serum ferritin:** Ferritin is normally present only in the tissue as stored iron, from where a small amount leaks into plasma. Estimation of serum ferritin is a sensitive index of iron stores of the body.

5. Red cell protoporphyrin: During normal erythropoiesis, protoporphyrin synthesis in the developing red cells is followed by incorporation of iron. In iron deficiency, this step is interfered with and hence red cell protoporphyrin concentration is increased.

6. Bone marrow iron: Presence of iron stored in the bone marrow can be visualized by examination of a marrow smear stained with Prussian blue stain.

Laboratory indices of iron deficiency

Decreased serum iron conc.
Increased TIBC
Decreased TIBC saturation
Decreased serum ferritin conc.
Increased red cell protoporphyrin conc.
Poor marrow iron stores

Haemochromatosis

A condition of iron overload of the body, may be classified as two types: Idiopathic and secondry.

1. Idiopathic Haemochromatosis It is a genetic disorder, in which excessive intestinal absorption of iron occurs even though the intake is normal. Actually, the absorption is 2–4 mg per day, only slightly above normal. But by 40–50 years age, when the disease manifests, the body contains about 20–40 g of iron. The excessive iron is stored as haemosiderin in various tissues, e.g. skin, exocrine and endocrine pancreas, liver, gonads, and cornea, leading to tissue necrosis. The disorder is characterized by:

(i) Yellowish-brown pigmentation of the skin
(ii) Diabetes due to damaged endocrine pancreas. These two features have led to the name, bronze diabetes for the disorder.
(iii) Sterility because of damage in gonads.

2. Secondary Haemochromatosis It is an acquired defect commonly seen in children suffering from thalassemia, who are treated by repeated blood transfusions.

Calcium

Total body calcium content is about 1 kg. Of this, approximately 99% is present in the skeleton. Plasma calcium level is maintained within a very narrow normal range of 9–11 mg%, of which approximately 50% is in ionic form. Ionic plasma calcium has notable effects on neuromuscular excitability and myocardial function. In addition, ionic calcium is involved in numerous intracellular biochemical reactions, excitation-contraction coupling in the skeletal and cardiac muscles and in coagulation of blood.

ICMR has recommended an intake of 400 mg calcium/day. It should be increased to 1 gm/day in pregnancy and lactation. Traditionally, in the western literature, an intake of 1gm calcium/day for adults and 1.5 gm/day in pregnant and lactating women is recommended. The lower recommended daily allowance (RDA) by ICMR is based on the knowledge that chronically low intake of dietary calcium induces adaptive changes in the body in the form of increased production of 1, 25-dihydroxy vitamin D_3.

Sources

Main dietary sources of calcium include milk and milk products, egg, fish, green leafy vegetables and cereals. Rice is a poor source of calcium. The presence of phytic acid and oxalates in cereals and in some leafy vegetables decreases the bioavailability of calcium by forming insoluble non-absorable calcium phytate and calcium oxalate.

Rickets in babies and osteomalacia in adults (usually women) are the disorders of bone metabolism primarily related to vitamin D deficiency rather than deficiency of dietary calcium.

Iodine

Iodine is an essential component of thyroxine, the important hormone regulating the basal metabolic rate of the body. Sea fish and other sea foods are very rich sources of iodine. Meat, eggs, some green leafy vegetables and cereals are other sources (Table 44.6). Recommended intake of iodine is about 150 μg/day.

Thyroxine has a crucial role in the growth and development of nervous tissue. In view of widespread prevalence of iodine deficiency goiter, only iodinated salt is allowed to be sold in India.

Table 44.6: Iodine content of foods

Food	*Iodine content (microgram/100 g weight)*
Sea fish	832
Fresh water fish	30
Meat	50
Eggs	93
Cereals	47
Legumes	29
Green vegetables	29
Fruits	18

VITAMINS

The sources, daily requirement, their role in the body and disorders caused by deficiency of the various vitamins are summarized in Table 44.7.

DISORDERS OF OVER-NUTRITION AND UNDER-NUTRITION

Obesity

Obesity is a fairly common problem in the affluent members of the society. Although there is an internal regulation of body weight and long-term intake of food, these individuals tend to be obese due to some genetic factors. Obesity attributable to endocrine disorders is relatively less common.

44

The pattern of fat distribution throughout the body affects metabolic consequences. A person with fat located predominantly in the abdominal region, the so-called apple-shaped or upper body obesity (Fig. 44.3), may be at greater risk cardiovascular diseases than another person with a greater total amount of adipose tissue that is located predominantly in the lower abdomen, hips and thighs (pear-shaped obesity). Upper body obesity is common in males, whereas pear-shaped obesity (Fig. 44.3) is common in females.

Even though the exact cause of obesity is not known, the basic fact remains that their energy intake exceeds the energy expenditure. Moreover, excess energy input needs to be present only when obesity is developing. Once a person has become obese, his energy intake is usually not more than that of a lean individual. Obesity is associated with increased incidence of diabetes mellitus, athero-

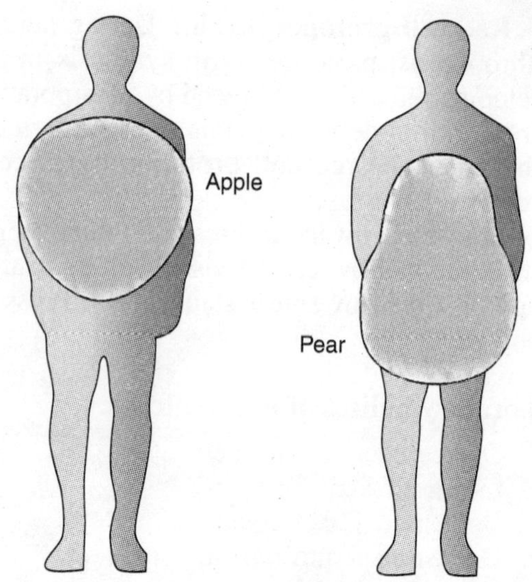

Fig. 44.3: Apple- and pear-shaped obesity.

sclerosis, coronary artery disease, hypertension, joint pains specially in knees, and psychological disturbances. A person is said to be obese if his body weight is 20% or more greater than the desirable weight for his age and sex. A rough guide to the diagnosis is the calculation of body mass index (BMI).

$$\text{Body mass index} = \frac{\text{Weight in kg}}{\text{Height in metres squared}}$$

BMI	
Normal:	18.5–24.9
Overweight:	25–29.9
Obese:	30 and over

In the treatment of obesity, dieting is commonly resorted to. Most often dieting can reduce the body weight only transiently. Moreover prolonged and severe dieting may lead to vitamin and mineral deficiency disorders. Moderate decrease in food intake especially of fats coupled with increased physical activity constitute a more effective regimen for the reduction of body weight. Increased physical activity should not be taken to mean paddling a bicycle for a few minutes every day. A change of lifestyle involving willingness to engage in physical activity at every available opportunity is required. In principle, the aim

Table 44.7: Vitamins, their sources, role in the body and deficiency disorders

Vitamin	*Sources*	*Actions*	*Deficiency disorders*
Fat soluble			
A	Fish liver oil, liver, butter, egg, cheese, carrot, amaranth spinch, mango, papaya, tomato	• Constituent of retinal photo-pigments • Maintenance of the integrity of glandular and epithelial tissues specially or the skin and eyes • Supports growth	• Night blindness • Conjunctival xerosis (dryness) • Bitot's spot • Corneal xerosis • Keratomalacia
D	Cutaneous synthesis, animal food like liver, egg yolk, butter, cheese, and fish liver and fortified vanaspati ghee	Intestine: Promotes calcium absorption Bone: Stimulates mineralization Kidney: Increases calcium reabsorptions	Rickets in children, osteomalacia in adults
E	Vegetable oils, sunflower seed, egg yolk and butter	An important antioxidant on cellular and subcellular membrane phospholipids	Anaemia in pregnancy and neurological disorders
K	Green vegetables synthesised by intestinal bacteria	Synthesis of clotting factors II, VII, IX and X	Clotting disorders
Water soluble			
B-complex group of vitamins			
B_1, Thiamine	Whole grain cereals, wheat germ, pulses, groundnut	Coenzyme for oxidative decarboxylation and transketolase reaction HMP shunt	Beri-beri Dry: neuropathy Wet: cardiovascular degeneration
B_2, Riboflavin	Milk, egg, liver, green vegetables	As cofactor in cellular oxidation in energy metabolism	Stomatitis, glossitis, chelosis
Niacin	Liver, meat, eggs, fish, groundnut	Coenzyme in NAD linked dehydrogenases	Pellagra: weight loss, diarrhoea, dermatitis, and dernentia
B_6, Pyridoxine	Milk, egg yolk, meat, cereals and vegetables	Role in metabolism of carbohydrate, fat and amino acids	Rare because of wide distribution in foods
Pantothenic acid	All foods	Present in cells as coenzyme-A	Deficiency never occurs
Folic acid	Leafy vegetables, meat, egg, milk, cereals	Role in nucleic acid synthesis	Megaloblastic anaemia, glossitis, diarrhoea
B_{12} Cyano-cobalamine	Liver, meat, fish, eggs, milk, and cheese, also synthesized by colonic bacteria	DNA synthesis	Pernicious anaemia, megaloblastic anaemia and subacute combined degeneration of spinal cord
Vitamin C	Citrus food and green leafy vegetables, amla, guava	Role in tissue oxidation, collagen synthesis absorption of iron	Scurvy, bleeding from gums, local haemorrhages, increased capillary fragility

should be to increase the energy expenditure so that it exceeds the energy intake.

Hypervitaminosis

Due to self-medication, excessive intake of vitamins is a common occurrence. Rapid urinary excretion prevents any toxic effects of water soluble vitamins. In contrast, fat soluble vitamins tend to be stored in the liver and adipose tissue and cannot be excreted. Hypervitaminosis A and D are well-recognized clinical disorders.

Hypervitaminosis A is characterized by anorexia, hepato-splenomegaly, dermatitis, loss of hair and bone pains.

Hypervitaminosis D is associated with hypercalcaemia, weight loss, and soft tissue calcification in the kidney and blood vessels. Renal failure may ultimately lead to death.

Undernutrition

Starvation

The effects of complete starvation may be studied in individuals who undertake fast unto death. Complete starvation may also occur in some psychiatric patients, or patients with later stages of cancer oesophagus, or very old bedridden individuals neglected by the family. Partial starvation used to be more common due to famines in India but even now it is not rare.

The body stores of glycogen are so little (200 g) that they are unable to maintain blood sugar level for more than 24 hours. After this, tissue fat and proteins are utilized to provide energy and maintain blood glucose level (gluconeogenesis). Free fatty acids released by lipolysis can be utilized as fuel by most of the tissues specially skeletal muscle and cardiac muscle. However, tissues like brain, retina, germinal epithelium and RBCs are purely glucose dependent for their energy requirements. Whereas lipolysis has glucose sparing action, enhanced breakdown of proteins helps in gluconeogenesis and maintenance of blood glucose level.

Within 3–4 weeks of complete starvation over 25% of the body weight may be lost. Of this, loss of fat is 5–6 kg, loss of protein 2.5–3 kg, and loss of body water about 5 kg. Loss of body water occurs mainly from intracellular compartment. Decreased plasma protein concentration leads to oedema especially in elderly individuals.

Deficiency of TSH secretion leads to marked atrophy of thyroid gland. Hence BMR falls. Decreased secretion of gonadotropins leads to loss of libido in males and menstrual disturbances in the female.

Severe Malnutrition

Severe malnutrition is not uncommon in India. It may be seen in extremely poor population of rural and urban India. It results in deficiency diseases like protein energy malnutrition, nutritional anaemias, vitamin deficiency disorders, goiter and nutritional oedema, etc.

Chronic Undernutrition

Chronic undernutrition is a national health problem in India and other under-developed countries. According to a study by WHO in 1998, about 50% of the population of India is underweight (as compared to only 2% in the UK). Subnormal body weight, without any positive sign of illness is an indication of mild chronic undernutrition.

Chronic undernutrition in childhood leads to physical and possibly mental growth retardation and more susceptibility to infections leading to greater childhood mortality. In adults, chronic undernutrition produces a significant reduction in work *capacity, easy fatigability, greater susceptibility to infections and premature ageing.*

Section XI

Endocrines

45 CHAPTER

Mode of Action of Hormones

Hormones and nervous system constitute the two important regulatory mechanisms of the body. Generally speaking, the nervous system controls the rapid activities in the body such as muscular contraction, whereas hormones regulate the metabolic activities. Nervous system often, but not always, regulates the secretion of some of the hormones directly (e.g. adrenal medullary hormones) or indirectly (e.g. adrenal glucocorticoids). On the other hand, hormones often influence the activity of nervous system, e.g. thyroxine, parathormone, etc.

ENDOCRINE, PARACRINE AND AUTOCRINE HORMONES

In the classical definition, a hormone is a chemical substance that is secreted directly into bloodstream by a group of cells and that exerts physiological control on some distant cells of the body. Some hormones such as secretin or cholecystokinin are released into bloodstream but exert their action on nearby tissues only. Such hormones are called *local hormones*. Hormones secreted by specific endocrine glands such as pituitary gland or thyroid gland are poured into blood and act on tissues far away from the site of secretion. Such hormones are known as *general hormones* or simply *hormone* or *endocrines.*

The classical definition of a hormone given above has now been found to be too restrictive. A hormone may not necessarily be poured into bloodstream. It may act on nearby cells only. Such hormones are called **paracrine hormones**. A paracrine hormone is conveyed over a short distance by diffusion through the interstitial fluid to act on neighbouring cells. For example, in the islets of Langerhans, somatostatin secreted by δ-cells regulates the activity of α- and β-cells of the islets. An **autocrine hormone** regulates the activity of the same cell which produced it, e.g. prostaglandins.

In other word, a hormone may have *endocrine, paracrine* or *autocrine* action (Fig. 45.1).

SOME PHYSICAL CHARACTERISTICS OF HORMONES

Chemical Classification The chemical classification of hormones is given in Table 45.1.

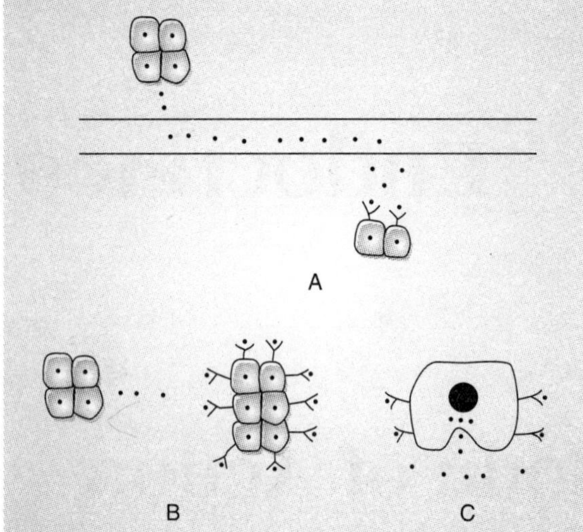

Fig. 45.1: Different types of hormone action. (A) Endocrine action, (B) Paracrine action, and (C) Autocrine action.

Post-secretory Modification A hormone may not be in the active form when secreted by the endocrine gland. It may undergo post-secretory structural modification in the bloodstream, liver, kidney or in the target tissues. Activation may occur by proteolytic cleavage in a peptide hormone or by enzymic modification in case of steroids or thyroid hormones.

Circulating Forms Some hormones circulate free in the plasma (e.g. protein and polypeptide hormones), whereas others circulate bound to specific plasma proteins (e.g. thyroxine, steroids). Protein binding of hormones :

(i) Protects them against excretion by the kidneys;
(ii) Slows the rate of degradation by the liver; and
(iii) Provides a circulating reservoir of the hormones from where they are slowly released into free form for biological activity.

Hormone Receptors These are unique protein molecular groups situated on the cell membrane or in the cytoplasm or even nucleus of the target cell. Interaction between the hormone and its specific receptor initiates the specific responses in the target cell. This property is responsible for specificity of a hormonal action. Endocrines circulate in the blood. Therefore, most of the tissues are exposed to all the endocrines. A hormone shall act only in the tissues which contain specific receptors for the hormone (Fig. 45.2). The effects of hormone-receptor interaction shall be discussed in detail later in this chapter.

Half-life Most hormones are metabolized rapidly after secretion. In general, peptides have shorter half-life than steroids (Table 45.2).

Intracellular Degradation The interaction of a hormone with its target cell is followed by intracellular degradation of the hormone.

Table 45.1: Classification of hormones

Amines
Epinephrine
Norepinephrine
Thyroxine (T_4)
Tri-iodothyronine (T_3)
Small peptides
Calcitonin
Glucagon
Growth hormone
Adrenocorticotropic hormone (ACTH)
Insulin
Malanocyte stimulating hormone (MSH)
Parathyroid hormone
Prolactin
Vasopressin (ADH)
Glycoproteins
Follicle stimulating hormone (FSH)
Luteinizing hormone (LH)
Thyroid stimulating hormone (TSH)
Human chorionic gonadotropin (hCG)
Steroids
Aldosterone
Cortisol
Oestradiol
Progesterone
Testosterone
Vitamin D

Table 45.2: Half-life of some of the hormones

Peptides		*Amines*		*Steroids*	
Hormone	*Half-life*	*Hormone*	*Half-life*	*Hormone*	*Half-life*
Oxytocin	1 min	Epinephrine	2 min	Aldosterone	30 min
Insulin	5 min	Norepinephrine	2 min	Cortisol	90 min
Prolactin	12 min	T_3	1–3 days	1,25(OH)2D_3	15 hours
ADH	18 min	T_4	5–7 days	25(OH)D_3	15 days
GH	20 min				
ACTH	20 min				
LH	30 min				
FSH	180 min				

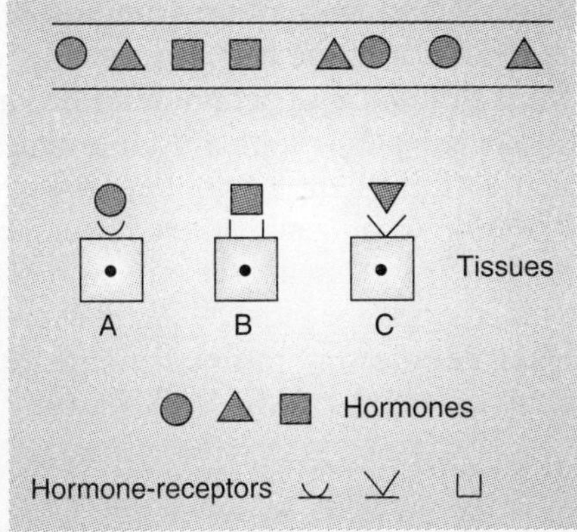

Fig. 45.2: Specificity of hormonal action.

Inactivation and Excretion Only a small fraction of circulating hormone is removed by its target tissues. The remainder is inactivated in the liver or the kidneys by various mechanisms like hydrolysis, oxidation, hydroxylation, methylation, decarboxylation, sulfation, glucuronidation, etc. A very small fraction (less than 1%) is excreted unchanged in the urine or faeces.

Feedback Control In our body, most of the physiological processes are regulated by a feedback control. Secretion of most of the hormones is regulated by a **negative feedback control** system. A negative feedback control is said to be present when *output* of a pathway *inhibits input* into the pathway. Negative feedback control is best illustrated by the anterior pituitary-target gland axis. Anterior pituitary gland secretes a trophic hormone, say ACTH. The trophic hormone acts on the target gland (adrenal cortex). The adrenal cortex secretes cortisol.When the plasma level of cortisol exceeds the physiological limit; it has an inhibitory action on the secretion of ACTH by anterior pituitary gland. When the plasma cortisol level begins to fall, inhibition is abolished and ACTH secretion starts once again. Thus the negative feedback control helps to maintain plasma cortisol level within the physiological range (Fig. 48.3).

In the example given above, the hormone secreted by the target gland exerted a negative feedback control. In case of some of the hormones, the plasma chemical constituent regulated by the hormone exerts a negative feedback control. For example, plasma glucose level exerts a feedback control over the secretion of insulin and glucagons, plasma ionic calcium level has a feedback control over the secretion of parathyroid hormone and calcitonin and plasma osmolality over secretion of antidiuretic hormone.

MECHANISM OF ACTION OF HORMONE-RECEPTOR COMPLEX

Hormones may regulate the metabolic function in a variety of ways. A hormone may:

- Regulate the rate of chemical reactions.
- Alter the rate of transport of a substance into the target cell.
- Regulate growth and development, or
- Regulate the secretory activity.

The binding of a hormone with a specific receptor results in the formation of a receptor-hormone complex. The hormone receptor complex once formed leads to conformational change in the receptor molecule resulting in one of the following consequences.

1. Action on Membrane Permeability

The activated receptor may directly alter the membrane permeability. Few hormones like insulin and possibly growth hormone act in this way.

2. Action through Genes (Transcription and Translation Effects)

Steroid Hormones Hormones secreted by the adrenal cortex and gonads as well as thyroid hormones act by producing an alteration in the protein synthesis in the target cell.

Steroids being hydrophobic molecules are soluble in lipid environment of the cell membrane. They enter the cell by passive diffusion and bind with the specific receptors present in the cytoplasm. The cells containing the specific receptors for the hormones become the target cells. The activated receptor diffuses into the nucleus and binds tightly to the specific sites on the nuclear chromatin. As a result, the rate of transcription (messenger RNA) is altered. The messenger RNA (mRNA) diffuses into the cytoplasm, where it promotes the translation process at the ribosomes. In this way, new proteins are produced which result in specific responses. Some of the proteins synthesized are enzymes (Fig. 45.3).

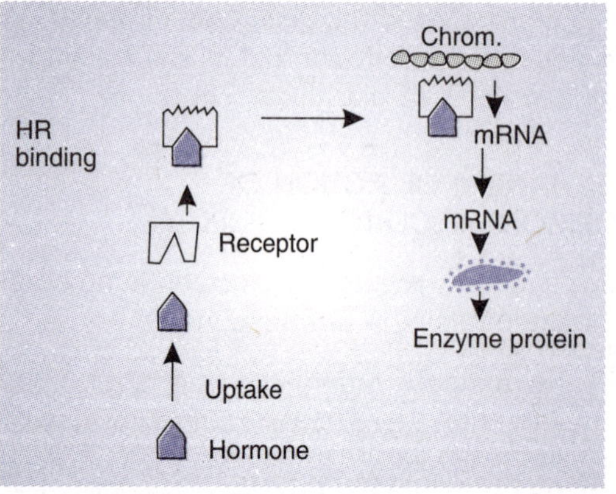

Fig. 45.3: Action of hormones through changes in protein synthesis.

Due to the time involved in the processes described above, there is a characteristic delay of about 45 minutes to several hours before the action of a steroid hormone manifests itself.

Thyroid Hormones They also increase the synthesis of mRNA but unlike the steroids, their receptor proteins are located in the nucleus bound to nuclear chromatin.

3. Action through "Second Messenger"

Peptides and biogenic amines are two principal classes of hydrophilic hormones that do not penetrate the cell membrane of the target cells. Receptors for such hormones are located in the cell membrane and the hormonal binding sites are expressed exterior to the cell surface (Fig. 45.4). In the first two modes of action described above, the hormone receptor complex itself produces the biological action of the hormone. However, in case of peptide or biogenic amine hormones, the hormone (the first messenger) exerts its biological effect by increasing the intracellular concentration of another regulatory molecule (the second messenger) like cyclic AMP (cAMP), Ca^{2+}, etc.

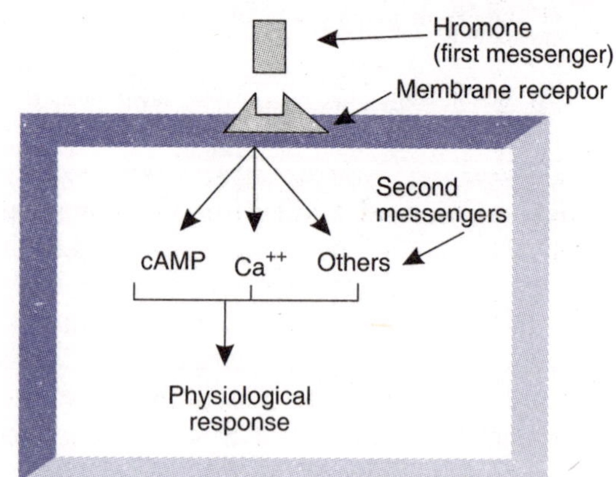

Fig. 45.4: The second messengers in hormonal action.

Cyclic AMP

When the hormone binds with the receptor in the cell membrane, the hormone-receptor complex activates an enzyme *adenyl-cyclase* which is also located in the cell membrane. A part of the enzyme protrudes through the inner surface of the cell membrane and, when activated, causes conversion of cytoplasmic ATP into cyclic AMP (adenosine monophosphate). The specific action occurring in the target cell in response to generation of cAMP depends on the intracellular machinery present in the cell (Fig. 45.5). Thus, in different tissues, cAMP may result in:

i. Alteration in cell membrane permeability,
ii. Initiation of secretion,
iii. Initiation of synthesis of specific intracellular enzymes,
iv. Activation of enzymes present in the cell.

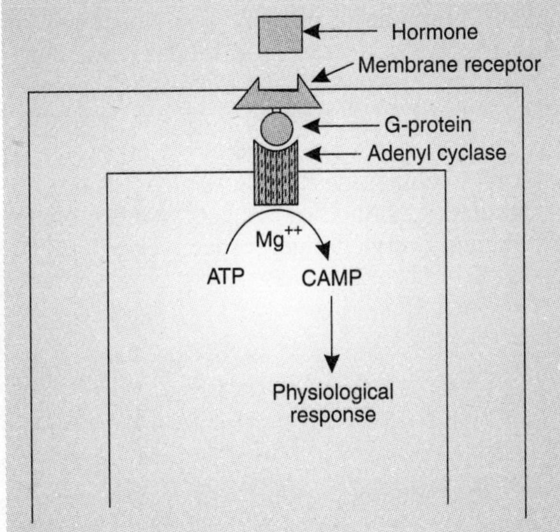

Fig. 45.5: Action of a hormone through cAMP as the second messenger.

Some of the important hormones which act by altering the concentration of intracellular cyclic AMP are listed in Table 45.3.

Table 45.3: Some important hormones that act by altering intracellular cAMP concentration

Increase cAMP
ACTH
TSH
FSH
LH
MSH
Parathormone
Calcitonin
Vasopressin (V_2 receptor)
Catecholamine (β_1, β_2 receptors)
Glucagon
Chorionic gonadotropic hormone
Decrease cAMP
Catecholamines (α_2 receptor)
Dopamine (D_2 receptor)
Somatostatin

Calcium Ions and Calmodulin

The hormone receptor complex may increase the intracellular Ca^{2+} concentration by opening Ca^{2+} channels in the cell membrane or by release of Ca^{2+} from intracellular calcium-pools notably endoplasmic reticulum. The Ca^{2+} bind with and activate an intracellular Ca^{2+} binding protein called calmodulin. The activated calmodulin (like cyclic AMP) can produce various types of biological responses (Fig. 45.6). Hormones which act by increasing intracellular Ca^{2+} are listed in Table 45.4.

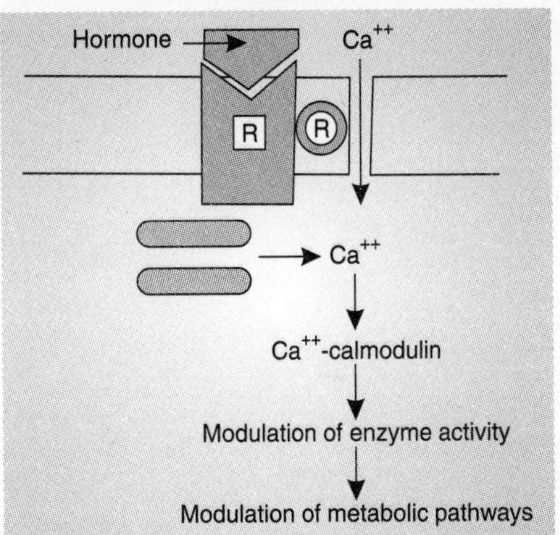

Fig. 45.6: Action of a hormone through Ca^{++} as the second messenger.

In contrast to the delayed biological response produced by the steroids, the hormone action through cyclic AMP or Ca^{2+} produces an almost instantaneous effect.

Tyrosine kinase or cyclic GMP are other well-known second messengers.

Table 45.4: Some of the hormones which act by increasing intracellular Ca^{++}

Catecholamines (α_1 receptor)	GnRH
Vasopressin (V_1 receptor)	Histamine (H_1 receptor)
Angiotensin-II	Serotonin
Oxytocin	CCK
TRH	Substance P.

Modulation of Hormone Receptors

Hormones not only bind with specific receptors and produce metabolic effects but also may produce alteration in the number or the sensitivity of the receptors. A hormone may regulate its own receptors in the target tissues or it may regulate receptors of another hormone. For example, exposure to high concentration of insulin decreases the number of insulin receptors on the target cells as well as responsiveness of the receptors to insulin (down regulation). Oestrogens increase the number of receptors for oxytocin in the pregnant uterine musculature (up regulation).

Receptor Diseases

A hormonal deficiency disorder is more often due to the deficiency of the hormone. However, in some disorders like nephrogenic diabetes insipidus or pseudo-hypoparathyroidism, the blood levels of vasopressin or parathormone respectively are normal but the patient suffers from the effects similar to those of hormone deficiency. Administration of the exogenous specific hormone in physiological concentration fails to produce any beneficial effect. Such disorders are believed to be due to deficiency or abnormality of the specific hormone receptors.

Certain diseases like diabetes mellitus (type II) and myasthenia gravis are caused by the presence of circulating antibodies against the receptors for insulin and acetylcholine, respectively.

46 CHAPTER

The Pituitary Gland

Pituitary gland (hypophysis) is the principal endocrine gland for the neuro-endocrine regulation of both metabolism and reproduction. It weighs only 500 mg, but its secretions produce widespread effects all over the body. Pituitary gland is located in the sella turcica of the sphenoid bone and connected to the hypothalamus by the pituitary stalk.

Pituitary gland consists of two different embryologically derived parts. The anterior lobe of the pituitary gland is a glandular structure and hence called **adenohypophysis**. It constitutes about 80% of the gland. The posterior lobe is a neural structure and hence called **neurohypophysis** (Fig. 46.1).

Neurohypophysis consists of the following three 3 portions: (i) the neural lobe, (ii) the pituitary stalk, and (iii) median eminence of the tuber cinereum, a part of hypothalamus.

Developmentally, the adenohypophysis arises from the Rathke's pouch whereas the neurohypophysis is derived from neural tissue in the floor of the third ventricle.

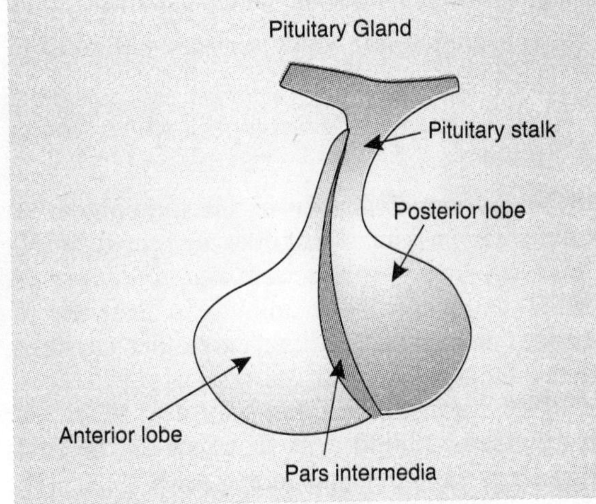

Fig. 46.1: Anatomical divisions of pituitary gland.

ADENOHYPOPHYSIS

The adenohypophysis secretes the following hormones:

1. Growth hormone (GH) accelerates body growth.

2. Thyroid stimulating hormone (TSH, thyrotropin) stimulates thyroid secretions.

3. Adrenocorticotropic hormone (ACTH corticotropin) stimulates adrenocortical secretion.

4. Follicle stimulating hormone (FSH) stimulates ovarian follicle growth in the female and spermatogenesis in the male.

5. Luteinizing hormone (LH) [also known as *interstitial cell stimulating hormone (ICSH) in males*] stimulates ovulation and luteinization of the ovarian follicle in females. In males, it stimulates the secretion of testosterone.

6. Prolactin (mammotropin) stimulates secretion of milk in the mammary gland.

Using ordinary staining techniques, about 40% of the cells in the adenohypophysis are acidophils, 10% are basophils and the rest are agranular chromophobes. The acidophils secrete GH and prolactin. The basophils secrete FSH, LH and TSH. The chromophobes secrete ACTH.

With modern techniques like *immunochemistry* and *electron microscopy*, it is possible to identify five types of cells in the adenohypophysis, namely:

1. **Somatotropes**, which secrete GH.
2. **Corticotropes**, which secrete ACTH.
3. **Thyrotropes**, which secrete TSH.
4. **Gonadotropes**, which secrete FSH and LH (ICSH).
5. **Mammotropes (lactotropes),** which secrete prolactin.

The *intermediate lobe* of the hypophysis is rudimentary in humans and does not secrete MSH. This lobe secretes *melanocyte stimulating hormone* (MSH) in certain lower animals in response to changes in exposure to light and other environmental factors. In humans, the clinical significance of MSH lies in the fact that a form of MSH has exactly same amino acid sequence as the first thirteen of the thirty nine amino acids in ACTH. Hence, ACTH has a weak MSH-like activity. That may be the reason why patients with hypersecretion of ACTH develop hyperpigmentation of the skin (e.g. in Addison's disease), whereas abnormal pallor is a hallmark of hypopituitarism.

REGULATION OF ANTERIOR PITUITARY FUNCTION

Hypothalamic Control

The nervous system receives information about changes in the internal or external environment. Appropriate neural and endocrinal adjustments are made so as to maintain the internal environment within the physiological range. Changes in secretion of hormones in response to threats like exposure to extremes of weather, hypoglycaemia or haemorrhage are some of such examples. Involution of gonads in winter and their regeneration in summer observed in some mammals like ferret (a polar cat), or occurrence of ovulation in response to the presence of a member of the opposite sex in certain birds, are further examples of the neural control of the anterior pituitary function. However, the absence of any direct neural link between the brain and the anterior pituitary gland made it difficult to understand the mechanism of such a control. Subsequently, it was shown that the peculiar blood supply of the anterior pituitary in the form of **hypothalamic-hypophysial portal vessels** was ideally suited for the neural control of the gland.

The superior hypophysial arteries form a capillary plexus in the median eminence of the hypothalamus. The capillaries converge to form long portal vessels which descend along the pituitary stalk and break up into a second set of capillary sinusoids in the adenohypophysis. The blood is finally drained into the veins (Colour Plate 6, Fig. 15; Fig. 46.2). Inferior hypophysial arteries supply blood directly to posterior pituitary gland.

Seven chemical agents called *releasing* and *release-inhibiting hormones (factors)* have been identified in the hypothalamic-hypophysial portal

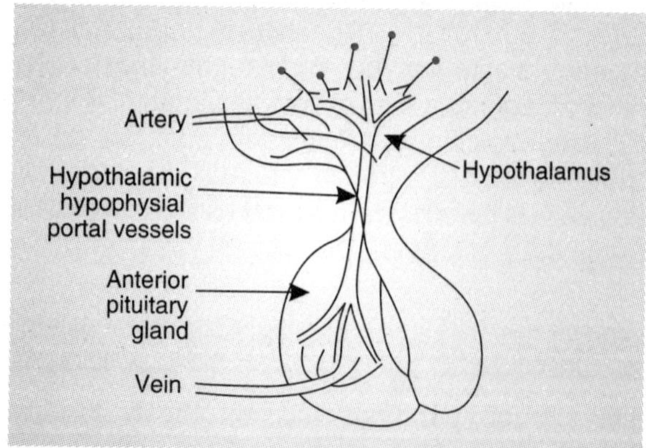

Fig. 46.2: The distribution of hypothalamic hypophyseal portal vessels.

vessels. Each of these factors regulates the secretion of one or more of the cells of the adenohypophysis.

Hypothalamic Hypophysiotropic Hormones

1. Growth hormone-releasing hormone (GRH)
2. Growth hormone-inhibiting hormone (GIH) also called somatostatin.
3. Corticotropin releasing hormone (CRH).
4. Thyrotropin releasing hormone (TRH).
5. Luteinizing hormone-releasing hormone (LHRH) (Gonadotropin releasing hormone, GnRH).
6. Prolactin releasing hormone (PRH).
7. Prolactin inhibiting hormone (PIH).

Besides regulating the secretion of the specific hormone, a hypothalamic hormone may influence the secretion of another anterior pituitary hormone. For example, TRH not only promotes the secretion of TSH but also of prolactin. GnRH promotes the release of both FSH and LH.

The cell bodies of the neurons secreting the hypothalamic hormones named above are situated in various regions of the hypothalamus but their axons terminate in the region of median eminence in close proximity to the capillary loops. In this manner, releasing or inhibiting hormones secreted by the hypothalamus in response to the neural stimuli are able to reach the adenohypophysis and regulate its secretion. Chemically, all the hypothalamic hypophysiotropic hormones have been identified as polypeptides except PIH which is dopamine.

Feedback Control

Experimental surgical removal of the pituitary gland results in atrophy of its target glands (adrenal cortex, thyroid and gonads) whereas administration of anterior pituitary extract causes hypertrophy of these glands. However, prolonged administration of the hormone of a target gland results in atrophy of the gland. For example, hypoplasia of adrenal cortex occurs in patients who have been on long-term corticosteroid therapy. Such observations led to the concept that anterior pituitary and its target glands are coupled in a negative feedback relationship (Fig. 46.3). The anterior pituitary secretes a tropic hormone which promotes the secretion of the target gland. When the plasma concentration of the target gland secretion exceeds a certain critical level, it inhibits the secretion its own tropic hormone by anterior pituitary. The feedback control helps to maintain a constant plasma level of the target gland hormone.

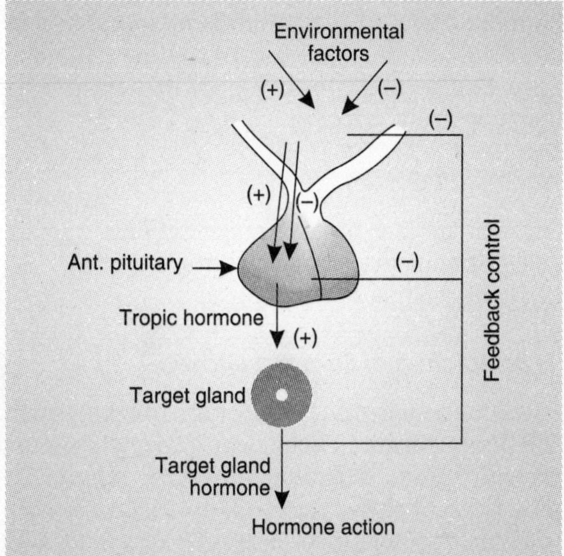

Fig. 46.3: The hypothalamus-anterior pituitary-target gland axis and the negative feedback control of anterior pituitary function.

Long- and Short-loop Control Systems

In the feedback system described above, secretion of a target gland regulates the secretion of the appropriate hypophysial hormone. Such a control system is called **long-loop feedback control**. Cartisol, thyroxin, oestrogen, progesterone and testosterone have a long-loop negative feedback control on the secretion of ACTH, TSH and gonadotropins respectively from the anterior hypophysis.

There are **short-loop control systems** also. In this case, the plasma level of a hypophysial hormone regulates its own secretion. For example, plasma levels of ACTH, TSH, LH, FSH, GH and prolactin have a direct inhibitory effect on their own secretion by the anterior hypophysis.

PHYSIOLOGY OF ANTERIOR PITUITARY HORMONES

Growth Hormone (GH)

This hormone is also known as somatotropic hormone (SH). Human growth hormone is a single polypeptide chain containing 191 amino acids and has a molecular weight of 21,500. Growth hormones obtained from different species show chemical and immunological variations. In man, only human and monkey growth hormone is therapeutically effective.

Actions of GH

Growth hormone has two major actions:

1. Stimulation of somatic growth.
2. Regulation of metabolism.

1. Stimulation of Somatic Growth

Growth hormone has an important role in growth and development. In young experimental animals and children, deficiency of GH results in retardation of physical growth (dwarfism). Timely treatment by administration of exogenous GH results in marked acceleration of growth and restoration of normal body size. Conversely, excessive secretion of GH by an anterior pituitary tumour produces growth acceleration resulting in giantism if it occurs before puberty and acromegaly in adults.

GH promotes acceleration of growth in skeletal and soft tissues. In the long bones, GH promotes chondrogenesis as well as calcification leading to an increase in the body stature. Most of the soft tissues notably skeletal muscles, abdominal and thoracic viscera, skin and connective tissue also participate in growth acceleration in proportion to the skeletal growth.

It was observed that when growth hormone was added to an excised cartilage *in vitro* there was no change in chondrogenesis. However, plasma obtained from an animal treated with growth hormone produced marked chondrogenesis and amono acid incorporation into collagen. This observation led to the concept that GH acts indirectly on the skeletal tissue. GH acts primarily on the liver to produce many types of small proteins (mol wt. 4500 to 7500) collectively called somatomedins. Somatomedins promote skeletal growth (by promoting chondrogenesis) as well as soft tissue growth. Somatomedins are nowadays known as **insulin-like growth factors (IGFs)**.

2. Regulation of Metabolism

Protein Metabolism GH increases the rate of protein synthesis in all the cells of the body. This is achieved by the following mechanisms:

(i) Increasing the rate of amino acid transport into the cells.
(ii) Increased protein synthesis in the ribosomes.
(iii) Increased synthesis of mRNA. In addition, GH decreases the protein breakdown as well as the rate of amino acid degradation for energy purposes.

Fat Metabolism GH causes mobilization of FFA from the adipose tissue resulting in an increase in the plasma FFA level. As a result, FFA becomes the predominant fuel for energy production.

Carbohydrate Metabolism GH decreases the uptake as well as utilization of glucose by the tissues for energy production. It results in an increase in the blood glucose level. Thus, GH has an anti-insulin action. Glycogen stores tend to increase because glycogen is not being utilized for energy production.

Anabolic Effect The anabolic effect of GH is reflected not only by a positive nitrogen balance but also by positive mineral balances. GH increases intestinal absorption of Ca^{2+} and decreases urinary excretion of Ca^{2+}, phosphate, Na^+ and K^+.

Regulation of GH Secretion

It may be assumed that plasma GH level would be very high during childhood and low in adults.

Actually basal fasting plasma GH concentration in adults (1–5 ng/ml) is almost similar to that in childhood. During sleep 2–3, bursts of GH secretion occur, each associated with stage III and IV of NREM sleep. These **nocturnal bursts** during sleep account for nearly 70% of the daily GH secretion. These secretory bursts are greater in childhood and decrease with age.

Hypoglycaemia It is an important stimulant for GH secretion. **Exercise, fasting**, various types of **stress**, and increased plasma concentration of certain amino acids like arginine also increase GH secretion. Most of these stimuli act on the hypothalamus to increase the secretion of growth hormone-releasing hormone (GRH). GRH reaches the anterior pituitary through hypothalamic hypophysial portal vessels.

GH secretion is *decreased* by the hypothalamic secretion of growth hormone-inhibiting hormone (GIH) (somatostatin). *Hyperglycaemia* and *high plasma FFA* concentration are important factors that decrease GH secretion.

Physiological plasma levels of thyroxine and cortisol are required for normal secretion of GH. Oestrogens also facilitate GH release. However, high concentrations of cortisol inhibit GH production. Thyroxine, cortisol and oestrogens influence the secretion of GH by a direct action on the pituitary cells (Table 46.1).

Table 46.1: Factors influencing growth hormone secretion

	Increased secretion	*Decreased secretion*
Metabolic	Hypoglycaemia Fasting Protein-rich meal	Hyperglycaemia High FFA level Obesity
Neurogenic	Deep NREM sleep Exercise Stress	REM sleep
Hormonal	Oestrogens Androgens Glucagon	Hypothyroidism Cushing syndrome

Pathophysiology

Pituitary Dwarfism Deficiency of GH during childhood results in growth retardation involving all parts of the body proportionately. Consequently, a pituitary dwarf has the body structure like that of a normal child of 7–10 years age even though his chronological age may be over 20 years (Fig. 46.4). Majority of such patients do not undergo puberty and sexual maturity since pituitary gonadotropin secretion is also decreased.

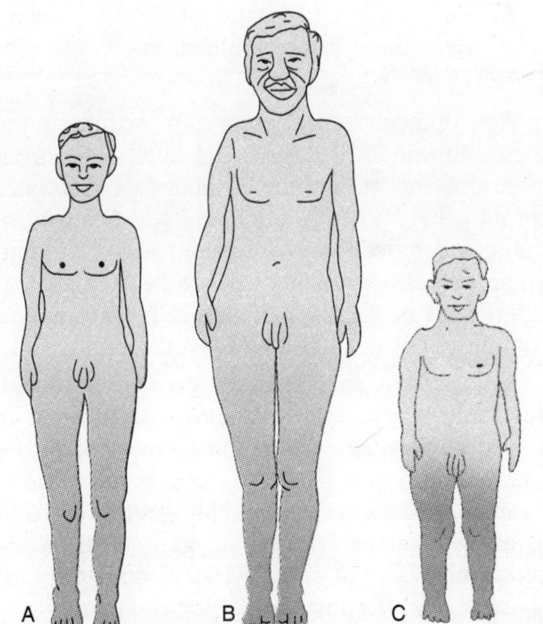

Fig. 46.4: Three individuals aged 25–30 years. (A) Normal adult; (B) A patient of giantism; (C) A patient of pituitary dwarfism.

Giantism and Acromegaly (Fig. 46.4) Acidophil-cell tumours of the anterior pituitary secrete large amounts of GH resulting in giantism if occurring in a child or acromegaly in an adult. In giantism, there is a rapid and excessive but proportionate growth of all parts of the body including long bones. The height of the patient may increase up to 8 or even 9 ft.

In adults, the epiphysial cartilages of long bones are already fused. Hence increased plasma concentration of growth hormone cannot produce increase in the length of long bones. Therefore, increase in the height of the body does not occur. However, small bones of the hands and feet, membranous bones of the face and soft tissues including skin and most of the viscera undergo excessive growth. Very large and thick hands and feet, protruding lower jaw, excessive development of supraorbital ridges and coarse facial features are characteristic features of acromegaly. Metabolic abnormalities including abnormal glucose tolerance can be demonstrated in about 25% of the patients.

Progressive increase in the size of acidophil tumour produces deficiency of other pituitary hormones by pressure on the other pituitary cells. The tumour also presses upon the overlying optic chiasma leading to characteristic visual field defects.

Function Tests

In view of the pulsatile nature of growth hormone secretion, random plasma GH level estimation often does not reflect the 24-hour GH secretion. On the other hand, plasma IGF-1 levels are more stable and reflect overall 24-hour GH secretion. Therefore, as a screening test for the diagnosis of acromegaly or giantism, plasma IGF-1 estimation is preferred over plasma GH level.

46

In a patient suspected of growth hormone deficiency, plasma GH level estimation is worthless because even in normal individuals, its concentration may be 1–5 ng /ml. In such cases, plasma GH level is estimated after administration of a provocative stimulus, e.g. insulin hypoglycaemia. Low plasma GH level during hypoglycaemia is diagnostic of hypopituitarism.

Prolactin

Prolactin is a single chain polypeptide with 198 amino acids (mol wt 22000).

Actions

The primary function of prolactin is stimulation of lactation after child-birth. During pregnancy, in concert with many other hormones, prolactin is involved in the development of the breast. However, in spite of many-fold increase in plasma prolactin concentration, lactation does not occur during pregnancy because of the inhibitory effect of oestrogens or progesterone. Only after parturition, prolactin can produce lactogenesis (when plasma oestrogen and progesterone levels fall).

In males, secretion of prolactin does occur but there seems to be no apparent function of the hormone. Hyperprolactinemia may occur due to presence of an anterior pituitary tumour or intake of certain drugs like reserpine or methyl dopa. In such patients, high plasma prolactin level causes impotence by interfering with the production of testosterone in the Leydig cells or by inhibiting the production of GnRH.

Regulation of Secretion

Normal plasma prolactin concentration is approximately 5 ng/ml in males and 9 ng/ml in females. During pregnancy, plasma prolactin concentration progressively increases and near the end of gestation, it may be 10 times the normal concentration. After parturition, plasma prolactin level falls but increases periodically with each session of suckling. The major regulator of prolactin secretion is the hypothalamic prolactin inhibiting hormone (PIH). Chemically, PIH has been found to be dopamine. Experimental resection of pituitary stalk leads to decreased synthesis of all the anterior pituitary hormones except prolactin whose secretion is increased. Thus, prolactin secretion is normally under the hypothalamic restraint.

Oestrogens increase the proliferation and secretion of lactotropes in the anterior pituitary gland by a direct action. That explains the progressive increase in plasma prolactin level during pregnancy.

Prolactin secretion is increased by suckling or sexual intercourse in the females. Many drugs which interfere with the production or the action of dopamine increase prolactin secretion which may cause impotence in the males and lactorrhoea in females.

High plasma concentration of prolactin inhibits the secretion of FSH and LH by a negative feedback mechanism. Therefore, in lactating mothers, ovarian cycle is suspended resulting in lactational amenorrhoea.

Other anterior pituitary hormones such as TSH, ACTH, FSH and LH are discussed on pages 516, 525, 566 and 577.

NEUROHYPOPHYSIS

Two hormones, namely, **antidiuretic hormone (ADH, vasopressin)** and **oxytocin** are secreted by the posterior pituitary gland. The posterior pituitary gland is also known as pars nervosa or the neurohypophysis. The posterior pituitary gland contains a large number of unmyelinated nerve fibres and modified glial cells called the pituicytes. The nerve fibres belong to the **hypothalamic-hypophysial tract**, whose cell bodies are located in the supraoptic and paraventricular nuclei of the hypothalamus. Their axons descend in the pituitary stalk and terminate in the posterior pituitary gland (Fig. 46.5). The hormones are synthesized in the cell bodies and transported in the axons to be stored in the axon terminals in the posterior pituitary as secretory granules (Herring bodies). In response to an appropriate stimulus, action potentials are generated in the hypothalamic nuclei and conducted down the axons. At the nerve terminals, the action potentials trigger the release of the appropriate hormone, through Ca^{++} dependent exocytosis of secretory granules.

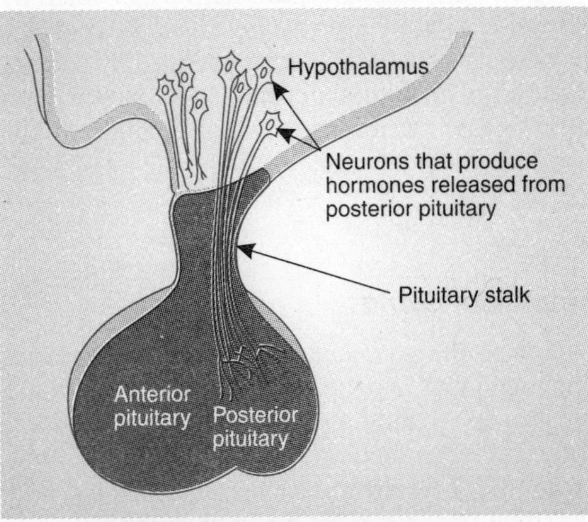

Fig. 46.5: The neurohypophysis.

Both the supraoptic and the paraventricular nuclei synthesize ADH as well as oxytocin. However, supraoptic nucleus predominantly contains ADH–forming neurons whereas paraventricular nucleus contains chiefly the oxytocin synthesizing neurons.

Chemically, both ADH and oxytocin are polypeptides containing nine amino acids each but they differ in the type and the sequence of amino acids. Both the hormones circulate in the blood in free form (unbound to any plasma protein) and have a short half-life (approximately 18 minute).

ANTIDIURETIC HORMONE (VASOPRESSIN) ACTIONS

Decreased Urinary Water Excretion

Kidney is the chief site of action of ADH where it decreases the excretion of free water. Of about 125 ml of glomerular filtrate formed per minute, only about 16 ml of hypotonic fluid (50 mOsm/kg) reach the distal tubule. ADH regulates the amount of water reabsorbed from the collecting ducts. In the absence of ADH, the collecting ducts become impermeable to water. Hence large volumes of urine, up to 16 ml/min with osmolality as low as 50 mOsm/kg may be excreted.

46

ADH acts via V_2 receptors and produces cyclic AMP-mediated opening of aquaporins (cellular water channels) in the epithelial cells of the collecting ducts (Fig. 46.6). Even with moderately high plasma concentrations of ADH, the collecting ducts become freely permeable to water. Consequently water moves along the osmotic gradient from hypotonic luminal fluid to hypertonic medullary interstitium. Thus, a small volume of highly concentrated urine (0.5 ml/min, 1200 mOsm/kg) is excreted. Changes in urinary volume from 0.5 to 16 ml/min are produced in response to changes in plasma ADH concentration from 1–10 picogram/ml.

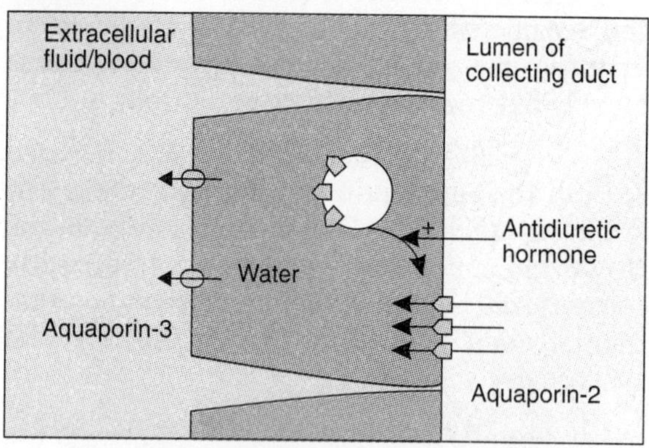

Fig. 46.6: Action of ADH on aquaporins.

Table 46.2: Stimuli influencing the secretion of antidiuretic hormone

Increased secretion	*Decreased secretion*
Increased plasma osmolality	Decreased plasma osmolality
Decreased ECF volume	Increased ECF volume
Standing posture	Alcohol
Pain	
Exercise	
Stress	
Nicotine	
Angiotensin II	
Nausea and vomiting	

Vasopressor Action

ADH also causes contraction of smooth muscle fibres of the blood vessels via V1 receptors, hence the name vasopressin. However, the *plasma concentration of ADH required to produce vasoconstriction is far higher than that for maximum renal water conservation.*

Regulation of Secretion

The secretion of ADH is chiefly regulated by changes in the plasma osmolality. Even 1% increase in plasma osmolality is sufficient to increase the secretion of ADH from the posterior pituitary. The consequent urinary water conservation restores the plasma osmolality to normal. The changes are mediated via osmoreceptors located close to the supraoptic nucleus.

Decreased extracellular fluid volume is another important stimulus for ADH secretion. When hypovolemia is very severe, ADH secretion is increased even in the face of hypotonicity of plasma. A change from recumbent to standing posture is sufficient stimulus for the volume receptors to increase the ADH secretion (due to decrease in central blood pool by approximately 400 ml). Volume receptors are believed to be located in the atria, great veins and the pulmonary circulation.

Pain, exercise, stress and nicotine are also important stimuli for increasing ADH secretion. ADH secretion decreases in response to decreased plasma osmotic pressure, increased ECF volume, or alcohol intake (Table 46.2).

Diabetes Insipidus (DI)

Diabetes insipidus is relatively rare disease produced by lesions of neurohypophysis. It is characterised by excretion of a large volume of dilute urine. About 10 litres of urine with osmolality of approximately 100 mOsm/kg is excreted every day. The polyuria, secondarily, leads to intake of large amount of water (polydipsia). This type of DI is known as **neurogenic (or central) diabetes insipidus.**

Nephrogenic Diabetes Insipidus It is a receptor disorder due to the inability of the kidneys to respond to normal levels of ADH. Clinical picture is similar to that of neurogenic DI.

The two types of DI can be differentiated by administration of a *physiological dose of ADH.* In case of a patient of neurogenic DI, urinary osmolality becomes normal. In a patient with nephrogenic DI, urinary osmolality remains low.

OXYTOCIN

Actions

Mammary Gland

In the *lactating mammary gland*, oxytocin causes contraction of myoepithelial cells which form a meshwork around the alveoli. As a result, milk is forced into the ducts and sinuses opening through the nipple. This phenomenon, called *milk ejection*, is reflexly triggered by suckling of the nipple of the breast by the baby.

Uterus

Oxytocin also causes powerful contraction of the smooth muscle of the *pregnant uterus*. The oxytocin receptors on the myometrium are markedly increased by high concentrations of plasma oestrogen and possibly by uterine distension in the later months of pregnancy. Once labour has started, dilatation of the cervix reflexly produces a marked rise in plasma oxytocin level, leading to more forceful contraction of the uterus and expulsion of the baby.

It has been suggested that oxytocin released during coitus may produce uterine contractions which facilitate the transfer of sperms from the vagina to the fallopian tubes where fertilization normally occurs.

CHAPTER 47

The Thyroid Gland

The human thyroid gland is the largest endocrine gland weighing 10–20 g. It consists of two large lobes joined together by a narrow isthmus wrapped around the upper part of the trachea. It is a highly vascular structure. Its rate of blood flow, 400–600 ml/100 g/min, is higher than even myocardium or kidneys.

Microscopically, the thyroid gland consists of a large number of follicles filled with a proteinaceous fluid known as the colloid (Colour Plate 7, Fig. 16). The wall of each follicle is lined by a single layer of epithelial cells whose shape varies from cuboidal to columnar, depending upon their functional state. The epithelial cells are tallest when the gland is most active. The major constituent of the colloid is thyroglobulin, a glycoprotein (Fig. 47.1).

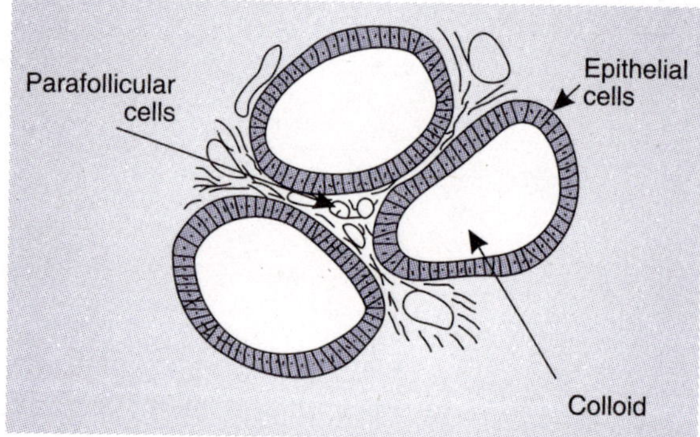

Fig. 47.1: Histological structure of the thyroid gland.

Thyroxine (T_4) and **triiodothyronine (T_3)** are principal thyroid hormones. These are stored in the colloid as components of thyroglobulin. In addition, parafollicular cells present between the follicles of thyroid gland synthesize and secrete another hormone called *calcitonin* (Chapter 50), but this hormone is not included under the term thyroid hormones.

BIOSYNTHESIS OF THYROID HORMONES (Fig. 47.2)

Thyroxine (T_4) and triiodothyronine (T_3) are iodinated derivatives of the amino acid tyrosine. The steps in the synthesis of T_3 and T_4 are briefly described below.

1. Iodide Trapping The first stage in the synthesis of thyroid hormone is the transfer of iodide from extracellular fluid into the follicular epithelial cells of the thyroid gland. The active transport mechanism, called the *iodide pump*, operates at the *basal membrane* of the epithelial cells (Fig. 47.3). By this process, the thyroid gland extracts iodide even when its plasma concentrations are very low. The transport mechanism is stimulated by thyroid stimulating hormone (TSH).

Ordinarily, the ratio of thyroid: plasma iodide concentration is 30. But, it may exceed 100 when the gland is maximally activated by TSH.

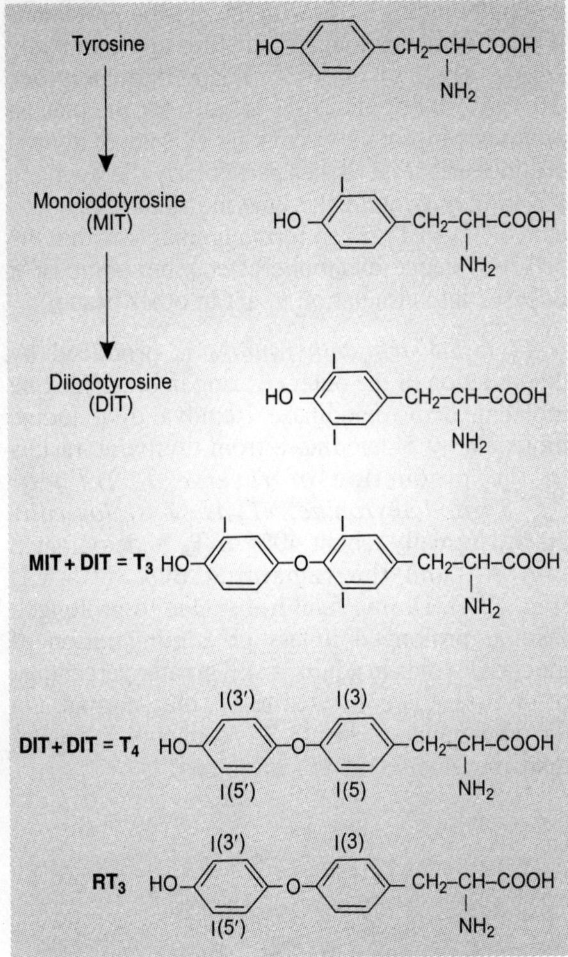

Fig. 47.2: Biosynthesis of thyroid hormones.

Certain other tissues of the body like salivary glands, gastric mucosa and mammary gland have the capacity to concentrate iodide, but T_3 or T_4 is not synthesized in these tissues. Moreover, the iodide uptake is not affected by TSH in these tissues.

2. Synthesis and Secretion of Thyroglobulin The protein portion of thyroglobulin is synthesized in the rough endoplasmic reticulum. In the Golgi apparatus, the carbohydrate moiety is added at the *apical border* of the cell. The secretory vesicles release the glycoprotein into the lumen of the follicle. Thyroglobulin is a large molecule with a molecular weight of 660,000. Each molecule contains 110 tyrosine residues. By iodination of tyrosine, thyroid hormones are formed within thyroglobulin molecule and remain there as storage form.

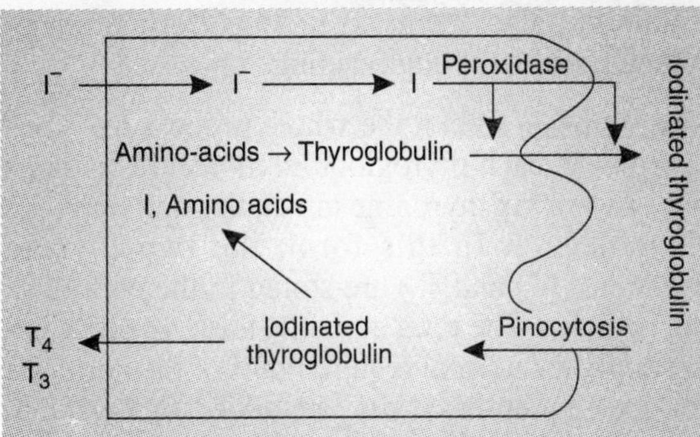

Fig. 47.3: Summary of synthesis, storage and release of thyroid hormones.

3. Oxidation of Iodide The enzyme thyroid peroxidase present near the apical border of the epithelial cell oxidises the iodide molecule to form iodine, which can combine with tyrosine. Hydrogen peroxide is also available at the apical border to accept the electrons.

4. Iodination of Tyrosine (Organification of Thyroglobulin) The binding of iodine with thyroglobulin molecule occurs within the lumen of the follicle or at the apical border of the epithelial cell. An enzyme iodinase required for this purpose is present at the apical border. As soon as thyroglobulin molecule is released by the secretory vesicles, within seconds about 1/6th of tyrosine residues present in it are iodinated. The initial product of iodination seems to be *monoiodotyrosine (MIT)*. Addition of another iodine molecule to MIT results in formation of *diiodotyrosine (DIT)*.

5. Coupling Reaction During the next few minutes or hours, two molecules of DIT gradually couple up to form a molecule of 3, 5, 3′, 5′ *tetra-iodothyronine or thyroxine (T_4)*.

One molecule of MIT may couple with a molecule of DIT to form *triiodothyronine (T_3)*. The enzyme thyroid-peroxidase not only oxidises iodide but also seems to produce iodination of tyrosine and coupling reaction.

6. Storage When the whole process has been completed, each thyroglobulin molecule contains only five or six thyroxine molecules and only one T_3 molecule. In this form, the two thyroid hormones (T_4 and T_3) are stored in the colloid of the follicles. The total amount stored is sufficient to supply the normal requirements of the hormone for 1 to 3 months. It may be added that a much larger number of tyrosine residues in the thyroglobulin molecule remain as MIT and DIT.

HORMONE SECRETION

For secretion of thyroid hormone, small droplets of colloid are taken up at the apical border of the epithelial cells, by the process of pinocytosis. The droplets fuse with the lysosome vesicles containing proteolytic enzymes. Proteinases digest the thyroglobulin molecule, releasing thyroxine (T_4) and T_3 into the cytoplasm of the epithelial cells, from where they diffuse through the basal border into the blood capillaries (Fig. 47.3). Proteolysis of colloidal droplets also releases large amounts of MIT and DIT and other amino acid constituents of the thyroglobulin molecule. An enzyme deiodinase removes iodine from MIT and DIT. Both the iodine and tyrosine are recycled into new thyroglobulin by the steps mentioned above.

It is interesting to note that the synthesis, and iodination of thyroglobulin, as well as, its digestion to release thyroid hormones, occur simultaneously in the follicular epithelial cells of the thyroid gland.

TRANSPORT AND METABOLISM

Normal plasma T_4 and T_3 levels are approximately 8 µg% and 0.15 µg%, respectively. Both are bound to plasma proteins, chiefly thyroxine-binding globulin (TBG), and to a lesser extent thyroxine-binding prealbumin (TBA). Only a small fraction of T_3 and T_4 circulates in the free form and this is the metabolically active form of the hormone. Binding of the hormone with plasma proteins serves to prevent renal losses of the hormone. It also constitutes a reservoir for the supply of free hormone.

Tight binding of T_4 with the plasma proteins is shown by its prolonged half-life, approximately 7 days. The half-life of T_3 is approximately one day only, due to its lesser affinity for the plasma proteins. Most of the circulating T_3 is not of thyroid origin. Peripheral tissues particularly the liver and the kidney contain the enzyme *deiodinase* and convert T_4 to T_3. T_3 so formed remains within the cell to produce metabolic effects but some of it diffuses into circulation to act in other tissues.

T_3 (3,5,3′-triiodothyronine) is produced by deiodination of the outer (B) ring in the thyroxine molecule by 5′-deiodinase. Removal of an iodine molecule by 5-deiodinase from thyroxine results in the production of *reverse T_3 (rT_3) or 3,3′,5′triiodothyronine. rT_3 is physiologically inert*. Normally, about 40% of T_4 is deiodinated into T_3, and the remaining 60% into rT_3 (Fig. 47.4). During fetal life or due to prolonged fasting, prolonged illness or administration of glucocorticoids in adults, a still greater percentage of thyroxine is converted to rT_3 than normal. On the other hand, in obesity, T_3 production is greater than the amount of rT_3 produced.

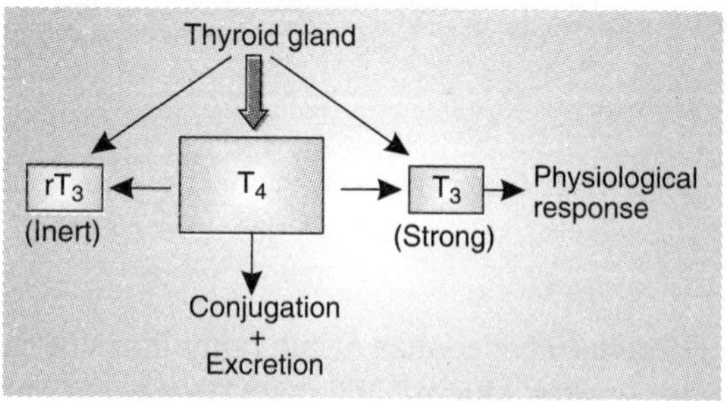

Fig. 47.4: T_4 metabolism.

Thyroxine and T_3 are also inactivated by conjugation with glucuronic acid or sulphuric acid in the liver followed by excretion of the metabolites in the bile.

ACTIONS OF THYROID HORMONE

Before discussing the detailed actions of the thyroid hormones, it would be pertinent to observe some general features of their actions. Firstly, thyroid hormones do not have any discrete target organs. Their actions manifest in almost all the organs of the body. Second important feature is the long delay in the onset of actions and a prolonged duration of their actions. After injection of a large dose of thyroxine in a hypothyroid patient, the basal metabolic rate begins to rise after an interval of 3–4 days, reaches its peak in 10–12 days and some effect can be observed up to 6–8 weeks. T_3 acts about four-times more rapidly than T_4. T_3 is also about four-times more potent than T_4. The following actions pertain to both T_3 and T_4.

1. Growth and Development Thyroxine is necessary for normal growth and development. *Congenital deficiency* of thyroxine results in growth retardation. Long bones remain infantile due to delayed appearance of the epiphyseal centres. Hence "bone age" lags behind the chronological age. Bones of the skull are particularly affected by thyroxine deficiency. Eruption of teeth is also delayed.

In cell cultures, T_3 stimulates proliferation of several types of cells indicating its direct growth promoting role. In addition, T_3 is required for the normal production of growth hormone and somatomedins.

T_3 seems to be necessary for proper axonal and dendritic development as well as normal myelination in the nervous system. That is the reason why mental retardation is a striking feature in a child with congenital hypothyroidism (a cretin). In such patients, the disorder must be detected at the earliest and replacement hormonal therapy started, otherwise the mental retardation becomes irreversible.

Absence of the metamorphosis of tadpoles into baby frogs after experimental removal of thyroid glands in the former is a dramatic evidence of the role of thyroxine in growth and maturation.

2. Metabolic Rate Thyroid hormone stimulates the basal metabolic rate, oxygen consumption and heat production in most of the tissues except adult brain, testis and uterus. Many of the actions of thyroxine to be described below can primarily be attributed to the calorigenic action. The magnitude of calorigenic action of thyroxine partly depends on the level of circulating catecholamines. Due to increased metabolic rate, thyroxine increases utilization of many hormones, vitamins and certain drugs. Therefore, patients with hyperthyroidism require a larger vitamin intake. On the other hand, patients with hypothyroidism may show toxic effects at usual doses of certain drugs.

3. Nervous System Besides its role during neonatal development of the nervous system, thyroxine seems to be required for the normal functioning of nervous tissue in adults. Impairment of memory, somnolence, and slowness of speech are characteristic features of hypothyroid adults. Hyperthyroid state results in hyperexcitability, irritability, restlessness and insomnia. Reaction time of stretch reflexes (e.g. ankle jerk) is prolonged in hypothyroidism and shortened in hyperthyroidism.

Thyroid hormones increase the number of ß-adrenergic receptors and hence potentiate the biological activity of circulating catecholamines.

4. Cardiovascular System In hyperthyroidism, increased body metabolism results in tachycardia (at rest, even during *sleep*) and increased cardiac output. There is generalized vasodilatation. Cutaneous vasodilatation is a particularly prominent feature, which helps in dissipation of excessive heat produced by increased metabolic rate. As a result of these factors, systolic blood pressure is increased whereas diastolic BP is decreased, leading to wide pulse pressure but normal mean blood pressure. These cardiovascular effects are produced by thyroxine partly by a direct action on the cardiac muscle and partly by potentiation of ß-adrenergic activity.

5. Carbohydrate Metabolism Thyroid hormones increase the rate of absorption of carbohydrates from the intestine. In addition, they seem to accelerate almost all aspects of glucose metabolism, i.e. rapid uptake of glucose by the cells, enhanced glycolysis, enhanced gluconeogenesis and increased insulin secretion.

6. Fat Metabolism Thyroid hormones cause mobilization of fat from the adipose tissue leading to increased plasma FFA concentration. Thus, thyroid hormones promote utilization of FFA for energy production. Plasma cholesterol level is lowered due to of greater degradation of cholesterol.

7. Protein Metabolism Physiological amounts of thyroid hormones have *anabolic effect*. Administration of thyroxine to a hypothyroid animal results in increased hepatic RNA synthesis, increased protein synthesis as well as decreased nitrogen losses in the urine and faeces. Excessive doses of thyroxine, however, produce greater protein *catabolism* as well as negative nitrogen balance. Muscle weakness and creatinuria are characteristic features of a hyperthyroid patient.

Deposition of a mucoprotein in the subcutaneous tissue and extracellular spaces is a prominent abnormality in hypothyroid patients. The abnormality is known as myxoedema.

8. GI Tract Thyroid hormones increase the rate of secretion of gastrointestinal juices as well as the rate of absorption of food stuffs in the intestine. Gastrointestinal motility is also increased. Diarrhoea is a common feature in patients with hyperthyroidism and constipation in patients with hypothyroid states.

9. Reproduction In females, the normal rhythmicity of ovarian cycles or normal lactation can occur only in the presence of normal circulating levels of thyroxine.

10. Relation to Catecholamines Many effects of catecholamines (e.g. on CNS, CVS and BMR) are similar to those of thyroxine. In general, thyroxine sensitizes the tissues to the effects of catecholamines.

11. Erythropoiesis Thyroxine is necessary for normal erythropoiesis. In hypothyroidism, mild anaemia is commonly observed. The haemoglobin level is elevated only on administration of thyroid hormone.

12. Vitamin Metabolism Thyroxine is essential for conversion of carotene to vitamin A. In hypothyroidism, this reaction is very slow and carotene accumulation in the blood and tissues (carotenemia) gives a yellow colour to the skin. Carotenemia can be clinically differentiated from jaundice by the fact that sclerae of the eyeballs are not affected in the former condition.

13. Lactation Thyroxine stimulates secretion of milk.

Mechanism of Action

No single mechanism of action can explain all the effects of thyroid hormones. Basically, they act through genes (transcription and translation effect). As the thyroid hormones enter the cell, T_4 is converted into T_3 in the cytoplasm of the target cell. T_3 diffuses into the nucleus and binds with the receptor proteins on the chromatin. As a result, the synthesis of mRNA is increased. This ultimately results in greater protein (enzyme) synthesis in the ribosomes .This mechanism can explain the anabolic action and other metabolic actions of thyroxine.

The calorigenic action of thyroxine seems to be due to increased synthesis of the enzyme Na^+-K^+ ATPase in many tissues. Increased metabolic rate has been attributed to increased energy consumption associated with increased Na^+ transport. Thyroxine also increases mitochondrial protein synthesis but this may be secondary to increased calorigenesis.

The mechanisms of action described above cannot explain many other actions of thyroxine, e.g. growth and maturation, metamorphosis at normal blood levels and catabolic action with excessive blood levels of the hormone.

Regulation of Secretion

The characteristic hypothalamus-anterior pituitary-thyroid gland axis along with negative feedback regulation maintains physiological levels of thyroid hormone in the blood (Fig. 47.5). In physiological conditions, unlike other hormones, marked variations in plasma level of T_4 and T_3 do not occur.

Role of Thyroid Stimulating Hormone (TSH)

Thyroid stimulating hormone, also called thyrotropin, is a glycoprotein with molecular weight of 28,000. It is secreted by thyrotropes (basophils) of the anterior pituitary. This hormone

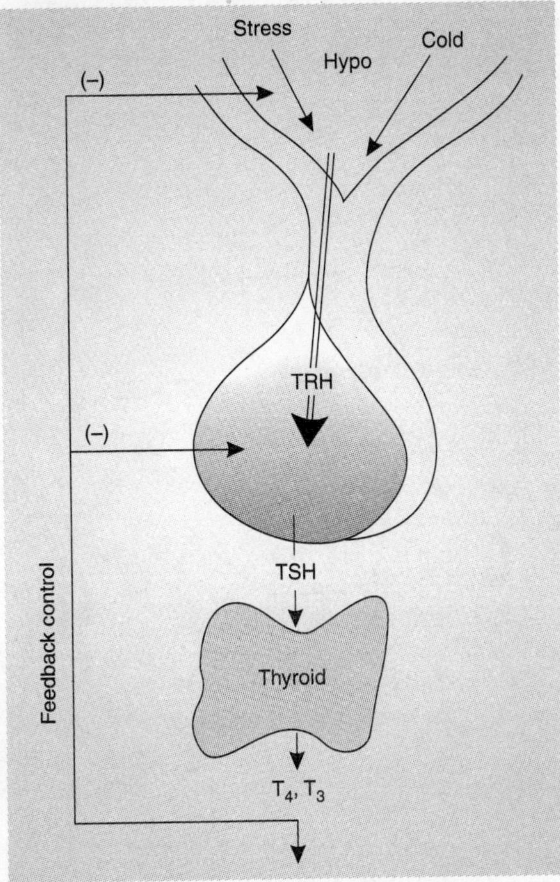

Fig. 47.5: The hypothalamus-anterior pituitary-thyroid gland axis. Hypo-hypothalamus.

increases the secretion of thyroid hormones by accelerating all the steps in the biosynthesis and release. TSH increases the rates of: (i) Iodide trapping, (ii) Synthesis of thyroglobulin, (iii) Organification of thyroglobulin, (iv) Coupling reaction, and (v) Proteolysis of thyroglobulin leading to increased secretion of T_3 and T_4. TSH also increases the number (hyperplasia) and the size (hypertrophy) of the follicular epithelial cells. All these effects of TSH on the epithelial cells are produced by cAMP mechanism. It also increases the vascularity of thyroid gland.

Role of Hypothalamus

Thyrotropin releasing hormone (TRH) is a polypeptide released by the hypothalamus. It reaches the anterior pituitary through the hypothalamic-hypophysial portal vessels and increases the release of TSH.

The negative feedback control of thyroid hormones operates both at the anterior pituitary as well as hypothalamic levels. In addition, hypothalamus may regulate the secretion of thyroid gland in response to some specific stimuli like emotional stress or exposure to cold. Increased secretion of TSH and thyroid hormones in response to cold has been demonstrated in infants. In human adults, the effect of cold on thyroid function occurs only after prolonged exposure. Plasma T_4 levels are slightly higher in winter than in summer.

PATHOPHYSIOLOGY OF THYROID HORMONE

Hyperthyroidism (Grave's Disease)

This clinical disorder is due to over-activity of thyroid gland leading to excessive secretion of thyroid hormones. Increased BMR, tachycardia (*even during sleep*), heat intolerance, excessive sweating, loss of weight in spite of increased appetite, diarrhoea, muscular weakness, nervousness and insomnia are some of the characteristic features of hyperthyroidism. Some patients develop protrusion of eyeballs due to oedematous swelling of retrobulbar tissue (exophthalmos) (Fig. 47.6).

Hyperthyroidism is believed to be an autoimmune disorder due to the presence of antibodies which bind with and stimulate the thyroid epithelial cells to secrete excessive thyroxine. The antibodies are known as *long-acting thyroid stimulator (LATS)* or *TSH receptor stimulating antibodies.*

47

Contrary to the earlier belief, hyperthyroidism is not due to excessive secretion of TSH by the anterior pituitary. Actually, plasma TSH level in hyperthyroidism is near zero because of negative feedback effect of increased levels of thyroxine.

In the medical (i.e. non-surgical) treatment of hyperthyroidism, antithyroid drugs are frequently used. These drugs decrease the secretion of thyroid hormones by blocking one or more steps in their biosynthesis. Monovalent anions, like perchlorate, inhibit iodide trapping by competitive blockade. Thiocarbamide inhibits organification of tyrosine.

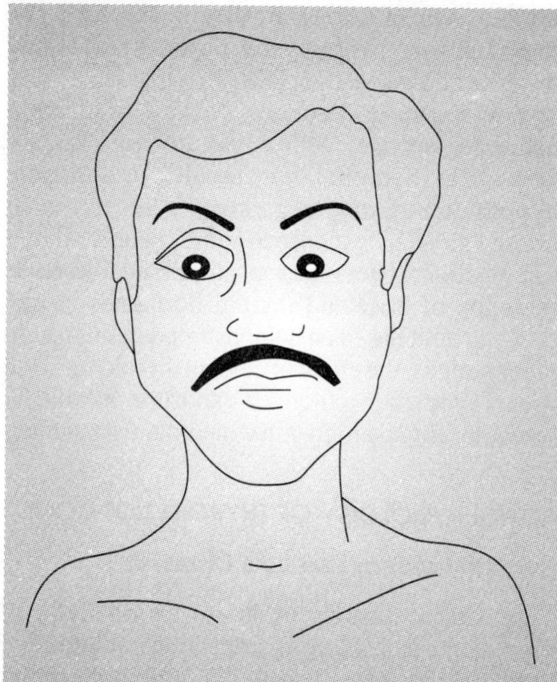

Fig. 47.6: A patient with hyperthyroidism showing exophthalmos.

Hypothyroidism

Decreased secretion of thyroxine may lead to one of the following clinical conditions.

Myxoedema

This condition is produced by severe hypothyroidism in adults. It is characterized by low BMR, slow heart rate, increased body weight, cold intolerance, mental sluggishness, constipation, decreased appetite, somnolence and muscular weakness. Accumulation of myxomatous gel in the subcutaneous tissue produces the characteristic puffiness of the face (Fig. 47.7). The skin is dry (due to absence of sweating) and yellowish (due to accumulation of carotene). The voice is husky and slow. Plasma cholesterol is elevated.

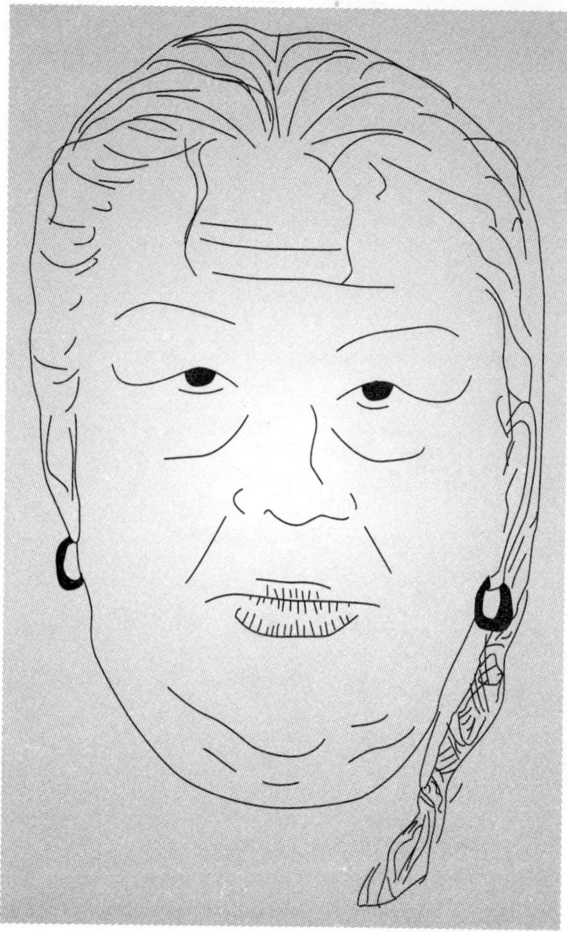

Fig. 47.7: A patient of myxodema.

Cretinism

This disorder results from congenital deficiency of thyroxine. The growth retardation in cretinism is characterized by retardation of physical and mental growth, potbelly and protuding tongue (Fig. 47.8). The most common cause of cretinism is maternal iodine deficiency. By the time the typical clinical picture develops in the infant, it is usually too late to reverse the mental retardation. Realization of this fact has led to wide-spread use of iodized salt.

Iodine-deficiency Goitre

Dietry intake of at least 100–150 μg of iodide per day is required for normal thyroid function.

Inadequate thyroid secretion occurs when iodide intake falls below 10 μg/day. Due to negative feedback mechanism, the secretion of TSH from the anterior pituitary is increased leading to hypertrophy of the thyroid gland. The

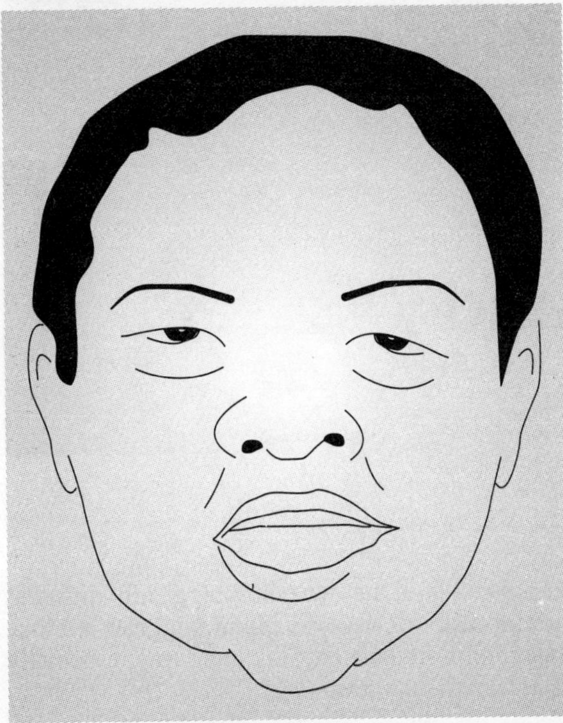

Fig. 47.8: A cretin.

enlarged hypertrophied thyroid gland so produced is known as iodine-deficiency goitre.

Goitrogens in Food

Excessive consumption of certain vegetables may produce enlargement of thyroid gland (goitre). Cabbage and turnips contain thiocyanates and certain other chemical agents with antithyroid activity called goitrogens. Consumption of these vegetables in usual amounts is not harmful. However, excessive intake of these vegetables, especially in areas with borderline iodine deficiency may result in goitre (cabbage goitre).

THYROID FUNCTION TESTS

1. Plasma T_3 and T_4 concentrations can be estimated by radioimmunoassay.

2. Plasma TSH estimation if available is also valuable. In hyperthyroidism, plasma T_3 and T_4 levels are elevated, whereas TSH is undetectable in the plasma. In hypothyroidism, plasma T_3, T_4 levels are low and plasma TSH level is elevated.

3. In hypothyroidism, ECG is also of diagnostic value (sinus bradycardia and low voltage QRS).

4. Estimation of protein bound iodine (PBI) or basal metabolic rate is now seldom used for the assessment of thyroid function. Normal plasma PBI level is 6 μg/100 ml. It reflects the level of circulating T_3 and T_4 bound to plasma proteins. Theoretically, BMR is the most physiological test of thyroid function, since it measures the tissue response (oxygen consumption). However, the value of BMR as a test of thyroid function is compromised by poor sensitivity, since it is influenced by many extraneous and uncontrollable variables.

CHAPTER 48

The Adrenal Gland

The adrenal glands are situated in the abdominal cavity, closely applied to the upper pole of each kidney. Each gland consists of an outer cortex of mesodermal origin and inner medulla of ectodermal origin. The adrenal cortex secretes a number of lipid-soluble steroid hormones, collectively called corticosteroids, whereas the medulla secretes a number of water-soluble hormones collectively known as catecholamines.

Histologically, the medulla consists of interlacing cords of densely innervated granule-containing cells which surround large venous sinusoids.

In the adrenal cortex, the cells are rich in lipids. Three distinct histological zones can be delineated (Colour Plate 7, Fig. 17). The outermost, (subcapsular) zona glomerulosa secretes mineralocorticoids. The next, zona fasciculata secretes glucocorticoids and the innermost, zona of recticularis secretes androgens.

Blood Supply

The blood is supplied to the adrenal gland by several small arteries which form a plexus in the capsule. From this capillary plexus, blood flows centripetally through fenestrated capillaries to zona glomerulosa, zona fasciculata, zona recticularis and finally into medulla to be drained by a single large vein on either side. The anatomical arrangement of the two embryologically different components of adrenal gland suggests a close integration in their physiological role, especially in adaptation to stress.

ADRENAL CORTEX

Corticosteroids may be classified into: *(i) glucocorticoids, (ii) mineralocorticoids and (iii) androgens.* Cortisol and corticosterone are the chief natural glucocorticoids. They are so called because of their widespread effect on glucose (and protein) metabolism. Aldosterone is the chief mineralocorticoid. It regulates sodium balance and ECF volume in the body. Dehydroepiandrosterone is the androgenic hormone secreted by the adrenal cortex.

Biosynthesis of Adrenal Cortical Hormones

All the corticosteroids are synthesized from cholesterol present in the adrenal cortical cells as cytoplasmic lipid droplets. The biochemical pathways involved in the biosynthesis of glucocorticoids are shown in Fig. 48.1, mineralocorticoids in Fig. 48.4 and adrenal androgens in Fig. 48.8.

Transport and Metabolism

Cortisol circulates in the blood mostly bound to an alpha-globulin known as *transcortin* or corticosteroid-binding globulin (CBG).

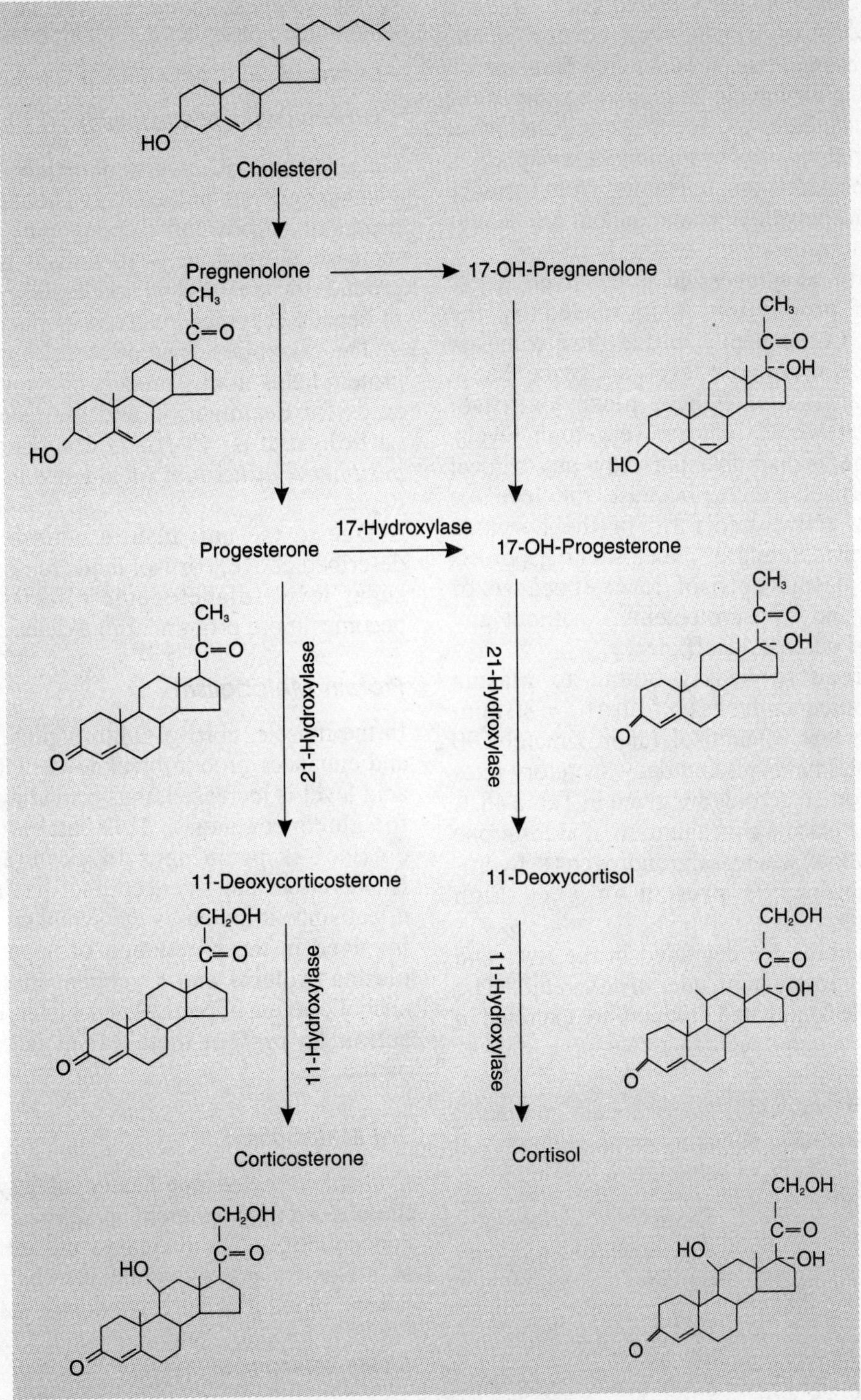

Fig. 48.1: Biosynthesis of glucocorticoids.

48

Corticosterone is similarly bound but to a lesser degree. Less than 10% of total cortisol in the plasma is in free form. It is the free form which is responsible for the physiological actions of the hormone including the feedback regulation of ACTH secretion. Protein binding in the plasma, not only protects the hormone from urinary excretion and hepatic degradation, but also serves as a circulating reservoir of the hormone.

Transcortin is synthesized in the liver, where its rate of production is increased by the oestrogens. Consequently, in the third trimester of pregnancy, transcortin levels are twice that in non-pregnant state. Hence, plasma cortisol measurement would indicate very high levels. Actually, the woman does not show any clinical sign of cortisol excess, because the level of biologically active free form of the hormone remains normal. Similarly, patients with nephrosis have low plasma cortisol level (because of proteinuria and hypoproteinemia) without any symptom of adrenal insufficiency.

Aldosterone is weakly bound to plasma proteins. Consequently, its half-life ($t_{1/2} = 30$ min) is less than that of cortisol (approximately 90 min). The plasma levels and daily secretory rates of adrenal corticosteroids are given in Table 48.1. Note that the plasma concentration of aldosterone is extremely low, whereas the androgen (dehydroepiandrosterone) is present in very high concentration.

Corticosteroids are degraded in the liver and conjugated mostly with glucuronic acid. The water-soluble conjugated products are excreted in the urine.

Table 48.1: Average plasma levels (morning values) and daily secretory rates of adrenal cortical hormones

Hormone	*Plasma concentration (μg/dl)*	*Daily secretion (mg)*
Cortisol	14.0	10
Corticosterone	0.4	3
Aldosterone	0.006	0.15
Dehydroepiandrosterone	175.0	20.0

GLUCOCORTICOIDS

Actions of Glucocorticoids

Carbohydrate Metabolism

Cortisol and other glucocorticoids stimulate *gluconeogenesis* in the liver. The rate of glucose production from non-carbohydrate sources may increase as much as 6–10 folds. Corticosteroids produce these effects by accelerating the synthesis of hepatic enzymes involved in gluconeogenesis.

The catabolic action of cortisol on the muscle protein helps in this process by providing amino acids for deamination and their conversion to carbohydrates. Cortisol also decreases the *peripheral utilization* of glucose to a moderate degree.

Due to the anti-insulin actions of cortisol described above, cortisol tends to raise the blood sugar level (diabetogenic effect). The effect becomes more prominent in a diabetic patient.

Protein Metabolism

In the muscle, cortisol inhibits protein synthesis and enhances protein breakdown. Plasma amino acid level is increased, thus providing a substrate for gluconeogenesis. This catabolic action of cortisol is prominent in skeletal muscles. However, in the liver, cortisol has an anabolic effect since it increases the synthesis of enzymes involved in the production of hepatic proteins, plasma proteins and glycogen. In spite of this anabolic action of cortisol in the liver, its dominant action on protein metabolism is catabolic in nature.

Fat Metabolism

Cortisol promotes mobilization of fatty acids from the adipose tissue, thereby increasing plasma FFA concentration. The increased utilization of FFA as a fuel for energy production helps in maintaining blood glucose level during starvation.

Stress Tolerance

A wide variety of non-specific stimuli increase the secretion of cortisol by the adrenal cortex.

These stimuli may vary from merely restraining an animal from making any movement to trauma, blood loss, surgery, infections, burns and exposure to intense heat or cold. These stimuli act on the hypothalamus and cause release of ACTH from the anterior pituitary. Within minutes, the plasma cortisol level may increase as much as 20-fold.

The increased plasma cortisol level during stress has a definite protective role. Adrenalectomized animals maintained on a fixed dose of glucocorticoids die when exposed to any type of stress mentioned above. However, they survive the stress if high doses of glucocorticoids are simultaneously administered. Similarly, patients with adrenal insufficiency (Addison's disease) have poor tolerance to stress. In such patients, even moderately prolonged fasting may result in fatal hypoglycemia. Such patients cannot tolerate any infection or haemorrhage. However, the exact mechanism by which glucocorticoids protect the body during stress is not yet clear.

Vascular Reactivity

In patients with deficiency of glucocorticoids, the vascular smooth muscle lose their normal responsiveness to epinephrine and norepinephrine. Blood vessels fail to undergo the expected vasoconstrictor response to hypovolemia. Hypovolemic shock is one of the important manifestations of Addison's disease.

Permissive Action

Normal circulating levels of cortisol are essential for the metabolic effects of many other hormones, even though cortisol does not directly produce these responses. Such action is known as permissive action of cortisol. Calorigenic, lipolytic, vasopressor and bronchodilator effects of catecholamines depend on the permissive actions of cortisol.

Effect on Water Metabolism

The normal response of the body to a water load (say ingestion of 1–1.5 litre of water) is increased urinary outflow (diuresis). All the water load is excreted within 3–4 hours. Patients with adrenal insufficiency have an inability to excrete the water load. The defect disappears after administration of a glucocorticoid. Low glomerular filtration rate (GFR) observed in patients with adrenal insufficiency can only partly explain the abnormalities in water metabolism.

Glucocorticoids have a very mild sodium-retaining action also. This action becomes clinically significant in patients with excessive secretion of cortisol (Cushing's disease), in whom marked degree of water and Na^+ retention occurs.

Effect on Blood Cells and Lymphatic Organs

Cortisol decreases the number of circulating eosinophils and basophils. In the lymphatic tissues, cortisol inhibits the proliferation of lymphocytes leading to decreased size of lymph nodes and thymus as well as decreased blood lymphocyte count. It increases red cell and neutrophil counts.

Central Nervous System

Cortisol receptors have been reported in various parts of CNS, especially in the limbic system. Personality changes (irritability, apprehension, inability to concentrate), increased sensitivity to olfactory and gustatory stimuli and EEG waves slower than α-rhythm can be observed in Addison's disease. These changes can be reversed only by administration of glucocorticoids. Euphoria (an unreal feeling of well-being) and insomnia are seen in patients with glucocorticoid excess.

Role in Fetal Life

Cortisol facilitates *in utero* maturation of CNS, retina, skin, gastrointestinal tract and especially the lungs. In the last week of gestation, cortisol increases the activity of key enzymes involved in the biosynthesis of pulmonary surfactant. This substance lowers the surface tension in pulmonary alveoli and thus permits proper inflation of lungs immediately after birth.

In fetal life, maternal glucose is transferred to the fetus through the placenta. In the late fetal life, digestive enzyme capacity of the intestinal mucosa changes from fetal pattern to postnatal pattern under the influence of cortisol. This change allows the newborn to digest disaccharides present in the milk.

Anti-inflammatory and Anti-allergic Actions

Anti-inflammatory and anti-allergic effects have been called the **pharmacologic actions of glucocorticoids,** since they are observed only when large doses of glucocorticoids are administered therapeutically. These two actions are not observed at normal physiological plasma levels of the hormone.

Glucocorticoids inhibit all the aspects of inflammatory response in the body. Glucocorticoids inhibit migration of polymorphonuclear leucocytes, monocyte-macrophages and lymphocytes at the site of inflammation. They also inhibit the release of vasoactive and proteolytic enzymes as well as growth of fibroblasts in the area of inflammation. All these effects seem to be produced by decreased formation of prostaglandins and leukotrienes, the two mediators of inflammation. Due to these actions, glucocorticoids have been extensively used in the treatment of autoimmune diseases like rheumatic heart disease, rheumatoid arthritis and acute glomerulonephritis.

48

Certain types of antigen-antibody reactions provoke the release of histamine from the mast cells present in various tissues like skin and lungs, resulting in the symptoms of allergy. Glucocorticoids do not prevent the antigen-antibody reaction but prevent the release of histamine. In this way, glucocorticoids help in the treatment of allergic states like asthma and life-threatening conditions of anaphylactic shock.

Undesirable (Side) Effects

Pharmacologic doses of glucocorticoids may have to be administered for several months, e.g. for treatment of rheumatoid arthritis. In such patients, many undesirable side effects of glucocorticoid therapy may be observed. Most of these complications are also present in patients of Cushing syndrome.

(a) Peptic Ulcer Cortisol damages the gastric mucosal barrier chiefly by decreasing the proliferation of gastric mucosal cells. Hence, such patients are predisposed to develop peptic ulcer.

(b) Osteoporosis Prolonged administration of glucocorticoids leads to osteoporosis by a number of mechanisms, which include increased bone resorption and inhibition of cellular proliferation and collagen synthesis in the bone. Glucocorticoids also decrease intestinal absorption of calcium and phosphate by an anti-vitamin D action.

(c) Growth Retardation Due to protein catabolic action, prolonged administration of glucocorticoids in children may inhibit somatic growth.

(d) Delayed Wound Healing It is due to excessive protein catabolism.

(e) Muscle Atrophy This results from excessive protein catabolism.

(f) Mental Symptoms Euphoria (an unreal feeling of well-being), insomnia and excessive appetite may occur.

(g) Susceptibility to Bacterial Infections Normally, bacterial infections produce inflammatory response in the involved tissue as well as systemic effects like fever, toxaemia and immunological response. If a patient on prolonged glucocorticoid therapy develops some bacterial infection, the protective inflammatory and immunological responses are suppressed. Consequently, the infection tends to spread quickly all over the body. Till it is too late, the patient may not even be aware of the gravity of situation since systemic effects of inflammation like fever and toxaemia are also absent.

(h) Adrenal Cortical Hypoplasia By negative feedback action, pharmacologic doses of glucocorticoids suppress ACTH secretion by anterior pituitary gland, leading to hypoplasia of adrenal cortex. The clinical implication of this action is given below (see feedback control).

Mechanism of Action of Glucocorticoids

Like other steroid hormones, glucocorticoids combine with the cytoplasmic receptors and thereby alter the protein-synthesizing machinery of the target cells through transcription and translation effects. Altered synthesis of different enzymes in different tissues produces the multiple effects.

Regulation of Secretion of Glucocorticoids

Anterior Pituitary Control

The secretion of glucocorticoids by the adrenal cortex is regulated by anterior pituitary gland through adrenocorticotropic hormone (ACTH).

ACTH or corticotropin is a single polypeptide chain containing 39 amino acids. Within minutes of its injection, the secretion of glucocorticoids by adrenal cortex increases. The secretion of adrenal androgens and aldosterone also increases but to a minor extent. ACTH is required not only for *regulation of secretion* of glucocorticoids but also for the *maintenance of normal morphology* of adrenal cortex. Experimental hypophysectomy results in atrophy of zona fasciculata and zona reticularis of adrenal cortex, sparing zona glomerulosa. Conversely, injection of large doses of ACTH produces hypertrophy of adrenal cortex. ACTH increases the secretion of glucocorticoids by cAMP mechanism.

Hypothalamic Control—Circadian Rhythm

The secretion of ACTH and consequently that of cortisol follows a circadian rhythm. ACTH secretion is minimum during night and maximum early in the morning (6–8 am). The biological clock responsible for the diurnal ACTH rhythm is located in the suprachiasmatic nucleus of the hypothalamus (Fig. 48.2).

Response to Stress Various types of physical or mental stressful stimuli promptly increase the secretion of ACTH. Within minutes, cortisol secretion may increase as much as 20-fold. All such stimuli primarily act on the hypothalamus and increase the secretion of corticotropin releasing hormone (CRH). CRH reaches the anterior pituitary through hypothalamic-hypophyseal portal system and acts by cAMP mechanism.

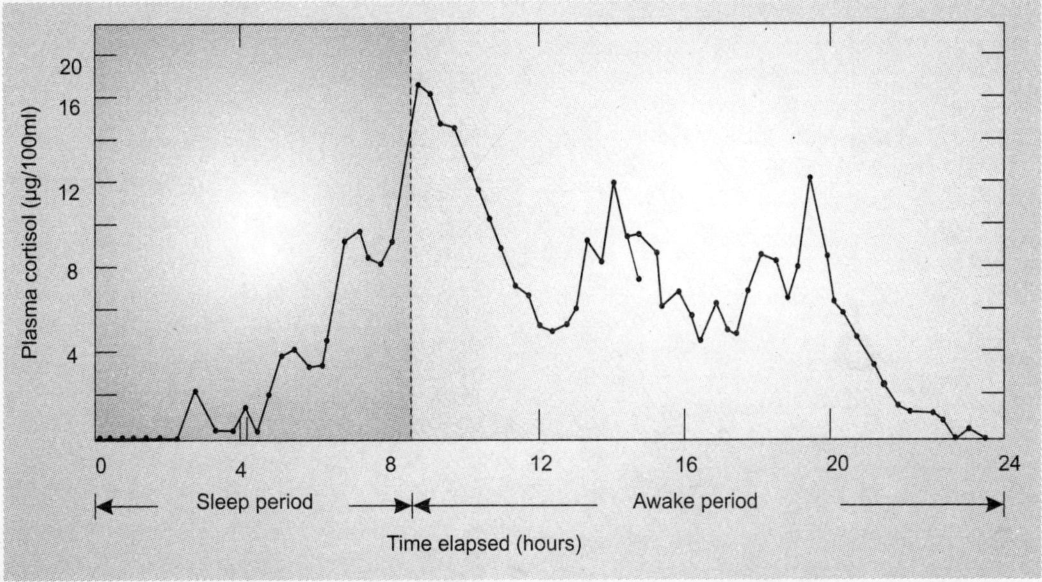

Fig. 48.2: The circadian rhythm of plasma cortisol level.

48

Feedback Control

High plasma levels of glucocorticoids inhibit ACTH secretion. Only the free (unbound to CBG) form of cortisol is responsible for this negative feedback action. The inhibitory effect is exerted both at anterior pituitary and hypothalamic levels (Fig. 48.3). As in many other endocrine glands, the feedback mechanism helps to stabilize the level of cortisol in the plasma. Stressful stimuli, however, can break through the feedback control and produce a marked increase in plasma cortisol level.

Knowledge of the negative feedback control of ACTH secretion has an important clinical implication. Prolonged administration of glucocorticoids in pharmacological doses results in almost complete inhibition of ACTH secretion, leading to the atrophy of adrenal cortex. For many weeks after the cessation of glucocorticoid therapy, the adrenal cortex as well as the anterior pituitary are not able to respond to stressful stimuli. During this period, exposure to any type of stress like infections or surgical trauma may prove fatal. The possible catastrophe can be avoided by tapering off the dose of glucocorticoids over a few weeks rather than suddenly withdrawing them.

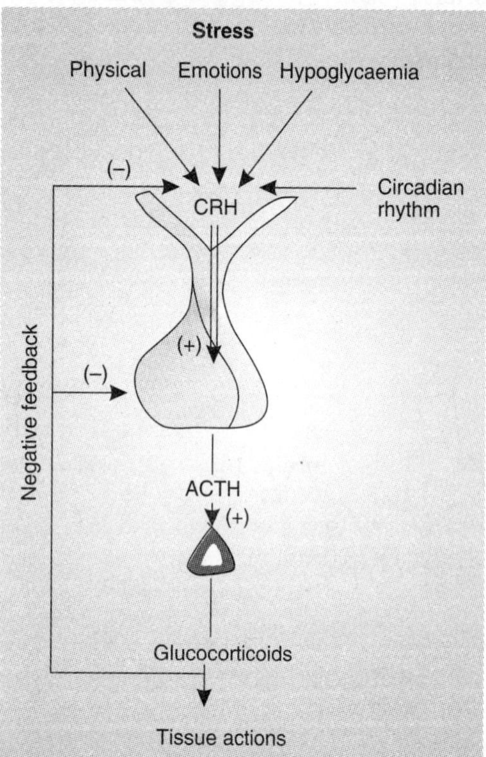

Fig. 48.3: The hypothalamus anterior pituitary-adrenal axis.

MINERALOCORTICOIDS

Aldosterone is the chief mineralocorticoid secreted by zona glomerulosa of adrenal cortex. Small amount of deoxycorticosterone (DOC) is also secreted but it has much less mineralocorticoid activity (Fig. 48.4).

ACTIONS OF MINERALOCORTICOIDS

Renal Tubular Reabsorption of Sodium and Secretion of Potassium

Aldosterone acts on the distal convoluted tubules and collecting ducts of the kidney. It produces active transport of Na^+ from the tubular fluid into the renal interstitial fluid and thereby into the ECF (Fig. 48.5). The Na^+-K^+ pump operates *at basolateral border* of the cell and not at luminal border.

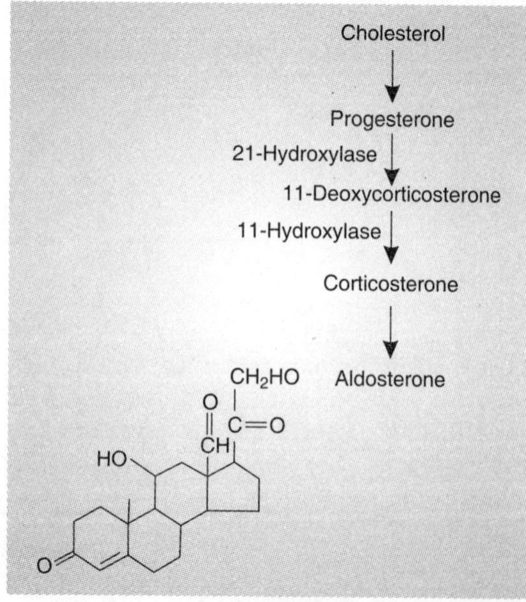

Fig. 48.4: Biosynthesis of aldosterone.

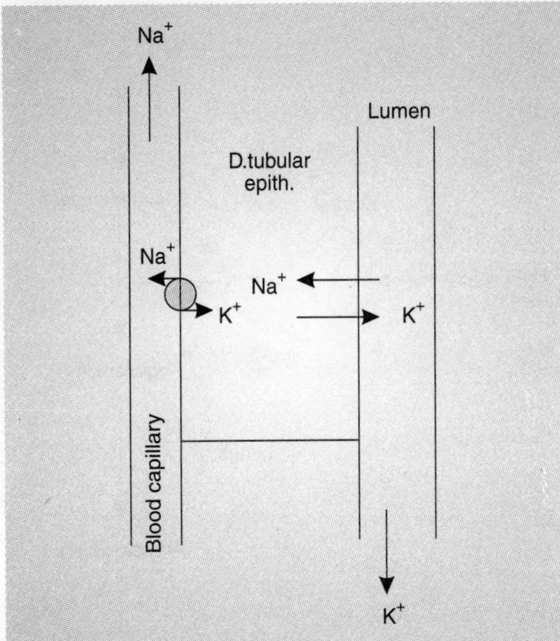

Fig. 48.5: Action of aldosterone on the distal renal tubules.

Under the effect of aldosterone, urinary sodium excretion may be reduced to only a few milligrams per day. Conversely, in adrenal insufficiency as much as 20 gm of sodium (chloride) may be lost in the urine every day.

At the *luminal border*, sodium transport involves passive Na^+ reabsorption *in exchange for K^+ and H^+*. Consequently, aldosterone not only increases renal conservation of Na^+ but also promotes greater excretion of K^+ and H^+ into the urine.

Sweat Glands

In salivary, sweat and gastric glands, aldosterone produces a similar increase in Na^+ reabsorption. The effect is of biological significance in sweat glands in adaptation to hot environment. Normally, sweat is hypotonic due to aldosterone-dependent reabsorption of Na^+ in ducts of the sweat glands. The effect becomes more prominent during adaptation to heat. Patients with adrenal insufficiency have a characteristic high Na^+ concentration in their sweat. They have an inability to restrict their salt losses both in urine and sweat. Therefore, such patients have very poor adaptability to hot environment.

Secondary Effects

Plasma Potassium Concentration

As mentioned above, Na^+ is reabsorbed in the renal tubules, in exchange of K^+ or H^+. Consequently, plasma aldosterone levels affect the plasma K^+ levels. In primary hyperaldosteronism (hypersecretion of aldosterone), excessive amount of aldosterone in plasma causes increased urinary potassium loss leading to a decrease in the plasma potassium concentration. When the K^+ concentration falls below 2.5 mEq/L, weakness or even paralysis of skeletal muscle may occur. Conversely, in adrenal insufficiency, hyperkalaemia occurs because of deficient aldosterone secretion. K^+ concentration may be raised to an extent that may cause cardiac toxicity.

Blood pH

The loss of H^+ into the tubular fluid in exchange for Na^+ may cause alterations in blood pH. In primary hyperaldosteronism mild, alkalosis occurs because of greater H^+ loss in the urine. Conversely, acidosis is commonly observed in adrenal insufficiency.

Body Water

Because Na^+ is the principal osmotically active substance in the extracellular fluid, changes in status of body Na^+ always lead secondarily to changes in body water. In adrenal insufficiency, hyponatremia is accompanied by decrease in ECF volume. Decreased blood pressure, hypovolemic shock and even death may occur.

Regulation of Secretion

Renin-Angiotensin System

This system serves as an important link between extracellular fluid volume, blood pressure and total body sodium on one hand and aldosterone secretion on the other.

Juxtaglomerular (JG) cells in the afferent arterioles in the kidney synthesize and secrete a proteolytic enzyme, known as renin. The secretion of renin is increased in response to a variety of stimuli, e.g. decreased renal perfusion pressure, ß-adrenergic stimulation, prostaglandins and fluid composition in distal convoluted renal tubules at the macula densa. Juxtaglomerular cells primarily monitor renal artery perfusion pressure. Renin secretion is increased whenever perfusion pressure falls. A decrease in the intravascular volume, e.g. because of haemorrhage or dehydration leads to not only decrease in renal perfusion pressure but also a reflex increase in sympathetic discharge to the renal vessels.

Renin acts as a proteolytic enzyme and splits angiotensinogen, a glycoprotein synthesized in the liver and circulating as an α_2-globulin. The splitting results in the formation of a decapeptide known as angiotensin-I. A converting enzyme further splits angiotensin-I into an octapeptide known as angiotensin-II. The angiotensin converting enzyme is widely distributed in the endothelium of the vascular beds, especially in the lungs. Angiotensin-II is an extremely potent vasoconstrictor. In addition, it binds with the zona glomerulosa cells and increases the secretion of aldosterone. The consequent retention of Na^+ and H_2O in the kidney helps to restore the intravascular volume to near normal (Fig. 48.6).

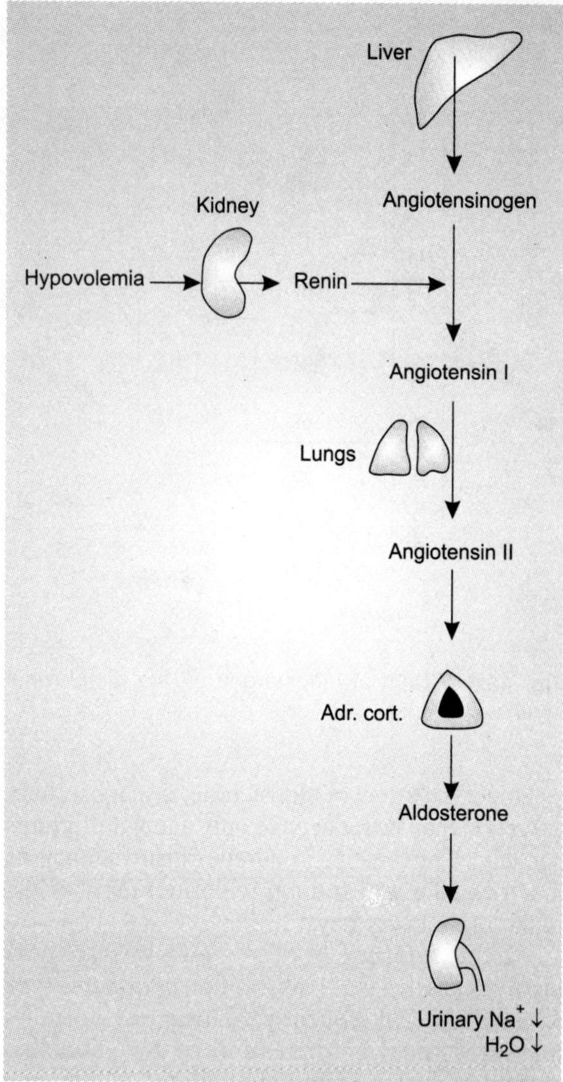

Fig. 48.6: The rennin-angiotensin II mechanism of aldosterone secretion.

48

Plasma Potassium Concentration

Plasma K^+ concentration is another important regulator of aldosterone secretion. The cells of zona glomerulosa of adrenal cortex are very sensitive to plasma K^+ concentration. Even a small increase in K^+ concentration, even though within the physiological range, increases the secretion of aldosterone. Conversely, even a small decrease in plasma K^+ concentration inhibits aldosterone.

Adrenocorticotropic Hormone (ACTH)

Primarily, zona glomerulosa of the adrenal cortex, unlike zona fasciculata and zona reticularis, is independent of the anterior pituitary control.

Increased plasma ACTH concentration produces a transient and very mild increase in aldosterone secretion.

Decrease in Dietary Intake of Sodium

A decrease in dietary intake of Na^+ or a *change from supine to standing posture* are also potent stimuli for aldosterone secretion. In either case, there is a decrease in the effective circulating blood volume which activates the renin-angiotensin-aldosterone system.

ADRENAL ANDROGENS

In adults, the adrenal cortex normally produces dehydroepiandrosterone, a hormone with very weak androgenic activity. It is secreted in both males as well as females and the secretion seems to be under ACTH control.

During fetal life, adrenal cortex is hyperplastic and secretes large amount of dehydroepiandrosterone which acts as the main precursor for synthesis of oestrogen by the placenta.

Although little androgen is secreted in childhood, its secretion increases dramatically at puberty and makes significant contribution to the body changes observed at puberty. Even in adults, plasma concentration of DHEA is more than 10 times the concentration of cortisol (Table 48.1). It is believed that DHEA is likely to have a physiological role other than its action as androgen (discussed below).

In adult females, adrenal dehydroepiandrosterone contributes to increased muscle mass, growth of pubic and axillary hair and libido. In males, similar but stronger action of testicular testosterone overshadows the action of adrenal dehydroepiandrosterone. The adrenal cortex secretes very small amounts of oestrogens also.

The secretion of sex hormones by the adrenal cortex assumes greater importance when certain tumours of the gland secrete huge amount of the sex hormones. Excessive androgen secretion by tumours of adrenal cortex produces *precocious pseudo-puberty* when occurring in prepubertal boys. Development of *male secondary sexual characteristics* (beard, muscular body, breaking of voice, etc.), occurs in prepubertal or adult females.

PATHOPHYSIOLOGY

Cushing's Syndrome

This disorder is produced by glucocorticoid excess due to:

(a) Prolonged therapeutic administration of high doses of the hormone, or

(b) Glucocorticoid secreting tumour of **adrenal cortex,** or

(c) ACTH-secreting tumour **of anterior pituitary**.

The characteristic features of Cushing's syndrome (Fig. 48.7) are:

(i) *Centripetal redistribution of body fat*. Fat collects in the abdominal wall, back and face, producing characteristic *moon face,* and *buffalo-hump*.

The extremities remain lean.

(ii) Due to excessive protein catabolism, the skin and the subcutaneous tissue become thin.

(iii) Muscles atrophy.

(iv) Hyperglycaemia and hyperlipidaemia are usually present.

(v) A significant degree of Na^+ and H_2O retention also occurs, and blood pressure tends to be elevated.

(vi) There is greater susceptibility to peptic ulcer, osteoporosis and bacterial infections.

(vii) Wound healing is delayed.

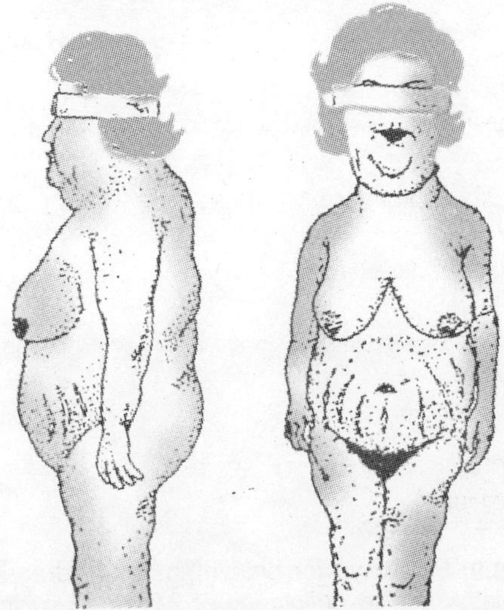

Fig. 48.7: A patient with Cushing's syndrome.

Addison's Disease

This disorder is usually produced by an atrophy of the adrenal gland due to an autoimmune disease or by tubercular infection of the gland. It is characterised by chronic deficiency of both mineralocorticoids as well as glucocorticoids. Hyponatraemia, hyperkalaemia, acidosis and decreased ECF volume are the characteristic features of Addison's disease. Due to feedback mechanism, ACTH production by anterior pituitary is massively increased causing diffuse pigmentation of the skin and mucous membranes. Fasting produces severe hypoglycaemia. The patient may die of circulatory shock because of hypovolemia. Exposure to any type of stress, e.g. even mild infection, may be fatal.

Primary Hyperaldosteronism

This disorder is due to hypersecretion of aldosterone by a tumour of zona glomerulosa of the adrenal cortex. It is characterised by hypokalaemia, muscular weakness, sodium and water retention, hypertension, alkalosis and tetany.

Gross hypernatraemia or oedema does not occur because Na^+ excretion is almost normal despite hypersecretion of aldosterone. This *escape phenomenon* is probably due to increased secretion of atrial natriuretic peptide (ANP) (page 555).

Congenital Adrenal Hyperplasia

This disorder is caused by congenital deficiency of one of the enzymes involved in the biosynthesis of glucocorticoids (Fig. 48.8). The most common defect is **21-hydroxylase deficiency**. It results in low plasma levels of cortisol and aldosterone but elevated levels of immediate precursors like 17 hydroxyprogesterone. Decreased plasma cortisol level leads to increased ACTH secretion (due to negative feedback effect). Excessive plasma ACTH level stimulates the open pathways and also causes immense hyperplasia of adrenal cortex.

Since 17-hyroxyprogesterone serves as a major precursor of adrenal androgens, 21-hydroxylase deficiency leads to excessive plasma levels of adrenal androgens like DHEA and testosterone. In female fetuses, high plasma adrenal androgen levels cause a masculanized pattern of development of external genitalia (*congenital adrenogenital syndrome*). If the enzyme deficiency is

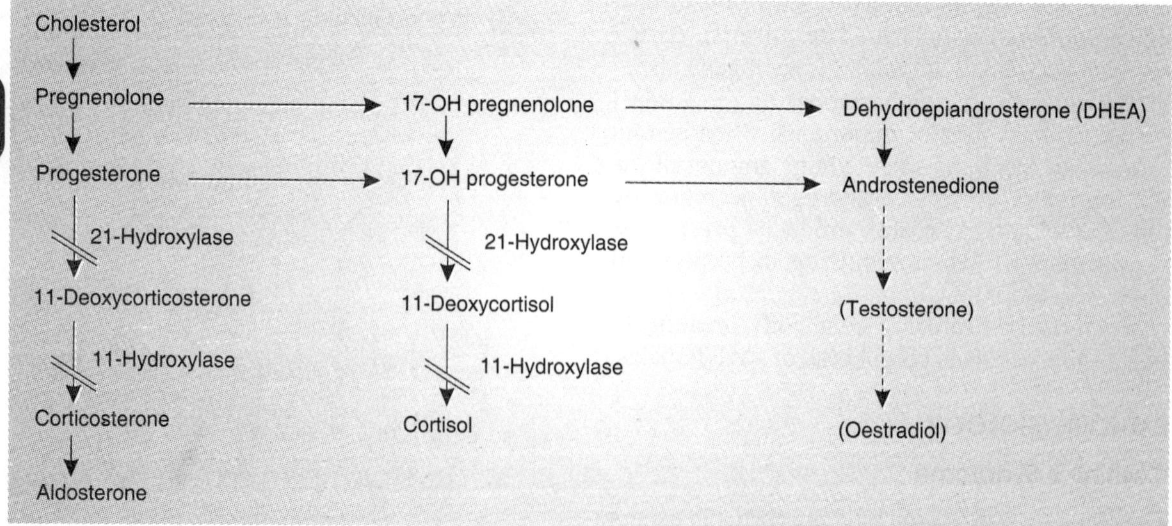

Fig. 48.8: Pathways for biosynthesis of adrenal corticosteroids. 1. Mechanism of virilism in congenital adrenal hyperplasia due to deficiency of 21- or 11-hydroxylase (——→). 2. Pathway through which adrenal tumour may produce oestradiol (---- →).

very severe, effects of deficiency of cortisol and aldosterone may also be observed.

Deficiency of 11-hydroxylase leads to deficiency of cortisol accompanied by excessive blood levels of adrenal androgens and deoxycorticosteroid (a mineralocorticoid) leading to virilization as well as salt and water retention. The condition is known as *hypertensive form of congenital adrenogenital syndrome.*

ADRENAL MEDULLA

Adrenal medulla consists of interlacing cords of densely innervated granule-containing cells. The nerve fibres are preganglionic fibres of sympathetic nervous system (T_6-T_{12}). The adrenal medulla secretes three catecholamines namely, epinephrine, norepinephrine and dopamine. They are synthesized from the amino acid tyrosine (Fig. 48.9).

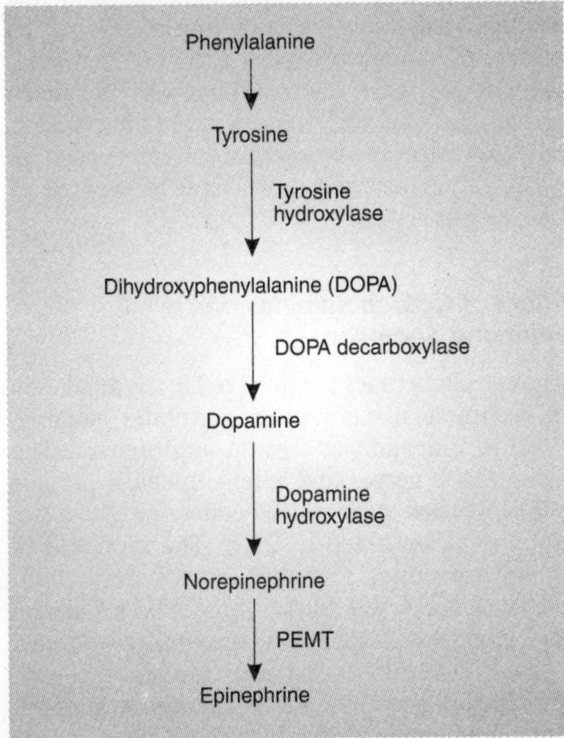

Fig. 48.9: Biosynthesis of catecholamines.

An enzyme, phenyl ethanolamine-n-methyl transferase (PEMT) is present in adrenal medulla and certain regions of CNS (but not in postganglionic sympathetic neurons). This enzyme converts norepinephrine into epinephrine. The activity of this enzyme in the adrenal medulla is increased by glucocorticoids.

The half-life of catecholamines in circulation is 2 minutes. They are methoxylated and then oxidized to 3-methoxy-4-hydroxy mandelic acid (Vanillyl mandelic acid, VMA), which is excreted in the urine.

Adrenal medulla secretes epinephrine and norepinephrine in the ratio of 4 : 1. In recumbent humans, normal plasma levels of free epinephrine and norepinephrine are about 30 picogram/ml and 300 picogram/ml, respectively.

After adrenalectomy, plasma epinephrine level falls to almost zero but norepinephrine level remains practically unchanged. This observation suggests that in humans, the chief source of epinephrine in the plasma is the adrenal medulla but circulating norepinephrine is mostly derived from postganglionic sympathetic nerve endings.

The physiological role of circulating dopamine is not clear. However, dopamine is an important pharmacologic agent in the treatment of circulatory shock. In pharmacologic concentrations, dopamine produces elevation of systolic blood pressure without any change in total peripheral resistance. Dopamine has a positive inotropic effect on the heart. It also produces vasodilatation in the renal and mesenteric vessels as well as vasoconstriction in skeletal and cutaneous vessels. In the treatment of circulatory shock, dopamine is preferred over norepinephrine.

Norepinephrine increases systolic blood pressure but it also increases total peripheral resistance by producing vasoconstriction in renal, mesenteric, cutaneous and skeletal blood vessels.

Adrenergic Receptors

Besides mimicking the actions of sympathetic nerve stimulation, circulating epinephrine and norepinephrine produce CNS stimulation as well as certain metabolic effects such as glycogenolysis, lipolysis and calorigenesis. The effects of the two catecholamines are brought about by action on two types of receptors, namely alpha (α) and beta (ß) adrenergic receptors. ß-adrenergic receptors are further divided into ß1 and ß2 receptors. Norepinephrine mainly excites the ß-adrenergic receptors whereas epinephrine can excite both α-as well as ß-adrenergic receptors. The effect of epinephrine on a given organ depends on the type of adrenergic receptors present in it.

Effects of **α-receptor stimulation** include vasoconstriction in coronary, pulmonary, cutaneous, skeletal, cerebral, and splanchnic vessels, dilatation of pupil, relaxation of gastrointestinal smooth muscle, constriction of intestinal sphincters, contraction of piloerector muscle and constriction of sphincter of urinary bladder.

ß1 receptor stimulation leads to increase in the rate and force of contraction of the heart. Stimulation of ß1 receptors present in the adipose tissue produces lipolysis.

ß2 receptor stimulation produces vasodilatation (in coronary, skeletal and pulmonary vessels), relaxation of smooth muscle of intestine, uterus, urinary bladder and bronchi. ß2 receptor stimulation also produces glycogenolysis and calorigenesis.

Actions of Adrenal Catecholamines

Supplementation of Sympathetic Neural Actions

48

The adrenal medulla is supplied by preganglionic sympathetic fibres through splanchnic nerves (T_6–T_{12}). Therefore, adrenal medullary secretion of epinephrine and to a minor extent norepinephrine occurs as a part of generalised sympathetic response. The actions of adrenal medullary secretions supplement those produced by increased sympathetic discharge by about 20%.

Metabolic Actions

Glycogenolysis Epinephrine and norepinephrine produce glycogenolysis both in the liver and skeletal muscle by activation of the enzyme phosphorylase. ß2 adrenergic receptors are involved in these actions. In addition, the two catecholamines increase the secretion of glucagon, thus further contributing to the elevation of blood glucose level. In humans, epinephrine produces far greater elevation of blood glucose level than norepinephrine.

Lipolysis Catecholamines combine with ß1receptors in the adipose tissue and activate cAMP mechanism. Thus, the enzyme hormone sensitive lipase is activated resulting in lipolysis. Both epinephrine and norepinephrine are equally potent in the mobilization of FFA from the adipose tissue.

Calorigenic Action The two catecholamines are equally potent in calorigenesis. The presence of thyroxine and glucocorticoids is essential for calorigenic effect of catecholamines.

Mental Alertness

Epinephrine and norepinephrine lower the threshold of neurons of reticular activating system in the brainstem. The result is increased mental alertness and arousal reaction in EEG. During an emergency which provokes a generalized sympathetic response, the usefulness of increased mental alertness for "fight or flight" response is obvious. Intravenous injection of epinephrine or norepinephrine produces a similar degree of mental stimulation.

Effect of Catecholamines on Hormone Secretion

The catecholamines are involved in the regulation of secretion of many other hormones, notably, insulin, glucagon and renin-angiotensin. The sympathetic nerves and adrenal medulla provide a link between the brain and endocrine glands not otherwise connected to CNS. The secretion of these hormones also has own independent feedback loops, e.g. blood sugar level for insulin and glucagon. Imposition of sympatho-adrenal system introduces the advantage of speed, anticipation and integration with other responses. Thus, it provides further help in the maintenance of homeostasis.

Role of Sympathoadrenal System in Various Physiological States

Cold Exposure Intact sympathoadrenal system is an absolute requirement for normal mammalian defence against exposure to cold. In experimental animals, if sympathetic nervous system and adrenal medulla are ablated, body temperature is not maintained in cold environment and the animal dies from hypothermia. However, either sympathetic nervous system or adrenal medulla can independently sustain life. Increased sympathoadrenal activity sets up two groups of responses: (i) Those concerned with heat conservation and (ii) Those concerned with heat production (thermogenesis).

Heat Conservation Exposure to cold produces graded cutaneous vasoconstriction. As a result, the skin practically becomes a bloodless sheet of tissue insulating the warmer deeper tissues from the cold environment. In animals with fur or feathers, the cold-induced piloerection is also mediated through sympathoadrenal system.

Thermogenesis Basal production of heat is regulated by thyroxine. Catecholamines do not have any significant role in the function. Shivering is one of the important mechanisms of increasing thermogenesis on exposure to cold. *Non-shivering thermogenesis* is another mechanism of heat production, in which sympathoadrenal system plays a critical role. Non-shivering thermogenesis occurs in the brown adipose tissue. Besides this, the catecholamines seem to stimulate the chemical metabolic processes in general, leading to greater production of heat (*chemical thermogenesis*). For example, catecholamines increase oxygen consumption in the skeletal muscle beyond that induced by muscular activity. Moreover, the lipolytic and glycogenolytic actions of catecholamines provide additional substrates like glucose and FFA for increased tissue metabolism.

Exercise Mild to moderate exercise mainly activates sympathetic nervous system. However, severe exercise increases adrenal medullary secretion as well. Adrenergic blockade or autonomic neuropathy impairs cardiovascular responses to exercise and diminishes exercise tolerance.

Increased sympathoadrenal discharge in exercise provides appropriate cardiovascular responses for massive blood flow to the actively contracting muscles. Increased blood flow is necessary for providing oxygen and fuel (glucose, FFA) for increased muscle metabolism. Catecholamines also contribute to the mobilization of stored fuel by promoting glycogenolysis and lipolysis.

Hypoglycemia Plasma epinephrine concentration increases when plasma glucose level falls below the normal range. It may rise 10–50 folds depending upon the severity of hypoglycemia. During hypoglycemia, adrenal medulla is strongly stimulated whereas sympathetic neural activity is not increased to any significant degree. The actions of epinephrine that contribute to rise of blood glucose level include: (a) enhancement of hepatic glucose output by glycogenolysis, (b) stimulation of lipolysis in the adipose tissue providing FFA as an alternate fuel, and (c) suppression of endogenous insulin secretion and release of glucagon. The cardiovascular signs of hypoglycemia (tachycardia, etc.) are due to the effects of adrenal medullary epinephrine on the heart.

Role in Stress

Exposure to any type of acute stress like excessive environmental heat or cold, hypoglycemia, haemorrhage, trauma, infections, anaesthesia, surgery, severe exercise or even psychological stress results in strong activation of sympathoadrenal system, i.e. increased sympathetic neural discharge as well as increased adrenal medullary secretion. Similar response occurs in fight or flight (flee) reaction of an animal faced with a life-threatening situation. The beneficial role of sympatho-adrenal discharge in severe exercise, hypoglycemia, cold exposure and haemorrhage is obvious. However, the physiological benefit of such a response in some conditions like psychological stress is not clear.

When the stress becomes chronic (e.g. in burns, multiple fractures, etc.), the elevated adrenal medullary secretion returns to normal but the increased sympathetic neural discharge usually continues as long as the stress persists.

Despite the important physiological role of adrenal medulla discussed above, (unlike adrenal cortex), it is not essential for survival. Following bilateral adrenalectomy, replacement therapy with glucomineralocorticoids is sufficient for maintenance of normal health. Sympathetic nervous system, without the help of adrenal medullary secretion, is able to produce adequate sympathetic responses.

Regulation of Adrenal Medullary Secretion: Neural Control

The secretion of adrenal medulla is entirely controlled by splanchnic nerves. These nerves are preganglionic sympathetic fibres and hence act by releasing acetylcholine close to the adrenal medullary chromaffin cells. Splanchnic neural acitivity is controlled by sympathetic centres in the medulla oblongata, which in turn, are controlled by the hypothalamus.

Generalized Sympathetic Alarm Reaction

48

As discussed above, adrenal medullary discharge occurs as a part of generalized sympathetic response to any emergency situation (any acute stress). This has been called sympathetic alarm reaction. Increased adrenal medullary discharge during hypoglycemia, cold exposure, haemorrhage and severe exercise produces appropriate cardiovascular and metabolic responses, and thereby helps in the maintenance of homeostasis.

Independent Stimulation of Adrenal Medulla

Adrenal medullary discharge does not always occur as a part of generalized sympathetic response. The sympathetic neural system and adrenal medullary system may operate relatively independently also. For example, in baroreceptor-mediated cardiovascular reflexes, sympathetic neural system is predominantly involved. On the other hand, hypoglycemia produces marked increase in adrenal medullary secretion without any significant increase in sympathetic neural discharge.

(c) Selective Secretion and Selective Actions

When adrenal medullary secretion increases, the secretion of norepinephrine and epinephrine usually increases in the same proportion. However, the threshold level at which circulating norepinephrine can produce physiological effects is five times (500%) the basal plasma level of the hormone. But the threshold level at which epinephrine produces its effects is only marginally above its basal plasma level. Hence, in most of the physiological and pathological conditions, increased adrenal medullary secretion results in selective *epinephrine-mediated effects*, in spite of increased secretion of both the catecholamines (Fig. 48.10).

Hypoglycemia is one condition which produces selective and massive epinephrine secretion from the adrenal medulla. On the other hand, secretion of norepinephrine is proportionately much more than that of epinephrine in response to asphyxia and hypoxia or in patients with pheochromocytoma (Fig. 48.10).

FUNCTION TESTS FOR ADRENAL CORTEX

Plasma levels of cortisol, ACTH and aldosterone can be estimated by radio-immunoassay.

Cushing's Syndrome The diagnostic investigations in Cushing's syndrome are as follows.

(i) Elevated plasma level of cortisol (8 AM sample).
(ii) Loss of circadian rhythm in the plasma cortisol level.
(iii) High plasma cortisol levels cannot be suppressed by administration of a low dose of a synthetic glucocorticoid (loss of normal negative feedback control).
(iv) Increased urinary free cortisol excretion.
(v) Absence of rise in plasma cortisol level following hypoglycaemia produced by insulin injection.

If the existence of Cushing's syndrome is confirmed by above mentioned tests, the estimation of plasma ACTH level can differentiate the two chief causes of Cushing's syndrome. In case of adrenal tumour, plasma ACTH level is

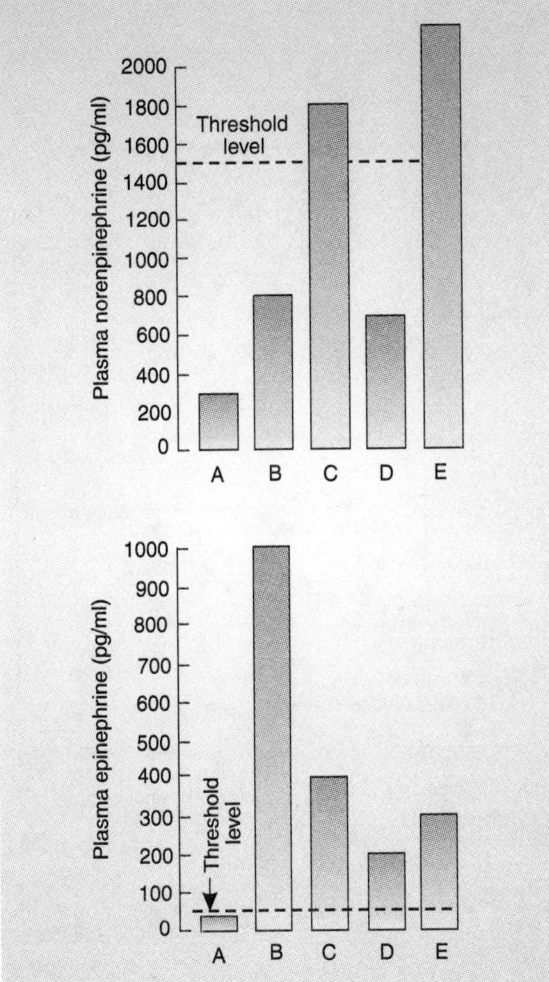

Fig. 48.10: Plasma norepinephrine and epinephrine levels in different conditions. (A) basal level; (B) hypoglycemia; (C) severe exercise; (D) surgery; (E) pheochromocytoma. Threshold level is the level at which physiological response can be observed.

almost zero. Plasma ACTH level is elevated if Cushing's syndrome is due to a pituitary tumour.

Primary Hyperaldosteronism It is characterised by elevation of plasma/urinary aldosterone level. It is further confirmed if plasma renin activity is suppressed.

Addison's Disease It is characterised by:

(i) Low basal (8 AM) plasma cortisol level.

(ii) Elevated plasma ACTH level.

(iii) Low plasma Na^+ concentration and elevated K^+ concentration.

(iv) Failure of plasma cortisol level to rise after injection of ACTH further confirms the diagnosis of Addison's disease.

TESTS FOR ADRENAL MEDULLARY FUNCTION

Pheochromocytoma It is a rare tumour of adrenal medulla. It is characterised by attacks of hypertension accompanied by palpitation, sweating and headache. Weight loss, constipation and glucose intolerance are other important clinical features.

Tests for pheochromocytoma include estimation of 24-hour urinary VMA excretion or 24-hour urinary free catecholamines excretion. Plasma epinephrine and norepinephrine levels can also be estimated.

NEUROENDOCRINE RESPONSE TO SURGICAL STRESS

Sudden exposure to any type of stress initially produces the sympathetic alarm reaction. The alarm reaction consists of a generalized and profuse sympathetic neural discharge as well as an increase in adrenal medullary secretion. If the stressful stimulus persists, the short-lived alarm reaction is followed by a complex neuroendocrine response which may last hours, days or even weeks. Such a sustained neuroendocrine response is typically seen in patients who undergo major abdominal surgery or in patients with multiple fractures or extensive burns. In uncomplicated surgery, it lasts only 2-4 days. However, in cases with multiple fractures, extensive burns or post-surgical complications, the response may continue for days or weeks. In view of the common occurrence, the metabolic effects of surgical stress are described below in detail. In other forms of stress, qualitatively similar metabolic changes occur but the degree and duration of metabolic disturbance vary in each case.

Following a surgical trauma or surgical operation, two distinct phases of tissue metabolism can be distinguished.

The Catabolic Phase It which lasts 2-4 days after major surgery, but longer in cases with multiple fractures or extensive burns. This is the stage of stress. During this phase there is increased oxygen consumption, severe protein catabolism leading to loss of lean body mass and negative nitrogen balance, loss of body weight, fluid retention and increased susceptibility to infections.

Anabolic Phase It follows the catabolic phase. It lasts 4-5 days in uncomplicated surgical operation but longer in patients with prolonged catabolic phase. This phase consists of a slow accumulation of proteins and fat. It is a slow process. Proteins lost in a few days of catabolic phase may be restored over a period of several weeks. Fat stores are replenished over several months.

Catabolic Phase

The causes of catabolic phase in surgical stress include fear, pain, anaesthesia, surgical trauma (tissue destruction and loss of blood and fluids from the operated site) and post-surgical complications like haemorrhage, hypoxia, shock and infections.

Neuroendocrine Response

The complex neuroendocrine response and the consequent metabolic disturbances are summarized in Fig. 48.11. The hypothalamus mediated neuro-endocrine response leads to increased secretion of ACTH, cortisol, growth hormone, adrenal medullary catecholamines, thyroxine and antidiuretic hormone. Increased sympathetic discharge to the renal vessels coupled with hypovolemia due to loss of blood, etc. increases the secretion of renin, angiotensin II and aldosterone. Increased sympathetic discharge to the pancreas depresses insulin secretion but promotes the secretion of glucagon. There is a decrease in the secretion of pituitary gonadotropins. The concentration of most of the hormones especially cortisol increases in proportion to the severity of surgery. However, the rise in plasma ACTH concentration is far in excess of the level required to produce maximum cortisol response. It seems, ACTH has some metabolic role other than increasing the cortisol secretion. The endocrine changes described above result in the following metabolic changes.

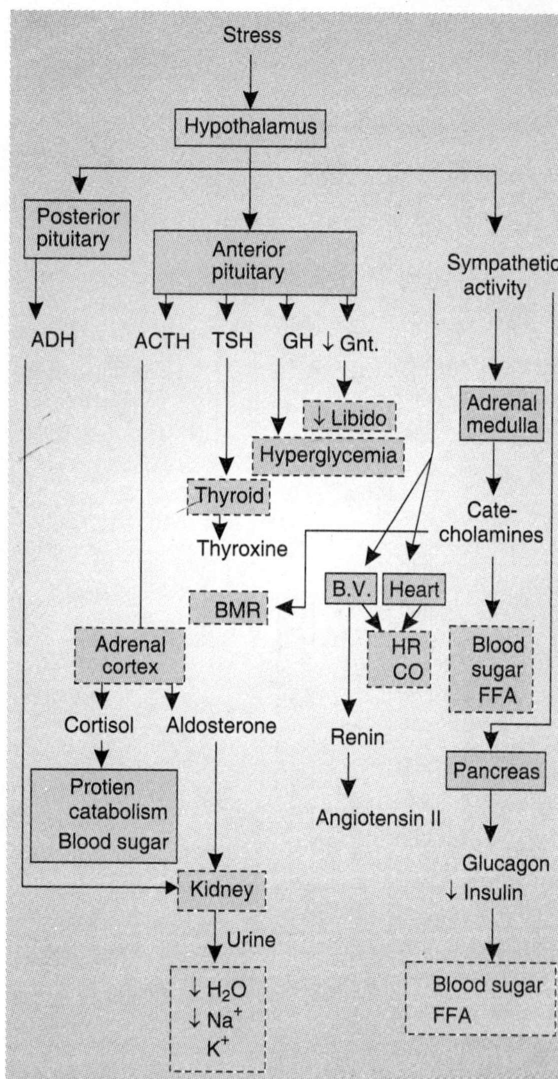

Fig. 48.11: Neuroendocrine response to surgical

Protein Catabolism This is the most important metabolic change in the catabolic phase. It results in anaemia, hypoproteinemia and loss of lean body mass (mainly muscle proteins). An average person loses 400 gm of wet lean tissue every day of the catabolic phase. Increased protein catabolism is reflected in increased urinary losses nitrogen and potassium.

The severity of protein catabolism can be decreased by:

(i) Minimizing tissue trauma during surgery.
(ii) Maintaining adequate analgesia during surgery and postoperative period.
(iii) Maintaining adequate supply of oxygen, fluids and electrolytes, and nutrition during the postoperative period.
(iv) Preventing postoperative complications such as infection and haemorrhage.

However, even the best medical care, during surgery and postoperatively, can only attenuate but cannot abolish the catabolic phase. Therefore, it is believed that the catabolic phase has some fundamental biological role in the body's response to tissue injury.

Hyperglycemia Suppression of insulin secretion coupled with increased secretion of glucagon, GH, cortisol and catecholamines leads to hyperglycemia, which may be severe enough to produce glycosuria. The glucose tolerance curve resembles that of a diabetic patient. The phenomenon is called "*traumatic diabetes*". These changes typically occur 3 days after a major surgical operation. This metabolic change seems to be very useful because large amount of glucose is utilized in the process of wound repair. Protein catabolism may help by providing extra glucose through gluconeogenesis.

Increased Plasma FFA Level Increased lipolysis leading to elevated plasma FFA level is the result of suppression of insulin secretion as well as increased secretion of cortisol, G.H. and catecholamines. Consequently, FFA rather than glucose becomes the chief fuel for energy production,particularly in the skeletal muscle.

Salt and Water Retention ADH secretion starts rising during surgery and remains elevated during the next 2 to 4 days. As a result, there is an inappropriate antidiuresis. At the same time, urinary excretion of Na^+ is drastically curtailed by activation of renin-angiotensin-aldosterone mechanism. Water retention is partly due to diminished (renal) excretion and partly due to increased production by catabolic processes. About 500 ml of water is released from the intracellular sources every day. This fact must be kept in mind while calculating water requirements of a surgical patient.

To some extent, water and salt retention helps to overcome hypovolemia caused by loss of blood and other body fluids.

Potassium Loss Peak urinary K^+ excretion occurs during the first 24 hours after an injury or surgery but increased urinary K^+ excretion continues during the next 2 to 3 days. However, positive K^+ balance is restored several days before the nitrogen balance returns to normal.

Sexual Function Sexual function fades immediately after injury. In males, the libido is decreased. In females, amenorrhoea may persist until convalescence is well established. All these changes are due to decreased secretion of pituitary gonadotropins.

CHAPTER 49

The Endocrine Pancreas

Scattered among the pancreatic exocrine acini are 1–2 million collections of endocrine cells called the islets of Langerhans. The islets constitute 1–2% of the total weight of the pancreas. Each islet has profuse blood supply (as in all ductless glands). The blood is drained into the portal vein. The islets are innervated by both vagal and sympathetic fibres. Histologically, the following types of cells can be identified in each islet (Colour Plate 7, Fig. 18).

(i) A cells (α cells) secreting glucagon.
(ii) B cells (β cells) secreting insulin
(iii) D cells (δ cells) secreting somatostatin
(iv) F cells (PP cells) secreting pancreatic polypeptide.

B cells, the most abundant cells, form a central mass in each islet whereas the A cells constitute the outer rim. D cells are interposed between the central mass of B cells and the outer rim of A cells. F cells are scattered amongst the A cells in the outer rim. The B cells secrete insulin, A cells glucagon and D cells somatostatin. Somatostatin acts in a paracrine fashion to modulate the secretion of A and B cells. The physiological significance of the secretion of pancreatic polypeptide is yet not clear. Insulin and glucagon are discussed below.

INSULIN

Chemically, insulin is a polypeptide containing two chains of amino acids linked by disulphide bridges. The molecular weight of human insulin is 5808. Insulin obtained from different species shows slight variations in amino acid sequence. Therefore, although insulin from one species is effective in another species, but it acts as a foreign protein. That is why diabetic patients who are commonly treated with the beef insulin gradually develop antibodies against the injected insulin. Therefore, resistance to exogenous insulin ultimately occurs in many diabetics on insulin therapy resulting in extremely high insulin requirements. Nowadays, recombinant human insulin is available. It has very low antigenicity, but it is more expensive than bovine insulin.

ACTION OF INSULIN

Due to easily recognizable effects of insulin deficiency on glucose metabolism, it is a common impression that regulation of blood sugar is the main function of insulin. As a matter of fact, insulin affects the metabolism of carbohydrates, fats and proteins and favours anabolism and storage of all the three foodstuffs in the body.

Although most of the tissues of the body are insulin sensitive, the liver, skeletal muscle and adipose tissue are the principal target tissues for the hormone.

Carbohydrate Metabolism

Insulin reduces plasma glucose level by stimulating the uptake of glucose by the tissues and by decreasing the production and release of glucose into circulation.

In the **liver,** insulin enhances the uptake of glucose by increasing the activity of glucokinase. It also increases the activity of glycogen synthetase.

It inhibits the activity of the enzyme phosphorylase, thus decreasing the breakdown of glycogen. Due to these actions, insulin increases the deposition of glycogen in the liver and less glucose is poured into the circulation.

In **the skeletal muscle**, insulin increases the rate of glucose transport into the cell by an action on the cell membrane. The hormone receptor complex activates the carrier system responsible for facilitated diffusion of glucose. Increased rate of glucose transport into the skeletal muscle leads to greater use of glucose for energy production (by glycolysis), as well as, deposition of glucose as muscle glycogen (Fig. 49.1).

From the above discussion, it would be obvious that increased transport of glucose across the hepatic cell membrane is secondary to greater utilization of glucose brought about by insulin mediated increase in the activity of glucokinase. On the other hand, insulin increases transport of glucose in the skeletal muscle directly by acting on the cell membrane. Greater availability of glucose in the muscle fibres secondarily leads to increased glucose utilization (by law of mass action).

Glucose transport in the nervous tissue, renal tubules, intestinal mucosa and RBCs is not insulin-dependent. This property is of critical importance in the nervous system because glucose is the only source of energy and insulin is present in the blood for about 2 hours after each meal. The transport of glucose into the nervous tissue depends on blood glucose level only. Severe hypoglycaemia results in convulsions, coma or even death.

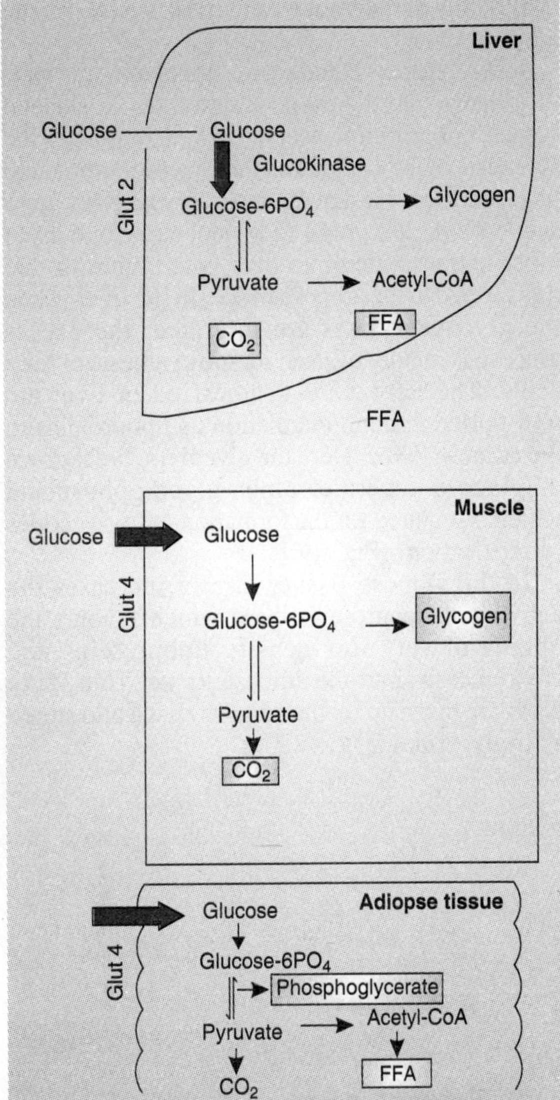

Fig. 49.1: Action of insulin on the carbohydrate metabolism in the liver, skeletal muscle and adipose tissue.

Fat Metabolism

In the adipose tissue, insulin inhibits the mobilization of FFA. Insulin brings about this effect at a lower plasma concentration than required for its hypoglycaemic effect. The rate of utilization of FFA by the peripheral tissues is regulated only by its plasma levels. Thus, by regulating the production of FFA, insulin provides a primary control on its utilization. The inhibition of lipolysis by insulin is brought about by

49

inhibition of hormone-sensitive lipase in the adipose tissue.

Insulin increases the carrier-mediated transport of glucose into the adipose tissue (as in skeletal muscle). By forming acetyl-CoA, it stimulates the synthesis of fatty acids and their incorporation into triglycerides. However, *most of the fatty acid synthesis occurs in the liver*, since the amount of glucose transported into liver is ten times of that transported to the adipose tissue. In the liver, when the glycogen stores are saturated, the excess glucose is rapidly utilized for the synthesis of fatty acids. The fatty acids synthesized in liver are transported through circulation as lipoproteins to the adipose tissue. Here the glycolytic breakdown of glucose generates alpha-glycerophosphate which is required for the formation of triglycerides (esterification) (Fig. 49.1).

In the adipose tissue, insulin increases the activity of lipoprotein lipase which favours the uptake of very low density lipoproteins and chylomicrons into the adipose tissue. Thus, fatty acids are taken up by the adipose tissue and stored as triglycerides (Fig. 49.2).

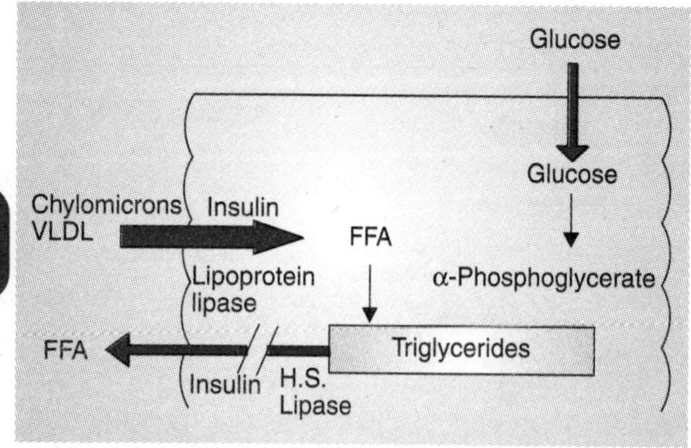

Fig. 49.2: Action of insulin on fat metabolism in the adipose tissue.

From its effects on carbohydrate and fat metabolism described above, it would be obvious that the secretion of insulin regulates the use of glucose or FFA for energy production. After a carbohydrate rich meal, blood insulin level rises and consequently glucose becomes the chief fuel in the muscle. FFA is not used at this time because of low plasma FFA concentration induced by insulin. In between the meals when the blood glucose level tends to fall, insulin secretion also decreases, resulting in greater lipolysis and increased production of FFA. Consequently, FFA becomes the chief fuel.

Protein Metabolism

For a few hours after a meal, large amounts of nutrients accumulate in the blood. Insulin promotes deposition of not only carbohydrates and fats but also proteins. Insulin increases the protein synthesis by a number of mechanisms. Insulin increases the active transport of many amino acids into tissues. In addition, insulin increases protein synthesis by increasing the rate of synthesis of mRNA.

Insulin decreases the catabolism of proteins by a direct action on the muscle cells. It also depresses the activity of enzymes involved in gluconeogenesis in the liver. Thus, insulin indirectly also decreases the protein catabolism since the amino acids are the chief substrate for gluconeogenesis (Fig. 49.3).

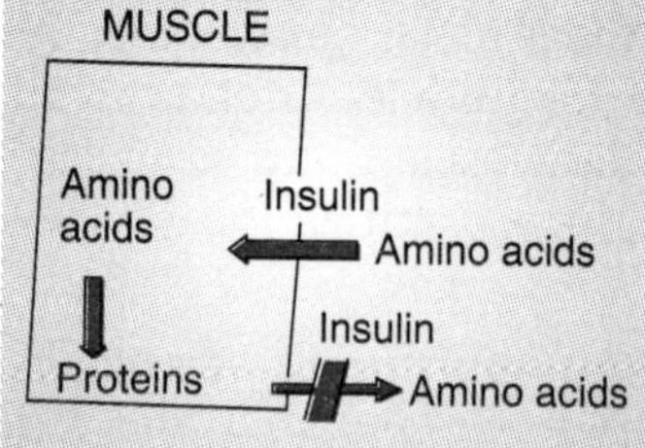

Fig. 49.3: Action of insulin on protein metabolism in the skeletal muscle and the liver.

Growth and Development

The anabolic action of insulin is as important as growth hormone for promotion of normal growth. Proper growth and development requires the presence of both the hormones because anabolic action of one hormone cannot compensate for the absence of the other (because of their different modes of action).

Ion Transport

Insulin increases the transport of K^+ from ECF into the skeletal muscle and hepatic cells. That is why hypokalaemia often develops in patients of diabetic acidosis treated with large doses of insulin.

Table 49.1 shows the list of actions of insulin.

Table 49.1: Actions of insulin

Liver
- Increased glycolysis.
- Increased glycogen synthesis.
- Increased protein synthesis.
- Increased fatty acid synthesis.
- Decreased gluconeogenesis.
- Decreased glucose output
- Decreased ketogenesis.

Skeletal muscle
- Increased glucose utilization.
- Increased glycogen synthesis
- Increased amino acid uptake.
- Increased protein synthesis
- Increased K^+ uptake.
- Decreased protein catabolism.

Adipose tissue
- Increased glucose uptake.
- Increased fatty acid synthesis.
- Increased glycerol phosphate synthesis
- Increased triglyceride deposition.
- Activation of lipoprotein lipase.
- Inhibition of hormone-sensitive lipase.
- Increased K^+ uptake.

General
- Increased cellular growth.

Mechanism of Action of Insulin

The binding of insulin with the receptor proteins is followed by a number of biological effects. The stimulation of glucose, amino acids and ion transport in the muscle seems to be a direct consequence of insulin receptor interaction. However, the effect on the activity of many intracellular enzymes would involve a second messenger whose identity is not yet established.

Metabolism of Insulin

The liver and the kidneys are chief sites for the degradation of insulin. The half-life of insulin in the circulation is about 5 minutes. For pharmacological administration, insulin is injected as protein-zinc insulin (PZI) which has relatively longer half-life because insulin is in a bound form.

Regulation of Insulin Secretion

Blood Glucose

This is the most important factor regulating the release of insulin. At the normal fasting blood glucose level of 70–110 mg%, the rate of insulin secretion is minimal. An increase of blood sugar level above 110 mg% promptly increases the insulin secretion. If blood sugar level is experimentally increased to 400–600 mg%, the rate of insulin secretion may increase by 10–30 times the basal level. Insulin secretion is cut off with similar promptness when blood sugar level falls below 110 mg%. The ß cells of the islets of Langerhans are believed to possess specific receptors which respond to changes in the blood glucose level and regulate the release of insulin.

Plasma Amino Acids

Plasma insulin level rises even after a meal consisting of proteins only. Certain amino acids like arginine, leucine, and lysine are more effective in promoting insulin release than others like valine and histidine. Like glucose, amino acids also regulate the insulin release by a direct action on the ß cells.

Gastrointestinal Hormones

Blood sugar level can be elevated to a similar degree by oral or intravenous administration of glucose in appropriate amounts. It would be seen that insulin secretion is greater when hyperglycaemia is produced by oral administration of glucose. Response to amino acids also is more effective when given orally than intravenously.

Several gastrointestinal hormones such as gastrin, secretin, cholecystokinin and gastric-inhibitory polypeptide (GIP) can stimulate the release of insulin from the ß cells. Of these, GIP seems to be most important. Since, these hormones are produced during the process of digestion of food stuffs, they seem to provide an *anticipatory release of insulin*, i.e. insulin secretion begins to increase after a meal, even before the blood sugar and amino acid levels have risen to a significant degree. Thus, it prevents marked rise in the levels of plasma glucose and amino acids by promoting their deposition in the tissue almost as quickly as they appear in the circulation.

Autonomic Nervous System

Insulin secretion is increased by vagal stimulation, and decreased by sympathetic stimulation. Administration of catecholamines also decreases the release of insulin. Decreased insulin secretion on exposure to stressful stimuli may be attributed to increased sympathetic discharge. In a life-threatening situation, the fight or flight response would require rapid mobilization of energy yielding substrates. This is provided by glycogenolytic and lipolytic action of catecholamines, on one hand, and by hyperglycaemia and lipolysis because of inhibition of insulin release, on the other.

GLUCAGON

Glucagon is secreted by A cells of islets of Langerhans. It is a polypeptide with 29 amino acids and a molecular weight of 3485. All mammalian glucagons seem to have similar structure.

Actions of Glucagon

Glycogenolysis in the Liver Liver is the principal target organ for the action of glucagon. Glucagon increases the blood sugar level by the following actions:

(i) Through cAMP mechanism, glucagon increases the activity of the enzyme *phosphorylase* and inactivates glycogen synthetase.

(ii) Glucagon also increases the activity of the enzymes involved in *gluconeogenesis* in the liver. It may be stressed that, unlike catecholamines, glucagon does not promote glycogenolysis in the skeletal muscle.

Lipolysis Glucagon promotes lipolysis and ketone-body formation.

Calorigenic Effect Glucagon has a calorigenic effect also. It is probably related to increased hepatic deamination of amino acids.

Besides islets of Langerhans, glucagon is produced in the gastric and intestinal mucosa by certain cells resembling the A cells of the islets. The physiological role of the extra-pancreatic glucagon secretion is not clear.

Regulation of Secretion

Blood Glucose Level A decrease in the blood glucose level is the most potent stimulus for the secretion of glucagon. The A cells begin to secrete large amount of glucagon even when the blood sugar level falls to just below 70 mg% (normal range 70–110 mg%). Conversely, hyperglycaemia inhibits glucagon release. Therefore, the secretion of glucagon increases during the period of fasting and decreases after a carbohydrate rich meal. The secretory patterns of glucagon and insulin, as well as, their actions in the liver are opposite to each other. Thus, proper ratio of the two hormones in the blood maintains the blood sugar level within a narrow normal range.

Plasma Amino Acids A protein rich meal or intravenous infusion of amino acids increases the secretion of glucagon. Since, the amino acids increase insulin secretion also, simultaneous release of glucagon along with insulin prevents the risk of hypoglycaemia, which otherwise might occur after a large protein meal.

Sympathetic Nervous System Increased sympathetic discharge to the pancreas causes inhibition of insulin release and stimulation of glucagon release. The consequent increase in blood sugar level is beneficial in various types of stress or in heavy exercise.

HORMONAL REGULATION OF BLOOD GLUCOSE LEVEL

Blood sugar level is normally maintained within a narrow range. In the morning (after an overnight fast), blood glucose level is normally between 70–

110 mg%. After a large carbohydrate meal or following oral administration of glucose in the dose, 1 gm/kg BW, blood glucose level transiently increases to about 140 mg% but prompt increase in insulin secretion brings it back to baseline value within two hours. The response, when plotted on a time scale, is known as glucose tolerance curve (Fig. 49.4).

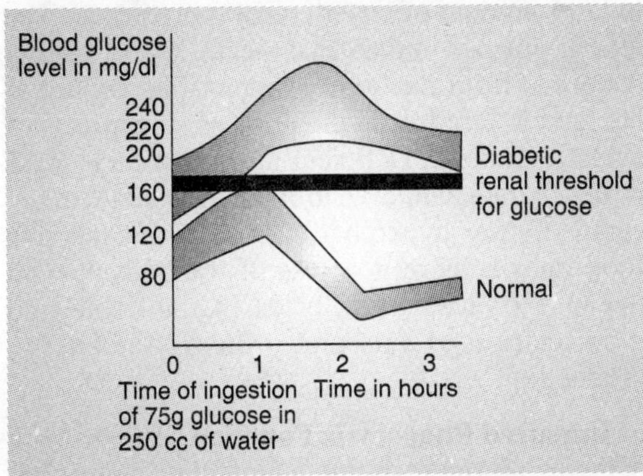

Fig. 49.4: Glucose tolerance curves.

During starvation, a number of hormones, which include glucagon, epinephrine, growth hormone and glucocorticoids, prevent any significant decrease in blood glucose level. It is obvious that there is only one hormone, insulin, which prevents hyperglycaemia, whereas at least four hormones are available for the prevention of hypoglycaemia. It may be correlated with the fact that moderate and transient increase in blood sugar is harmless and occurs after every meal. However, even moderate hypoglycaemia may lead to serious complications. The brain, retina and germinal epithelium of the gonads are particularly vulnerable to the effects of hypoglycaemia, since they cannot use any fuel other than glucose. During *normal pattern of food intake, consisting of 2–3 meals/day, insulin and glucagon are able to maintain blood glucose level within the normal range.*

After food intake, increase in blood glucose level promotes the release of insulin. Due to multiple actions of insulin, glucose becomes the chief fuel in the muscles and is also stored as glycogen in the liver and as triglycerides in the adipose tissue. During the succeeding hours, when the glucose level tends to decrease, insulin secretion stops, and instead, glucagon is poured into the bloodstream. Absence of insulin promotes lipolysis and therefore FFA becomes the chief fuel for the muscles. Glucagon promotes hepatic glycogenolysis and gluconeogenesis and thus, glucose is poured into the circulation from the liver (Fig. 49.5).

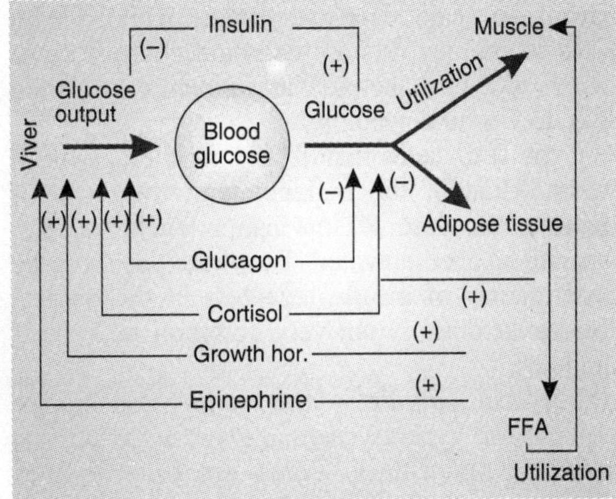

Fig. 49.5: Hormonal regulation of blood sugar level.

When food intake is curtailed for many hours, the blood glucose level begins to fall. The consequent hypoglycaemia stimulates the sympathetic nervous system through hypothalamus to promote the release of epinephrine from the adrenal medulla. Epinephrine not only supplements the action of glucagon (glycogenolysis and gluconeogenesis) but also promotes lipolysis.

When fasting is more prolonged (say for a few days) the secretion of growth hormone and cortisol is also increased. These hormones not only promote gluconeogenesis but also decrease the peripheral utilization of glucose, thereby sparing glucose for neural tissue. They also promote lipolysis, providing FFA as the alternative fuel for the other tissues specially skeletal muscles.

DIABETES MELLITUS

This is a fairly common metabolic disorder. Type-I or insulin-dependent diabetes mellitus (IDDM) is juvenile-onset diabetes. Type-II or non-insulin-dependent diabetes (NIDDM) is maturity onset diabetes mellitus. The term diabetes when used alone, is meant for "diabetes mellitus". The disorder caused by deficiency of ADH is always expressed by the full name 'diabetes insipidus'.

In Type-I diabetes, there is an absolute deficiency of insulin. It is believed to be an autoimmune disease, which manifests before the age of 40 years. The patients are usually lean. Ketosis and acidosis are common complications of this type of diabetes. Plasma insulin levels are very low or undetectable.

Type-II diabetes manifests after the age of 40 years. Most of the patients with this type of diabetes are obese. Plasma insulin levels are often normal or even elevated. But there seems to be a deficiency of insulin receptors in the tissues. Ketotic-acidosis is not very common in Type-II diabetes.

Polyuria, polydipsia and weight loss despite polyphagia, hyperglycaemia, glycosuria, ketosis, acidosis and finally coma are the cardinal symptoms and signs of diabetes mellitus.

Besides the risk of ketotic coma, non-ketotic hyperosmolar coma and predisposition to infections, patients with long-standing uncontrolled diabetes mellitus are liable to develop many other complications like neuropathy, retinopathy, cataract, nephropathy, hypertension and atherosclerosis leading to coronary artery disease or cerebral strokes.

Pathophysiology of Diabetes Mellitus (Fig. 49.6)

Hyperglycemia and its Consequences

Hyperglycemia is one of the cardinal features of diabetes mellitus. It is due to decreased peripheral utilization coupled with increased hepatic production of glucose (gluconeogenesis). Mild transient hyperglycemia is harmless and occurs after every meal. But when the blood glucose level is chronically elevated, numerous complications arise.

Glycosuria and Polyuria When the blood glucose level exceeds the renal threshold, glucose appears in the urine (glycosuria). Renal excretion of osmotically active glucose molecules leads to the loss of large amount of water in the urine (polyuria, osmotic diuresis). The resultant dehydration activates the thirst mechanism leading to large amount of water intake (polydipsia). The loss of glucose in the urine means loss of energy (calories) from the body. Appreciable amount of Na^+ and K^+ are lost in the urine as side effects of osmotic diuresis. Deficient utilization of glucose in the hypothalamic ventromedial nuclei (satiety centre) causes hyperphagia. In spite of excessive food intake, there is a loss of the body weight because of loss of calories in the urine and mobilization of fats and proteins for energy production.

Impaired Phagocytic Function Patients with diabetes are more prone to infection than non-diabetic individuals. All aspects of leucocytic phagocytic function (adherence, diapedesis, phagocytosis and intracellular killing) seem to be impaired by hyperglycemia. Infection is one of the factors which precipitate diabetic ketoacidosis.

Hyperosmolar Effects As the plasma glucose level increases above the renal threshold, progressively increasing degree of glycosuria occurs. As a result, plasma glucose level usually does not exceed 300–500 mg%. An intercurrent illness increases glucose production due to release of stress hormones as well as impairs capacity to ingest fluids. As extracellular fluid volume and plasma volume shrinks, urinary volume falls leading to decreased excretion of glucose. As a result of increased production and decreased urinary excretion, plasma glucose level may increase up to 1000 mg %. At such blood glucose level, plasma osmolality is over 375 mOsm/kg. Such hyperosmolality causes cellular dehydration especially in the central nervous system leading to impairment of cerebral function. The condition is called **non-ketotic hyperosmolar coma,** which may be fatal.

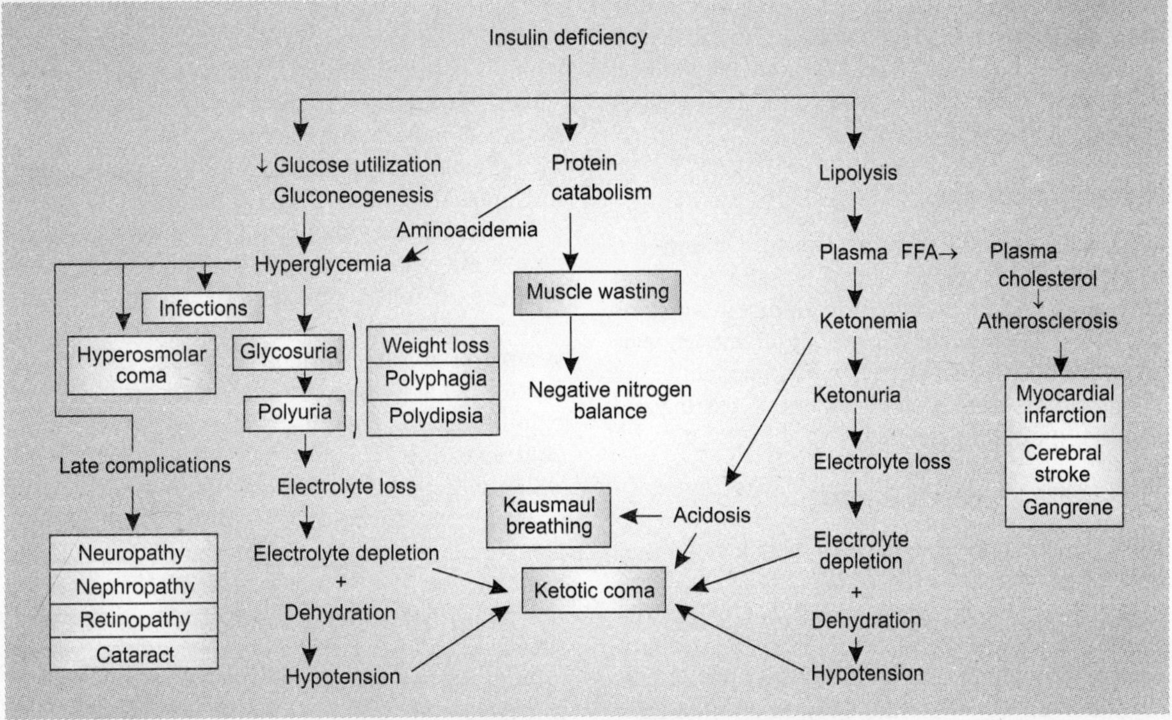

Fig. 49.6: Pathophysiology of diabetes mellitus.

Glycosylation of Haemoglobin In a normoglycemic subject, glucose molecules get *non-enzymatically* attached to a small proportion (< 7%) of haemoglobin A (Hb A_1). Three varients of Hb A_1 have been isolated by chromatographic or electrophoretic techniques, namely Hb A_1a, HbA_1b and Hb A_1c. In Hb A_1c, glucose is attached to terminal valine of each β-chain. Glycosylation blocks the reaction of 2,3-DPG with haemoglobin causing slight but clinically insignificant increase in its affinity for oxygen. In case of sustained hyperglycemia, such as in diabetes mellitus, greater proportion (10–20%) of haemoglobin A is glycosylated. The concentration of Hb A_1c has been found to reflect average blood glucose level during the previous 6–8 weeks. Therefore, measurement of Hb A_1c has become an important tool for proper regulation of insulin therapy, i.e. to find out whether the given dose of insulin has been able to maintain blood glucose level within the physiological range.

When blood glucose level is chronically elevated, even tissue proteins are glycosylated, leading to irreversible changes in their chemical structure. These chemical changes are believed to be responsible for many long-term complications of diabetes mellitus, e.g. diabetic nephropathy, retinopathy, etc.

Ketosis and its Consequences

Deficiency of insulin causes great reduction in lipogenesis and accelerates the process of lipolysis. As a result, plasma level of FFA is more than doubled. Free fatty acids provide energy to the glucose-starved insulin-sensitive tissues like skeletal muscle. However, FFA mobilization also causes formation of ketone bodies. The ketone bodies formation exceeds the rate of their utilization leading to ketosis and metabolic acidosis. Acidosis results in rapid, deep respiration (dyspnoea, Kussmaul breathing). Patient's breath smells of acetone. The urine becomes highly acidic. When the capacity of kidney to replace plasma cations accompanying the organic anions with H^+ and NH_4 is exceeded,

Na^+ and K^+ are lost in the urine. The electrolyte and water loss leads to dehydration, hypovolemia and hypotension. Finally acidosis and dehydration may depress the consciousness to the level of (ketotic) coma and death.

Protein Catabolism

In diabetes, protein anabolism is suppressed and catabolism is increased. Large amount of amino acids are used for energy production. Amino acids also act as substrate for enhanced gluconeogenesis promoted by insulin deficiency. Consequently, the patient suffers from protein depletion, wasting and negative nitrogen balance.

Glucose Tolerance Test (GTT)

This is a test for the diagnosis of diabetes mellitus. After an overnight fast, a venous blood sample is taken. Then, the patient is given 75 g of glucose orally and four blood samples are collected half-hourly for estimation of plasma glucose levels. Plasma glucose levels are plotted against time scale and the graph so obtained is known as glucose tolerance curve (Fig. 49.4). The results are interpreted as follows:

	Plasma glucose concentration (mg %)		
	Normal	*Impaired glucose tolerance*	*Diabetes mellitus*
Fasting	< 110	110–125	> 126
At 2h	< 140	140–200	> 200

Note: Glucose level can be estimated in the plasma or in whole blood. Plasma glucose values are 10–15% higher than blood glucose values.

Hypoglycemia

As noted above, hyperglycemia is a cardinal feature of diabetes mellitus. However, because of difficulty in adjusting the requirement of antidiabetic drugs, hypoglycemia occurs frequently in such patients. About 4% of deaths of IDDM are said to be due to hypoglycemia. In a diabetic patient, on antidiabetic treatment, hypoglycemia may occur following an overnight fast, missing a meal or heavy exercise.

In normal individuals, fall of blood sugar level below 80 mg% shuts off insulin secretion. At level of 70 mg%, glucagon secretion begins to increase. At still lower level, CNS-mediated sympatho-adrenal discharge is activated. This results in a non-specific sense of arousal, anxiety, palpitation, tachycardia, shakiness, hunger and cold sweating.

In many patients of IDDM, both glucagon and epinephrine secretory response is deficient. Hence, the above mentioned warning symptoms fail to occur. The **hypoglycemic unawareness** is potentially dangerous because blood glucose level may fall so low that *cerebral manifestations of hypoglycemia* occur. These include impaired mentation, lethargy, confusion, tremor, vertigo, paraesthesias, incoordination of movements, slurred speech, diplopia and other visual defects. At still lower level (<30 mg%) convulsions, coma and even death may occur.

Hypoglycemia may also be observed in patients with hepatic failure. Insulin secreting tumour of pancreatic islets (insulinoma) is a rare but potentially lethal cause of hypoglycemia.

The hypoglycemia described above is classified as **post-absorptive (fasting) hypoglycemia.** Another type is **post-prandial (reactive) hypoglycemia**. In this case, hypoglycemia occurs exclusively after meals, typically within 4 hours after ingestion of food. Post-prandial hypoglycemia is common in patients who have undergone gastric resection. In such patients, rapid movement of swallowed food into the intestine leads to sudden and marked increase in insulin secretion which produces hypoglycemia.

50

CHAPTER

Hormonal Control of Calcium Metabolism

Three hormones, namely, parathyroid hormone (PTH), calcitonin and cholecalciferol (vitamin D_3) are involved in the regulation of extracellular calcium ion concentration. Plasma calcium level needs to be regulated within a very narrow range because of its marked effect on neuromuscular and cardiac excitability. In addition, normal ionic calcium level in the plasma is essential for bone mineralization and maintenance of cell membrane integrity. Ionic calcium (Ca^{2+}) is also involved in many intracellular biochemical reactions, excitation-contraction coupling in muscles and in blood coagulation.

CALCIUM METABOLISM

Normal adult human body contains about one kg of calcium. Of this, about 99% is present in the skeleton as hydroxyl-apatite [$Ca_{10}(PO_4)_6(OH)_2$] and the rest 1% in the soft tissues and extracellular fluids. Normal plasma calcium level is about 10 mg% (normal range 9–11 mg%). Calcium is present in the plasma both as ionic and non-ionic form (Table 50.1)

Table 50.1: Distribution of calcium in human plasma

Diffusible	
Ionized (Ca^{++})	50%
Complexed (to bicarbonate and citrate)	10%
Non-diffusible (Protein bound)	40%

The amount of calcium bound to proteins varies with the total protein concentration as well as pH of the plasma. In hypoproteinaemia, the total plasma calcium level is low but the symptoms of tetany (ionic calcium deficiency) do not occur because only the protein bound component is affected but plasma ionic calcium (Ca^{2+}) concentration is normal.

On the other hand, in alkalosis, symptoms of hypocalcaemic tetany occur even though the total plasma calcium level is normal. It is because with increase in pH, more of plasma proteins are ionized which bind with ionic calcium, decreasing the concentration of plasma free ionic calcium.

Calcium Balance (Fig. 50.1)

On a normal diet, the daily intake of calcium may vary from 200–1500 mg, depending mainly on the amount of milk and milk products consumed.

With an average intake of 1000 mg of calcium, its net intestinal absorption is only 175 mg/day. Calcium is absorbed mainly in the duodenum by an active transport mechanism regulated by $1,25(OH)_2D_3$. Parathormone indirectly promotes absorption of calcium by increasing the renal synthesis of $1,25(OH)_2D_3$. Dietary lactose promotes intestinal calcium absorption by some

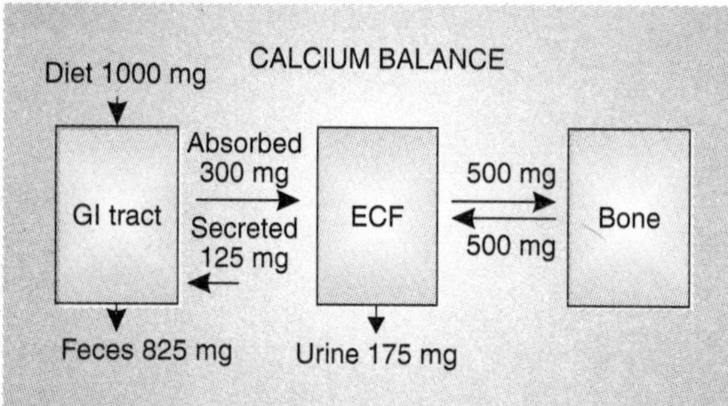

Fig. 50.1: Calcium metabolism in an adult.

unknown mechanism. When the dietary intake of calcium is chronically low, relatively greater percentage of dietary calcium is absorbed. The adaptation seems to be produced through greater synthesis of $1,25(OH)_2D_3$. Intestinal calcium absorption is decreased by substances that form insoluble salts with calcium ion, e.g. phosphates and oxalates. On the other hand, a high protein diet promotes calcium absorption.

Total extracellular fluid space contains about 900 mg of calcium, which is in dynamic equilibrium with skeleton. About 1% of the skeletal calcium (10 g) is readily exchangeable with calcium in extracellular fluid and constitutes a fairly large reservoir. The remaining 99% of bone calcium is only slowly exchangeable. Nearly 500 mg of calcium is deposited into and mobilized from the bone daily in a continuous process of remodelling.

Calcium is secreted into the intestine through bile, pancreatic juice and intestinal secretions but is completely reabsorbed.

Renal Handling of Calcium

About 60% of plasma calcium is ultrafiltrable. However, about 98–99% of the filtered calcium is reabsorbed in the renal tubules. About 60% of the reabsorption occurs in the proximal convoluted tubules and the remaining in the loop of Henle and distal tubules. *Distal tubular reabsorption of calcium is regulated by parathormone.*

In a normal healthy adult, the excretion of calcium in the urine and faeces exactly equals the daily intake of calcium.

BONE METABOLISM

Bone is a living tissue, consisting of tough organic matrix impregnated by calcium salts. The organic matrix is composed of collagen fibres and a small amount of homogeneous ground substance. The collagen fibres give tensile strength to the bone. The inorganic component of bone consists primarily of calcium and phosphate in the form of hydroxy-apatite crystals $[(Ca_{10}(PO_4)_6(OH)_2]$. Each crystal is about 400 Å units long, 100 Å units wide, 10–30 Å units thick. It is shaped like a long, flat plate. Small amounts of magnesium, sodium, potassium and carbonate are also present in the bone adsorbed on the surface of hydroxyapatite crystals.

Remodelling of Bone

Deposition and resorption of bone are continual processes occurring throughout the life. By this process, bone can adjust to the changes in the degree of bone stress. The thickness or even the shape of a bone can change according to the mechanical forces acting on it.

Bone Formation

Bone is continuously deposited by the **osteoblasts**. These cells are found in the periosteum and endosteum. The osteoblasts secrete collagen and the ground substance. The collagen polymerizes to form collagen fibres. The resultant organic tissue is known as the osteoid. As the osteoid is being formed, some of the osteoblasts get entrapped in it and that are now called **osteocytes**. Soon after the osteoid is formed, hydroxyapatite crystals are deposited on the surface of collagen fibres. The factors causing precipitation of calcium phosphate from the ECF are not exactly known. Osteoblastic activity is associated with increased concentration of alkaline phosphatase. The enzyme hydrolyses phosphate esters to increase the concentration of phosphate. As a result, calcium phosphate solubility product ($Ca^{2+} \times PO_4^{3-}$) increases to such a critical value that the salt precipitates out. Some unknown property of the bone collagen may also be helping in binding the calcium salts.

Long fine cytoplasmic processes extend from one osteocyte to the next throughout the bone, ultimately connecting all the osteocytes and osteoblasts. Thus, osteoblasts present outside the compact and spongy bone and osteocytes present within the bone form a system of interconnected cells that spread over all the bone surfaces.

Bone Resorption

Bone mineral may be removed from the bone by a rapid mechanism, taking a few minutes called *osteolysis* or by a slow process taking several days or weeks known as *osteoclastic resorption.*

Parathormone is the chief hormone responsible for the resorption of bone. When a large dose of parathormone is injected, plasma calcium level rises within a few minutes due to activity of already existing osteocytes and osteoclasts. If parathormone level is chronically elevated, a slower phase of bone resorption takes several days or weeks to develop fully. It results from activation and proliferation of osteoclasts.

VITAMIN D

Besides dietary intake, cutaneous synthesis is the other and more important source of vitamin D (cholecalciferol) in the body. In the skin, it is produced in the inner layers of the epidermis by the action of ultraviolet rays on 7-dehydrocholesterol. Although the cutaneous production of vitamin D is restricted in individuals with poor solar exposure, excessive exposure to the sun, e.g. in fishermen, does not produce vitamin D toxicity, because of blockade in the synthetic reactions (Fig. 50.2) and conversion of previtamin D_3 to inert metabolites like lumisterol and tachysterol.

Vitamin D_3 is transported in the plasma bound to a specific globulin called vitamin D-binding protein (DBP). In the liver, vitamin D_3 is converted to 25-OH-cholecalciferol [25(OH)D_3]. Another enzyme 1-α-hydroxylase present in the cells of proximal convoluted tubules of the kidney converts 25(OH)D_3 into 1,25-dihydroxy cholecalciferol [1,25(OH)$_2$$D_3$].

The steps in the biosynthesis and degradation of vitamin D metabolites are shown in Fig. 50.2.

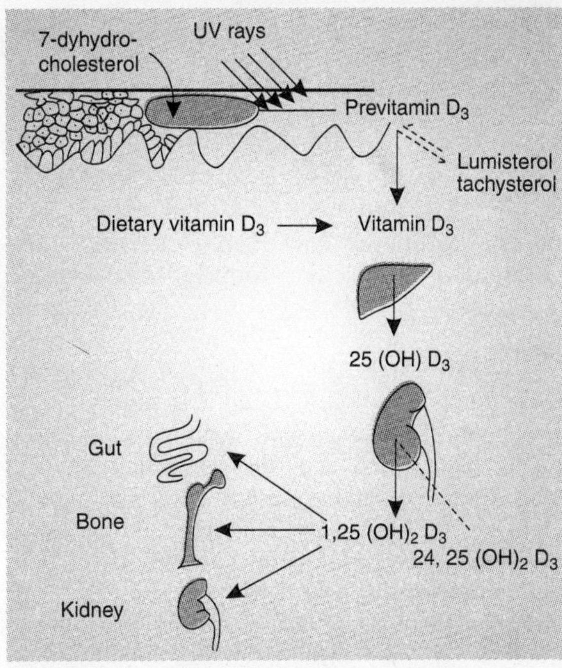

Fig. 50.2: Synthesis, activation and sites of action of vitamin D.

Actions

Since 1,25(OH)$_2$$D_3$, the active metabolite of vitamin D, is produced in the kidney and acts on many tissues away from the site of its production, it is often called a hormone. The endogenous synthesis and feedback control over its synthesis are other important reasons for labelling cholecalciferol a hormone rather than a vitamin. Further, in the target cells 1, 25(OH)$_2$$D_3$ acts like a steroid hormone and increases the synthesis of mRNA to increase the concentration of calcium-binding protein in many tissues especially in intestinal mucosa. The intestine, kidney and the bone are its chief target organs.

Intestine

In the intestinal mucosa, 1,25(OH)$_2$$D_3$ increases the absorption of dietary Ca^{2+}. As mentioned above, it is done by increasing the synthesis of calcium-binding protein in the intestinal epithelium and thereby increasing the transport of calcium from intestinal lumen to the epithelium. The rate of calcium absorption appears to be directly proportionate to the amount of calcium-binding protein present in the mucosal cells.

Kidney

In the kidney, $1,25(OH)_2D_3$ increases the reabsorption of calcium from the renal tubules.

Bone

Deficiency of vitamin D in the body due to inadequate solar exposure, coupled with inadequate dietary intake of the vitamin, results in well-known disorders called rickets in young children, and osteomalacia in adults. In these two disorders, failure of mineralization of osteoid can be demonstrated. However, the exact role of vitamin D or its metabolite, $1,25(OH)_2D_3$ in the process of *bone mineralization* is not clear. Vitamin D might have a direct action on osteogenesis or it could influence the mineralization by increasing the Ca^{2+} concentration in the extracellular fluid.

In pharmacological toxic doses, vitamin D promotes *mobilization of calcium* from the bone leading to hypercalcaemia and pathological deposition of calcium in many soft tissues like kidney, arteries and heart.

50 Receptor sites for $1,25(OH)_2D_3$ have been observed in many other tissues such as brain, various endocrine glands, placenta, testis, and monocytes, etc. The physiological role of vitamin D in these tissues is under investigation.

Feedback Control on Synthesis of $1,25(OH)_2D_3$

The formation of $1,25(OH)_2D_3$ is tightly regulated whereas that of $25(OH)D_3$ is not so. Excessive dietary intake of vitamin D_3 leads to proportionate increase in the level of plasma $25(OH)D_3$, but plasma level of $1,25\ (OH)_2D_3$ is not increased.

The activity of the enzyme 1-α-hydroxylase is increased by parathormone, oestrogens and prolactin. The last two stimulators help to provide more calcium to the pregnant and lactating mother.

In normal individuals, a decrease in plasma calcium level results in increased secretion of PTH from the parathyroid gland. The consequent increase in the activity of 1-α-hydroxylase, and hence in the synthesis of $1,25(OH)_2D_3$, leads to restoration of plasma calcium level to normal.

When plasma calcium levels are adequate, most of the $25(OH)D_3$ is converted to metabolically inert $24,25(OH)_2D_3$ in the kidney rather than $1,25(OH)_2D_3$ due to suppression of 1-α-hydroxylase.

PARATHYROID GLANDS

There are four parathyroid glands, embedded in the superior and the inferior poles, on the posterior surface of the thyroid gland. Each parathyroid gland measures only 6 mm × 3 mm × 2 mm. The small size and the location of the parathyroid glands make them vulnerable to their accidental removal during thyroidectomy.

Histologically, majority of the cells of parathyroid gland are small and have agranular (clear) cytoplasm. These cells, known as the **chief cells**, secrete parathyroid hormone (PTH or parathormone). Some large cells containing acidophilic granules called oxyphil cells are also present among the chief cells but their function is not known.

Actions

Human parathormone is a polypeptide with a molecular weight of 9,500.

Parathormone acts on the bone and the kidney by cAMP mechanism to increase plasma calcium and decrease plasma inorganic phosphate levels.

Bone

Several days of increased parathyroid activity are required to demonstrate the actions of the hormone. Parathormone causes:

(a) Activation of the osteoclasts already present in the bone, and

(b) Formation of new osteoclasts from osteoprogenitor cells. Osteoclasts are multinucleated giant cells which produce resorption of bone surfaces in contact with them. Osteoclasts are believed to send out finger-like projections towards the bone which release proteolytic digestive enzymes, as well as, acids like citric acid and lactic acid. The proteolytic enzymes digest the organic matrix, whereas the acids dissolve the bone minerals. Small fragments of the bone may be phagocytosed as such and digested within the cytoplasm of the osteoclasts. Calcium and phosphate released by the osteoclastic activity are poured directly into the extracellular fluid.

Kidney

Parathormone *increases the distal tubular reabsorption of calcium* in the kidney. However, hypercalciuria is one of the characteristic features of primary hyperparathyroidism. This paradoxical effect can be explained by the fact that in hyperparathyroidism, hypercalcaemia produces such a large load of filtered calcium in glomerular filtrate that in spite of increased distal tubular calcium reabsorption, the net excretion of urinary calcium is increased.

Parathormone *decreases the reabsorption of inorganic phosphate* in the proximal convoluted tubules of the kidney. By this action, parathormone produces phosphaturia and hypophosphatemia.

In the kidney, parathormone also increases the synthesis of the enzyme 1-α-hydroxylase which converts $25(OH)D_3$ to $1,25(OH)_2D_3$. Thus, parathormone indirectly increases the intestinal absorption of calcium.

Regulation of PTH Secretion

Circulating levels of ionized calcium act directly on the parathyroid glands in a feedback fashion to regulate the secretion of parathormone. Even slight decrease in plasma calcium ion concentration increases the secretion of PTH, whereas increase in calcium ion concentration decreases its secretion.

The readily exchangeable calcium pool of the bone also influences the plasma calcium ion concentration. After an intravenous injection of a large dose of calcium salts, plasma calcium concentration rises to a high level. However, within one hour, deposition of calcium in the bones restores the plasma calcium levels to normal. Conversely, calcium can be easily withdrawn from the readily exchangeable pool, in case of depletion of plasma ionic calcium. The exchangeable pool of calcium in the bone can maintain total plasma calcium level at nearly 7 mg%. Parathormone is required to maintain it at the normal level of 9–11 mg%. Inadvertent parathyroidectomy during thyroid surgery produces hypocalcaemia and tetany but the plasma calcium level seldom falls below 7 mg%.

An acute decrease in plasma Mg^{2+} concentration is another stimulant for secretion of parathormone.

CALCITONIN

Calcitonin is a polypeptide containing 32 amino acids. It has a molecular weight of 3,500. Calcitonin is secreted by the parafollicular cells of the thyroid gland. These cells, also known as clear cells or C cells, are large, secretory granule-containing cells lying in the interstitium between the thyroid follicles.

Actions

Bone is the only well-established target organ for calcitonin. It prevents formation of new osteoclasts from the osteoprogenitor cells. Thus, it tends to lower the plasma calcium concentration by shifting the balance in favour of deposition of calcium salts in the bone.

Regulation of Secretion

The secretion of calcitonin is regulated by plasma Ca^{2+} concentration. An increase of plasma total calcium level above 9.5 mg% stimulates the secretion of calcitonin. A linear relation can be demonstrated between plasma calcium level and the secretion of calcitonin.

As mentioned above, the parathormone and calcitonin secretion is regulated by plasma Ca^{2+} level in a reciprocal manner. However, in adults, the secretion of calcitonin is of minor importance. Normal plasma Ca^{2+} concentration is maintained chiefly by parathormone. Thyroidectomy removes the calcitonin secreting cells also, but plasma calcium level remains normal if the parathyroid glands are intact.

It is believed that calcitonin may have a more significant role in children, in whom the rate of turnover of bone is high. It may also protect the bones of the mother from excessive calcium loss during pregnancy when plasma parathormone and $1,25(OH)_2D_3$ levels are physiologically elevated.

PATHOPHYSIOLOGY

Hypocalcaemia

Dietary deficiency of calcium alone usually does not produce hypocalcaemia, because certain adaptive mechanisms in the intestine help to absorb completely the small amounts of calcium ingested.

On the other hand, vitamin D deficiency, due to inadequate intake or inadequate solar exposure, results in not only hypocalcaemia, but also metabolic bone disease in the form of rickets in young children and osteomalacia in adults. In both these metabolic disorders, there is softening and deformities of bone due to a failure of mineralization of osteoid. Osteomalacia is more commonly observed in "pardah" observing women in whom the problem manifests specially during pregnancy and lactation.

Parathormone deficiency is another cause of hypocalcaemia. It may be produced by inadvertent removal of all the four parathyroid glands during total thyroidectomy (hypoparathyroidism). In another related disorder, a receptor defect results in parathormone deficiency effects even though plasma parathormone levels are normal (pseudo-hypoparathyroidism).

Tetany The neuromuscular effects of hypocalcaemia, called *hypocalcaemic tetany,* are characterized by neuromuscular irritability, muscle cramps especially in the extremities known as carpopedal spasm (hand and feet spasm) (Fig. 50.3), laryngospasm, paraesthesias and even convulsions. Laryngospasm may produce fatal asphyxia.

Subclinical tetany can be unmasked by the following clinical tests.

(i) Chvostek's Sign (pronounced "vostek's sign"): Spasm of ipsilateral facial muscles elicited by tapping over the facial nerve at the angle of the jaw.

(ii) Trousseau's Sign (pronounced "troosoz's sign"): Spasm of the muscles of the forearm leading to flexion of the wrist and thumb and extension of the fingers (Fig. 50.3) induced by occluding the blood circulation of the forearm with blood pressure cuff up to three minutes.

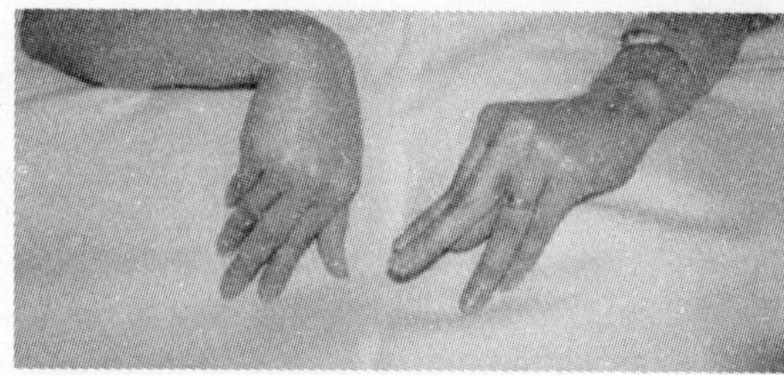

Fig. 50.3: Position of the hands in tetany (Trousseau's sign).

Ionized calcium is required for clotting of blood. However, the level of plasma Ca^{2+} at which fatal tetany occurs is much above the level at which blood clotting is affected. In other words, hypocalcaemia is seldom a cause of bleeding disorders.

A more common cause of *tetany* in adults is *alkalosis* (metabolic or respiratory type). In alkalosis, plasma proteins undergo greater degree of ionization and bind with ionic calcium. Thus though total plasma calcium level is normal, there is a decrease in the plasma concentration of ionized calcium, leading to tetany.

Hypercalcaemia

Hypercalcaemia results from excessive secretion of parathormone (e.g. primary hyperparathyroidism) or from excessive intake of pharmacological doses of vitamin D. Hypercalcaemia produces muscle weakness, lethargy, constipation and even coma. Increased load of filtered calcium predisposes the patient to renal stone disease. Metastatic calcification in the soft tissues may also occur.

Primary hyperparathyroidism is characterised by hypercalcaemia leading to hypercalciuria, hyperphosphaturia leading to hypophosphataemia; renal stones and bone fractures (due to excessive osteoclastic activity).

Metabolic Bone Disease

This term is used to include a group of generalized disorders of the bone like rickets and osteomalacia, hyperparathyroidism and osteoporosis.

Nutritional Rickets

It is caused by nutritional deficiency of vitamin D coupled with inadequate solar exposure. Vegetarian diet including milk is a poor source of vitamin D. This disorder usually manifests between the age of 6 months to 2 years, when the growth of bones is vary rapid and the baby is kept mostly indoors. The disorder is particularly common in industrial areas where environmental pollution (smoke) prevents the solar ultraviolet rays from reaching the earth. The most characteristic feature of this disorder is failure of mineralization of organic matrix of bone. The organic component of bone is normal or somewhat excessive (Fig. 50.4). Hence, the bones become soft and deformed. There is frontal bossing and posterior flattening of the skull, bulging of costochondral junctions and enlargement of wrists. Deformities of the legs (bow-legs or knock-knee) may occur (Fig. 50.5). There is severe muscular weakness leading to inability to stand without

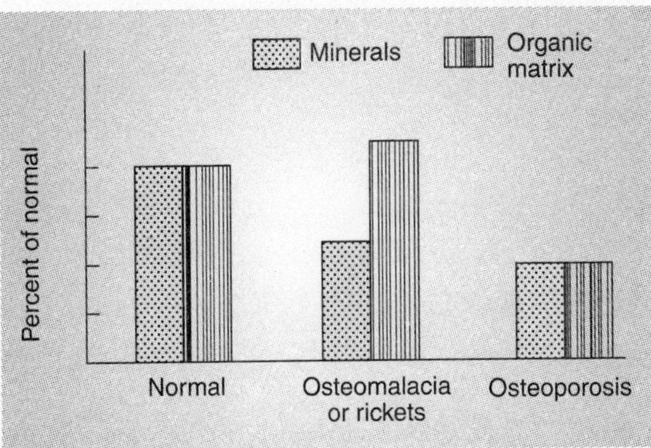

Fig. 50.4: Changes in organic component and mineral content of bone in osteomalacia and osteoporosis.

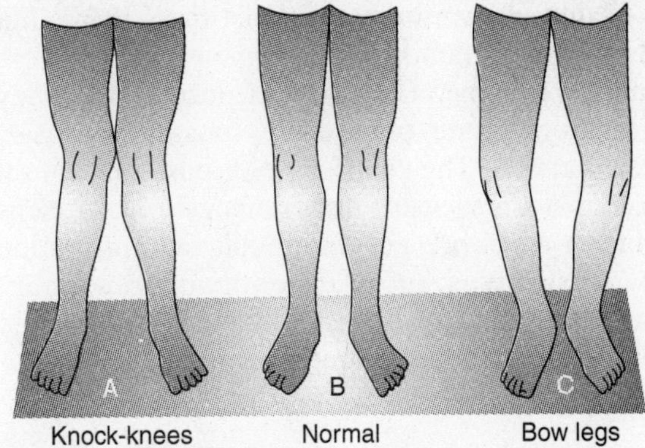

Fig. 50.5: Effects of rickets. A, knock knees; B, normal child; C, bow-legs.

support. Characteristic biochemical features include hypocalcaemia, hypophosphataemia, hypocalciuria and elevated plasma alkaline phosphatase level. Plasma 25(OH)D_3 level is low.

Vitamin D deficiency in adults also produces softness of bone. The disorder called **osteomalacia** occurs more commonly in purdah-observing poor women living in industrial areas. The characteristic features include severe pain and deformities of spine and pelvis. Biochemical features are similar to those seen in rickets.

Osteoporosis

This disorder is characterized by a reduction of bone mass per unit volume with normal ratio of mineral to organic matrix, i.e. there is loss of both organic and inorganic components of bone (Fig. 50.4). Osteoporotic bone is liable to fracture with minimum trauma.

All individuals gain bone mass during adolescence. After a plateau, all of us begin to lose bone mass after the age of 40 years. Consequently, some degree of osteoporosis can be seen in all individuals over the age of 50 years, especially in women after menopause. In most cases, the osteoporosis is said to be primary, senile osteoporosis, since it cannot be attributed to any particular cause.

Cushing's disease or hyperthyroidism also produce osteoporosis (secondary osteoporosis).

Adult women have less bone mass than adult men. After menopause, women lose it more rapidly than men (Fig. 50.6). Consequently, they are more prone to develop (postmenopausal) osteoporosis. The chief cause of postmenopausal osteoporosis seems to be deficiency of oestrogens since it can be prevented by regular administration of oestrogens in postmenopausal women. However, the mechanism by which oestrogen deficiency produces bone loss is not known.

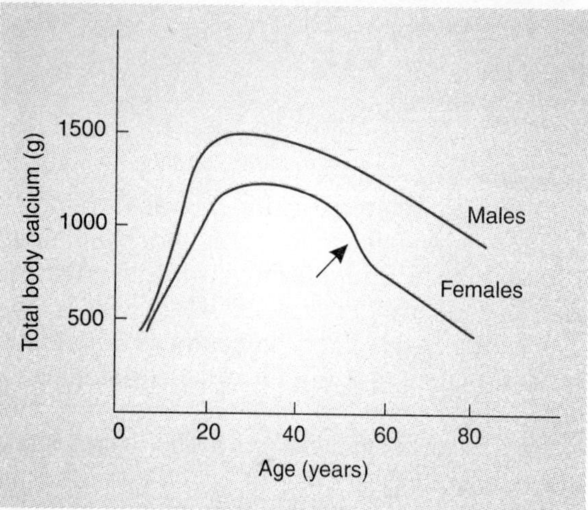

Fig. 50.6: Effect of age and sex on total body calcium (bone mass). Arrow points to the postmenopausal rapid bone loss.

Immobilization is another cause of osteoporosis. Weight-bearing and muscular activity seem to be essential for maintenance of normal bone mass. When a limb is placed in plaster of Paris cast, the bones undergo rapid osteoporosis. Weightlessness in space travel produces significant osteoporosis within few months. It has been suggested that adequate calcium intake and moderate exercise may prevent or slow down the progress of senile or postmenopausal osteoporosis.

In senile osteoporosis, plasma and urine calcium levels are usually normal. Radiological evidence is seen only in advanced cases of osteoporosis (Fig. 50.7). Bone biopsy provides definitive diagnosis of various types of metabolic bone disease.

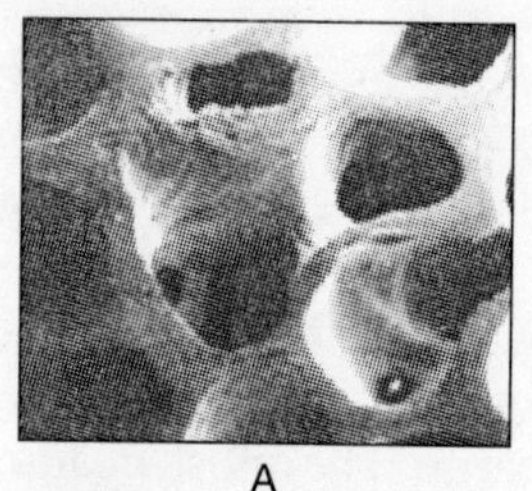
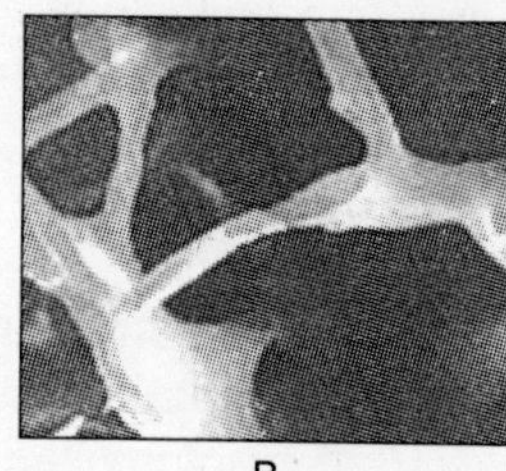

A B

Fig. 50.7: Spongy bone in a normal adult (left) and a patient with severe osteoporosis (right).

FUNCTION TESTS

Vitamin D deficiency disorders are characterized by hypocalcaemia along with low plasma 25 hydroxycholecalciferol [25(OH)D] level. In hypoparathyroidism, plasma calcium level is low, but plasma 25(OH)D level is normal.

Laboratory investigations for primary hyperparathyroidism include estimation of plasma calcium and parathyroid hormone levels.

Endocrine Function of the Heart, Kidneys and Pineal Gland

CHAPTER 51

The chief endocrine glands have been described in the previous chapters. In addition, many other tissues of the body contain isolated cells or groups of cells with endocrine function. The gastrointestinal hormones have been discussed earlier. Cytokines, interleukins, prostaglandins and various growth factors, described elsewhere in this book, have hormone-like actions. In this chapter, the hormonal functions of the heart, kidney and pineal gland shall be discussed.

ENDOCRINE FUNCTION OF HEART: ATRIAL NATRIURETIC PEPTIDE

The atrial muscle cells synthesize and store a polypeptide called atrial natriuretic peptide **(ANP)** which increases the urinary excretion of Na^+. Under electron microscope, granules of ANP precursors can be seen in the atrial myocytes. The circulating form of ANP has 28 amino acid residues. Distension (stretch) of the atrial wall is the physiological stimulus for the release of ANP. The secretion of ANP has been found to increase under the following conditions:

(i) Ingestion of high sodium diet which increases ECF volume.
(ii) Infusion of isotonic saline which increases ECF volume.
(iii) Immersion of the body in water up to the neck. This procedure counteracts the effect of gravity on the circulation leading to an *increase in central venous pressure*.
(iv) Stretch of isolated strips of atrial muscle (*in vitro*).

Decreased central venous pressure as occurs on rising from supine to standing posture leads to a small *decrease in plasma ANP levels.*

In view of the observations discussed above, it has been concluded that the atria act as low pressure volume receptors and the rate of ANP secretion is proportionate to the degree of distension of the atria.

Actions of ANP

1. Increased GFR ANP causes vasodilatation of afferent and efferent arterioles of the kidney leading to increased renal blood flow and increased GFR. As a result, there is an increase in filtered load of Na^+ (Filtered load = GFR × Plasma Na^+ concentration).

2. Decreased Renin Secretion The secretion of renin from the afferent arterioles is decreased.

3. Decreased Aldosterone Secretion ANP causes decreased secretion of aldosterone from the adrenal cortex by two mechanisms. (i) Reduced plasma renin activity decreases plasma angiotensin II levels. (ii) ANP decreases aldosterone secretion by a direct action on the zona glomerulosa of the adrenal cortex.

4. Decreased NaCl Reabsorption ANP reduces NaCl reabsorption in the collecting ducts of the kidney. This action is partly due to a reduction in plasma aldosterone level and partly due to a direct action of ANP on the ductal epithelial cells.

5. Decreased ADH secretion from the posterior pituitary gland.

6. Blood Pressure ANP lowers blood pressure by: (a) decreasing renin-angiotensin II levels and (b) by decreasing the responsiveness of vascular smooth muscle to many vasoconstrictor substances.

ENDOCRINE FUNCTION OF KIDNEYS

Renin-Angiotensin System

Renin

The tunica media of the afferent arterioles of the kidney contains epitheloid cells. These cells synthesize and store secretory granules of an enzyme called renin. The afferent arterioles act as baroreceptors and respond to the afferent arteriolar blood pressure. Renin secretion is increased by the following factors:

(i) **A fall in the afferent arteriolar blood pressure** This is the most important mechanism of renin release. In addition, renin release is increased by the following other mechanisms.

(ii) **Increased sympathetic neural discharge** to the renal vessels or increased circulating catecholamine levels.

(iii) **Decreased delivery of NaCl to the distal convoluted tubules** This action is mediated through the macula densa cells.

(iv) **Prostaglandins** also increase renin release.

Acting through one or more of the four factors named above, renin secretion is increased in:

Hypotension,
Haemorrhage,
Dehydration,
Upright posture,
Sodium depletion,
Trauma,
Surgery
Anxiety.

Renin secretion is also increased in *pathological conditions* such as:

Renal artery stenosis,
Congestive heart failure and
Cirrhosis of the liver.

As discussed below, increased renin secretion leads to increased plasma angiotensin II level which inhibits renin secretion in a negative feedback manner. Increased afferent arteriolar pressure and increased delivery of NaCl to the macula densa cells also inhibit renin secretion.

Angiotensin

Angiotensinogen, a glycoprotein, is the only substrate of renin. It is synthesized in the liver and circulates in the plasma as an α_2-globulin.

Renin splits angiotensinogen to form a physiologically inactive decapeptide, angiotensin I. Angiotensin I is further split by an enzyme called **angiotensin converting enzyme (ACE)** into a physiologically active octapeptide, angiotensin II (Fig. 48.6). The converting enzyme is widely distributed in the endothelial cells of the vascular beds, especially in the lungs. Hence, most of the conversion of angiotensin I to angiotensin II occurs in the pulmonary circulation. Angiotensin II has half-life of 1–2 minutes. It is degraded by an enzyme angiotensinase, present in the red blood cells and many other tissues, into angiotensin III. Of many actions of angiotensin II, only aldosterone stimulating activity seems to be retained by angiotensin III. Angiotensins II and III are degraded into inactive metabolites.

Actions of Angiotensin II

1. Increased Aldosterone Secretion Angiotensin II acts on the zona glomerulosa cells of adrenal cortex and stimulates the secretion of aldosterone. Consequently, there is retention of NaCl (and water) in the kidneys. Renin-angiotensin II-aldosterone axis constitutes the most important mechanism for the maintenance of ECF volume.

2. Vasoconstriction Angiotensin II is very potent vasoconstrictor. Weight for weight it has

4 to 8 times greater vasopressor activity than norepinephrine. However, its vasopressor activity is reduced in states of sodium depletion. In such circumstances, it is more effective as a salt retaining hormone than a vasoconstrictor hormone. Its pressor effect seems to be more important in hypotensive conditions like haemorrhage.

3. Thirst Angiotensin II acts on circumventricular organs of the brain to increase thirst, thereby promoting water intake.

4. ADH Secretion It promotes secretion of ADH by the posterior pituitary gland.

5. NaCl Reabsorption It enhances NaCl reabsorption by the proximal convoluted tubules of the kidney.

6. Decreased GFR It decreases GFR by causing contraction of the mesangial cells of the renal glomeruli.

7. Norepinephrine Release It facilitates the release of norepinephrine by a direct action on the postganglionic sympathetic nerves.

Erythropoietin

It is discussed on page 28.

1,25-Dihydroxycholecalciferol

It is discussed on page 549.

Endocrine Function of Pineal Gland

The pineal gland is a small cone-shaped structure (like the cone of a pine tree, hence the name). It lies in the centre of the brain behind the third ventricle (Fig. 30.5). It consists of two types of cells:

(i) Pinealocytes which predominate and produce a hormone melatonin (N-acetyl-5-methoxytryptamine), and
(ii) Neuroglial cells.

The gland is highly vascular. In children, the pineal gland is rather large in size but before puberty it involutes and becomes calcified.

The mammalian pineal gland is a neuroendocrine transducer. Photopic information from the retina is transmitted through the retino-hypothalamic tract to the suprachiasmatic nucleus, and then it passes to the superior cervical ganglion. From here, postganglionic sympathetic fibres carry the impulses to the pineal gland. The neuronal system is activated by darkness and suppressed by light. The daily rhythm of melatonin secretion is also controlled by an endogenous circadian pace maker located in the suprachiasmatic nucleus.

Actions of Melatonin

The name melatonin is derived from its ability to aggregate melanin granules and thereby lighten the colour of the frog's skin. This does not happen in mammals. Based largely on the information obtained in experimental animals and some clinical studies in humans, the following actions of melatonin have been proposed.

1. Sleep Plasma melatonin level begins to rise soon after sunset and reaches the peak at middle of the night and then declines in early hours of the morning. Peak night time melatonin concentration is six times the day time concentration. Administration of melatonin in physiological doses produces reduced alertness, increased fatigue and early onset of sleep. Therefore, it has been suggested that melatonin has a role in the production of sleep-wakefulness cycles.

2. Circadian Rhythms Administration of exogenous melatonin has been shown to produce beneficial effects on the symptoms of jet-lag. Melatonin seems to hasten the adaptation to the new day-night cycle by resynchronization of circadian rhythm.

3. Sexual Maturation and Reproduction In humans, peak night time plasma melatonin concentration declines progressively throughout childhood and adolescence. It has been proposed that the onset of puberty is related to the decline in melatonin secretion. Some children with precocious puberty have lower plasma melatonin levels for their age.

4. Free Radical Scavenging In pharmacologic doses, melatonin is more potent scavenger of highly toxic free radicals than other known antioxidants (glutathione or vitamin E).

Section XII

Reproduction

CHAPTER 52

The Male Reproductive System

FUNCTIONAL ANATOMY

The male reproductive system consists of:

(i) Paired gonads, the testes which produce spermatozoa and secrete androgens, the male sex hormones,

(ii) A series of ducts which lead from the testis to the copulatory organ, the penis, and

(iii) Several male accessory glands namely, the prostate, seminal vesicles and bulbourethral glands.

Each testis is composed of about 100 coiled tubules, each about 3/4th metre long, called the seminiferous tubules lined by germinal epithelium.

Both ends of the tubules empty into a network of passages called the rete-testes. From here, vasa-efferentes lead the sperms into about six-metre long and coiled tube called the epididymis, where the sperms undergo further maturation. Further on, the sperms enter a thick-walled duct, the vas deferens, where they are stored specially in its terminal part called the ampulla. The ampulla of the vas deferens is joined by the seminal vesicle, a tortuous, sacculated tubular gland. The common duct so formed is called the ejaculatory duct which opens into the prostatic part of the urethra. Semen ejaculated during the male sexual act is composed of fluids from vas deferens, the seminal vesicles, the prostate gland and mucus derived from a large number of urethral glands located all along the urethra and from bilateral bulbo-urethral glands (Fig. 52.1).

Besides the production of sperms, the testes have an endocrine function also. Certain large polyhedral cells situated in the connective tissue between the seminiferous tubules are called the Leydig cells or the interstitial cells of Leydig. These cells secrete androgens, chiefly the testosterone (Fig. 52.2).

SPERMATOGENESIS

In the male, gametogenesis, the production of sperms, the male gametes, begins at puberty and continues throughout the remainder life. Spermatogenesis occurs continuously in all the seminiferous tubules. Two types of cells can be recognized histologically in the seminiferous tubules:

i. Those in the process of becoming sperms.

ii. Large supporting cells, the *Sertoli cells* that extend from the basement membrane to the lumen of the tubules (Fig. 52.3).

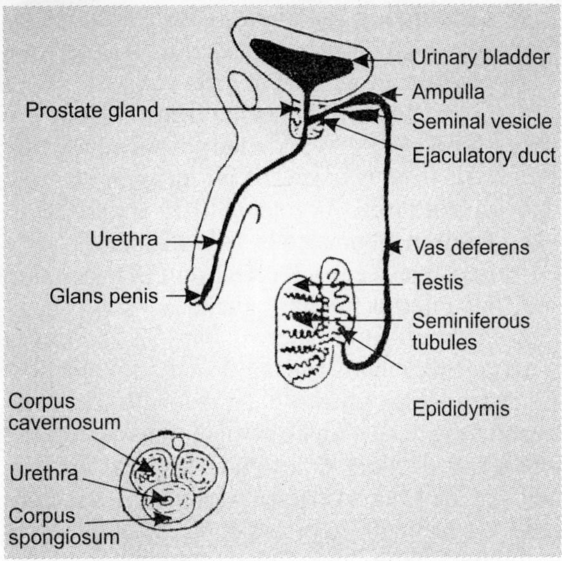

Fig. 52.1: The male reproductive tract.

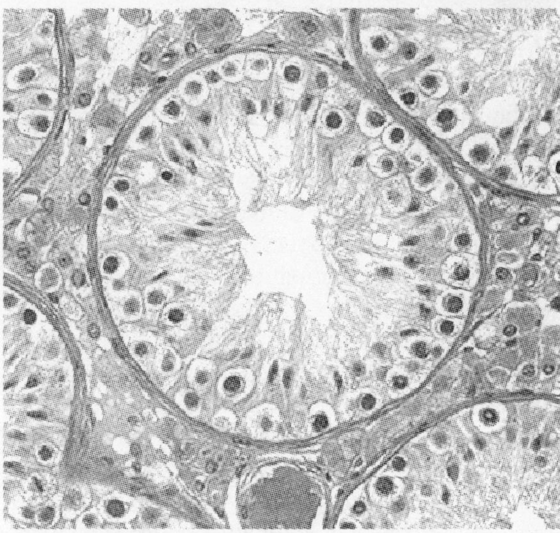

Fig. 52.2: Histological structure of the testis, showing a seminiferous tubule. Note polyhedral interstitial cells of Leydig outside the tubule.

The sperms develop from medium sized, spherical cells called *spermatogonia,* which form a single layer of cells, next to the basement membrane of the seminiferous tubule. These germ cells continually proliferate to replenish themselves, and some of them pass through the various stages leading to the formation of sperms.

The first step in the process of spermatogenesis is the formation of *primary spermatocytes* (Fig. 52.3). These cells are considerably larger than

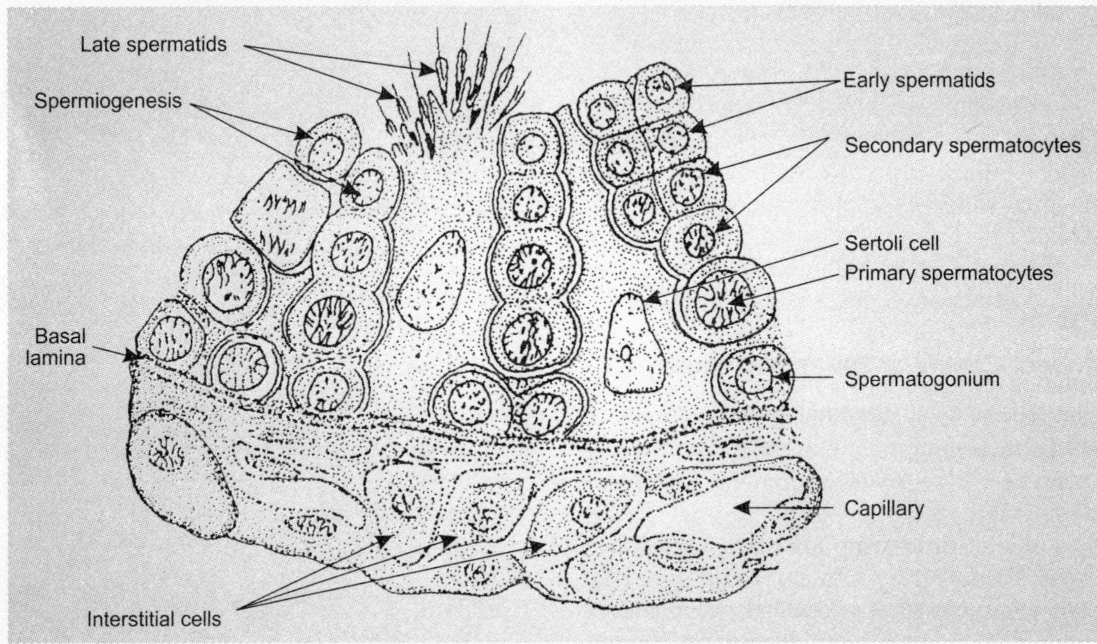

Fig. 52.3: Different stages in spermatogenesis.

52

spermatogonia. Each primary spermatocyte divides into two *secondary spermatocytes* by *a meiotic division* so that each secondary spermatocyte and all the subsequent stages contain haploid number (23) of chromosomes. Secondary spermatocytes divide by mitotic division to give rise to *spermatids*. By a series of mitotic divisions and one meiotic division mentioned above, each spermatogonium gives rise to 512 spermatids. The spermatids do not divide any further. It takes several weeks for the maturation of a spermatid into a spermatozoon. In humans, the transformation of a spermatogonium to spermatozoon takes about 74 days.

Thus, **spermatogenesis** can be divided into three parts:

a. **Spermatocytogenesis**—proliferative phase of germ cells to generate more of such cells.
b. **Meiosis—production of the haploid cells:** The first meiotic division produces two *secondary spermatocytes.* Division of the secondary spermatocytes completes meiosis and produces the *spermatids.*
c. **Spermiogenesis:** Morphological conversion of round spermatid into spermatozoa without a division. Events associated with spermiogenesis are:
   (a) Condensation of nuclear material
   (b) Removal of extraneous cytoplasm
   (c) Formation of the acrosome, and
   (d) Formation of tail structures.

Throughout spermiogenesis, spermatozoa are embedded in the Sertoli cells. Spermiogenesis ends in the testis with release of the spermatozoa from the *Sertoli cell*. The process by which spermatozoa are shed into the lumen of the seminiferous tubule for transport out of the testis is **spermiation.**

Hormonal Control of Spermatogenesis

Hormones that affect spermatogenesis are:

a. **Testosterone** This is an androgen produced by Leydig cells which promotes Sertoli cell function.
b. **Follicle stimulating hormone (FSH)**
   i. Produced by anterior pituitary, FSH regulates each stage of spermatogenesis.
   ii. FSH is necessary during development: required to establish Sertoli cell function.
c. **Luteinizing hormone (LH)** Produced by anterior pituitary, it increases testosterone production by Leydig cells.
d. **Gonadotropic releasing hormone (GnRH)** A hypothalamic hormone that controls release of anterior pituitary gonadotropic hormones (LH and FSH).
e. **Inhibin** Produced by Sertoli cells. It has a negative feedback effect on FSH secretion by anterior pituitary gland.

A **spermatozoon (sperm)** (Fig. 52.4) consists of a head, neck, body and tail. The head is elliptical in shape and measures 4–5 μm in length. The head contains the nuclear material of the sperm required for the fertilization of the ovum. The anterior two-thirds of the head is covered with a small structure called acrosomal cap or acrosome. The acrosome is derived from the Golgi apparatus of the spermatid and contains enzymes like hyaluronidase and proteases, which play an important role in the entry of the sperm into the ovum. The centrioles are aggregated in the neck of the sperm.

The body of the sperm contains a large number of mitochondria arranged in the form of a spiral. The tail contains two paired microtubules in the middle and nine pairs of microtubules around the

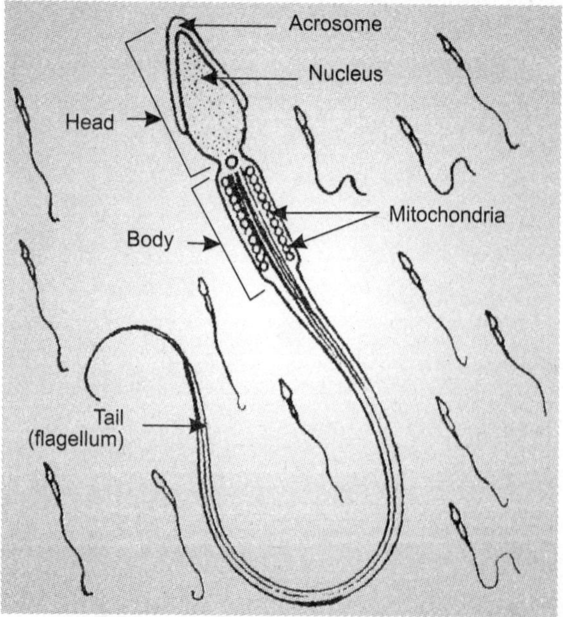

Fig. 52.4: Structure of a human sperm.

periphery extending throughout the tail. The tail is a flagellum. It provides motility to the sperm. The energy for the movements of the sperm is provided by the mitochondria present in the body of the sperm. To and fro movement of the tail of the sperm provides motility to it at the rate of 1–4 mm/ minute. (The body and tail are 50 μ long).

"Male" and "Female" Sperms

Each primary spermatocyte, like any other cell in the male, contains 22 pairs of autosomes along with an X and a Y chromosome. During the meiotic division, one secondary spermatocyte will contain the X chromosome along with 22 autosomes and the other secondary spermatocyte would contain Y chromosome along with 22 autosomes. Consequently, 50% of the sperms contain X-chromosomes, which are known as the "female" sperms. The remaining 50% contain Y chromosomes, and these are known as the "male sperms". The sex of the offspring is determined by the type of sperm with which the ovum (23, X) is fertilized. Fertilization of the ovum (23, X) with female sperm (23, X) results in the formation of a female offspring (46, XX). Fertilization of the ovum (23, X) with a male sperm (22, Y) results in a male baby (46 XY).

Sertoli Cells

The Sertoli cells extend from the basement membrane across the entire thickness of the germinal epithelium to the lumen of the seminiferous tubules. The spermatids attach themselves to the luminal folds of the Sertoli cells and undergo morphological changes leading to the formation of spermatozoa. The Sertoli cells provide *nutrients, hormones and enzymes* necessary for the maturation of spermatids. They also remove the excessive cytoplasm as the epitheloid spermatids are gradually converted into long and thin spermatozoa. This transformation process is called *spermiogenesis*.

Sertoli cells secrete an *androgen binding protein* (ABP) which helps to maintain a high concentration of androgens in the seminiferous tubular fluid.

Androgens are required for the maturation of sperms in the seminiferous tubules and in the epididymis.

Sertoli cells also secrete a hormone called *inhibin*. It is a polypeptide and inhibits FSH secretion from the anterior pituitary by feedback inhibition.

During fetal life, Sertoli cells secrete *Muller regression factor (MRF*).

Tight junctions between the adjacent Sertoli cells near the basement membrane constitute a barrier that prevents the passage of proteins and other large molecules from the blood to the lumen of seminiferous tubules. Thus, the tight junctions constitute a *blood-testis barrier*, which also prevents the antigenic products of germ cell division and maturation from entering the circulation and generating an autoimmune response.

To summarize, the Sertoli cells serve a number of functions during spermatogenesis:

- Maintain the environment necessary for development and maturation via the blood-testes barrier.
- Secrete substances initiating meiosis.
- Secrete supporting testicular fluid.
- Secrete androgen-binding protein, which concentrates testosterone in close proximity to the developing gametes. Testosterone is needed in very high concentrations for maintenance of the reproductive tract, and ABP allows a much higher level of fertility.
- Secrete hormones affecting pituitary gland control of spermatogenesis, particularly the polypeptide hormone, inhibin.
- Phagocytose residual cytoplasm left over from spermiogenesis.
- They release anti-mullerian hormone MRF which prevents formation of the Mullerian duct / oviduct during development of a male fetus.

Effect of Temperature on Spermatogenesis

In most of the mammals, the testes descend out of the abdomen into the scrotum during the perinatal period. In the scrotum, the testes are maintained at a temperature of about 32°C, i.e. at about 5°C below the intra-abdominal temperature. Lower testicular temperature seems to be an important requirement of proper spermatogenesis. Failure of testicular descent *(cryptorchidism)* causes defective spermatogenesis and infertility. However, the Leydig cell function remains unaffected.

The peculiar vascular supply to the testes and the anatomical structure of the scrotum help in maintaining the testes at a lower temperature. The testicular artery is highly tortuous and convoluted. Its convolutions are intimately intermingled with those of the testicular veins in the spermatic cord. This vascular arrangement is ideal for heat loss from the arterial blood by counter-current exchange system. Moreover, relaxation of dartos muscle of the scrotum in response to heat exposure lowers the testes further away from the body. In cold weather, contraction of dartos muscle brings the testes closer to the body.

Role of Epididymis

Epididymis is the site of extra-testicular **maturation** of sperms. When the sperms arrive in the epididymis, they are non-motile. By the time, they reach the tail of epididymis, taking 18 hours to 10 days, they become *motile* and *capable of fertilization*. The epididymal secretions required for this maturation are androgen dependent.

The non-motile spermatozoa are transported to the epididymis in *testicular fluid* secreted by the Sertoli cells with the aid of peristaltic contractions. Whilst in the epididymis, they acquire motility. However, transport of the mature spermatozoa through the remainder of the male reproductive system is achieved via contractions of smooth muscle rather than the spermatozoon's recently acquired motility.

Storage of Sperms

Vas deferens, particularly its **ampulla**, is the chief site of storage of sperms, although some sperms are stored in the epididymis also. The duration of storage in the vas deferens depends on the frequency of sexual activity. Sperms remain viable in these stores for several months.

Role of Seminal Vesicles and Prostate Gland

The seminal vesicles secrete a mucoid material containing an abundance of fructose and other nutrients, fibrinogen and large quantities of prostaglandins.

The secretion of the prostate gland is a thin, milky, mildly acidic fluid containing citric acid, calcium, Na^+, acid phosphatase and pre-fibrinolysins, as well as, a clotting enzyme. About 60% of the total volume of semen is contributed by seminal vesicles and 20% by the prostate gland.

Semen (Table 52.1)

Semen is the name given to the fluid ejaculated during the male sexual act. It is composed of fluids from the vas deferens (containing sperms) and from the seminal vesicles, the prostate gland, and mucous glands particularly from the bulbourethral gland. The average pH of semen is 7.5. The seminal fluid provides nutrition in the form of fructose to the sperms. The alkaline semen brings

Table 52.1: Composition of normal human semen

Colour: white opalescent
pH: 7.35–7.50
Volume per ejaculate: 2.4–3.5 ml
Sperm count: 35 to 200 million/ml, average 100 million/ml
Sperm morphology: > 60% normal
Sperm motility: > 60% of sperms show forward progression

Chemical Composition

Fructose (1.5–6.5 mg/ml) Ascorbic acid Prostaglandins Fibrinogen Mucus	from seminal vesicles (60% of total volume)
Citric acid Ca^{++} Acid phosphatase Phosphates Bicarbonate Hyaluronic acid	from prostate gland (20% of total volume)

the vaginal pH (3.5–4) to about 6–6.5, the pH at which sperms show optimum motility. The prostatic fluid contains a clotting enzyme, as well as, prefibrinolysins. These two enzymes cause the fibrinogen of seminal vesicle fluid to undergo clotting, followed 15 minutes later by fibrinolysis. The clotting of semen soon after ejaculation helps to retain it in the vagina for some time. Lysis, later on, would release the sperms for their free movement into the uterine cavity for fertilization.

During ejaculation, the seminal vesicles are last to contract. Therefore, besides other functions of its constituents, its secretion serves to flush the sperms out of the ejaculatory duct and urethra.

The average volume of semen per ejaculate is 2.5–3.5 ml. The normal sperm count varies from 35 to 200 million per ml of semen, average being 100 million/ml.

Male Sexual Act

The male sexual act consists of three stages, namely, the erection of penis, the emission and the ejaculation. It is a reflex response with its integration centres located in the L_1, L_2 and S_2, S_3, S_4 segments of the spinal cord.

The glans penis contains sensory nerve endings that transmit into the central nervous system a special modality of sensation called the sexual sensation. The afferent impulses are carried to the spinal cord through pudendal nerves (somatic S_2, S_3, S_4) and transmitted to the cerebrum. Appropriate psychic stimuli can also initiate the sexual reflex or at least enhance the effect of genital afferent stimulation. The cerebral cortex has an inhibitory control over the spinal centres, which is vital for the normal social behaviour of the human male.

Erection of Penis

Erection of the penis is essential for its introduction into the vagina during sexual intercourse.

The penis contains erectile tissue in the form of two corpora cavernosa and a corpus spongiosum (Fig. 52.1). The erectile tissue consists of large cavernous venous sinusoids which are normally empty and the penis is flaccid. Appropriate genital or psychic stimulation result in discharge of parasympathetic impulses from S_2, S_3, S_4 spinal segments, through nervi erigentes to the penile arterioles. Increased blood flow to the erectile tissue, coupled with compression of penile veins under the strong fibrous tunica albugenia, makes the penis hard and elongated.

Parasympathetic discharge also increases the secretion of urethral and bulbourethral glands. The mucus flows through the urethra during the early stages of the coitus (sexual intercourse) and helps to lubricate the vagina.

Emission and Ejaculation

During sexual intercourse, the massaging action of the vagina on the glans penis stimulates the sensory end organs in the latter. When the sexual stimulation becomes extremely intense, the spinal integration centre increases the sympathetic discharge from L_1, L_2 spinal segments to the genitalia, which result in emission. Rhythmic contraction of smooth muscle of vas deferens, seminal vesicles and prostate gland expel the sperms and other seminal fluids into the urethra. The process up to this point is called *emission.* The semen is propelled out of the urethra by contraction of bulbo-cavernosus muscle, a skeletal muscle, supplied by somatic S_2, S_3, S_4 spinal segments. This step is called *ejaculation.*

Orgasm As mentioned above, increased sympathetic discharge causes emission and ejaculation. It also produces contraction of internal sphincter of urinary bladder. Hence retrograde ejaculation (transfer of sperms into urinary bladder) does not occur. A feeling of intense pleasure arises with ejaculation and the event is called an orgasm. Simultaneously, there is noticeable skeletal muscle contraction throughout the body which is followed by psychological and muscular relaxation.

Cardiorespiratory Changes During sexual intercourse, there is a marked increase in heart rate, blood pressure and respiratory rate, both in males and females. Peak values are reached during orgasm, when heart rate may increase up to 150 beats per rate minute for a few moments. Respiratory rate as high as 40 per minute has been recorded. Systolic blood pressure may increase by 30–80 mmHg. Diastolic blood pressure may increase by 20–40 mmHg. Flushing of the face and sweating also occur. These changes are equivalent to the effects of mild muscular exercise. The cardiovascular changes during coitus mentioned above may be kept in mind when a patient with coronary artery disease or severe hypertension seeks medical advice regarding continuation of sexual activity.

ENDOCRINE FUNCTION OF TESTES

The testes secrete several male sex-hormones which are collectively called *androgens*. Of these, testosterone is the most abundant and most potent androgen.

TESTOSTERONE

It is a steroid synthesized by the interstitial cells of Leydig (Leydig cells) from cholesterol. The Leydig cells are large polyhedral cells lying as cords or groups of cells around large blood capillaries in the interstitial connective tissue between the seminiferous tubules.

Dehydroepiandrosterone (DHEA) It is another important androgen present in the blood of not only males but also females. This androgen originates from the adrenal cortex. When secreted in normal amounts, it has very little masculinizing effect. It is of little metabolic importance in males, but it has important anabolic effect in the females. Secretion of large amount of dehydroepiandrosterone by certain tumours of adrenal cortex may produce masculinizing effect in prepubertal and adult females or precocious puberty in prepubertal boys (precocious pseudopuberty).

Biosynthesis

The biochemical pathways involved in the synthesis of androgens are shown in Fig. 52.5.

Plasma testosterone level in adult males is about 0.65 mg%. Most of it is bound to the various plasma proteins [32% to albumin, 65% to gonadal steroid binding globulin (GBG) and only 3% is in free form]. Within 15–30 min of its entry into circulation, testosterone is either fixed to the target tissues or degraded in the liver. In the target cells, it is converted into *dihydrotestosterone* which can combine with the cytoplasmic hormone receptors and modify the synthesis of mRNA in the nucleus. Plasma testosterone level declines with age (Fig. 52.6). The degradation products of testosterone include androsterone, epiandrosterone and etiocholanolone. These three products are grouped together *as 17-ketosteroids*. These are conjugated with glucuronic acid or sulphuric acid in the liver and excreted in the bile and urine. About two-thirds of the urinary 17-ketosteroids are of adrenal origin (derived from DHEA) and only one-third are of

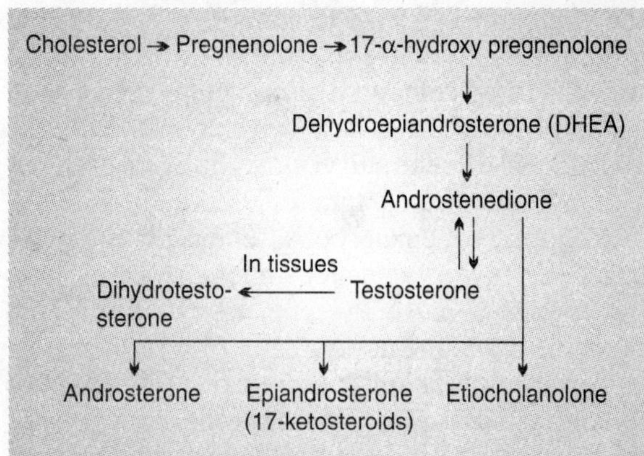

Fig. 52.5: Biochemical pathways involved in synthesis of androgens.

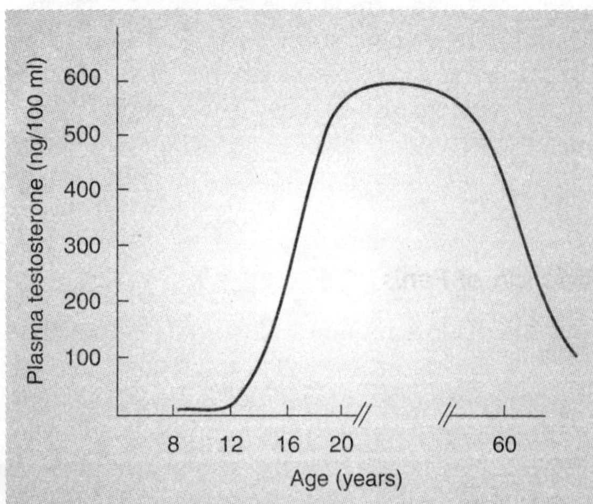

Fig. 52.6: Plasma testosterone level at various ages in the male.

testicular origin. Excessive secretion of 17-ketosteroids in the urine is an important sign of masculinizing tumours of adrenal cortex.

Actions of Testosterone

Growth of Genitalia and Accessory Sexual Organs

The increased secretion of testosterone is responsible for the growth of the testes, scrotum and penis at puberty. Testosterone also increases the growth of accessory sexual organs like epididymis, seminal vesicles, prostate and bulbourethral glands. It also produces pigmentation in the external genitalia.

Development of Secondary Sexual Characteristics

The secondary sexual characteristics of the male are produced by increased plasma concentration of testosterone at puberty.

(i) Body Hair It increases the growth of hair on the face, chest and other parts of the body. It also causes a particular pattern of growth of pubic hair which extend up to umbilicus. The recession of hair line on the temples produces the characteristic male type of baldness (Fig. 52.7).

(ii) Voice Enlargement of larynx, and thickening of vocal cords lowers the pitch of the voice, making it characteristically masculine.

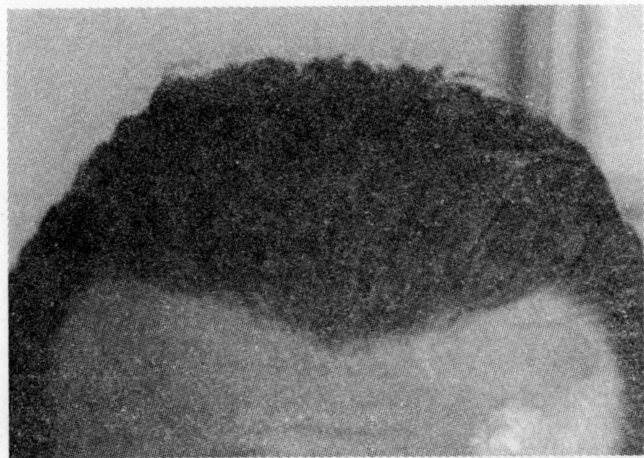

Fig 52.7: The characteristic male baldness.

(iii) Shoulder Girdle It produces pronounced development of the shoulder girdle.

(iv) Muscle Mass Greater muscular development in the males than females is an effect of testosterone.

(v) Skin The skin becomes thicker all over the body. There is increase in the amount and thickness of the secretions of the sebaceous glands, predisposing the young males to acne.

(vi) Libido The male sexual drive (libido) is due to the effect of testosterone on the hypothalamus.

(vii) Aggressive Behaviour Testosterone produces aggressive behaviour and interest in the opposite sex.

Anabolic Effects

Testosterone causes increased synthesis and decreased breakdown of tissue proteins leading to accelerated growth of the body in general and skeletal muscle in particular. Pronounced development of musculature at puberty is one of the most important characteristics of the male. This action of testosterone has led to the misuse of synthetic androgens by athletes to improve their muscular performance.

Testosterone also increases the rate of linear growth of the bones causing a rapid increase in stature at puberty (pubertal spurt of growth). There is considerable deposition of calcium salts in the bones. The bones grow not only in length but also become thicker. However, testosterone also causes early fusion of the epiphysis in the long bones, putting an end to any further increase in height.

Renal retention of calcium, phosphate, sodium, potassium and water are other anabolic effects of testosterone.

Erythropoiesis

Greater haemoglobin concentration and RBC count in males are due to the effect of testosterone on the production of erythropoietin.

Prenatal Development

Male fetuses start secreting testosterone during the second month of embryonic life. Leydig cell proliferation and the secretion of testosterone, at this stage, is an effect of chorionic gonadotropin. Secretion of testosterone by genital ridges and subsequent development of testes is responsible for the development of male sexual organs like penis, scrotum, prostate, seminal vesicles, etc. In the absence of testosterone, the genital ridges develop into female sex organs.

The descent of testes, during the last two months of fetal life, or soon after birth, is also testosterone dependent.

During childhood, the testicular Leydig cells revert to an undifferentiated state, to be reactivated at puberty, with the onset of secretion of pituitary gonadotropins.

Regulation of Testicular Function

Anterior Pituitary Control

Testicular function is regulated by two gonadotropic hormones secreted by the anterior pituitary. Follicle stimulating hormone (FSH) and luteinizing hormone (LH) were originally named after their function in the female. Since, the two gonadotropic hormones regulating spermatogenesis and Leydig cell function respectively have the chemical structure similar to FSH and LH, the same names have been used for the male gonadotropic hormones also. In males, LH is also known as interstitial cell stimulating hormone (ICSH).

Regulation of Spermatogenesis

52

Administration of FSH to immature or hypophysectomized experimental male animals for several days results in testicular enlargement and proliferation of germinal epithelium in the seminiferous tubules. Moreover, at puberty, the onset of spermatogenesis can be correlated with the onset of secretion of FSH by the anterior pituitary. Conversely, in adult male animals, hypophysectomy results in almost complete cessation of spermatogenesis and atrophy of the testes and accessory sexual organs.

The exact role of FSH in spermatogenesis, however, is not yet clear. Proliferation and function of Sertoli cells seems to be controlled by FSH. High concentration of testosterone in the seminiferous tubular fluid is also essential for proper spermatogenesis. Testosterone diffuses freely through the blood-testicular barrier to reach the lumen of the seminiferous tubules. Since LH regulates the secretion of testosterone by the Leydig cells, LH also has an indirect role in spermatogenesis. The secretion of androgen-binding protein (ABP) by the Sertoli cells is also FSH dependent.

Feedback Control of Spermatogenesis Plasma FSH levels are elevated in patients with atrophied seminiferous tubules but normal Leydig cell function. This observation shows a feedback control on the secretion of FSH. Recently, it has been demonstrated that the seminiferous follicular fluid contains a polypeptide named **inhibin** which acts directly on the anterior pituitary and inhibits the secretion of FSH. It has been presumed that the feedback control of FSH secretion maintains the normal rate of spermatogenesis (Fig. 52.8).

Testosterone Secretion

The pituitary gonadotropin, LH, is required for initial proliferation of Leydig cells at puberty and for their continual secretory activity in later life. In experimental animals, it has been observed that hypophysectomy produces atrophy of the Leydig cells, which can be restored to normal by administration of exogenous LH. LH binds to specific receptors on the surface of Leydig cells to activate cAMP synthesis which triggers testosterone synthesis and secretion.

Feedback Control Plasma testosterone level is maintained at a constant level by a feedback control exerted by testosterone on the secretion of LH by the anterior pituitary. Testosterone produces feedback inhibition by mainly acting on the hypothalamus (Fig. 52.8).

Hypothalamic Control

The hypothalamus regulates the secretion of gonadotropins through gonadotropin-releasing

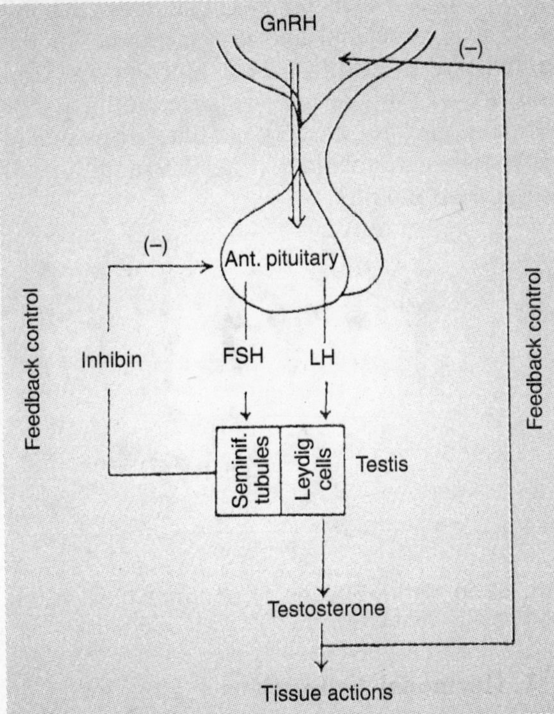

Fig. 52.8: Regulation of testicular function.

hormone (GnRH), which reaches the anterior pituitary through hypothalamic-hypophysial portal vessels. During surgical stress, libido is markedly depressed. The effect of psychic stimuli on gonadal function is more apparent in the female as shown by disturbed menstrual cycles in women under mental stress. Experimentally, temporary sterility has been observed in bulls during transport under uncomfortable conditions.

Puberty In a male child, the sex organs are small in size, since the anterior pituitary does not secrete the gonadotropins. At 12–14 years of age, anterior pituitary begins to secrete progressively increasing amounts of gonadotropins, leading to initiation of testicular function and enlargement of primary and accessory sexual organs. The initiation of puberty is primarily because of the maturation in hypothalamus rather than anterior pituitary, because anterior pituitary can start secreting gonadotropins if GnRH is available even in childhood.

Role of Prolactin in Male

The hormone prolactin is named after its well-known role of production of milk in the mammary gland. Recent studies have demonstrated that even in males, plasma prolactin levels are comparable to those in the female. In certain animals, prolactin potentiates the effect of LH on Leydig cells. However, men with prolactin-producing pituitary tumours are impotent, even if plasma testosterone levels are normal. It has been speculated that prolactin may have an inhibitory action on the brain centres concerned with the sexual desire in the male.

Role of Oestrogens in Male

In the peripheral tissues, most of the circulating testosterone is converted into its active metabolite dihydrotestosterone, which produces the androgenic effects. However, small amount of testosterone is converted into oestradiol and oestrone. Thus, even in males, the blood contains small amounts of female sex hormones. Now, it is believed that the physiological effects of testosterone are the result of combined effects of testosterone itself plus those of its metabolites dihydrotestosterone and oestrogens. In some tissues, oestrogens seem to act in concert with androgens to influence the physiological processes. However, oestrogens may have independent effects or effects opposite to those of androgens. Very small amounts of oestrogens are also produced by the Leydig cells of the testes. In normal men, there is high blood androgens: oestrogens ratio and hence virilization is the dominant effect. In pathological states, the ratio may be disturbed by decreased secretion of testosterone (e.g. Klinefelter's syndrome). In liver cirrhosis, hepatic degradation of testosterone is reduced and hence greater percentage of testosterone is metabolized to oestrogens. Hence, in such patients, the androgens: oestrogens ratio becomes low. All such conditions may lead to enlargement of the breasts (*gynecomastia*) and other signs of feminization. In old age, gynecomastia is physiological. It is caused by reduced testosterone secretion which results in reduction in blood androgens: oestrogens ratio.

PATHOPHYSIOLOGY

Impotence

It is defined as the inability to attain an erection of sufficient rigidity for vaginal penetration. The prevalence of impotence increases rapidly after the age of 50 years, especially in those with diabetes mellitus or atherosclerosis.

Impotence may be due to severe hypogonadism which causes erectile failure as well as loss of libido (sexual interest and initiative). However, in most of the cases, the erectile dysfunction can be attributed to atherosclerosis of the penile blood vessels or autonomic neuropathy involving nervi erigentes. In some cases, impotence may be psychological.

Infertility

The failure to conceive after one year of unprotected intercourse is called infertility. It affects about 10% of married couples. The problem may be in the husband or the wife or both.

The congenital causes of male infertility are not common. These include Klinefelter's syndrome, isolated gonadotropin deficiency (Kallmann's syndrome) and cryptorchidism. More common causes of male infertility are acquired defects of the testes which include viral orchitis (mumps virus) and testicular trauma. Hyperprolactinemia is also a cause of secondary testicular dysfunction leading to infertility and impotence.

FUNCTION TESTS

1. Semen Analysis For analysis, semen is collected by masturbation into a clean glass container. A sperm count of less than 20 million/ml with total sperms per ejaculate lower than 60 million is abnormal and may account for the infertility. In addition, the morphology and motility of the sperms is also examined. For normal fertility, at least 60% of the sperms should show normal morphology (Fig. 52.9) and forward progressive motility.

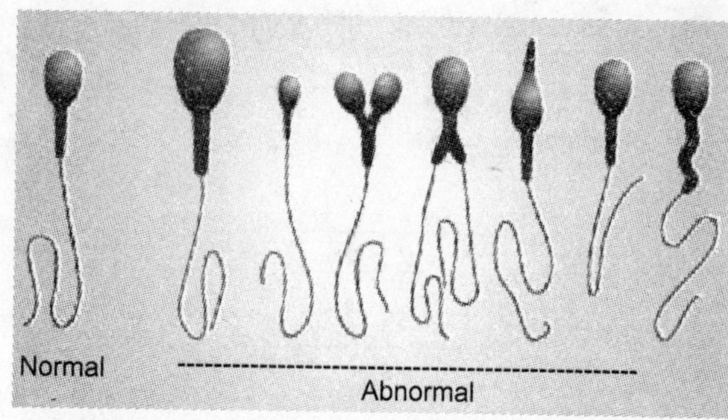

Fig. 52.9: Various types of abnormalities in the morphology of sperms.

2. Hormonal Estimations Plasma levels of FSH, LH, testosterone and prolactin are usually determined. Plasma FSH, LH and testosterone levels are low in Kallmann's syndrome. In Klinefelter's syndrome, the patients have azoospermia with low plasma testosterone and elevated plasma FSH and LH levels.

3. Chromosomal Analysis It is essential for the diagnosis of Klinefelter's syndrome.

4. Testicular Biopsy If semen shows zero sperm count (azoospermia), testicular biopsy helps to know whether there is absence of production of sperms or there is a blockade in the reproductive tract. The latter disorder can be surgically corrected.

53

CHAPTER

The Female Reproductive System

FUNCTIONAL ANATOMY

The ovaries, fallopian tubes, uterus and vagina constitute the organs of female reproductive tract (Fig. 53.1).

The Ovaries The adult human ovaries are paired flattened ellipsoid structures measuring 5 cm in length. They are attached to the uterus by the broad ligament and round ligament of ovary on each side.

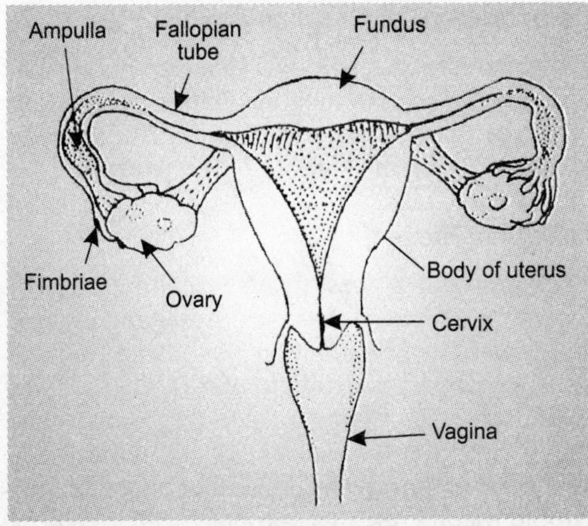

Fig. 53.1: The female reproductive tract.

The Uterus The uterus is a hollow, pear-shaped structure. It is divided anatomically and functionally into two parts, the body and the cervix. The cavity of the uterus communicates above and laterally with a fallopian tube on either side. Below, it opens into the vagina at the external os of the cervix. The part of the body of the uterus above the opening of fallopian tubes is called *fundus* (Fig. 53.1).

The wall of uterus consists of three layers, the outermost peritoneal layer called *perimetrium*, the middle smooth muscle layer called *myometrium* and the innermost mucous membrane called the *endometrium*. Myometrium is the thickest of all the three layers. The smooth muscle fibres tend to interlace with each other. Myometrium plays the most important role during parturition.

Endometrium of the body of the uterus, i.e. above the level of the internal os of the cervix, consists of surface epithelium, glands and stroma. The superficial two-thirds of the endometrium undergoes monthly cyclic changes in preparation for the implantation of the fertilized ovum. This layer of the endometrium is known as *stratum functionale*.

The deeper one-thirds layer of the endometrium or the *stratum basale* does not participate in these cyclic changes. The stratum functionale is supplied by long and coiled spiral arteries, whereas the stratum basale is supplied by short and straight basilar arteries.

Vagina The vagina is about 10 cm long, muscular tube. The cervix projects into its upper end. It opens outside at the vaginal orifice. In adult female, the vaginal mucosa is lined by stratified squamous epithelium. No glands open into vagina. The small amount of secretion present in the vagina is derived partly from the mucus discharge from the cervix and partly from the transudation of fluid from the vaginal epithelium. The epithelial cells are rich in glycogen and this property is oestrogen-dependent. Action of certain bacteria on the glycogen present in the vaginal secretion produces lactic acid, which maintains the vaginal pH around 4.0. Acidic environment of vagina prevents the growth of pathogenic organisms.

Fallopian Tubes Each fallopian tube is approximately 10 cm in length and 8 mm in diameter. Anatomically, it can be divided into four parts: (i) the interstitial portion which traverses the myometrium of the uterus; (ii) the isthmus, the next lateral 2.5 cm length; (iii) the ampulla, the widest and the longest (7 cm) part; and (iv) the fimbriated end or the infundibulum, which opens into the peritoneal cavity. The infundibulum is surrounded by a number of radiating fimbriae, one of which is longer than the rest and is attached to the outer pole of the ovary.

The mucous layer of the fallopian tubes is thrown into folds. It is lined by ciliated columnar cells with few goblet cells interspersed within them. The cilia help to propel a fluid current towards the uterus along which the non-motile ovum can be transported. The peristaltic activity of the smooth muscle of the fallopian tube also helps in the transport of the ovum.

Menarche and Menopause The cyclic activity in the ovary changes the hormonal environment in the uterus in such a way that there is a periodic proliferation, followed by partial shedding of the endometrium (menstrual bleeding). The average length of the ovarian and menstrual cycles in human female is 28 days. Traditionally, 1st day of the menstrual bleeding is taken as the 1st day of the menstrual and ovarian cycles.

The menstrual cycle begins at the age of 10–14 years and the onset of the cycles is known as menarche. At the age of 45–50 years, the ovarian and the menstrual cycles cease. The cessation of reproductive cycles in the female is known as the menopause. Thus, the reproductive period in human female is limited to about 35 years, i.e. from age of 15 to 50 years.

THE OVARIAN CYCLE

Histologically, the outer or the cortical portion of the ovary contains the primordial follicles containing the ova. Each primordial follicle consists of the primary oocyte (the female germ cell) surrounded by a single layer of spindle-shaped cells called the *granulosa cells* (Fig. 53.2). The primary oocyte is in prophase of the meiotic division since fetal life. The reduction division is completed only after ovulation, when expulsion of the 1st polar body produces the secondary oocyte. After another nuclear division, second polar body is extruded during its passage in the fallopian tube.

At menarche, the two ovaries contain about 3,00,000 ova. Since only one ovum is expelled from one or the other ovary every month, not more than 450 ova are expelled during the entire reproductive period. The rest of the primordial follicles undergo atresia (atrophy).

Development of Graafian Follicle

Every month, in each ovary, many primordial follicles start undergoing maturation process but only one reaches maturity and the rest undergo atresia at different stages of development.

Follicular Phase

The maturation process involves multiplication of the granulosa cells into many layers and gradual accumulation of fluid within the follicle. With the enlargement of the follicle, the *follicular fluid* collects in such a large amount that it surrounds the ovum all around except at one point. As a result, the ovum covered by a layer of cells called *corona radiata* remains in contact with granulosa cells only at a hillock-like area called *cumulus*

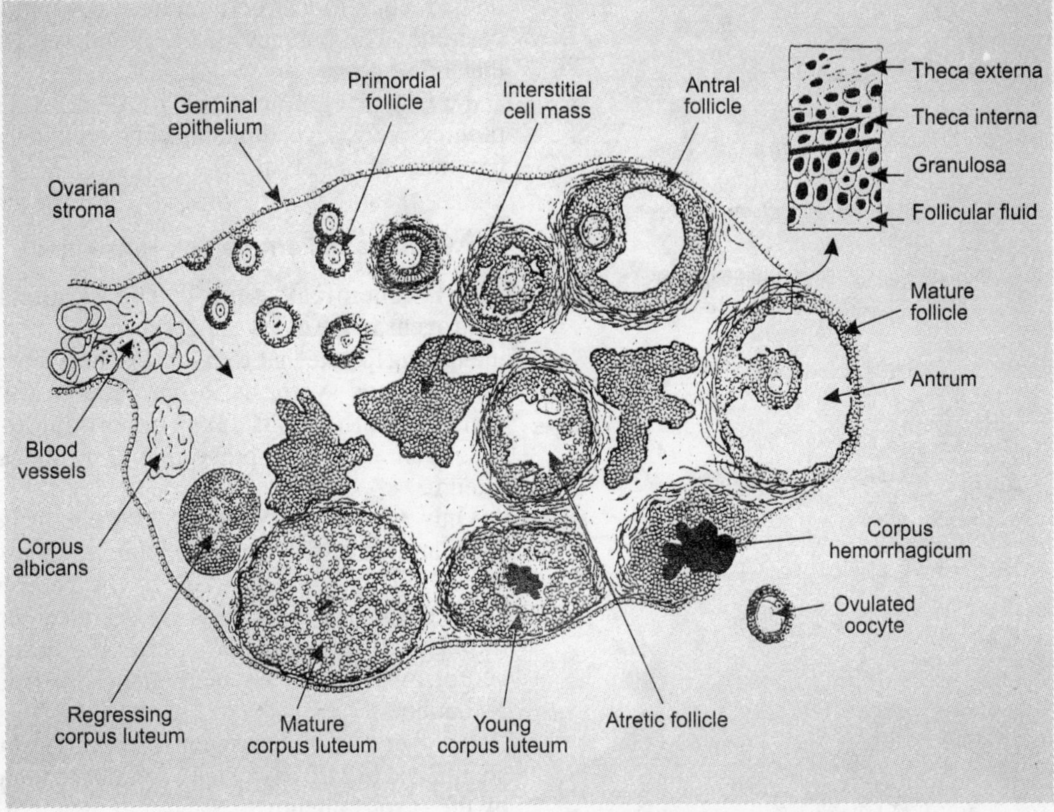

Fig. 53.2: Histological section of human ovary.

oophorus (Fig. 53.3). A transparent muco-protein envelope, the *zona pellucida* can be seen between the ovum and the corona radiata.

The mature follicle is now called a *Graafian follicle*. It partly bulges out of the surface of the ovary into the peritoneal cavity. The Graafian follicle is surrounded by the *theca folliculi*, which arises from the ovarian stroma. The theca consists of an inner rim of secretory cells called the *theca interna* and an outer rim of fibrous tissue, the *theca externa*.

Ovulation At about 14th day of the cycle, the distended Graafian follicle ruptures and the ovum surrounded by corona radiata is released into the peritoneal cavity, close to the open end of the fallopian tube. This process is called the ovulation. The ovum is the largest cell in the human body (120 μ diameter).

Luteal Phase

Following ovulation, the outer wall of the Graafian follicle collapses and the follicle becomes filled with blood (*corpus haemorrhagica*). The cavity is soon filled up by proliferation and modification of the granulosa cells into large *polyhedral cells containing large amount of lipid and a yellow pigment, the lutein.* The theca interna cells also undergo a similar transformation called *luteinization*. The whole structure, so formed, is called the *corpus luteum*. By 22nd day of the cycle, the corpus luteum attains a diameter of about 1.5 cm.

Unless pregnancy occurs, the corpus luteum begins to regress rapidly after 24th day of the ovarian cycle, ultimately ending as a whitish scar tissue, called the *corpus albicans*. In the mean time, the next ovarian cycle begins once again.

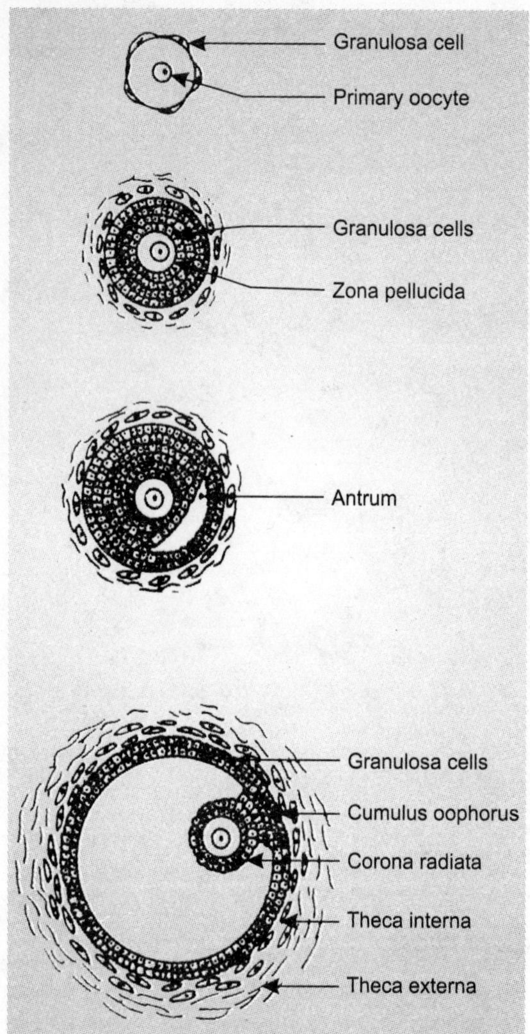

Fig. 53.3: Development of graafian follicle.

Ovarian Hormones

The two most important groups of female sex hormones secreted by the ovary are the oestrogens and the progesterone. Both of them are steroids.

Oestrogens

In the adult female, blood contains three types of oestrogens, namely, oestradiol, oestrone and oestriol. Oestradiol is the chief oestrogen secreted by the *ovary*, although small amount of oestrone is also secreted. Oestriol is an oxidative degradation product derived from oestradiol and oestrone. The potency of oestradiol is 12-times that of oestrone.

During pregnancy, the *placenta* secretes progressively larger amounts of oestriol in the last 6 months of gestation.

Biosynthesis of Female Sex Hormones

The biochemical steps in the synthesis of oestrogens in the ovary are given in Fig. 53.4. It is interesting to note that pathway I is the major route for oestrogen synthesis in the graafian follicle, whereas pathway II leads to production of oestrogen as well as progesterone in the corpus luteum.

Only 3% of the circulating oestradiol is in free form, and the rest is bound to albumin and gonadal steroid binding globulin (GBG). On the average, about 0.3 mg of oestrogens are secreted per day throughout the menstrual cycle. The oestrogen secretion reaches its peak near the time of ovulation.

Another rise of oestrogen secretion occurs on about 22nd to 24th day of the cycle due to secretion by the corpus luteum.

During the last 6 months of pregnancy, oestrogens (mainly oestriol) are secreted by the placenta in progressively increasing amounts.

Oestrogens are metabolized in the liver by oxidation to oestriol followed by conjugation with glucuronic and sulphuric acids. The water soluble conjugation products are excreted in the urine.

Actions of Oestrogens

Reproductive Organs

Organs of reproduction are the chief target organs for oestrogens. Oestrogens promote the growth and development of: (i) uterus, (ii) fallopian tubes, (iii) vagina, (iv) external genitalia, and (v) mammary glands at puberty. Subsequently, maintenance of these organs in functional stage is also oestrogen-dependent. A decrease in the plasma oestrogen level due to menopause, or ovariectomy in young females, results in involution and atrophy of these organs.

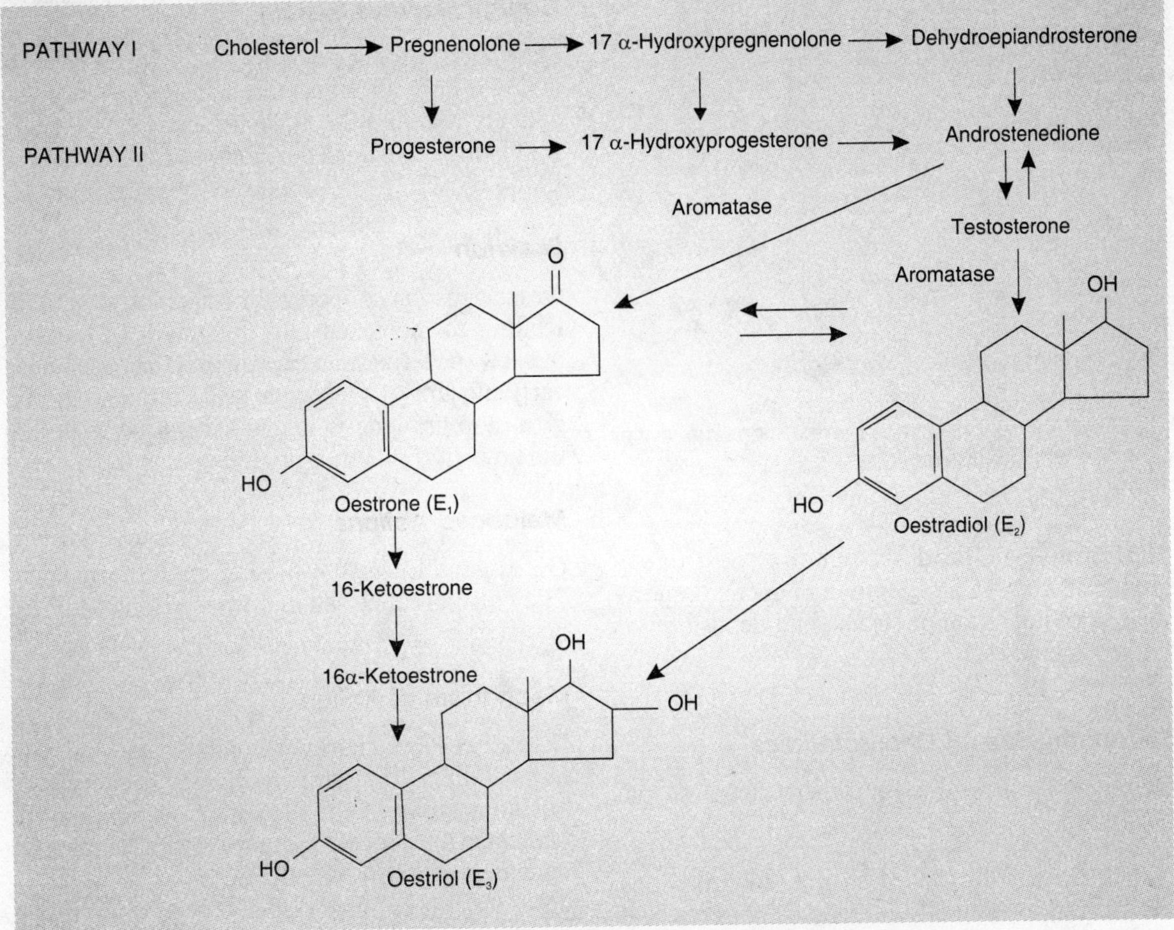

Fig. 53.4: Biosynthesis of female sex hormones.

Utreus In the uterus, during normal reproductive cycles, the oestrogens increase the thickness of the endometrium two-three folds. They cause proliferation of the endometrial stroma and increase the number and the length of the endometrial glands. They also cause rapid growth of the spiral arteries in the endometrium. Oestrogens also increase the spontaneous activity of the myometrial fibres, particularly increasing its sensitivity to oxytocin.

Cervical Mucus Under the influence of oestrogens, the cervical glands secrete thin watery mucus which facilitates the movement of sperms into the uterine cavity. When the mucus is spread on a glass slide and allowed to dry, a characteristic fern-like pattern is observed under the microscope (Fig. 53.5).

Fallopian Tubes Oestrogens increase the activity of both the secretory as well as the ciliated cells of the epithelium of the fallopian tubes. The contractility of its smooth muscle is also increased, which may be helpful in the transport of the ovum towards the uterus.

Vagina Oestrogens produce thickening of the mucosa and cornification of the superficial vaginal epithelial cells. There is heavy deposition of glycogen in the vaginal epithelium.

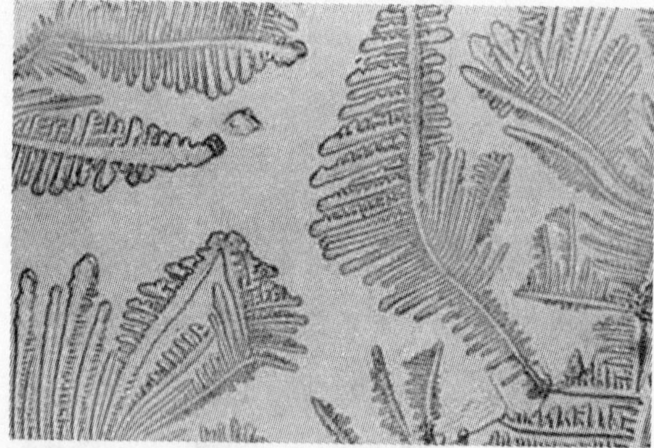

Fig. 53.5: Microscopic appearance of a dried smear of cervical mucus on 12th day of the menstrual cycle. Note the fern-like pattern.

Mammary Gland At puberty, oestrogens produce extensive proliferation of ductal tissue as well as proliferation of stroma and deposition of fat in the breasts.

Secondary Sexual Characteristics

Oestrogens produce many other effects on the body such as:

(i) Deposition of fat in the subcutaneous tissues specially in breasts, buttocks and thighs.

(ii) Narrow shoulders and broad hips, thighs that converge.

(iii) Less body hair, more scalp hair, flat topped pubic hair pattern.

(iv) High pitched voice.

The secondary sexual characteristics mentioned above are chiefly due to the actions of oestrogens, but some of them are more because of the absence of testosterone rather than the direct effect of oestrogens. These characteristics are called secondary sexual characteristics, since they make a female attractive to the male.

Growth of pubic and axillary hair is due to the action of adrenal androgens but the typical pattern of pubic hair is oestrogen dependent.

Central Nervous System

Oestrogens produce oestrus behaviour in animals (female animals under the effect of oestrogen actively seek out the male and become receptive for mating). In human females, oestrogens increase libido by acting on the anterior hypothalamus.

Skeleton

Oestrogens cause increased osteoblastic activity leading to increased rate of growth of bone at puberty (pubertal spurt of growth). They also cause early closure of the epiphyseal cartilage so that girls stop growing in height several years before the boys of the same age group.

Metabolic Actions

Oestrogens lower the plasma cholesterol level. They also produce salt and water retention in the body.

Mechanism of Action

Like other steroid hormones, oestrogens bind with intracellular cytoplasmic receptors. The receptor-hormone complex moves into the nucleus to stimulate the process of transcription leading to increased synthesis of mRNA.

Progesterone

Progesterone is synthesized by *corpus luteum* during the second half of the menstrual cycle and the first three months of pregnancy. Progressively, larger amounts of progesterone are produced by the *placenta* during the last 6 months of pregnancy.

Progesterone is synthesized from cholesterol (Fig. 53.4). It is transported in the blood bound to plasma proteins, chiefly albumin and only 1–2% of it is in free form. In the liver, progesterone is inactivated by the process of reduction to pregnanediol, which is further conjugated with glucuronic acid to be excreted in the urine.

During the follicular phase of the ovarian cycle, very little progesterone is secreted. But during the luteal phase of the ovarian cycle, progesterone secretion is increased by about 20-folds.

Plasma oestradiol and progesterone level in different phases of menstrual cycle are given in Table 53.1.

Table 53.1: Plasma oestradiol and progesterone level in different phases of menstrual cycle

Phase of menstrual cycle	*Plasma gonadal steroid concentration (ng/100 ml)*	
	Oestradiol	*Progesterone*
Early follicular	6	0
Late follicular	50	100
Middle luteal	20	1000

Actions of Progesterone

Progesterone is essential for preparation of the endometrium for implantation of the fertilized ovum and the maintenance of pregnancy (gestation), hence the name. In the endometrium and the mammary glands, the effects of progesterone can be demonstrated only after prior administration of oestrogens. In other words, progesterone is effective only in oestrogen-primed tissues.

Uterus

In oestrogen-primed endometrium, progesterone is responsible for the secretory phase of the menstrual cycle. Under the effect of progesterone, the endometrium proliferates further and becomes oedematous. The glands elongate further and become tortuous. They produce carbohydrate-rich secretion which nourishes the blastula until implantation has been completed.

In the myometrium, progesterone increases the membrane potential of the smooth muscle cells leading to *decreased excitability and sensitivity to oxytocin.* Progesterone also decreases the number of oestrogen receptors in the myometrium.

Cervical Mucus

Under the effect of progesterone, the secretions of cervical glands become thick and viscous (which help to prevent entry of sperms into the uterine cavity). When spread on a glass slide and allowed to dry, the ferning effect is no more observed. Thus, the presence of ferning (Fig. 53.5) in the first-half of the ovarian cycle and its disappearance in second-half is taken as a strong evidence of ovulation having occurred. Persistent ferning throughout the menstrual cycle suggests anovulatory cycle.

Cessation of progesterone secretion by the ovary produces dramatic effects like menstrual bleeding/termination of pregnancy.

Mammary Gland

In the oestrogen-primed mammary gland, progesterone promotes the growth of acini.

Thermogenic Effect

Progesterone has a thermogenic effect. The basal body temperature is higher by ½°C in the luteal phase of the ovarian cycle as compared to that in the follicular phase (Fig. 53.6). Measurement of basal body temperature (in early morning before the patient leaves the bed) is often clinically used to find out whether ovulation is occurring or not. The information is important when conception is desired in cases of infertility.

Respiration

Acting on the brainstem, progesterone stimulates respiration. Alveolar pCO_2 is lower in women during the luteal phase than in men. In later months of pregnancy also pCO_2 decreases.

Mechanism of Action

Progesterone produces its effects by binding with intracellular cytoplasmic receptors, leading to increased transcription in the nucleus.

Other Ovarian Hormones

Relaxin It is a polypeptide secreted by the corpus luteum and the placenta. During pregnancy, it relaxes pubic symphysis and other pelvic joints which is helpful during the parturition. Its function in non-pregnant female is not known.

Inhibin This polypeptide hormone is secreted by the corpus luteum. It inhibits FSH secretion.

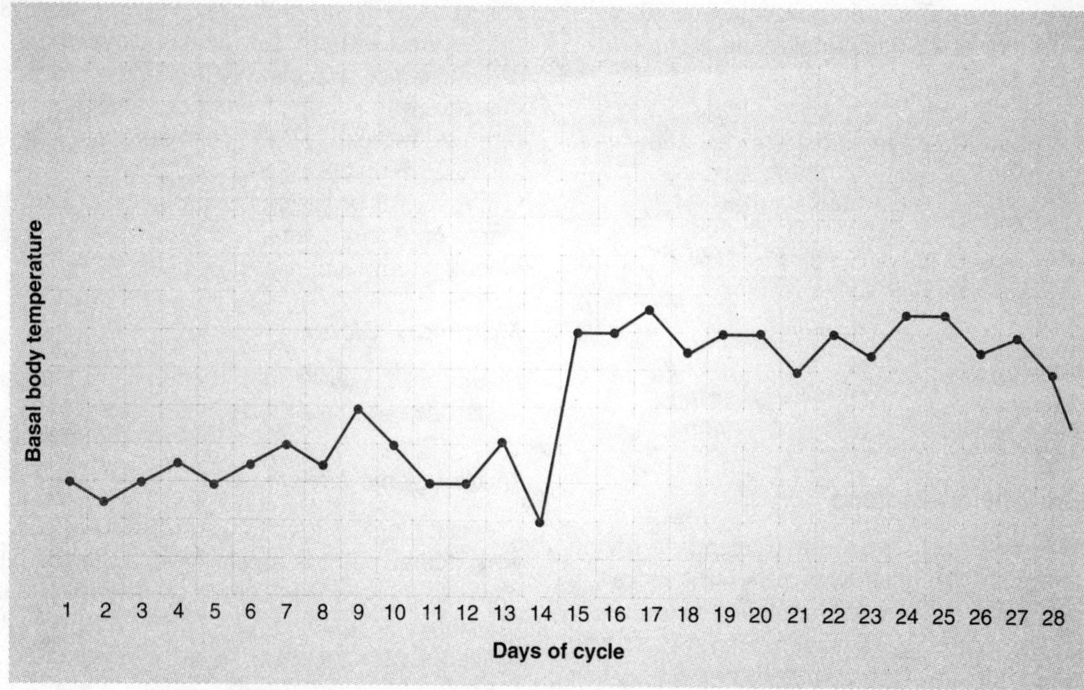

Fig. 53.6: Basal body temperature in the two phases of ovarian cycle.

Testosterone Small amount of testosterone is produced by the theca cells of the ovarian follicles and released into bloodstream. In the peripheral tissues, some of the adrenal androgen (DHEA) is converted to testosterone which also enters blood circulation. Function of the small concentrations of testosterone in the female is not clear. Probably at such low concentrations, testosterone helps in protein anabolism without producing masculinizing effects.

MENSTRUAL CYCLE

The cyclic production of oestrogens and progesterone by the ovary produces cyclic changes in the uterine endometrium terminating in sloughing of the endometrium and bleeding per vaginum (menstruation). On the average, each cycle lasts for 28 days. Conventionally, 1st day of the bleeding is considered to be the 1st day of menstrual cycle. The endometrial changes may be described under three phases, i.e. menstruation (0–5th day), proliferative phase (6th–14th day), and secretory phase (15th–28th day).

For better understanding, the phase of menstruation shall be described last of all.

Proliferative (Follicular) Phase (6th–14th day)

After menstruation, only a thin basal of layer of the original endometrium is left. Under the influence of oestrogens secreted by the developing graafian follicle in the ovary (follicular phase of the ovarian cycle), the glandular epithelial cells proliferate and re-epithelize the endometrial surface. The endometrium gradually thickens due to proliferation of stromal cells and the endometrial glands. The endometrium, which is less than 2 mm thick at the end of menstruation, becomes 3–4 mm thick at the end of the proliferative phase.

Secretory (Luteal) Phase (15th–28th day)

This phase coincides with the luteal phase of the ovarian cycle, when the corpus luteum secretes both the oestrogens and progesterone. Oestrogens produce further proliferation of the endometrial stroma. Progesterone produces marked enlargement and thickening of the endometrial glands.

The glands become coiled and tortuous and secrete small quantities of endometrial fluid.

The endometrium also becomes highly vascularized. The endometrium is supplied by two types of arteries. The superficial two-thirds of the endometrium (stratum functionale) is supplied by long and coiled, spiral arteries whereas the deeper one-third of it (stratum basale) is supplied by short and straight basilar arteries. The coiled arteries become more spiral and form perpendicular columns through the mucosa. The stroma cells become oedematous. Prominent cork-screw-shaped glands and increased vascularity are the two characteristic features of the endometrium in secretory phase. By the end of secretory phase, the endometrium is 4–6 mm thick (Fig. 53.7).

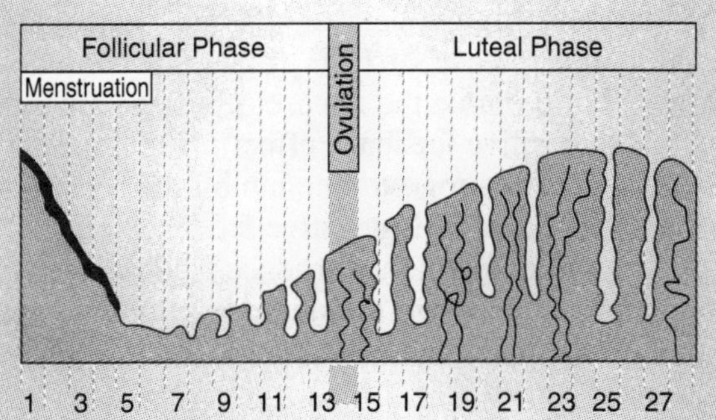

Fig. 53.7: Diagrammatic representation of changes in the endometrium during the menstrual cycle.

Menstruation (0–5th day)

About two days before the end of the menstrual cycle, involution of the corpus luteum causes a sharp decline in the plasma levels of oestrogen and progesterone (Fig. 53.8). The sudden decline in the plasma levels of the two ovarian hormones produces necrotic changes in the stratum functionale of the endometrium, which is ultimately shed along with some amount of blood and mucus.

During 24 hours preceding the onset of menstruation, the spiral arteries undergo intense spasm leading to hypoxia and necrosis in the endometrium, including the walls of the spiral arteries. Blood seeps out of the necrotic vessels into the adjoining stroma. Gradually, the necrotic tissue separates from the remaining viable part of the endometrium to be shed per vaginum. The necrosis and shedding of the endometrium occur in small patches over a period extending from 3–5 days. During this period, approximately 35 ml of blood and another 35 ml of serous fluid are lost along with the necrotic endometrial tissue.

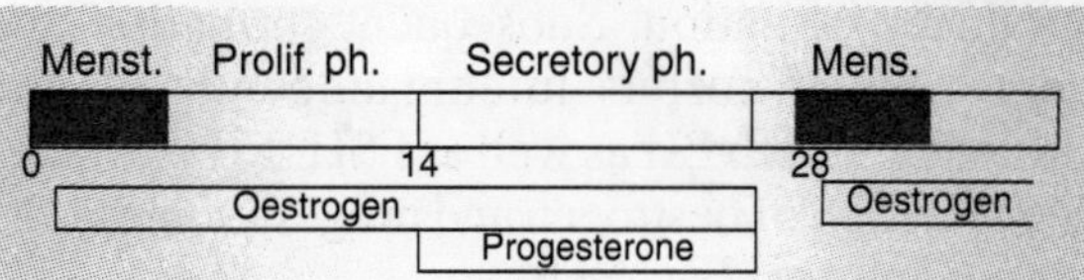

Fig. 53.8: Correlation of different phases of menstrual cycle with the secretion of ovarian hormones.

Changes in the hormonal environment of the endometrium described above, seem to produce large quantities of prostaglandins in the endometrium. Prostaglandins, not only produce vasospasm and necrosis of the endometrium, but also produce contractions of the myometrium which help in the expulsion of the necrotic material.

The menstrual blood is primarily arterial in origin. It does not normally clot because of the fibrinolysins released along with the necrotic endometrial tissue.

Hormonal Regulation of Female Reproductive Cycles

Anterior Pituitary Control Gonadotropins

Two gonadotropins, namely, **follicle stimulating hormone** (FSH) and **luteinizing hormone** (LH), secreted by the anterior pituitary, regulate the ovarian cycle. Both of these hormones are glycoproteins, with molecular weights around 30,000.

FSH is responsible for the development of graafian follicle, as well as, corpus luteum. During the follicular phase, FSH produces proliferation and hypertrophy of granulosa cells, secretion of follicular fluid and differentiation of ovarian stroma into theca interna.

A burst of LH secretion (LH surge) on approximately 14th day of the ovarian cycle produces ovulation. Subsequent formation and secretion of corpus luteum depends on the presence of both LH as well as FSH. LH promotes the secretion of oestrogen and progesterone by the corpus luteum (Fig. 53.9).

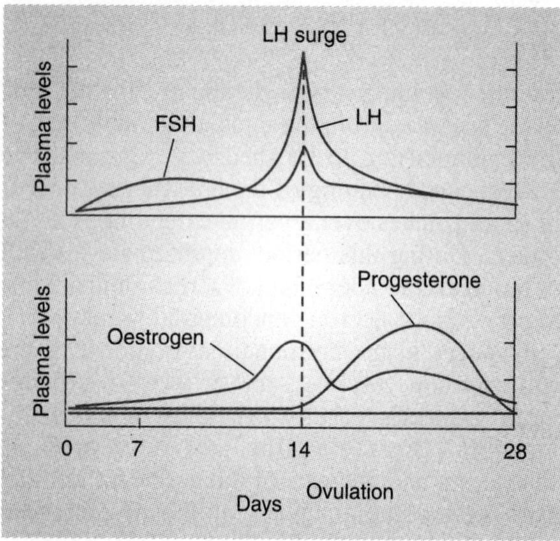

Fig. 53.9: Correlation of blood levels of pituitary gonadotropins with ovarian hormones in different stages of menstrual (ovarian) cycle.

Chorionic Gonadotropin It is produced by the placenta during the first 12–16 weeks of pregnancy. It acts like LH. If the ovum is fertilized and implanted in the endometrium, the secretion of chorionic gonadotropin maintains the corpus luteum in functional state in spite of the deficiency of anterior pituitary gonadotropins. Due to its action, the corpus luteum continues to secrete oestrogen and progesterone during the 1st 3–4 months of pregnancy.

53

Hypothalamic Control

The hypothalamus regulates the secretion of both FSH and LH by a single hormone, the gonadotropin releasing hormone (GnRH). GnRH reaches the anterior pituitary through the hypothalamic-hypophysial portal vessels. In human female, the hypothalamic influence is easily demonstrated by the fact that various types of mental stress commonly disturb the ovarian and menstrual cycles.

Many lower animals are seasonal breeders. The polar cat breeds only in summer. In winter, her gonads are atrophied due to deficient secretion of pituitary gonadotropins. But experimentally, they may be made to breed even in mid-winter by exposure to gradually increasing periods of artificial light. Rabbits and cats ovulate only after mating (reflex ovulation). These examples demonstrate the neural (hypothalamic) control over the anterior pituitary.

Feedback Control

The ovarian hormones oestrogen and progesterone influence the secretion of gonadotropins by the anterior pituitary by a feedback control. Depending on their relative plasma concentrations, they can exert both positive and negative feedback action. Moderately high levels of plasma oestrogens inhibit the release of FSH (negative feedback effect) but promote the release of a large amount of LH (a positive feedback effect). High levels of oestrogens and progesterone inhibit the secretion of both FSH and LH (negative feedback effect).

The ovarian hormones produce feedback effect by acting directly on the anterior pituitary, and through the hypothalamus.

Control of Ovarian Cycle

When the corpus luteum degenerates at the end of ovarian cycle, decreased plasma oestrogen and progesterone levels increase the secretion of FSH, which initiates the development of next ovarian follicle. As the new follicle matures, the oestrogen secretion by the ovary increases. Moderately high levels of oestrogen near the mid-cycle trigger a burst of LH secretion by its positive feedback action. Ovulation occurs approximately 9 hours after the LH surge. After an initial drop in the plasma oestrogen level, it rises once again to a moderate degree during the luteal phase, when progesterone level is also elevated to a more marked degree. The markedly elevated progesterone and oestrogen levels inhibit the release of both FSH and LH from the anterior pituitary. Hence unless pregnancy occurs, the corpus luteum degenerates and the next cycle begins once again (Fig. 53.9).

Control of Endometrial Cycle

The steroid hormones, secreted by the ovary, prepare the endometrium for implantation of the fertilized ovum. The endometrium proliferates by the action of oestrogen during the follicular phase. The further thickening and increased secretory activity during the luteal phase is due to the combined action of oestrogen and progesterone. As a result, the endometrium becomes suitable for nourishment and implantation of the fertilized ovum.

If pregnancy does not occur, the degeneration of corpus luteum leads to a sharp decline in plasma oestrogen and progesterone levels. The withdrawal of hormonal support leads to necrosis and shedding of the superficial layers of the endometrium.

If the ovum is fertilized and implanted, the secretion of chorionic gonadotropin maintains the corpus luteum in secretory state. Consequently, instead of necrosis, the endometrium undergoes further growth and development to form decidua (Fig. 53.10).

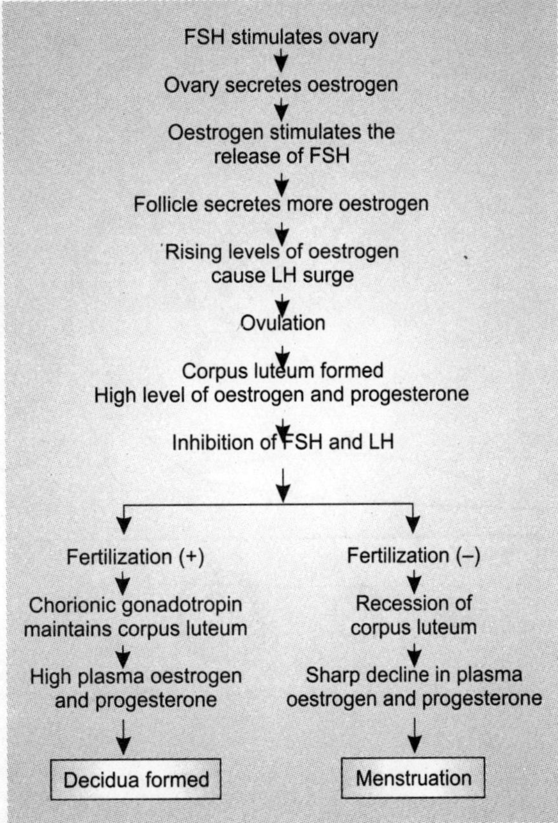

Fig. 53.10: Summary of hormonal control of ovarian and menstrual cycle.

Inter-relationship between Ovarian and Menstrual Cycles

The inter-relationship of different events in the ovarian and menstrual cycles is depicted in Fig. 53.11. The proliferative phase of the menstrual cycle corresponds to the follicular phase of the ovarian cycle. The secretory phase of the menstrual cycle corresponds to the luteal phase of the ovarian cycle (Fig. 53.11).

Each woman has a fairly fixed duration of ovarian and menstrual cycles. However, the duration of menstrual (ovarian) cycle in different women may vary from 25 to 30 days (average 28 days). Of these, the duration of secretory (luteal) phase is remarkably constant at about 14 days. Therefore the variations in the duration of menstrual cycles are mostly due to variations in the length of the proliferative phase. In other words, ovulation occurs approximately on 11th, 14th and 16th day of the menstrual cycles of 25, 28 and 30 days duration, respectively.

Mechanism of Puberty

Puberty means the onset of adult sexual life. It is caused by a gradual increase in the gonadotropin secretion by the anterior pituitary. It begins approximately at the age of 10–14 years in females and at the age of about 12–16 years in males. In childhood, the gonads and the anterior pituitary are capable of function, if appropriately stimulated. However, the hypothalamus does not secrete GnRH. It is believed that the process of maturity basically occurs somewhere in the limbic system, which sends signals to the hypothalamus to start the secretion of GnRH.

Mechanism of Menopause

After the age of 45–50 years, the ovarian cycles and the associated menstrual cycles become initially irregular and ultimately cease altogether. The cessation of reproductive cycles is called the menopause.

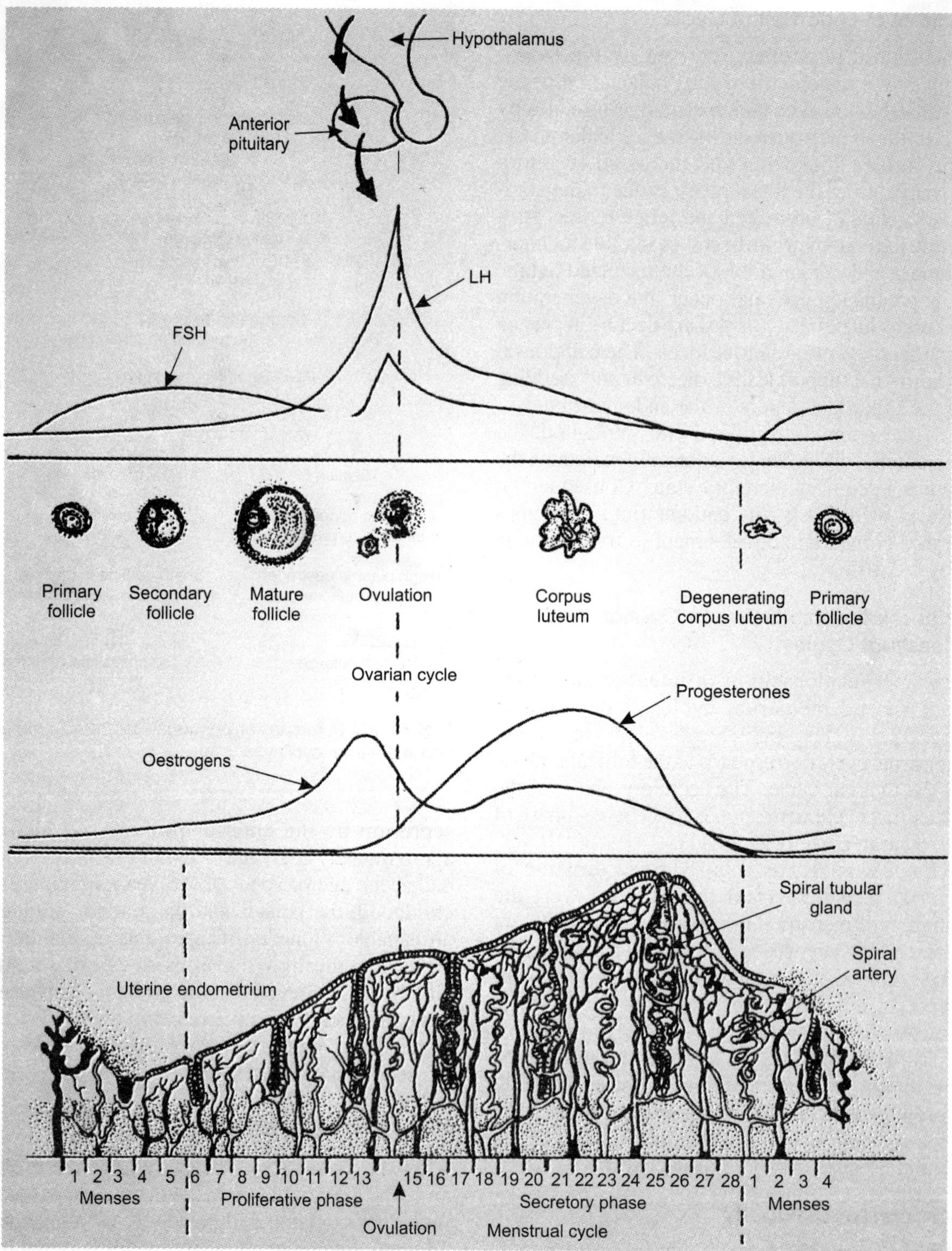

Fig. 53.11: Inter-relationship of different events in the ovarian and menstrual cycles.

As discussed earlier, during each ovarian cycle, many primordial follicles begin to grow, of which only one matures to be ovulated. In this fashion, by the time a woman reaches 45–50 years of age, the number of primordial follicles is reduced to zero and the ovaries become small and fibrosed. The consequent decrease in oestrogen secretion results in persistent and marked increase in FSH secretion. To some extent, LH secretion is also increased (feedback effect).

Thus, the menopause is because of ovarian failure rather than deficiency of pituitary gonadotropins.

Female Sexual Act

The sexual desire in the female is partly produced by the effect of oestrogen on the hypothalamus. The sexual desire is believed to be increased near the time of ovulation, probably because of high levels of oestrogens secreted by the ovary. Erotic thoughts also increase the sexual desire.

In the female, the sexual sensation is aroused from massage or irritation of the external genitalia and the perineal region. The clitoris is specially sensitive for initiating sexual sensation. The sensory signals are transmitted to the sacral segments of spinal cord through pudendal nerve (somatic S_2, S_3, S_4) for onward transmission to the cereberal cortex. Local reflexes are integrated in the S_2, S_3, S_4 and L_1, L_2 spinal segments.

In the initial stages of sexual stimulation, parasympathetic discharge to the external genitalia causes rapid accumulation of blood in the introitus and clitoris. Parasympathetic discharge also increases the secretion of mucus by Bartholin's gland, just inside the introitus.

Upper part of vagina is sensitive to stretch produced by glans penis. In addition, tactile stimulation of labia minora and clitoris adds to the sexual excitement. These stimuli are reinforced by tactile stimulation of the breasts. When the sexual stimulation reaches maximum intensity, sexual reflexes produce rhythmic contractions of vaginal wall and bulbocavernosus and ischio-cavernosus muscles. These contractions produce the sensation called the female orgasm, which gives a feeling of sexual satisfaction.

Indicators of Ovulation

In clinical practice, it is often important to know whether ovulation is occurring or not or to know the day of ovulation, e.g. in cases of female infertility.

1. Basal Body Temperature The woman is asked to record her basal body temperature each morning of the menstrual cycle. The body temperature is elevated by 0.2–0.5°C during the luteal phase as compared to that in the follicular phase (Fig. 53.6). The elevation of temperature begins 1–2 days after ovulation, corresponding to the elevated plasma progesterone level.

2. Changes in Cervical Mucus When a smear of cervical mucus is examined under a microscope, a characteristic fern-like pattern is seen during the follicular phase which is absent in the secretory phase. In anovulatory cycles, the fern-like pattern persists throughout the menstrual cycle (Fig. 53.5).

3. Endometrial Biopsy An endometrial biopsy is taken during the third week of menstrual cycle. Histological evidence of secretory endometrium indicates that the menstrual cycles are ovulatory.

4. Ultrasonography of the Ovaries Serial ultrasonographic study of the ovaries can reveal the development and the day of rupture of the Graafian follicle. This is by far more accurate and less cumbersome method to find out the day of ovulation than the measurement of basal body temperature.

5. Plasma Progesterone Level Elevation of plasma progesterone level on 21st day of 28 days menstrual cycle is the easiest, most accurate and non-invasive method to confirm the ovulatory nature of the ovarian cycles.

Female Infertility

Absence of ovulation (anovulation) during the reproductive age of the female may result from isolated gonadotropin deficiency, prolactin secreting tumour of anterior pituitary, abnormalities of thyroid or adrenal glands or due to primary ovarian failure.

Blockade of fallopian tubes by pelvic inflammation is a fairly common cause of female infertility in the face of normal ovulatory ovarian cycles.

Function Tests

1. At first, it is important to establish whether ovulation is occurring or not. One or more of the five tests for this purpose described above may be used.

2. Hormonal studies can help in the diagnosis of the cause of anovulation. Plasma levels of FSH, LH, oestradiol and prolactin are estimated. The function of thyroid and adrenal gland is also investigated. Low plasma FSH, LH and oestradiol levels are seen in patients with pituitary disorders.

High plasma FSH and LH levels and low plasma oestradiol are seen in patients with primary ovarian failure.

3. Hysterosalpingography. Radiological examination of uterus and fallopian tubes after injection of a radio-opaque aqueous solution through the cervix is the most useful investigation for testing the patency of the fallopian tubes.

4. Chromosomal analysis. It is essential for the diagnosis of Turner's syndrome.

IN VITRO FERTILIZATION— EMBRYO TRANSFER (IVF-ET)

A woman with infertility due to bilateral tubal blockade may be helped to conceive by IVF-ET. In this method, the woman is given drugs which induce hyperovulation (hCG; clomiphene). Just before the expulsion, all the mature ova are retrieved from the ovaries and incubated *in vitro* with the husband's sperms. The fertilized ova are transferred to the woman's uterine cavity for implantation and further development.

Artificial Insemination

In a couple with infertility due to poor quality of sperms, the woman can be made to conceive by artificial insemination by a donor's sperms. The semen is introduced into the vagina on the day of ovulation.

CHAPTER 54

Physiology of Human Pregnancy and Lactation

PREGNANCY

TRANSPORT OF SPERMS

During coitus, the sperms are released in the upper part of vagina. Within 30 minutes, sperms can be detected in the lateral one-third of the fallopian tubes.

The rapidity of sperm transport cannot be explained merely on the basis of sperm motility (1–4 mm/min). It is believed that the stimulation of female genitalia during coitus leads to secretion of oxytocin by the posterior pituitary gland. Oxytocin induces propulsive movements in the uterus and fallopian tubes. Seminal prostaglandins also seem to be involved in the production of retrograde uterine motility. High concentration of oestrogen in the plasma at the time of ovulation also helps in sperm transport by production of thin, watery and copious amounts of mucus by the cervical glands. Even then, of the several million sperms released into the vagina, only 100–300 sperms manage to reach the fallopian tubes and only one would be required for the fertilization of the ovum.

TRANSPORT OF OVUM

After expulsion from the ovary, the ovum surrounded by corona radiata enters the fimbriated end of the fallopian tube. Oestrogen induced increase in the ciliary movement of the fimbriae helps to guide the ovum into the fallopian tube.

The fertilization usually occurs in the ampulla of the fallopian tube. The ovum is viable for 6–24 hours after it is shed from the ovary. The sperms can survive for 1–2 days in the female genital tract. Therefore, pregnancy occurs only if sexual intercourse takes place some time between one day before and one day after the ovulation.

FERTILIZATION

Although many sperms surround the corona radiata, only one of them can manage to enter the ovum and fertilize it. The penetration of the ovum is aided by the proteolytic enzymes present in the acrosome of the head of the sperm. The chemical structure of the zona pellucida is such that, after the entry of one sperm, the change in its molecular structure makes it non-penetrable by another sperm. Soon after the sperm enters the ovum, the 2nd polar body is extruded and the fertilization occurs. The fertilized ovum begins to divide and proceed through the fallopian tube towards the uterine cavity. It takes about 3 days for the fertilized ovum to reach the uterus; by this time, it has undergone several divisions and is called *blastocyst*. Once the blastocyst comes in contact with the endometrium, it becomes surrounded by an outer layer of syncytiotrophoblast and an inner layer of cytotrophoblast. The syncytiotrophoblast cells secrete proteolytic enzymes that digest the endometrium and the blastocyst burrows into the endometrium. This process is called the *implantation* of the blastocyst. Thus, the blastocyst spends about 3 days in the fallopian tube and another 3 days in the uterine cavity before implantation. During this period, it is nourished by the secretions of the fallopian tube and the uterine glands. Ultimately, the placenta takes up the nutritive, hormonal and immunological functions.

A textbook of embryology may be consulted for the details of embryogenesis and development of the placenta.

FUNCTIONS OF PLACENTA

Hormone Secretion

The placenta secretes a large number of hormones, such as human chorionic gonadotropin (hCG), oestrogens, progesterone, human chorionic somatomammotropin and relaxin. All these hormones are secreted predominantly into the maternal circulation but they have an important role in fetal physiology also.

Human Chorionic Gonadotropin (hCG)

Human chorionic gonadotropin is a glycoprotein with a molecular weight of 39,000. Its chemical structure and functions are similar to those of LH secreted by the anterior pituitary. It can be detected in the maternal blood as early as 8 days after fertilization, i.e. just after the implantation of the blastocyst in the endometrium. The blood levels of hCG gradually increase and reach a peak approximately 8 weeks after fertilization (Fig. 54.1) and then decline to very low levels by 12–16 weeks. The placenta continues to produce small amount of hCG throughout pregnancy. Its most important function is to prevent the involution of corpus luteum which normally occurs about 2 weeks after the ovulation, because of decreased gonadotropin secretion by the anterior pituitary.

(i) HCG maintains the corpus luteum viable for 3–4 months after the onset of pregnancy. The corpus luteum, in fact, enlarges further and secretes larger amounts of oestrogens and progesterone required

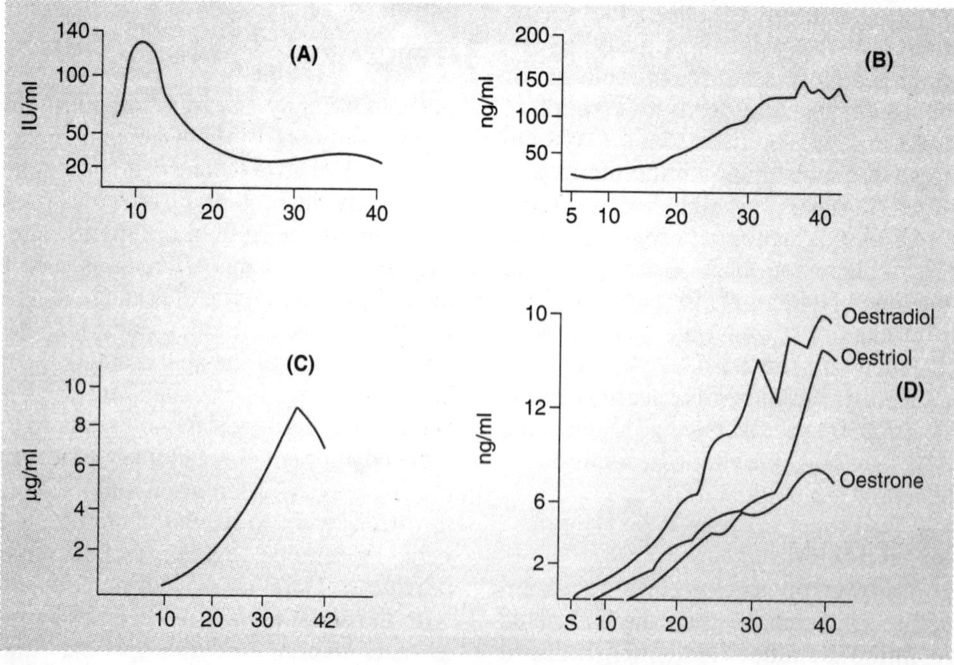

Plasma levels of hCG (A), progesterone (B), hCS (C) and oestrogens (D) during different weeks of human pregnancy.

for the development of decidua and myometrium. The removal of the corpus luteum in the first 12 weeks leads to termination of pregnancy (abortion).

(ii) In the male fetus, hCG serves an additional function. It causes proliferation of Leydig cells in the fetal testes and causes secretion of testosterone. In the male fetus, testosterone is essential for the development of male sex organs in the early embryonic life, and the descent of testis out of the abdomen in the later stages of gestation.

(iii) hCG is excreted by the kidney in the urine, as such. The presence of hCG in the urine can be detected by a sensitive immunological test and hence can be used to establish the diagnosis of pregnancy at a very early stage of gestation.

Oestrogens

After the first three months of pregnancy, placenta becomes the chief site of synthesis and secretion of oestrogens. Oestrogen secretion increases progressively throughout the later months of pregnancy (Fig. 54.1). Near term, 24-hour urinary oestrogen excretion may exceed 30 mg as compared to 0.1–0.5 mg in non-pregnant state. In the synthesis of oestrogen (and progesterone), the fetus and the placenta are so intimately involved that these hormones are said to be synthesized by the feto-placental unit rather than by placenta alone.

Besides oestradiol, the placenta produces large amount of oestriol. Its major precursor is dehydroepiandrosterone sulphate (DHEAs). DHEAs is synthesized by the fetal adrenal cortex from acetate. It is hydroxylated in the fetal liver and the product is passed on to the placenta where α-hydroxydehydroepiandrosterone is converted to oestriol. In the mother, oestriol is excreted into urine after conjugation with glucuronic acid. In view of this fundamental role of feto-placental unit in the synthesis of oestrogens, urinary oestriol level is clinically used as an index of the health of the fetus. Fetal growth retardation or death results in a decline in the urinary excretion of oestriol in the mother (Fig. 54.2A). The importance of this function of fetal adrenal cortex is shown by the fact that the size of adrenal cortex is larger in fetus than in adults.

During pregnancy, the high level of plasma oestrogens produce enlargement of the uterus and breast. Oestrogens also produce relaxation of pelvic ligaments, so that the sacroiliac joints and the pubic symphysis are softened. These changes facilitate the passage of the baby out of the birth canal.

The purpose of secretion of oestriol in large amounts during pregnancy is not clear. According to one hypothesis, large amounts of oestriol, produced during human pregnancy, ensure a quiescent uterus during prelabour pregnancy. By combining with most of the myometrial nuclear receptors, oestriol leaves an inadequate number of receptors for the excitatory action of oestradiol on the myometrium.

Progesterone

The placental secretion of progesterone also increases progressively during the last 6 months of pregnancy. At term, the urinary excretion of progesterone is approximately 45 mg/day as compared to 5 mg/day in the luteal phase of the ovarian cycle. Cholesterol from the maternal compartment is the chief substrate for the placental synthesis of progesterone. After synthesis in the placenta, progesterone passes to the mother as well as to the fetus. In the fetal adrenal cortex, it is used for the synthesis of corticosteroids (Fig. 54.2B). In the mother, the initial (1–3 months) development of decidua and maintenance of pregnancy is due to progesterone secreted by the corpus luteum. In subsequent (4–9) months, progesterone secreted from placenta is essential for decreasing the spontaneous contractions of the uterine myometrium. Progesterone also promotes the alveolar growth in the breasts and thus prepares them for lactation.

Human Chorionic Somatomammotropin (HCS)

The placenta also secretes large amounts of a protein that is lactogenic in nature. It has a small degree of growth promoting activity also. This hormone has been called human chorionic

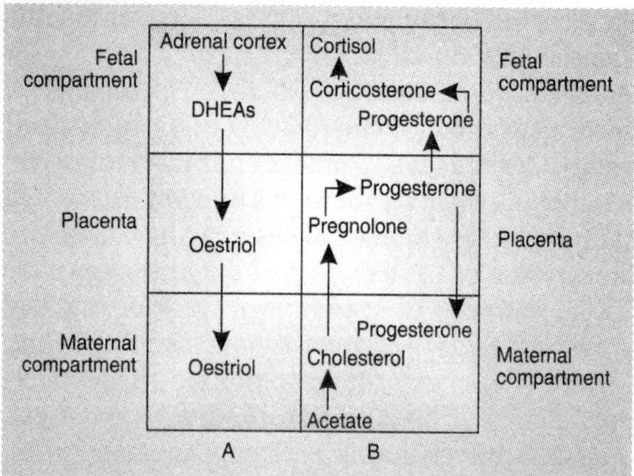

Fig. 54.2: Synthesis of steroid hormones by feto-placental unit.

somatomammotropin or chorionic growth hormone prolactin. Large quantities of this hormone are found in the maternal blood but very little amount reaches the fetus. It seems to produce retention of nitrogen, calcium and potassium in the mother. It also decreases maternal glucose utilization and promotes lipolysis, thereby sparing more glucose for the fetus.

Relaxin

It is believed to soften pelvic ligaments, particularly the pubic symphysis. Thus, it helps in the delivery.

Other Functions of Placenta

Gas Transfer

The placenta acts as the fetal-lung. Respiratory gases are transferred between the maternal and the fetal blood across the villus membrane.

The diffusion across the villus membrane is not as efficient as is across the pulmonary alveolar membrane. Even otherwise, the mean pO_2 of the maternal blood in the placental sinuses is only about 50 mmHg (cf. 100 mmHg in the alveolar air). The mean pO_2 of the fetal blood leaving the chorionic villi is not more than 30 mmHg (cf. 100 mmHg in the arterial blood). Low pO_2 of the fetal arterial blood would have been a serious problem for oxygen transport, but for the presence of fetal-haemoglobin (HbF) in the fetal RBCs. Since HbF has far greater affinity for O_2 than the adult haemoglobin (p. 194), fetal blood can become fairly well saturated with O_2 even at this low pO_2 value. The oxygen carrying capacity is further increased by greater haemoglobin concentration in the fetal blood. Moreover, fetal tissues are more resistant to hypoxia than the adult tissues.

CO_2 diffuses from the fetal blood to the maternal blood across the placental membrane. Due to greater solubility coefficient of CO_2, the diffusion of CO_2 is more efficient than O_2.

Nutritive Function

The placenta provides for all the nutritive needs of the fetus. Many substances like glucose, FFA, potassium, sodium and chloride diffuse rapidly from maternal to the fetal blood. Amino acids, calcium and inorganic phosphate are transferred to the fetus by an active transport mechanism. Their concentrations in the fetal blood are greater than those in the maternal blood.

The maternal proteins do not traverse the placental barrier, with the exception of immunoglobulin **(IgG)**, which passes over from the mother to the fetus by receptor mediated endocytosis. Thereby the fetus obtains a passive immunity against various infectious diseases. The other immunglobulins, mainly IgM proteins, do not pass through the placental barrier.

Transferrin It is another important maternal protein that, as the name indicates, transports iron. On the surface of the placenta, specific receptors exist for this protein, which, by means of active transport, enters into fetal tissue.

Protein can also be transferred from the fetus to the mother; **alpha-fetoprotein** (the concentration of which is elevated in several fetal abnormalities) can be detected in the maternal blood.

It may be remembered that Rh-agglutinins are transferred easily from the mother to the fetus but ABO agglutinins are not. That is why Rh incompatibility between the fetus and the mother results in far more serious complications than the ABO incompatibility.

54

Many drugs including nicotine and barbiturates can pass through the placental barrier. That is how maternal smoking can harm the fetus.

Excretory Function

Excretory products like urea, uric acid and creatinine, etc. are removed from the fetal blood by diffusion into the maternal circulation.

Immunosuppression

The fetus is not rejected even though its set of chromosomes differs from that of its mother and halfway represents an allogenic transplantation to the maternal organism (two individuals of the same kind, but genetically only half identical). This phenomenon remains an enigma. After birth, the maternal organism rejects any tissue of the newborn, even though the same tissue ("natural allogeneic transplantation") was accepted, protected and nourished for 9 months. During pregnancy, the mother developed a tolerance to her child. This phenomenon is based on the specific antigenic property of the embryo and the placenta as well as on the transitory changes of the maternal immune system during pregnancy.

PREGNANCY TESTS

All the tests for the diagnosis of pregnancy at an early stage are based on the detection of hCG in the urine of the pregnant female. The *biological tests* used earlier consisted of injecting mother's urine in immature female mice or virgin rabbit or male toad. Presence of hCG in the urine resulted in ovulation in the immature female mice or virgin rabbit. In the male toad, the release of sperms indicated the presence of hCG in the urine.

Nowadays, biological tests have been replaced by *immunological test* of pregnancy because of the greater sensitivity, convenience and immediate results.

In the immunological test, the urine sample is mixed with anti-serum against hCG and then latex particles coated with hCG are added. Absence of flocculation is taken as evidence of pregnancy since hCG antibodies have been neutralized by hCG present in the urine.

With the urine sample from a non-pregnant subject, the hCG antibodies produce flocculation of the hCG-coated latex particles (Fig. 54.3).

Immunological test for pregnancy can give positive results just 2 weeks after conception, i.e. just when menstrual period is missed for the first time and suspicion of pregnancy arises.

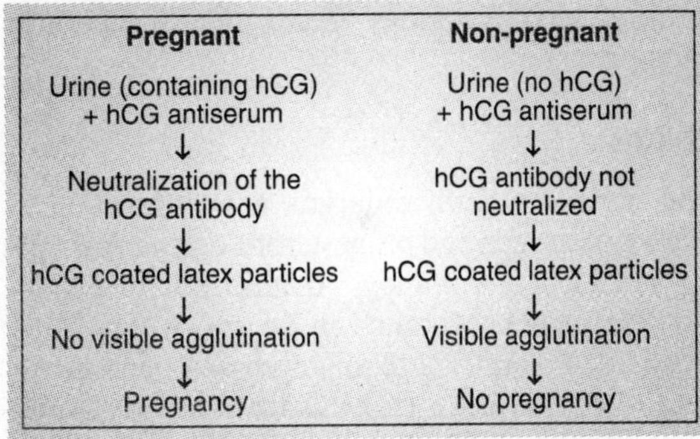

Fig. 54.3: Principle of immunological test for pregnancy.

PHYSIOLOGICAL CHANGES DURING PREGNANCY

The progressive growth of the fetus from a single-celled ovum to a three kilogram baby imposes various types of extra demands on the body of the mother. These additional demands are met with by tremendous adaptations in almost all the organ-systems of the body.

Genital Organs

Uterus

The uterus undergoes a gradual enlargement from 7.5 cm length in non-pregnant state to 35 cm length at term. Its weight also increases from 50 gm to 1 kg at term. The initial enlargement of the uterus is chiefly because of the hypertrophy of the myometrial smooth muscle fibres, although some hyperplasia also occurs specially during the first trimester of pregnancy (0–12 weeks). Enlargement of the uterus during 2nd and 3rd trimesters (12–24 weeks, and 24–36 weeks respectively) is mainly because of the stretching of the muscle fibres by the enlarging fetus. The non-pregnant uterine wall is about 1.25 cm thick. It becomes thicker during the initial stages of hypertrophy and hyperplasia. By term, the stretching of the muscle fibres makes it as thin as 5 mm only. The muscle fibres of the myometrium form an interlacing network around the uterine blood vessels. Contraction of these muscle fibres after delivery of the placenta limits the blood loss from the raw placental site by acting as 'living ligatures'. Failure of firm contraction of the myometrium may lead to fatal postpartum haemorrhage.

Ovary

The corpus luteum enlarges and continues to secrete oestrogen and progesterone during first 12–16 weeks of pregnancy. Around 8th week, its diameter may be as much as 2.5 cm. After 12–16 weeks, the corpus luteum regresses because of decreased secretion of hCG from the placenta. Throughout pregnancy, and initial 6 weeks postpartum, the ovarian cycles (menstrual cycles) remain suspended.

Breasts

Enlargement of the breasts starts early in pregnancy. Increased secretion of various hormones is responsible for hyperplasia of the ductal and alveolar tissue. The nipple becomes larger and deeply pigmented. The pigmentation is prominent in the areola also. Many sebaceous glands become prominent in the areola (Montgomery's tubercles).

Weight Gain

In normal pregnancy, the mother gains 10–12 kg of body weight. Of this, the fetus accounts for 3 kg only. The rest of the weight gain is due to increased weight of the uterus (1 kg), placenta and amniotic fluid (1.5 kg), increased blood volume (1.3 kg), increased interstitial fluid (1.2 kg) and maternal deposition of fat (3.5 kg).

Increased secretion of oestrogens, progesterone, aldosterone and ADH is responsible for NaCl and H_2O retention in pregnancy.

During antenatal examination, body weight of the expectant mother is regularly monitored. Absence of weight gain in 2nd or 3rd trimester is an important sign of fetal growth retardation or fetal death. Conversely, excessive and rapid weight gain (because of excessive fluid retention) should raise the suspicion of toxaemia of pregnancy. In the 1st trimester, significant gain in body weight may not occur because of severe anorexia and vomiting (*morning sickness*).

Skin Changes

Excessive pigmentation on the face in butterfly pattern (chloasma), in areola, nipple and midline of abdomen extending from xiphisternum to symphysis pubis are prominent skin changes which occur during pregnancy. In most of the cases, the pigmentation regresses after delivery.

Stria gravidarum are slightly depressed linear scars on the lower abdominal wall. They are cutaneous scars produced by mechanical stretching of the abdominal wall. (Besides pregnancy, such scars may occur in ascites, severe obesity and Cushing's syndrome, i.e. whenever the abdominal wall is over-stretched).

Blood

The blood volume begins to increase after 12 weeks of pregnancy and by 32nd week, it is about 30% above the non-pregnant level. This increased blood volume is maintained till delivery and returns to normal by the end of 2nd week postpartum. The extra blood volume helps to fill up the additional placental circulation.

The increase in the blood volume is produced by relatively greater increase in plasma volume than the red cell volume. The consequent haemodilution accounts for slight decrease in haemoglobin concentration (by 1–2 gm%) even though the total red cell mass has actually increased (Fig. 54.4).

The total plasma protein concentration decreases from the normal 7.5 gm% to about 6 gm%. The decrease is only partly because of haemodilution because there are quantitative differences in different plasma proteins. The concentration of albumin is decreased, whereas that of globulins, and especially fibrinogen is

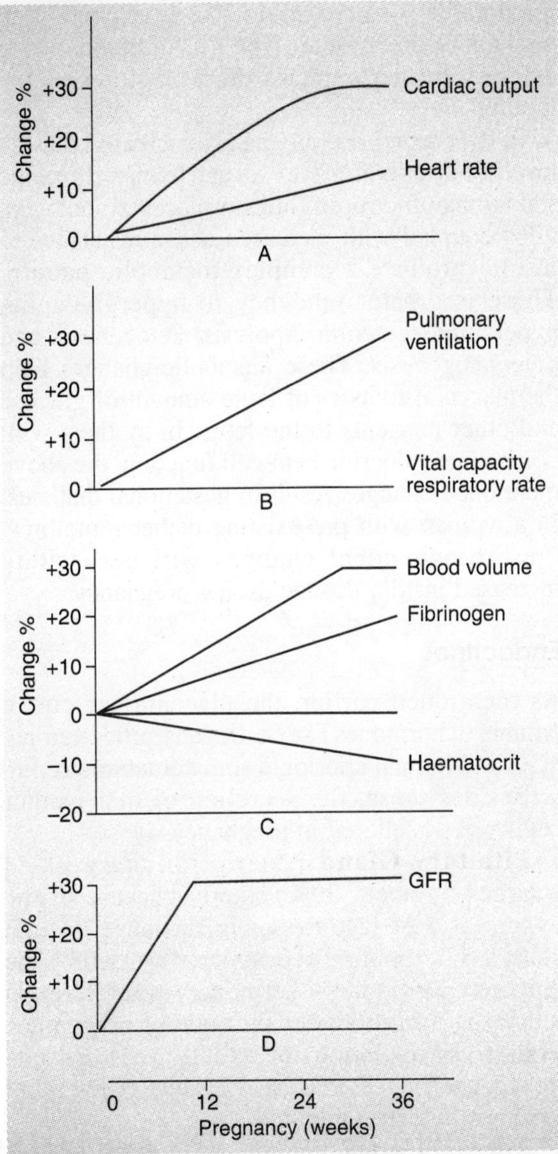

Fig. 54.4: Physiological changes during pregnancy. (A) Cardiovascular; (B) Respiratory; (C) Haematological; (D) Renal.

increased. The increased fibrinogen concentration explains the raised ESR during pregnancy.

Total leucocyte count may increase to 15,000–20,000/mm³. It is mainly because of increased neutrophil count.

Cardiovascular System

In the later months of pregnancy, enlarged uterus presses upon the diaphragm and displaces the heart into a more horizontal position. Clinically, the apex beat may be detected 2.5 cm outside the mid-clavicular line. Equally misleading is the left-axis deviation observed in ECG. Both these findings may mislead one to diagnose left ventricular hypertrophy, although the findings are merely because of horizontal position of the heart.

The cardiac output increases progressively throughout pregnancy and at 32nd week it is approximately 30% above normal (Fig. 54.4). The normal value of cardiac output is restored during the first week postpartum. The additional cardiac output is distributed mainly to the uterus, and kidneys. The circulation to these regions may increase by 750 ml/min, and 400 ml/min, respectively.

Blood pressure remains normal in spite of marked increase in blood volume and cardiac output. Obviously, this is because of decrease in the peripheral resistance. In the 2nd trimester of pregnancy, the diastolic blood pressure may actually be lower by 5–10 mmHg, than in the non-pregnant state. The peripheral resistance is decreased by the action of progesterone on the vascular smooth muscle.

Femoral venous pressure is increased by the effect of gravid uterus on the inferior vena cava. As a result, prolonged period of standing commonly produces oedema of the feet. The increased abdominal venous pressure predisposes the pregnant women to varicose veins, piles, and peripheral venous thrombosis.

Respiratory System

In spite of increased pressure of the uterus on the diaphragm, the vital capacity remains unchanged during pregnancy. Tidal volume and pulmonary ventilation are, however, increased (Fig. 54.4) due to increased sensitivity of respiratory centres to CO_2. Arterial pCO_2 may be as low as 33 mmHg (cf. 40 mmHg normally). Progesterone seems to be responsible for the altered sensitivity of the respiratory centres.

Gastrointestinal Tract

Hypochlorhydria is fairly common in pregnancy. The motility of the stomach, gut and bile duct is decreased under the effect of progesterone. Anorexia, nausea and vomiting, especially in the morning are commonly seen during the 1st trimester of pregnancy. The condition is called "morning sickness".

The disturbance in the glucose tolerance curve is commonly observed in pregnancy. It nearly approaches the prediabetic pattern. It is partly because of rapid glucose absorption in the intestine. The glycosuria is also common, but its chief cause is increased GFR and consequent greater glucose load on the renal tubules.

Kidney

The glomerular filtration rate is increased by about 25% (Fig. 54.4). Consequently, the clearance of many substances, including useful nutrients, is increased. Slight hypercalciuria, glycosuria and amino aciduria commonly occur in pregnancy.

Metabolism

Oxygen consumption is increased by approximately 30% in pregnancy. This may be attributed to increased metabolism in the fetus and the uterus.

There is a positive nitrogen balance. The abnormality in glucose tolerance has been mentioned above. Plasma concentrations of cholesterol, phospholipids and triglycerides are increased. Fat is stored in the adipose tissue to serve as a reservoir of energy for lactation.

During normal pregnancy, the mother retains an extra 50 g of calcium and 30–40 g of phosphorus. Of this, over 30 g of calcium and phosphorus each are deposited in the fetus and the rest in the maternal stores in the skeleton. Skeletal stores act as reservoir for the additional demands of calcium during lactation.

Iron requirements of the body are markedly increased during pregnancy, as well as, during lactation. Iron is required for the synthesis of increased red cell mass of the mother, as well as, red cell production in the fetus. Hypertrophy and hyperplasia of the uterus also increase the requirement of myoglobin (the iron containing pigment of the muscle). The loss of blood during delivery further depletes the iron stores of the mother.

In later months of pregnancy, increased plasma levels of insulin, free cortisol and human chorionic somatomammotropin (human placental lactogen, hPL) coupled with increased tissue resistance to insulin produce a complex metabolic pattern. These is greater tendency to hyperglycemia, hyperaminoacidemia, lipolysis, ketogenesis and gluconeogenesis. These metabolic changes help the placental transfer of large amount of glucose and other nutrients to the fetus. In mothers with borderline endocrine beta-cell function, the above mentioned changes result in gestational diabetes. In a woman with pre-existing diabetes mellitus, these biochemical changes will necessitate increased insulin dosage during pregnancy.

Endocrines

As mentioned earlier, the placenta secretes a number of hormones like oestrogens, progesterone, hCG and human chorionic somatomammotropin.

Besides these, the secretion of many other endocrines is altered in pregnancy.

Pituitary Gland Anterior pituitary gland enlarges by about 30%, chiefly because of the hyperplasia of lactotropes in response to high plasma concentration of oestrogen. Prolactin is the only anterior pituitary hormone whose secretion increases progressively throughout pregnancy. Plasma concentrations of ACTH, TSH and GH remain unchanged. Plasma FSH and LH levels fall to almost undetectable levels.

Adrenal Cortex Plasma total cortisol level is elevated to 3 times the normal level, mainly because of oestrogen induced increase in cortisol-binding globulin. However, plasma free cortisol level also rises but to a moderate degree only. Enhanced glucocorticoid level may contribute to deposition of fat in the adipose tissues, including the breasts. It may contribute to plethoric face, thin skin, appearance of striae, etc. in pregnancy.

Pancreas During pregnancy, ß cell hyperplasia leads to increased size of the islets. Plasma insulin levels are elevated during the 2nd and 3rd trimesters of pregnancy. However, maternal tissue sensitivity to insulin is depressed, as shown by elevated blood glucose levels during glucose tolerance test. Thus, insulin hypersecretion may be considered compensatory in nature.

Aldosterone Secretion of aldosterone increases progressively during pregnancy, reaching 6–8 folds the non-pregnant level by term. This is because of the increased plasma renin and angiotensin levels. Increased renin secretion seems to occur in response to a decrease in effective circulating volume resulting from the large placental blood pool. The plasma concentration of the other mineralo-corticoid, the deoxycorticosterone (DOC) is increased thousand fold. It is synthesized in the maternal kidney by 21-hydroxylation of pro-gesterone. Maternal hyperaldosteronism serves to maintain positive Na^+ balance and high maternal plasma volume.

Parathormone and 1,25(OH)$_2$D$_3$ Large fetal demand of calcium requires increased intestinal calcium absorption. This is met with by hyper-plasia of parathyroid glands and increased plasma PTH levels. Plasma 1, 25(OH)$_2$D$_3$ level is also elevated in pregnancy.

Thyroid Maternal thyroid gland increases in size during pregnancy. Increased iodide uptake, BMR and resting pulse rate are indicative of increased thyroid gland activity, even though plasma *free* T_4 level remains normal. Total plasma T_4 level is elevated because of the oestrogen-induced increase in thyroxin-binding globulin.

PARTURITION

This is the process by which the products of conception, which include fetus, membranes and the placenta, are expelled out of the uterus per vaginum.

The average duration of human pregnancy is 270 days from the day of fertilization of the ovum. Since this day cannot be accurately determined, the first day of the last menstrual period (LMP) is the day from which the duration of pregnancy is conventionally calculated. When counted in this way, the average period of gestation is 284 days (Fig. 54.5).

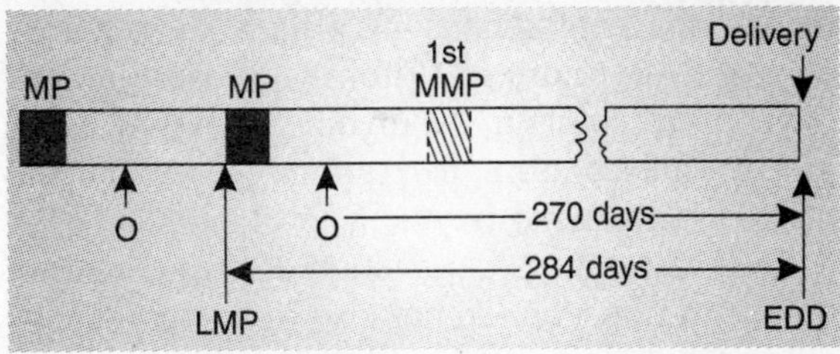

Fig. 54.5: Calculation of expected date of delivery (EDD). O, ovulation; MP, menstrual period; MMP, missed menstrual period; LMP, last menstrual period.

Throughout pregnancy, the myometrium has been practically quiescent, although it becomes progressively more excitable near the term (end of normal duration of pregnancy). The onset of parturition (labour) is difficult to predict. It may start any time between 37th–40th weeks of gestation.

At the onset of labour, mild contractions of the myometrium begin, which become progressively stronger during the next 10–12 hours. Ultimately, the uterine contractions become so powerful that the baby as well the other products of conception are expelled. Although, the exact cause of the onset of labour is not known, a number of hormonal mechanisms seem to be involved.

Oestrogen-Progesterone Ratio The excit-ability of uterine smooth muscle is increased by oestrogens and decreased by progesterone. Throughout later months of pregnancy, both the hormones are secreted in progressively increasing amounts by the placenta. However, in the last few weeks of pregnancy, the secretion of oestrogens increases more than that of progesterone. Therefore, it has been suggested that finally, oestrogens to progesterone ratio increases to such an extent that the uterus begins to contract.

Oxytocin The number of oxytocin receptors in the myometrium and decidua increase by more than 100-fold by the end of pregnancy. Increased plasma oestrogens concentration seems to be responsible for this increase in the number of oxytocin receptors.

The oxytocin concentration in the maternal plasma is found to increase only in later stages of labour, when the cervix begins to dilate. Then, the uterine contractions may be at least partly oxytocin-dependent. Increased number of oxytocin receptors in the myometrium may cause uterine musculature to respond even to mild increase in plasma oxytocin level.

Oxytocin causes contraction of the uterus not only by a direct action but also by increasing the formation of prostaglandins in the decidua. Prostaglandins enhance the force of oxytocin-induced uterine contractions. Administration of drugs like aspirin or indomethacin, which inhibit prostaglandin synthesis, may interfere with the process of labour.

Spinal Reflexes and Voluntary Contraction of abdominal muscles during labour help in the expulsion of the baby but are not absolutely essential.

Role of Fetus It is also possible that some hormones of fetal origin may play a role in initiating the onset of labour. Experimental destruction of fetal pituitary gland has been shown to delay the onset of labour in sheep. In sheep, the fetal pituitary gland secretes larger amount of ACTH a few days before parturition. ACTH causes fetal adrenal gland to secrete larger quantities of adrenal cortical steroids which reach the placenta via the umbilical cord. In the placenta, the adrenal steroids increase the synthesis of oestrogens and prostaglandins, which initiate the first stage of labour.

Mechanics of Parturition (Labour)

54 During pregnancy, the uterus can be divided into three segments, namely: (i) upper uterine segment, (ii) lower uterine segment and (iii) the cervix. During pregnancy, the upper uterine segment undergoes greatest degree of myometrial hyperplasia and hypertrophy. During labour, this segment shows strong contractions which push the fetus along the birth canal. The cervix is comprised mostly (90%) of collagen tissue and very small amount of smooth muscle fibres. In the last few weeks of pregnancy, various hormonal changes result in chemical changes in the collagen fibres leading to softening of the cervix. Moreover, the cervix is gradually incorporated into the lower uterine segment.

By the end of pregnancy, in about 90% of the cases, the head of the fetus occupies the lower uterine segment whereas the hips with folded legs occupy the fundus of the uterus (Fig. 54.6).

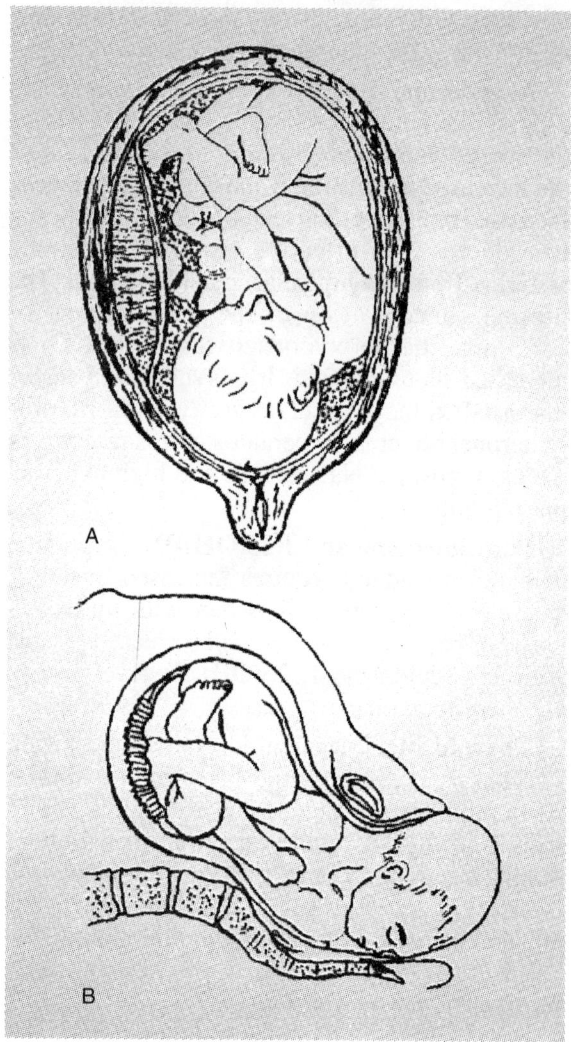

Fig. 54.6: Fetus in the last month of pregnancy (A), and 2nd stage of delivery (B).

Uterine Contractions

After 36 weeks of pregnancy, a uterine contraction may occur after about every 30 minutes. These contractions are painless but can be palpated over the abdomen. The first stage of labour is said to have begun when *painful contractions* occur every 10 minutes and the cervix begins to dilate. As the labour progresses, the frequency and intensity of contractions increases. In the second stage of labour, each contraction lasts 60–90 seconds and the contractions occur at 2–5 minutes intervals. Thus, throughout labour, the uterine contractions remain intermittent. (A continued strong uterine contraction would stop the blood flow through the placenta leading to fetal hypoxia and death).

There is another important feature of uterine contractions. In other organs, contraction of a muscle fibre is followed by its relaxation to the original length. During labour, uterine muscle fibres undergo *contraction and retraction*. After each contraction, the muscle fibre undergoes permanent shortening, i.e. the muscle fibre relaxes but not to the previous length.

Stages of Labour

First Stage

The upper uterine segment undergoes strongest contractions. Hence, the fetus is driven downward with each uterine contraction. The cervix begins to dilate and merge with the lower uterine segment. The first stage of labour is said to be over when the external os (cervix) is large enough (about 10 cm diameter) to allow the head of the fetus to pass into vagina. The first stage of labour lasts from 8 to 24 hours in the first pregnancy.

Second Stage

During this stage, strong and more frequent uterine contractions push the baby out of the uterus and vagina. Voluntary contractions of the diaphragm and abdominal muscles help to propel the baby through the dilated vagina (Fig. 54.6). Second stage of labour lasts about one hour. This stage ends with the delivery of the baby.

Third Stage

During the next 10–45 minutes, the uterus contracts and retracts to a very small size resulting in separation of placenta from its attachment to the uterus followed by its expulsion through the vagina. Separation of the placenta leads to opening of uterine blood vessels at the placental site leading to profuse bleeding. However, the blood rapidly clots in the ruptured vessels. Moreover, the uterine smooth muscle fibres form "figures-of-8" around the uterine blood vessels. Therefore, uterine contraction and retraction during this stage has throttling effect (living ligature action) on the uterine vessels. In this way, the uterine bleeding is usually limited to about 350 ml only. In some women, the uterus fails to contract strongly in the third stage of labour, leading to a risk of severe uterine bleeding. In such cases, the uterus can be induced to contract by injection of synthetic oxytocin and ergometrine.

During the next 6 weeks following delivery (puerperium), there is a remarkable involution of the uterus to the almost pre-pregnant size. The cervix is formed again. The vagina also regains its tonicity.

LACTATION

The mammary glands begin to develop at puberty. The breasts begin to enlarge gradually, due to the action of oestrogens secreted during each ovarian cycle. However, it is only during the first pregnancy that the glandular tissue develops fully. The marked enlargement of the breast may be correlated with the tremendous amounts of oestrogens and progesterone secreted by the placenta during the last 6 months of pregnancy. Oestrogens cause further development of stroma, ductal tissue and deposition of fat in the breasts. Acting along with oestrogens, progesterone produces marked glandular development. Elevated plasma levels of prolactin and chorionic somatomammotropin also promote glandular hyperplasia. Growth hormone, cortisol and thyroxine also seem to be essential for the growth and development of mammary glands during pregnancy.

Milk Secretion (A Function of Prolactin)

Prolactin promotes secretion of milk by the alveolar cells of the mammary gland. The secretion of this hormone by the anterior pituitary gland gradually increases during pregnancy, and by term, its plasma concentration is ten times that of non-pregnant level. (High plasma oestrogens level causes proliferation and secretion of lactotropes in anterior pituitary gland by a direct action.) During pregnancy, prolactin causes *development of mammary gland*. However, during pregnancy, its *secretory action* on the mammary gland is inhibited by high concentration of plasma oestrogens and progesterone. After the expulsion of baby and the placenta, there is a sharp decline in the level of circulating oestrogens and progesterone (secreted by the placenta during pregnancy). As a result, the lactogenic effect of prolactin becomes prominent within 2–3 days after delivery, and large amount of milk secretion starts.

After a few weeks, the basal plasma level of prolactin falls to the non-pregnant level. But each time the mother breastfeeds the baby, the neural impulses arising from the nipple and reaching the hypothalamus (via spinal cord and brainstem) cause manyfold increase in prolactin secretion by the anterior pituitary. Consequently, plasma prolactin level rises sharply during each feeding session (Fig. 54.7).

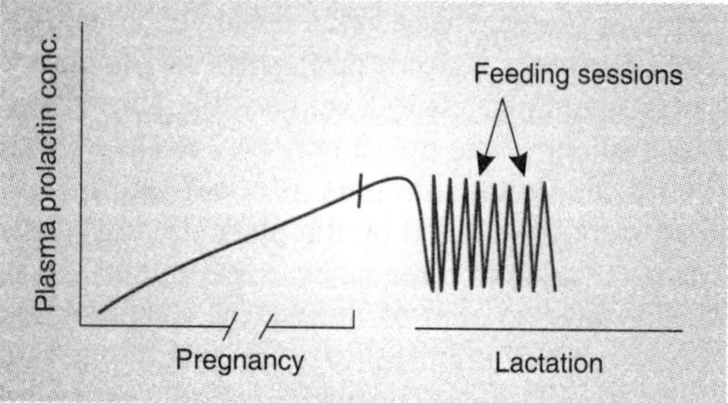

Fig. 54.7: Plasma prolactin level during feeding sessions.

54

The neural pathway involved in the reflex increase in secretion of prolactin is illustrated in Fig. 54.8. It is not yet clear whether the impulses arising from the nipple merely decrease the secretion of prolactin inhibitory hormone (PIH; dopamine) during the feeding session, or whether a prolactin releasing hormone (PRH) is also secreted by the hypothalamus.

Milk Ejection (A Function of Oxytocin)

Milk is secreted continuously into the alveoli of the breasts, but it does not enter the ducts on its

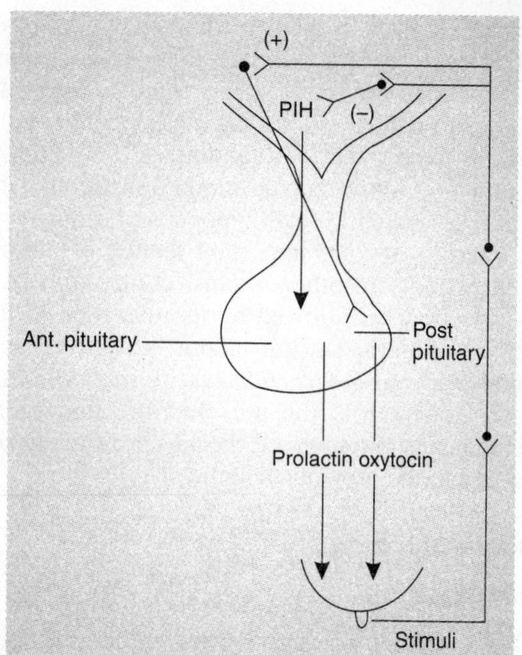

Fig. 54.8: Mechanism of secretion of prolactin and oxytocin during each feeding session.

own. Milk is ejected out of the alveoli by oxytocin secreted by the posterior pituitary gland. Sensory signals arising from the nipple during suckling reach the hypothalamus and cause secretion of oxytocin from the posterior pituitary (Fig. 54.8). Oxytocin causes contraction of myoepithelial cells surrounding the outer walls of the alveoli as a basket of cells. Contraction of the myoepithelial cells expels milk from the alveoli into the ducts and finally out of the nipple.

Milk

When the lactation is fully developed, approximately 1.5 litre of milk is secreted each day. The composition of human milk has been compared with the cow's milk in Table 54.1. It would be obvious that cow's milk is not similar in composition to human milk. The cow's milk has higher protein, particularly casein, as well as, higher mineral content and relatively less lactose.

Milk from other species shows still greater differences in the composition. For example, buffalo's milk contains 7% fat. It appears that the composition of milk in each species is such that

Table 54.1: Composition (g%) of human milk and cow's milk

	Human milk	*Cow's milk*
Fat	3.0–5.0	4.1
Protein	1.0–2.0	3.2
Lactose	6.5–8.0	4.4
Ash	0.2	0.8
Calcium	0.03	0.12

it is ideal for the nutritional requirements of the young ones of that species only. The recent tendency of the "modern" mothers to avoid breast feeding, and raise the infant on cow's milk, or commercial milk preparations should be discouraged, not only because the mother's milk is ideally suited for the newborn, but also because it provides immunoglobulins (antibodies) for the defence mechanisms against many infections. This is important in particular because the newborn's own defence mechanisms are not fully developed. The breast-milk, secreted during the first few days after parturition, is called colostrum. It is thicker and more yellowish. It contains more proteins and NaCl and less lactose and K^+. The importance of colostrum lies in the fact that it is particularly important source of antibodies for the neonate.

The high electrolyte content of the cow's milk can become a serious problem, especially in the premature infant. At this stage, the newborn's kidneys are unable to handle larger electrolyte load. Moreover, larger amounts of casein, present in the cow's milk, form large masses of calcium caseinate which are difficult to digest.

An additional benefit of breast feeding is that during the period of full-lactation, the mother remains relatively infertile due to the negative feedback effect of prolactin on the secretion of pituitary gonadotropins. Consequently, the ovarian cycle and menstrual cycles remain suspended (**lactational amenorrhoea)** for approximately 3 months after the parturition, provided the mother breast feeds the baby. However, this cannot be considered as an efficient and reliable measure of contraception.

Contraceptives

Contraceptives are measures, temporary or permanent, designed to prevent pregnancy in spite of coital acts.

Contraceptives are being used not only for limiting the size of the family, but also for spacing the pregnancies. A cycle of pregnancy-lactation followed by another pregnancy can jeopardize the health of the mother, as well as, of the offspring. One or more of the following contraceptive measures can be recommended, depending on the specific requirements of each couple.

Condom and Diaphragm (Mechanical Barriers)

Condom is probably the most widely accepted method of contraception used by the males. It is very effective, simple and cheap. An additional advantage of the method is that it protects the individual against sexually transmitted diseases like AIDS, hepatitis-B and other venereal diseases like syphilis and gonorrhoea.

A similar mechanical barrier for the sperms is provided by a rubber diaphragm which is fitted in the vagina over the cervix. As an extra precaution, a spermicidal jelly is used along with the diaphragm.

Safe Period

If the menstrual cycles are regular, the day of ovulation can be predicted by the study of basal body temperature. The possibility of pregnancy is very little if coitus is avoided 4 days before and 3 days after the predicted day of ovulation. It is probably the most physiological method of contraception, but also the least reliable one.

Oral Contraceptives

Administration of orally effective synthetic oestrogens and progesterone for 21 days in each cycle of 28 days is a very effective method of contraception. High concentration of progesterone in the plasma:

(i) Prevents ovulation by inhibiting the LH surge (negative feedback action).

(ii) Renders the cervical mucus hostile to sperm penetration.

(iii) Induces changes in the fallopian tubes and endometrium which are not conducive to fertilization and implantation, even if ovulation occurs by chance.

The use of oral contraceptive is not free from its inherent risks. There are reports of thrombo-embolic disorders, hypertension, fluid retention and oedema in women taking oral contraceptives.

Intrauterine Contraceptive Devices (IUCDs)

Two types of intrauterine contraceptive devices, known as the loop and copper-T, are the commonly used. IUCD is introduced and left in the uterine cavity. The foreign body action of the IUCD causes "aseptic inflammation" of the uterine endometrium and makes it unfit for the implantation of the fertilized ovum. It is a safe, effective and reversible method. IUCD can be easily pulled out when contraception is no more required (Fig. 54.9).

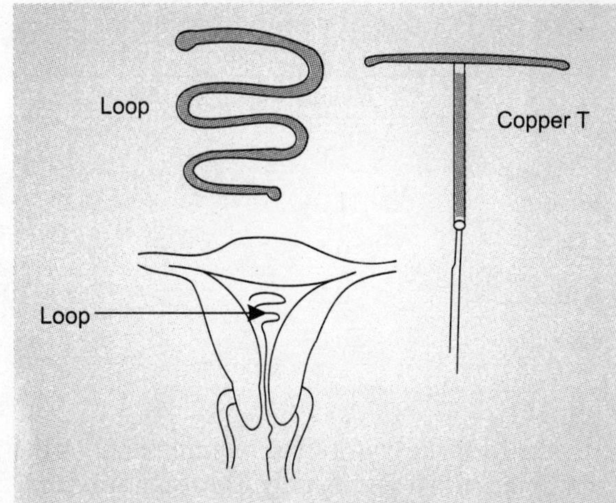

Fig. 54.9: Intrauterine contraceptive devices.

Vasectomy or Tubectomy

These are almost completely irreversible methods of contraception because, even if needed, the patency of the ducts cannot be restored with certainty. Of the two, vasectomy is a simpler outpatient procedure. Since the ligation of vas deferens does not interfere with the Leydig cell function, there is no risk of impotency at all. This imaginary risk makes many a male afraid of vasectomy.

54

Section XIII

Pediatric Physiology

CHAPTER 55

Growth and Development

The terms growth and development are commonly used together because both the processes occur simultaneously in a growing child. Growth refers to an increase in the physical size of the tissue or an organ. It is due to hyperplasia or hypertrophy of the tissue cells. The term development is used to indicate a change in the tissue for the better, i.e. an improvement in the capability of the tissue. For example, *development* of gonads occurs during fetal life and further *development* occurs at puberty. During puberty, the increased size of the liver, heart, spleen, etc. also occurs and this change would be called growth. During growth and development of a child, various periods can be recognised (Table 55.1).

Table 55.1: Periods of growth and development of a child

	Growing period	*Age*
Antenatal	Ovum	d 0-d 14
	Embryo	d 14–9 weeks
	Fetus	9 weeks–birth
Postnatal	Neonate	1–4 weeks
	Infant	1 month–1 year
	Early childhood	1–6 years
	Late childhood	6–10 years
	Puberty	10–14 years

GENERAL GROWTH

Measurements of weight and height are commonly used to monitor the rate of growth of the child. Increase in body weight is a better index of growth in childhood because it represents an increase in the body mass (provided obesity is excluded). The rate of growth varies during various phases of childhood. Maximum growth occurs during the 1st year of postnatal life. As compared to the birth weight, the weight of the baby is doubled at 6 months, tripled at 1 year and quadrupled by the end of 2nd year. After this, the increase in the body weight occurs at the rate of nearly 2 kg/year. With the onset of adolescent (puberty) spurt, the body weight may increase by 4–5 kg per year till the age of 14–16 years. After this, the rate of growth again slows down. The weights of some of the organs during different stages of childhood are given in Table 55.2.

Table 55.3 shows the mean weight and height of Indian children of different age groups.

Table 55.2: Weights (g) of some of the organs in relation to age

Age	*Brain*	*Heart*	*Kidneys*	*Lungs*	*Liver*	*Thymus*
Newborn	350	24	25	60	150	12
1 year	910	45	70	130	300	20
5 years	1200	95	120	260	550	24
15 years	1300	150	170	410	1500	30
Adult	1350	300	300	1200	1600	0–15

Table 55.3: Mean weight and height of Indian children

Age (years)	*Weight (kg)*		*Height (cm)*	
	Boys	*Girls*	*Boys*	*Girls*
5	17.5	17.0	107.0	10.6.0
6	19.0	18.5	113.5	113.0
7	21.0	20.5	118.5	118.0
8	23.5	23.0	124.0	122.5
9	26.5	26.0	130.5	128.5
10	28.5	29.5	134.5	135.0
11	32.0	34.0	139.5	141.0
12	35.5	38.5	144.5	146.5
13	39.5	42.6	150.0	151.5
14	44.5	45.5	158.0	153.5
15	51.0	48.0	164.5	155.0
16	55.0	49.0	167.0	156.0
17	56.5	49.0	168.0	157.0
18	59.5	51.0	169.5	157.0

GROWTH CURVES

General Type of Growth Curve The pattern of growth described above for height and weight also involves the growth of the skeletal muscles, blood volume, respiratory system, cardiovascular system, GIT and excretory system. This type of growth curve, i.e. rapid growth in infancy followed by a second growth spurt at puberty is called the general type of growth curve (Fig. 55.1A).

Neural Type of Growth Curve Brain, spinal cord, visual apparatus (and many head dimensions) grow very rapidly in infancy and early childhood. By the age of 4-5 years, over 90% of the growth of the tissues is completed (Fig. 55.1B).

Lymphoid Type of Growth Curve This is characterized by rapid growth in infancy and childhood followed by partial involution at puberty (Fig. 55.1C).

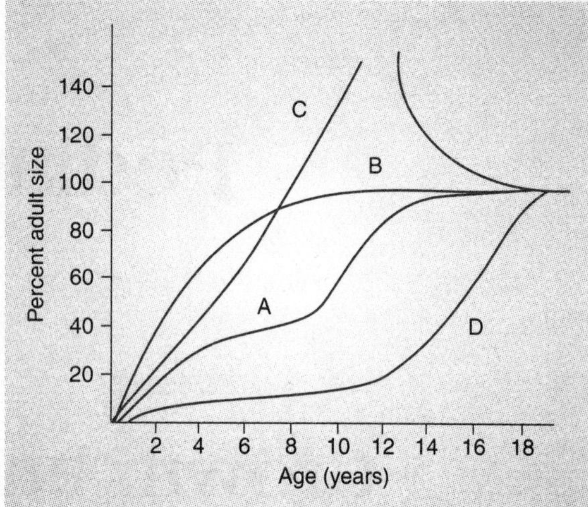

Fig. 55.1: Different types of growth curves

This type of growth is seen in tonsils, adenoids, thymus, spleen, lymph nodes and lymphoid tissues of the intestine.

Genital Type of Growth Curve The gonads and accessory organs of reproduction do not grow to any significant degree during childhood. Their growth coincides with the onset of puberty (Fig. 55.1D).

REGULATION OF GROWTH

The general pattern of growth has been described above. However, there is a difference in the rate of growth in different races or even different individuals of a community. A number of genetic, hormonal and nutritional factors regulate the rate of growth. An acute or chronic illness may retard growth temporarily or even permanently.

Genetic Factors

Racial differences in the height and body-built are well known. The Dinkas of Sudan are among the tallest races of the world, whereas pygmies of Congo are the smallest. No hormonal difference can be detected in these races. It may, therefore, be assumed that the difference in the rate of growth is genetically determined.

It is a common observation that children of tall parents tend to be taller than other children of the same age group. Similarly, small stature runs in some families. All these observations reflect a genetic control over the rate of growth and development.

Hormonal Factors Normal growth and development depends on the optimum secretion of a number of hormones.

Growth Hormone Plasma growth hormone levels are elevated during the neonatal period. Subsequently during childhood, the basal levels remain low but many peaks of elevated growth hormone level can be observed in the 24-hour cycle, specially during non-REM sleep. These peaks become more frequent and taller during adolescence, showing an elevation of mean plasma growth hormone level.

Although significant elevation of growth hormone cannot be demonstrated in childhood, the plasma level of insulin-like growth factor I (IGF-I) is definitely elevated during childhood, reaching a peak at 13-17 years of age.

IGF-I is one of the polypeptides collectively known as somatomedins. Chemically, IGF-I resembles insulin hence the name. IGF not only has insulin-like activity on glucose metabolism, but also has a number of other actions like promotion of protein synthesis, epiphyseal growth, and antilipolytic activity. Some of the effects of IGF-I are opposite to those of growth hormone (Fig. 55.2).

Deficiency of growth hormone produces growth retardation called pituitary dwarfism.

Sex Hormones The growth spurt at puberty is due to anabolic effect of the sex hormones. The secretion of adrenal androgens is also increased in both the sexes during puberty. The anabolic actions of sex hormones, adrenal androgens, growth hormone and IGF-I seem to potentiate each other producing a marked growth spurt.

Thyroxine The importance of thyroxine for normal growth and development in perinatal period cannot be over emphasized. Congenital deficiency of thyroxine produces retardation of physical, as well as, mental growth (cretinism). The mental retardation is an irreversible defect. Besides a direct action on the growth and differentiation of tissues, thyroxine promotes growth by potentiating the release of growth hormone and somatomedins.

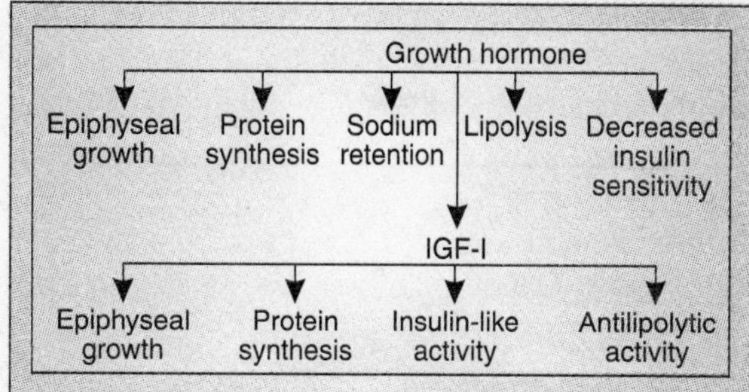

Fig. 55.2: Showing actions of growth hormone and IGF-I.

Insulin

Being an anabolic hormone, normal secretion of insulin is required for normal growth. Retardation of growth is one of the characteristic features of juvenile diabetes mellitus.

The relative importance of different hormones at various stages of growth is shown in Fig. 55.3. The presence of thyroxine is of critical importance in late fetal life and first few years of postnatal life. On the other hand, G.H. does not seem to be essential for normal growth *in utero* and early postnatal life. Infants with congenital deficiency of G.H. have normal weight and length at birth but a decrease in the velocity of growth becomes apparent during the first 2 years of life. Insulin is the primary mediator of somatic growth in the fetus. It causes stimulation of uptake and utilization of substances involved in growth. This action remains essential throughout the post-natal growth also. The mutual importance of growth hormone, adrenal androgens and gonadal hormones in growth spurt at puberty has been discussed earlier.

Nutritional Factors

Growth primarily involves increase in size or mass of tissues. Even if all the factors like genetic factors and hormones are normal, growth would not occur unless the caloric supply is over and above the requirement for the basal metabolism and physical activity. Formation of soft tissues and bones necessitates intake of larger amounts of proteins, vitamins and minerals in the diet. Under-nutrition during childhood is fairly common in all the under-developed countries. It is responsible for smaller stature, poor muscular built, generalized

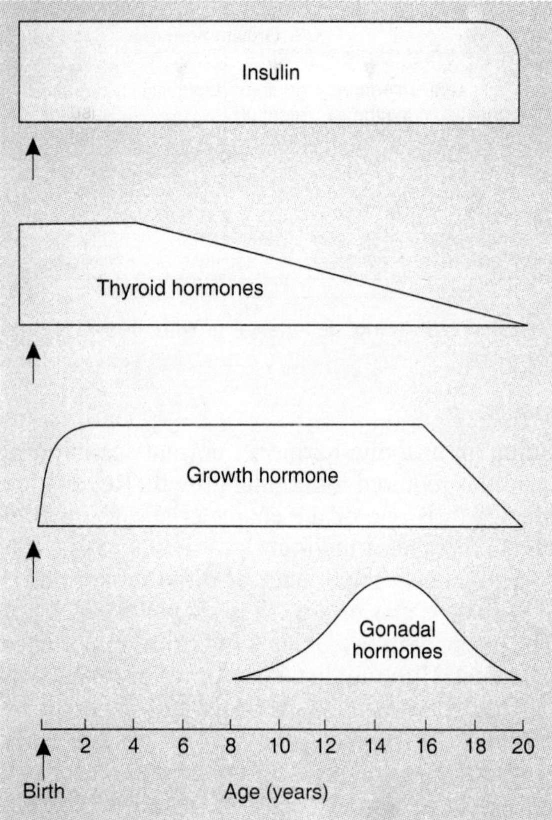

Fig. 55.3: Relative importance of different hormones in the growth of various stages of pre- and post-natal life.

apathy and reluctance to engage in any type of severe physical activity, even sports.

Acute and Chronic Diseases

An acute illness temporarily depresses growth. Once cured, the child soon recovers the growth deficit. Chronic cardiac disorder or renal tubular defects, etc. can produce a permanent growth retardation.

GROWTH FACTORS

The proliferation of cells in the embryonic and post-natal life seems to be regulated by a number of polypeptides called growth factors. Some of these growth factors are released into the circulation and act at a distant site (endocrine mechanism). Erythropoietin and growth hormone are examples of growth factors acting by this mechanism. Secondly, a cell may release a growth factor into the extracellular environment and it acts on the nearby cells (paracrine mechanism). Platelet derived growth factor or fibroblast growth factor acts in this fashion. Thirdly, the growth factor may act on the cell which produced it (autocrine mechanism).

The knowledge of these growth factors is not of academic interest only. A number of diseases result from hyper- or hypo-proliferation of certain cells. Cancer is produced by uncontrolled cell division. Atherosclerosis, psoriasis, etc. are other examples of hyperproliferative disorders. In chronic renal disease, anaemia results from the deficiency of erythropoietin leading to hypoproliferation of red cell precursors.

Some of the growth factors like growth hormone, erythropoietin, insulin-like growth factor, etc. have been mentioned before. The actions of these and other growth factors are presented in Table 55.4.

Table 55.4: Names and actions of various growth factors

Growth factor	*Action*
Growth hormone	General tissue growth
Insulin-like growth factor-I	General tissue growth
Erythropoietin	Proliferation of red cell precursors
Thrombopoietin	Proliferation of platelet precursors
Colony stimulating factors	
(i) Granulocyte stimulating factor	Proliferation of granulocytes and monocytes
(ii) Macrophage stimulating factor	
(iii) Granulocyte macrophage	
Lymphokines	Proliferation of lymphocytes
Epidermal growth factor	Proliferation of epithelial cells, fibroblasts and glial cells
Platelet derived growth factor	Growth of vascular smooth muscle, glial cells, fibroblasts
Fibroblast growth factor	Proliferation of fibroblast, endothelial cells and vascular smooth muscle
Nerve growth factor	Growth and maintenance of neurons

CHAPTER 56

Systemic Physiology of Fetus, Neonate and Childhood

During fetal life, the placenta supplies nutrients and oxygen, and removes the waste products like CO_2, urea, bilirubin, etc. The amniotic fluid provides not only a cushion against physical trauma but also provides a constant thermal environment. From this protected and ideal environment, the fetus passes through the most hazardous event, the process of birth. The hazard becomes more pronounced in premature babies than in full-term babies. This stressful event is followed by exposure to extrauterine environment, where the neonate's body suddenly takes over all the functions hitherto performed by the placenta. This sudden change requires complex cardiorespiratory, renal, hepatic and endocrine adjustments. Consequently, physiology of the newborn baby is much more complex than that of a mature adult.

At birth, many organs are in state of full functional capacity while others like brain and kidney reach full maturity after months or years of postnatal life. Gonadal maturity is delayed for 10–15 years after birth.

Just after birth, the fetus is exposed to a large number of stimuli like cold, light, sound, touch, pain, gravity, hypoxia and hypoglycaemia. The neonate does not respond to this stressful period like an adult. The neonate's response is characterized by *tolerance.* A neonate can tolerate hypoxia, hypoglycaemia and hypothermia to an extent not possible in later life. By rendering these stresses ineffective, tolerance helps the neonate from exhaustion of energy reserves.

It is worth remembering that an infant or a child is not a miniature adult. Some of the organs develop during different stages of infancy or childhood. In other organs, the function is not as well developed as in an adult.

NERVOUS SYSTEM

Most of the development of the brain occurs in fetal life, but it continues postnatally also. All the six layers of the cereberal cortex are completely differentiated by the 7th month of fetal life. At birth, all the primary fissures and sulci are present, but secondary folds continue to appear for several months after birth, indicating an increase in the thickness of cortical grey matter. At birth, the thickness of the cereberal cortex is only half of the thickness in an adult.

Nearly 50% of the postnatal growth in the nervous tissue is completed by the end of 1 year age, 75% by 3 years age and 90% by the end of 5th year. The relation between CNS weight over body weight is 1/10th at birth, 1/20th at 5 years age and 1/50th in an adult.

Myelination begins during fetal life, but continues for several years postnatally. The blood-brain barrier is not well-developed at birth. This accounts for kernicterus in an infant, whereas a similar degree of increase in serum bilirubin is harmless in an adult. The protein and sugar contents, and white cell count of CSF are considerably higher during neonatal period, specially in a premature baby, than in later infancy or childhood. The visual apparatus is not fully functional at birth. The structural and functional differentiation of macula and fovea of the retina is completed 4 months after birth. Colour perception also seems to develop by this time. However, pupillary response to light can be elicited even at birth.

Throughout infancy, the eyeball is small and the baby is therefore hypermetropic. The adult size of the eyeball is attained at 2–4 years of age. Due to hypermetropia, the visual acuity is 6/18 at the age of 2 years, 6/12 at the age of 5 years and 6/6 after 7 years of age.

The internal ear is almost fully developed at term. The response to loud noise can be elicited just after birth. Sensation of taste is present at birth, but becomes sharper by 2–3 months of age.

Visceral reflexes involved in swallowing, micturition, defaecation, sneezing, coughing are fully developed at birth. All the deep reflexes (tendon jerks) can be elicited except the ankle jerk. The Babinski's sign appears only a few weeks after the birth and can be elicited during the next 1–2 years.

Many recent researches have demostrated the beneficial effects of exposure to larger sensory inputs on the development of brain in infancy and childhood. Rats brought up in an interesting environment (big cages with lots of companions) developed denser, more complex brains than rats that always lived in boring environment (small cages, few companions). An interesting environment is good for the brain at any stage of life. Even elderly rats, within a month of moving to a new and more interesting cage, show a thickening of parts of their brains—although the effect is smaller for old rats than for young ones. The more synapses a brain has per nerve cell, the more likely it is that the brain will be able to process and respond to new information. Rats that live in more complex environment do indeed develop more synapses between their nerve cells. In animals living in interesting places, glial cells get bigger and become more active, wrapping themselves snugly around nerve cells. When stimulated by an interesting environment, brain also acquires more numerous capillaries.

RESPIRATORY SYSTEM

The placenta acts as the site of gas exchange for the fetus. The umbilical artery carries venous blood to the placenta. The chorionic villi containing capillaries dip directly into the large intervillous spaces containing maternal blood. The maternal and fetal circulations are separated by three thin layers, the fetal endothelium, the connective tissue of the villous and the trophoblast layer covering the villous. Table 56.1 shows the values of gaseous interchange in the placenta.

Table 56.1: Values of pO_2 and pCO_2 in the maternal and umbilical blood vessels

Blood vessel	*pO_2 mmHg*	*pCO_2 mmHg*
Uterine artery	95	36
Uterine vein	50	40
Umbilical artery	20	50
Umbilical vein	35	43

Oxygen Transport in Fetus

It would be obvious from Table 56.1 that even after full oxygenation, pO_2 value of the blood in umbilical vein is only one-third of the maternal arterial blood. Such low pO_2 value would produce severe hypoxia in adults. However, several adaptations in the fetus ensure adequate oxygen supply to the tissues.

Fetal Haemoglobin The fetal red cells contain haemoglobin F (Fetal haemoglobin, HbF). This type of haemoglobin has greater affinity for oxygen as shown by the shift of haemoglobin-oxygen dissociation curve to the left (Fig. 17.8). Chemically, haemoglobin-F contains two alpha (α) chains and two gamma (γ) chains (HbF = α_2 γ_2), in contrast to α_2 β_2 pattern of HbA (adult haemoglobin). The absence of β-chains in HbF reduces its affinity for 2,3-DPG, a constituent of fetal and adult red cells. DPG competes with oxygen for the binding sites on haemoglobin molecule. Therefore, less affinity of Hb-F for DPG results in its greater affinity for oxygen. This is the major factor helping in oxygen transport in the fetus. In addition, some other relatively minor, but still important, factors help to improve the oxygen uptake by the fetal blood from the maternal sinuses:

Haemoglobin Concentration Haemoglobin concentration of fetal blood is usually about 16–17 g% but may be up to 20 g%. Thus, in combination with the factor mentioned above, the total oxygen content of fetal blood is much higher than the maternal blood at similar value of pO_2 (Fig. 56.1).

Double Bohr Effect This is another factor helping in the uptake of oxygen. An increased value of pCO_2 of blood shifts the haemoglobin-oxygen dissociation curve to the right, whereas decreased pCO_2 shifts the curve to the left. This is called Bohr effect. In the adults, these two changes in the pCO_2 occur in the tissues and the lungs, respectively. In the fetus, both the changes occur simultaneously in the placenta, hence the term double Bohr effect. The transfer of CO_2 from the fetal blood to the maternal blood increases the latter's pCO_2. It leads to shift of the curve to right, and greater unloading of oxygen from the *maternal blood.* At the same time, loss of CO_2 from the fetal blood shifts the curve in the *fetal blood* to the left, resulting in greater uptake of oxygen.

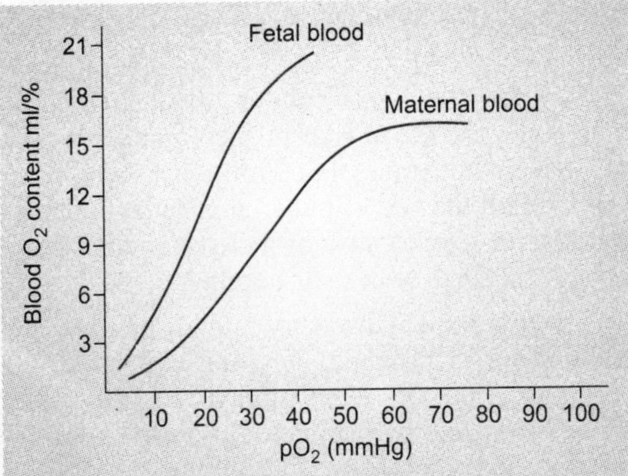

Fig. 56.1: Difference in the oxygen content of fetal and maternal blood at similar values of pO_2.

Due to all the factors mentioned above, fetal tissues seem to receive adequate amounts of oxygen and there seems to be no hypoxia in the fetal tissues. Moreover, lower pO_2 value of the fetal blood may be a physiological (developmental) necessity since higher pO_2 in the fetal and neonatal tissues seems to produce serious cardiovascular and retinal disturbances like closure of ductus arteriosus, vasodilatation in the lungs, and retrolental fibroplasia in the retina.

Carbon Dioxide Transport

Because of greater solubility, the transfer of CO_2 from the fetal blood to the maternal sinuses is not difficult.

Fetal Respiratory Movements

Since there is no gaseous exchange in the fetal lung, it may be assumed that there are no respiratory movements in fetal life. Actually, numerous research workers have demonstrated mild rhythmic respiratory movements during fetal life. The fetal lung is full of fluid which is mainly secreted by the pulmonary parenchyma. The mild respiratory movements merely move the fluid in and out of the respiratory passages, but it helps to exercise and train the respiratory muscles for their function immediately after birth.

Peripheral chemoreceptors are also fully developed before birth, but due to some unknown reason, there is no chemoreceptor discharge in spite of very low pO_2 in the fetal blood.

During fetal life, pulmonary blood flow is a fraction of the right ventricular outflow. Due to high pulmonary vascular resistance, most of the right ventricular output is diverted to the aorta through the ductus arteriosus.

Pulmonary Surfactant

The secretion of pulmonary surfactant, a phospholipid with surface tension-lowering action, begins in the middle of gestation and increases markedly near the term. Surfactant is secreted by type II alveolar cells of the pulmonary parenchyma. Increased secretion of corticosteroids by the fetal adrenal gland seems to be necessary for proper secretion of pulmonary surfactant. In premature deliveries, the deficiency of pulmonary surfactant produces a serious problem in the inflation of the lungs after birth. This condition is called the *fetal respiratory distress syndrome* (page 182).

Initiation of Breathing

During its passage through the birth canal, all parts of the fetus including the thorax are subjected to intense pressure. As a result, most of the fluid present in the lungs and upper respiratory passages is expelled out through the mouth. Whatever little fluid is left behind is absorbed into the blood and lymph capillaries.

After birth of the baby, the umbilical cord is ligated. Within a few seconds, or at the most a couple of minutes after ligation of the cord, the neonate takes the first breath. The exact mechanism of the sudden onset of respiration is not known. After birth, the neonate is exposed to a large number of stimuli:

(i) Asphyxia: Ligation of the cord cuts off placental exchange of gases. Consequently, a gradually increasing fetal asphyxia develops resulting in intense peripheral chemoreceptor discharge.
(ii) Cold.
(iii) Tactile and painful stimuli.
(iv) Sound.
(v) Light.
(vi) Gravity.
(vii) Increased sympathetic discharge.

Of all the factors, factor number (i) and (vii) seem to be most important and related to the ligation of the cord. When the baby is born, it is in extreme obtunded state untill the cord is ligated. Soon after ligation, the neonate makes movements of the limbs and trunk and the first breath follows. At this period, the circulating catecholamine level is seen to increase 10-fold. The intense sympathetic discharge seems to be a consequence of asphyxia. It results in a generalized arousal of the CNS, which becomes responsive to the increased chemoreceptor discharge. Within hours, the neonate recovers from hypoxia, hypercapnea and acidosis present throughout fetal life and aggravated by the process of birth, and subsequent ligation of the cord. After the first gasping breath, normal breathing pattern is gradually established.

It may be mentioned that even when the breathing does not start up to 10 minutes, the neonate shows normal growth and development. Resistance to such prolonged and severe hypoxia is a peculiar feature of neonatal physiology and does not occur in later life.

The first breath is a result of a severe inspiratory effort resulting in a marked decrease in the intrapleural pressure (–30 to –50 mm Hg). The result is expansion of partially opened fluid-filled alveoli. The presence of pulmonary surfactant in the alveolar fluid is critically important for the gradual expansion of most of the alveoli in the next few minutes. Since surfactant is mostly synthesized in the later months of gestation, premature infants are more prone to suffer from the effects of pulmonary surfactant deficiency. In such newborn babies, high surface tension at the water-air interface prevents full expansion of the alveoli. Even partially opened alveoli tend to collapse gradually, resulting in severe hypoxia and hypercapnea. The condition is called fetal respiratory distress syndrome.

The onset of normal breathing improves the pO_2, pCO_2 and pH values of the neonate's blood to the adult values. The loss of peripheral resistance, due to interruption of placental circulation, and increased arterial pO_2 produce marked cardiovascular changes like decreased pulmonary vascular resistance, increased systemic vascular resistance, closure of foramen ovale and closure of ductus arteriosus.

At birth, the lungs contain about 20 million alveoli. By the age of 8 years, their number increases to the adult value of 300 million alveoli. After this age, till the end of pubertal growth, the lungs increase in size because of increase in the size of alveoli rather than in their number.

A newborn baby has very high respiratory rate (30-80/min). During infancy and childhood, the respiratory rate decreases gradually and the adult value is reached by the age of 10 years. Tidal air volume and vital capacity continue to increase throughout childhood, till the pubertal growth is completed (Table 56.2).

Table 56.2: Some of respiratory values in relation to age

Age	Respiratory rate/min	Tidal air (ml)	Vital capacity (L)
Premature	40–90	12	?
Full-term newborn	30–80	19	?
1 year	20–40	48	?
2 years	20–30	90	?
5 years	20–25	175	1.2
10 years	15–20	400	2.0
15 years	15–20	400	3.3

CARDIOVASCULAR SYSTEM

During fetal life, the two ventricles have almost similar thickness. If anything, the right ventricle is slightly thicker than the left ventricle. This is related to the fact that the pressure in the pulmonary artery is slightly greater than the aortic pressure. Due to high resistance in the pulmonary vessels, very little blood enters the pulmonary circulation, and most of the right ventricular output is diverted to the aorta through the ductus arteriosus. Another difference between the fetal and the adult circulation is that the two ventricles do not have the similar cardiac output. The left ventricular output is approximately 20% greater than the right ventricular output. The disparity between the outputs of two ventricles does not produce any haemodynamic complications because, unlike in adults, the two ventricles work in parallel and not in series.

The combined output of the two ventricles is approximately 360 ml/kg fetal weight (at birth) as compared to 140 ml/kg BW in adults. The autonomic innervation of the heart, as well as, baroreceptor and chemoreceptor reflexes are well developed at birth. Even during late fetal life, cardiovascular reflexes are operational. This is demonstrated by the observation of fetal bradycardia in response to maternal hypoxia. In the later months of gestation, the fetal heart rate normally varies from 120–160 beats/min. Values above or below this range are considered abnormal.

The deoxygenated blood enters the right atrium through the superior vena cava. It is diverted through the tricuspid valve into the right ventricle and then into the pulmonary artery. Due to high pulmonary arteriolar resistance, it is diverted through the ductus arteriosus into the descending aorta. Thus, poorly oxygenated blood is supplied to the lower limbs and the placenta through two umbilical arteries. As much as 40% of the total cardiac output of the fetus reaches the placenta. The oxygen saturation of blood is about 60% in the umbilical artery and 80% in the umbilical vein.

The inferior vena cava carries oxygenated blood from the umbilical veins, as well as, deoxygenated blood from the abdomen and the lower limbs. In the right atrium, the crista dividens diverts most of this (pure) blood to the left atrium through the foramen ovale. Rest of blood, along with that of superior vena cava, enters the right ventricle.

Change at Birth (Fig. 56.2)

Closure of the placental circulation, foramen ovale, and ductus arteriosus are the three important circulatory changes which occur just after birth.

Inflation of the lungs, just after birth, causes a significant increase in the arterial pO_2 in the newborn. The physical expansion of the pulmonary vessels (due to alveolar inflation) coupled with effect of higher arterial pO_2 on the pulmonary vascular smooth muscle result in a marked decrease in the pulmonary vascular resistance. On the other hand, increased arterial pO_2 causes contraction of the smooth muscle in the wall of ductus arteriosus, leading to its closure. It is also believed that, during fetal life, patency of the ductus arteriosus is maintained by a vasodilator prostaglandin released from the placenta. (Inhibitors of prostaglandin synthesis like aspirin and indomethacin have been used clinically to promote closure of patent ductus arteriosus in premature infants). Whatever the mechanism, the closure of ductus arteriosus leads to a marked increase in the pulmonary circulation.

The cessation of placental circulation, an area of low vascular resistance causes elevation of the aortic pressure. This change, along with increased pulmonary blood flow, increases the left atrial

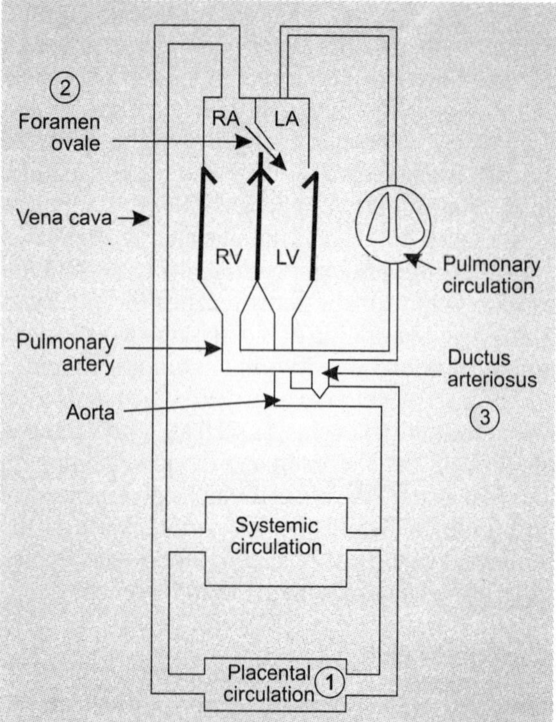

Fig. 56.2: Fetal circulation. Birth is accompanied by closure of (1) placental circulation (2) foramen ovale and (3) ductus arteriosus.

pressure, reversing the pressure gradient present earlier between the two atria. Higher pressure in the left atrium presses upon the flap to close the foramen ovale.

Functional closure of the ductus arteriosus is complete within 24 hours of birth. During this transient period, some blood may flow from the aorta to the pulmonary artery through incompletely obliterated ductus arteriosus because of the reversal of the pressure gradients between the aorta and pulmonary trunk.

Anatomical closure of the foramen ovale and ductus arteriosus may take several weeks.

Just after birth, the heart rate is approximately 140 beats/min. During infancy and childhood, the heart rate decreases gradually. Adult value of the heart rate is reached only at puberty (Table 56.3).

During infancy and childhood variations in heart rate during the two phases of respiration can be observed even during normal quiet breathing.

Table 56.3: Heart rate values in relation to age

Age	*Heart rate (beats/min)*
Birth	140
1 month	130
1 year	110
5 years	105
10 years	95
15 years	80

This variation in heart rate, called sinus arrhythmia, occurs in adults only during deep breathing.

At birth, the mean blood pressure is approximately 80 mmHg. During the next few hours, it declines to approximately 65 mmHg. Throughout infancy and childhood, the blood pressure gradually increases to reach the adult values by the end of pubertal growth (Table 56.4).

Table 56.4: Blood pressure values in relation to age

Age	*BP (mmHg)*	
	Systolic	*(Diastolic)*
1 month	90	60
1 year	96	65
5 years	100	70
15 years	120	80

ECG

Even at birth, electrocardiographic record shows all the normal waves of ECG. The right ventricular preponderance is indicated by mild right-axis deviation in the ECG. Within a few months of postnatal life, the right axis deviation is no more evident. Left ventricular preponderance is established by the age of 7 years.

BLOOD

Erythropoiesis begins in the mesenchymal tissue of the yolk sac as early as 2 weeks after the conception. The red cells produced at this stage are large nucleated cells with low haemoglobin concentration. During the 2nd and 3rd month of gestation, the liver and spleen are the chief sites of erythropoiesis, leucopoiesis and thrombopoiesis. After 4 months of gestation, the bone marrow is the chief site of erythropoiesis. In the postnatal life, bone marrow remains the only site of erythropoiesis. However, extramedullary organs like liver and spleen remain the potential sites of erythropoiesis when the entire bone marrow has been damaged (myelosclerosis).

High concentration of erythropoietin can be demonstrated in the cord blood. It is related to the low pO_2 of the fetal blood. This factor is responsible for the higher concentration of the Hb (16–18 g%) and red cell count (5.5–6.5 million/mm^3) observed in the fetus at birth. At birth, the total white blood cell count is nearly 20,000/mm^3 with preponderance of (70%) neutrophils.

In fetal life, the red cells contain HbF which has higher affinity of oxygen than the adult Hb (Hb-A). Hb-A begins to be synthesized in low concentration after 32 weeks of gestation. At 36 weeks of gestation, 90% of the Hb in the fetal red cells is Hb-F and only 10% is Hb-A. After birth, synthesis of Hb-F practically ceases and all the newly formed red cells contain Hb-A. The concentration of Hb-F in the neonatal blood declines linearly, and at 3–4 months of age, it is completely absent from the blood.

Physiologic Anaemia

After the 1st week of life, the red cell count and haemoglobin concentration begin to decline rapidly. At 10–12 weeks, haemoglobin concentration may be as low as 10 g% or even lower in the premature infants. This decrease in Hb concentration is known as the physiologic anaemia of the newborn, because it occurs in most of the infants and does not seem to produce any ill-effects. The fall in the red cell number or haemoglobin concentration cannot be prevented even by administration of haematinics. Physiologic anaemia of the newborn is due to almost complete cessation of red cell production in the bone marrow. It seems to be related to disappearance of hypoxic stimulus present throughout the intrauterine life. This explanation is supported by disappearance of erythropoietin and reticulocytes from the baby's blood. Shorter lifespan of the red cells containing Hb-F is another contributory factor for rapid decrease in the red cell count.

From an average of 20,000 leucocytes/mm^3 with 70% neutrophils, the total count falls to about 12,000 cells per mm^3 and 30% neutrophils by the end of the first month. Lymphocytes predominate from the 1st month to one year of life (Table 56.5).

Table 56.5: Values of red and white blood cells in relation to age

Age	*RBC count million/mm³*	*Hb conc. g%*	*TLC per mm³*	*DLC Poly(%)*	*DLC Lymph(%)*
1 day	6.0	18	20,000	70	20
1 month	4.7	16	12,000	30	60
1 year	4.6	12.5	10,000	45	50
5 years	4.7	13.0	8,000	55	40
10 years	4.7	13.0	8,000	60	35

Coagulation Factors

At birth, all the clotting factors and fibrinolysins are present in the plasma. However, plasma levels of prothrombin and factor V, VII and X are subnormal and levels decline further during the next 2–4 days. Subsequently, their level begins to rise to reach the adult value between 2–12 months of age. During the 1st week of postnatal life, the levels of these clotting factors may decline to such an extent that bleeding may occur from the umbilicus, GIT and other internal organs. The condition is called the haemorrhagic disease of the newborn.

Deficiency of the vitamin K-dependent clotting factors in the first week of postnatal life is primarily due to their insufficient synthesis by immature hepatic cells. Deficiency of vitamin K seems to be equally important because the disorder can be prevented by a single injection of 1 mg of vitamin K at birth. Premature infants are more prone to develop haemorrhagic disease of the newborn. In such neonates, the plasma prothrombin level is still lower. Moreover, immaturity of hepatic cells is so severe that even the administration of vitamin K does not help.

Immunologic Function

At birth, the infant is competent to produce T lymphocyte as well as B lymphocyte-mediated response. At birth, the neonate's plasma level of IgG is even higher than the maternal plasma level (Table 56.6).

Table 56.6: Plasma concentration of different immunoglobulins in the maternal and fetal blood (mg%)

	Maternal blood	*Fetal blood*
IgG	1000	1230
IgA	350	7
IgM	125	15

During intrauterine life, IgG are transferred from the maternal blood to the fetus by active transport mechanism. In contrast, IgA and IgM are not transferred to the fetus. That explains extremely low levels of these two types of immunoglobulins in the cord blood. However, IgG levels begin to decline very rapidly and within one week, the IgG level may fall to 400–500 mg% as compared to over 1200 mg% at birth. After 3 months of age, the immunological apparatus of the baby begins to manufacture IgG and adult levels are reached in the plasma by the age of 8 months.

From very low plasma levels at birth, IgM begin to rise rapidly reaching about 30 mg% by the end of one week and 45 mg% at 6 months of age. IgA levels also begin to rise in infancy but adult levels are reached by the age of 12–16 years.

56

Immunization at birth produces an antibody response which is slower than in adults. For example, an injection of typhoid vaccine increases plasma IgM levels after 10–20 days and IgG levels 6–10 weeks later. In adults, both the immunoglobulins begin to increase just after 4 days.

GASTROINTESTINAL SYSTEM

Gastrointestinal function is fairly well developed at birth. Salivary secretion can be observed soon after birth, but the rate of salivary secretion increases during the next 3–4 months, due to maturation of the salivary glands. At about 6 months of age, drooling of saliva becomes prominent. It is more because of infrequent swallowing of the saliva rather than excessive production. Eruption of teeth may, however, accentuate the problem because of reflex stimulation of salivary secretion.

On the first postnatal day, the stomach contains high concentration of hydrochloric acid, but within next 10–15 days, the gastric acid secretion almost ceases. At 3–4 months of age, the gastric acid secretion starts once again. The pepsinogen secretion continues throughout this period. The physiological significance of increased acidity of the stomach at birth, followed by a phase of achlorhydria for the next 2–3 months, is not clear.

At birth, the pancreatic juice contains adequate concentration of lipase and proteolytic enzymes but the concentration of α-amylase is very low. α-amylase begins to appear in the pancreatic juice a few months later. Consequently, administration of starch during early postnatal life may produce severe diarrhoea. The intestinal mucosa can absorb disaccharides very efficiently due to the presence of disaccharidases. Similarly, monosaccharides are well absorbed right from birth.

Liver

Constant and plentiful supply of maternal glucose is a characteristic feature of fetal life. Just after birth, this supply is suddenly cut off. Moreover, the newborn has to fulfil his caloric requirements from carbohydrate-poor, fat-rich milk. A number of adaptive changes in the hepatic enzymes help in this transition.

During fetal life, the blood glucose level is regulated by the maternal blood glucose levels. Due to deficiency of enzymes like glucokinase and those for glycogenolysis and gluconeogenesis, the fetus is incapable of regulating the blood sugar level on its own. Large amounts of free fatty acids and amino acids are transported to the fetus across the placenta but they are used for tissue formation rather than for energy production.

As the term approaches, the activity of glycogen synthetase in the fetal liver increases. As a result, the fetal liver is very rich in glycogen at birth. With the ligation of cord, the blood sugar level begins to fall and may reach 60 mg% within one hour. Hypoglycaemia induces the secretion of glucagon, catecholamines and glucocorticoids. Presence of hepatic glucose-6-phosphatase in high concentration in the full-term infant helps to convert glycogen into glucose and therefore the blood glucose level recovers very soon. The enzymes involved in gluconeogenesis take a few days to develop fully. The problem of neonatal hypoglycaemia is more pronounced in premature babies.

The increased utilization of FFA during early postnatal period is reflected in the plasma FFA levels at birth and during the next 24 hours (Table 56.7).

Table 56.7: Average plasma FFA level in the neonate during the first 24 hours of postnatal life (maternal level 1.2 mEq/L)

	Plasma FFA (mEq/L)
Fetus	0.4
Birth	0.5
1 hour	1.3
24 hours	1.5

The increase in the plasma FFA level seems to be due to increased secretion of hormones like catecholamines and glucocorticoids because of neonatal hypoglycaemia.

It would be obvious that some of the hepatic enzymes are fully operational at birth while activity of some other enzymes is induced by metabolic changes after birth.

Hepatic Bilirubin Excretion

The lifespan of fetal red cells is approximately 70 days. Therefore, about 1.4% of circulating red cell mass is destroyed everyday leading to production of a large amount of bilirubin. In pathological states like Rh-incompatibility, the production of bilirubin is further increased. In spite of all this, the fetal plasma bilirubin level usually remains below 1 mg% and does not exceed 5 mg% even during pathological states like Rh incompatibility.

Soon after birth, plasma bilirubin level rises moderately in most of the babies. This condition has been called *physiological jaundice of the newborn*. In some neonates, bilirubin may rise to toxic levels either due to over-production of bilirubin or failure of conjugation and excretion by the liver or both.

During fetal life, the lipid soluble unconjugated bilirubin can cross the placental barrier whereas water-soluble conjugated bilirubin cannot. That is why plasma bilirubin level in the fetus remains low even in the face of massive haemolysis.

During fetal life, the hepatic conjugation enzyme UDP-glucuronyl transferase is not utilized and its activity in the hepatic liver is very low. After birth, the enzyme activity begins to rise rapidly, and by the age of 15 days, it even exceeds the adult level (Fig. 56.3). There seems to be some variation in the rate of increase of the hepatic conjugation enzyme activity. That is why some babies develop more severe physiological jaundice than others.

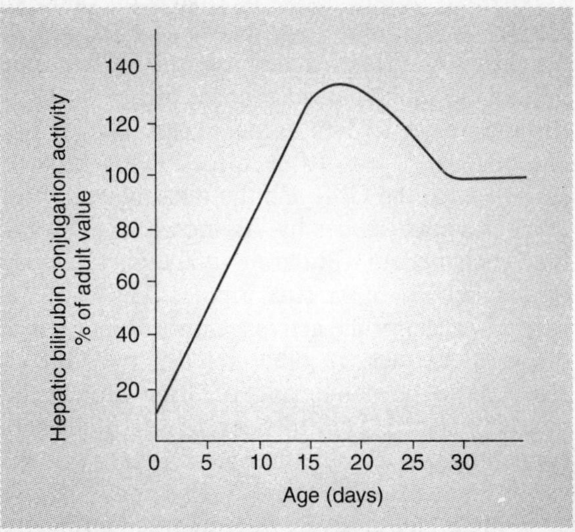

Fig. 56.3: Changes in rate of hepatic conjugation of bilirubin during the neonatal period.

In some babies, the physiological jaundice of the newborn may lead to rise of plasma bilirubin beyond 18 mg%. This risk is greater in case of premature babies or those suffering from Rh-incompatibility. Such babies are under the risk of development of kernicterus. In infants with congenital hypothyroidism, the neonatal increase in the activity of glucuronyl transferase may be delayed for several weeks.

KIDNEY

During fetal life,kidney forms urine which is passed into the amniotic sac. At birth, the anatomical development of nephrons is fairly complete and no new nephrons are formed in postnatal life. During childhood, the length of the nephron gradually increases. At birth, 20% of the loops of Henle fail to reach the medulla in contrast to 1-2% in adults. This explains the poor power of urinary concentration in infants. Besides the anatomical difference, the lower urinary concentration is also due to low excretion of urea leading to only mild osmolar gradient in the medullary pyramids. In turn, low urea excretion of the neonate is because of the fact that the rate of deamination is low and more amino acids are utilized for tissue formation. During infancy, the maximum urinary specific gravity may be only 1.008. Normal adult values of urinary concentration are reached by the age of 5-6 years. At 15th postnatal day, the GFR is only 50% of the adult value after correction of the body surface area to 1.73 m^2. Renal plasma flow is also proportionately less. After correction for the body surface area, the GFR and the renal plasma flow reach the adult values by 7th month of postnatal life. The smaller GFR during infancy is related to the smaller size of the renal tubules. The low GFR is appropriate for the active transport functions of the renal tubules. In other words, low GFR is essential for the maintenance of proper glomerulo-tubular balance. Due to poor power of urinary concentration, the infant up to 1 year of age continues to pass iso-osmolar urine or even dilute urine in the face of severe dehydration. During this period, the kidney has poor power of hydrogen ion excretion as well. It is related to the fact that there is lesser glomerular filtration of phosphates, as well as, inadequate synthesis of ammonia by the tubular cells. The infant is equally incapable of excreting an excessive water load during the 1st month of life. The clinical implication of all the facts about renal function in infancy is that the functionally immature kidney can manage to maintain normal blood chemistry only as long as there is no homeostatic disturbance, i.e. there is very little margin of safety. Any disturbance in haemodynamic function due to diarrhoea, infection or solute overload may lead to dehydration or the opposite, oedema. Average daily urinary volume at different age groups is shown in Table 56.8.

Table 56.8: Average daily excretion of urine in relation to age

Age	*Urinary volume (ml)*
D 1	15–50
D 10	50–300
1 month	250–400
1 year	400–500
5 years	600–750
10 years	700–1500
15 years	1500

The extracellular fluid volume of the newborn infant per kilogram body weight is nearly double that of an adult. An average adult takes and excretes about 2000 ml of water every day. It represents nearly 15% of ECF volume. An infant excretes about 500 ml of water per day representing nearly 50% of ECF volume. (The water loss in stools is rather high during infancy.) All these facts underline the risk of dehydration during infancy and the need for urgent treatment.

TEMPERATURE REGULATION

Throughout childhood, the basal metabolic rate is relatively higher than the adult values. Moreover, as compared to the body mass, the surface area is rather high specially during infancy. These factors tend to make the temperature regulation of the infant more difficult than in an adult. Moreover, during infancy the sweating mechanism is not fully developed.

Thermoneutral zone is the range of ambient temperature within which the metabolic rate is at a minimum and temperature regulation is achieved by non-evaporative physical processes alone. For an unclothed adult, the thermoneutral zone is 26–28°C, but for a naked newborn infant, it is 32–34°C and 35°C for a premature infant (Fig. 56.4). These facts underline the poor tolerance of the infant to cold. Moreover, the thermoneutral zone of the infant should be kept in mind while adjusting the temperature of the incubator for premature babies and temperature of the labour room in general.

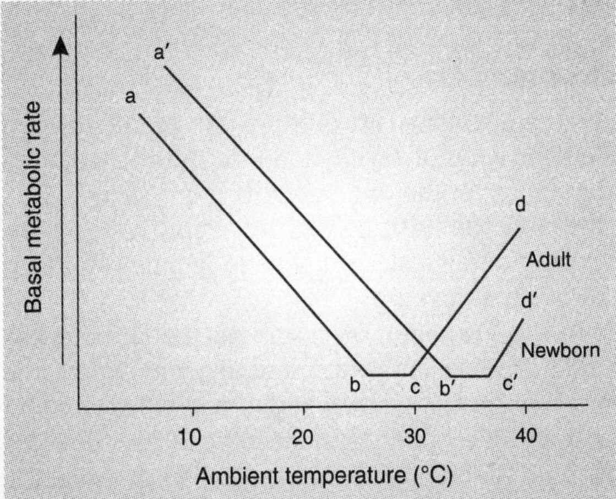

Fig. 56.4: Thermoneutral zone of the newborn (b'–c') as compared to that of an adult human (b–c).

On exposure to cold, heat generation in the body can be increased by: (i) voluntary muscle activity, (ii) involuntary muscle activity called shivering and (iii) non-shivering thermogenesis. Of these, shivering is the most important mode of heat generation in adults as well as children. However, in infants, although shivering does occur, non-shivering thermogenesis is most effective mechanism against cold.

Brown adipose tissue is the chief site of non-shivering thermogenesis. This type of adipose tissue is distributed in the human neonate around the neck, interscapular region, axilla and on the surface of the heart and the kidney. In hibernating animals, the brown adipose tissue is brown in colour and hence the name. In non-hibernating mammals, including human infants, this tissue is reddish-yellow in colour rather than brown.

Ordinary white adipose tissue contains fat cells which are large in size and a single large fat droplet fills the whole cytoplasm, pushing the nucleus to an eccentric position. In the brown adipose tissue, the fat cell is smaller in size and has a centrally situated nucleus. It contains many small droplets of fat and a large number of mitochondria among the fat droplets. Sympathetic nerve endings make close contact with each fat cell (Fig. 56.5).

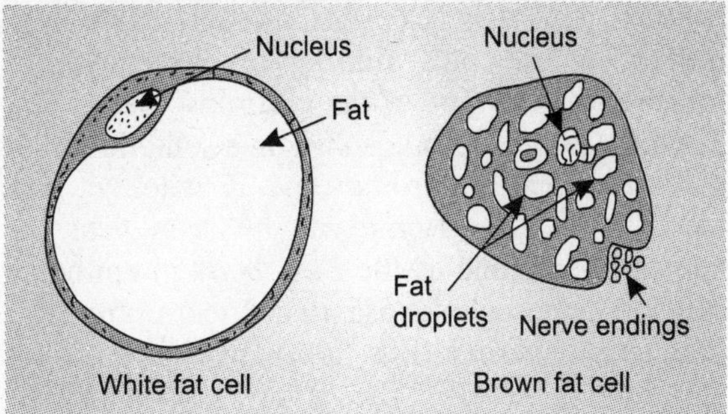

Fig. 56.5: Histological structure of brown adipose tissue cell as compared to ordinary (white) adipose tissue cell.

On exposure to cold, the increased sympathetic discharge to the brown adipose tissue causes marked increase in the oxygen consumption and heat production. Sympathetic stimulation seems to activate a lipase which releases FFA for oxidation within the fat cells.

SEXUAL GROWTH AND DEVELOPMENT

Sexual Differentiation in Fetus

Sexual differentiation begins at the time of fertilization and continues into early adult life. Sex of an individual has genetic (chromosomal), gonadal, genital and psychological components. In a vast majority of individuals, all the four components are similar, i.e. a person is a male or a female with all the four components mentioned above. However, due to hormonal or environmental factors, the last two may not tally with the first two components.

56

Genetic (Chromosomal) Sex

The genetic sex is determined at the time of fertilization by the type of sperm (X or Y) uniting with the ovum. All the ova contain X-chromosome, but a sperm may have an X-chromosome (female sperm) or a Y-chromosome (male sperm). If the ovum is fertilized by a female sperm the zygote shall have XX-chromosomal pattern and a female embryo develops. On the other hand, a male embryo is produced when a male sperm fertilizes the ovum and the zygote has XY-chromosomal composition. The karyotype (chromosomal pattern of a cell) is designated as 46, XX in a normal female, and 46, XY in a normal male, i.e. indicating the total number of chromosomes followed by the type of sex chromosomes.

Of the two X-chromosomes in a somatic cell of a female, one X-chromosome is inactive. The inactive X-chromosome can be seen near the nuclear membrane as the *Barr body* in epithelial cells of the buccal mucosa. In the neutrophils, it is seen as a *drumstick* (Fig. 56.6).

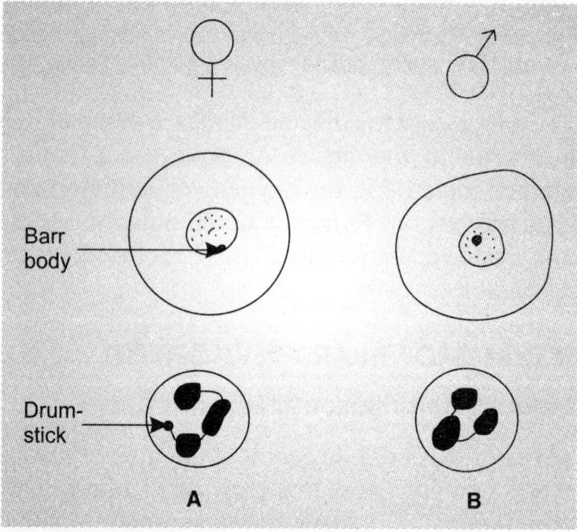

Fig. 56.6: Barr body and a drumstick chromatin in the epithelial cell of buccal mucosa and neutrophil of the female, respectively.

56

Due to certain abnormalities during the meiotic division, the karyotype of a female may be 47, XXX. In that case, the somatic cells show two Barr bodies or two drumsticks.

Abnormalities in sex-chromosomes can occur due to disordered cell division during gametogenesis. In the most common sex-chromosomal abnormality, the chromosomal pattern is 45, XO (ovarian dysgenesis, Turner's syndrome). In another type of disorder, the chromosomal pattern may be 47, XXX ("Super females") or 47, XXY (Klinefelter's syndrome or seminiferous tubule dysgenesis).

Sex-chromosomal abnormalities mentioned above occur due to a failure of the separation of the sex-chromosomes (non-dysjunction) during the meiotic division during gametogenesis. Similar non-dysjunctional abnormalities may also occur in autosomal chromosomes. Down's syndrome (mongolism) is produced by trisomy 21 (the cells have an extra chromosome 21).

Gonadal Sex

Primitive gonads arise from the genital ridges. Until 6th week of development the primitive gonads are similar in the two sexes. If the zygote has Y-chromosome (46, XY), the primitive gonads develop into a testes. In genetic female (46, XX), the ovaries develop.

In the 7th week of gestation, the embryo has both male and female primordial genital ducts (the Wolffian duct system and the Mullerian duct system, respectively). In the male fetus, the testes become functional and secrete testosterone and a Mullerian regression factor (MRF). MRF is a polypeptide and acts unilaterally. MRF not only causes regression of the Mullerian duct but also, with the help of testosterone, causes development of Wolffian ducts into vas deferens and other related structures. The development of male external genitalia is also dependent on the presence of testosterone.

In the absence of testosterone, i.e. in a female fetus, Wolffian duct system regresses automatically. The Mullerian duct system develops into external and internal genitalia of the female.

Genital Sex

From the above discussion, it is apparent that the development of female genitalia occurs in the absence of embryonic gonadal hormones whereas testosterone and MRF are required for the development of male genitalia. It is also clear that the gonadal sex is determined by the chromosomal sex and both are same in almost all the individuals. However, genital sex and secondary sexual characteristics are determined by the hormonal environment and may be disturbed by abnormal hormonal secretions.

In individuals with XO chromosomal pattern, the gonads are rudimentary or absent. The female internal and external genitalia develop but there is no sexual maturity at puberty.

In the Klinefelter's syndrome, the individual has XXY chromosomal pattern and genitalia like that of a normal male. Testosterone is secreted in normal amounts at puberty and therefore the secondary sexual characteristics of the male develop normally. However, the seminiferous tubules are highly abnormal and mental abnormality is often associated.

Male genital development may occur in a genetic female exposed to androgens during 8th-13th week of gestation, e.g. due to congenital virilizing hyperplasia of adrenal cortex or due to administration of androgens to the pregnant female. Such an individual is called a *female-pseudohermaphrodite.* Male-pseudohermaphrodite is produced when the fetal testes are defective and do not secrete normal amounts of testosterone and MRF. Consequently, female internal genitalia develop although the external genitalia are male type.

Growth and Development at Adolescence and Puberty

Adolescence has been defined as the period between childhood and adulthood. Puberty is the period of growth and development leading to completion of sexual and physical maturity. Since the two phases of growth are almost overlapping the two terms are used interchangeably.

Physical Development

Due to adolescent spurt in growth the height increases by 7–12 cm in boys and 6–11 cm in girls. Peak growth spurt occurs at about 14 years of age in boys and at about 12 years in girls (Fig. 56.7). Greater part of increase in height is due to increase in the length of the trunk rather than the limbs. The growth spurt is genetically timed but mediated through the hormones.

Muscle Mass The increase in the muscle mass and muscle strength is far greater in boys than in girls (Fig. 56.8). Greater muscle mass, as well as, increase in haemoglobin concentration (Fig. 56.9) at puberty in boys can be attributed to the secretion of testosterone.

The first sign of puberty in boys is the acceleration of growth of testes and scrotum. Axillary hair growth appears about 2 years after the onset of puberty. In girls, the appearance of

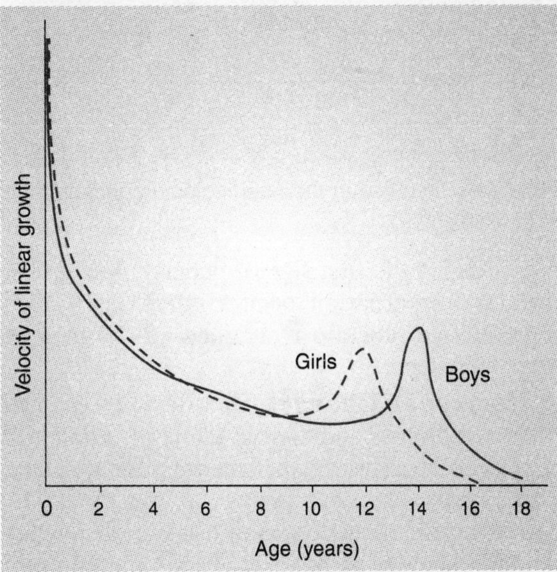

Fig. 56.7: Adolescent spurt in the velocity of growth.

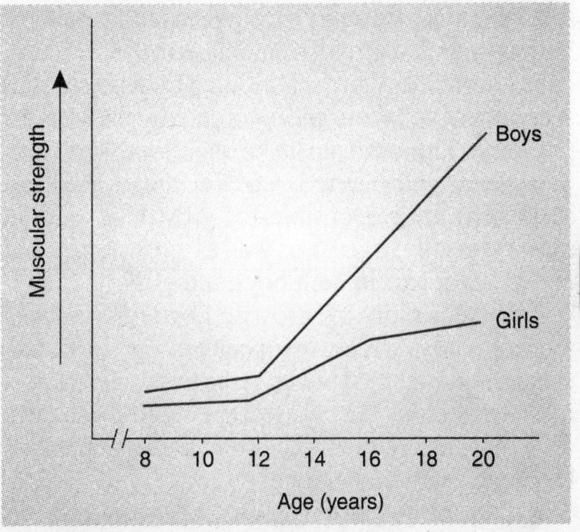

Fig. 56.8: Increase in the muscle mass and strength at puberty in boys and girls.

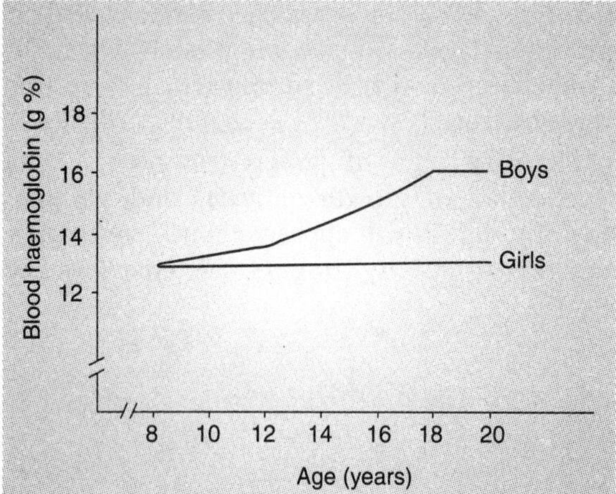

Fig. 56.9: Increase in the haemoglobin concentration at puberty in boys.

breast bud is the first sign of puberty. Menarche, the 1st menstruation occurs much later. Full reproductive function is attained 12–18 months after menarche.

Hormonal Changes Besides testes and ovaries, adrenals and thyroid gland also undergo adolescent spurt in growth. Anterior pituitary gland also increases in size, more so in the girls. The secretory rate of oestrogens or testosterone begins to increase at about 10 years in girls and 14 years of age in boys, reaching the peak level in the next 3–4 years (Fig. 56.10A, B). The secretion of adrenal androgens is also markedly increased at puberty both in boys and girls. The increase in the secretion of sex hormones can the attributed to the increased secretion of gonadotropic hormones by the anterior pituitary. The mechanism of increased secretion of adrenal androgens is not yet clear. Adrenal androgens are responsible for growth of muscle mass (specially in girls), as well as, growth of pubic and axillary hair in both boys and girls.

The secretion of growth hormone occurs intermittently, with a few peaks every 24 hours, specially at night. At puberty, the basal secretion is not elevated but the peaks occur more frequently and reach higher levels. The mechanism of puberty has been discussed earlier.

Effect of Protein Caloric Malnutrition in Childhood The incidence of protein caloric malnutrition or protein energy malnutrition (PEM)

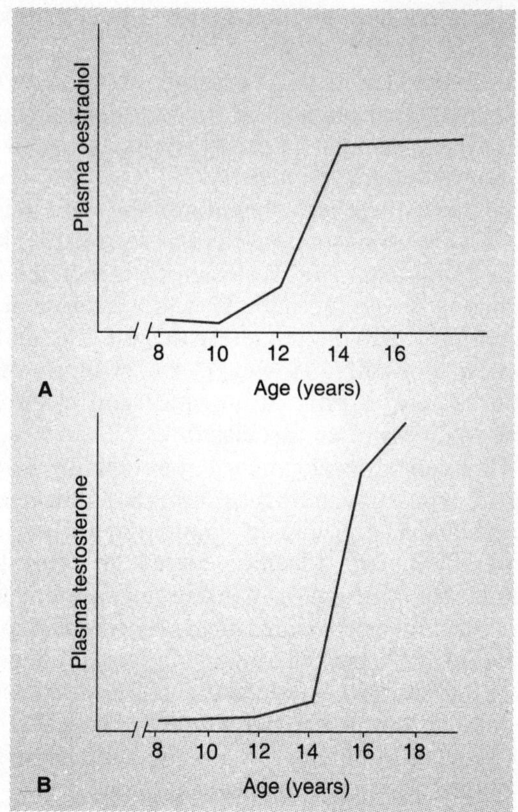

Fig. 56.10: Puberty-related increase in plasma oestrogen level in girls (A) and testosterone level in boys (B).

is fairly high in India and other third world countries. It may take the form of nutritional marasmus or kwashiorkor. Nutritional marasmus is more common type of nutritional deficiency disorder in childhood. It is caused by deficiency of calories in the diet at 6-12 months of age. The child is very thin and the muscles are wasted. The limbs look like sticks. Diarrhoea and other infections are common complications which worsen the disorder.

Kwashiorkor is caused by deficiency of proteins when the diet is adequate in calories. It usually occurs at about 2 years of age, when the child is weaned to a diet consisting of carbohydrates only. Low body weight, generalized oedema, apathy, pigmentation, thick and cracked skin are characteristic features. The colour of hair changes from black to reddish or grey. Plasma albumin level is very low.

Section XIV

The Kidneys and The Body Fluids

CHAPTER 57

The Kidney

FUNCTIONAL ANATOMY

The two kidneys are the chief excretory organs of the body. In addition, they regulate the concentrations of most of the constituents of the body fluids. The cut surface of the kidney (Fig. 57.1) is characterized by an outer cortex and an inner medulla. The medulla contains 5–10 pyramids whose tips project into the renal pelvis, the dilated upper end of the ureter.

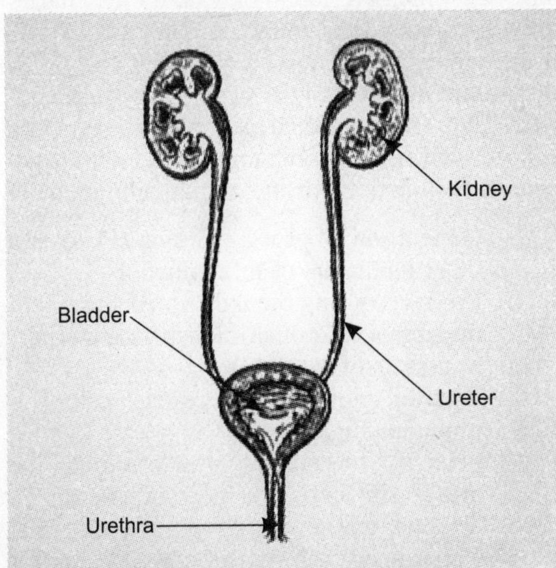

Fig. 57.1: Anatomical structure of the urinary tract.

Each kidney contains approximately 1.2 million nephrons. A nephron is a thin (20–50 μ diameter), elongated, (50 mm long) tube. It consists of a dilated blind end, the Bowman's capsule followed by segments known as the proximal convoluted tubule (PCT), loop of Henle and the distal convoluted tubule (DCT). Many distal convoluted tubules open into a collecting duct, which drains into the renal pelvis (Fig. 57.2). An anastomosing network of capillaries, called the glomerulus invaginates into the Bowman's capsule to constitute a malpighian corpuscle (Colour Plate 7, Fig. 19). The glomerulus is about 200 μm in diameter. The blood enters the glomerular capillaries through the afferent arterioles and leaves through the slightly narrower efferent arterioles. The glomeruli, PCT and DCT, are present in the cortex only. The medulla contains the loops of Henle and the collecting ducts.

Glomerulus

The glomerular capillaries are unique in the sense that they are interposed between two arterioles.

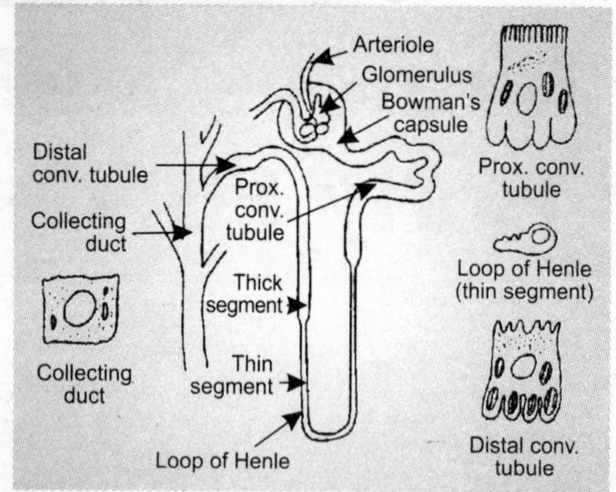

Fig. 57.2: Diagram of a nephron. Ultramicroscopic features of the constituent cells are also depicted.

This arrangement serves to maintain high hydrostatic pressure in the capillaries necessary for massive glomerular filtration (vide infra).

The glomerulus is made up of the fenestrated type of capillaries having very high permeability. The epithelial cells of the inner layer of Bowman's capsule are called **podocytes**, since they have feet-like processes which rest on the outer aspect of the capillary basement membrane.

The fluid that filters through the glomerular membrane is known as glomerular filtrate. The *glomerular membrane* (Fig. 57.3) consists of three layers:

(i) The endothelial cells lining the capillaries;
(ii) The common basement membrane; and
(iii) The epithelial cells of the Bowman's capsule.

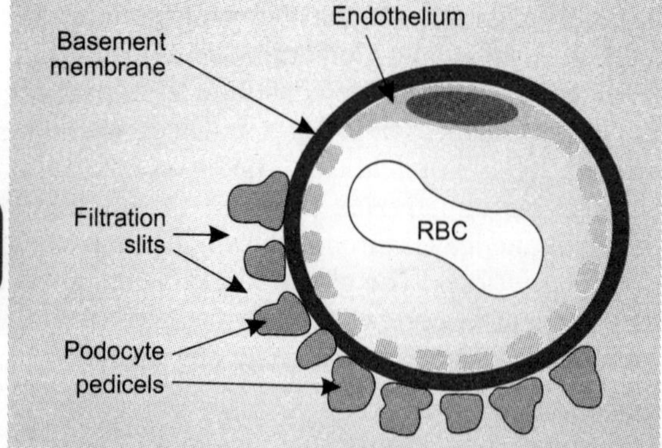

Fig. 57.3: The glomerular membrane.

The feet of the podocytes form an interdigitating network separated by *slit pores* which are bridged by a thin membrane called the filtration slit membrane. From the blood in the capillaries, the fluid passes through: (i) fenestra of the endothelial cells, (ii) the basement membrane, and finally through (iii) the filtration slit membrane.

In spite of tremendous permeability of the glomerular membrane, it has high degree of selectivity regarding the molecules that are allowed to pass through it. Substances like albumin and other plasma proteins with molecular weight of 69,000 and above are completely excluded whereas haemoglobin (mol. wt. 64,000), if present free in plasma, is allowed to pass through. Substances with diameter less than 40 Å (4 nm) can pass through most freely. Passage of the molecules across the glomerular filter is not determined solely be the molecular size; its charge is equally important. A positively-charged particle is allowed to pass more freely than a negatively-charged particle of the same size.

Mesangial cells

They that are modified smooth muscle cells, are also present around the capillaries. The intraglomerular mesangial cells are similar to cells called pericytes which are found outside the capillaries elsewhere. They are contractile. They play a role in the regulation of renal blood flow and GFR. Intraglomerular mesangial cells are also phagocytic. They are an unusual example of phagocytic cells derived from smooth muscle and not monocytes. The functions of mesangial cells include:

(i) Generation of prostaglandins (PGs) and other mediators of inflammation.
(ii) Production and breakdown of basement membrane and other biomatrix material;
(iii) Synthesis of cytokines;
(iv) Uptake of macromolecules, including immune complexes.
(v) In terms of its smooth muscle activity, the mesangial cell contracts or relaxes in response to a number of vasoactive agents. This ability allows the cells to modify glomerular filtration locally.

Proximal Convoluted Tubule (PCT)

The proximal convoluted tubule, approximately 15 mm in length, constitutes the major portion of the nephron and bulk of the renal parenchyma. The tubule is lined by a single layer of epithelial cells that exhibit a prominent brush border at the luminal surface, and a large number of mitochondria in the cytoplasm (Fig. 57.2). These characteristics of the epithelial cells may be correlated with extensive reabsorptive activity of the PCT.

Loop of Henley

It consists of a thick descending segment, followed by a thin descending segment forming a loop, with a thin ascending segment in the medulla and a thick ascending segment that enters the cortex once again. The thin segment of the loop of Henle (2–14 mm long) is lined with squamous epithelial cells with a few microvilli and mitochondria. The thick descending segment of the loop of Henle resembles, structurally and functionally, the PCT. Similarly, the thick ascending segment of the loop of Henle has structural and functional similarity to DCT (vide infra).

Each thick ascending segment of loop of Henle (12 mm in length) returns to the cortex and comes in close contact with its own glomerulus. The point of contact is called the **macula densa**, since here the epithelial cells of the tubule are narrower and their nuclei are crowded together.

The loops of Henle penetrate the medulla to a varying extent. The loops arising from the deeper region of the cortex (juxtamedullary glomeruli) descend deeper into the medulla than those arising from the glomeruli located in the superficial cortical region. In humans, only about 15% of the glomeruli have longer loops.

Distal Convoluted Tubule (DCT)

The distal convoluted tubule is only 5 mm in length. It is lined by epithelial cells with no distinct brush border but having many mitochondria near the basal border.

Collecting Duct

The collecting duct is about 20 mm long and passes through the renal cortex and medulla to empty into the renal pelvis at the apex of the medullary pyramid. Most of the epithelial cells of the collecting ducts are tall and have few organelles. These cells, called principal cells (P cells), are involved in *Na^+ reabsorption* and *ADH-induced water reabsorption*. In between P cells are present a few intercalated cells (I cells) having more microvilli, cytoplasmic vesicles and mitochondria. They are concerned with *acid secretion*.

Blood Vessels of Kidney

(Colour Plate 7, Fig. 20)

Each renal artery is a major branch arising from the aorta. It subdivides progressively into smaller branches. The smallest branch is called interlobular artery. Each interlobular artery gives off a series of *afferent arterioles*. Each afferent arteriole breaks up into a bunch of capillaries, the *glomerular capillaries* which join together again forming another arteriole, *the efferent arteriole*. The efferent arteriole again divides to form *peritubular capillaries* that surround the various portions of the renal tubules (Fig. 57.4).

The efferent arterioles of the *cortical glomeruli* break up into a network of microvessels, *the*

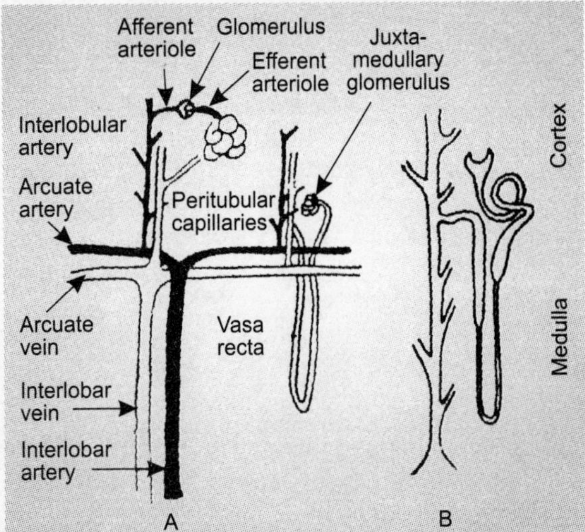

Fig. 57.4: The renal microcirculation. A nephron is juxtaposed on the right.

peritubular capillaries, which surround chiefly the PCT and DCT in the cortex. Efferent arterioles of the *juxtamedullary glomeruli* form a special type of peritubular capillaries called the *vasa recta*. The vasa recta are relatively straight and long capillary loops that descend into the renal medulla and form hair-pin loops along side the loops of Henle. The vasa recta, as well as, the peritubular capillaries in the cortex form an anastomosing network with the capillaries from the adjacent efferent arterioles.

Innervation of Renal Vessels

Renal vessels have rich sympathetic noradrenergic innervation. The sympathetic discharge is minimum at rest, but can increase markedly during states of cardiovascular stress (like severe exercise or haemorrhage), leading to intense renal vasoconstriction.

Juxtaglomerular Apparatus

The tunica media of the afferent arterioles of the kidney consists of cells containing prominent granules. The granules consist of a proteolytic enzyme called renin. These cells are called juxtaglomerular cells (JG cells) (Fig. 57.5). They act as baroreceptors. They monitor the vascular volume and are stimulated by hypovolemia or decreased renal perfusion pressure. These cells are innervated by noradrenergic sympathetic fibres.

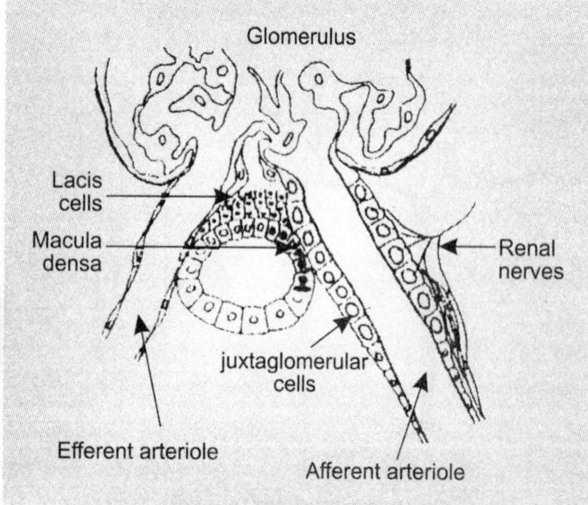

Fig. 57.5: The juxtaglomerular apparatus.

The cells of **macula densa** of the distal convoluted tubules act as chemoreceptors and are stimulated by decreased sodium load in the DCT.

A collection of *extraglomerular* **mesangial cells (Lacis cells)** are present between the JG cells and the macula densa.

The JG cells, the macula densa and the mesangial cells constitute the **juxtaglomerular apparatus.** Lacis cells are believed to transfer information about sodium chloride tubular load to the granular cells and may be involved in tubuloglomerular feedback regulation. Its role in sodium homeostasis is discussed elsewhere in this chapter.

Renal Blood Flow (RBF)

The two kidneys together receive approximately 1.2 litres of blood per minute (over 20% of total cardiac output). The extremely high blood flow in terms of tissue weight (400 ml/100 g/min) is related to its excretory function rather than its metabolic requirements.

Autoregulation of Renal Blood Flow

Variations in mean blood pressure between 70 and 200 mmHg do not produce any change in the rate of renal blood flow. This phenomenon called autoregulation of renal blood flow persists even after denervation of the kidney, but can be abolished by papaverin, a drug which relaxes smooth muscle or by administration of an inhibitor of prostaglandin synthesis.

The autoregulation of blood flow represents an intrinsic mechanism that maintains renal blood flow (and GFR, vide infra) constant in the face of normal or high perfusion pressure.

Variations of Renal Blood Flow

Renal blood flow is strongly affected by extrinsic regulatory factors like **sympathetic innervation, circulating catecholamines and angiotensin-II.**

(i) Baroreceptor mediated reflexes (e.g. during erect posture, haemorrhage) may produce from mild to most intense renal vasoconstriction. These effects are produced by an increase in the sympathetic nerve discharge to the renal vessels, as well as, through renin-angiotensin-II mechanism.

(ii) Circulating norepinephrine also constricts the renal vessels specially the afferent arterioles.

(iii) Angiotensin-II has a selective vaso-constrictor action on the efferent arterioles.

(iv) **Renal prostaglandins** are produced during circulatory stress like standing posture or haemorrhage. They have a local *vaso-dilatory* action on the renal vessels. They tend to counteract the renal vasoconstrictor effect of generalized increase in sympathetic nerve discharge or increased angiotensin-II secretion. Thus, they help in the autoregulation of RBF and GFR.

Intra-renal Difference in RBF

Approximately 90% of the total renal blood flow perfuses the renal cortex and only 10% perfuses the medulla. The marked regional difference in the cortical and medullary blood flow is due to relatively high vascular resistance in the vasa recta. Low medullary blood flow plays an important role in the urinary concentrating mechanism.

Clinically, total renal blood flow is estimated by measurement of para-amino-hippuric acid (PAH) clearance (page 623).

Hydrostatic Pressure in Renal Vessels

The *glomerular capillaries* have relatively high hydrostatic pressure (approximately 45 mmHg), which is an important factor in the formation of glomerular filtrate. In the *peritubular capillaries,* the mean hydrostatic pressure is about 8 mmHg only, which facilitates the reabsorptive function of the proximal and the distal convoluted tubules.

FUNCTIONS OF KIDNEY

Excretory Functions

Kidneys constitute the most important excretory organs of the body. They are the site of removal of non-volatile excretory products of protein metabolism such as urea, uric acid, creatinine, oxalates, phosphates, etc.

Non-excretory Functions

Besides the excretory function, the kidneys serve many important non-excretory functions also.

(i) Regulation of water and electrolyte balance.

(ii) Regulation of acid base homeostasis.

(iii) Regulation of blood volume.

(iv) Regulation of blood pressure.

(v) Synthesis of erythropoietin.

(vi) Activation of vitamin D_3: $25(OH)D_3$ is hydroxylated to $1,25(OH)_2D_3$

(vii) Under unusual circumstances, such as prolonged starvation, gluconeogenesis can also occur in the kidney.

Non-excretory functions (i), (iii) and (iv) are mediated through the release of renin, and thereby activation of renin-angiotensin mechanism.

GLOMERULAR FILTRATION

Of the 650 ml of plasma (1250 ml of blood) passing through the two kidneys each minute, about 125 ml of fluid is filtered out through the glomerular membrane into the Bowman's capsule. Thus, the normal glomerular filtration rate (GFR) is 125 ml/min. In women, the value is 10% lower. Normal filtration fraction is approximately 0.2 (125 ml/650 ml). In other words, approximately 180 litres of fluid are filtered daily from the glomerular capillaries. In contrast, only 20 L of fluid is filtered out per day in the rest of the systemic capillaries of the body. These figures demonstrate the massive scale at which glomerular filtration occurs. As the glomerular filtrate passes through the remaining parts of the nephron, and subjected to various reabsorptive and secretory processes, over 99% of the filtered fluid is reabsorbed and only 1 ml of the fluid is excreted per minute as urine.

Composition of Glomerular Filtrate

The composition of glomerular filtrate is similar to that of the interstitial fluid filtered out of the systemic capillaries. It contains all the electrolytes and solute constituents, in same concentrations as present in the plasma except that it is practically devoid of proteins (nor it contains any of the blood cells).

Factors Affecting GFR

The factors governing the filtration across the glomerular capillaries are the same as governing the filtration across any other capillary, i.e.:

(i) Hydrostatic pressure gradient across the capillary walls,
(ii) Osmotic pressure gradient across the capillary walls,
(iii) Size of the capillary bed and,
(iv) Permeability of the capillaries.

$$GFR = Kf\,[P_{GC} - P_T) - (\Pi_{GC} - \Pi_T)$$

where Kf, the glomerular filtration coefficient, is the product of glomerular capillary wall permeability and the effective filtration surface area :

P_{GC} = hydrostatic pressure in the glomerular capillaries

P_T = hydrostatic pressure in the Bowman's capsule

Π_{GC} = osmotic pressure of plasma in the glomerular capillaries

Π_T = osmotic pressure of filtrate in the Bowman's capsule.

Measurement of these forces has been made in the rat. Values of P_{GC} and P_T were found to be 45 mmHg and 10 mmHg, respectively. **ΠGC** was found to be 20 mmHg at the afferent arterial end and 35 mmHg at the efferent end. The increase in the osmotic pressure of plasma at the efferent end is explained by the increase in plasma protein concentration due to loss of fluid by ultrafiltration in the glomerulus. The value of Π_T was practically zero. Thus at the afferent arterial end, the net filtering force is 15 mmHg [+ 45 – (10 + 20)] but practically zero at the efferent end [+ 45 – (10 + 35)]. Therefore, the net filtering force in the glomerular capillary is almost similar to that at the arteriolar end of any other systemic capillary. Under these conditions how can the massive rate of glomerular filtration be accounted for? The permeability of the glomerular capillaries is approximately 50–100 times that of the capillaries in the skeletal muscle. Thus, many-fold increased value of Kf accounts for the proportionately increased volume of GFR as compared to the volume of filtrate from the other systemic capillaries.

The value of Kf is under a regulatory control. The contraction of the mesangial cells decreases the value of Kf by decreasing the number of patent capillaries. Angiotensin-II, vasopressin, norepinephrine and histamine decrease GFR by causing contraction of the mesangial cells. Renal prostaglandins and dopamine increase RBF and GFR by causing relaxation of mesangial cells.

Effect of Renal Blood Flow on GFR

Regarding the Starling forces, there is an important difference between an ordinary extra-renal capillary and a renal glomerular capillary.

In *an ordinary capillary*, the amount of fluid filtered is so small that the concentration of plasma proteins and hence their osmotic pressure does not practically vary over the entire length of the capillary. However, the capillary hydrostatic pressure gradually decreases. Consequently, filtration of fluid occurs in the proximal half (arteriolar half) of the capillary where the hydrostatic pressure exceeds the plasma protein colloidal osmotic pressure. In the distal half (venular half) of the capillary, tissue fluid is reabsorbed because colloidal osmotic pressure exceeds the capillary hydrostatic pressure (Fig. 57.6A).

In a *glomerular capillary*, efferent arteriolar resistance helps to maintain a constant hydrostatic pressure throughout the length of the capillary. On the other hand, massive filtration of fluid causes a gradual increase in the colloidal osmotic pressure. Hence filtration ceases when the colloidal osmotic pressure becomes equal to the hydrostatic pressure. In other words, roughly speaking, there is no filtration of fluid in the distal 25% of the glomerular capillary (Fig. 57.6B). However, if the rate of capillary blood flow is increased, the equilibrium between the hydrostatic pressure and the colloidal pressure would be reached more slowly, i.e. filtration would continue over a larger length of the glomerular capillary. That is why, besides other factors (Starling forces), rate of renal

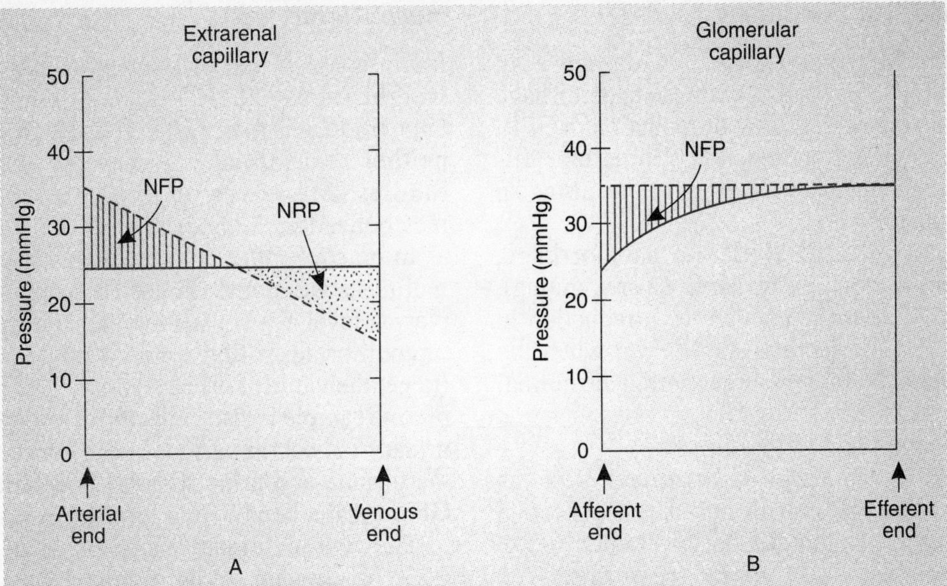

Fig. 57.6: Interaction of capillary hydrostatic pressure (- - - -), and colloidal osmotic pressure (——) in an extrarenal and a glomerular capillary. NFP, net filtration pressure; NRP, net reabsorption pressure.

blood flow is an important factor determining the glomerular filtration rate.

Variations in GFR

Theoretically, variation in GFR may occur because of a change in any one or more of the factors mentioned above, e.g. P_{GC}, P_T, Π_{GC}. However, under physiological conditions, the last two factors remain almost constant. In other words, variations in GFR can occur due to variation in P_{GC}. Besides this, renal blood flow is another important factor which can affect the GFR. Basically, both renal blood flow and GFR are under an intrinsic autoregulatory control so that variations in blood pressure from 70 to 200 mmHg do not produce any significant change in the renal blood flow or GFR (Fig. 57.7).

Extrinsic regulatory mechanisms (neural and humoral), however, can override the intrinsic regulatory mechanism and affect RBF and GFR.

Increased GFR

Pregnancy is a physiological condition in which GFR is markedly increased. It is related to the increase in total blood volume leading to increased RBF.

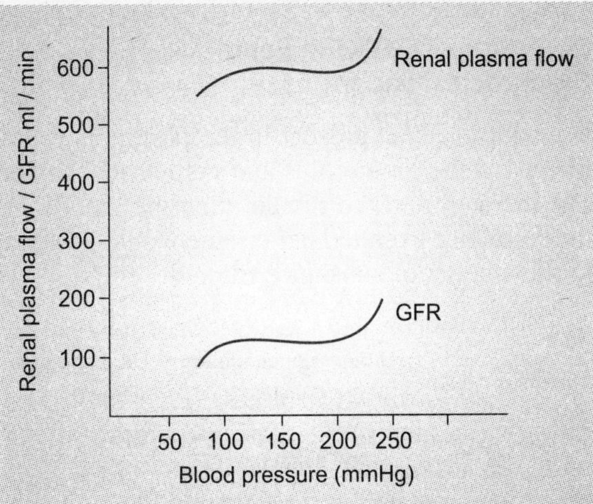

Fig. 57.7: The autoregulation of GFR and renal blood flow.

Decreased GFR

(A) Physiological Conditions RBF and GFR may decrease in varying degrees in physiological conditions like upright posture and exercise.

57

(B) Pathological Conditions

(i) *Arterial hypotension:* A decrease in arterial blood pressure due to haemorrhage is an important cause of reduction in GFR. In severe hypotension, glomerular filtration may cease altogether resulting in anuria.
(ii) *Hypovolemia:* Moderate haemorrhage, dehydration (due to diarrhoea or vomiting), burns. In these conditions, a reduction in RBF may decrease GFR even when the arterial blood pressure is within the normal range.
(iii) *Congestive heart failure*
(iv) *Renal parenchymal disorders* such as chronic glomerulonephritis, where a decrease in the number of glomeruli (i.e. decreased Kf) leads to progressive decrease in GFR.
(v) *An acute obstruction* of the ureter or renal pelvis (e.g. by a renal stone) decreases GFR by increasing the value of P_T.

Estimation of GFR: The Renal Clearance Concept

If a substance (x) present in the plasma is freely filtered at the glomerulus and neither reabsorbed nor secreted into the tubule, then the amount of the substance excreted per minute would be equal to the amount of substance filtered.

$$\text{Amount excreted} = \text{Urinary concentration of the substance } (U_x) \times \text{Urinary volume per minute } (V)$$

$$\text{Amount filtered} = \text{Plasma concentration of the substance } (P_x) \times \text{GFR}$$

Since, amount excreted = Amount filtered (x is freely filterable; neither reabsorbed nor secreted)

$$U_x \times V = P_x \times GFR$$

$$GFR = \frac{U_x \times V}{P_x}$$

Therefore, GFR can be known if we know: (i) The concentration of the substance in the plasma, (ii) Concentration of substance in the urine and (iii) Urinary volume per minute.

Inulin Clearance

Inulin is a polymer of fructose with a molecular weight of 5,400. If injected into the blood circulation, it is freely filtered in the glomeruli and neither reabsorbed nor secreted in the renal tubules. Moreover, it is non-toxic, and not metabolized in the body.

In practice, after an intravenous loading dose, inulin is continuously infused so as to maintain its plasma level at a constant value. During this state of equilibrium, a timed urine sample is collected (to get the value of urinary volume per minute). A plasma sample is also collected at mid-point of the urinary collection period. Inulin concentration in the plasma and urine samples is determined and GFR is calculated by the formula given above.

The rate of urinary excretion of a substance ($U_x \times V$) divided by its plasma concentration is a measure of the minimum amount of plasma required to supply the amount of substance excreted in the urine in the given time. This is termed as clearance of the substance (C_x).

$$C_x = \frac{U_x \times V}{P_x}$$

In other words, the **renal clearance** value of a plasma constituent *is the volume (in ml) of plasma which contains the amount of the constituent which is excreted in the urine in one minute.* Clearance of any substance, appearing in urine, can be calculated by this method. Because of the special property of inulin mentioned above, its clearance value equals the rate of GFR.

Clearance of a substance partially reabsorbed by the renal tubules is less than the GFR.

If a substance is freely filtered and also secreted by the renal tubular cells, its clearance value shall be greater than GFR. Clearance values of some of the substances present in the plasma are given in Table 57.1.

Creatinine Clearance

Creatinine is an endogenous product of muscle metabolism. Its rate of production in the body is almost constant. Creatinine is freely filtered by the glomeruli and neither reabsorbed nor secreted

Table 57.1: Clearance values of some of the plasma constituents

Substance	*Clearance value (ml/min)*
Na	0.9
K	12.0
Glucose	0.0
Urea	70.0
Uric acid	14.0

by the renal tubules. Therefore, the estimation of its clearance value is a simple and practical method for the clinical estimation of GFR in patients with renal diseases. Simplicity is the chief advantage of this method. Inulin clearance reflects GFR far more accurately, but the necessity of its continuous infusion precludes its use as a routine test for estimation of GFR.

Determination of Renal Plasma Flow (RPF) (PAH Clearance)

Renal plasma flow can be measured by Fick's principle.

$$\text{RPF (per minute)} = \frac{Q_x}{RA_x - RV_x} \qquad \text{(i)}$$

where Q_x is the amount of substance x taken up or removed by the kidney per minute; RA_x and RV_x are the plasma concentrations of the substance in the renal artery and the renal vein, respectively.

Para-amino-hippuric (PAH) acid is continuously infused so as to keep its plasma concentration at a constant low level. PAH is freely filtered by the glomeruli and also secreted by the proximal convoluted tubules to such an extent that it is completely removed during its renal circulation.

Consequently, its concentration in the renal vein is practically zero. Therefore, the equation given above is reduced to

$$\text{RPF} = \frac{Q_x}{RA_x}$$

$$= \frac{\text{Amount of PAH excreted per minute}}{\text{Plasma conc. of PAH in renal artery}}$$

$$= \frac{U_{PAH} \times V}{P_{PAH}} \qquad \text{(ii)}$$

Equation (ii) is nothing else but an equation for PAH clearance. Therefore, renal plasma flow can be determined by estimation of PAH clearance.

During constant infusion of PAH, peripheral venous blood sample is used for estimation of P_{PAH}, since its concentration is similar to that of renal arterial blood.

About 10% of the total renal plasma flow perfuses the non-excretory portions of the kidney, e.g. renal capsule, perirenal fat and renal pelvis. Therefore, such plasma is not cleared off the PAH since it does not undergo filtration and secretion. Therefore, PAH clearance value actually gives *effective renal plasma flow* (ERPF) rather than the *actual RPF*. The latter is approximately 10% higher than the estimated ERPF. From the value of renal plasma flow, value of *renal blood flow* can be easily determined, if haematocrit value (HCT) is known.

$$\text{RBF} = \text{RPF} \times \frac{1}{1 - \text{HCT}}$$

Normal values of ERPF are 650 ml/min/1.73 m^2 BSA in males and 600 ml/min/1.73 m^2 BSA in females. Accordingly, renal blood flow is approximately 1200 ml/min.

TUBULAR MECHANISMS

The glomerular filtrate (125 ml/min) contains all the constituents of plasma except proteins. This fluid passes through the remaining parts of the nephron (i.e. PCT, loop of Henle, and DCT) and the collecting ducts, where it is subjected to various *reabsorptive and secretory processes*. The end result is that a small volume (1 ml/min) of highly concentrated fluid containing the waste products, called urine, enters the renal pelvis.

The **renal handling** of a substance may involve:

(a) Glomerular filtration only, or

(b) Glomerular filtration followed by partial tubular reabsorption, or

(c) Glomerular filtration followed by complete tubular reabsorption, or

(d) Glomerular filtration followed by tubular secretion (Fig. 57.8).

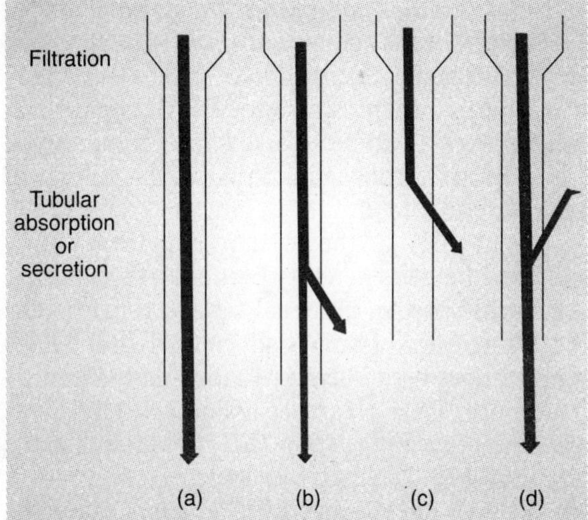

Fig. 57.8: Different patterns of tubular handling of substances in the glomerular filtrate.

Reabsorption occurs in the renal tubules mostly through transcellular pathway, e.g. glucose, Na^+, etc. but may occur through paracellular pathway also , e.g. Cl^- (Fig. 57.9).

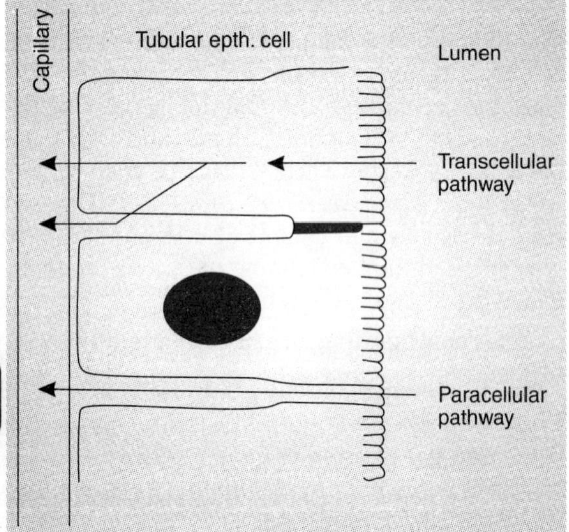

Fig. 57.9: The two absorptive pathways in the renal tubules.

Tubular Reabsorption

Complete Reabsorption

Substances of nutritive value such as glucose, amino acids, electrolytes (Na^+, K^+, Cl^-, HCO_3^-) and vitamins are completely or almost completely reabsorbed, mostly in the PCT. Most of these substances are reabsorbed *actively by Na^+-cotransport or exchange* mechanisms.

The proximal tubular cells are characterized by the presence of brush border on their luminal surface. The brush is composed of thousands of microvilli which increase the absorptive surface area of each cell by 20 folds. From the basal border of the epithelial cell, the absorbed substances are transferred into the peritubular capillaries. It is interesting to note that the active transport mechanism for sodium operates at the basal border of the proximal tubular cells and not at the luminal surface. Sodium crosses the luminal border by passive diffusion (Fig. 57.10).

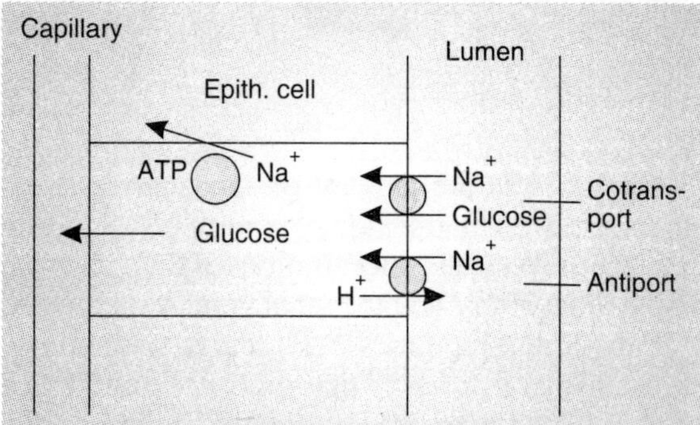

Fig. 57.10: Active transport mechanism in the renal tubular cells.

Reabsorption of Proteins

Although the glomerular membrane is said to be impermeable to proteins, as in capillaries elsewhere, small amount of proteins (3 mg/100 ml, mostly albumin) manage to escape into the glomerular filtrate. Even this extremely small concentration of protein would mean urinary loss of as much as 30 g of protein per day. Hence, proteins need to be completely reabsorbed in the renal tubules. Protein molecules are too large to be reabsorbed by ordinary active transport mechanisms operating at the renal epithelial cells. Instead, proteins are reabsorbed in the PCT by the process of *pinocytosis,* operating at the brush border. Once inside the epithelial cell, the proteins are digested into its constituent amino acids, which are reabsorbed into the circulation from the basal border.

Water is reabsorbed in various segments of the nephron except the ascending limb of the loop of Henle. However, 7/8th of the glomerular filtrate-water is reabsorbed in the PCT alone by the process of osmotic diffusion (passively).

Poor Reabsorption of Metabolic Waste Products

Creatinine is not reabsorbed at all in the renal tubules. (In fact small amount of creatinine is actually secreted by the proximal tubular cells into the lumen. That is why creatinine clearance is slightly greater than inulin clearance.) Most of the other waste products like urea, uric acid, sulphates, phosphates, etc. are only partially reabsorbed. For example, 90% of phosphates and only 50% of urea and uric acid are reabsorbed in the tubules. Since, 99% of filtered water is reabsorbed, the urinary concentrations of all these substances are considerably higher than in the plasma. Some of the substances are reabsorbed by active cotransport, e.g. glucose, amino acids, while others like urea, Cl^-, HCO_3^-, etc. are reabsorbed passively (Table 57.2).

Tubular Secretion

The process of tubular secretion is just opposite to that of tubular reabsorption. In tubular reabsorption, substances are recovered from the tubular fluid whereas in tubular secretion, substances are added to the tubular fluid (Fig. 57.8).

Only two natural constituents of plasma are secreted by the distal tubular cells namely, K^+ and H^+ ions. Secretion occurs by active transport mechanism. Secretion of H^+ occurs in the PCT, DCT and collecting ducts by an active transport pump operating at the luminal surface. In contrast, active transport mechanism for secretion of K^+ operates at the basal surface of the epithelial cells in the DCT and collecting ducts.

The proximal tubular cells may secrete uric acid, many drugs (e.g. penicillin, sulpha drugs), PAH, and iodinated contrast media. Uric acid is the only organic substance which can be both reabsorbed and secreted. K^+ is the only inorganic substance which can be both reabsorbed and secreted (Table 57.2).

Table 57.2: Summary of proximal and distal tubular function

Reabsorption		*Non-reabsorption*	*Secretion*
Active	*Passive*		
PCT			
Na^+	Cl^-	Inulin	H^+
K^+	HCO_3^-	Creatinine	Urate
Ca^{2+}	HPO_4^-	Sucrose	PAH
Mg^{2+}	Water	Mannitol	Penicillin
HPO_4^{2-}	Urea		Sulphonamide
SO_4^{2-}			Creatinine
NO_3^-			
Glucose			
Amino acid			
Protein			
Urate			
Vitamins			
Acetoacetate			
β-Hydroxybutyrate			
DCT			
Na^+	Cl^-	Urea	K^+
Ca^{2+}	HCO_3^-		H^+
Mg^{2+}	Water		
Urate			

RENAL TRANSPORT OF SOME SPECIFIC SUBSTANCES

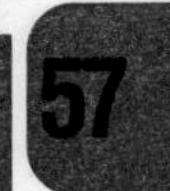

GLUCOSE

Glucose is reabsorbed in the proximal tubule by a secondary active transport mechanism. The energy for the active transport is provided by the Na^+-K^+.

ATPase that pumps Na^+ out of the cells at their basolateral border. At the luminal membrane, glucose and sodium bind to a common carrier called SGLT-1 (sodium dependent glucose transporter-1). Both sodium and glucose are carried into the cell as sodium moves down the electrochemical gradient. This process is an example of secondary active transport.

Then sodium is pumped out of the cell by Na^+-K^+ pump operating at the basolateral surface. Glucose is separately transported into the interstitial fluid by GLUT-2 (Fig. 57.11).

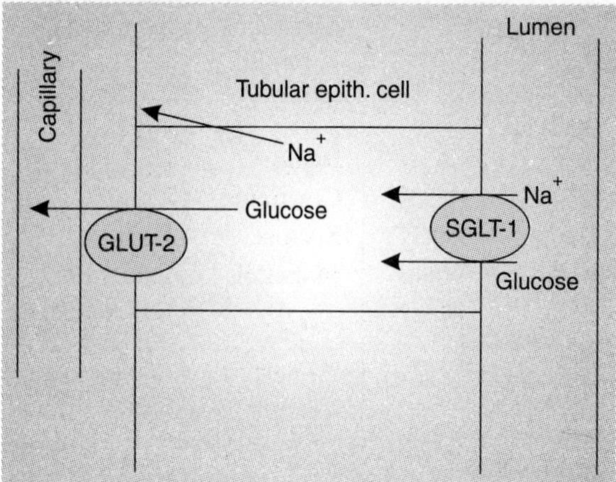

Fig. 57.11: Transport of glucose in the proximal renal tubules.

At normal plasma glucose level, all the filtered load of glucose (125 mg/min if GFR is 125 ml/min and plasma sugar level is 100 mg%) is reabsorbed into the proximal tubule and glucose is totally absent from the urine.

If blood sugar level is gradually increased (e.g. by intravenous glucose infusion), the filtered load of glucose gradually increases. At a certain plasma glucose level, glucose begins to appear in the urine because the filtered load of glucose exceeds the transport maximum for glucose (TmG). TmG can be defined as the maximum amount of glucose that can be transported (reabsorbed) in the renal tubules per minute. The plasma level of glucose at which glucose begins to appear in the urine is called the renal threshold for glucose. Its normal value is 180 mg%.

TmG of an individual can be found by plotting the curves of filtered glucose load (GFR × plasma glucose level) and the amount of glucose excreted in urine (Fig. 57.12). As the plasma level of glucose is increased in small steps, there is a linear increase in filtered load of glucose. Small amount of glucose starts appearing in the urine above plasma glucose level of 180 mg%. At about 300 mg% of blood glucose level, the transport mechanism for glucose is completely saturated. At still higher plasma levels of glucose, the urinary excretion of glucose increases linearly with increase in plasma glucose level. At this stage, the difference between the filtered load of glucose (GFR × PG) and the amount of glucose excreted in the urine per minute (U × V), gives the value of TmG. Normal value of TmG is 370 mg/min in males and 300 mg/min in females.

According to the normal value of TmG, the renal threshold for glucose should be approximately 300 mg%. But actually it is 180 mg% because some of the nephrons have lower reabsorptive capacity than others. Such nephrons start excreting glucose while others are still reabsorbing all the glucose load they receive. This difference in the behaviour of different types of nephrons is the cause of splay (a rounded part of the curve of excreted glucose) in the glucose titration curve (Fig. 57.12).

Many other substances like amino acids, uric acid, phosphates are absorbed by an active carrier-

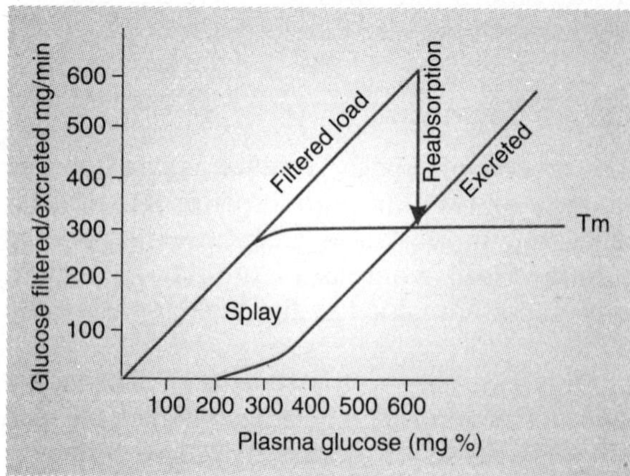

Fig. 57.12: Estimation of transport maximum for glucose (TmG). The filtered load of glucose = GFR (inulin clearance) X PG (plasma glucose).

57

mediated processes. They too also have a transport maximum (Tm). However, there is no Tm for absorption of Na^+ and secretion of K^+.

Renal glycosuria is a congenital defect characterized by urinary excretion of glucose even at normal blood glucose levels. The condition is caused by an inborn tubular defect involving decreased value of TmG.

Sodium Transport

Over 99% of filtered sodium is reabsorbed in the renal tubules. About two-thirds is reabsorbed in the PCT and the rest in the thick ascending limb of loop of Henle, DCT and collecting ducts. To maintain electrical neutrality, approximately 75% of the Na^+ reabsorption is accompanied by Cl^- and the rest by HCO_3^-.

Proximal Tubule

In the PCT, part of the Na^+ is reabsorbed by unidirectional Na^+ transport. In this process, Na^+ passively enters the tubular epithelial cell due to chemical and electrical gradients. Active extrusion of Na^+ occurs at the basolateral border by the Na^+-K^+ ATPase pump. In other words, the pump maintains very low concentration of Na^+ in the cell which allows passive diffusion of Na^+ from the tubular lumen (Fig. 57.13A). Passive transport of chloride through the tight junctions prevents development of transepithelial potential difference (potential difference between the luminal fluid and the peritubular fluid).

In the PCT, Na^+ reabsorption also occurs by Na^+-H^+ antiport mechanism. The electrochemical gradient for the passive movement of Na^+ from the tubular fluid into the epithelial cell provides the driving force for extrusion (secretion) of H^+ into the tubular fluid (Fig. 57.13B). The energy for Na^+-H^+ antiport is again provided indirectly by ATPase operating at the basolateral border which maintains intracellular Na^+ concentration low. Further, generation and secretion of H^+ indirectly lead to HCO_3 reabsorption.

A minor fraction of filtered sodium is reabsorbed through the transcellular pathway in company with chloride (Fig 57.13C).

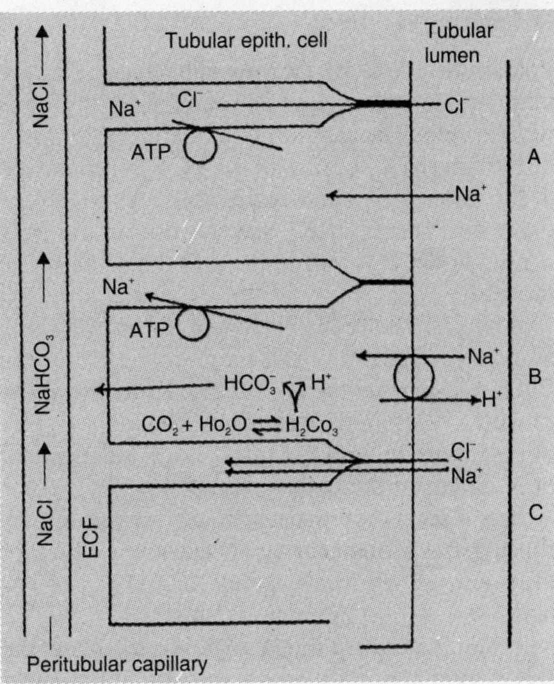

Fig. 57.13: Mechanism of sodium reabsorption in the proximal tubules.

Loop of Henle, Distal Tubule and Collecting Ducts

Reabsorption of Na^+ occurs in all segments of the nephron except thin segment of the loop of Henle. In the thick ascending limb of loop of Henle, DCT and collecting ducts, Na^+ reabsorption occurs by unidirectional transport mechanism, as well as, Na^+-H^+ antiport mechanism described above.

In the thick ascending limb, Na^+ reabsorption is accompanied by Cl^- reabsorption. On the other hand, **in DCT and collecting ducts**, Na^+ reabsorption is not only hormone **(aldosterone) dependent** but also occurs *as Na^+-K^+ antiport or Na^+-H^+ antiport system,* i.e. increased Na^+ reabsorption is accompanied by increased urinary excretion of K^+ and/or H^+. The regulation of urinary Na^+ excretion is mainly achieved through aldosterone. In the presence of high concentration of aldosterone in the plasma, urinary Na^+ excretion may be as low as 0.1 g/day. On the other hand, in the absence of aldosterone, over 20 g of Na^+ may be lost per day.

Potassium Excretion

Potassium is one of the few substances that are both reabsorbed as well as secreted by the renal tubular cells. The reabsorption of about two-thirds of the filtered K^+ occurs in the PCT in proportion to the volume of water reabsorbed. Although the exact mechanism of K^+ reabsorption in the PCT is not known, it is independent of the K^+ status of the body.

After further reabsorption of K^+ in the thick ascending segment of the loop, only 10% of the filtered K^+ reaches the DCT. Here, K^+ reabsorption as well as secretion takes place. The reabsorption of potassium in the DCT also occurs independent of K^+ status of the body.

It is a **secretory process** that is **regulated by the plasma aldosterone** concentration which in turn depends on the K^+ (and Na^+) status of the body.

When the dietary intake of K^+ is adequate, the secretory rate of K^+ exceeds the rate of its absorption in the DCT, i.e. there is a net secretion of K^+.

With high dietary K^+ intake, K^+ secretion is markedly increased.

The secretory mechanism of K^+ is linked with the Na^+ pump operating at the basolateral border (Fig. 57.14). The Na^+-K^+ ATPase pump actively transfers K^+ from the peritubular fluid into the epithelial cell. From the cell, K^+ diffuses passively into the lumen of the DCT and collecting ducts.

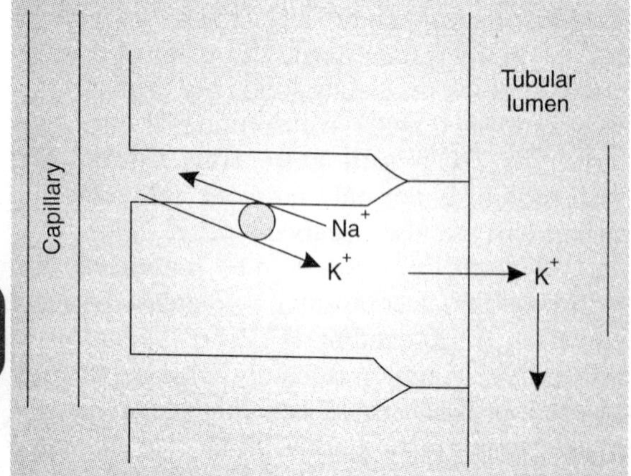

Fig. 57.14: Mechanism of distal tubular secretion of K^+.

Aldosterone markedly increases the secretion of K^+ in these cells by increasing the activity of Na^+-K^+ ATPase.

Besides the dietary intake of K^+, many **other factors** influence the secretion of K^+ in the distal nephron.

(a) Na^+ Reabsorption in the Distal Nephron Since K^+ secretion in the distal nephron is linked with Na^+-K^+ ATPase system, any factor increasing Na^+ reabsorption in the distal nephron increases K^+ secretion e.g.

(i) Decreased dietary intake of Na^+ or
(ii) Increased delivery of Na^+ to the DCT and collecting ducts by certain diuretics. Diuretic drugs such as furosemide or thiazide tend to produce hypokalaemia.

(b) Acid-base Balance Potassium and hydrogen ions have a reciprocal relationship in the maintenance of electrical neutrality within the cells. Acute alkalosis causes increased entry of K^+ in all the cells including renal tubular epithelium. It results in increased urinary secretion of K^+. Chronic alkalosis may actually cause depletion of total body K^+.

URINARY WATER EXCRETION

Maintenance of the osmolality of body fluid is one of the most important functions of the kidney. With glomerular filtration rate of 125 ml/min, approximately 180 litres of fluid is filtered into the Bowman's capsule per day. Of this, about 1.5 L/day (1 ml/min) reaches the renal pelvis as urine and the rest is reabsorbed in various segments of the nephron. However, the urinary volume excreted per day may vary from 500 ml to several litres per day. When the plasma osmolality is high, small volume of urine containing large concentration of solutes (i.e. highly concentrated urine) is excreted. When the plasma osmolality is low, large volume of urine with low concentration of solute (dilute urine) is excreted.

The kidney's ability to concentrate or dilute urine is related to two factors:

(i) Hyperosmolality of renal medullary interstitium and
(ii) Plasma level of antidiuretic hormone (ADH).

Hyperosmolality of Renal Medullary Interstitium

The osmolality of renal cortical interstitial fluid is approximately 300 mOsm/kg (285 mOsm/kg H_2O to be precise). However, the osmolality of the renal medullary interstitium progressively increases from 300 mOsm/kg H_2O near the cortex to 1200 mOsm/ kg H_2O at the tip of the pyramid (Fig. 57.15). The gradient of hyperosmolality is produced by the operation of **countercurrent multiplier system** *in the loop of Henle* and **the countercurrent exchanger system** *in the vasa recta*.

A countercurrent system is a system, in which the outflow runs parallel to, in close proximity to inflow for some distance. The effect of such a system is best illustrated by studying the effect of a heater on a straight water pipe and a pipe bent in U shape (Fig. 57.16). If the heater gives 100 calories of heat per minute and water flows at the rate of 10 ml/min, it will raise the temperature of water flowing through the straight tube by 10°C, e.g. from 30°C to 40°C. If the pipe is bent in U shape and the two limbs are brought in close proximity, the temperature at the outlet is again 40°C but at the tip of the U-tube (B) the temperature is 100°C. This is because the outgoing fluid warms the incoming fluid and sets up the countercurrent system.

The thick ascending limb of loop of Henle is impermeable to water but it actively reabsorbs

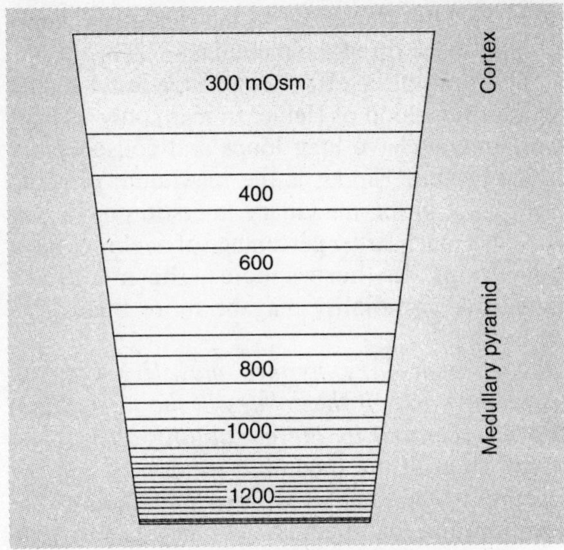

Fig. 57.15: Osmolality (mOsm) of renal medullary interstitium.

sodium chloride (NaCl). The thin descending limb of loop of Henle is relatively impermeable to solutes but highly permeable to water.

Active transfer of NaCl from the ascending limb increases the osmolality of medullary interstitium. Consequently, the osmolality of the fluid in the descending limb increases by passive loss of water into the medullary interstitium (Fig. 57.16C). At any one horizontal level, a segment of the ascending limb can create an osmotic gradient of 200 mOsm/L but the total effect of the countercurrent multiplier system results in an osmolality

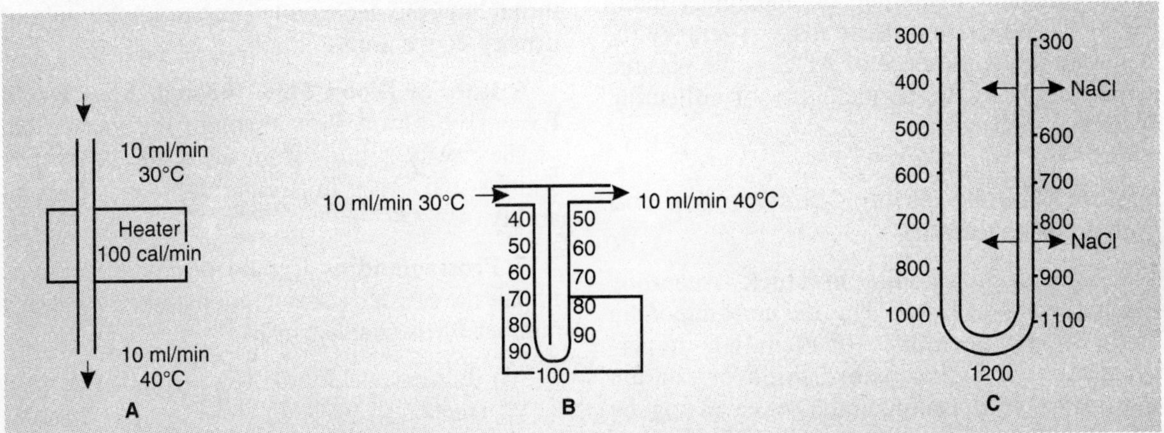

Fig. 57.16: The principle of countercurrent multiplier system.

57

of 1200–1400 mOsm/kg in the medullary interstitium, at the tip of the medulla.

The multiplier effect is proportional to the length of the loop of Henle. In man, only 15% of the nephrons have long loops and consequently 1200–1400 mOsm/kg is the maximum possible osmolality in the medullary interstitium. In dog and rat, a much larger percentage of nephrons have long loops. In these species, the medullary interstitial osmolality may be more than 2500 mOsm/kg.

The medullary hyperosmolality can be maintained only if the solutes in the interstitium are not removed by the circulating blood. The blood flow in the medullary region is a small fraction of the total renal flow. This permits the creation and maintenance of medullary hyperosmolality. Further, the close proximity of ascending and descending limbs of the vasa recta permit them to act as *countercurrent exchangers*. Water diffuses out of the descending vessels into the ascending vessels whereas solutes diffuse out of the ascending vessels into the descending vessels. In this fashion, solutes tend to recirculate within the medulla. It may be added that the countercurrent exchange is a passive process and only has to sustain the medullary hyperosmolality generated by the active countercurrent multiplier system operating in the loop of Henle.

Besides *NaCl*, *urea* is another important solute involved in the creation of hyperosmolality of medullary interstitium. Urea diffuses passively out of the collecting ducts into the medullary interstitium. The diffusion of urea is markedly increased in the presence of ADH in the plasma, which increases the permeability of collecting ducts to water and urea.

Factors Affecting Urinary Concentration and Dilution Mechanisms

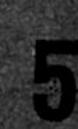

1. Normal Functioning of Thick Ascending Limb of Loop of Henle This the most important factor for the generation of medullary hyperosmolality. If active reabsorption of sodium chloride in the ascending limb is blocked (e.g. by loop diuretics), the entire medullary gradient of hyperosmolality disappears within minutes. As a result, the urine can neither be concentrated nor diluted.

2. Length of the loop of Henle Long looped juxtamedullary nephrons are involved in the countercurrent multiplier system. Therefore animal species with a larger percentage of long looped nephrons (cat, dog) have higher power of urinary concentration.

3. Availability of Urea Besides NaCl, urea is another solute present in the medulla in high concentration. Intake of protein deficient diet results in a decrease in the osmolar gradient of medullary interstitium.

4. Rate of Flow in the Loop of Henle A rapid flow of fluid through the loop of Henle causes greater reabsorption of water from the thin descending limb, which dilutes the solutes in the medullary interstitium. As a result, there is a decrease in the urinary concentration ability. Conversely, a decreases in the rate of flow (e.g. due to decreased GFR) tends to cause increased urinary concentration even in the absence of ADH.

5. Rate of Flow of Fluid in Collecting Ducts Excessive flow of fluid in the collecting ducts dilutes the solutes in the medullary interstitium. It also decreases urinary concentration ability. Osmotic diuretics (like mannitol or excessive glucose) when present in the proximal convoluted tubules interfere with reabsorption of NaCl and water. Therefore, intratubular flow rate is increased throughout the nephron leading to impairment of urinary concentration ability.

6. Rate of Blood Flow through Vasa Recta Excessive blood flow through the vasa recta washes away solutes from the medullary interstitium, and hence impairs urinary concentration ability.

7. Prostaglandins Certain renal prostaglandins impair the urinary concentration ability through a number of mechanisms:

(i) Increased blood flow through the vasa recta.

(ii) Inhibition of active transport of NaCl in the thick ascending limb.

(iii) Inhibition of the enzyme adenyl cyclase in the collecting ducts. Adenyl cyclase is involved in the genesis of cAMP. Since ADH acts through cAMP mechanism, prostaglandins inhibit reabsorption of water from the collecting ducts leading to urinary dilution even in the presense of ADH.

Role of ADH

The glomerular filtrate has an osmolality of 300 mOsm/kg. In the PCT, about 70% of the solutes are reabsorbed but the fluid remains iso-osmotic because a similar proportion of water also accompanies passively. The descending limb of loop of Henle is permeable to water but relatively impermeable to solutes. Therefore, the fluid in the descending limb becomes progressively hyperosmolar as water moves out into the hyperosmolar interstitium.

The active transport of NaCl in the ascending limb of loop of Henle progressively decreases the osmolality of the tubular fluid. By the time it reaches DCT, the osmolality of the fluid is about 100 mOsm/kg. Moreover, out of 125 ml of the fluid filtered by the glomeruli each minute only about 15 ml reach DCT. *The fate of this 15 ml of fluid with an osmolality of 100 mOsm/kg depends on the presence or the absence of ADH in the plasma.*

Absence of ADH—Formation of a Large Volume of Dilute Urine

A decrease in plasma osmolality, e.g. by drinking large volume (1–2 litres) of water or a hypotonic fluid, result in the inhibition of ADH secretion from the posterior pituitary gland. About 30 minutes after the intake of water, the urinary volume may increase to 10–15 ml/min and its osmolality varies from 30–100 mOsm/kg (**water diuresis**). In the absence of ADH, the distal convoluted tubules and the collecting ducts become impermeable to water but NaCl reabsorption continues. Therefore, most of the fluid reaching the DCT is excreted out. Reabsorption of NaCl in the collecting ducts further reduces the osmolality of the fluid from 100 mOsm/kg to as low as 30 mOsm/kg (Fig. 57.17).

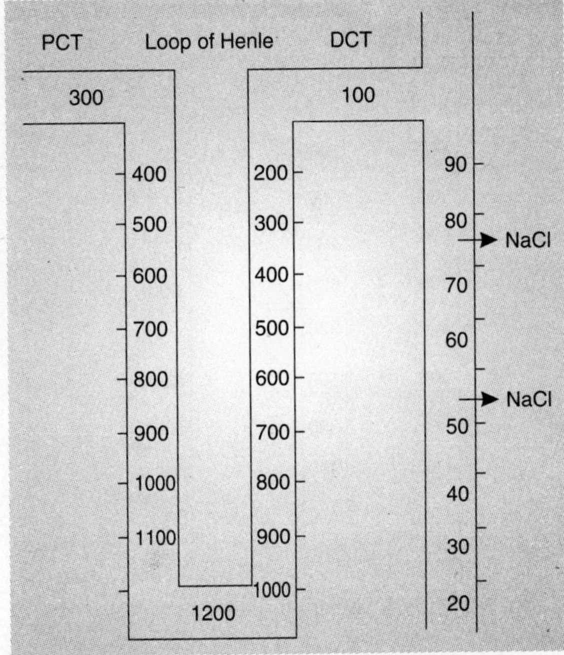

Fig. 57.17: Mechanism of urinary dilution.

Presence of ADH—Formation of a Small Volume of Concentrated Urine

An increase in the plasma osmolality (e.g. by dehydration) stimulates the secretion of ADH from the posterior pituitary gland. The antidiuretic hormone increases the permeability of *DCT and the collecting ducts* to water by translocation of aquaporins (*see* Fig. 46.6) in its epithelial cells. Therefore, water leaves the tubular fluid passively. In the DCT, osmosis results in raising the osmolality of the tubular fluid to 300 mOsm/kg, i.e. equal to the osmolality of the cortical interstitium. On the other hand, as the fluid passes through the collecting ducts, it becomes progressively more and more concentrated, since water is progressively reabsorbed into the hyperosmolar medullary interstitium. When enough ADH is present in the plasma, urinary osmolality may increase up to 1200–1400 mOsm/kg (Fig. 57.18).

It may be emphasized that the tubular response to ADH is *not* an all or none phenomenon. Varying grades of plasma ADH concentrations can produce

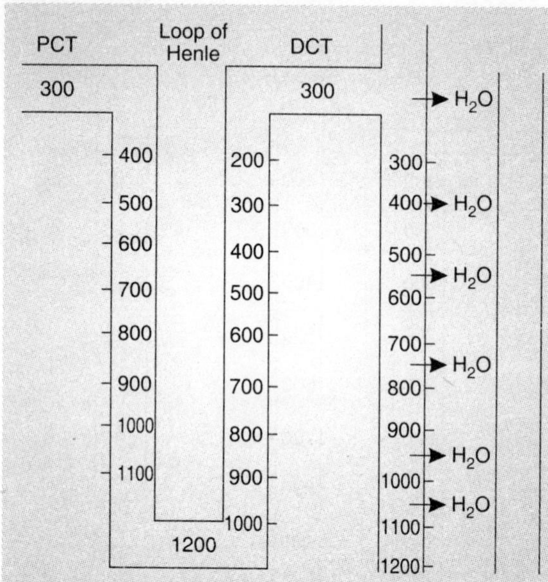

Fig. 57.18: Mechanism of urinary concentration.

proportionate increase in the permeability of collecting ducts to water. Consequently, depending on the status of body water and plasma osmolality, considerable variations in the rate of urine flow and urinary osmolality normally occur in different parts of the day. After an overnight fast, the morning urine samples tend to be relatively more concentrated.

Clinical Measurement In clinical laboratories, it is far simpler to measure the **specific gravity** of urine by a hydrometer than to measure the urinary osmolality which requires a very expensive instrument called osmometer. The specific gravity of urine is usually around 1.020. But, it can vary from 1.002 to 1.040. It may be clarified that whereas osmolality depends on the number of solute particles in a fluid, the specific gravity depends on the weight of the particles. When the urine contains normal constituents, the correlation between its osmolality and specific gravity is very close. But in the presence of glucose or proteins in the urine, the specific gravity would be far greater than the osmolality of the urine sample.

Osmotic Diuresis and Water Diuresis The term diuresis means an increased urinary output. As explained above, excessive intake of water increases the urinary volume because of the absence of ADH in the plasma and the consequent *decreased reabsorption of water in the DCT and collecting ducts*. The condition is called **water diuresis**. During water diuresis, *water reabsorption in the PCT is not affected.*

Presence of a larger amount of solutes in the renal tubular fluid also causes an increase in the volume of urinary excretion of water because of an osmotic effect. Unabsorbed glucose (e.g. in diabetes mellitus), mannitol, or presence of excessive NaCl (due to administration of certain diuretics) *prevent normal water reabsorption in the PCT and loop of Henle*. Therefore, urinary volume increases. This type of diuresis is known as **osmotic diuresis**. Osmotic diuresis can be differentiated from water diuresis by observation of osmolality/specific gravity of urine. In case of water diuresis, urinary osmolality is always low (below 300 mOsm/kg; specific gravity below 1.010). On the other hand, in osmotic diuresis the osmolality of the urine is higher than 300 mOsm/kg (specific gravity over 1.010).

The mechanism of action of some of the diuretic agents is given in Table 57.3.

HYDROGEN ION SECRETION: ACIDIFICATION OF URINE

Proximal convoluted tubule, thick ascending limb of loop of Henle, distal convoluted tubule and collecting duct are capable of H^+ secretion.

As much as 60 mEq of H^+ are added to the body every day from non-volatile acids produced by protein metabolism. These acids are buffered by HCO_3^- and other buffers in the blood.

$$H_2SO_4 + 2NaHCO_3 \longrightarrow 2H_2CO_3 + Na_2SO_4$$
$$\downarrow$$
$$2CO_2 + 2H_2O$$

The kidney is the only organ which can eliminate the fixed acids by active secretion of H^+. During H^+ secretion, bicarbonate (HCO_3^-) is generated, which replaces the HCO_3^- lost while buffering the fixed acids.

Over 4000 mEq of HCO_3^- are filtered out into the glomerular filtrate each day. All of it is

Table 57.3: Different diuretics and their mechanism of action

Diuretic agent	*Mechanism of action*
1. Water	Inhibition of ADH secretion
2. Alcohol	Inhibition of ADH secretion
3. Glucose (e.g. in diabetes mellitus)	Osmotic diuresis
4. Caffeine	Increased GFR (water load) and probably decreased renal tubular Na reabsorption
5. Drugs used as diuretics	
(a) Acetazolamide (Diamox)	Inhibition of H^+ secretion and therefore increased Na^+ and K^+ excretion
(b) Thiazide	Inhibition of NaCl reabsorption in early part of DCT
(c) Furosemide	Inhibition of NaCl reabsorption in thick ascending segment of loop of Henle
(d) Spironolactone (K^+-sparing diuretic)	Inhibition of Na^+-K^+ exchange in the collecting duct

reabsorbed in the renal tubules by a mechanism which depends on H^+ secretion in the tubules.

Generation of H^+ Ions in Tubular Epithelial Cells

In the renal tubular epithelial cells, H^+ are generated by hydration of CO_2 produced locally or diffusing from the blood.

$$CO_2 + H_2O \overset{CA}{\rightleftharpoons} H_2CO_3 \rightleftharpoons H^+ + HCO_3^-$$

The enzyme carbonic anhydrase (CA), which catalyses the hydration of CO_2, is present in the epithelial cells throughout the renal tubules. In addition, the enzyme is also present in the brush border of the PCT. Administration of acetazolamide, a carbonic anhydrase-inhibitor results in inhibition of H^+ secretion as well as reabsorption of HCO_3^- in the renal tubules.

In the proximal convoluted tubule, H^+ are secreted in exchange for Na^+ as Na^+-H^+ antiport. The driving force for the H^+ secretion is provided by the passive (downhill) movement of Na^+ at the luminal surface of the epithelial cell. The energy for Na^+-H^+ antiport is indirectly provided by Na^+-K^+ ATPase pump operating at the basolateral border which maintains intracellular Na^+ concentration low.

In the DCT and collecting ducts, H^+ secretion occurs independent of Na^+ reabsorption from the luminal surface. In this part of the tubule, *H^+ are secreted by an ATP driven proton-pump*, which can increase H^+ concentration of the luminal fluid 1000 times the plasma concentration.

The secretion of H^+ in the renal tubule can continue only if free H^+ is immediately buffered in the luminal fluid. In the *PCT, the filtered HCO_3^-* buffers the secreted H^+. In the *DCT and collecting ducts, Na_2HPO_4 and NH_3* act as buffers and neutralize the secreted H^+.

Effect of H^+ Secretion in Proximal Tubule: Bicarbonate Reabsorption

The renal tubular cells are not very permeable to HCO_3^-. Therefore, the large amount of HCO_3^- filtered into the Bowman's capsule is reabsorbed in an indirect manner. The H^+ secreted into the lumen of the PCT combines with the filtered HCO_3^- to form carbonic acid which is further dissociated into CO_2 and H_2O. H_2O becomes a part of tubular fluid whereas CO_2 diffuses into the tubular cell or the blood. Presence of carbonic anhydrase on the microvilli (brush border) of the proximal tubular epithelial cell catalyzes the hydrolysis of H_2CO_3 into CO_2 and H_2O (Fig. 57.19A).

As shown in Fig. 57.19, the secretion of H^+ simultaneously generates HCO_3^- in the epithelial cell which enters the peritubular capillaries. In other words, for each H^+ secreted into the lumen of PCT, one HCO_3^- disappears from the tubular fluid but at the same time, one HCO_3^- enters the blood circulation. Thus, in the PCT, H^+ secretion leads to reabsorption of filtered HCO_3^-, although the HCO_3^- which enters the blood is not the same ion which was removed from the tubular fluid.

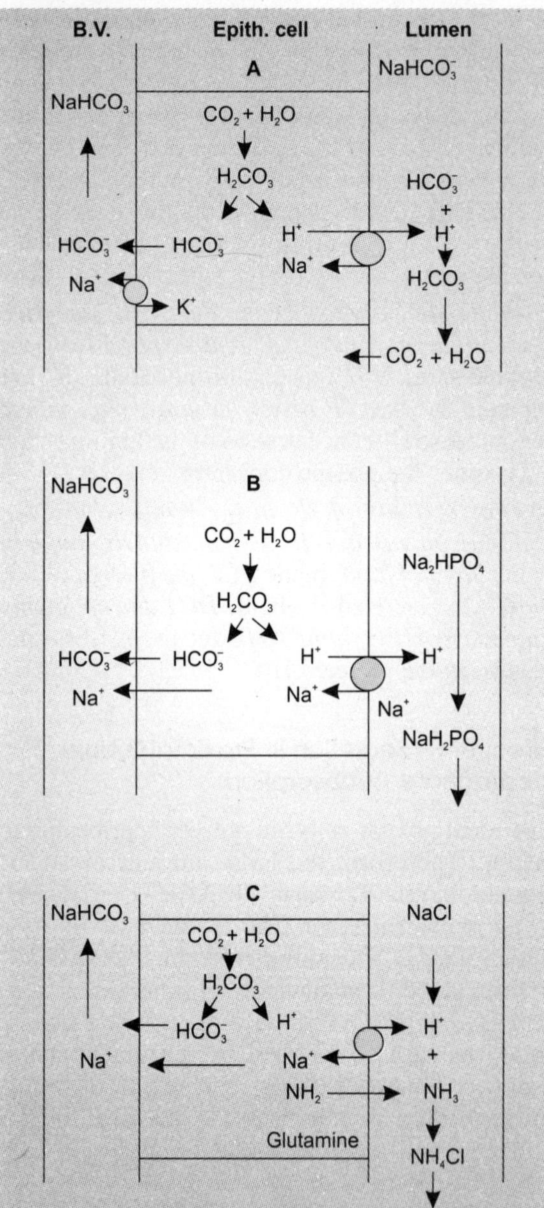

Fig. 57.19: Fate of H^+ secretion in the kidney. (A) Reabsorption of filtered bicarbonate; (B) Increase in titrable acidity; (C) Formation of ammonium.

57

By the process described above, H^+ secretion in the PCT leads to almost total (over 90%) reabsorption of the filtered HCO_3^-. But there is no net secretion of H^+ from the body. Only when the secreted H^+ are trapped by phosphate buffers or ammonia, i.e. in distal tubular segments, that net secretion of H^+ takes place. Even though tubular cells secrete over 4000 mEq of H^+ per day, most of it is used for reabsorption of bicarbonate in the proximal tubule. Only about 60 mEq of H^+ are excreted from the body per day—20 mEq with phosphate buffer and 40 mEq with ammonia, as described below.

Effect of H^+ Secretion in Distal Tubular Segments: Acidification of Urine

(a) Role of Phosphate Buffers

In the plasma, the phosphate buffers consist of a mixture of Na_2HPO_4 (basic phosphate) and NaH_2PO_4 (acid phosphate) in the ratio of 4 : 1. In the plasma, the concentration of phosphates is too low to be effective as a blood buffer. However, the phosphates filtered into the Bowman's capsule are only partially reabsorbed. By the time the tubular fluid reaches the DCT and collecting duct, the reabsorption of water increases the concentration of phosphates to such an extent that they constitute a very efficient urinary buffer.

Hydrogen ion secreted into the distal tubule combines with Na_2HPO_4 to form NaH_2PO_4 and Na^+ which is reabsorbed in exchange for the H^+ secreted. NaH_2PO_4 is excreted into the urine.

$$Na_2HPO_4 \xrightarrow{H^+} NaH_2PO_4 + Na^+$$

In the urine, the ratio of Na_2HPO_4 to NaH_2PO_4 increases to 1 : 4. As a result of the change in the ratio, the urinary pH decreases sharply. The lowest pH of urine achieved by human kidney is approximately 4.5, i.e. H^+ concentration of urine is approximately 1000 times the concentration of H^+ in the plasma. The secretion of H^+ is accompanied by generation of HCO_3^- which diffuses into the circulation and replenishes the HCO_3^- buffer of the blood (Fig. 57.19B).

Titrable acidity of the urine is equal to the amount of N/10 NaOH that must be added to the urine to raise its pH to 7.4 (i.e. pH of the plasma). The amount of NaH_2PO_4 present in the urine determines the titrable acidity of the urine.

It may be repeated that although nearly 4,000 mEq of H^+ are secreted into the PCT, the pH of the fluid does not change because almost all the H^+ secreted into the PCT leads to reabsorption of filtered bicarbonate only.

(b) Role of Ammonia Secretion

Ammonia (NH_3) and ammonium ion (NH_4^+) constitute another important buffer system in the tubular fluid. Ammonia can be synthesized by all segments of the nephron except the thin descending limb of loop of Henle. Ammonia diffuses into the tubular lumen and immediately binds with H^+ to form ammonium (NH_4^+), a non-diffusible ion.

$$NH_3 + H^+ \longrightarrow NH_4^+$$

Ammonium is excreted in the urine mostly as NH_4Cl. One HCO_3 generated for each H^+ secreted enters the circulation (Fig. 57.19C). The mechanism of production of ammonia from the amino acid glutamine is given below :

$$\text{Glutamine} \xrightarrow[\text{Glutaminase}]{NH_3} \text{Glutamic acid} \xrightarrow[\text{Glutamic acid dehydrogenase}]{} \alpha\text{-Keto glutaric acid} + NH_3$$

About 60% of the NH_3 is derived from glutamine while the remaining 40% is derived from the deamination of the amino acids glycine and alanine.

The ammonium content of urine is negligible until the urinary pH falls below 6. Below this urinary pH, the ammonium secretion increases linearly with the fall in pH. Therefore, under normal circumstances ammonia secretion mainly occurs in the DCT and collecting ducts. But as mentioned above, PCT and ascending limb of loop of Henle are also capable of synthesizing NH_3.

The importance of NH_3 as a urinary buffer lies in the fact that, unlike phosphate buffer, the capacity of ammonia buffer is not limited by the amount filtered in glomerular filtrate. In states of chronic acidosis (diabetic ketoacidosis, respiratory acidosis), the amount of H^+ excreted as NH_4^+ may increase by 10-fold, as compared to 5-fold increase in excretion with phosphate buffer.

Since the pK value of this buffer system is 9, H^+ captured as NH_4 does not contribute to the titrable acidity of the urine. *The total H^+ excretion by the kidney equals the amount of titrable acidity plus the urinary NH_3 excretion.*

Factors Regulating Urinary Acid Secretion

Arterial pH

The changes in arterial pH produce corresponding changes in the intracellular pH of all the tissues including the renal epithelial cells. Renal H^+ secretion is increased by acidosis and decreased by alkalosis. Renal adaptations to changes in the arterial pH take 4–5 days to develop fully. Since, renal H^+ secretion is mediated through hydration of CO_2 which can diffuse freely through the cell membranes, urinary H^+ secretion is more sensitive to pH alterations caused by changes in pCO_2 (respiratory acidosis/alkalosis) than caused by changes in HCO_3^- (metabolic acidosis or alkalosis) (Henderson-Hasselbach equation). This fact can be experimentally proved; if pCO_2 is elevated whereas arterial pH is kept constant, or even elevated, urinary secretion of H^+ is found to be increased.

Plasma K^+ Concentration

K^+ and H^+ have reciprocal relationship in the maintenance of intracellular neutrality. Consequently, K^+ depletion enhances urinary H^+ excretion, whereas hyperkalaemia decreases urinary H^+ excretion. The effects of changes in plasma K^+ concentration are produced through changes in the rate of aldosterone secretion.

Aldosterone and Adrenal Glucocorticoids

Aldosterone, the chief mineralocorticoid, increases Na^+ reabsorption and thereby increases secretion of H^+ or K^+ through Na^+-H^+ antiport or Na^+-K^+ antiport system.

At high plasma concentrations of glucocorticoids (e.g. when administered in pharmacological doses for treatment of certain diseases or in Cushing's syndrome), increased urinary excretion of H^+ may lead to metabolic alkalosis.

Carbonic Anhydrase

Certain diuretics (acetazolamide) inhibit the activity of carbonic anhydrase. As a result, urinary H^+ secretion is markedly decreased and urinary HCO_3^- excretion is elevated.

Renal Tubular Acidosis (RTA)

This name is given to a group of congenital or acquired renal disorders characterized by *inadequate H^+ secretion in the face of normal or adequate GFR*. Two well, known types of RTA are briefly described below.

1. Distal (Type I) RTA In this disorder, collecting ducts of the kidney cannot produce adequate H^+ gradient. Consequent decrease in H^+ excretion leads to: (a) failure to lower the urinary pH adequately, and (b) decreased renal production of HCO_3^-. The fall in plasma HCO_3^- leads to metabolic acidosis.

2. Proximal (Type II) RTA In this disorder, the proximal renal tubules have a reduced capacity of HCO_3^- reabsorption leading to a reduction in plasma HCO_3^- and hence metabolic acidosis.

In both types of RTA, since bicarbonate reabsorption is decreased, Na^+ reabsorption in the renal tubules is accompanied by excessive chloride reabsorption. Hence in both types, plasma Cl^- level is elevated, i.e. **both types of RTA result in hyperchloremic metabolic acidosis.**

CHLORIDE TRANSPORT

Chloride is the chief anion to accompany Na^+ through the renal tubular epithelium. Hence, its reabsorption varies with reabsorption of Na^+. Some Cl^- is also excreted with ammonia.

57

There is a reciprocal relationship between HCO_3^- reabsorption and Cl^- reabsorption. Hence, when HCO_3^- reabsorbed is decreased, e.g. in alkalosis, Cl^- reabsorption is increased.

Chloride is actively reabsorbed in the *thick ascending segment of the loop of Henle* and Na^+ follows Cl^- passively (Fig. 57.13C). In other segments of the nephron, Cl^- reabsorption is a passive process.

UREA TRANSPORT

About 50% of the filtered urea is reabsorbed passively in the tubules. Most of the reabsorption occurs in the PCT due to the concentration gradient created by reabsorption of water. The rest of urea reabsorption occurs passively in the collecting ducts following reabsorption of water.

Urates, sulphates, phosphates and **nitrates** are only partly reabsorbed in the tubules. Their urinary concentration is larger than their concentration in the plasma.

URINE

Normal Urine

The rate of formation of urine and its composition are subjected to diurnal variations, as well as, influenced by diet, muscular activity on even emotions. Therefore, it is better to analyze a 24-hour urine sample than a random or short time collection.

Volume Average 24-hour urinary volume is 1.5 litres (normal range: 0.6–2.5 L). Physiologically, urinary volume varies with the intake of fluids (water, tea, coffee, alcohol, etc.), on one hand, and non-renal losses of fluid (sweating, etc.) on the other. Normally, nocturnal urine is more concentrated and hence smaller in volume than urine passed in day time. (say 10 PM to 6 AM versus 10 AM to 6 PM collection). In diabetes mellitus, and in early stages of renal failure, there is a failure of nocturnal urinary concentration. **Oliguria (less than 500 ml urinary excretion per day), and anuria** may be due to *severe renal failure* or more commonly due *to extrarenal uraemia*, (in severe dehydration, haemorrhage and shock).

Colour The light yellow colour of normal urine is due to the presence of urochrome pigment (a compound of urobilin and urobilinogen with a peptide). On standing, the colour deepens due to oxidation of urobilinogen to urobilin. In hepatic and post-hepatic types of jaundice, urine is brownish yellow in colour due to the presence of conjugated biliruin.

Osmolality (specific gravity) Normal urinary osmolality may vary from 50 to 1200 mOsm/kg

(Sp. gr. 1.003 to 1.040), depending on the state of hydration of the body. *Fixed urinary osmolality* of 300 mOsm/kg (Sp. gr. 1.010) is an evidence of fairly advanced renal failure. It indicates failure of both urinary concentration and dilution mechanisms.

Ordinarily, estimation of urinary specific gravity (by using a cheap urinometer) is sufficient. However, fallaciously high specific gravity is recorded if the urine contains large amount of glucose or albumin. In such cases, accurate results are obtained by estimation of urinary osmolality. Persistently low urinary osmolality (less than 100 mOsm/kg) even after 8 hours of fluid deprivation is diagnostic of *diabetes insipidus*.

pH Urinary pH normally varies from 4.5 to 8. Except for a short post-prandial alkaline tide, urinary pH remains acidic for most of the day.

Intake of high protein diet shifts the urinary pH towards the lower side of normal range, whereas vegetarian food shifts it towards alkaline side. In certain congenital renal tubular disorders, there is failure of urinary acidification.

The inorganic and organic constituents of normal urine are given in Table 57.4.

Microscopic examination of a contrifuged sediment of normal urine often reveals crystals of calcium oxalate, calcium phosphate, calcium-ammonium-magnesium phosphate (triple phosphate) or uric acid (Fig. 57.20).

Table 57.4: Composition of normal urine

Constituent	*Total excreted in 24 h urine*
Water	1.5 L
Na^+	5 g
Cl^-	9 g
K^+	2.2 g
PO_4^{2-}	1.2 g
HCO_3^-	0.1 g
Ca^{2+}	0.2 g
SO_4^{2-}	2.7 g
Mg^{2+}	0.1 g
Urea	30 g
Uric acid	0.8 g
Creatinine	1.5 g
Oxalate	20 mg

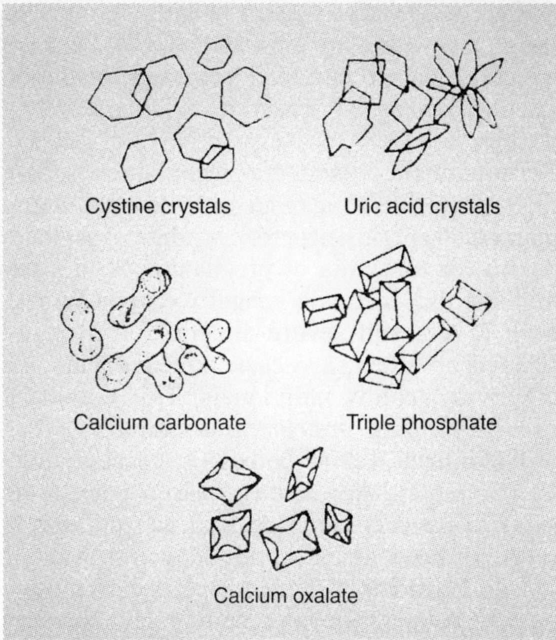

Fig. 57.20: Various types of crystals found in normal urine.

Abnormal Constituents of Urine

In patients with certain renal or non-renal (metabolic) disorders, the urine may contain some abnormal constituents like glucose (glycosuria), proteins, chiefly albumin (proteinuria or albuminuria), bile pigments, ketone bodies (ketonuria), or blood (haematuria). Such abnormal constituents can be detected by chemical analysis of the urine. Microscopic examination of the contrifuged sediment of urine may reveal red blood cells, pus cells, or casts.

Glycosuria This term is used to indicate the presence of a reducing sugar in the urine. In clinical practice, it practically means glucosuria, because other sugars (fructose, galactose, or lactose) are rarely present in the urine. Diabetes mellitus is the most frequent cause of glycosuria. In this disorder, glucose appears in the urine when the blood glucose level exceeds the renal threshold for glucose (180 mg%). In some patients with congenital renal tubular defects, glucose may appear in the urine at relatively normal blood glucose levels. Such a disorder, known as renal glycosuria, is due to decreased renal threshold (TmG) for glucose.

Glycosuria also occurs in later months of pregnancy (due to increased GFR), severe hyperthyroidism, and after general anaesthesia. Lactosuria may be observed in some lactating women.

Proteinuria Proteinuria (albuminuria) is more frequently due to a renal disorder like acute glomerulonephritis, nephrotic syndrome, pyelonephritis, or toxaemia of pregnancy. Mild albuminuria also occurs in congestive heart failure, high fevers and severe anaemia. Prolonged standing or walking may cause proteinuria in some otherwise healthy individuals. This condition called *orthostatic proteinuria* is harmless.

Ketonuria Ketone bodies (acetoacetic acid, hydroxybutyric acid, and acetone) appear in the urine in patients suffering from ketosis due to severe diabetes mellitus or prolonged starvation.

Bile Pigments Bilirubin appears in the urine in patients with elevated conjugated bilirubin levels, i.e. in hepatic or post-hepatic jaundice. Excessive urinary excretion of urobilinogen is one of the characteristic features of haemolytic jaundice.

Haemoglobinuria and Haematuria Haemoglobin may be present in the urine in patients suffering from intravascular haemolysis, or due to haemolysis of red blood cells when present in hypotonic urine. Haemoglobin imparts reddish brown colour to the urine. Haematuria is seen in acute glomerulonephritis, renal stone disease and in malignancy of the urinary tract. Gross haematuria imparts red colour to the urine.

Amino Aciduria Amino aciduria is seen in a variety of congenital renal tubular disorders.

Casts Casts are formed by coagulation of proteins in the renal tubules. Hence they have cylindrical shapes. Red blood cells, white blood cells and desquamated tubular epithelial cells often adhere to the casts; such casts are called red cells casts, leucocyte casts, and epithelial casts, respectively.

PATHOPHYSIOLOGY OF RENAL DISORDERS

Renal Failure

Renal failure or *renal insufficiency* may be a result of acute or chronic inflammatory process chiefly involving the glomeruli (acute or chronic glomerulonephritis). When approximately 75% of the nephrons are damaged, the excretion of waste products like urea, uric acid, creatinine, phosphates, H^+ and K^+ are affected to an extent that their concentrations in the blood begin to rise. At this stage of the renal disease, **uraemia** is said to have set in. The most characteristic features of uraemia are:

1. Accumulation of nitrogenous waste products (urea, creatinine,uric acid, etc.) in the blood.
2. Metabolic acidosis (due to failure of H^+ excretion).
3. Hyperkalaemia (due to failure of K^+ excretion).
4. Anaemia (deficiency of erythropoietin).
5. Uraemic coma: It is the terminal event in chronic renal disorders. It has been attributed chiefly to acidosis and hyperkalaemia. Accumulation of nitrogenous waste products contribute relatively less to the loss of consciousness in uraemic coma.

Haemodialysis of the uraemic patient can keep him alive for months or even years. Haemodialysis can be a life-saving measure in many types of acute renal failure produced by reversible pathological processes. During haemodialysis, the patient's radial artery is connected to a long and coiled cellophane tube immersed in a dialyzing fluid. The chemical composition of dialyzing fluid is similar to that of plasma except that it is free of the waste products like urea, uric acid, etc. (Table 57.5).

The patient's blood passes through the dialyzing system and returns to a peripheral vein. The semipermeable cellophane membrane permits free diffusion of all the constituents of plasma except proteins. In this way, the dialysis of patient's blood removes the toxic waste products and restores normal electrolyte concentration in the plasma. The dialyzing system is also known as the artificial kidney (Fig. 57.21).

The haemodialysis is an expensive procedure and needs to be repeated almost every week. Therefore, it cannot be regarded as a remedy for irreversible renal failure caused by chronic renal diseases. With the recent advances in medical

Table 57.5: Composition of dialyzing fluid as compared to that of a typical uraemic plasma

	Uraemic plasma	*Dialysate*
Electrolyte (mEq/L)		
Na^+	142	142
K^+	7	4
Ca^{++}	2	3
Mg^{++}	1.5	1.5
Cl^-	107	107
HCO_3^-	14	27
Lactate	1.2	1.2
HPO_4^{2-}	9	0
Urate	2	0
SO_4^{2-}	3	0
Non-electrolyte (mg/%)		
Glucose	100	125
Urea	200	0
Creatinine	6	0

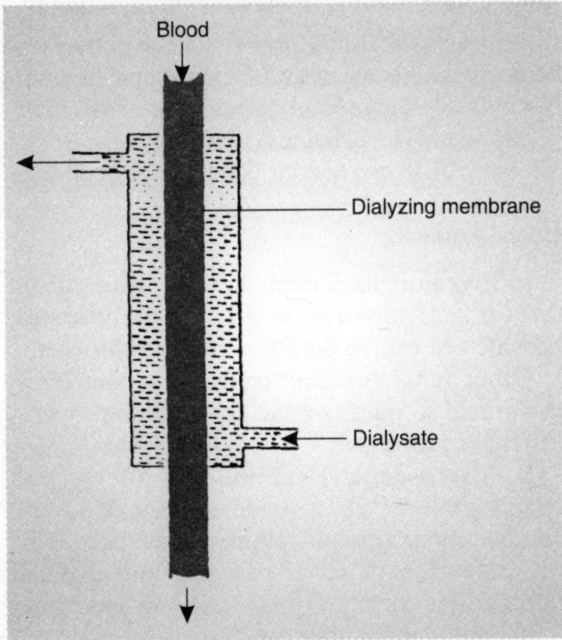

Fig. 57.21: Basic principle of artificial kidney.

technology, such patients are treated by renal transplantation.

In another type of renal disease, called pyelonephritis, the infective organisms invade chiefly the renal medulla, and only in the later stages of the disease the renal cortex is damaged. Therefore, in the early stages, tubular function is relatively more affected. But ultimately, glomerular insufficiency supervenes.

Congenital renal tubular disorders are characterized by evidence of impaired tubular function with relatively intact glomerular function. Glycosuria, aminoaciduria, phosphaturia and renal tubular acidosis may be present together or as isolated renal defects.

Renal Stones

Normal urine is supersaturated with respect to many inorganic and organic constituents. This is shown by common occurrence of crystals of calcium oxalate, phosphates and uric acid in the urine of normal individuals (Fig. 57.20). These crystals normally do not grow in size or become aggregated since the urine contains certain glycoproteins known as *crystal growth inhibitor*. Due to a variety of reasons like excessive urinary concentration (e.g. during dehydration), excessive excretion of calcium or uric acid or gross changes in urinary pH, solid masses of calcium oxalate, calcium phosphate or uric acid may be formed in the urinary tract (renal pelvis, ureter or urinary bladder). These masses called renal stones (Fig. 57.22) may grow into a large size and cause attacks of severe pain (renal colic) accompanied by haematuria. Infection or obstruction of the urinary tract may also occur.

KIDNEY FUNCTION TESTS

A number of tests are available for the assessment of different renal functions.

Test of Glomerular Function

Endogenous Creatinine Clearance Test

Estimation of 24-hour or 4-hour creatinine clearance is the most convenient method for clinical assessment of glomerular filtration rate. A 24-hour (or 4-hour), accurately timed, urine sample is collected and a blood sample is taken at

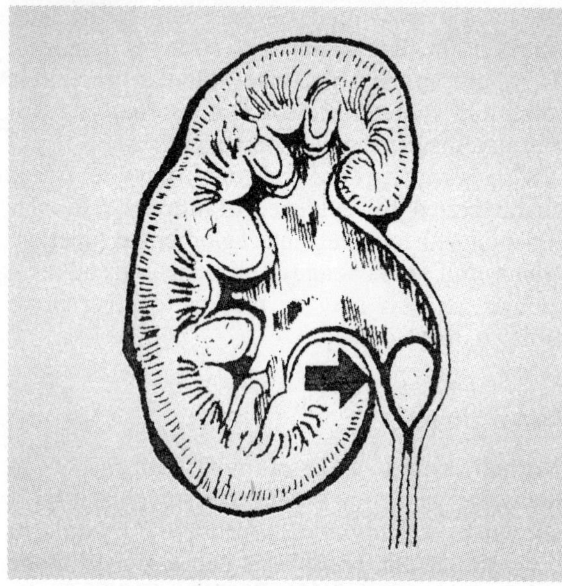

Fig. 57.22: Renal stone.

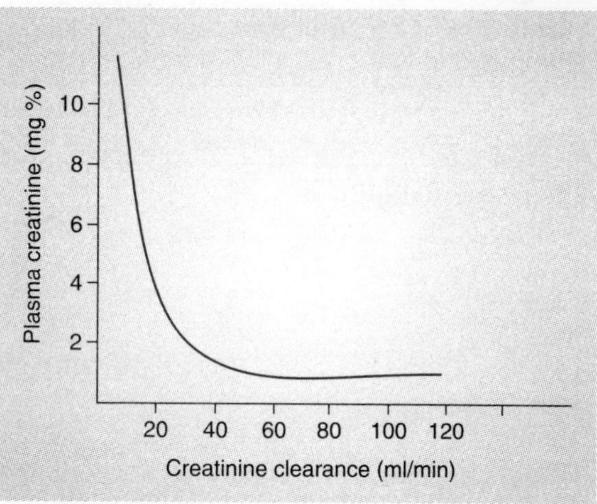

Fig. 57.23: Relation between plasma creatinine level and creatinine clearance.

midpoint of the urinary collection period. The concentration of creatinine in plasma and urine samples is estimated. The creatinine clearance is calculated by the usual formula (U × V/P).

$$\text{Creatinine clearance (ml/min)} = \frac{\text{Urinary creatinine concentration} \times \text{Urinary volume (ml/min)}}{\text{Plasma creatinine concentration}}$$

The normal range of creatinine clearance is 97 to 137 ml/min in males and 88 to 128 ml/min in females.

For the estimation of GFR, estimation of inulin clearance is far more accurate method than estimation of creatinine clearance. However, continuous infusion of inulin is required for the estimation of inulin clearance. The inconvenience of the procedure precludes its use in the clinical setting. Inulin clearance is estimated for research purposes only.

57

Plasma Creatinine Concentration

Normal plasma creatinine concentration is 0.2–1.4 mg%. In progressive renal disease, plasma creatinine concentration begins to rise after more than 50% glomerular function has been lost (Fig. 57.23). In other words, elevation of plasma creatinine level indicates fairly advanced glomerular insufficiency.

Blood Urea

Like plasma creatinine, blood urea level may also be estimated as an index of glomerular function. Normal blood urea level ranges from 15–40 mg%.

Blood urea level begins to rise only after approximately 50% glomerular damage has occurred.

Urine Analysis

a. Proteinuria Examination of urine for the presence of albumin is an extremely simple bedside test for the detection of renal disorder.

Other renal function tests are subsequently performed to diagnose the type and the severity of renal dysfunction.

b. Microscopic Examination Microscopic examination of centrifuged urinary deposit is another component of routine urine analysis for the detection of renal parenchymal disease. Glomerular damage often leads to leakage of RBCs and WBCs from the glomeruli.

Test for Tubular Function

A large number of reabsorptive and secretory functions are performed by the renal tubules, some of which can be easily tested.

Urinary Concentration Test

This test is performed by estimation of urinary specific gravity after 12 hours of water deprivation. In very hot weather, the period of water deprivation may be reduced to 8 hours only because of the risk of dehydration. To avoid this risk, urinary specific gravity may be measured 12 hours after injection of vasopressin. In either case, urinary specific gravity below 1.020 indicates inability of the kidney to concentrate the urine.

Urinary Dilution Test

The patient is asked to drink 1 litre of water and subsequently four 1 hour urine samples are collected. Normally, the patient can excrete at least 75% of the volume ingested within 4 hours and at least one of the urine samples has a specific gravity below 1.004.

Urinary Acidification Test

This test is used for assessing the ability of the tubules to excrete the acid (H^+). Ammonium chloride (NH_4Cl) in the dose of 0.1 g/kg BW is administered orally. Six hours later, the urinary pH should fall below 5.3. In renal tubular acidosis, urinary pH remains above 5.3.

The principle behind the test is that in the liver NH_4Cl yields NH_3 and HCl.

$$NH_4Cl \longrightarrow NH_3 + HCl$$

NH_3 is metabolised to urea whereas HCl is excreted by the kidney leading to a fall in urinary pH.

Glycosuria

Glycosuria occurring at relatively normal blood glucose level is sufficient evidence for defective renal tubular reabsorption of glucose. TmG need not be determined for clinical assessment of renal tubular function.

Intravenous Pyelography

This investigation provides information about the size, shape and position of the kidney, as well as, the size and the configuration of pelvicalyceal system. A radio-opaque dye like urographin is injected intravenously and radiograms (X-ray pictures) of the abdomen are taken at short intervals (at 1, 5, 10 and 30 minutes) after injection of the dye. The dye is filtered into the Bowman's capsules and concentrated by the tubules. The concentrated dye casts a radio-opaque shadow in the renal pelvis, ureters and urinary bladder. Calcium-containing renal stones (calculi) can be detected by plain X-ray of the abdomen. Translucent renal stones (e.g. pure uric acid stones) can be detected by intravenous pyelography as filling defects.

Indications

(i) **Detection of renal stones** is the commonest indication for IVP (Fig. 57.24).

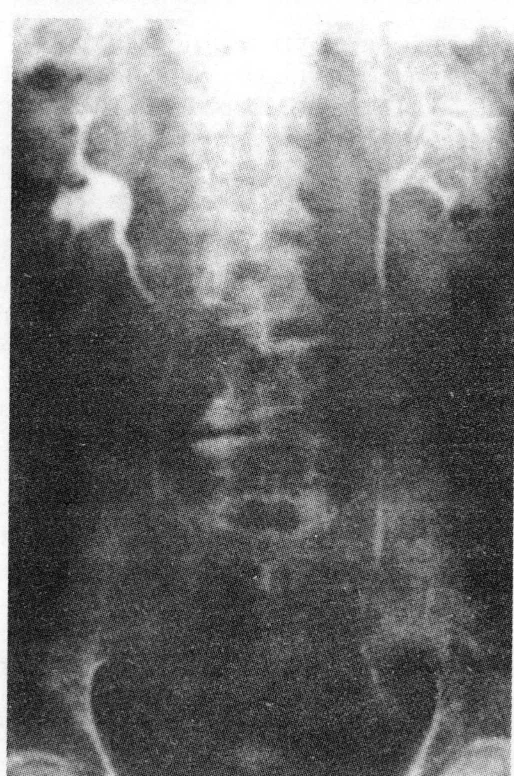

Fig. 57.24: Intravenous pyelogram.

(ii) Intravenous pyelography is also an important investigation for the detection of **developmental abnormalities of the kidney**, e.g. horseshoe-shaped kidney.

CHAPTER 58 Physiology of Micturition

The formation of urine in the kidney is a continuous process. It is carried by the ureters to the urinary bladder where it is stored. The bladder is evacuated at intervals of several hours.

Structure of Urinary Bladder

Smooth muscle of the urinary bladder, called the **detrusor muscle**, is arranged in interlacing longitudinal, circular and spiral bundles. When full of urine, two portions of the bladder can be identified, i.e. the body containing the urine and a funnel-shaped neck, as an extension of the body. The neck continues as the posterior urethra (Fig. 58.1). The **smooth muscle of the neck constitutes the internal sphincter** of the bladder. Natural tone of the internal sphincter muscle normally keeps the bladder neck closed, preventing any passage of urine into the urethra.

As the urethra passes through the urogenital diaphragm, it is encircled by a **ring of voluntary muscle** called the **external sphincter** of the bladder. External sphincter provides voluntary control over micturition.

The terminal 1–2 cm portion of the ureters passes obliquely through the detrusor muscle before opening into the lumen of the urinary bladder. The oblique passage acts as a valve and prevents reflux of urine into the ureters when the bladder pressure rises.

Innervation

Parasympathetic Innervation

(i) The **pelvic nerves** contain parasympathetic efferents from S_2 and S_3 spinal segments. These fibres carry motor impulses to the urinary bladder which cause contraction of detrusor muscle and emptying of urinary bladder. Pelvic nerves also carry **sensory fibres** from the bladder to S_2 and S_3 spinal segments.

(ii) Sympathetic Innervation The sympathetic supply to the urinary bladder arises from $L_{1,2}$ spinal segments. These nerves have a weak inhibitory action on the detrusor muscle, and cause contraction of internal sphincter.

(iii) Somatic Innervation The external sphincter of the bladder is innervated by somatic efferent fibres from $S_{2,3}$ spinal segments through the pudendal nerve.

Filling of Urinary Bladder

Fairly large volume of urine accumulates in the urinary bladder without any significant increase in the intravesical pressure. This is because of the property of plasticity of the smooth muscle, as well as, the law of Laplace. The relation between the intravesical pressure and volume can be studied experimentally by cystometry. The bladder is catheterized and connected to a T-tube. One limb

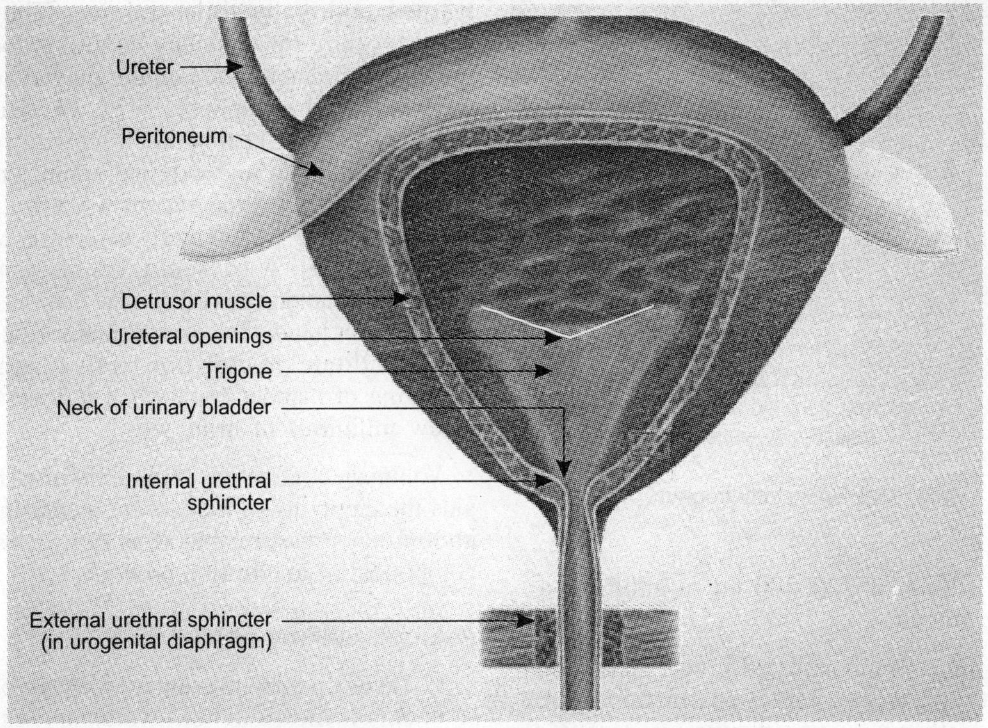

Fig. 58.1: The structure of lower urinary tract.

of T-tube is connected to a bottle of normal saline and the other limb to the pressure transducer of a polygraph (Fig. 58.2). The bladder is filled with 50 ml increments of saline and at each volume, the intravesical pressure is recorded. The record

Urinary bladder

Saline

To pressure transducer

Fig. 58.2: Procedure to demonstrate pressure-volume relationship in the urinary bladder.

is called **cystometrogram.** When the bladder is empty, the pressure is practically zero. Addition of 50 ml of water raises the pressure to only 10 cm H_2O. Additional filling of 200–300 ml of saline does not produce any significant increase in the intravesical pressure. Beyond 400 ml volume, the pressure begins to rise markedly, triggering the micturition reflex (Fig. 58.3).

Under natural circumstances, the first urge to empty the bladder occurs at approximately 150 ml of the urinary volume but it can be easily suppressed.

Beyond 600 ml, the urge to void urine becomes almost unbearable.

Emptying of Urinary Bladder

Micturition Reflex

Spinal Reflex Micturition is basically a reflex action. It is initiated by stimulation of the stretch receptors situated in the wall of the urinary bladder.

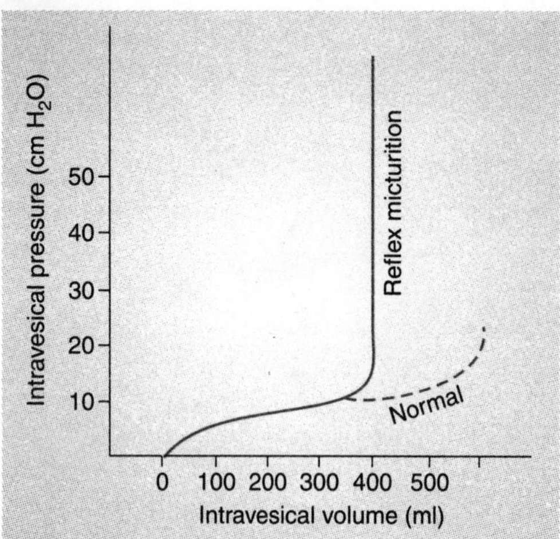

Fig. 58.3: A cystometrogram.

Bladder filling of 300–400 ml in adults is an adequate stimulus.

Once the reflex is initiated it becomes a self-regenerating process. Initial contraction of the bladder further activates the stretch receptors causing stronger reflex contraction and a marked rise of intravesical pressure which opens the bladder neck. The external sphincter is reflexly inhibited and thus the urine escapes through the urethra. The integration centre of the micturition reflex lies in $S_{2,3}$ spinal segments. The pelvic nerves contain both the sensory and the motor (parasympathetic) fibres of the reflex arc.

Role of Pontine Micturition Centre Although, basically a spinal reflex, micturition reflex is influenced by both the inhibitory and the facilitatory impulses from centres situated in the brainstem. The higher influences can alter the threshold of micturition reflex, i.e. the bladder volume which initiates the reflex. Pontine micturition centre is a modulator centre for micturition. It coordinates contraction of detrusor by parasympathetic discharge, and relaxation of internal sphincter by inhibition of sympathetic discharge.

Voluntary Control In infants and young children, micturition is purely a reflex action. The voluntary control is gradually acquired as a learned ability by toilet-training. The higher cortical centre for voluntary control is located at the top of the motor area on the medial aspect of the cerebral hemispheres. The **cortical micturition centre** keeps the micturition reflex partially inhibited and external sphincter tightly contracted all the time except when micturition is desired. The higher cortical centre can also inhibit micturition by strong contraction of the external sphincter, even after urine flow has begun. On the other hand, the cortical micturition centres may facilitate micturition reflex and cause emptying of bladder even when it contains only a few millilitres of urine.

Voluntary contraction of the abdominal muscles aids the emptying of bladder by increasing intra-abdominal pressure, but it is not an essential component of micturition process.

Pathophysiology of Micturition

- **Incontinence** involuntary leakage of urine.
- **Stress incontinence** involuntary leakage of urine on exertion, coughing, sneezing, laughing—an act which raises intra-

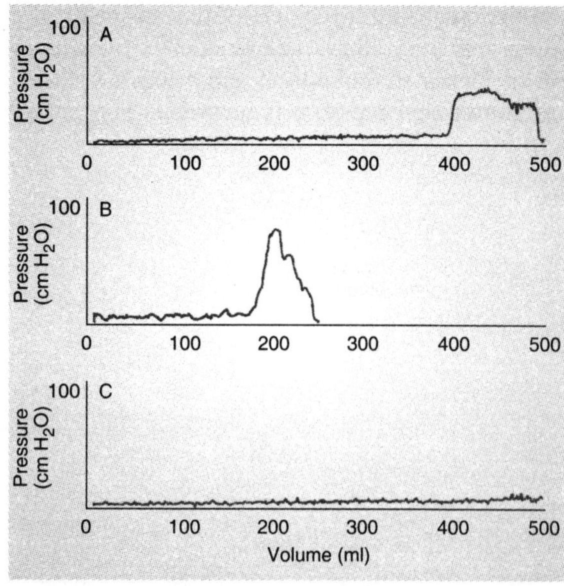

Fig. 58.4: Cystometrogram. (A) normal, (B) a patient with urge incontinence, and (C) a patient with overflow incontinence.

58

abdominal pressure. The problem is due to poor tone of external sphincter.

Urge incontinence leakage of urine whenever urge to pass urine arises (Fig. 58.4B).The problem lies in the lack of cortical or pontine control over micturition. Common causes include *cerebral stroke, brain tumor and Parkinson disease or spinal cord injuries above the sacral segments.*

Overflow incontinence Urinary bladder overfills and overflows because of a loss of sensations in the bladder. The patient has no sensation of bladder fullness. Bladder overfills but does not contract even when it overflows (Fig. 58.4C). Causes include *diabetic autonomic neuropathy, tabes dorsalis, spinal cord tumor, herniated disc, spina bifida and traumatic injury at sacral segments.*

CHAPTER 59 Regulation of Extracellular Fluid Composition and Blood Volume

Sodium chloride is the most abundant solute in the ECF. Since, chloride exchange is mostly secondary to sodium exchange, the regulation of extracellular volume is mediated mostly through regulation of sodium balance in the body. In addition, ECF volume is partly maintained by regulation of water balance.

EFFECTIVE CIRCULATING VOLUME (ECV)

Extra-cellular fluid (14 L) is distributed between interstitial compartment (10.5 L) and vascular compartment (3.5 L). Sensors for the regulation of extracellular fluid volume, however, are located entirely within the vascular tree. Even here, it is not the actual plasma volume which is sensed. The volume sensory receptors sense what is called the effective circulating volume (ECV). Sensation of ECV is related to "fullness" or pressure within the vascular tree. In normal individuals, ECF volume and ECV vary in parallel. However in pathological conditions, they may not be related. For example, in congestive heart failure, ECV is reduced even though ECF volume is markedly increased. Kidneys regulate the excretion of NaCl in response to changes in ECV rather than in ECF volume.

ECV Sensors

Sensors of ECV act as baroreceptors. They respond to the degree of stretch of the vessel wall and not to the volume of the vessel. Effective circulating volume receptors can be divided into two categories: (*i*) low pressure volume receptors (*ii*) high pressure volume receptors. The two types of receptors are located on the venous side and the arterial side of the circulation respectively.

1. Low Pressure Volume Sensors

(a) Cardiac atria
(b) Pulmonary vessels

2. High Pressure Volume Sensors

(a) Carotid sinus baroreceptors
(b) Aortic arch baroreceptors
(c) Afferent arterioles of the kidney (Juxtaglomerular apparatus).

Low pressure volume sensors respond to fullness of the vascular tree. The afferent input reaches the brain via the vagus nerve and reflexly alters the sympathetic discharge and release of antidiuretic hormone (ADH) and atrial natriuretic peptide (ANP).

The sinoaortic baroreceptors respond to the arterial blood pressure and reflexly regulate the sympathetic discharge to the heart and resistance vessels including the renal arterioles. Renal afferent arterioles have a particular important role in the renal excretion of NaCl through renin-angiotensin mechanism.

Effector Mechanisms

Neural Regulation of Urinary NaCl Excretion

Sympathetic fibres innervate afferent as well as efferent arterioles of the kidney. When ECV is reduced, decreased discharge from the low pressure and high pressure volume receptors increases sympathetic discharge to the kidney which decreases urinary NaCl excretion by the following mechanisms.

(i) **Reduction of GFR** Reduced GFR leads to a decrease in the filtered load of sodium. However, changes in the filtered load of sodium are not reflected in parallel changes in the urinary sodium excretion because of the following reasons.

(a) **Glomerulotubular Balance** Any decrease in filtered load of Na^+ decreases reabsorption of Na^+ in the proximal tubule. In this way, the percentage of Na^+ reabsorbed in the proximal tubule is held constant. This phenomenon is called glomerulotubular balance (Fig. 59.1)

(b) **Tubuloglomerular Feedback** Signals from the renal tubules may affect GFR. Decreased filtered load of Na^+ decreases the concentration of Na^+ reaching the macula densa region of distal convoluted tubule (DCT). This results in an increase in GFR through prostaglandins.

(ii) **Stimulation of Renin Secretion** It results in increased plasma concentration of angiotensin II and aldosterone.

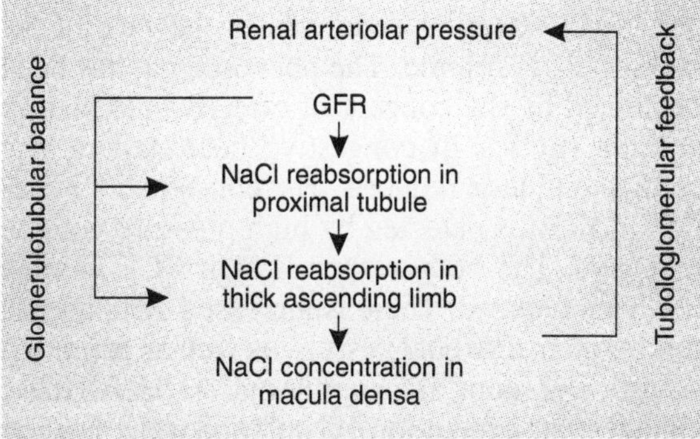

Fig. 59.1: Phenomenon of glomerulotubular balance and tubuloglomerular feedback.

Hormonal Regulation of Urinary NaCl Excretion

(i) **Renin-angiotensin II-aldosterone System** Renin secretion from the afferent arterioles of the kidney is increased by: (a) decreased perfusion pressure, (b) increased sympathetic discharge to the afferent arterioles, (c) decreased delivery of NaCl to the macula densa cells of DCT. Renin acts on the circulating angiotensinogen and ultimately results increased plasma concentration of angiotensin II and aldosterone. Aldosterone increases NaCl reabsorption from the DCT and collecting ducts of the kidney.

(ii) **Atrial Natriuretic Peptide (ANP)** Increased ECV causes release of ANP from the atrial myocytes. ANP increases urinary excretion of NaCl by a number of mechanisms (Ch. 51).

(iii) **Antidiuretic Hormone** In response to decreased ECV, secretion of ADH is increased, leading to retention of water by the kidneys. Conversely, increased ECV inhibits ADH secretion.

RESPONSE TO VARYING SALT INTAKES

A normal individual is able to maintain normal ECF volume and normal ECV over wide range of NaCl intake. This is possible because certain homeostatic mechanisms help to maintain salt balance of the body, i.e. daily urinary Na^+ excretion almost exactly matches the amount ingested. If the amount of salt intake is suddenly altered, the appropriate response of the kidneys occurs after 2-3 days. During the transitional period, the individual's salt balance may be positive (intake > excretion) or negative (excretion > intake) depending on whether the intake has suddenly increased or decreased. For example, if NaCl intake is suddenly increased (Fig. 59.2), the individual remains in positive balance during the first 2-3 days, i.e. the excretion does not match the enhanced intake and extra NaCl remains in the ECF. The consequent retention of water is shown by parallel increase in body weight. After a few days, the daily urinary excertion of NaCl matches the amount ingested. When the salt intake is abruptly decreased, the individual remains

59

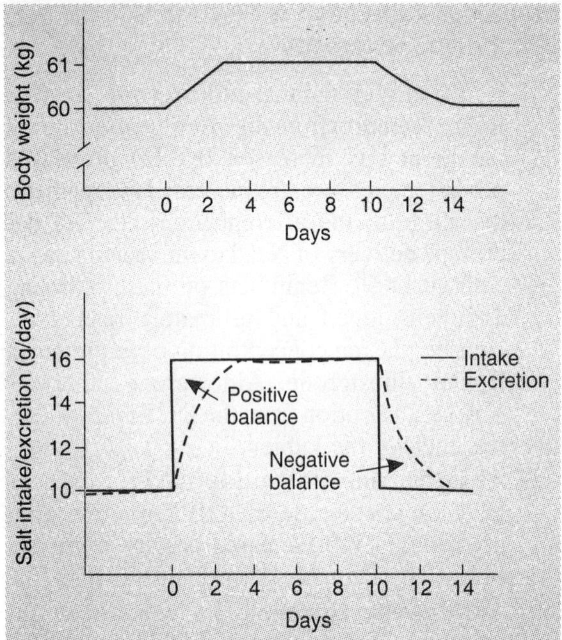

Fig. 59.2: Effect of sudden increase and decrease in dietary salt intake on the salt balance.

in a negative salt balance for a few days because NaCl excretion remains elevated. Consequent loss of water is shown by parallel loss of body weight. A few days later, urinary salt excretion falls to match the amount ingested.

Mechanism With moderate changes in salt intake, aldosterone is a main regulator of NaCl excretion. Small changes in ECF volume and hence in ECV are detected by low and high pressure volume receptors mentioned above. The consequent change in renin-angiotensin system is able to produce appropriate changes in aldosterone secretion. Aldosterone secretion has been shown to decrease with high salt intake and increase with low salt intake.

59

Very Large Increase in ECF Volume

Very large increase in ECF volume may occur due to excessive salt intake or excessive administration of intravenous saline. The change is detected by low- and high-pressure volume receptors. Urinary salt excretion is increased by the following mechanisms :

(a) Decreased discharge in renal sympathetic nerves.

(b) Increased ANP secretion from atrial myocytes.

(c) Decreased renin secretion leading to decreased plasma aldosterone levels.

(d) Inhibition of ADH release

Very Large Decrease in ECF Volume

Very large decrease in ECF volume may occur due to severe extrarenal losses of NaCl, e.g. due to heavy sweating or diarrhoea. The change is detected by low- and high-pressure volume receptors. The following mechanisms help to decrease the urinary NaCl excretion.

(a) Increased discharge in renal sympathetic nerves.

(b) Increased secretion of renin leading to increased plasma level of aldosterone.

(c) Stimulation of ADH secretion.

(d) Decreased ANP secretion from atrial myocytes

Pathophysiology

Congestive Heart Failure In certain pathological conditions like congestive heart failure, the normal regulatory mechanisms of NaCl excretion breakdown. As a result, urinary salt excretion remains less than salt intake. Consequent retention of NaCl and water leads to oedema. In this disorder, NaCl retention continues in the face of increased ECF volume. The phenomenon has been explained by the concept of effective circulating volume (ECV). In congestive heart failure, the cardiac output is reduced. The consequent reduction in ECV is detected by high pressure volume receptors. The body responds as if ECF volume has been reduced. There is increased sympathetic discharge in the renal vessels, as well as increased secretion of renin, aldosterone and ADH. All these changes cause retention of NaCl and water leading to expansion of interstitial body fluid volume (oedema).

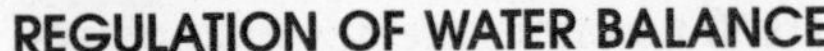

REGULATION OF WATER BALANCE

Water Input

Water is added to the body fluids mainly by ingestion of water and as content of the food. Water generated by oxidation of food stuffs also contributes to the water content of the body. Depending on the environmental conditions, ingestion of water may vary from 1–20 litres/day. A decrease in body water induces the sensation of thirst, promoting ingestion of water.

Water Output

Water is lost from the body by four routes, i.e. the skin, the faeces, urine and the respiratory tract. In the skin, water is lost as **insensible water loss** and **sweating (perspiration)**. The amount of water lost as sweat may vary from a negligible amount in winter to over 10 L/day in very hot weather (Table 59.1).

The regulation of output of water occurs only in the kidney. Urinary water loss is usually 1.5 L/day. But, it may vary from 0.5 L to over 20 L/day depending primarily on the ADH concentration in the plasma.

The regulation of both the input (thirst) and output (urinary excretion) of water is controlled by (i) plasma osmolality and (ii) blood volume.

PLASMA OSMOLALITY

Plasma osmolality is sensed by osmoreceptors located in the anterior hypothalamus. These receptors are stimulated by cellular dehydration which causes them to shrink. Cellular dehydration may occur because of:

(a) Deficiency of total body water.
(b) Excessive intake of NaCl which causes water to shift from intracellular compartment to extracellular compartment.

Even small increase in plasma osmolality increases thirst as well as increases the secretion of ADH.

Blood Volume

A decrease in blood volume also stimulates thirst, as well as, release of ADH from the posterior pituitary. Decreased blood volume is sensed by low pressure receptors in the atria and the pulmonary vessels. Under normal circumstances, the water balance of the body is mainly controlled by the osmoreceptors. Significant changes in the ADH secretion occur by less than 1% change in plasma osmolality. In contrast, more than 10% decrease in blood volume is required for stimulation of ADH-release. When there is a conflict between plasma osmolality and blood volume, the latter is maintained at the cost of plasma osmolality. If blood volume is markedly decreased, ADH release is stimulated even if plasma osmolality is low.

REGULATION OF HYDROGEN ION BALANCE

Under normal circumstances, tremendous amounts of hydrogen ions (H^+) are being continuously added to the body fluids. Carbon dioxide accounts for the addition of over 12,000 mEq H^+ per day. Non-volatile (fixed) acids account for another 60 mEq/day. Almost all the CO_2 is excreted by the lungs, whereas the kidney is responsible for the excretion of non-volatile acid products of protein metabolism. Lactic acid produced during severe

Table 59.1: Typical water balance in normal humans

Source	*Water intake ml/day* Obligatory	Elective	Source	*Water output ml/day* Obligatory	Elective
(i) Ingested water	400	1000–2000	(i) Urine	500	1000
(ii) Water content of food	850	—	(ii) Skin	500	0–1000
(iii) Water of oxidation	350	—	(iii) Respiratory tract	400	—
			(iv) Stools	200	—
Total	1600	1000–2000		1600	1000–2000

exercise or keto acids produced in severe diabetes are also excreted by the kidney.

Fruits are the main dietary source of the alkali. They contain sodium and potassium salts of weak organic acids, whose metabolism produces $NaHCO_3$ or $KHCO_3$ (and CO_2). Normally, the alkali content of the diet is very small and all the normal individuals excrete an acidic urine except for transient post-prandial alkaline tide.

Role of Respiration

In spite of addition of 12,000 mEq H^+ per day to the blood, the pH of arterial blood remains remarkably constant at 7.4. Similarly pCO_2 of the arterial blood is kept constant at 40 mmHg. This is made possible by two factors :

(i) In the venous blood, CO_2 is converted to H_2CO_3 and further to H^+ and HCO^-_3. Hydrogen ions are immediately buffered by the blood buffers, chiefly haemoglobin and plasma proteins.

(ii) As the venous blood passes through the lungs, CO_2 is regenerated by reversal of the reactions mentioned above and excreted very efficiently. The pulmonary ventilation is so delicately adjusted that it exactly matches the CO_2 produced is the body. Even during severe exercise, when CO_2 production increases 20 folds, CO_2 excretion is so efficient that arterial pCO_2 does not increase at all. Such a delicate control is made possible by the fact that ventilation is controlled by both CO_2 as well as H^+ concentration through central and peripheral chemoreceptors.

(a) **Effect of CO_2** CO_2 is a highly diffusible gas. It can easily cross the blood-brain-CSF barriers, and stimulate the medullary central chemoreceptors. In constrast, H^+ cannot cross these barriers easily. Therefore, central chemoreceptors are most sensitive to changes in arterial pCO_2 and less so to changes in H^+ concentration.

(b) **Effect of pH** An increase in H^+ concentration of arterial blood also stimulates pulmonary ventilation, chiefly through the peripheral (sino-aortic) chemoreceptors. Therefore, the respiratory system helps in regulation of acid-base balance of the body even when the increase in H^+ concentration is not due to CO_2 but due to non-volatile acids like sulphuric acid, phosphoric acid or lactic acid.

Role of Kidneys

As mentioned above, about 60 mEq of H^+ is added to the blood every day as non-volatile acids. They cannot be excreted by the lungs. They are excreted by the kidneys in an indirect manner. In the kidneys, most of the excretory products are initially filtered into the glomerular filtrate. All that is necessary for their excretion is that renal tubules reabsorb them partially or not all. In contrast, the concentration of H^+ in the blood is so small, that they cannot be excreted in this manner. Actually, most of the H^+ produced in the body do not remain as such. They are immediately buffered by HCO_3^- and other buffers. The kidney generates new hydrogen ions equivalent to the amount metabolically produced and actively secretes them into the urinary tubules, where they are buffered by phosphate and ammonium ions. The generation of H^+ in the renal tubules is accompanied by production of HCO_3^- which diffuses into the blood circulation and replenishes the amount of HCO_3^- lost during initial buffering of the acids.

In case excess of base ($NaHCO_3$) is ingested, it is excreted by the kidney by filtration followed by partial or complete non-reabsorption.

In primary pulmonary diseases like emphysema, pulmonary excretion of CO_2 is diminished and therefore arterial pCO_2 and H^+ concentration tend to rise (respiratory acidosis). In such circumstances, renal excretion of H^+ is the only means of maintaining body pH near normal (renal compensation). Similarly in chronic renal failure, renal excretion of H^+ is diminished leading to metabolic acidosis. In such a condition, excessive loss of CO_2 by hyperventilation is the only means of maintaining body pH near normal (respiratory compensation).

Some common types of disturbance in body pH along with renal and/or respiratory compensations for each type are described below.

Respiratory Acidosis

Respiratory acidosis is commonly due to hypoventilation produced by narcotic poisoning or a pulmonary disorder like emphysema. The primary event is increased arterial pCO_2.

$$\downarrow pH = pK + \log \frac{NaHCO_3}{pCO_2\downarrow} \quad \text{(Uncompensated respiratory acidosis)}$$

Renal Compensation Since CO_2 easily diffuses across the cell membrane, the increased pCO_2 causes increased intracellular pCO_2 in the renal tubules. The resulting increase in H^+ excretion not only eliminates more H^+ from the body but also generates more HCO_3^- which enters the circulation. Consequently, elevation of plasma HCO_3^- level restores the HCO_3^-/H_2CO_3 ratio to *near normal.* Thus, the acidosis is mostly but not completely compensated by the kidneys.

$$pH = pK + \log \frac{HCO_3\uparrow}{pCO_2\uparrow} \quad \text{(Compensated respiratory acidosis)}$$

Example: A fairly typical pattern of concentrations of electrolytes in a patient with chronic respiratory acidosis:

Na^+	137 mEq/L
K^+	4.5 mEq/L
HCO_3^-	40 mEq/L
Cl^-	90 mEq/L
pH	7.31
pCO_2	75 mmHg

Respiratory Alkalosis

It is produced by hyperventilation, e.g. due to high altitude hypoxia or some psychological disorder. The primary change is a decrease in the arterial pCO_2.

$$\uparrow pH = pK + \log \frac{HCO_3^-}{pCO_2\downarrow} \quad \text{(Uncompensated respiratory alkalosis)}$$

Renal Compensation

Decreased intracellular pCO_2 in the renal tubules decreases the renal secretion of H^+. Consequently, the new HCO_3^- is not generated. More importantly, even the filtered bicarbonate is not fully reabsorbed in the renal tubules. The resulting decrease in plasma HCO_3^- level restores the pH of blood to almost (but not completely) normal value.

$$pH = pK + \log \frac{HCO_3\downarrow}{pCO_2\downarrow} \quad \text{(Compensated respiratory alkalosis)}$$

Example: A fairly typical pattern of concentrations of electrolytes in the serum of a patient with acute respiratory alkalosis:

Na^+	135 mEq/L
K^+	3.2 mEq/L
HCO_3^-	19 mEq/L
Cl^-	105 mEq/L
pH	7.55
pCO_2	22 mmHg

Metabolic Acidosis

Uncontrolled diabetes mellitus (diabetic ketocidosis), hypovolemic and other forms of circulatory shock (lactacidosis), and renal failure are common causes of metabolic acidosis. The primary change in metabolic acidosis is a decrease in plasma HCO_3 level since it is used up in buffering excess of H^+.

$$\downarrow pH = pK + \log \frac{HCO_3\downarrow}{pCO_2} \quad \text{(Uncompensated metabolic acidosis)}$$

When metabolic acidosis is produced by nonrenal factors, respiratory and renal compensatory mechanisms tend to minimise the change in pH of blood. In renal failure, only respiratory compensation is possible.

Respiratory Compensation Hyperventilation produced by the action of increased H^+ on the peripheral chemoreceptors decrease the arterial pCO_2 value and minimises the degree of acidosis.

$$pH = pK + \log \frac{HCO_3\downarrow}{PCO_2\downarrow} \quad \text{(Compensated metabolic acidosis)}$$

Renal Compensation In metabolic acidosis, the renal excretion of H^+ is markedly increased, except when the acidosis is due to renal failure. There is tremendous increase in the urinary titrable acid and NH_3 excretion. Increased renal excretion of H^+ is accompanied by increase in generation of HCO_3^- which partially restores the depleted plasma HCO_3^- stores. Although the respiratory compensatory mechanism is very prompt and renal compensation is slow, the latter is far more effective compensatory mechanism. To some extent, the respiratory compensatory mechanism tends to inhibit the renal compensation by decreasing arterial pCO_2. However, intracellular acidosis is such a strong stimulus for renal H^+ secretion that the effect of decreased pCO_2 is practically ignored by the tubular cells.

Example: A fairly typical pattern of concentrations of electrolytes in the serum in a patient with diabetic acidosis and renal failure are given below.

Diabetic patient		*Uraemic patient*	
Na^+	125 mEq/L	Na^+	135 mEq/L
K^+	3.5 mEq/L	K^+	5.4 mEq/L
HCO_3^-	5 mEq/L	HCO_3^-	12 mEq/L
Cl^-	90 mEq/L	Cl^-	101 mEq/L
pH	7.01	pH	7.32
pCO_2	20 mmHg	pCO_2	24 mmHg

Hyperchloraemic Metabolic Acidosis The metabolic acidosis described above is caused by addition of an acid like lactic acid or a keto acid to the blood. The acid is buffered by bicarbonate resulting in a decrease in plasma HCO_3^- level. There is another type of metabolic acidosis in which the decrease in plasma HCO_3^- level is accompanied by an increase in plasma Cl^- and hence called hyperchloraemic metabolic acidosis. This type of acidosis may be caused by diarrhoea or renal tubular acidosis (RTA). In diarrhoea, HCO_3^- is lost from the gut in exchange for Cl^-. In RTA, failure of HCO_3^- reabsorption in kidney is accompanied by excessive reabsorption of Cl^-. A typical pattern of electrolyte concentration in the serum of a patient with RTA is given as follows.

Na^+	140 mEq/L
K^+	2.5 mEq/L
HCO_3^-	15 mEq/L
Cl^-	115 mEq/L
pH	7.30
pCO_2	30 mmHg

Anion Gap Concept Metabolic acidosis may be divided into two broad groups, namely, hyperchloraemic and normochloraemic metabolic acidosis. The two groups can be easily differentiated by calculation of anion gap.

In the plasma, the total cations (Na^+, K^+) are always counterbalanced by total anions (Cl^-, HCO_3^-, plasma proteins and other organic anions, PO_4^{2-}, SO_4^{2-}). Of these ions, only Na^+, K^+, Cl^- and HCO_3^- are routinely measured. Hence, total concentration of **measured anions** is found to be less than the total concentration of measured cations :

$$\text{Anion gap} = [Na^+ + K^+] - [Cl^- + HCO_3^-]$$

Example:

$$[140 + 4] - [100 + 28] = 16 \text{ mEq/L}$$

Since K^+ concentration does not vary grossly in clinical situations, the anion gap is usually calculated as follows :

$$\text{Anion gap} = Na^+ - [Cl^- + HCO_3^-]$$

When calculated in this way, the normal anion gap is 12 + 4 mEq/L. In metabolic acidosis due to ketoacidosis or lactacidosis, there is a decrease in plasma HCO_3^- without any significant change in plasma Cl^-. Hence, the anion gap becomes higher. Therefore, it is called high anion gap or normochloraemic metabolic acidosis. In diarrhoea or RTA, the fall in plasma bicarbonate is compensated by an increase in plasma Cl^-. Hence the anion gap remains normal. Therefore, it is known as hyperchloraemic (normal anion gap) metabolic acidosis (Fig. 59.3).

Metabolic Alkalosis

Metabolic alkalosis is commonly due to loss of acidic gastric juice, or ingestion of large amount of $NaHCO_3$ (as an antacid in patients with peptic

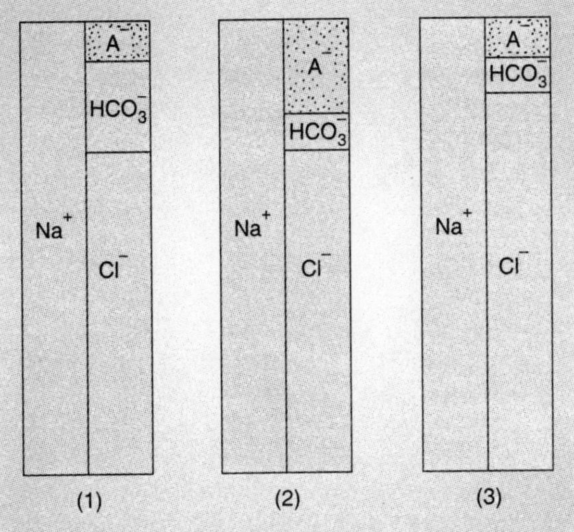

Fig. 59.3: Anion gap (A^-) in normal individuals (1); a patient with diabetic acidosis (high anion gap acidosis) (2); and a patient of RTA (hyperchloraemic, normal anion gap acidosis) (3).

ulcer). The primary change in the blood chemistry is an increase in the level of plasma HCO_3^-.

$$\uparrow pH = pK + \log \frac{HCO_3 \uparrow}{pCO_2} \quad \text{(Uncompensated metabolic alkalosis)}$$

Respiratory Compensation The alkalosis ($\uparrow$pH) inhibits the peripheral chemo-receptors, the resulting hypoventilation restores the blood pH to near normal by elevating arterial pCO_2 value.

$$pH = pK + \log \frac{HCO_3 \uparrow}{pCO_2 \uparrow} \quad \text{(Compensated metabolic alkalosis)}$$

However, the magnitude of respiratory compensation is limited by the fact that hypoventilation results in decreased arterial pO_2 which stimulates the respiratory centres via peripheral chemo-receptors.

Renal Compensation Metabolic alkalosis results in decreased H^+ secretion by the renal tubules. Therefore the filtered HCO_3^- is not completely reabsorbed. The urinary loss of HCO_3^- decreases level of plasma HCO_3^-, thereby restoring the pH of blood to near normal.

Metabolic alkalosis may be due to persistant vomiting which causes not only loss of acid but also fluids from the stomach. The resulting hypovolemia becomes a strong stimulus for Na^+ reabsorption by increased H^+ secretion (because of Na^+-H^+ antiport system). Thus, when metabolic alkalosis is accompanied by hypovolemia, the renal response tends to aggravate alkalosis rather than correct it.

Example: A fairly typical pattern of concentrations of electrolytes in the serum of patient with metabolic alkalosis due to vomiting is given below.

Na^+	140 mEq/L
K^+	3.2 mEq/L
HCO_3^-	42 mEq/L
Cl^-	84 mEq/L
pH	7.52
pCO_2	52 mmHg

Section XV

Physiology of Exercise and Sports

CHAPTER 60

Physiology of Exercise and Sports

In physiological terms, any activity involving muscular contraction is an exercise. So, it includes not only athletic sports but also routine daily activities like walking or lifting a bag of groceries, etc. Exercise not only involves neuromuscular coordination but also produces a considerable disturbance of internal environment. As result, almost all the body systems undergo readjustments. Study of exercise physiology gives an excellent scope to discuss the interplay of different organ systems in the maintenance of constant internal environment. Another reason for this detailed discussion lies in the growing awareness of the importance of physical fitness in the general population. A doctor would be required to guide a patient or even a healthy person in selecting the type of exercise suitable to his age and condition of health.

MUSCULAR PERFORMANCE

Basically, a muscle may undergo an isometric contraction and generate a force or it may undergo isotonic contraction and shorten to bring about a movement. Any type of manual work or athletic sport depends upon one or more of the following three characteristics of muscle contraction : (1) Strength, (2) Power, and (3) Endurance.

1. Strength It is measured as maximum contractile force in kilograms per cm^2 of cross-sectional area of the muscle. Maximum isometric strength can be measured by a dynamometer. Maximum isotonic strength can be measured by testing how heavy a barbell one can move through a complete range of elbow flexion. Strength of a muscle is determined by its size. World class weight lifters have muscle strength of 3.5 kg per cm^2 of muscle cross-sectional area. If the quadriceps have cross-section area of 150 cm^2, maximum contractile strength would be 525 kg.

Strength Sports Wrestling, weightlifting.

2. Power Power is the measure of total amount of work that muscle can perform in a given time. Power is determined not only by the strength of muscle contraction but also by the speed of contraction. It is measured in kilogram-meters (kg-m) per minute (or per second).

Power Sports Sprints, long jump, shot put, pole vault, football, hockey, tennis, table tennis, etc.

3. Endurance Endurance or staying capacity in physical work is limited not so much by muscle strength as by the capacity of the cardiopulmonary system to deliver oxygen and nutrition to the muscles and remove chemical waste products away from them. Aerobic endurance can be tested by measure of maximum oxygen uptake ($VO_{2\,max}$) in litres per minute. An individual is made to perform gradually increasing grades of physical work on a treadmill or a bicycle ergometer. At each work load, his oxygen consumption is estimated. The oxygen consumption increases to a limit and then a plateau is reached. The oxygen consumption at the plateau gives the value of $VO_{2\,max}$ (Fig. 60.1).

Endurance Sports Long distance running, long distance cycling, swimming, etc.

FAST AND SLOW MUSCLE FIBRES

Skeletal muscle are composed of two types of muscle fibres: (1) Red or slow muscle fibres; and (2) white or fast muscle fibres. Red muscle fibres are red because of higher myoglobin content. They also have longer (75 msec) twitch time. White muscle fibres have low myoglobin content and shorter (25 msec) twitch time. The two types of muscle fibres differ in many other histological and metabolic aspects (Table 60.1).

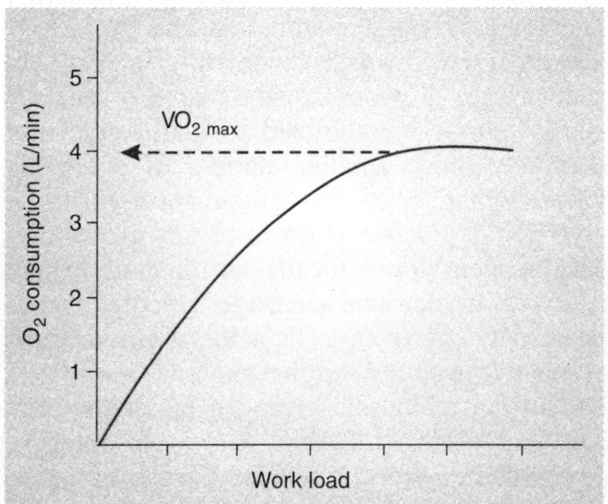

Fig. 60.1: Estimation of $VO_{2\,max}$.

Table 60.1: Some characteristics of fast and slow types of skeletal muscle fibres

Characteristics	*Slow type*	*Fast type*
Myoglobin content	High	Low
Colour	Red	White
Muscle fibre diameter	Smaller	Larger
Twitch time (msec)	75	25
Nerve activity	Continous, low frequency	Intermittent, high frequency
Glycogen content	Low	High
Mitochondrial density	High	Low
Capillary density	High	Low
Aerobic oxidative enzyme conc.	High	Low
Glycolytic enzyme conc.	Low	High
Myosin ATPase activity	Low	High
Fatty acid oxidative enzyme conc.	High	Low

Muscles involved in slow postural movements have higher percentage of slow muscle fibres, e.g. soleus. Muscles involved in fast phasic movements have higher percentage of fast muscle fibres, e.g.. gastrocnemius. The percentage of the two types of muscle fibres in a given muscle also varies in different types of athletic champions. Muscle biopsy has revealed higher percentage of slow type of fibres in long distance runners. Sprinters have higher percentage of fast type of muscle fibres. Due to the metabolic differences mentioned above, fast muscle fibres are more suited for short explosive bursts of contractions whereas slow types are more suited for subminimal work. The variation in the two types of muscle fibres is genetically determined. Thus, each athlete is genetically determined to be good in a particular kind of sport. Training can give further boost to the performance.

Myoglobin

The red colour of the muscle is due to the presence of a pigment myoglobin. Myoglobin is synthesized in the muscle fibre itself. It is present in higher concentration in red (slow) type of skeletal muscle fibres than in white (fast) type of fibres. Myoglobin differs from haemoglobin in many aspects:

(i) Myoglobin contains only one haem (iron-porphyrin) moiety per molecule whereas haemoglobin contains four haem moieties per molecule.
(ii) Molecular weight of myoglobin is 16,700 (i.e. 1/4th of haemoglobin).
(iii) The globin component of myoglobin has different amino acid residues as compared to haemoglobin.
(iv) Myoglobin has greater affinity for oxygen than haemoglobin. The myoglobin-oxygen dissociation curve is shifted far to the left than Hb-O_2 dissociation curve (Fig. 60.2). It has the shape of hyperbola as compared to sigmoid shape of Hb-O_2 curve.

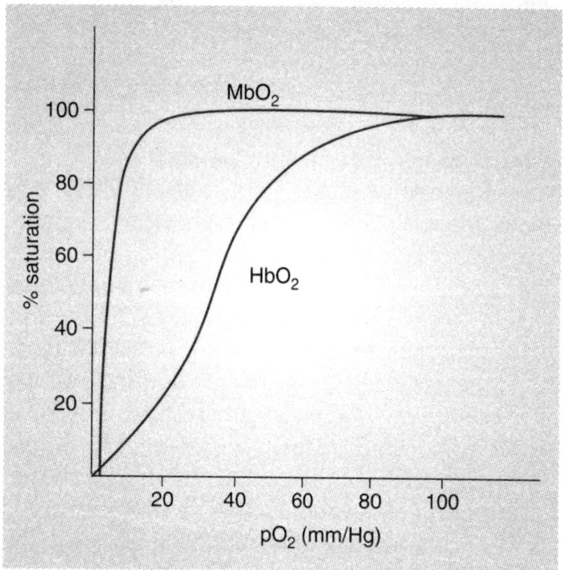

Fig. 60.2: Oxygen dissociation curves for myoglobin and haemoglobin.

However, myoglobin loads and unloads oxygen at a greater speed than haemoglobin. Myoglobin is 50% saturated with O_2 at pO_2 value of 5 mmHg, which is closer to intracellular pO_2 of contracting muscle fibre. Myoglobin serves as a temporary intracellular oxygen storage mechanism. It helps to supply oxygen when blood flow is temporarily interrupted during phasic muscular contractions.

SOURCES OF ENERGY FOR MUSCULAR WORK

During muscular contraction, the energy for actin-myosin sliding movement is provided by ATP. However, total amount of energy stored as ATP in the skeletal muscle is sufficient for severe contractions for one second only. Hence, an additional source of energy must be available to replenish ATP stores, if muscular centractions are to continue any further. Energy is also stored in the muscle in another form, namely, creatine phosphate. Hydrolysis of one molecule of creatine phosphate releases one high energy phosphate bond resulting in conversion of one molecule of ADP to ATP. In this fashion, energy is passed from creatine phosphate to ATP and from ATP to the myofilaments. Creatine phosphate stores allow strenuous muscular contractions for another 5–7 seconds. In all, energy rich phosphagen stores (ATP and creatine phosphate) permit severe muscle contractions for 8–10 seconds only. After this, energy is obtained from metabolism of glycogen stored is the muscle or from circulating glucose and free fatty acids diffusing into the muscle. Metabolism of glycogen, glucose and free fatty acids (FFA) varies depending on whether enough oxygen is available to the muscle or not

Anaerobic Muscular Work

In exhaustive but short exercise, e.g. 400 metres dash, the cardio-respiratory system cannot provide enough oxygen for aerobic oxidation of food stuffs. Therefore, glycogen stored in the muscle is metabolized through anaerobic glycolytic pathways to provide a ready source of energy. Glygcogen is metabolized to lactic acid and relatively much smaller amount of energy is released than given by aerobic metabolism of glycogen or glucose. However, ready availability of glycogen stored locally in the muscle and relatively shorter time needed for glycolytic processes make glycogen-lactic acid system ideal for exhaustive exercise lasting about 1–5 minutes. Exhaustion of muscle glycogen is not the only limiting factor for this source of energy. Accumulation of lactic acid in high concentration in the muscle may stop further glycolysis even if glycogen is present in the muscle.

Aerobic Muscular Work

Aerobic metabolism of food stuffs in the mitochondria is possible when oxygen is freely available to the skeletal muscle, e.g. during jogging, marathon run, cross country cycling, etc. In aerobic system, food stuffs are metabolized through Krebs citric acid cycle, which takes relatively longer time than glycolysis but provides very large amount of energy (ATPs). Under this system of energy, exercise may continue for many hours.

Out of three possible sources of energy, namely carbohydrates, fats and proteins, only the first two are utilized during exercise. Muscle glycogen is an important source but soon exhausted. Subsequently, glucose and free fatty acids, brought to the muscle through the bloodstream, become the chief fuel for muscular work. Of the two sources, proportionately more carbohydrates are utilized at the initial stages. But as the exercise is prolonged, free fatty acids become the predominant fuel (Fig. 60.3). The shift in the type of fuel seems to be created by hormonal changes in exercise. Moderately severe but prolonged exercise not only inhibits insulin secretion but also causes increased secretion of glucagon, growth hormone, cortisol and catecholamines. These hormonal changes promote lipolysis and increase FFA level in the blood. Utilization of FFA rather than glucose helps to prevent hypoglycemia which otherwise might occur.

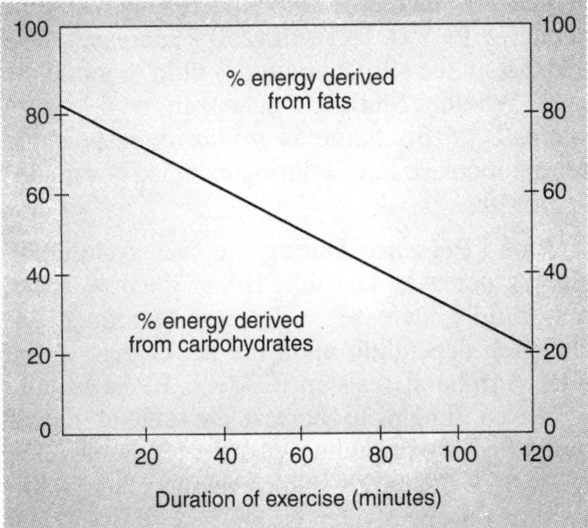

Fig. 60.3: Effect of duration of exercise on the utilization of fuel.

At the end of exercise, products of anaerobic metabolism, chiefly lactic acid, are metabolized at first. Muscle glycogen is fully replenished in about two days. In view of these facts, it is important for an athlete to: (i) consume high carbohydrate diet for a few days before an athletic event and (ii) not to participate in exhaustive exercise during the 48 hours preceding the event. High carbohydrate diet, mixed diet and high fat diet result in storage of 40 g, 20 g and 6 g of glycogen per kg muscle, respectively.

CARDIOVASCULAR ADJUSTMENTS IN EXERCISE

In muscular exercise, oxygen demand of the body increases in proportion to the severity of exercise. Severe exercise is the most stressful physiological condition that the cardiovascular system faces. Consequently, many cardiovascular, respiratory and metabolic adjustments take place.

Skeletal Muscle Blood Flow

At rest, the blood flow to the skeletal muscle is approximately 3–4 ml/100 gm/min or a total of 750 ml/min to the whole of the skeletal muscle mass. During maximal exercise, it may increase to 50-80 ml/100 gm/min or a total blood flow of over 20 L/min (to the whole of the skeletal muscle mass). During exercise, the blood flow to the muscle is intermittent, because during each contraction, muscle fibres squeeze the blood vessels passing through them. During a sustained and severe contraction, the blood flow to the muscle may cease altogether. Marked increase in the blood flow between the contractions ensures adequate oxygen supply to the muscle fibres.

Neural Control of Blood Flow to Skeletal Muscles Skeletal vessels are supplied with noradrenergic sympathetic nerve fibres. Under resting conditions, these nerve fibres have a moderate degree of tonic discharge. A decrease in the vasomotor discharge can only double the blood flow to the skeletal muscles. Therefore, the tremendous increase in the blood flow (nearly 20-

fold) observed in exercising muscle must be due to some other more important mechanisms (local metabolites). Sympathetic vasoconstrictor mechanism assumes physiological importance during circulatory shock or other types of circulatory stress when increased sympathetic discharge increases peripheral resistance in the skeletal blood vessels. This diverts the blood from the muscles to the vital organs.

The skeletal blood vessels are also supplied with sympathetic cholinergic vasodilator nerve fibres. The physiological significance of this type of innervation is not yet clear.

Skeletal blood vessels contain not only α-adrenergic receptors in proximity of the terminals of vasoconstrictor sympathetic nerve fibres but also β-adrenergic receptors (independent of any innervation). During strenuous exercise, epinephrine released into the general circulation from the adrenal medulla produces vasodilatation by acting on the β-adrenergic receptors.

Local Metabolites Local mechanisms are chiefly responsible for the tremendous increase in skeletal blood flow during muscular exercise. The stimuli may include a fall in tissue pO_2, a rise in tissue pCO_2, accumulation of K^+ and lactic acid. The rise of tissue temperature due to muscular activity may also contribute to the dilatation of the arterioles and the pre-capillary sphincters. As a result, there is a 10 to 100-fold increase in the number of open capillaries in the skeletal muscle.

Systemic Circulatory Changes during Exercise

As mentioned earlier, the skeletal muscle total blood flow during maximal exercise may be more than 20 L/min as compared to only 750 ml/min at rest. Such a large increase in the skeletal blood flow is achieved by two mechanisms:

(i) The cardiac output increases from a resting value of 5 to 30–35 L/min, in proportion to the severity of exercise.

(ii) The cardiac output is redistributed in such a way that the blood flow is diverted towards the active tissues (skeletal muscle and the myocardium) at the cost of other tissues where it can be temporarily curtailed (e.g. splanchnic and renal vessels). In the cutaneous vessels, the blood flow is initially decreased, but in sustained exercise it tends to increase when the body temperature rises. The cerebral blood flow remains unchanged during muscular exercise (Table 60.2).

Table 60.2: Distribution of cardiac output in standing posture and during exercise

	Quiet standing	*Heavy exercise*
CO	5.2 L	24 L
Blood flow per minute to		
Heart	250 ml	1000 ml
Brain	750 ml	750 ml
Skeletal muscle	750 ml	20 L
Abdominal viscera	3100 ml	600 ml
Skin	500 ml	Initially 400 ml; later on 1000 ml.

The mechanism of increased CO in exercise has been discussed in detail elsewhere (page 102). The prompt increase in the HR at the beginning or even before the start of exercise is very well known. Many studies have revealed a linear relation between the HR and the total body O_2 consumption (a measure of work load) (Fig. 60.4).

The HR increases from the resting value of about 75 to 150–180/min (250% increase). The increase in the stroke volume is mild to moderate only. Whether Starling mechanism, or increased sympathetic discharge is *primarily* responsible for the increase in CO during exercise is a matter of debate.

Blood Pressure During exercise, systolic BP always increases. Diastolic BP, on the other hand, may mildly increase or decrease or remain unchanged, depending upon the net change in the total peripheral resistance. Mean BP is usually increased. It helps to increase the skeletal muscle blood flow by providing greater pressure head in the face of dilated resistance vessels (Fig. 60.4).

After the end of exercise, the heart rate, CO and O_2 consumption do not return to be resting level immediately. These values decrease gradually over

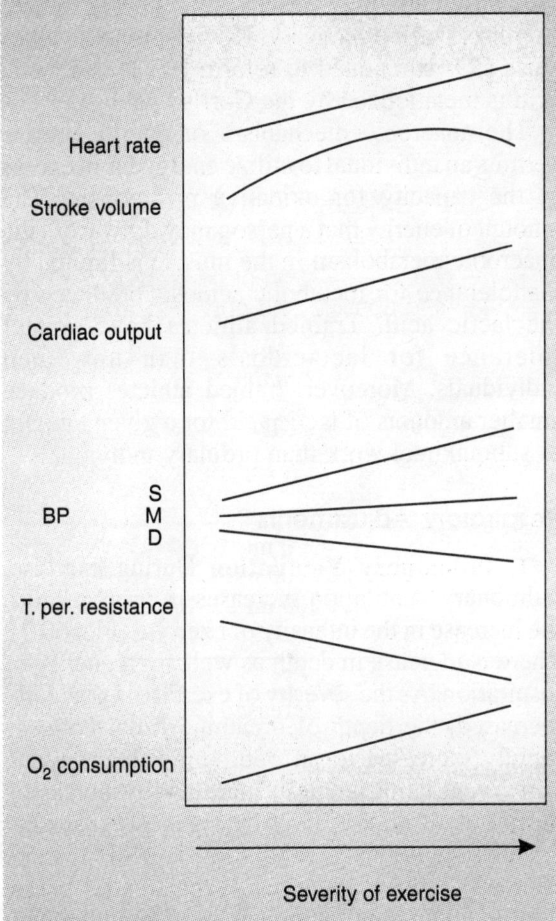

Fig. 60.4: Effect of severity of muscular exercise on the oxygen consumption and various cardiovascular parameters.

a period of 2–5 minutes depending upon the severity of exercise. During this period, the O_2-debt, incurred during the exercise, is paid back.

RESPIRATORY ADJUSTMENTS IN EXERCISE

The energy for muscular work is provided by increased fuel consumption, which is reflected in greater O_2 consumption and CO_2 production. The relation between the severity of work performed and the consumption of O_2 has been found to be linear (Fig. 60.5). Therefore, the severity of exercise (work) has been usually defined in terms of O_2 consumption as follows:

Degree of work	*O_2 consumption (L/min)*
Light	0.4-0.8
Moderate	0.8-1.6
Hard	1.6-2.4
Severe	> 2.4

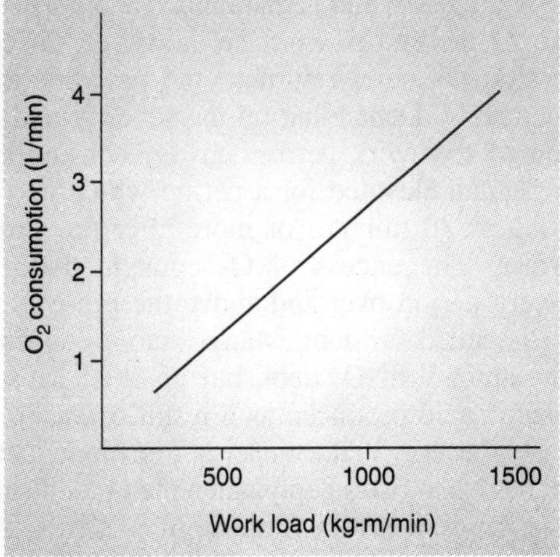

Fig. 60.5: Relation between work load and oxygen consumption.

For experimental or clinical studies, a person can be subjected to a gradually increasing work load on a bicycle ergometer or a treadmill.

The maximal O_2 consumption of an individual refers to his maximal rate of aerobic energy released for work. Average normal maximal O_2 consumption ($VO_{2\ max}$) in adult is 3 L/min. In trained athletes the $VO_{2\ max}$ may be 5 L/min. Maximal O_2 consumption is probably the best physiological indicator of a person's capacity to continue severe work.

Increased O_2 delivery to the tissues during exercise is achieved by the following mechanisms:

(a) Larger volume of O_2 is delivered to the lungs by increased pulmonary ventilation.
(b) Increased rate of O_2 diffusion.
(c) Increased rate of O_2 transport by the circulation. This factor depends upon the cardiac output and O_2 carrying capacity of blood.

The maximal O_2 consumption of a normal individual is limited by the degree to which cardiac output can increase (factor c) and not by the ventilatory capacity (factor a) or oxygen diffusion capacity of the lungs (factor b).

Blood Lactate

If a person performs work on a treadmill at a steady rate for a given period, the oxygen consumption rapidly increases and is maintained at a particular level. At the end of exercise, however, O_2 consumption does not return to the prework level immediately. Depending on the severity and duration of the work performed, O_2 consumption may remain elevated for a period which may be as long as 30 minutes or more after the end of exercise. The excess of O_2 consumed during recovery period over and above the pre-exercise level is called O_2 debt. Many factors contribute to the amount of O_2 debt, but its chief cause is the lactic acid produced as a result of anaerobic release of energy in the muscles. The blood lactate level begins to rise steeply when the O_2 consumption exceeds 2 L/min (Fig. 60.6).

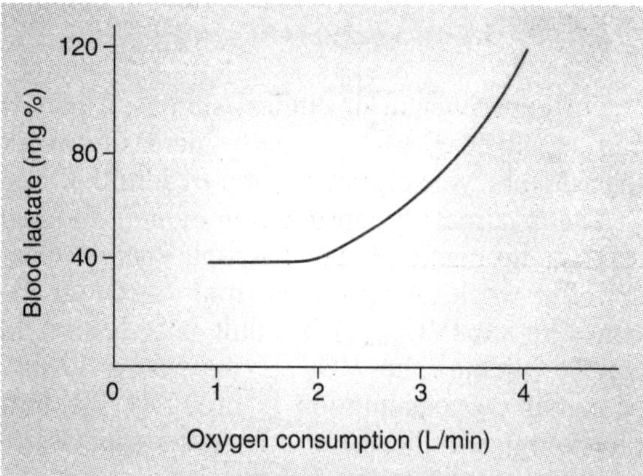

Fig. 60.6: The relation between the rise in blood lactate and severity of exercise.

In the blood, lactic acid is buffered by the bicarbonate buffer as follows :

$$H^+ + HCO_3^- \Leftrightarrow H_2CO_3 \Leftrightarrow CO_2 + H_2O$$

The extra CO_2 so evolved is removed by hyperventilation. Since, CO_2 evolved is more than O_2 consumed, the respiratory quotient (CO_2 evolved/ O_2 consumed) may reach 1.5-2 during severe exercise. During recovery, RQ falls to low values since CO_2 is retained to reform HCO_3^- and lactic acid is metabolized by the Cori's cycle.

The anaerobic mechanism of energy release permits an individual to utilize energy far in excess of the capacity for oxidative metabolism. The amount of energy that a person may draw from the anaerobic metabolism in the muscle is limited by his tolerance for metabolic acidosis produced by the lactic acid. Trained athletes have greater tolerance for lactacidosis than untrained individuals. Moreover, trained athletes produce smaller amounts of lactic acid for a given amount of submaximal work than ordinary individuals.

Respiratory Adjustments

1. Pulmonary Ventilation During exercise, pulmonary ventilation increases in proportion to the increase in the intensity of exercise (Fig. 60.7). There is increase in depth as well as frequency of respiration. As the severity of exercise is gradually increased, the depth of breathing (tidal volume) rapidly increases to an optimum value, beyond which ventilation is chiefly increased by increasing the rate of respiration. Even during most exhausting exercise, pulmonary ventilation is seldom more than 100-120 L/minute, i.e. it remains far below the maximum breathing capacity of the individual.

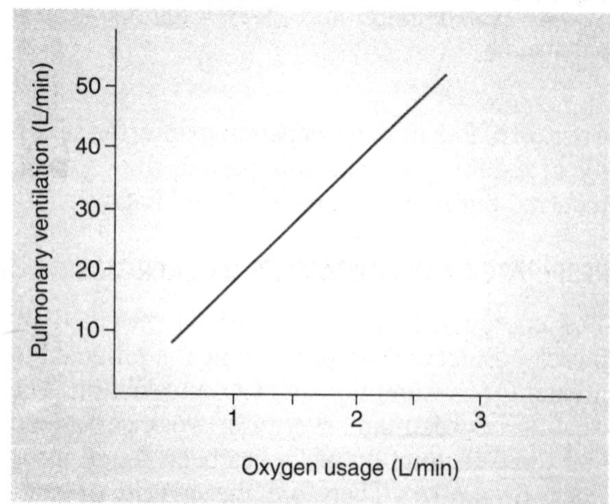

Fig. 60.7: The relation between oxygen consumption and pulmonary ventilation.

In spite of extensive research, the mechanism of increased pulmonary ventilation during exercise remains obscure. One may imagine that because of increased O_2 utilization and CO_2 production, decreased arterial pO_2 and increased arterial pCO_2 are the most likely causes of increased pulmonary ventilation. No doubt, during exercise the venous blood has lesser O_2 content (and pO_2) and greater CO_2 content (and pCO_2) but the receptors sensitive to pO_2 and pCO_2 are situated in the *arterial side* of the circulation. Pulmonary ventilation is so well matched with the metabolic demand, that even during the most strenuous exercise, the arterial pO_2 and pCO_2 values are practically normal.

If a person performs work steadily on a treadmill or a bicycle ergometer, it would be seen that there is an abrupt increase in pulmonary ventilation, just at the beginning of exercise, followed by a gradual further increase as the exercise is continued. At the end of exercise, there is an equally abrupt moderate decrease, followed by further decline during the recovery period (Fig. 60.8). The abruptness with which the pulmonary ventilation increases and decreases, at the beginning and the end of exercise, suggest that some neural rather than chemical mechanism is responsible for it. It is believed that psychic stimuli and afferent impulses from proprioceptors in the muscles and joints are at least partly responsible for increase in the pulmonary ventilation during exercise.

In severe and sustained exercise, lactic acid accumulates in the blood and the pH of blood may drop to as low as 7.2. The acidosis causes further increase in the pulmonary ventilation out of proportion to the O_2 consumption. During this period, the arterial pCO_2 may drop significantly.

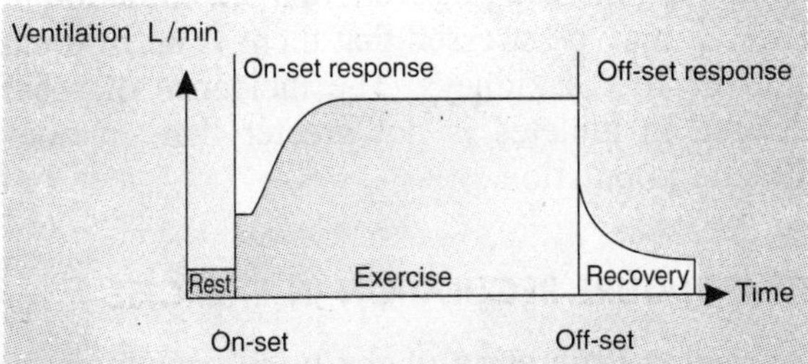

Fig. 60.8: Pulmonary ventilation during exercise, showing an abrupt change in ventilation at the beginning and the end of exercise.

During sustained exercise, the rise of body temperature may also contribute to the increase in pulmonary ventilation.

Oxygen Uptake in the Lungs Greater O_2 uptake by the blood in the lungs is due to the following factors :

a. Because of greater extraction of O_2 by the muscles, the O_2 content of mixed venous blood reaching the lungs may be as low as 3 ml/100 ml of blood (as compared to 14-15 ml% at rest). Moreover, due to increased cardiac output (30-35 L/min) larger volume of blood passes through the lungs per minute. In this way during exercise, the blood can carry much larger volume of O_2 from the lungs to the tissues.
b. During exercise, the diffusion capacity of the lungs for O_2 increases to about 90 ml/min/mmHg as compared to 25 ml/min/mmHg at rest. The increase in diffusion capacity is due to opening up of many previously closed pulmonary capillaries, and increased pulmonary blood flow.

As a result of factors (a) and (b), the O_2 uptake in the lungs increases from 0.25 L/min at rest to 4 L/min during exercise.

HAEMATOLOGICAL CHANGES IN EXERCISE

A transient increase in red blood cell count and haemoglobin concentration can be observed after a bout of strenuous exercise. In the dog, the changes can be attributed to the discharge of blood with high haematocrit value from the spleen. It is caused by the contraction of splenic capsule, under the effect of circulating adrenaline. In man, any effective contraction of the splenic capsule does not occur. Therefore, the increase in red cell count and haemoglobin concentration seems to be an effect of haemoconcentration caused by loss of plasma fluid in sweat. A bout of exercise also causes neutrophilic leucocytosis by adrenaline-induced mobilization of neutrophils from the marginated pool. The above mentioned haematological change as well as changes in blood gases content after a bout of heavy exercise are shown in Table 60.3.

Table 60.3: Effect of a bout of heavy exercise on haematological parameters and blood gases

Parameter	*Before exercise*	*After exercise*
Total blood volume (L)	5.7	5.5
Haemoglobin conc. (g%)	16.0	17.6
Haematocrit (%)	47.0	50.0
RBC count (million/cmm)	5.4	5.7
Total leucocyte count (thousand/cmm)	7.0	15.0
Arterial pO_2 (mmHg)	100.0	100.0
Arterial pCO_2 (mmHg)	40.0	38.0
Arterial O_2 content (ml/100 ml)	19.5	19.5
Femoral venous blood pO_2 (mmHg)	30.0	13.0
Blood lactate (mg%)	12.0	100.0
Body temperature (°C)	37.5	40.0

HORMONAL CHANGES IN EXERCISE

Mild exercise or a brief bout of heavy exercise may not produce any significant hormonal changes. Prolonged heavy exercise produces a substantial increase in plasma levels of growth hormone, glucagon, ACTH, cortisol and catecholamines. Plasma insulin level is significantly reduced. All these hormonal changes are effects of exercise stress. The metabolic effects of the above mentioned hormonal changes include an increase in plasma FFA level leading to greater utilization of FFA and decreased glucose utilization in the skeletal muscle. Increased gluconeogenesis helps to prevent hypoglycemia during exercise. Exercise stress also causes increased plasma aldosterone level leading to decreased NaCl losses in the sweat and urine. The secretion of aldosterone is more prominent when endurance type of exercise is performed in hot environment, especially in athletes acclimatized to heat. Exercise stress also causes increased secretion of ADH.

RENAL CHANGES IN EXERCISE

The effect of exercise on renal function is highly variable. It depends upon the intensity and duration of exercise, as well as, on the environmental conditions, degree of prior hydration and training of the individual. With work load less than 50% of $VO_{2\,max}$ and exercise lasting less than 15 minutes, there may be no change in the renal blood flow (RBF), GFR and urinary volume. Sustained exercise with work load more than 50% of $VO_{2\,max}$ may produce intense renal vasoconstriction leading to about 70% reduction in RBF and 50-60% reduction in GFR. Urine flow may be markedly reduced. These changes are still more severe if the exercise is performed in hot and humid environment. Neural cardiovascular regulatory mechanisms and increased secretion of renin-aldosterone and catecholamines account for the above mentioned renal changes. After the end of exercise, as sympathetic discharge abates, RBF is restored to normal within a few minutes, followed by recovery of GFR. The urine flow rate may remain subnormal even one hour after the end of exercise. This may be correlated with the persistence of ADH secretion following loss of fluid in the sweat.

Athletic Pseudonephritis Following prolonged heavy exercise, protein and red blood cells may be observed in the urine of most of the healthy athletes. Since these changes, typical of renal disorder (nephritis), are seen in normal individuals, the term athletic pseudonephritis has been used to describe the phenomenon. The exact mechanism of athletic pseudonephritis is not clear. It is apparently due to an increase in the permeability of glomerular capillary membrane possibly due to renal hypoxia resulting from marked reduction in RBF. It may be stressed that there is no residual damage to the kidneys. The incidence of renal disease in athletes is not greater than in nonathletic population.

TEMPERATURE REGULATION IN EXERCISE

Oxygen consumption of the body may increase 20-25 folds during strenuous exercise, resulting in a proportionate increase in heat production. The extra heat is efficiently dissipated by activation of heat loss mechanisms of the body, particularly sweating. Sweating may start within a minute of the start of exercise, much before an increase in cutaneous or core temperature occurs. Similarly, at the end of exercise in cool environment, sweating may cease before rectal temperature begins to fall to normal. In view of this observation, it has been suggested that during exercise, besides thermal stimuli, proprioceptive stimuli may also be involved in the regulation of sweating. From this account, one may presume that body temperature would not increase during exercise, especially if it is performed in cool environment. Actually, when moderately heavy exercise is continued, there is a rise in core (rectal) temperature even in cold environment, when dissipation of heat is not a problem. In endurance type of exercise, rectal temperature up to 40°C may be recorded. Apparently, physical exercise raises the hypothalamic thermostat to a higher set point until the exercise stops. The exact mechanism of resetting of thermostat is not known. The raised core temperature improves the physical performance by accelerating the metabolic processes, dissociation of oxyhaemoglobin and decreasing the viscous resistance in the joints and muscles.

Role of Environmental Temperature

When heavy exercise is performed in cool environment, the extra heat production does not create any problems. Enhanced heat production makes skiing over snow or swimming in ice-cold water an enjoyable experience. There is no risk of failure of temperature regulatory mechanisms while exercising in cold environment. On the other hand, in hot weather, heavy exercise puts an extra load on the heat loss mechanisms of the body. Consequently, the body temperature tends to increase even beyond the elevated set point. Prolonged exercise or heavy work, performed in hot and humid climate by unacclimatized individuals, may lead to failure of thermoregulatory mechanisms known as heat stroke. The risk of heat stroke is minimized if :

(i) The athlete or the manual worker is given enough time to acclimatize to the hot environment and

(ii) Proper hydration is maintained by intake of water or hypotonic saline during prolonged exercise.

BODY FLUIDS IN EXERCISE

Prolonged exercise in hot and humid climate may produce severe salt and water deficit. Athletes may lose 2-4 kg body weight in one hour of endurance type of exercise. Most of the weight loss is due to loss of water (and NaCl) in sweat. Salt loss in sweat is decreased if an athlete has been given 1-2 weeks to acclimatize before participating in the athletic event. Acclimatization mainly involves greater secretion of aldosterone which decreases NaCl excretion in sweat and urine. Greater aldosterone secretion, however, promotes K^+ excretion in the urine and sweat. Therefore, nowadays, athletes engaged in endurance type of exercise are encouraged to consume water with proportionate Na^+ and K^+ during the event.

EXERCISE AND IMMUNE SYSTEM

Moderate exercise has an overall beneficial effect on general health and reduces the incidence of minor infections. However, exhaustive exercise reduces T and B lymphocyte function and predisposes the athlete to infectious diseases. It could be due to exercise-induced release of ACTH and cortisol.

EFFECT OF GENDER

Adult males and females differ in their body size, muscle mass, subcutaneous fat content and temperament. These differences appear chiefly after puberty due to secretion of testosterone in the male. Before puberty, the muscle strength of boys is only slightly better than girls. After puberty, generally speaking, women have about two-thirds strength as men. VO_{2max} of females is also less than males. Fat constitutes about 25% of total body weight in females as compared to about 15% in males. The extra fat in females does not contribute to muscle strength but may be helpful in endurance type of exercise. That may be the reason why women are only 12% poorer than men in endurance exercises.

FATIGUE

Fatigue is a state of discomfort or weariness in the muscles produced by a steady prolonged exercise. It is produced by a number of ill-understood factors. It has been mainly attributed to changes in the cerebral synapses resulting from slight hypoxia and acidosis. Afferent impulses set up in the muscle by local chemical changes may contribute to the muscular discomfort. There is a correlation between the feeling of exhaustion and the degree of depletion of muscle glycogen. Some of the stiffness of the muscles may be due to accumulation of interstitial fluid.

TRAINING OF AN ATHLETE

It is a well-known observation that muscular strength can be improved by training. Use of a muscle for usual isotonic movements, e.g. walking or flexion and extension of the elbow would not improve muscle strength. For improvement of strength, a muscle must be made to contract against a resistance or a load (Fig. 60.9). Strength of a muscle increases when it is made to contract with maximum or near maximum force. Following are the general guidelines for training of an athlete:

(i) Training programme should provide a progressively increasing overload. The load should be slightly more than what the muscle can lift. As the athlete adapts to a particular load, it must be further increased to provoke further adaptation.

(ii) Allow adequate recovery time between training sessions. It is useless to train a fatigued muscle. Therefore, different groups of muscles may be trained in each session, allowing 1-2 days of rest between the training sessions.

(iii) Aerobic endurance can be increased by fast running, or training on a bicycle ergometer or a treadmill. In this case, the exercise should increase the heart rate to at least 130 beats per minute to begin with. The intensity of exercise should be gradually increased. Aerobic endurance exercise improves VO_{2max} of the individual by producing changes in cardiorespiratory system described below.

(iv) Besides general training to build up the muscles and VO_{2max}, each athlete must have special training in the particular sport the athlete is interested in.

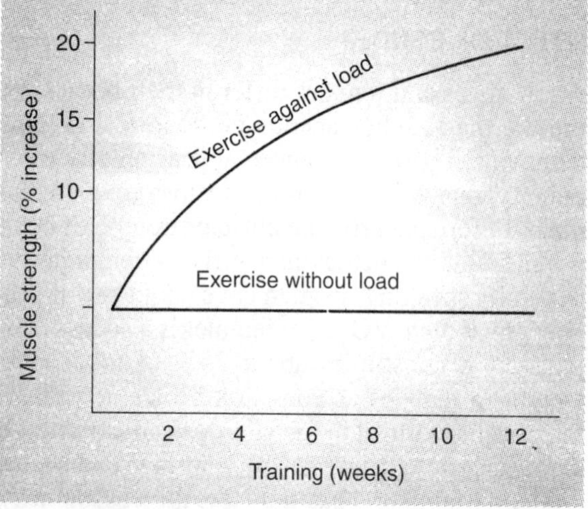

Fig. 60.9: Effect of load on the benefits of exercise training.

Effects of Training

Skeletal Muscle After a few weeks of strength training programme, an increase in the size of the muscles can be observed. The increase in muscle mass is due to hypertrophy of the existing muscle fibres and not due to formation of new muscle fibres. The improvement in the strength is far more than what can be explained by the hypertrophy. At the same time, there is an improvement in the power of contraction, i.e. the stronger muscles not only contract more forcefully but also more quickly. In the hypertrophied muscle the following changes can be observed :

(i) Increased fibre diameter.

(ii) Up to 120% increase in mitochondrial enzyme concentration.

(iii) 60-80% increase in phosphogen energy stores.

(iv) 50% increase in stored glycogen.

(v) 75–100% increase in stored triglycerides.

Cardiovascular System In aerobic endurance type of training, the heart is subjected to increased work load. Therefore, it hypertrophies like skeletal muscle. Cardiac muscle mass may increase by 50–75%. In addition, athletic training causes increased parasympathetic tone to the heart. As a result, the resting heart rate may decrease to 50–60 beats/minute. Since resting cardiac out put remains normal, the resting stroke volume must be increased in trained athletes. Typical values of heart rate, stroke volume and cardiac output in non-athletes and athletes during rest and maximum work are as follows :

		Heart rate (beats/min)	*Stroke volume (ml)*	*Cardiac output (ml/min)*
Resting	Non-athlete	70	70	4,900
	Athlete	50	100	5,000
Max.	Non-athlete	180	110	19,800
work	Athlete	180	160	28,800

During exercise, there is an increase in the heart rate as well as stroke volume. As a result, the cardiac output increases to 20–25 L/min in non-athletes and 35–40 L/min in athletes. In non-athletes, under maximum work, there is about 250% increase in heart rate (from 70 to 180 beats per minute) and about 60% increase in stroke volume (from 70 to 110 ml). In trained athletes, the heart rate increases from 50 per minute at rest to 180 beats per minute under maximal work, an increase of about 360%. More importantly the stroke volume can increase up to 160 ml (130% increase).

Respiratory System Average normal oxygen consumption at rest is about 250 ml per minute. During maximal work, it may be 2.5–4 L/min ($VO_{2\ max}$) in untrained male individuals. World class male athletes may have $VO_{2\ max}$ of about 6 L/min. The substantial increase in $VO_{2\ max}$ is chiefly due to the effect of training on cardiovascular system and in oxygen diffusion capacity. There is only mild increase in vital capacity or maximum breathing capacity. During maximal exercise, trained athletes have pulmonary ventilation of 100–120 litres per minute whereas their maximum breathing capacity (MBC) is 150–170 litres per minute. Thus, respiratory system is not called upon to utilize fully the MBC. In other words, the availability of oxygen is always more than what can be taken up by the circulatory system.

Maximum diffusing capacity of oxygen in endurance athlete is about 80–90 ml/min/mmHg as compared to 50 ml/min/mmHg in untrained individuals.

Effect of Age and Gender Athletic training can increase strength of the muscles at any age, but the effect is maximum around 25 years of age. In childhood or old age, very little improvement in strength may be expected. Female athletes have lesser improvement with training than males.

BENEFITS OF REGULAR EXERCISE

Lifespan It is widely believed that those who exercise regularly lead a healthier life than those who lead a sedentary life. However, there are conflicting reports on the possible beneficial effects on the longevity of life. Part of the difficulty of such studies arises because there are so many variables affecting longevity; and exercise is only one of them. Unless all other variables are eliminated, the beneficial effect of exercise cannot be assessed accurately. Therefore, lifespan of a large number of persons with similar socio-economic status but jobs involving different degree of physical activity was compared. It was found that postmen and bus conductors had longer lifespan than postal clerks and bus drivers. In laboratory animals, dietary and other variables can be rigidly controlled. One such study showed that lifespan of rats who were made to do exercise regularly was 35% longer than rats who led a sedentary life in their cages.

Besides longevity, quality of life is also important. There is no doubt that those who exercise regularly have better quality of life than those who do not. Day to day activities like climbing stairs, running to catch a bus or lifting a bag of groceries, etc. are enjoyable to those who exercise regularly but an unbearable burden to sedentary persons.

Prevention of Disease In bed-ridden patients, hypokinetic degeneration can be observed in most of the organs, especially in bones, skeletal muscle, tendons and ligaments. There is a deterioration in cardiorespiratory, bladder and bowel function. All such problems are less common even in persons who are just up and about and not engaged in any regular exercise. Further, it has been established that regular exercise definitely lowers the incidence of obesity, coronary artery disease and atherosclerosis. In elderly individuals, even regular walking helps to decrease the degree of osteoporosis and incidence of fracture neck femur.

Therapeutic Effects of Exercise Regular exercise programme is an important adjunct to treatment of many disorders like coronary artery disease, hypertension, occlusive arterial disease, chronic obstructive lung disease, obesity and diabetes mellitus.

POTENTIAL HARMFUL EFFECTS OF EXERCISE

In view of the numerous beneficial effects of exercise mentioned above, one may be tempted to advise vigorous exercise to all the persons. Actually for a middle-aged person, a thorough medical check-up is absolutely essential before the start of any exercise programme. Sedentary persons should increase the intensity of exercise slowly over many weeks. Vigorous exercise does present some risk of coronary ischemia or cerebrovascular accident in middle-aged and aged individuals. A safe limit of aerobic exercise is that which produces a heart rate of 170 minus age of the subject (i.e. 130 beats per min for 40 years old; 120 beats per min for 50 years old).

Even in young adults participating in competitive sports, injuries to muscles, bones, joints, tendons and ligaments are not uncommon.

Drug and Other Adjuvents in Sports: Doping

The term doping is derived from the ancient African custom of using a local liquor called dope as a stimulant during sports. Doping is defined as administration or use by a competing athlete of any substance foreign to the body or any physiological substance taken in abnormal quantity with the sole intention of increasing in an unfair manner his/her performance in competition. Some of the adjuvents used by the athletes do not provide any physiological benefit while others are effective to a varying degree but are potentially harmful.

Mostly Useless Adjuvents

(i) Eating sugar before the event.
(ii) Use of extra vitamins and minerals.
(iii) Dehydration (in order to compete with persons with lower body weight).
(iv) Water intake before the event.
(v) Oxygen inhalation.
(vi) Alcohol intake.
(vii) Tobacco.
(viii) Training at high altitude.
(ix) Blood transfusion.

Effective but potentially Dangerous Adjuvents

Use of the following drugs is forbidden by athletic regulations. In Olympic games, many athletes have lost their medals because their blood was found to contain one of the following drugs.

(i) Amphetamines Sympathomimetic drugs like benzedrine or dexedrine delay the sense of fatigue and hence allow the athlete to prolong activities like marathon run or cross-country cycling. There is no improvement in the physical performance in shorter events. Continuous and excessive use of these drugs may produce addiction, circulatory failure or even death.

(ii) Cocain This drug also inhibits sense of fatigue and hence helps to prolong the endurance type of exercise. The drug is highly addictive and dangerous. It causes serious psychotic disorders.

(iii) Caffeine Caffeine causes cerebral stimulation. About 500 mg of caffeine (more than 3 cups of coffee or 4 cups of tea) are required to produce any significant reduction in fatigue. It is useful only during endurance type of exercise.

(iv) Anabolic Steroids Testosterone has androgenic as well as anabolic effects. Certain synthetic steroids like Dianabol have strong anabolic effect with minimal androgenic activity. Anabolic steroids are normally used in patients recovering from debilitating illness. Some male as well as female athletes use testosterone or synthetic anabolic steroids to build up greater muscle mass and muscle strength. No doubt, there is definite improvement in muscle mass but their use is not only unethical but also dangerous. These drugs suppress spermatogenesis and endogenous testosterone production. In females, there is varying degree of masculinization. Long-term use of these drugs predisposes to atherosclerosis, liver damage, aggressive psychotic behaviour and cancer of liver and prostate.

Section XVI

Geriatric Physiology

CHAPTER 61

Geriatric Physiology (Physiology of the Aged)

All living animals undergo a series of changes after birth. There is an initial period of growth till adulthood is reached. With the passage of time, the involution sets in, and after a varied lifespan, all animals ultimately die. No particular time can be set at which ageing starts. Ageing is a composite part of one's life. Ageing includes all the changes which occur in the body with passage of time. The process of ageing may be hastened in some individuals and delayed in others, but it must occur in each one of us. Abnormal wear and tear may hasten the process, e.g. repeated traumas, infections, excessive emotional excitement, dietary abuse and exhaustive activities may lead to premature ageing. There may be some genetic difference also. In some families, individuals tend to age rather early in life. Others may look young till sixth or seventh decade of life.

In old age, many pathological disorders are also prevalent. Hence, a physician should know whether the apparent abnormality is a normal physiological process or a disease. Further, the knowledge of effect of age on different organ systems may be important in the treatment of the diseases. The tolerance or excretion of a drug may be altered and hence a different dose schedule may have to be used. A relatively new speciality of medicine called *geriatrics* deals with the curative, preventive and social aspects of illnesses of the elderly.

In the next few pages, the important changes of the ageing process in different organ systems shall be discussed.

CARDIOVASCULAR SYSTEM

Histological examination of the myocardium reveals accumulation of yellowish brown lipofuscin pigment. Under electron microscope, degenerative changes in the myofibrils and mitochondria and vacuolization have been observed in the myocardium. How far these anatomical changes can be related to the physiological changes remains controversial.

The left ventricular wall may be 25% thicker at the age of 75–80 years than in young adults. There is a thickening of the valves of the heart. Large areas of fibrosis, especially in the subendocardial region, may be observed. The capillary density of the myocardium may be decreased.

The resting heart rate is not affected in the aged. But stroke volume is decreased. In response to exercise, the maximum cardiac output is decreased at the rate of 1% per year after the age of 40 years (Fig. 61.1).

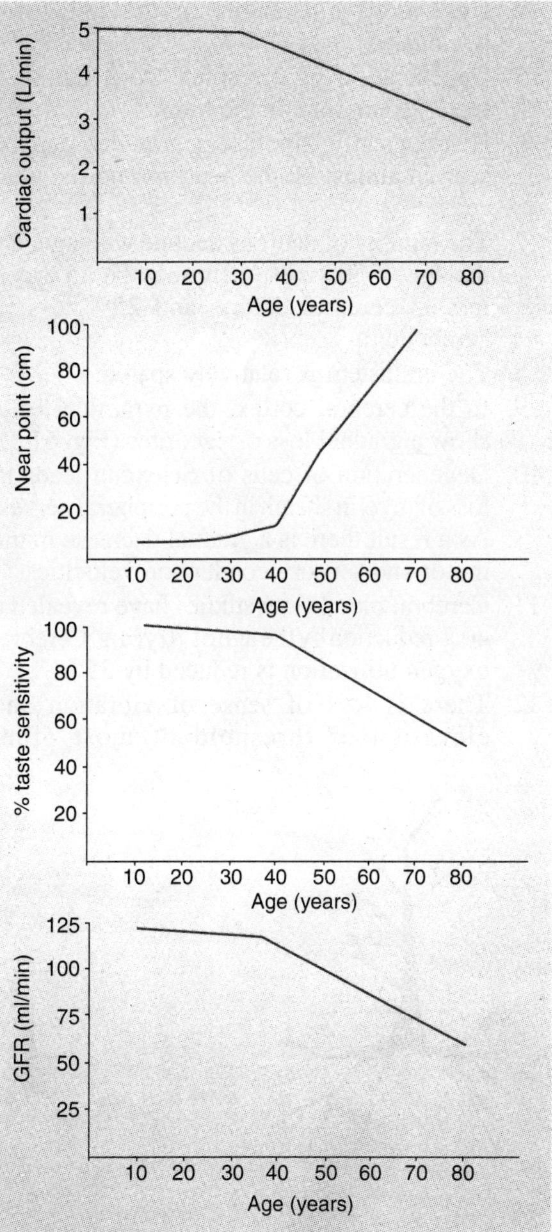

Fig. 61.1: Effect of age on cardiac output, power of accommodation in the eye, taste sensitivity and GFR.

The electrocardiogram does not change significantly with age. Therefore, any significant change in ECG of an elderly individual should be considered pathological. In the blood vessels, there is a gradual decrease in the number of elastic fibres. Accumulation of calcium salts in the elastic and muscular type of arteries, as well as, deposition of more collagen fibres decrease the distensibility of the blood vessels. Loss of elasticity in the aorta and its major branches accounts for the systolic hypertension and wide pulse pressure observed in the aged individuals (Fig. 61.2). The blood flow to the heart, brain, liver and especially to kidney is decreased.

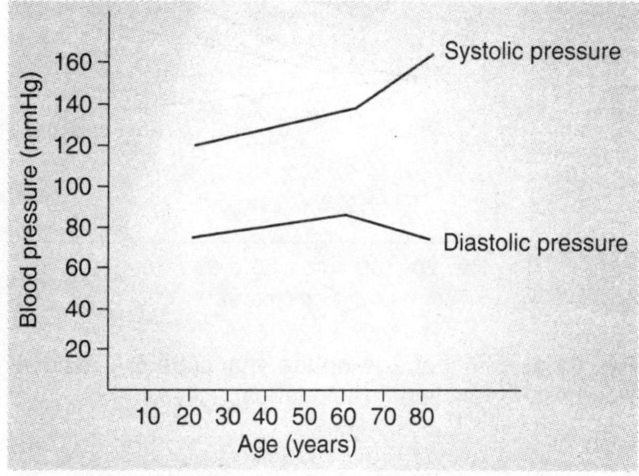

Fig. 61.2: Effect of age on blood pressure.

RESPIRATORY SYSTEM

There is a gradual decline in the number of alveoli due to progressive loss of interalveolar septa. The residual alveoli and alveolar ducts are dilated (Fig. 61.3). The elasticity of the lungs is decreased leading to increased pulmonary compliance. On the other hand, calcification of costal cartilages decreases the mobility of the ribs, as well as, the compliance of the thoracic cage. There is a progressive kyphosis due to osteoporosis and vertebral collapse. As a result of all these changes, there is a 50% increase in the functional residual capacity of the lungs, and 100% increase in the residual volume (Fig. 61.4). Partial hyperinflation

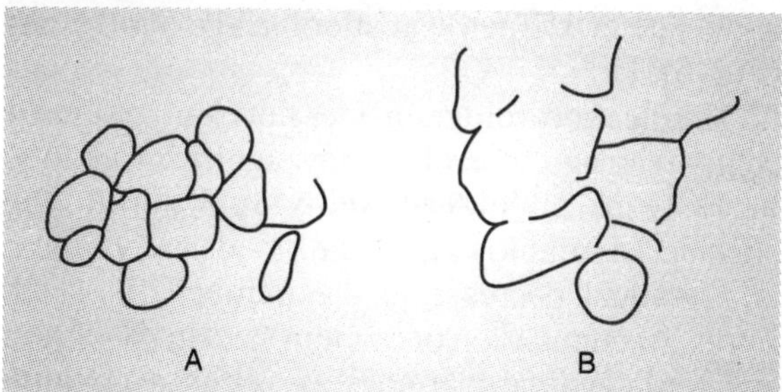

Fig. 61.3: Pulmonary parenchyma in adult (A) and old age (B).

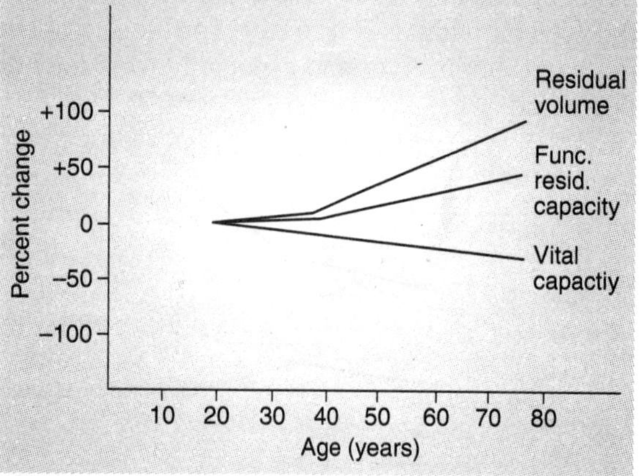

Fig. 61.4: Effect of age on the vital capacity, residual volume and functional residual capacity.

of the lungs gives barrel shape to the chest. Vital capacity, FEV_1, MBC, and diffusion capacity for oxygen are significantly decreased in the aged individuals. However, all these changes are not so detrimental because the respiratory system is seldom subjected to excessive demands. There is no change in the arterial pCO_2. Arterial pO_2 is decreased by 10–15% due to an increase in physiological dead space. But it has no serious detrimental effect on the body. Impairment of bronchiolar escalator function is a serious problem, more so, in smokers.

CENTRAL NERVOUS SYSTEM

Postmortem examination of the aged individuals who died from non-neurological disorders and *in vivo* studies have revealed a number of changes.

1. Atrophy of the brain especially involving frontal lobes leading to shrinkage of gyri and enlargement of sulci.
2. Enlargement of the ventricles.
3. Depigmentation and other degenerative changes in the substantia nigra.
4. Degenerative changes in the lentiform nucleus.
5. Degeneration of the spinal cord but to a lesser extent than in the brain.
6. Histologically, lipofuscin granules can be seen in almost all the neurons and the glial cells.
7. The number of neurons decline with age. By the age of 70 years, there may be 45% cell loss in cerebral cortex, and 25% loss in cerebellum.
8. The brainstem is relatively spared.
9. In the cerebral cortex, the pyramidal cells show a gradual loss of dendrites (Fig. 61.5).
10. Degeneration of cells of Schwann leads to loss of myelin sheath in the peripheral nerves. As a result there is a gradual decrease in the motor and sensory conduction velocities.
11. Cerebral blood flow studies have revealed a 40% reduction by the age of 70 years. Cerebral oxygen utilization is reduced by 25%.
12. There is loss of sense of vibration and elevation of threshold of most other

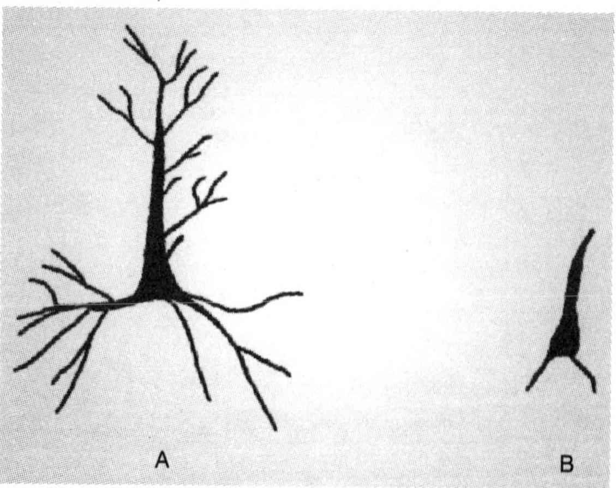

Fig. 61.5: Histological structure of a pyramidal cell of the cerebral cortex in an adult (A) and an aged individual (B).

sensations. Sense of two point discrimination is also affected.
13. Reflexes: Ankle jerk is lost in most of the elderly individuals. Other deep and superficial reflexes tend to be sluggish or absent.
14. Skeletal muscle atrophy gradually increases with age.

Total sleep time is not actually decreased in old age, but there is a gradual decrease in the stage 3 and 4 of the non-REM sleep. Very old individuals may not go into stage 4 at all. Numerous brief arousals do occur and form the basis of the complaints of sleeplessness. Another cause for this complaint is that with not much to do, the elderly individuals sleep for a considerable period in daytime. Hence, the duration of sleep during night is curtailed.

Senile dementia and Alzheimer's disease are very serious disorders of the nervous system, because they affect the higher cortical functions. Basically, both are similar in nature and caused by degeneration of cholinergic neurons in the forebrain. The onset of Alzheimer's disease is in the 5th-6th decade, whereas senile dementia is a name given when the disorder occurs in the 7th-8th decade of life. Parkinsonism is another disorder of the aged involving the basal ganglia. It is caused by degeneration of dopaminergic neurons of the substantia nigra.

AUTONOMIC NERVOUS SYSTEM

Progressive disturbance of temperature regulation is an evidence of autonomic disturbances in the aged. In young adults, exposure to cold is well tolerated. Hypothermia occurs only in victims of shipwrecks or mountaineers lost in snow. Many elderly individuals go into hypothermia in their own home, sometime even when the weather is not so cold. Investigations in the elderly reveal that exposure to moderate cold or hot environment does not produce the expected vasoconstriction and shivering or vasodilatation and sweating, respectively. The threshold for sweating is elevated. Therefore, exposure to heat may produce hyperthermia or even heat stroke.

Postural hypotension is a fairly common problem faced by the elderly. It is attributed to partial failure of the baroreceptor mechanism.

SPECIAL SENSES

Eyes

Besides graying of the hair, presbyopia or the loss of accommodation is the most well-known and obvious sign of ageing. This change sets in rather early, and by the age of 50 years, most of the normal individuals need reading glasses. Age-related loss of elasticity of the lens results in failure to increase the curvature of the lens while focusing on a near object. After 8th decade, degenerative changes in the muscles of accommodation further accentuate the problem (Fig. 61.1).

Gradual opacification of the lens (cataract) also occurs almost *universally*. However, it is difficult to say whether it should be considered a physiological or pathological change. The appearance of white (opaque) circle at the edge of the cornea, called arcus senilis, is another sign of ageing. However, it may be seen even in younger individuals, especially if hyperlipidemia is present.

A gradual decrease in the depth of anterior chamber, and deterioration in the reabsorptive mechanism of aqueous humour at the angle of the eye, predispose the aged individuals to chronic glaucoma. The pupillary responses to light and accommodation also decline with age.

The visual acuity gradually decreases in old age. It may be partly due to cataractous changes in the lens. However, surgical removal of the cataract often does not restore normal vision because of degenerative changes in the retina.

Reduced secretion of the tears causes the dryness of cornea and conjunctiva.

Ears

Degenerative changes in the organ of Corti (hair cells), ganglion cells, as well as, temporal cortex produce impairment of hearing (presbycusia), especially for higher frequencies (Fig. 61.6). In addition, elasticity of the basilar membrane is also decreased. The localization of sound is also compromised in old age. Another cause of deafness in old age is the otosclerosis.

Atrophy of the stria vascularis causes impairment of endolymph production. Degeneration of hair cells of the cristae ampullaris further contrib-

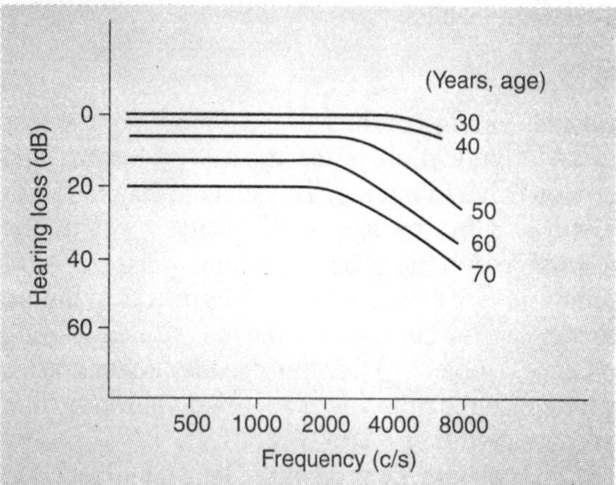

Fig. 61.6: Effect of age on the sensation of hearing of different sound frequencies.

utes to the impairment of postural reflexes. This is one of the reasons why the aged individuals feel difficulty in moving about in the dark.

Taste and Smell

The number of taste buds per papilla decreases from an average of 250 in childhood to 90 by the age of 80 years. Hence, the taste threshold is elevated in old age. The sensitivity of the sense of smell is also impaired. The impairment of the sensation of smell and taste may be partly due to cellular loss in the cerebral cortical centres (Fig. 61.1).

GASTROINTESTINAL TRACT

Dryness of mouth is a common complaint in old age. The secretion of saliva under basal state and after reflex stimulation is only one-third of normal adult values. Salivary amylase secretion is drastically reduced but it does not affect the digestion of starch.

Gastric secretion falls to l/5th the adult value by the age of 60 years. Achlorhydria occurs fairly commonly resulting in deficiency of iron and B_{12} vitamin. The secretion of pancreatic amylase is not affected in old age. Thus, as a whole digestion and absorption of foodstuffs does not seem to be affected in old age except for deficiency of iron and vitamin B_{12} due to achlorhydria. Since of digestibility and absorption of carbohydrates, fats and proteins in the aged individuals shows no apparent deterioration, nutritional deficiency in an elderly individual cannot be attributed to malabsorption and actually reflects deficient intake of the nutrients.

The hepatic weight declines significantly after the age of 70 years. But the hepatic function is maintained at normal level. All the hepatic function tests show normal results except for a decrease in albumin/globulin ratio. Bile pigment excretion also remains normal.

ENDOCRINES

The anterior pituitary hormone secretion is not reduced in old age. In females, the gonadotropin secretion from anterior pituitary is actually increased due to ovarian failure and negative feedback effect of ovarian hormones on the gonadotropin secretion. As compared to adult level, there is 15-fold increase in secretion of FSH and 3-fold increase in LH. In males, the increase in FSH and LH secretion is not very significant. There is definite decrease in the secretion of thyroid hormones.

Basal plasma insulin levels seem to be unaffected but there is impairment of insulin response to a glucose load. Two hours after administration of glucose load, plasma glucose level is about 30 mg% higher at the age of 70 years than in younger adults. Plasma adrenal cortical level and glucagon level remain normal. Plasma oestrogens and progesterone levels are markedly decreased. After the age of 70 years, there is a significant decline in the plasma testosterone level.

BLOOD

Total blood volume, and total leucocyte count remain normal in old age. However, anaemia tends to be more common due to deficiency of iron and vitamin B_{12}. Polymorphonuclear cells seem to be hypersegmented. Immunological function is markedly depressed. Immune surveillance by T lymphocytes is reduced and may, at least in part, explain the greater incidence of malignancy in old age. B lymphocyte function is also depressed, as shown by lesser immunoglobulin production following an antigenic challenge. Due to all these factors, old people are more prone to infections.

The function of coagulation of blood and platelet count remain normal in old age. Senile purpura is due to a defect in the capillary endothelium.

ESR value tends to be markedly elevated (up to 40 mmHg 1st hour) without evidence of any disease. It is probably related to increased plasma fibrinogen level observed in old age.

MUSCULOSKELETAL SYSTEM

Progressive loss of muscular power is a characteristic feature of ageing. The loss of muscle fibres is much greater than the number explained by the loss of motor neurons in central nervous system. Deposition of lipofuscin and many other degenerative changes can be observed under electron microscope.

The physiological studies reveal a prolongation of latency, contraction period and relaxation period of a muscle twitch. The maximum tension development in a muscle is much less than in young adult.

Degenerative changes in joints start by the age of 30 years and become well marked by the age of 60-70 years.

Osteoporosis is an essential component of ageing. It becomes especially prominent in women after menopause, although no definite cause for osteoporosis can be detected in males or females. Thinness of bones predisposes to fracture. A fracture leads to immobility, which further aggravates osteoporosis.

Stature and Posture

A progressive decline in height sets in by the middle age, and becomes prominent by the age of 70-80 years. In addition, kyphosis, as well as, slight flexion at hip and knee make an aged person look still smaller. In a longitudinal study of a group of people, the mean height decreased from 169 cm at the age of 20 years to 164 cm by the age of 80 years, and 161 cm at the age of 90 years.

Long bones of the limbs do not undergo any significant decrease in length with age. So the decrease in height must be due to a change in the vertebral column. Initially, there is thinning of intervertebral discs only. After the age of 50-60 years, osteoporotic changes cause a decrease in height of individual vertebrae.

SKIN AND HAIR

Wrinkling of skin and graying are hallmark of ageing. The graying of hair is due to loss of melanin pigment. In females, there is loss of axillary and pubic hair due to a decrease in the plasma level of adrenal androgens. On the other hand, almost complete deficiency of oestrogens leads to unopposed action of the residual adrenal androgens causing increased facial hair growth. In males, baldness is very common but the growth of beard is not affected.

Sweat glands decrease in size and number. There is decrease in secretion of sweat glands, as well as, sebaceous glands. The thinning of epidermis and dermis and increased capillary fragility produce senile purpura.

KIDNEYS

By the age of 80 years, there is 30-40% decrease in the number of renal glomeruli, leading to a corresponding decrease in GFR (Fig. 61.1). Both concentration and dilution mechanisms of the kidneys are affected. Maximum urinary osmolality is about 750 mOsm/kg (specific gravity 1.024) at the age of 80 years. The ability to excrete acid is also diminished. Because of large renal reserves, plasma concentrations of creatinine and other nitrogenous waste products are not elevated. However, the renal function is only borderline normal. Any type of circulatory stress may precipitate renal failure. Decreased urinary excretion of certain drugs may produce toxicity at doses well tolerated in younger individuals.

THEORIES OF AGEING

A number of theories have been presented to explain the mechanism of ageing. None of them can answer all the questions. The following theories are accepted to some extent.

Waste Product Theory

Lipofuscin, the yellow brown pigment can be observed in most of the tissues of an aged individual. The pigment is especially prominent in the neurons and the cardiac muscle. The exact site of origin of lipofuscin in the cells is controversial. The ageing pigment is believed to arise from the breakdown of mitochondria or endoplasmic reticulum. Others believe it to be remnants of lysosomes. Whatever the intracellular site of production, there is no doubt that its concentration is directly proportionate to the age of the person. It is believed that *lipofuscin granules disrupt the cellular mechanism leading to a gradual death of the cells.*

Cell Replication Theory

In adults, the cells can be divided into three categories:

(a) Cells in which replication is a continuous process, e.g. blood cells, epidermis and gastrointestinal cells.
(b) Cells which replicate only under stress like injury, e.g. endothelial cells, hepatocytes and fibroblasts.
(c) Cells which do not replicate at all, e.g. neurons, myocardial and skeletal muscle cells.

The replicating cells seem to have a definite replicating limit. For example, fibroblasts obtained from a young individual may undergo replication (doubling) about 50 times. However, fibroblasts obtained from aged individuals stop replicating much earlier. Moreover, fibroblast cells obtained from an old person are less sensitive to growth factors.

In different species there is a difference in the maximum lifespan. In the tortoise, the maximum lifespan is 175 years. It is 120 years in man, 30 years in chickens. There is a corresponding difference in the limit of replication of fibroblasts in cell culture. As compared to 50 times in man, the cellular doubling can occur 115 times in tortoise and 25 times in chicken. Therefore, ageing may represent a stage of life when replication of cell ceases.

Gene Regulation Theory of Aging

This theory proposes that senescence results from changes in gene expression. Studies of human centenarians and their relatives have identified a significant genetic aspect of the ability to survive to exceptional ages. In one study, the mortality rate of centenarian siblings was shown to be, on average, half the mortality rate of contemporaries.

Free Radical Theory of Aging

The free radical theory of aging was first proposed in 1957. It is one of the best-known theories and remains controversial to this day. The free radical theory supposes that free radical reactivity is inherent in biology and results in cumulative damage and senescence. In fact, elevated levels of both oxidant-damaged DNA and protein are found in aged organisms. Although it is clear that oxidative damage accumulates with aging, it is not clear whether this process contributes to aging in all organisms. Dietary antioxidants can reduce the accumulation of oxidized molecules in mice, yet they fail to extend life span.

Neuroendocrine Theory

An important component of this theory is the perception of the hypothalamo-pituitary-adrenal axis as the master regulator, the "pacemaker" that signals the onset and termination of each life stage. During lifespan, chronic exposure to severe stress from a multitude of physical, biological, or emotional stimuli may exhaust or weaken the capacity to adapt and lead to the so-called "diseases of adaptation" and death. Aging would then result from "a decreasing ability to survive stress," one of the many definitions of aging that suggests a close relationship between stress and longevity.

Index

Reader's Notes

Reader's Notes